Cancer Biomarkers

Minimal and Noninvasive Early Diagnosis and Prognosis

Cancer Biomarkers

Minimal and Noninvasive Early Diagnosis and Prognosis

Edited by

Debmalya Barh
Angelo Carpi
Mukesh Verma
Mehmet Gunduz

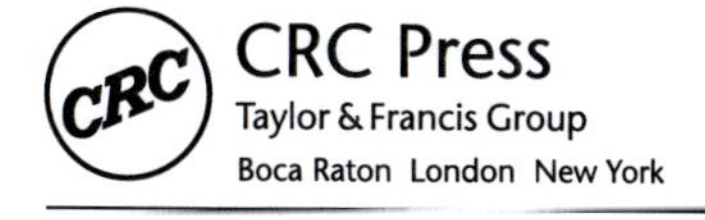

CRC Press is an imprint of the
Taylor & Francis Group, an **informa** business

CRC Press
Taylor & Francis Group
6000 Broken Sound Parkway NW, Suite 300
Boca Raton, FL 33487-2742

Printed on acid-free paper
Version Date: 20131122

International Standard Book Number-13: 978-1-4665-8428-0 (Hardback)

Visit the Taylor & Francis Web site at
http://www.taylorandfrancis.com

and the CRC Press Web site at
http://www.crcpress.com

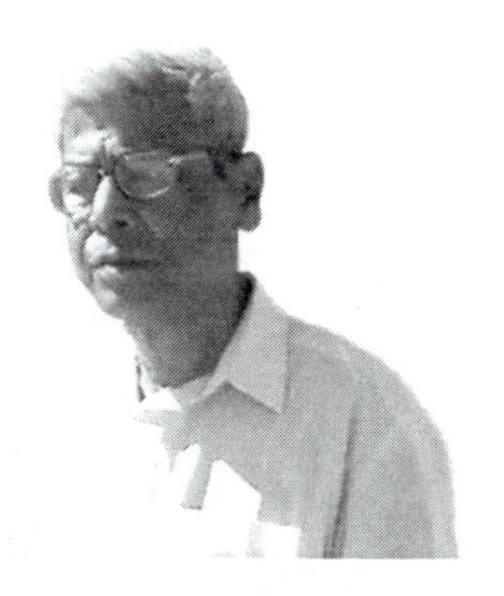

Purnendu Bhusan Barh

(February 22, 1940–February 28, 2008)

This book is dedicated to Purnendu Bhusan Barh, an eminent academician, philosopher, and visionary who is the inspiration behind the Institute of Integrative Omics and Applied Biotechnology (IIOAB) and all its activities.

Contents

Foreword

This book, *Cancer Biomarkers: Minimal and Noninvasive Early Diagnosis and Prognosis* edited by Debmalya Barh, Angelo Carpi, Mukesh Verma, and Mehmet Gunduz, covers an important and rapidly evolving topic. It is informative, comprehensive, and timely. The chapters have been contributed by international scholars. Topics are presented principally by cancer type (covering most common cancers) with introductory chapters on such topics as biomarker discovery, quality control, imaging techniques, innovative tools, nanodiagnostics, and mitochondrial DNA, stem cell, salivary, and miRNA biomarkers.

This book is particularly timely because the field of biomarkers will see explosive growth over the next decade. There are several reasons for this: (1) the various "omics" revolutions (genomics, proteomics, metabolomics, etc.) have provided comprehensive parts lists, thus enabling biomarker discovery; (2) advances in information technology and in particular our ability to gather, store, mine, and transmit large data sets (from which biomarkers will be identified) has exploded; and (3) technologies for probing human pathophysiologic processes both invasively and noninvasively are becoming smaller, cheaper, and more robust. Finally, patients are more engaged, informed, and empowered with regard to their medical care than they have ever been. They may well contribute important information on disease processes from the "field." Thus, biomarkers for disease diagnosis, prognosis, prediction, and treatment will likely increase rapidly in the near future. There will nevertheless be important challenges. These include funding for biomarker discovery research, the need for close industry–academic–health center collaborations, barriers to commercialization, regulatory requirements, and so on. Such issues are highlighted in many of the chapters in this book.

A few other general pointers about biomarkers, and cancer biomarkers in particular, are worth mentioning. The source of the biomarker may reside in the cancer cell but may equally well be in cancer stroma, that is, in cancer-associated fibroblasts, invading immune cells, endothelial cells, etc. It may also be that certain biomarkers will be produced in organs far from the tumor, for example, by liver, fat, or muscle tissue or by immune cells in lymph nodes or spleen, and that these may reflect various facets of cancer biology. Particular attention should be paid to biomarkers that are pathophysiologic, that is, ones that not only reflect the underlying disease process but that, if countered, would impact disease progression. These biomarkers would then be drug targets.

This book focuses on noninvasive or minimally invasive molecular cancer markers that are in use or under development. The significance of these is that they generally pose relatively minimal risk to patients and could thus be assessed multiple times in the course of the disease. Finding biomarkers of this type that are also pathophysiology related, as defined earlier, would be a particularly laudable goal. Thus, the book is a unique effort and a readily available resource for next-generation cancer diagnosis, prognosis, and therapy.

This book will benefit scientists working in the field of biomarkers in academia, in industry, and in regulatory affairs as well as clinicians, including medical oncologists, radiation therapists, surgeons, internists, and others who care for cancer patients. At the end of the day, biomarkers will foster the more rapid introduction of drugs and that too for the right patients, at the right time, and in the right doses—personalized/precision medicine at its best.

Vikas P. Sukhatme, MD, PhD
Victor J. Aresty Professor of Medicine
Beth Israel Deaconess Medical Center
Harvard Medical School
Boston, Massachusetts

Preface

According to the American Cancer Society report, "By 2030, the global cancer burden is expected to nearly double, growing to 21.4 million cases and 13.2 million deaths." Early diagnosis improves treatment efficacy and quality of life as well as reduces the cost for disease management. However, the development of molecular markers for early cancer diagnosis is always a challenge. Some fundamental principles in medical practice are (a) *primum non nocere*, a Latin phrase that means "first, do no harm," and (b) even when a patient's prognosis is poor, the physician must do his or her best for improving quality of the patient's life. Therefore, noninvasive or minimally invasive cancer diagnostic methods are of choice that can avoid complications of biopsy and other unfavorable impacts on patients' health. In this context, patients' easily collectable biospecimens such as blood, serum, plasma, urine, stool, sputum, saliva, etc., based molecular markers having high specificity and sensitivity in early diagnosis are emerging rapidly, and in many instances such markers are also emerging as next-generation prognostic indicators and personalized therapeutics and precision medicine. Several patents have been filed and/or granted on such markers, and a number of health-care companies and authorities currently use or focus on the development of such markers. The significance of clinical validation approaches of several markers has been discussed in different chapters.

This book, *Cancer Biomarkers: Minimal and Noninvasive Early Diagnosis and Prognosis*, reflects the rapid expansion of important scientific, technological, clinical, and translational aspects of noninvasive or minimally invasive molecular cancer biomarkers and their applications along with other conventional markers. It presents the most recent data and almost all promising current and upcoming early diagnostic noninvasive molecular markers for the majority of the common cancers. Furthermore, sensitivity and specificity of markers, biomarker market, test providers, and patent information have been provided. Therefore, the book is a readily available resource for doctors, clinicians, scientists, researchers, and all those working in the health-care industry to recommend or develop early diagnostics, at-risk tests, and prognostic biomarkers for various cancers.

The book is an international effort coordinated and headed by Debmalya Barh, the principal member of the editorial board, who has brought together more than 100 experts (clinicians, doctors, and scientists) in the field of cutting-edge cancer diagnosis, prognosis, and therapy from 23 countries to contribute and share their knowledge. It is divided into eight parts that include 32 chapters covering almost all commonly prevalent cancers. Part I describes the general and technical aspects of noninvasive cancer markers. It consists of nine chapters that cover imaging as well as cutting-edge molecular technologies for biomarker development, noninvasive or minimally invasive sources of molecular markers, and even quality control and ethical issues in cancer biomarker discovery. Part II consists of three chapters that provide a detailed account of brain, head and neck, and oral cancer markers. Part III consists of five chapters that provide comprehensive information on various gastrointestinal cancers. Part IV deals with lung cancer and mesothelioma markers. An entire chapter on promising exhaled volatile markers for early lung cancer diagnosis is included to emphasize the importance of volatile markers in early cancer diagnosis. Part V covers noninvasive early molecular markers in urological cancers. It consists of three chapters that describe kidney, bladder, and prostate cancers. Part VI consists of five chapters that describe gynecological and endocrine cancer markers. It also discusses noninvasive markers of breast, ovarian, cervical, and thyroid cancers. Part VII deals with hematological malignancies. It consists of four chapters that cover noninvasive molecular markers in myelodysplastic syndromes, acute myeloid leukemia, Hodgkin's lymphoma, and multiple myeloma. Part VIII provides comprehensive information on diagnostic and prognostic biomarkers in cutaneous melanoma.

We hope that the book will be worthwhile for our readers, and we highly appreciate your opinion to improve its next edition.

Debmalya Barh
Angelo Carpi
Mukesh Verma
Mehmet Gunduz

Editors

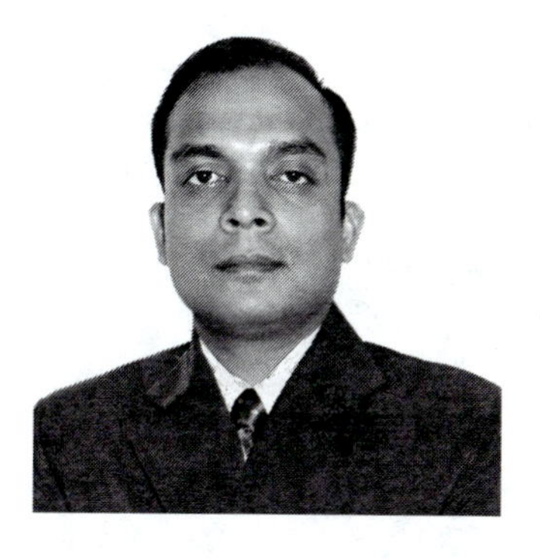

Debmalya Barh (MSc, MTech, MPhil, PhD, PGDM) is the founder and president of the Institute of Integrative Omics and Applied Biotechnology (IIOAB), India, a global platform for multidisciplinary research and advocacy. He is a consultant biotechnologist and an active researcher in integrative omics–based biomarkers, targeted drug discovery, and personalized medicine in cancer, neurodisorders, and cardiovascular, infectious, and metabolic diseases. He works with nearly 400 esteemed researchers from 30–35 countries and he has more than 100 high-impact publications. He has edited ten books in the field of omics such as *OMICS: Biomedical Perspectives and Applications*; *OMICS: Applications in Biomedical, Agricultural, and Environmental Sciences*; *Omics for Personalized Medicine*; and *Omics Approaches in Breast Cancer*, among others, published by renowned international publishers. He also serves as an editorial and review board member for several highly respected international journals.

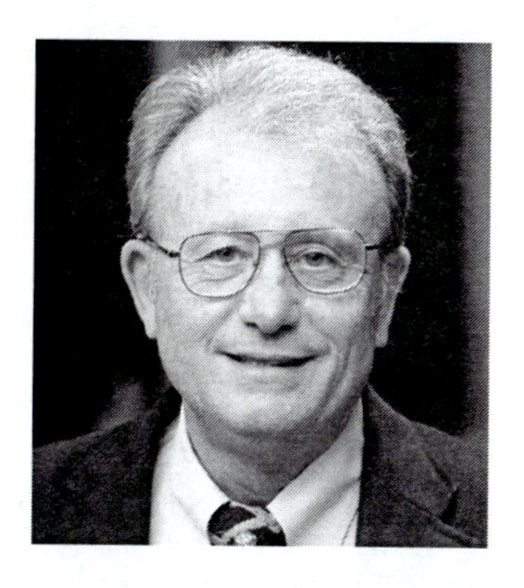

Dr. Angelo Carpi is a clinical professor of medicine at the Pisa University Medical School, Pisa, Italy. He received his MD and postgraduate diplomas in internal medicine and nuclear medicine from the University of Pisa and his diploma of qualification on peptide hormones from the Collegio Medico Giuridico-Scuola Normale Superiore and the Scuola Superiore Sant'Anna, Pisa, Italy. His clinical practice and research included thyroid and breast tumors. He has authored close to 300 publications included in PubMed. He is also a member of the editorial boards of international journals such as *Biomedicine & Pharmacotherapy* and *Frontiers in Bioscience.*

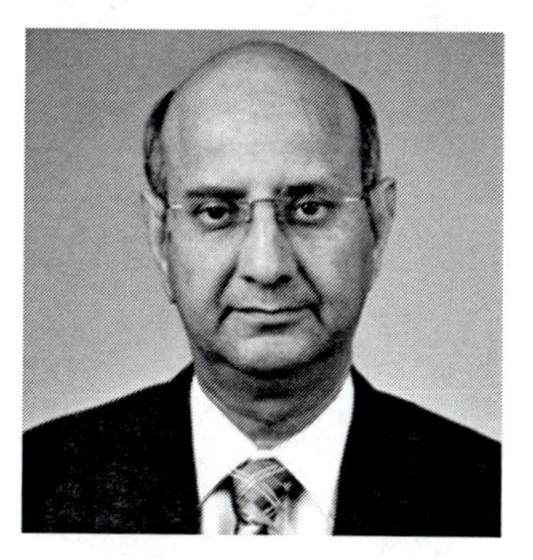

Dr. Mukesh Verma is a program director and chief in the Methods and Technologies Branch (MTB), Epidemiology and Genomics Research Program (EGRP) of the Division of Cancer Control and Population Sciences (DCCPS) at the National Cancer Institute (NCI), National Institutes of Health (NIH). Before coming to the DCCPS, he was a program director in the Division of Cancer Prevention (DCP), NCI, providing direction in the areas of biomarkers, early detection, risk assessment, and prevention of cancer and cancers associated with infectious agents. Dr. Verma received his MSc from Pantnagar University and his PhD from Banaras Hindu University. He did postdoctoral research at George Washington University and was a faculty member at Georgetown University. He has published 128 research articles, book chapters, and reviews. He has also edited three books in the field of cancer epigenetics and epidemiology.

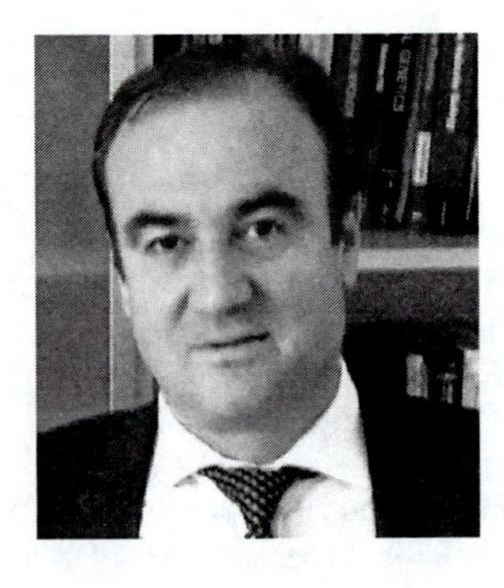

Mehmet Gunduz, MD, PhD, is a professor of otolaryngology and medical genetics, Faculty of Medicine, Turgut Ozal University, Turkey. He graduated from Medical School Hacettepe University, Turkey, as the top fourth student in 1990. Dr. Gunduz completed his residency in otolaryngology, head and neck surgery, at the same university. He did his PhD from Okayama University and Wakayama Medical University, Japan, and is medical board certified from both the Turkish and Japanese certification authorities. From 2003 to 2004, he worked as a visiting scientist at MD Anderson Cancer Center, Texas University in Houston, United States. Dr. Gunduz is one of the pioneers in identifying ING family tumor suppressors. He has more than 150 international publications and 3000 citations, several book chapters, and over 200 presentations in national and international conferences.

Contributors

Neelesh Agarwal
National Cancer Institute
National Institutes of Health
Rockville, Maryland

Eugen Ancuta
Research Department
Cuza-Voda Obstetrics and Gynecology Clinical Hospital
Iasi, Romania

Cuneyd Anil
Department of Endocrinology and Metabolism
Baskent University
Ankara, Turkey

Mumtaz Ahmad Ansari
Department of General Surgery
Institute of Medical Sciences
Banaras Hindu University
Varanasi, India

Debmalya Barh
Centre for Genomics and Applied Gene Technology
Institute of Integrative Omics and Applied Biotechnology
Nonakuri, India

H. Barr
Department of Upper GI Surgery
Gloucestershire Royal Hospital
Gloucester, United Kingdom

Saroj K. Basak
David Geffen School of Medicine
Wadsworth Stem Cell Institute
University of California, Los Angeles
Los Angeles, California

Miroslava Bilecová-Rabajdová
Faculty of Medicine
P. J. Šafárik University in Košice
Košice, Slovakia

Jan Bornschein
Department of Gastroenterology, Hepatology and Infectious Diseases
Otto-von-Guericke University
Magdeburg, Germany

and

MRC Cancer Cell Unit
Hutchison-MRC Research Centre
University of Cambridge
Cambridge, United Kingdom

Michael Byrne
Department of Medicine
Division of Hematology/Oncology
College of Medicine
University of Florida
Gainesville, Florida

Dolores J. Cahill
Conway Institute of Biomedical and Biomolecular Research
University College Dublin
Dublin, Ireland

Danielle Resende Camisasca
Section of Oral Medicine and Pathology
Fluminense Federal University
Nova Friburgo, Brazil

Marisa Cañadas-Garre
Pharmacogenetics Unit
Provincial Unit for the Clinical Management of Pharmacy of Granada
Bio-Health Research Institute of Granada
Hospital Universitario Virgen de las Nieves
Granada, Spain

Angelo Carpi
Department of Clinical and Experimental Medicine
University of Pisa
Pisa, Italy

Alistair J. Cochran
Department of Pathology and Laboratory Medicine
and
Department of Surgery
David Geffen School of Medicine
and
Jonsson Comprehensive Cancer Center
University of California, Los Angeles
Los Angeles, California

Pablo Conesa-Zamora
Department of Pathology
Santa Lucía General University Hospital
Cartagena, Spain

Brian W. Cross
Department of Urology and Winship Cancer Institute
Emory University
Atlanta, Georgia

Vasco Ariston de Carvalho Azevedo
Department of General Biology
Institute of Biological Sciences
Federal University of Minas Gerais
Minas Gerais, Brazil

Mohammed Dehbi
Department of Biomedical Research
Dasman Diabetes Institute
Dasman, Kuwait

and

Qatar Biomedical Research Institute
Education City
Doha, Qatar

Esin Demir
Faculty of Medicine
Department of Medical Genetics
Turgut Ozal University
Istanbul, Turkey

Said Dermime
Department of Biomedical Research
Dasman Diabetes Institute
Dasman, Kuwait

and

King Fahad Specialist Hospital
Dammam, Saudi Arabia

Dipali Dhawan
Institute of Life Sciences
Ahmedabad University
and
Department of Cellular and Molecular Biology
B. V. Patel Pharmaceutical Education and Research Development Centre
Ahmedabad, India

Ruhi Dixit
Department of General Surgery
Institute of Medical Sciences
Banaras Hindu University
Varanasi, India

Zhizhen Dong
Research Center of Clinical Medicine
Affiliated Hospital of Nantong University
Nantong, Jiangsu, People's Republic of China

Eman El-Abd
Department of Radiation Sciences
Medical Research Institute
Alexandria University
Alexandria, Egypt

and

Faculty of Science
Department of Biology
Hail University
Hail, Saudi Arabia

Mohamed Abd El-Salam
Faculty of Science
Department of Physics
Suez Canal University
Ismailia, Egypt

and

Department of Physics
College of Arts and Sciences
King Khalid University
Abha, Saudi Arabia

José Antonio Ferrón Orihuela
Department of General and Digestive Surgery
Division of Endocrine Surgery
Hospital Universitario Virgen de las Nieves
Granada, Spain

Ota Fuchs
Department of Molecular Genetics
Institute of Hematology and Blood Transfusion
Prague, Czech Republic

Abel García García
Faculty of Medicine and Dentistry
Department of Oral Medicine, Oral Surgery and Implantology
University of Santiago de Compostela
Galicia, Spain

Mario Pérez-Sayáns García
Faculty of Medicine and Dentistry
Department of Oral Medicine, Oral Surgery and Implantology
University of Santiago de Compostela
Galicia, Spain

Melvin George
Department of Cardiology
SRM Medical College and Hospital Research Centre
Chennai, India

Esra Gunduz
Faculty of Medicine
Department of Medical Genetics
Turgut Ozal University
Istanbul, Turkey

Mehmet Gunduz
Faculty of Medicine
Department of Medical Genetics
Turgut Ozal University
Istanbul, Turkey

Alptekin Gursoy
Department of Endocrinology and Metabolism
Guven Hospital
Ankara, Turkey

Hossam Haick
Department of Chemical Engineering and Russell Berrie Nanotechnology Institute
Technion—Israel Institute of Technology
Haifa, Israel

Meggie Hakim
Department of Chemical Engineering and Russell Berrie Nanotechnology Institute
Technion—Israel Institute of Technology
Haifa, Israel

Amal Hasan
Department of Biomedical Research
Dasman Diabetes Institute
Dasman, Kuwait

Jonathan Huang
Department of Urology
and
Winship Cancer Institute
Emory University
Atlanta, Georgia

Serife Mehlika Isıldak
Department of Endocrinology and Metabolism
Baskent University
Ankara, Turkey

Eijun Itakura
Department of Pathology and Laboratory Medicine
David Geffen School of Medicine
University of California, Los Angeles
Los Angeles, California

Yusuf Izci
Department of Neurosurgery
Gulhane Military Medical Academy
Ankara, Turkey

Neha Jain
Institute of Integrative Omics and Applied Biotechnology
Purba Medinipur, India

Joseph Katz
Department of Oral Diagnostic Sciences
College of Dentistry
University of Florida
Gainesville, Florida

Ruchika Kaul-Ghanekar
Interactive Research School for Health Affairs
Medical College
Bharati Vidyapeeth Deemed University
Pune, India

Abdelkrim Khadir
Department of Biomedical Research
Dasman Diabetes Institute
Dasman, Kuwait

Anand Kumar
Department of General Surgery
Institute of Medical Sciences
Banaras Hindu University
Varanasi, India

Suresh Kumar
Department of Clinical Pharmacology
JIPMER
Puducherry, India

Juozas Kupcinskas
Department of Gastroenterology
Lithuanian University of Health Sciences
Kaunas, Lithuania

Ream Langhe
Department of Obstetrics and Gynaecology
Trinity Center
and
Central Pathology Laboratory
Sir Patrick Duns Research Laboratory
Department of Histopathology
Trinity College Dublin
St. James's Hospital
and
Coombe Womens & Infants University Hospital
Dublin, Ireland

Marcis Leja
Faculty of Medicine
University of Latvia
Riga, Latvia

and

Digestive Diseases Centre GASTRO
Otto-von-Guericke University
Magdeburg, Germany

and

Riga East University Hospital
Lithuanian University of Health Sciences
Kaunas, Lithuania

Lance Liotta
Center for Applied Proteomics and Molecular Medicine
George Mason University
Manassas, Virginia

José Manuel Llamas-Elvira
Nuclear Medicine Department
Hospital Universitario Virgen de las Nieves
Granada, Spain

Néstor L. López Corrales
Department of General Biology
Institute of Biological Sciences
Federal University of Minas Gerais
Minas Gerais, Brazil

Salwa Lotfi
Faculty of Science
Department of Biology
Hail University
Hail, Saudi Arabia

Simone de Queiroz Chaves Lourenço
Department of Pathology
Fluminense Federal University
Rio de Janeiro, Brazil

Peter Malfertheiner
Department of Gastroenterology, Hepatology and Infectious Diseases
Otto-von-Guericke University
Magdeburg, Germany

Mária Mareková
Faculty of Medicine
P. J. Šafárik University in Košice
Košice, Slovakia

Anastasios Markopoulos
Department of Oral Medicine and Pathology
Aristotle University
Thessaloniki, Greece

Cara Martin
Central Pathology Laboratory
Sir Patrick Duns Research Laboratory
Department of Histopathology
Trinity College Dublin
St. James's Hospital
and
Coombe Womens & Infants University Hospital
Dublin, Ireland

Viraj A. Master
Department of Urology
and
Winship Cancer Institute
Emory University
Atlanta, Georgia

Lynda McEvoy
Department of Obstetrics and Gynaecology
Trinity Center
and
Central Pathology Laboratory
Sir Patrick Duns Research Laboratory
Department of Histopathology
Trinity College Dublin
St. James's Hospital
and
Coombe Womens & Infants University Hospital
Dublin, Ireland

Hana Mlcochova
Masaryk Memorial Cancer Institute
and
Central European Institute of Technology
Masaryk University
Brno, Czech Republic

Simon J.W. Monkhouse
Department of Bariatric Surgery
North Tyneside Hospital
Northumbria, United Kingdom

Jan S. Moreb
Department of Medicine
Division of Hematology/Oncology
College of Medicine
University of Florida
Gainesville, Florida

Umut Mousa
Department of Endocrinology and Metabolism
Baskent University
Ankara, Turkey

J. Muhlschlegel
Department of Surgery
Royal United Hospital
Bath, United Kingdom

Nuria Muñoz Pérez
Department of General and Digestive Surgery
Division of Endocrine Surgery
Hospital Universitario Virgen de las Nieves
Granada, Spain

Anjana Munshi
Department of Molecular Biology
Institute of Genetics and Hospital for Genetic Diseases
Osmania University
Hyderabad, India

Mairead Murphy
Central Pathology Laboratory
Sir Patrick Duns Research Laboratory
Department of Histopathology
Trinity College Dublin
St. James's Hospital
and
Coombe Womens & Infants University Hospital
and
Conway Institute of Biomedical and Biomolecular Research
University College
Dublin, Ireland

Nigel P. Murray
Department of Hematology
Carabineros Hospital
and
Faculty of Medicine
University Mayor
and
Institute of Bio-Oncology
Santiago, Chile

Vincent Nagy
Faculty of Medicine
P. J. Šafárik University in Košice
Košice, Slovakia

Aleksandra Nikolic
Institute of Molecular Genetics and Genetic Engineering
University of Belgrade
Belgrade, Serbia

John J. O'Leary
Department of Obstetrics and Gynaecology
Trinity Center
Trinity College Dublin
St James's Hospital
Dublin, Ireland

Sharon A. O'Toole
Department of Obstetrics and Gynaecology
Trinity Center
and
Central Pathology Laboratory
Sir Patrick Duns Research Laboratory
Department of Histopathology
Trinity College Dublin
St. James's Hospital
and
Coombe Womens & Infants University Hospital
Dublin, Ireland

Harish Padh
Department of Cellular and Molecular Biology
B. V. Patel Pharmaceutical Education and Research Development Centre
Ahmedabad, India

Emmanuel Petricoin
Center for Applied Proteomics and Molecular Medicine
George Mason University
Manassas, Virginia

Prerna Raina
Interactive Research School for Health Affairs
Medical College
Bharati Vidyapeeth Deemed University
Pune, India

Sonia Reda
Department of Physics
Zakazik University
Sharkeya, Egypt

and

Faculty of Science
Department of Physics
Hail University
Hail, Saudi Arabia

Martina Redova
Masaryk Memorial Cancer Institute
and
Central European Institute of Technology
Masaryk University
Brno, Czech Republic

Tamer Refaat
Faculty of Medicine
Alexandria University
Alexandria, Egypt

and

Feinberg School of Medicine
Northwestern University
Chicago, Illinois

Sandhiya Selvarajan
Department of Clinical Pharmacology
JIPMER
Puducherry, India

Vandana Sharma
Institute of Genetics and Hospital for Genetic Diseases
Osmania University
Hyderabad, India

Orla Sheils
Department of Obstetrics and Gynaecology
Trinity Center
Trinity College Dublin
St James's Hospital
Dublin, Ireland

Vijay Kumar Shukla
Department of General Surgery
Institute of Medical Sciences
Banaras Hindu University
Varanasi, India

Ondrej Slaby
Masaryk Memorial Cancer Institute
and
Central European Institute of Technology
Masaryk University
Brno, Czech Republic

Cathy Spillane
Department of Obstetrics and Gynaecology
Trinity Center
Trinity College Dublin
St James's Hospital
Dublin, Ireland

Vivek Srivastava
Department of General Surgery
Institute of Medical Sciences
Banaras Hindu University
Varanasi, India

Eri S. Srivatsan
David Geffen School of Medicine
Wadsworth Stem Cell Institute
University of California, Los Angeles
Los Angeles, California

Antonella Stefanelli
Institute of Nuclear Medicine
Catholic University of Rome
Rome, Italy

Snehal Suryavanshi
Interactive Research School for Health Affairs
Medical College
Bharati Vidyapeeth Deemed University
Pune, India

Silvia Taralli
Institute of Nuclear Medicine
Catholic University of Rome
Rome, Italy

Ulrike Tisch
Department of Chemical Engineering and Russell Berrie Nanotechnology Institute
Technion—Israel Institute of Technology
Haifa, Israel

Ali Tiss
Department of Biomedical Research
Dasman Diabetes Institute
Dasman, Kuwait

Giorgio Treglia
Department of Nuclear Medicine
Oncology Institute of Southern Switzerland
Bellinzona, Switzerland

Michael Unger
Pulmonary Division
Department of Medicine
Fox Chase Cancer Center
Philadelphia, Pennsylvania

Peter Urban
Faculty of Medicine
P. J. Šafárik University in Košice
Košice, Slovakia

Mudit Verma
National Cancer Institute
National Institutes of Health
Rockville, Maryland

Mukesh Verma
National Cancer Institute
National Institutes of Health
Rockville, Maryland

Jesús María Villar del Moral
Department of General and Digestive Surgery
Division of Endocrine Surgery
Hospital Universitario Virgen de las Nieves
Granada, Spain

Li Wang
Research Center of Clinical Medicine
Affiliated Hospital of Nantong University
Nantong, Jiangsu, People's Republic of China

Xiaodi Yan
Research Center of Clinical Medicine
Affiliated Hospital of Nantong University
Nantong, Jiangsu, People' Republic of China

Dengfu Yao
Research Center of Clinical Medicine
Affiliated Hospital of Nantong University
Nantong, Jiangsu, People's Republic of China

Min Yao
Research Center of Clinical Medicine
Affiliated Hospital of Nantong University
Nantong, Jiangsu, People's Republic of China

Burak Yılmaz
Faculty of Medicine
Department of Medical Genetics
Turgut Ozal University
Istanbul, Turkey

Part I

General and Technical Aspects

1

Quality Control and Ethical Issues of Cancer Biomarker Discovery

Anjana Munshi and Vandana Sharma

CONTENTS

ABSTRACT Biomarkers have gained immense clinical importance because of their wide spectrum in early detection, diagnosis, prevention, and treatment of cancer. Before diagnosis, biomarkers are used for risk assessment, screening, and follow-up prevention. During diagnosis, biomarkers are used for staging and grading of tumor/cancer, and during prognosis (the course of treatment), biomarkers play an important role for determination of initial therapy, treatment response, and clinical outcome. With recent advances in genomics, epigenomics, and proteomics and with the use of high-throughput technologies, a plethora of new candidate biomarkers have been recognized. Despite major scientific achievements, only a few of these biomarkers have been translated into clinical practice especially in the field of carcinogenesis. A number of barriers such as poor quality control and lack of samples for validating and testing procedures during the development and validation (analytical and clinical) of biomarkers result in less efficient diagnostics and unpredictability in clinical outcome in cancer.

Regulatory and ethical issues depend on the intended use of biomarkers. The Food and Drug Administration (FDA) regulates the issues relating to the development of biomarkers. One of the recent examples is that FDA has encouraged pharmaceutical industry to share pharmacogenomic data. FDA has a role in working with pharmaceutical firms and biotechnology laboratories for developing new evaluation methods and paradigms for specimen storage and data collection after consideration of ethical and legal issues. FDA also streamlines the approval process with clarity, coordination across centers, cooperation and collaboration with other stakeholders. The present chapter provides an insight into the biomarker development and importance of quality control and validation process in the area of cancer so that these biomarkers can be used in clinics.

KEY WORDS: *biomarkers, detection, diagnosis, prevention, treatment, cancer, Food and Drug Administration, genomics, quality control, validation, ethical and legal issues, stakeholders.*

Abbreviations

AACR	American Association for Cancer Research
AUC	Area under the curve
BRCA1, BRCA2	Breast cancer 1, breast cancer 2
CA 125	Carbohydrate antigen 125
CA 15.3	Carcinoma antigen 15.3
caHUB	Cancer Human Biobank
CBC	Cancer Biomarkers Collaborative
CBER	Center for Biologics Evaluation and Research
CDER	Center for Drug Evaluation and Research
CDKN2A	Cyclin-dependent kinase inhibitor
CDRH	Center for Drug Evaluation and Radiological Health
CEA	Carcinoembryonic antigen
CK18	Cytokeratin 18
CMS	Center for Medicaid and Medicare Services
DNA	Deoxyribonucleic acid
EDRN	Early Detection Research Network
ELISA	Enzyme-linked immunosorbent assay
FDA	Food and Drug Administration
GCP	Good Clinical Practice
GINA	Genetic Information Nondiscrimination Act
HER2	Herceptin2
HIPAA	Health Insurance Portability and Accountability Act of 1996
IDSC	Investigational Drug Steering Committee
KRAS	v-Ki-ras2 Kirsten rat sarcoma viral oncogene homolog
LC	Liquid chromatography
(mi)RNA	microRNA
MS	Mass spectrometry
NCI	National Cancer Institute
OBBR	Biorepositories and Biospecimen Research
PSA	Prostate-specific antigen
RNA	Ribonucleic acid
SNPs	Single-nucleotide polymorphisms
SOPs	Standard operating procedures
TCGA	The Cancer Genome Atlas
TP53	Tumor protein 53

1.1 Introduction

The last two decades have observed a significant exponential growth in the knowledge of cancer treatment at molecular and cellular levels due to tremendous advances in the area of cancer research. In spite of this, cancer still continues to be a major cause of morbidity and mortality globally. The detection of various forms of cancers at an early stage is an important measurable step for physicians as well as for patients. Biomarkers play a central role in this and act as catalysts in the process of identification of new targeted and effective therapeutics. The range of disease biomarkers varies widely in type. These include biochemical and immunological molecular markers and metabolites or processes such as apoptosis, angiogenesis, or proliferation (Hayes et al., 1996; Diamandis, 2010). These biomarkers can be detected from plasma, serum, cerebrospinal fluid, urine, saliva, and cyst fluid, which serve as important sources of noninvasive biomarkers for the detection and diagnosis of cancers. The premise behind the use of biomarkers in clinical practice for cancer is that it can be used as an indicator for the presence or absence of the disease or treatment outcome (Diamandis, 2010).

Based on their use, biomarkers can be divided into different categories. The first one includes biomarkers for early detection or for screening of patients; the second category consists of diagnostic biomarkers used to detect the presence/absence of cancer; the third one includes prognostic biomarkers to assess the survival probabilities of patients or to detect the aggressive phenotype. The fourth category includes predictive biomarkers to predict the effectiveness of drug treatment and the fifth consists of a target that is used to identify the molecular targets of novel therapies and to know which molecular markers are expressed and affected by therapy (Manne et al., 2005). The validated biomarkers provide an accurate tool for guiding the best treatment and provide the resources or early *proof of concept* for developing novel drug molecules (Frank and Harhreaves, 2003). The era of detecting malignant disease using biomarkers started with the discovery of alpha-fetoprotein and carcinoembryonic antigen (CEA) detected by using the technique of radioimmunoassay. In the year 1980, hybridoma technology enabled the development of the marker carbohydrate antigen (CA 125) in ovarian epithelial cancer (Bast et al., 1981). There are a handful of cancer biomarkers that are currently recommended for monitoring treatment response among cancer patients with advanced disease (Diamandis, 2010). Some other biomarkers that have been effectively used in the diagnosis and prognosis of different types of cancers are prostate-specific antigen (PSA) for prostate cancer, alpha-fetoprotein for hepatocellular carcinoma, BRCA1 and BRCA2 for breast cancer, and heat shock proteins for gastric and prostate carcinomas, osteosarcomas, and uterine, cervical, and bladder carcinoma (Bhatt et al., 2010). Till date, approximately 15 biomarkers have been approved by the Food and Drug Administration (FDA) for monitoring drug response, surveillance, or recurrence of cancer. This chapter reviews the major bottlenecks in the development of biomarkers and a need for the adoption of tight quality control and regulatory structure in cancer diagnosis and drug development.

1.2 Sensitivity and Specificity of Cancer Biomarkers

The characteristics of an ideal biomarker are safety, accuracy, reliability, reproducibility, low cost, consistency across gender and ethnic groups, and quantifiable in an accessible biological fluid and clinical sample. A biomarker ideally should possess 100% specificity and sensitivity (Manne et al., 2005). None of the biomarkers established so far in cancer has 100% specificity and sensitivity. One of the best serum biomarkers (PSA) is used for the detection of prostate cancer. PSA has been found to have high sensitivity (more than 90%) but low specificity (25%). Another serum biomarker, like CA 15.3 for breast cancer, has only 23% sensitivity and 69% specificity, which is used in monitoring therapy for the recurrence of breast cancer. Receiver operating curve is used to represent the relation between specificity and sensitivity. This curve helps to evaluate the efficacy of tumor markers at various cutoff points (Kulasingam and Diamendis, 2008). The area under the curve (AUC) is taken into consideration.

1.3 Phases of Biomarker Development

The National Institutes of Health has initiated and supported the Early Detection Research Network (EDRN), for the early detection of cancer biomarkers and to predict cancer risk and prognosis (Feng et al., 2004). The biomarker evaluation and development is an orderly process wherein one step follows the other after meeting the prescribed criteria. These phases have been mentioned under the following sections.

1.3.1 Preclinical Phase or Phase 1

The preclinical studies are conducted on animals in search of biomarkers comparing tumor tissues with nontumor tissues, and the lead compound is also tested on these animal models (Mauro et al., 2002; Brodie, 2003). The preclinical phase can explain in vitro and in vivo pharmacological mechanism of action of the lead compound with the help of biomarkers. Nowadays, biomarkers in this phase are discovered using advanced tools such as knowledge-based gene selection, gene expression profiling, or protein profiling. These exploratory studies are meant to identify the clinical tests using biomarkers for detecting disease or cancer. The biomarkers are further prioritized according to their diagnostic, prognostic, and therapeutic values, which help in their evaluation process (Manne et al., 2005). Although not necessary, it is preferred that the specimen for this phase comes from cohorts, tissue banks (biological fluid), or a clinical trial with active follow-ups (Kumar and Sarin, 2009).

PSA, a routine marker for human prostate cancer, has been adapted for the monitoring of treatment response in prostate cancer from preclinical studies (Chau et al., 2008). A few examples of the biological fluids that provide as source/specimen for biomarkers have been summed up in Table 1.1.

1.3.2 Phase 2 Studies

Phase 2 studies include clinical studies based on the development of a clinical bioassay. A clinical assay (e.g., ELISA) is developed based on a specimen obtained noninvasively, for example, a protein expressed uniquely by tumor and is measured with serum antibodies. The clinical assay is meant to identify subjects with cancer and those without cancer. Conventional clinical assays are still used routinely in the diagnosis of a particular type of cancer or for monitoring treatment response, for example, CA-125 antigen for ovarian cancer (Beshara et al., 2002). The evaluation of standard assays in preclinical studies using appropriate tumor models demonstrates the correlation between biomarkers and inhibition of tumor growth, which further increases the confidence for the use of a particular biomarker in subsequent clinical trials. The assay developed should be simple and reproducible in case of phase 3 studies.

1.3.3 Phase 3

Phase 3 studies are also known as retrospective longitudinal repository studies. These studies evaluate the sensitivity and specificity of the test, which has yet to surface clinically (Feng et al., 2004).

TABLE 1.1

Specimens and Their Use for Detection of Cancer

Biological Fluid (Specimen)	Indicates Type of Cancer
Blood (plasma/serum)	A number of cancers (ovarian, prostate, lung, breast)
Cerebrospinal fluid	Brain tumor
Aspirated fluid from breast	Breast cancer
Stool	Colorectal cancer
Pleural fluid	Lung cancer
Saliva	Oral cancer
Pancreatic fluid	Cancer of pancreas
Seminal plasma	Prostate/testicular cancer
Urine	Cancer of urinary tract

At this phase, biomarker validation studies will end and the biomarker will be ready for clinical use. The specimens should be collected from cancer case subjects before their clinical diagnosis with active follow-up and are compared with control subjects to ascertain clinical outcome (Pepe et al., 2001; Feng et al., 2004). Therefore, these studies should be attached to large cohort studies or intervention trials if possible. Control subjects are the individuals who have not developed the cancer during a given follow-up period. The three important things that are required to be confirmed during designing a phase 3 study are (1) number of control subjects, (2) number of case subjects, and (3) number of clinical specimens per subject. Phase 3 studies are meant to develop an algorithm for screening positivity based on combination of markers (Pepe et al., 2001; Feng et al., 2004). Most of the clinical studies end up here and provide biomarker to be used in clinical service.

1.3.4 Phase 4

The retrospective studies in phase 3 determine whether tumors can be detected with the help of biomarker early before clinical diagnosis, but it does not establish the stage or nature of cancer. Phase 4 studies are different from phase 1, phase 2, and phase 3 studies, because they directly deal with patients. Therefore, utmost care should be taken of ethical considerations. Adequate planning of phase 4 studies is very important with inclusion/exclusion criteria and compliance potential. The main objectives of phase 4 studies are (1) to identify the characteristics of the biomarker-based screening test in a relevant population by determining the detection rate and false referral rate and (2) to make preliminary assessments of the effects of screening on costs and mortality associated with cancer (Pepe et al., 2001).

1.3.5 Phase 5 Studies/Cancer Control Studies

This final phase explains whether screening decreases the burden of cancer in a population. This phase evaluates the benefit/risk of the newly developed diagnostic assay on the screened population. These types of studies require a large-scale study of long period and are expensive. The samples for this type of studies are randomly selected from the screening population. A standard parallel arm randomized clinical trial is undertaken in phase 5 with one arm consisting of subjects undergoing the screening protocol and the other arm consisting of unscreened subjects (Pepe et al., 2001). Phase 5 studies include survival analysis methods for censored data, which are used in order to compare the study arms with overall mortality and cause-specific mortality (Pepe et al., 2001). Phase 5 studies evaluate the benefits and risks of the assay/test/biomarker developed, costs of screening, and treatment and cost of per life saved (Pepe et al., 2001).

1.3.6 Biomarker Discovery Using High-Throughput Technology

The field of early detection in cancer has been plagued by problems such as overdiagnosis (e.g., PSA), inadequate specificity of individual markers (CEA), low-compliance colonoscopy, and lack of fresh analytical measures. High-throughput technologies have provided a platform for investigators to assess genomic data, transcriptomics data, proteomic data, and fluxomic data. Genomic studies are valuable in cancer research because cancer cells show damage at the level of DNA, which might not be present in normal cells. Microarray techniques allow for the simultaneous identification of thousands of single-nucleotide polymorphisms (SNPs) in an individual's DNA (Feng et al., 2004). The genomic biomarkers may provide important information concerned with etiology of disease and identification of individuals having a favorable benefit versus risk profile of an intervention or treatment (Feng et al., 2004).

Contrary to genetic markers, phenotypic expression markers such as RNA/protein vary among cell types and change over time because of posttranslational and posttranscriptional modifications (Kumar and Sarin, 2009). Protein, peptides, and metabolites are accessible easily in body fluids for measuring disease status and clinical outcome. Increased DNA concentrations have been found to be associated with various types of cancers. Mutations in oncogenes, tumor suppressor genes, and mismatch repair genes can serve as biomarkers for the identification of different types of cancers, for example, v-Ki-ras2 Kirsten rat sarcoma (KRAS) gene mutations predict the metastatic spread in various tumor tissues. Similarly, germ line inheritance of TP53 mutation in case of Li–Fraumeni syndrome has been reported to confer a risk of developing many types of the cancers. Mutations in other genes, for example, cyclin-dependent kinase inhibitor (CDKN2A), adenomatous polyposis coli gene, and retinoblastoma gene, have the potential as markers for prognosis or selection of therapy. Other biomarkers are pattern-based RNA-expression analysis and proteins in case of clinical breast cancer.

A noncoding short single-stranded RNA molecule micro (mi)RNA has emerged as a new class of cancer biomarkers in the last decade. The identification of miRNA expression signatures in cancers has explored its applications in (1) specific cancer type (2) to predict tumor subtypes (stage, hormonal status), (3) drug resistance, (4) chemotherapy response, and clinical outcome (Semenuk et al., 2011). A number of patents have been filed claiming the utility of miRNA as biomarkers for cancer diagnostics followed by cancer detection, predictions of response to therapy, and clinical outcome in case of drug resistance (Semenuk et al., 2011). miRNAs like miR-21, miR-126, and miR-205 are used for the diagnosis of lung cancer, and miR-204 and miR-510 are used for the detection of breast cancer or prostate cancer. miRNAs like miR-17–92 and miR-106a92 clusters are used for the treatment of gastric cancer. miR-26 is used in the diagnostics of hepatocellular carcinoma. miR-21, miR-92, and miR-93 have been used for the diagnostics of ovarian cancer.

1.4 Quality Control

Quality control is a scientific approach that consists of a framework of operational techniques and activities for better planning and conducting a study and drawing valid conclusions from it. Quality is a degree to which a set of inherent characteristics fulfills requirements. The main purpose of quality control is to control the quality of products or services by detecting problems and defects. Quality assurance (QA) involves implementation of these techniques to provide adequate confidence that an entity will fulfill requirement for quality. QA is aimed at preventing problems and defects. Quality control is very important in any organization or biomarker laboratory and its management. Quality check and SOPs are important in biomarker development because there is a lack of definition to guarantee the reproducibility of new procedures (Bensalah et al., 2007). A set of guidelines of quality control are applicable to each stage and phase of biomarker development in cancer. Planning of study with a significant sample size and clear goals, taking consent from recruited subjects followed by sample storage at specified conditions, should be taken into consideration while developing a biomarker.

The quality control starts from the very first step of specimen collection for the development of biomarkers. Biospecimens provide raw materials for further discovery. The absence of high-quality biomarker is considered to be one of the most significant barriers in developing and validating the biomarkers. Therefore, quality improvement in biospecimen resources has been identified as one of the top priorities of Cancer Biomarkers Collaborative (CBC) consortium. The biospecimens are affected by a number of factors such as preacquisition, acquisition, and postacquisition (sample processing, storage, and analysis) (Khleif et al., 2010). At present, there is little QA and control on newly archived/collected samples. Although there exist a number of guidelines and recommendations for biospecimen collection and processing, the standards have not been adopted uniformly. This problem was highlighted when The Cancer Genome Atlas (TCGA) project of the National Cancer Institute (NCI) surveyed specimens for its large sequencing effort. In this project, a large collection of biospecimens that was considered to be of quality was found to be unacceptable for use in this pilot project (http:/biospecimens.cancer.gov/practices/forum/boston2007/pdf; Khleif et al., 2010). Universal uptake of best practices of quality control in specimen collection/biospecimen repositories requires an international accreditation program.

To achieve this goal, the NCI Office of Biorepositories and Biospecimen Research (OBBR) has developed a national, standardized human biospecimen resource called the cancer Human Biobank (caHUB). The availability of high quality of biospecimens would provide a new and better analytical platform for the researchers in the field of cancer biomarkers (Khleif et al., 2010).

All the assays used in biomarkers development should be subjected to an appropriate level of validation prior to analysis. Assays conducted should incorporate quality control samples along with acceptance criteria in order to minimize the risk of errors leading to misreporting of data. Research studies that are carried out in laboratories without defined quality measures in order to validate biomarkers provide inconsistent results leading to reduced level of confidence in assays (Khleif et al., 2010). Standard operating procedures (SOPs) should be followed at all the technical levels of biomarker development. The role of quality control appears once the biomarker is validated in an assay procedure and comes in the market for routine use. In a nutshell, the analysis and evaluation of biomarkers in the field of cancer are the result of a number of processes (including managerial, technical, data interpretation, and analytical phases), which need to be monitored and controlled to prevent errors so as to provide a satisfactory level of quality (Paradiso et al., 2002).

1.5 Quality Assurance

QA is concerned with the validity of all the analytical processes (from collection of the specimens to result interpretation). It is not an abstract concept but must be adapted to the different situations such as the different exposure levels, the different analytical methods, and the context of use (risk assessment procedures, research, routine determinations).

1.6 Biomarker Method Validation

Method validation is an important component in biomarker research. Sometimes a biomarker fails in the clinical settings not because of underlying scientific rationale but due to poor assay choice and lack of robust validation (Pepe et al., 2001; Baker and Kramer, 2005). The main areas to be emphasized during method validation include utmost care during specimen collection, handling, storage, and processing in order to maintain sample integrity. Optimization and processing control are required depending upon the type of biomarker and source of analyte.

Since the ultimate aim of developing a biomarker is to transfer the assay into clinical practice or from benchside to bedside, therefore all the key components should be assembled in a validated method such as consistent supply of reagents, certificated standard of the target molecule to use as a calibration standard, and a control matrix free from the target molecule that replicates closely the clinical sample to be investigated (Cummings et al., 2008). The lack of resources can result in compromised analytical technique and can lead to failure of biomarker qualification (Bast et al., 2005). However, during the development of biomarkers, the laboratories must follow the regulations and Good Clinical Practice (GCP) guidelines before starting any clinical trial investigations. Ideally, biomarker validation has three stages; first is the development of method, with an aim of performing feasibility studies, assessing reagent availability, and so on, followed by second stage of prestudy method validation with the aim to perform feasibility studies. At the third stage, the plan is put into effect and is conducted using validation samples. The objective of validation process is (1) to produce a body of data that proves that method meets acceptable standards of performance, (2) formalize these data into analytical report, and (3) draft a method SOPs, which is then directed to specimen analysis. Finally, during the sample analysis part, quality control is incorporated in order to confirm that method is performing in accordance to the specifications (Cummings et al., 2008). As a result of this, the patient-derived data are confidently accepted as valid. The performance parameters studied in the second stage of validation include selectivity, sensitivity, calibration response, choice of quality control samples, analyze recovery, precision, accuracy, and reproducibility of the biomarker or assay developed (Shah et al., 1991, 2000; Nowatzke and Woolf, 2007; Cummings et al., 2008).

The international recognized standards have been established for the various parameters of bioanalytical method validation (Shah et al., 1991, 2000; Peters et al., 2007). These standards were devised by the pharmaceutical firms for small molecule analysis using the techniques of liquid chromatography (LC) or LC–mass spectrometry (MS) but nevertheless been endorsed by national agencies and regulatory authorities (FDA, 2001). Selectivity is demonstrated as lack of interference in six independent samples of drug-free matrix. A calibration curve is acceptable if 75% or a minimum of six different standard concentrations fall within ±15% of their nominal values except at lower limit of quantitation when ±20%

is acceptable (Cummmings et al., 2008). Precision or accuracy in repeat analysis is expected to vary by less than ±15% (Cummmings et al., 2008). The analytical run is accepted valid when at least 67% (4/6) of the QCs fall within 15% of their nominal values (Shah et al., 1991, 2000; Bansal and DeStefano, 2007).

There are certain critical issues in the development of biomarkers that impose challenges to the quality control and validation methods. Since the biomarkers are the endogenous substances, an analyte-free matrix to perform specificity studies or to be used as resource to make a calibration curve is often not available (Cummings et al., 2008). Biomarker analytical methods often lack sensitivity and dynamic range and are prone to be labor intensive and variability. The analytical phases of biomarkers depend on the integrity of reagents, for example, antibodies (often derived from biological source), and are subjected to their own problems of QC and stability. In many cases, researchers have to use noncertified standards, for example, a recombinant protein and a variety of surrogate matrices, to construct a validation curve. Parallel studies are needed to perform where the response of the assay to a range of calibration standard is made up of a surrogate matrix and is compared to serial dilutions of patient samples (Smolec et al., 2005). In this case, dilution linearity can create problems because antibody and ligand binding affinities can vary in different media.

There are some specific examples of biomarker validation. MS is an absolute quantitative technique for biomarker research, which is a platform of choice in proteomics (Zhang et al., 2007). Other examples of validated biomarker assays include M30 and M65 ELISA assays that fall into the category of quantitative analysis, which determine different circulating forms of protein cytokeratin 18 (CK 18) and are proposed to be the surrogate markers of different mechanisms of cell death in cancer. The M30 ELISA assay is based on the use of M5 antibody as a catcher and M30 to detect the CK18 fragments that contain a neoepitope at positions 387–396 generated by caspases 3, 7, and 9 activated during apoptosis (Leers et al., 1999; Schutte et al., 2004). The cancer cells contain a substantial pool of cytokeratins (CK 8, 18, 19) which increase in response to stress (Ditzel et al., 2002; Schutte et al., 2004). Both these techniques have been employed extensively in clinical trials as pharmacodynamic biomarkers of cell death induced by a variety of chemotherapeutic agents (Ueno et al., 2003).

Cancer is a heterogeneous disease; therefore, the disease has biologically different phenotypes with varied response to intervention (screening and treatment) (Manne et al., 2005). The treatment is evaluated in randomized controlled clinical trials. Heterogeneity and admixture of patients (belonging to different ethnicity and racial groups) can lead to sample bias affecting the study outcome. To avoid sample biasing, heterogeneity and effect of other confounding factor studies are conducted using observational and clinical epidemiology. In case of use of high-throughput technology, overfitting of the data is another problem when there are large numbers of potential indicators among a small number of outcome events (Manne et al., 2005). For example, a study on RNA microarray analysis showed overfitting data with a small number of samples. *Omics*-derived approaches have this problem of data overfitting in case the training and validation sets are small and not randomized. To avoid this, information on samples should be blinded and should be sent to several laboratories for assay and analysis to be conducted under fixed protocol. The data obtained should be analyzed by an independent manager to see the variation/similar results reproduced by each laboratory. Splitting the samples randomly between validation set and training set has been found to be an important technique to minimize the overfitting (Ranshoff et al., 2004; Manne et al., 2005).

Quality control measures should be undertaken to document analytical performance during clinical studies and to determine selection/rejection of an analytical procedure during sample analysis. In addition to this, biomarker analysis and validation requires stability in calibration standards. With the progress of drug development or biomarker assay development, validation should keep pace with the required precision and reliability, which is needed to achieve expected study objectives (Chau et al., 2008).

1.7 Standardization/Validation through Collaboration

Researchers have recognized the impact of biomarkers on drug discovery and clinical outcome phases and, therefore, have joined forces in an effort to integrate it into the system. The most recent is a consortium known as CBC composed of AACR, FDA, and NCI with a focus on facilitating the use of validated bioinformatics and information sharing. The goal of CBC is to develop guidelines in the area of biospecimens and how to conduct drug trials. The CBC recommends standards and specifications regarding the development of biomarkers in the area of cancer research. CBC collects the inputs from distinguished experts (more than 120 experts in the area of cancer research) and key stakeholders such as government agencies, academia, pharmaceutical industries, regulators, and patient advocates worldwide (Khleif et al., 2010). In addition to CBC, other alliances include industry, partnership with government, patient advocacy groups (ethical committees), and nonprofit sector organizations. It verifies, qualifies, and validates biomarkers and formalizes their use in research and regulatory approval to guide the clinical practice.

The EDRN of NCI has come into existence to foster collaboration among independent institutions and laboratories to facilitate standardization and validation of candidate cancer biomarkers (Srivastava, 2007). EDRN has four components: biomarker reference laboratories, biomarker developmental laboratories, and clinical epidemiology and validation centers. EDRN is responsible for the development of biomarker validation, to develop QA regimens, SOPs, to conduct early clinical epidemiological studies to evaluate predictive value of biomarkers (EDRN, 2002).

1.8 Biomarkers into Drug Development

Traditionally, cancer patients were treated with drugs having less toxicity or high tolerance, most often accompanied with drug-induced side effects. However, the development of basic and clinical sciences has facilitated and improved the cancer treatment strategies in the form of personalized medicine. A successful example of integration of integrating biomarkers into drug development in the field of cancer is of HER2 (Herceptin2). HER2 is a proto-oncogene that becomes a potential biomarker when studies observed that its overexpression in breast cancer found to be associated with poor prognosis. As a result of this, trastuzumab was subsequently approved in 1998 by FDA as second-/third-line monotherapy or first-line therapy with paclitaxel for the treatment of HER2-overexpressed breast cancer (Baselga et al., 1996; Cobleigh et al., 1999; Slamon et al., 2001; Vogel et al., 2002). Another example is of imatinib mesylate. This molecular targeted drug has proved to be highly effective in chronic myeloid leukemia and gastrointestinal stromal tumor.

With these few examples, it is evident that biomarkers provide a key rationale endpoints in the development of targeted anticancer drug molecules. The need for standardized pathway approach for the quality control and validation of biomarkers is gaining more importance given the recent surge in biomarker development pipeline. The development and integration of effective biomarkers for diagnosis, detection, and treatment of cancer depends on understanding host and tumor biology, consensus definitions of biomarkers, high-quality specimen, data repositories, surrogate endpoints, stringent analytical criteria for assay, and management system for these resources.

The future of drug and biomarker development resides in following all the ethical and regulatory issues along with stringent quality control methods. This will eliminate the failures of biomarkers in clinical settings and would explain the role of biomarkers as surrogate endpoints and diagnostic indicators for disease screening, monitoring of disease progression, and treatment efficacy and to predict clinical outcome.

1.9 Ethical Considerations in the Development of Cancer Biomarkers

The consideration of ethical and regulatory issues in the development of a biomarkers is a very important step as these belong to human subjects to be treated or under diagnosis. Although there is enormous potential for biomarker studies to influence the clinical strategies designed by trials, it has been observed that the practical measures to achieve this goal are slow, uncoordinated, and, at times, misdirected (Dancey et al., 2010). NCI and Investigational Drug Steering Committee (IDSC) have developed Biomarker Task Force in 2007, which provides recommendations for the conduct of biomarker studies in early clinical trials (Dancey et al., 2010). Ethical and social implications have been widely acknowledged in the area of cancer research, particularly issues relating to patient privacy, data collection and storage, specimen storage, and interpretation of results that require careful handling by researchers and policy makers.

1.9.1 Informed Consent

Persons (volunteers/patients) recruited for sample collection should be informed about the study and informed about all the risks and benefits of participating in the study. The informed consent should be taken prior to their recruitment as study subjects. At present, there is lack of common informed consent document for the use of biospecimen collection in cancer research (Khleif et al., 2010). The informed consents vary substantially because no consensus is available to define the biomarkers and terms related to biospecimen collection (Khleif et al., 2010). There is no agreement among stakeholders regarding the detail to be incorporated to address issues relating to research and to explain coding and confidentiality. Adopting a simple, standard, and efficient informed consent document clarifies authorized research and protects the confidentiality and confidence of the study subjects, thus facilitating research and development of cancer biomarkers. A clear explanation of the study, samples to be used (tissues/serum), duration of study period, risks/benefits from the study, reimbursements and their voluntary withdrawal, etc., should be mentioned in the informed consent document.

1.9.2 Sample Collection

Study subjects should not be misguided by providing false expectations and pressurizing them for recruitment. Being a part of the study, the subjects generally don't provide consent for the dissemination of the data to any other parties, for example, employers, unions, insurers, credit agencies, and lawyers. The dissemination of results or observations, beyond the explicit purposes for which specimens were collected, interferes with study subject's privacy. Labeling of a subject as "abnormal" or as "in the extremes of a distribution of marker assay results" could have a potentially deleterious impact on the person's social life (Schulte et al., 1995). It could lead to risk of not obtaining insurance, job, or credit.

The people hesitate or refuse to participate in genetic research, for example, in a study carried out in year 2003 on hereditary colon cancer, 39% of patients did not undergo genetic testing (Hadley et al., 2003). How the samples/biospecimen will be used and stored (temperature specifications, cryopreservation) and who will be provided access to these are other issues to warrant the high quality of samples to be used in the research/study. Published guidelines for the blood shipment, processing, and timing should be followed strictly.

1.9.3 Biospecimen Annotation

The lack of standards for biospecimen annotation that meets the diverse need of various stakeholders results in compromising the biomarker validation process (Khleif et al., 2010). At present, there are no established standards and terminology for the amount of clinical data to be collected for biospecimens. A template document defining the minimal and comprehensive data sets should be generated and provided to the institutes/laboratories (Khleif et al., 2010). There should be a system for the legible, durable, and coded label that should be provided for biospecimen identification and tracking. There are websites, which provide information regarding biospecimen collection for the development of biomarkers. The Office of Technology Assessment has addressed some problematic questions in the storage and handling of biospecimens. These include certain issues, for example, who will own the cell line, should the biological materials be sold, and if so, then define the implications for equity of distribution. According to Office of Technology Assessment, 1987, "Should disclosure, informed consent, and regulatory requirements be modified to cope with the new questions raised by the increased importance and value of human biological materials" are the issues to which no single policy or law is applicable. The law pertaining to the research studies involving genomic analysis as a part of biomarker development, the Genetic Information Nondiscrimination Act known as "GINA," was signed into law in the year 2008. The Act has provisions of nondiscrimination for employers, against individuals on the basis of their genetic information (Rothstein, 2008).

1.9.4 Data Storage and Sharing

The records of government-sponsored or government-funded research studies are to be maintained according to the *Privacy Act of 1974 (PL93-579)*. Title 5 in the *Code of Federal Regulations* explains the *ethical issues and uses of human monitoring data conditions* for which records held by the federal government can be disclosed (5CFR 297.401) (Schulte and Sweeney, 1995). There are 12 such situations written into the Privacy Act that permit releasing information in identifiable form from records maintained (Schulte and Sweeney, 1995). The data should be stored in specifically designed software and should be retrievable as and when needed by the competent person. Most of the stakeholders are ready to work in collaboration by sharing data and resources, because this can accelerate the development of biomarkers in oncology. A protected environment is needed to share the data between researchers, pharmaceutical firms, and stakeholders.

1.9.5 Incentives

Incentives should be developed to encourage the collaborations among drug developers, clinical research sponsors, and regulatory authorities. The incentives vary depending on the risk of sharing data. There should be a priority list of defining incentives generated along with recommendations for implementation.

1.9.6 Codevelopment of Diagnostics and Therapeutics

The codevelopment of a biomarker as diagnostics and therapeutics involves a complex interaction between principal investigators and different regulatory groups, for example, FDA, Center for Drug Evaluation and Radiological Health (CDRH) and the Center for Drug Evaluation and Research or Center for Biologics Evaluation and Research (CBER). There are certain areas of concern such as the interaction of sponsors with FDA for the clearance and approval of an assay or biomarker developed (Khleif et al., 2010), especially the application of administrative and evidentiary standards to the development of biomarkers. Evidentiary standards include best practices for labeling and developing drugs and diagnostics. Best practices in the use of adaptive clinical trial design applicable to both drugs and diagnostics used in the process of codevelopment should be defined.

1.9.7 Stakeholder Education and Communication

There is an urgent need to communicate about information generated, new standards developed, and new guidance released to the stakeholders. They should be educated about the compliance of ethical guidelines and encouraged to adopt the new standards. Educate patients and healthcare providers for the value of participation in the studies for the development of biomarkers. A number of organizations are addressing the issues of assay validation and analytical quality control; however, considerable education is still required for stakeholders in order to implement the good laboratory practices and data reporting by cancer researchers (Khleif et al., 2010).

1.9.8 Regulatory Policy

The scientific area of development of biomarkers and theranostics is responsible for the advancement of biomarker use in drug development. It is vital to develop policies cultivating innovation and on the other side safeguarding people by providing quality care to patient community. The CBC has defined many areas where the developing biomarkers have some potential barriers. CBC has suggested that relevant federal agencies should be involved in the process of addressing these areas and should take necessary action through regulatory and statutory changes (Khleif et al., 2010). Before entering into the market, FDA reviews the processes to ensure that new method or assay developed should be validated for analytical and clinical performance and should have adequate instructions for its use (Khleif et al., 2010). The reimbursement process should be improved for diagnostic tests. By providing stakeholders and setting precedent for third-party payers, the coverage and reimbursement decisions would accelerate the use of biomarker assays in clinical settings (Khleif et al., 2010).

1.9.9 Health Insurance Portability and Accountability Act of 1996

Hospitals, health plans, and other US organizations handling medical records and samples must comply with the Privacy Rule of the Health Insurance Portability and Accountability Act (HIPAA) of 1996. HIPAA provisions have influenced the development of cancer biomarkers. The law provides the

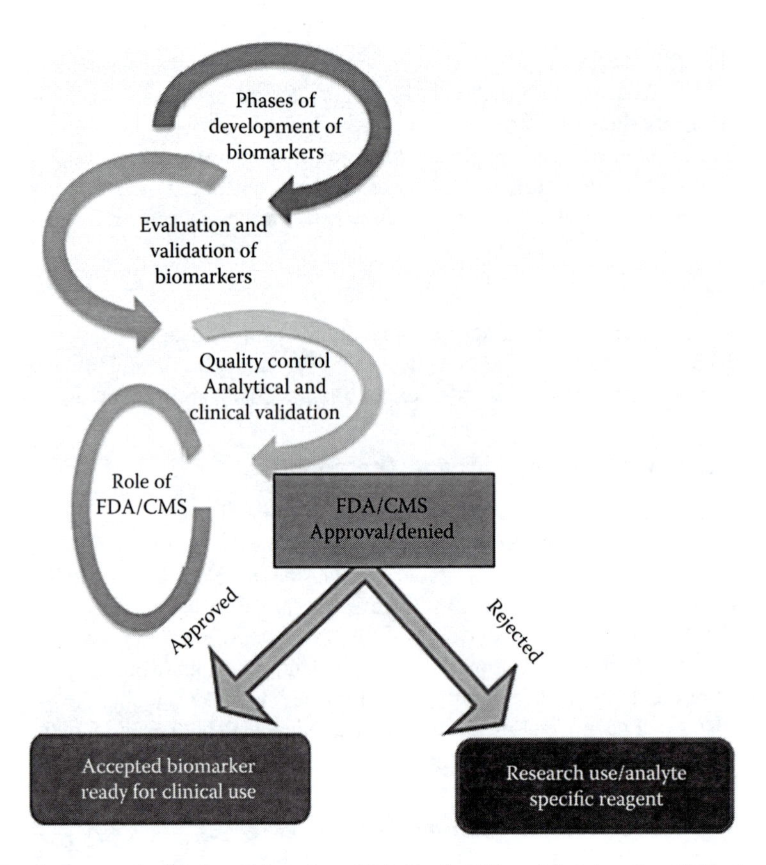

FIGURE 1.1 Development and validation of biomarkers. FDA, Food and Drug Administration; CMS, Center for Medicaid and Medicare Services.

protection of an individual's health information. In many cases, the access to existing biospecimen collections and acquisitions of new biospecimens has been hampered by HIPAA law. The need is to amend the law through proper evaluation of the impact of HIPAA provisions on biomarker research. The stages and validation of biomarkers in cancer have been summed in Figure 1.1.

1.10 Future Perspectives

There is enormous potential of biomarkers in early detection, diagnosis, and effective treatment of various types of cancers. The discovery of high-throughput technologies has proved to be instrumental in substantially reducing the burden of cancer providing quality diagnostics and treatment with the help of biomarkers. Despite this, very few biomarkers have been successfully translated into clinical practice in the area of oncology. The critical lynchpins are study design bias, artifacts during sampling, storage and processing, data analysis, and quality insufficient of methods adopted during various developmental and evaluation phases of biomarkers. The key enablers for the development of effective cancer biomarkers include a focused approach of identifying and selecting potential biomarkers with surrogate endpoints, stringent quality control, analytical and validation criteria, cost-effectiveness, and above all ethical regulations. The development of biomarkers is an imperative and can be achieved by collaboration between pharmaceutical firms, diagnostic companies, and academics including scientific researchers. The patient community will be served in a better way if better quality control, appropriate regulatory, and safety measures are considered along with cost-effectiveness during the development and validation of cancer biomarkers.

References

Baker SG, Kramer BS. Simple maximum likelihood estimates of efficacyin randomized trials and before-and-after studies, with implications for meta-analysis. *Stat Methods Med Res* 2005;4(4): 1–19.

Bansal S, DeStefano A. Key elements of bioanalytical method validation for small molecules. *AAPS J* 2007;9: E109–E114.

Baselga J, Tripathy D, Mendelsohn J, Baughman S, Benz CC, Dantis L, Sklarin NT et al. Phase II study of weekly intravenous recombinant humanized anti-p185HER2 monoclonal antibody in patients with HER2/neu-overexpressing metastatic breast cancer. *J Clin Oncol* 1996;14: 737–744.

Bast RC Jr, Feeney M, Lazarus H, Nadler LM, Colvin RB, Knapp RC. Reactivity of a monoclonal antibody with human ovarian carcinoma. *J Clin Invest* 1981;68: 1331–1337.

Bast RC Jr, Lilja H, Urban N, Rimm DL, Fritsche H, Gray J et al. Translational crossroads for biomarkers. *Clin Cancer Res* 2005;11: 6103–6108.

Bensalah K, Montorsi F, Shariat SF. Challenges of cancer biomarker profiling. *Eur Urol* 2007;52(6): 1601–1609.

Beshara N, Fung MFK, Faught W. The role of topotecan as a second-line therapy in patients with recurrent ovarian cancer. *Eur J Gynaecol Oncol* 2002;23: 287–290.

Bhatt AN, Mathur R, Farooque A, Verma A, Dwarakanath BS. Cancer biomarkers—Current perspectives. *Indian J Med Res* 2010;132: 129–149.

Boston, MA. http://biospecimens.cancer.gov/practices/forum/boston2007/pdf/FINAL_11-05-07_NCI_BPs_Forum_Boston_Summary_Rev1-24-08_Ed.pdf (accessed on June 7, 2013).

Brodie A. Aromatase inhibitor development and hormone therapy: A perspective. *Semin Oncol* 2003; 30: 12–22.

Chau CH, Rixe O, McLeod H, Figg WD. Validation of analytic methods for biomarkers used in drug development. *Clin Cancer Res* 2008;14: 5967–5976.

Cobleigh MA, Vogel CL, Tripathy D, Robert NJ, Scholl S, Fehrenbacher L, Wolter JM et al. Multinational study of the efficacy and safety of humanized anti-HER2 monoclonal antibody in women who have HER2-overexpressing metastatic breast cancer that has progressed after chemotherapy for metastatic disease. *J Clin Oncol* 1999;17: 2639–2648.

Cummings J, Ward TH, Greystoke A, Ranson M, Dive C. Biomarker method validation in anticancer drug development. *Br J Pharmacol* 2008;153: 646–656.

Dancey JE, Dobbin KK, Groshen S, Jessup JM, Hruszkewycz AH, Koehler M, Parchment R et al. Biomarkers Task Force of the NCI Investigational Drug Steering Committee. Guidelines for the development and incorporation of biomarker studies in early clinical trials of novel agents. *Clin Cancer Res* 2010;16(6): 1745–1755.

Diamandis EP. Cancer biomarkers: Can we turn recent failures into success. *J Natl Cancer Inst* 2010;102(19): 1462–1467.

Ditzel HJ, Strik MC, Larsen MK, Willis AC, Waseem A, Kejling K, Jensenius JC. Cancer-associated cleavage of cytokeratin 8/18 heterotypic complexes exposes a neoepitope in human adenocarcinomas. *J Biol Chem* 2002;277: 21712–21722.

Early Detection Research Network. 2002. Translational research to identify early cancer and cancer risk, second report. http://www3.cancer.gov/prevention/cbrg/edrn/publications.html (accessed on June 10, 2013).

Feng Z, Prentice R, Srivastava S. Research issues and strategies for genomic and proteomic biomarker discovery and validation: A statistical perspective. *Pharmacogenomics* 2004;5: 709–719.

Food and Drug Administration. 2001. Guidance for Industry: Bioanalytical Method Validation. Rockville, MD: US Department of Health and Human Services, Food and Drug Administration, Center for Drug Evaluation and Research.

Frank R, Hargreaves R. Clinical biomarkers in drug discovery and development. *Nat Drug Discov* 2003;2: 566–580.

Hadley DW, Jenkins J, Dimond E, Nakahara K, Grogan L, Liewehr DJ, Steinberg SM, Kirsch I. Genetic counseling and testing in families with hereditary nonpolyposis colorectal cancer. *Arch Intern Med* 2003;5(163): 573–582.

Hayes DF, Bast RC, Desch CE, Fritsche H Jr, Kemeny NE, Jessup JM, Locker GY et al. Tumor marker utility grading system: A framework to evaluate clinical utility of tumor markers. *J Natl Cancer Inst* 1996;88: 1456–1466.

Khleif SN, Doroshow JH, Hait WN. AACR-FDA-NCI cancer biomarkers collaborative consensus report: Advancing the use of biomarkers in cancer drug development. *Clin Cancer Res* 2010;16(13): 3299–3318.

Kulasingam V, Diamandis EP. Strategies for discovering novel cancer biomarkers through utilization of emerging technologies. *Nat Clin Pract Oncol* 2008;5: 588–599.

Kumar M, Sarin SK. Biomarkers of disease in medicine. *Curr Trends Sci*, Platinum Jubilee Special Issue, 2009;403–417.

Leers MP, Kölgen W, Bjorklund V, Bergman T, Tribbick G, Persson B, Björklund P et al. Immunocytochemical detection and mapping of a cytokeratin 18 neo-epitope exposed during early apoptosis. *J Pathol* 1999;187: 567–572.

Manne U, Srivastava RG, Srivastava S. Review, recent advances in biomarkers for cancer diagnosis and treatment. *Drug Discov Today* 2005;10(14): 965–976.

Mauro MJ, O'Dwyer M, Heinrich MC, Druker BJ. ST1571: A paradigm of new agents for cancer therapeutics. *J Clin Oncol* 2002;20: 325–334.

National Cancer Institute. Office of Biorepositories and Biospecimen Research. National Cancer Institute best practices for biospecimen resources. http://biospecimens.cancer.gov/global/pdfs/NCI_

Nowatzke W, Woolf E. Best practices during bioanalytical method validation for the characterization of assay reagents and the evaluation of analyte stability in assay standards, quality controls, and study samples. *AAPS J* 2007;9: E117–E122.

Office of Technology Assessment. New developments in biotechnology: Ownership of human tissues and cells—Special report, OTA-BA-337, Washington, DC: U.S. Government Printing Office, March 1987.

Paradiso A, Volpe S, Iacobacci A, Marubini E, Verderio P, Costa A, Daidone MG et al. Italian Network for Quality Assessment of Tumor Biomarkers. Quality control for biomarker determination in oncology: The experience of the Italian Network for Quality Assessment of Tumour Biomarkers (INQAT). *Int J Biol Markers* 2002;17: 201–214.

Pepe MS, Etzioni R, Feng Z, Potter JD, Thompson ML, Thornquist M, Winget M, Yasui Y. Phases of biomarker development for early detection of cancer. *J Natl Cancer Inst* 2001;93: 1054–1061.

Peters FT, Drummer OH, Musshoff F. Validation of new methods. *Forensic Sci Int* 2007;165: 216–224.

Ransohoff DF. Rules of evidence for cancer molecular marker discovery and validation. *Nature Rev Cancer* 2004;4: 309–314.

Rothstein MA. GINA, the ADA, and genetic discrimination in employment. *J Law Med Ethics* 2008 Winter;36(4): 837–840.

Schutte B, Henfling M, Kölgen W, Bouman M, Meex S, Leers MP, Nap M et al. Keratin 8/18 breakdown and reorganization during apoptosis. *Exp Cell Res* 2004;297: 11–26.

Schulte RA, Sweeney MH. Ethical considerations, confidentiality issues, rights of human subjects, and uses of monitoring data in research and regulation. *Environ Health Perspect* 1995;103: 69–74.

Semenuk MA, Veenstra TD, Georgevich G, Rochman M, Gusev Y, Hannes EJ, Bogunovic BM et al. Translating cancer biomarker discoveries to clinical tests: What should be considered. *Recent Pat Biomark* 2011;1: 222–240.

Shah VP, Midha KK, Dighe S, McGilveray IJ, Skelly JP, Yacobi A, Layloff T et al. Analytical methods validation: Bioavailability, bioequivalence and pharmacokinetic studies. Conference report. *Eur J Drug Metab Pharmacokinet* 1991;16: 249–255.

Shah VP, Midha KK, Findlay JW, Hill HM, Hulse JD, McGilveray IJ, McKay G et al. Bioanalytical method validation—A revisit with a decade of progress. *Pharm Res* 2000;17: 1551–1557.

Slamon DJ, Leyland-Jones B, Shak S, Fuchs H, Paton V, Bajamonde A, Fleming T et al. Use of chemotherapy plus a monoclonal antibody against HER2 for metastatic breast cancer that overexpresses HER2. *N Engl J Med* 2001;344: 783–792.

Smolec J, DeSilva B, Smith W, Weiner R, Kelly M, Lee B, Khan M et al. Bioanalytical method validation for macromolecules in support of pharmacokinetic studies. *Pharm Res* 2005;22: 1425–1431.

Srivastava S. Cancer biomarker discovery and development in gastrointestinal cancers: Early detection research network—A collaborative approach. *Gastrointest Cancer Res* 2007;1(4): S60–S63.

Ueno T, Toi M, Biven K, Bando H, Ogawa T, Linder S. Measurement of an apoptotic product in the sera of breast cancer patients. *Eur J Cancer* 2003;39: 769–774.

Vogel CL, Cobleigh MA, Tripathy D, Gutheil JC, Harris LN, Fehrenbacher L, Slamon DJ et al. Efficacy and safety of trastuzumab as a single agent in first-line treatment of HER2-overexpressing metastatic breast cancer. *J Clin Oncol* 2002;20: 719–726.

Zhang X, Wei D, Yap Y, Li L, Guo S, Chen F. Mass spectrometry-based "omics" technologies in cancer diagnostics. *Mass Spectrom Rev* 2007;26: 403–431.

2

Imaging Techniques in Cancer Diagnosis

Mohamed Abd El-Salam, Sonia Reda, Salwa Lotfi, Tamer Refaat, and Eman El-Abd

CONTENTS

ABSTRACT Medical imaging includes diagnostic and therapeutic imaging applications. Therapeutic imaging deals with treatment planning, guidance, assessment of tumor treatment response, palliation, and expansion of new therapeutics. Diagnostic imaging plays an important role in prediction, screening, detection, localization, differential diagnosis, staging, and prognosis of cancer. It includes invasive and noninvasive techniques. Noninvasive (i.e., the imaging modalities do not penetrate the skin physically) techniques use the full breadth of electromagnetic (EM) and acoustic spectrum. They range from plain to 3D+ modalities and can be classified into anatomical, functional (metabolic, physiological, and molecular), and combined or hybrid techniques. Imaging techniques differ in sensitivity, resolution, and contrast (due to the tissue nature or the agent used).

The current chapter focuses on the scientific advances in early detection of cancer using the noninvasive diagnostic imaging techniques such as x-ray, nuclear magnetic resonance (NMR), ultrasonography (USG); etc.

KEY WORDS: *cancer, diagnostic imaging, early detection, noninvasive techniques.*

2.1 Physics of Diagnostic Imaging

Images result from the interaction of energy at the molecular or atomic levels with human tissues. Energy forms can be radiation, magnetic or electric fields, or acoustic. A method for acquiring an image is called modality. Imaging modalities can be categorized according to the amount of energy applied to the body into ionizing (x-rays, computed tomography [CT], SPECT, and positron emission tomography [PET]) and nonionizing (magnetic resonance [MR] and ultrasound [US]) modalities. Ionizing modalities produce sufficient energy to ionize atoms or molecules (Bushberg et al., 2012). Currently, modalities are classified into four schemes: x-ray transmission, radionuclide emission, MR, and US (Morris and Perkins, 2012).

2.1.1 X-Ray Transmission

X-rays (Röntgen rays) are characterized as electromagnetic (EM) radiations (EM spectrum). X-ray particles are called photons and are delivered in packets called quanta with specific energy "E" that depends on the frequency "f." If the particle energy is greater than about 2–3 eV, then the photons are capable of ionizing atoms. Diagnostic x-rays are typically in the range of 12 eV–125 keV (100 nm to about 0.01 nm) (Bushberg et al., 2012; Dove, 2004).

The incident x-rays interact with matter in different ways (coherent [Rayleigh] scattering, photoelectric effect, Compton scattering, pair production, and photodisintegration) depending on many factors such as the energy of the incident photon, configuration of the electrons around the atom, atomic number, and mass of the target tissue (Bushberg et al., 2012; Dove, 2004). Understanding these interactions is important for understanding the development of image contrast in medical images and in understanding how x-ray detectors work.

Coherent (Rayleigh) scattering is not an ionizing interaction, and it is only important for thyroid scans using ^{125}I where it affects its resolution. It describes the deflection of a low-energy photon into new direction due to collision of a photon with an electron.

Photodisintegration results in the transformation of one element into a different one. Thus, it is extremely damaging to human tissue. The highly energetic incident photons (>1 MeV) interact with or are absorbed by the nucleus of the target atoms giving rise to ejection of one or more nuclear particles.

Photoelectric effect results in the production of photoelectrons, Auger electrons, and characteristic x-ray. The highly energetic interacting photon disappears after imparting all of its energy into core electron. If the binding energy of the electron is equal or less than that of the incident energy, then the electron can escape as a photoelectron. The electron vacant place is then filled by an electron from a higher energy level losing the energy difference as characteristic x-ray radiations. The emitted x-rays can cause emission of secondary electron, which is called an Auger electron.

Compton scattering (inelastic scattering) represents the main source of the background noise in x-ray images and tissue damage. High- or low-energy incident photon imparts only part of its energy to the emitted electron then continues its path with less energy and longer wavelength. The change in energy and wavelength depends on the rest mass of the electron, the speed of light, Planck's constant, and the angle of the scattered (recoiled) photon.

Pair production describes the formation of antimatter used in PET scanning. Highly energetic incident photon (>10 MeV) is absorbed by the nucleus releasing electron and its antiparticle positron (positive electron).

2.1.2 X-Ray Imaging Process

X-ray imaging (Bushberg et al., 2012; Dove, 2004) is an anatomical imaging modality. Heterogeneous or polychromatic photons generated by x-ray generator interact with tissues by photoelectric effect and Compton scattering. Part of the x-rays is filtered through the glass that surrounds the x-ray tube and aluminum filter, which is placed between patient and x-ray tube. As the body almost absorbs all the low-energy photons and thus they did not reach the detector, filters eliminate those photons and decrease patient exposure. The filtered incident photons then traverse the body where they are attenuated differently according to their energies and the half-value layer "HVL; the thickness required to attenuate the beam intensity by 50%." A grid is placed under the patient and before the detector to decrease scattering and hence decrease noise in the image. In order to correct for the nonideal nature of the x-ray source and detectors, an intensifying screen is placed beneath the patient and before the detector. Detectors then transform the transmitted x-rays into a visible form.

Detectors can be photographic film, viewed directly on a fluorescent screen (fluoroscopy), photostimulable phosphors, an ionization chamber, a scintillation detector (NaI), a semiconductor (silicon drift and pin diodes), or hybrid (scintillation plus semiconductor, for e.g., Medipix and flat panel [FP]) detectors. X-rays excite the silver halide crystals on the exposed photographic film leaving a viewable photo. Recently, films were replaced by a photostimulable phosphor (PSP) plate or computerized and digital radiography (DR). In photostimulated luminescence (PSL), the excited electrons in the phosphor material remain "trapped" in "color centers" in the crystal lattice until stimulated by a laser beam passed over the plate surface. The light given off during laser stimulation is collected by a photomultiplier tube, and the resulting signal is converted into a digital image by computer technology, which gives this process its common name, computed radiography (CR) (also referred to as DR). The PSP plate can be reused, and the existing x-ray equipment requires no modification to use them. Computer-processed x-rays can be utilized to produce slices of specific areas of the body (computed axial tomography, CAT or CT scanning). A 3D image can be generated from a large series of 2D x-ray images taken around a single axis of rotation using digital geometry processing.

Mammography, fluoroscopy, and xeroradiography are miscellaneous x-ray procedures. Mammography requires low-energy x-rays (typically 20 keV) and no contrast medium. Traditional fluoroscopy requires injection of a contrast medium to visualize real-time moving images of the internal structures of a patient. However, recent fluoroscopes that couple the screen to an x-ray image intensifier and CCD video camera allowing the image to be recorded and played on a monitor require contrast mediums. Xeroradiography uses electrostatic technique similar to the Xerox photocopy machine and x-ray energies from 35 to 45 keV.

In the ionization chamber (Geiger–Müller counter), x-rays ionize a gas, and the ions are attracted to electrodes under voltage difference. The most efficient detector (85%) is the scintillation detector coupled with photomultiplier tube. The x-ray photons are transformed into visible photons, which is amplified with a photomultiplier tube, and viewed. The solid-state detectors are built so that the incident photons generate electron–hole pairs in the semiconductor chip where the current flows proportional to incident photon density. The resulted electrons are collected under a high voltage and recorded as a negative pulse by a multichannel analyzer (MCA). In hybrid detectors, the incident radiation makes an electron/hole cloud on a semiconductor sensor layer. The charge is then collected and processed by a complementary metal-oxide semiconductor (CMOS) electronics layer, which counts the number of events in each pixel. Using discriminators allows counting events within a selected energy range.

2.1.3 Radionuclide Emission

Radionuclide emission (National Research Council [US] and Institute of Medicine [US] Committee on State of the Science of Nuclear Medicine, 2007) (e.g., PET) retrieves functional information via measuring the uptake and turnover of target-specific radiotracers, which is produced in a cyclotron, in tissue noninvasively. In PET, tiny amount of a biological compound labeled with a positron-emitting radionuclide that has a very short half-life is injected intravenously. The radionuclide emits positrons that annihilate after encountering an electron and produce a pair of photons that are then detected and measured in tissue by a PET scanner. The PET scan can construct tomography images representing quantitative physiological, pathological, or pharmacological information (McQuade et al., 2005).

Cancer cells particularly consume larger amounts of glucose due to defective mitochondrial oxidative phosphorylation what is known as the "Warburg effect." Based on this distinguished character, fluorine-18-fluorodeoxyglucose (FDG)-PET with relatively long half-life (110 min) is commonly used. It is transported by the same cell-surface hexose transporters and phosphorylated to FDG-6-phosphate, which cannot be further metabolized and remains trapped in the cells. Thus, its uptake and accumulation are higher in malignant regions. It can be used to differentiate between malignant and benign tumors and localize metastasis that is important in tumor staging and designing therapeutic strategies. It also helps in monitoring treatment response, which reduces the side effects and costs of ineffective therapies (Wieder et al., 2005; Juweid and Cheson, 2006; Weber and Wieder, 2006). However, some drawbacks of using FDG-PET were observed in imaging prostate and liver tumors (due to their low metabolic activities), brain tumors (as brain normally uses glucose), and under damage response conditions such as inflammatory response where body consumes higher glucose level. It is also affected by the tumor histological type, rate of growth, and intensity of metabolic activity (Figueiras et al., 2010).

The advancement in molecular oncology stimulated the identification of tumor factors influencing growth, metastasis, and cell death. Several targets have been identified and used in molecular imaging for diagnostic and therapeutic purposes (Haberkorn et al., 2011). Thymidine analogs were used in the measurement of DNA synthesis and in vivo cell proliferation reflecting accurate measure of tumor growth (Shields et al., 1998; Shields, 2006). Tumor hypoxia, O_2 partial pressure <2.5 mm Hg (Mottram, 1936), which characterizes aggressive tumors, was probed using fluorine-18-fluoromisonidazole 2-nitroimidazole derivatives, 18 F-azomycin arabinoside, and 64 Cu-methyl-thiosemicarbazone (Rajendran et al., 2006; Evans et al., 2011). Radiolabeled peptides, antibody fragments, and, more recently, nanoparticles targeting different cell-surface molecules also hold promise for tumor imaging and for targeted radionuclide therapy (Sharkey and Goldenberg, 2005; Haberkorn et al., 2011).

PET can be combined with anatomical imaging technique (PET/CT, SPECT/CT, and PET/magnetic resonance imaging [MRI]) to enhance its utility and accuracy (Lardinois et al., 2003; Cherry, 2006). Image fusion can be visual (by physician), hardware (using a single detector), or software (using software-based algorithm) fusion.

2.1.4 Nuclear Magnetic Resonance

Nuclear magnetic resonance (NMR) (Hornak, 2011) refers to a physical principal response of nuclei to a magnetic field (Kenyon et al., 1995). The technique depends on both magnetism and electricity. If a sample is placed in a magnetic field and is subjected to radio frequency (RF) radiation (energy) at the appropriate frequency, nuclei in the sample can absorb the energy. The frequency of the radiation necessary for absorption of energy depends on three things. First, it is characteristic of the type of nucleus (e.g., ^{1}H or ^{13}C). Second, the frequency depends on chemical environment of the nucleus (i.e., the CH_3 and OH protons of methanol absorb at different frequencies and amide protons of two different tryptophan residues in a native protein absorb at different frequencies since they are in different chemical environments). The NMR frequency also depends on spatial location in the magnetic field if that field is not everywhere uniform. This last variable provides the basis for MRI, for self-diffusion coefficient measurements, and for coherence selection—topics (James, 1998). If the object to be imaged, such as the human body, is divided into small cuboidal volume elements (i.e., voxels), the task in MR imaging is to distinguish the signal contributions of the voxels to the detected summation signal from one another and to present them in the form of sectional images (tomograms) (Hornak, 2011).

The technique is noninvasive and can generate high-resolution 3D images of any organ of the human body with excellent soft tissue contrast. Signals acquired from water and/or fat are utilized to generate an image, and image contrast depends on intrinsic properties of the tissue, for example, relaxation properties (T1- and T2-weighted images). The ability to modify image contrast simply by altering the parameters used for image acquisition is a major strength of MRI. Alternatively, image contrast can be improved by the administration of an external gadolinium-based contrast agent (Tafreshi et al., 2010).

Most clinical MRI machines operate between 5,000 and 15,000 G (Gauss) or 0.1 and 1.5 T, some lower, for example, at 0.3 T, some higher, for example, at 3.0 T (tesla). At low fields, one finds permanent magnets; at medium and high fields, the equipment is resistive or superconducting; both of them are different kinds of electromagnets (Rinck, 2012). To detect weak signals from metabolites, higher-strength field is required ($\geq$1.5 T). Higher field strength units have the advantage of higher signal-to-noise ratio (SNR), better resolution, and shorter acquisition times making the technique useful in sick patients and others that cannot hold still for long periods of time (Bertholdo et al.; Rinck, 2012).

Phosphorus (^{31}P), fluorine (^{19}F), carbon (^{13}C), and sodium (^{23}Na) nuclei may be used to obtain magnetic resonance spectroscopy (MRS). Protons are mostly used for clinical MRS (H-MRS) due to the abundance of hydrogen nucleus in human tissues. As motion affects MRS, abdomen and thorax cannot be imaged without very sophisticated motion-reduction techniques, while metabolic status of the brain is ideally imaged with H-MRS as it is nearly motionless. Abnormal spectral alterations are dependent on patient age and brain region (Bertholdo et al.). It is also important to know the normal brain spectra and their variations according to each technique. H-MRS requires only standard RF coils and a dedicated software package (Bertholdo et al.). The H-MRS acquisition usually starts with anatomical images, which are used to select a volume of interest (VOI), where the spectrum will be acquired. For the spectrum acquisition, different techniques may be used including single- and multivoxel imaging using both long and short echo times (TE). Each technique has advantages and disadvantages, and choosing the right one for a specific purpose is important to improve the quality of the results (Bertholdo et al.). A wide variety of CT- and MRI-based perfusion imaging techniques were developed and applied in both diagnostic and prognostic fields (Lin and Jackson, 2012).

2.1.5 MR Imaging Process

The imaging process includes several steps:

1. Patient is placed in a static magnetic field.
2. Magnetized protons (spinning H nuclei) in the patient align in this field like compass needles.
3. RF pulses then bombard the magnetized nuclei causing them to flip around.
4. The nuclei absorb the RF energy and enter an excited state.
5. When the magnet is turned off, excited nuclei return to normal state and give off RF energy.
6. The energy given off reflects the number of protons in a "slice" of tissue.
7. Different tissues absorb and give off different amounts of RF energy (different resonances).
8. The RF energy given off is picked up by the receiver coil and transformed into images.

2.1.6 Ultrasound

Unlike x-rays, sound waves (Chan and Perlas, 2011) constitute mechanical longitudinal waves, which can be described in terms of particle displacement or pressure changes. The term ultrasound is applied to mechanical pressure waves with frequencies above 20,000 Hz, beyond the audible range. A medium is required for US propagation to occur. US is a safe, relatively cost-effective, portable, and minimally invasive means of creating cross-sectional images of the human body. There is no discomfort apart from a cold probe. It is more effective than x-ray techniques in producing images of soft tissue (Chan and Perlas, 2011). The technology is enabling us to see the movement of organs (see their structure in 3D) and image their microvasculature.

In biological tissues, ultrasonic energy is propagated mainly in the form of longitudinal waves, as it is in fluid (Chan and Perlas, 2011). Frequency, propagation speed, pulsed US, interaction of US with tissue, angle of incidence, and attenuation are important measures in US imaging (USI). The frequency (cycles per second or hertz) of a US wave consists of the number of cycles or pressure changes that occur in 1 s. Frequency is determined by the sound source only and not by the medium in which the sound is traveling. Diagnostic medical US devices utilize high-frequency US waves at the frequency of 1–15 MHz to construct an image. Propagation speed is the speed at which sound can travel through a medium and is typically considered 1540 m/s for soft tissue. The speed is determined solely by the medium characteristics, especially those of density and stiffness. Pulsed US describes a means of emitting US waves from a source. To achieve the depth of resolution required for clinical uses, pulsed beams are used. Typically, the pulses are a millisecond or so long, and several thousands are emitted per second.

The transmitted US wave, mainly in the form of a train of short pulses, propagates in the tissue where the structures are reflected and returned to the head as echoes. A reflection occurs at the boundary between two materials provided that a certain property of the materials is different. If a beam of US strikes a boundary obliquely, however, then the interactions are more complex than for normal incidence. The echo will return from the boundary at an angle equal to the angle of incidence. The transmitted beam will be deviated from a straight line by an amount that depends on the difference in the velocity of US at either side of the boundary. This process is known as refraction, and the amount of deviation is given by the relations, and this actually helps to produce images of irregularly shaped objects. Rough surfaces have features that are the same sort of size as the wavelength of the US and produce echoes in many directions. In practice, this enables sound to get back to the transducer from oblique surfaces. Although the challenge of overcoming the problem of weakly reflected pulses is significant in itself, the intensity of the US beam is further reduced by attenuation due to various processes such as reflection, refraction, scattering, and absorption. All these processes divert energy from the main beam. Reflection and refraction occur at surfaces that are large compared with the wavelength of the US. For objects that are small in comparison with the wavelength, energy is scattered in many directions, and the eventual fate of the US is to be absorbed as particle vibration and the production of heat. The amount of attenuation varies with the frequency of US. A high-frequency beam will be attenuated more than a lower frequency. This means that to penetrate and subsequently image deep into the body, a lower-frequency transducer has to be used. Unfortunately, because higher frequencies enable finer detail to be resolved, there must therefore be a compromise between resolution and penetration for different imaging applications (Aldrich, 2007).

The signal of echoes is initially amplified and filtered in an analog chain and, next, digitally processed using analog–digital converter (ADC) with 8–14 bit of resolution (Thomenius, 2006). The received high-frequency signal (called RF) of the echoes is amplitude- and phase-modulated carrier frequency signal. The signal is demodulated in the device to obtain baseband frequency. The demodulated echo signal is further processed, depending on the application (Ali et al., 2008). Photoacoustic or optoacoustic imaging (PAI) bridged the gap between the higher resolution of optical imaging techniques and high detection sensitivity of other modalities (Mallidi et al., 2011). The technique combines optical (laser; generally a tunable, nanosecond pulsed laser) with USI (with US algorithms or equations). It can be combined with various USI and other modalities to provide simultaneous structural, functional, and molecular evaluations.

2.1.7 US Imaging Techniques

The echo principle forms the basis of all of the commonly used diagnostic US techniques. These are A-scan, B-scan, M-scan, and Doppler techniques (Chan and Perlas, 2011).

A-scan (amplitude modulation) is a 1D technique. The echoes received are displayed on a screen as vertical deflections. This technique is rarely used today except for measurements.

B-scan (brightness modulation) is a technique in which the echo amplitude is depicted as dots of different brightness (gray scale). It is mostly used as a 2D B-scan to form a 2D US image by multiple US beams, arranged successively in one plane. The images are built up by mechanically or electronically regulated scanning in a fraction of a second. The image rate of more than 15 per second enables an impression of "permanent" imaging during the examination (real time).

M-scan (also sometimes referred to as TM-scan) is a way to display motion, for example, of parts of the heart. The echoes produced by a stationary US beam are recorded over time, continuously.

Doppler techniques use the Doppler effects as a further source of information: if the US waves are reflected by an interface moving toward the transducer or away from it, the reflected frequency will be higher or lower respectively than the transmitted frequency. The difference between the emitted and received frequencies is proportional to the speed of the moving reflector. This phenomenon is called the Doppler effect, and the difference is called the Doppler frequency or Doppler shift.

In PAI, the absorbed laser stimulates rapid thermoelastic expansion of tissue leading to the generation of a wide-band US wave, which can be detected with a transducer that converts the US wave to electric signals then processes it to produce the image. Both endogenous agents (melanin, hemoglobin, PO_2, circulating tumor cells) and exogenous (nanoparticles, photoactivatable probes, fluorescence) chromophores can be used as contrast agents (Mallidi et al., 2011).

2.2 Applications in Cancer Imaging

Imaging modalities are an important part of cancer care and management. They operate over a wide range of size and time scales, allow real-time monitoring, have high accessibility without tissue destruction, and are minimally invasive or noninvasive (Fass, 2008). Combined imaging modalities provided complementary information that improved early diagnosis and prognosis of cancer. Metabolic, molecular (genetic, epigenetic, transcriptomic, and proteomic) markers as well as nanoprobes have been recently integrated to various imaging modalities (Czernin et al., 2010; McDonnell et al., 2010; Gore et al., 2011; Chi et al., 2012; Kircher et al., 2012; Pinker et al., 2012; Rosen et al., 2012).

2.2.1 Breast Cancer

Several imaging modalities are used currently for screening, detecting, and staging of breast cancer. Low-dose mammography (Figure 2.1) still remains the gold standard for breast cancer screening in asymptomatic individuals for breast cancer although it is less accurate in patients with dense breast tissue or implants. Positron emission mammography (PEM) enabled capture of sharp detailed, localized images of small breast tumors apart from the patient's menopausal/hormonal status or breast density (Moadel, 2011). It was recommended as an alternative presurgical option to MRI (Schilling et al., 2011). Recently, a high-resolution PEM/PET imaging guided biopsy was developed (Raylman et al., 2008) and proved safety and effectiveness in sampling breast lesions (Kalinyak et al., 2011). CT (Figure 2.2) techniques are useful in diagnosing breast cancer lesions (spiral CT), detecting intraductal extension of breast cancer (dynamic contrast-enhanced CT), and monitoring metastasis and nodal involvement (3D helical CT) (Ternier et al., 2006; Yamamoto et al., 2006).

Electric impedance tomography (EIT) relies on the fact that breast cancer cells have higher electric conductivity than normal cells due to biochemical and pathological changes. The technique is cost-effective but is limited by low resolution, inaccurate modeling, skin contact impedance, and poor SNR (Halter et al., 2007). Thermography (Mital and Scott, 2007) is another technique that has not proved useful in breast cancer screening. It relies on the temperature variation between normal cells and cancer and precancerous lesions due to angiogenesis. Temperature variations are captured using ultrasensitive infrared cameras and PCs to generate high-resolution diagnostic images. Galactography (Figure 2.3) (Prasad and Houserkova, 2007) is an x-ray procedure that enables visualizing the inside of the breast's milk ducts to determine the cause of nipple discharge (Schwab et al., 2008). It helps in the detection of

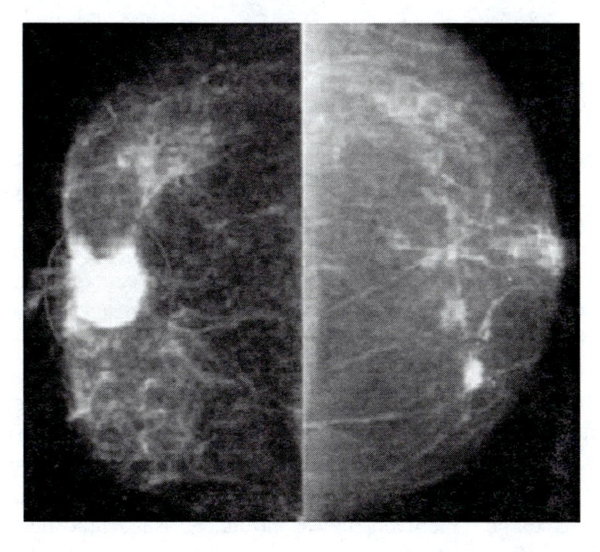

FIGURE 2.1 **(See color insert.)** A mammogram showing cancer in both breasts. (Reprinted from Weinstein Imaging Associates, Pittsburgh, PA.)

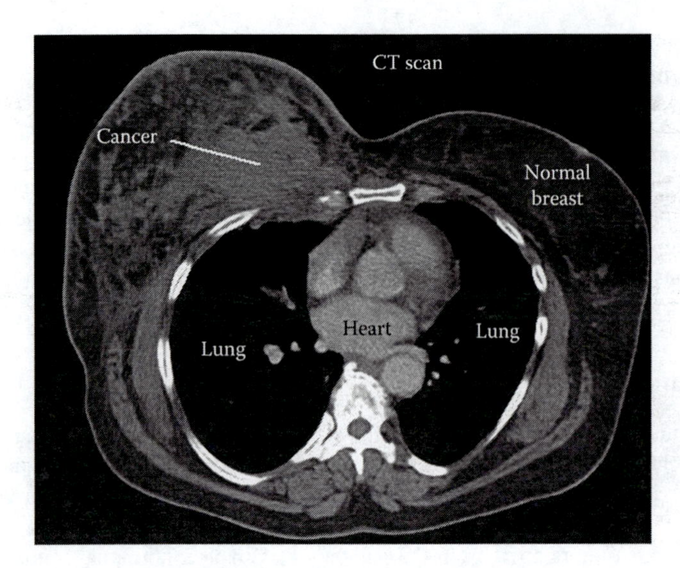

FIGURE 2.2 **(See color insert.)** CT scan of advanced inflammatory breast cancer (cancer of the right breast invading into chest wall). (Reprinted with permission from Dr. Robert Miller.)

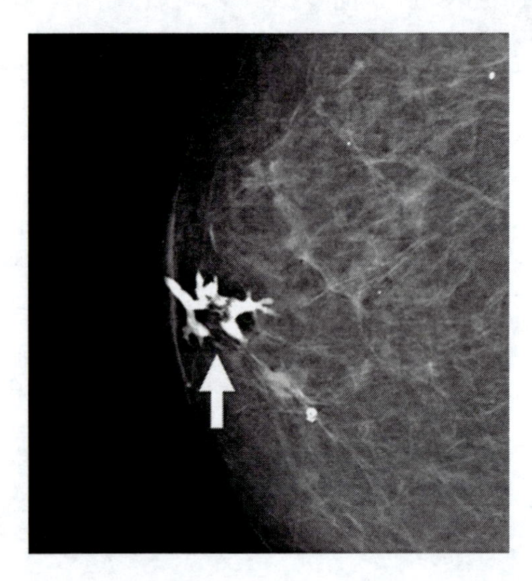

FIGURE 2.3 **(See color insert.)** Conventional craniocaudal galactogram (in a 76-year-old woman with pathologic nipple discharge) shows a retromammillary, solitary intraductal papilloma (arrow). (Reprinted from Schwab, S. et al., *Radiobiology,* 249(1), 54, 2008. With permission.)

small malignant and benign tumors that cannot be detected by other imaging modalities. Ductoscopy and endoscopy were used in diagnosing, locating, and defining the extent of duct excision (Holloway et al., 2010).

Ultrasonography (USG) (Figure 2.4) (Nothacker et al., 2009) enables differentiating cysts from solid breast masses with high specificity based on shape, margins, and echogenicity of a breast mass. USG advanced to differentiate benign/malignant solid breast lesions and to guide interventional procedures such as needle aspirations, core-needle biopsies, and prebiopsy needle localizations of breast masses or calcifications as an easy and real-time imaging technique. It is also a sensitive safe modality especially in women with dense breast tissue. Color Doppler was introduced as a diagnostic tool to assess the blood flow of breast tumors. Elasticity coupled with USI was used to detect breast tumors with high specificity and sensitivity without need for biopsy (Zhi et al., 2007).

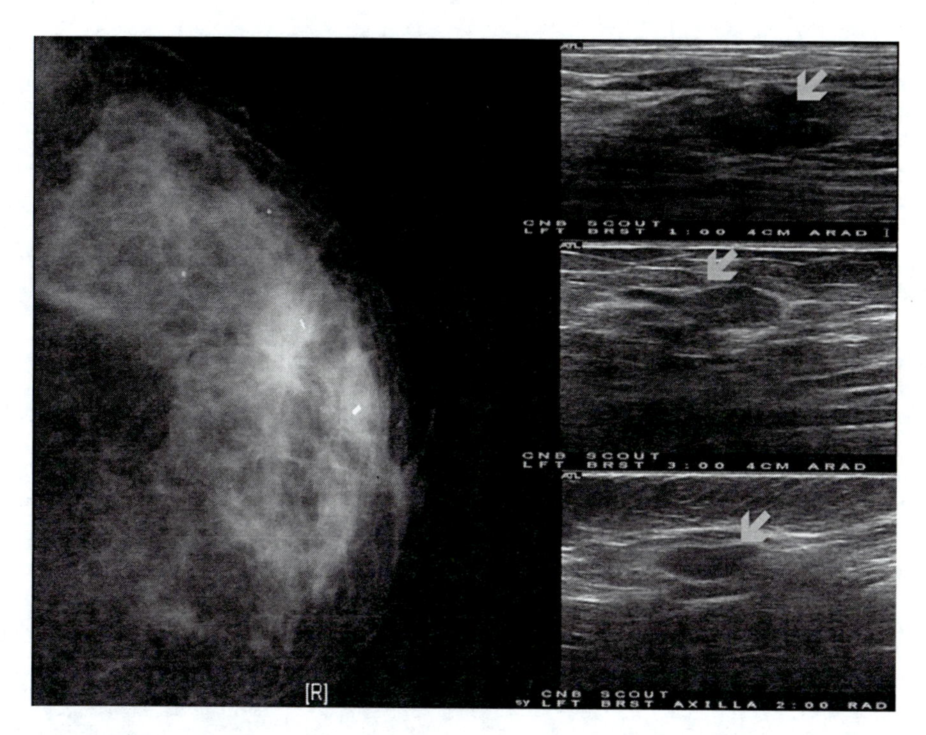

FIGURE 2.4 **(See color insert.)** Sonogram of left breast at 1 o'clock demonstrates a hypoechoic lesion with angular margins highly suspicious for malignancy. Sonogram of left breast at 3 o'clock shows a hypoechoic lesion with what appears to be a duct leading into it. Sonogram of the left axilla shows a lymph node with very prominent cortex highly suggestive of tumor involvement.

Sentinel lymph node (SLN) scintigraphy is another new technique that uses ^{99m}Tc-labeled colloids that are generally engulfed by macrophages and subsequently carried to lymphatic drainage. It showed high effectiveness in preoperative evaluation of lymphatic basin and detection of SLN (Tanaka et al., 2007). SPECT/CT SLN scintigraphy was developed to obtain 3D information about the involvement of SLN (Ibusuki et al., 2010). ^{99m}Tc-sestamibi is taken by active mitochondria and accumulates in breast cancers. Subsequently, breast cancers can be imaged using high-resolution γ-camera detector and positron detector to detect breast cancer. However, the technique showed poor sensitivity for small tumors <1 cm. Improvements such as using camera that utilizes a semiconductor-based γ-camera or position-sensitive photomultiplier tubes in molecular breast imaging (MBI) (Rhodes et al., 2005; O'Connor et al., 2007; Hampton, 2008) or breast-specific γ-imaging (BSGI) (Brem et al., 2008) enabled detection of breast tumors as small as <1 cm and 0–3 mm, respectively. MBI was successfully used in screening of women with family history of breast cancer or who had prior exposure to chest or mantle irradiation. It also helped in the follow-up after breast surgery. Both techniques were suggested to be used as an adjunct to MRI when the sensitivity of mammography is decreased by the density of the breast parenchyma.

^{18}FDG-PET/CT proved useful in detecting recurrent and metastatic breast cancer (Warning et al., 2011). High sensitivity was observed in detecting osteolytic bone metastasis, but Na-^{18}F-fluroride PET showed higher sensitivity in detecting bone metastasis. ^{18}FDG-PET/CT showed limited sensitivity in detecting micrometastasis so it cannot replace SLN technique. However, it can indicate LN involvement better than MRI. It has poor detection rate for smaller tumors (≤10 mm) than larger tumors (>10 mm) perhaps due to combined effect of limited metabolic activity of small tumors and low spatial resolution. It is promising for monitoring response to chemotherapy (Warning et al., 2011).

Contrast-enhanced MRI (CEMRI) and dynamic contrast-enhanced MRI (DCEMRI) are widely used in detection and characterization of breast lesions. DCEMRI of breast is routinely used in screening women at high risk for breast cancer such as BRCA1, BRCA2, and TP53 mutation carriers. Its power is limited in breast cancer staging due to its low specificity and lack of evidence-based benefits in the clinical management. It is also used in the detection of breast cancer and monitoring treatment response (Tafreshi et al., 2010). Chemical shift imaging (CSI) or magnetic resonance spectroscopic imaging (MRSI) is used to distinguish malignant from benign breast lesions and to monitor response to chemotherapy via total choline (tCho) level (Bolan et al., 2005; Gillies and Morse, 2005). Diffusion MRI is another technique that can differentiate malignant from benign breast lesions (Sinha et al., 2002). Apparent diffusion coefficient (ADC), which is significantly reduced in malignancy, was used as a biomarker to indicate early therapeutic response before measurable changes in tumor size (Tafreshi et al., 2010).

Her-2 expression and 16α-18F-fluoro-17-β-estradiol (FES) were used to predict targeted therapy (Slamon et al., 2001; Mankoff et al., 2008).

2.2.2 Liver

Contrast-enhanced US has been used to predict response in liver, renal, and stromal tumors (De Giorgi et al., 2005; Williams et al., 2011). Sonazoid-enhanced 3D US (Sugimoto et al., 2009) is a new promising imaging modality in differential diagnosis of hepatic lesions (sensitivity $\geq$ 83%, specificity $\geq$ 87%, PPV $\geq$ 71%, Az 0.89, $\kappa \geq 0.76$) and evaluation of the vascular characteristics of liver (Numata et al., 2011). It involves an early vascular phase and a late parenchyma-specific phase. Sonazoid is highly stable, allows prolonged imaging, and has a stronger contrast effect, but it has some side effects including diarrhea (1.6%), albuminuria (1.6%), and neutropenia (1%), and it is contraindicated in patients with history of egg allergy. Contrast-enhanced 3D CT has higher specificity ($\geq$92) and Az (0.92) than Sonazoid-enhanced 3D US.

2.2.3 Prostate

Low- and high-grade prostate cancers can be distinguished by MRS (Seitz et al., 2009) using choline and creatine apoptotic markers (Kobus et al., 2011). Acute hypoxia is detected in prostate cancer using blood oxygen level-dependent MRI (BLOD-MRI). The technique depends on the endogenous deoxyhemoglobin as a paramagnetic molecule that shortens the transverse relaxation allowing sensitive measurement of PO_2 in vessels and near tissues. BLOD-MRI should be performed concurrently with tumor perfusion to indicate the origin of the signal (Figueiras et al., 2010).

2.2.4 Pediatric

In pediatric oncology, combined ^{18}F-FDG-PET/CT (Nannia et al., 2006) is being used more often. However, it is necessary to recognize the physiologic variants, artifacts, and potential pitfalls in children in order to avoid misinterpretation, enhance accuracy, diminish the unnecessary follow-up, and improve treatment (Shammas et al., 2009). It is also recommended to take a complete clinical history of the patient, to consider special procedures for patient preparation, and to perform correlation with anatomical imaging.

2.2.5 Gastrointestinal

In gastrointestinal stromal tumors (GISTs) (Kalkmann et al., 2012), CT (Figure 2.5) represents the standard imaging technique in tumor detection, staging, and monitoring treatment response. In cases where CT is contraindicated, MRI is recommended. MRI also has higher sensitivity toward detection of small tumors so it is required in detection and follow-up of metastasis (liver, pelvis, and pulmonary) or progressive disease. In case of unclear CT and MRI results, ^{18}F-FDG-PET/CT is an alternative. For T staging of esophageal tumors, endoscopic US (EUS) is the imaging modality of choice, while PET/CT is used to detect primary tumors and assist invasion (Karaosmanoğlu and Blake, 2012).

Mesorectal nodal involvement was investigated using ultrasmall superparamagnetic iron oxide (USPIO)-enhanced MRI and proves to improve specificity compared to standard MRI (Koh et al., 2004). Primary colon cancer staging is performed using CT with spiral acquisition through the chest, abdomen, and pelvis following intravenous (IV) contrast administration (Brush et al., 2011). For suspected

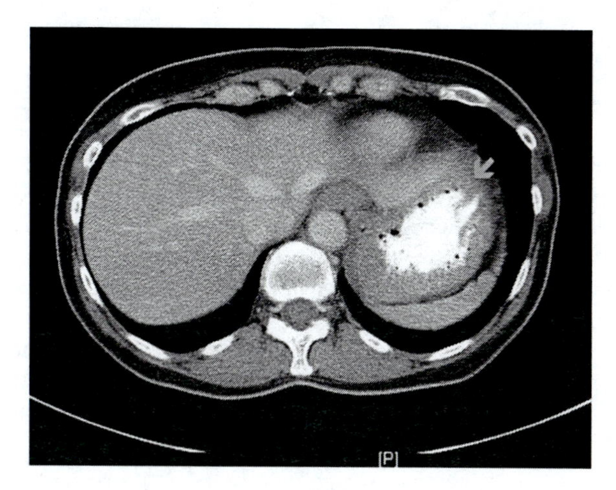

FIGURE 2.5 A case of gastric cancer, CT upper abdomen reveals a heterogeneous diffuse thickening of the stomach wall. A gastric cancer diagnosis was established in this patient.

recurrence of CRC (especially liver metastasis) and in preoperative staging, FDG-PET/CT is recommended. Based on lymph node size analysis, FDG-PET/CT showed a sensitivity of 30% and a specificity of 85% for tumors >10 mm. When recurrence is suspected, combinations of MRI, CT, chest radiography, US, and if available FDG-PET/CT are used for confirmation and reclassification of the disease status. MRI is regarded by many as the best method to image the rectum.

2.2.6 Lung

Although chest radiograph identified patients with early lung cancer, the technique was limited by poor sensitivity in identifying faint nodules and relatively high false-positive rate. Recent studies proved the effectiveness of CT in high-risk patients. However, increased false positivity, unnecessary additional testing and surgical intervention for benign lesions, radiation exposure, and cost-effectiveness remain major concerns in lung screening programs (Mazzone, 2012). PET/CT provides accurate prediction of TNM staging of NSCLC (non-small-cell lung cancer) (Chao and Zhang, 2012; Li et al., 2012), and thus it plays an important role in surgical and therapeutic interventions.

2.2.7 Gynecological

The Radiology Diagnostic Oncology Group (RDOG) proposed that solidity on MRI and a high-resistance index (RI) of the tumor on color Doppler US be used as the diagnostic features of a metastatic ovarian neoplasm (Lee et al., 2011). Multilocularity on MRI and US has been considered as a characteristic of primary ovarian cancer by the RDOG study. Metastasis from gastric cancers (Krukenberg tumor) is characterized by a (1) presence of signet-ring cells with mucin, (2) presence of stromal invasion, and (3) sarcomatoid proliferation of ovarian stroma as proposed by WHO. Bilaterality, slightly enlarged size, lobulation, and solidity are important radiological imaging findings. The solid area of the ovary can often be observed as a homogeneous enhancement on T1-weighted MRI and as heterogeneous intensity on T2-weighted MRI. Metastasis from colon cancer often exhibits a cystic nature and bilateral involvement. A stained glass appearance and multicystic chamber can be noted in CT and MRI. However, the increased density and prominently large amount of ascites compressing the bowels and liver due to metastasis from appendix can be observed on US and CT.

Presurgical MRI was considered an accurate predictor of cervical involvement in endometrial cancer and an important factor in decision about the type of hysterectomy (Nagar et al., 2006). Transvaginal US showed high specificity in diagnosing ovarian tumors (Bharwani et al., 2011). The combination of morphological US with power Doppler enhances sensitivity and specificity. To detect the origin of adnexal mass (benign or malignant), US represents the most appropriate initial imaging investigation.

Additional imaging investigation such as MRI (gadolinium-enhanced MRI) is required for further characterization of adnexal mass in women with RMI > 25 (risk of malignancy index = US score × menopausal status × CA 125 level). Patients with RMI > 1000 are considered to have malignant tumors and referred to CT (contrast-enhanced helical CT) evaluation. CT and MRI are used for tumor staging, planning patient management, and follow-up. When CT is negative or in areas that are difficult to assess by CT or MRI, FDG-PET/CT is used to assess metastatic ovarian tumors. Biopsy can be guided by imaging techniques. Currently, DWI is evaluated for monitoring therapeutic response, and optical imaging is holding a promise for improving intraoperative tumor detection and achieving maximal cytoreduction.

DW-MRI (diffusion-weighted MRI) showed high specificity and sensitivity in differentiation of cervical tumors from benign due to reduced tumor ADC (Kundu et al., 2012). Moreover, primary tumors and secondary nodal deposits can be identified due to high average of ADC of large infiltrative tumors. Stromal invasions >3 mm can be diagnosed with high specificity, sensitivity, and accuracy using DC-PWI (dynamic contrast perfusion-weighted MRI). PWI gives rational evaluation of cervical cancer oxygenation and angiogenesis.

2.2.8 Head and Neck

Only in head and neck and uterine cervix, perfusion CT and MRI showed a correlation with tumor hypoxia. Complex studies revealed variable results about the relationship between hypoxia, blood flow, and glucose metabolism, yet information about tumor functionality using angiogenic, metabolic, cellular, and molecular markers is of potential value in tumor mapping, new drug design, and monitoring tumor response (Figueiras et al., 2010).

2.2.9 Brain

Radiotracers such as 18F- or 11C-labeled amino acids and amino acid analogs have been used successfully for imaging brain tumors (Pirotte et al., 2004; Nariai et al., 2005; Chen et al., 2006). MRS is superior to MRI (Figures 2.6 through 2.8) in detecting brain metabolic changes, which often precede structural abnormalities (Fayed et al., 2006). Combining optical imaging (fluorescence imaging) with PAI enabled localization of brain tumors in vivo (Lungu et al., 2007).

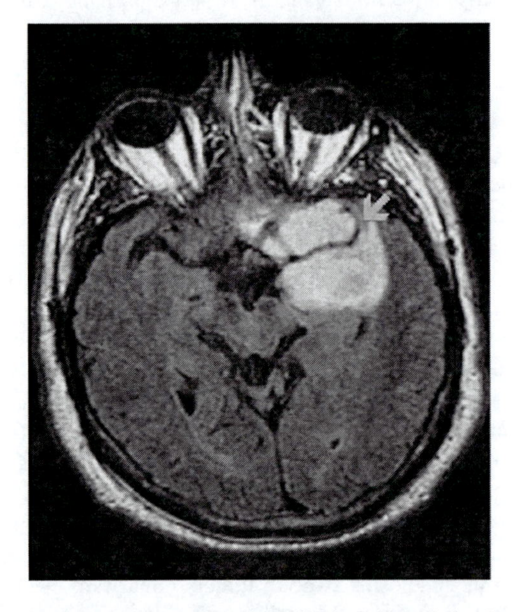

FIGURE 2.6 Brain MRI scan shows a hyperintense T2-weighted lesion with indistinct borders and minimal surrounding edema, a picture consistent with low-grade brain tumor (astrocytoma).

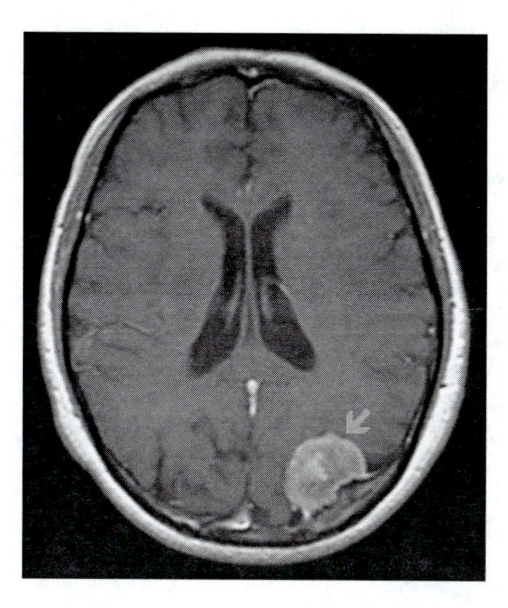

FIGURE 2.7 MRI scan shows heterogeneous hypo- to isointensity on T1 weighted with avid enhancement postgadolinium. "Dural tail"—curvilinear area of enhancement tapering off from margin of tumor along dural surface and notable hyperostosis of adjacent bone. The patient was diagnosed with meningioma.

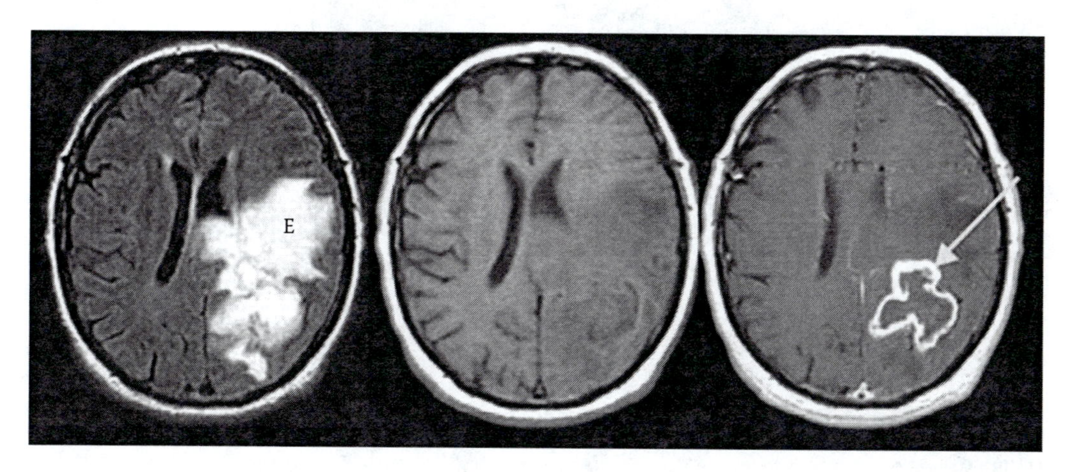

FIGURE 2.8 A case of glioblastoma multiform MRI T1 pregadolinium contrast shows a hypointense lesion. The T1 post-gadolinium contrast image shows heterogeneous enhancement with irregular, ring-like configuration that may surround a central area of necrosis, a picture that enhancement implies malignant tumor. The T2-weighted/FLAIR image shows edema (E) surrounding the tumor that is hyperintense.

2.2.10 Pancreatic

CT scan (Figures 2.9 and 2.10) is widely used for evaluation, diagnosis, and surgical staging of solid pancreatic malignancies (Iglesias-García et al., 2012). Chronic pancreatitis can be differentiated from pancreatic adenocarcinoma by triple-phase helical CT scan and MRI. EUS is an accurate method for the diagnosis and staging of inflammatory, cystic, and neoplastic diseases of the pancreas. It can be combined with FNA, Tru-Cut, Quick-Core, and other needles to obtain tumor samples for pathological assessments. EUS elastography-based modalities were used to differentiate between benign and malignant pancreatic tumors. Autoimmune pancreatitis can be distinguished from pancreatic cancer using CT and MRI.

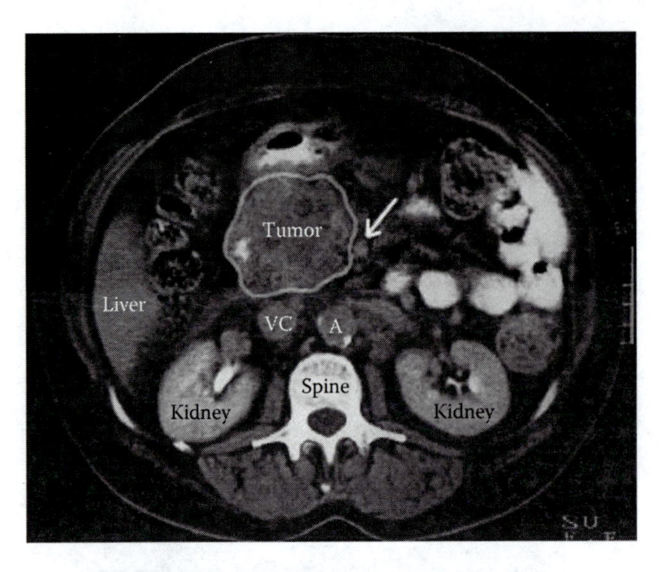

FIGURE 2.9 CT of upper abdomen reveals a heterogeneous mass replacing the pancreatic head that was diagnosed as pancreatic cancer.

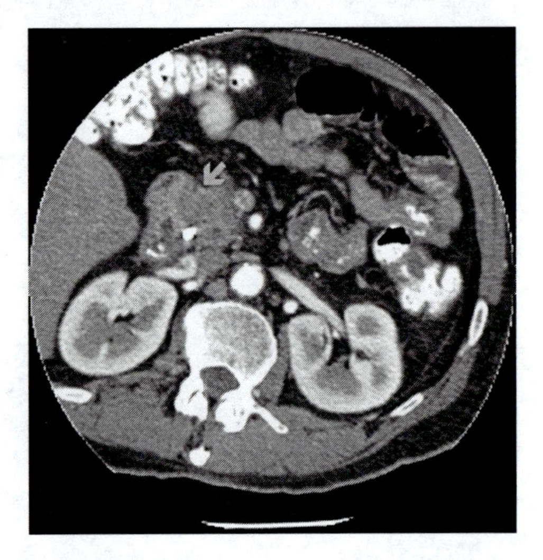

FIGURE 2.10 CT of upper abdomen reveals a heterogeneous mass replacing the pancreatic head that was diagnosed as pancreatic cancer.

2.2.11 Oral

Light-based detection systems, chemiluminescence, and tissue fluorescence imaging have been used to detect malignant oral lesions (Lestón and Dios, 2010). Primary tumor and regional lymph nodes are often assessed by dental panoramic tomography (DPT), CT (for bone invasion), and MRI (to evaluate the extent of soft tissue invasion, neurovascular bundle infiltration, and cervical lymph node involvement). Preoperative cone beam CT (CBCT) is used to determine the degree of invasion and extension of the lesion toward the jaw bones, staging oral cancers, and planning of the surgical resection. Optical coherence tomography (OCT) allows the detection and diagnosis of oral premalignant lesions.

2.2.12 Pelvis

Bone tumors (Girish et al., 2012a) such as osteogenic sarcoma (OGS) are initially assessed and diagnosed by radiographs. Relevant history including age, rate of onset, and duration of symptoms is necessary in assessing osseous pelvic tumors. For assessment of bone tumor characteristics and in classifying matrix mineralization, multidetector-row computed tomography (MDCT) is used. MRI is better than CT in assessing the involvement of soft tissue, marrow, and neurovascular structures. Bone destruction that is a major feature of Ewing's sarcoma (ES) is best characterized by CT. Multiple myeloma is characterized by osteopenia and punched-out lytic lesions on the plain film, while on MRI, it can present as distinct multifocal small intramedullary lesions, diffuse marrow abnormality, a variegated appearance of the marrow, or a combination. Whole-body MRI is useful in tumor staging and identification of any complications. Lymphoma and chondrosarcoma have characteristic findings on MRI, while enchondroma is best characterized by calcification on CT, which varies according to the tumor grade. Combination of CT and MRI are important in detecting primary bone tumors. They reveal the soft tissue component, calcifications, and epidural extension of chordomas (Girish et al., 2012a).

Detection of metastatic bone tumors depends on the site of metastasis. Renal metastasis is specifically detected by MDCT, while lytic pelvic metastases are more easily detected by MRI. Bone scans are very sensitive in the detection of osteoblastic metastasis, still valuable in detecting thyroid bone metastases and less accurate in detecting lytic metastasis (Girish et al., 2012a).

Bone scan is used to diagnose insufficiency fracture. MRI and CT identify additional findings that help in making the correct diagnosis. Relevant history, bone scan, and MRI are important in diagnosing a bone graft donor site (Girish et al., 2012a).

Pelvic osteochondroma can be diagnosed by plain film and CT. Osteochondroma may be large and lead to soft tissue displacement, bursitis, or nerve compression or prone to trauma-induced fracture depending on its anatomical location. Malignant transformation might be indicated by the onset of pain; a large, poorly defined cap, containing irregular or incomplete calcification; and any increase in the thickness of the cartilage cap after puberty (>2 cm). Malignant osteoblastoma is characterized by bone sclerosis and an exuberant periostitis. Osteoblastomas may show secondary aneurysmal bone cyst (ABC) formation, which makes it resembles the giant cell tumor (GCT); however, it can be distinguished by the high signal of the solid portion of tumor on T2-weighted images. About 5%–10% of GCTs are malignant. Pelvic GCTs are generally lytic with aggressive features and high vascularity. Pelvic fibrous dysplasia is lytic and occurs specifically in the iliac bone. Definitive diagnosis of ABC is achieved by using CT, MRI, and open biopsy by frozen section. Chondroblastoma is characterized by an extensive bone marrow edema on MRI and can show increased uptake on bone scan (Girish et al., 2012b).

2.2.13 Thyroid

Several imaging modalities including neck US, CT, MRI, FDG-PET, CT/MRI, FDG-PET/CT, DMSA (V) scintigraphy, and bone scan are used in diagnosing and follow-up of thyroid cancers. GLUT-1 (glucose transporter 1) and hypoxia-inducible factor 1 (HIF-1) that act as a signaling molecule in glucose metabolism in thyroid cancer are highly expressed on aggressive thyroid carcinoma cells. Thus, PET imaging is indicated in the assessment of patients with differentiated thyroid carcinoma and papillary thyroid carcinoma after surgery. FDG-PET/CT showed more accuracy than PET alone. Usually, diffuse uptake assigned chronic thyroiditis, whereas 25%–50% of focal uptake signified malignant lesions. It is suggested to consider thyroglobulin levels and ^{131}I WBS findings, as well as the clinical and histopathologic features. It is recommended to perform FDG-PET/CT after recombinant human thyroid-stimulating hormone (rhTSH) stimulation (0.9 mg intramuscularly on 2 consecutive days, with PET imaging late on day 2 or in the morning of day 3). It is also advisable to conduct the PET scan just before the administration of ^{131}I for diagnostic assessment or therapy. To detect metastasis in patients with medullary thyroid cancer and elevated calcitonin and carcinoembryonic antigen (CEA), FDOPA PET/CT should be performed whenever possible. ^{124}I PET/CT imaging detects more lesions and is promising in treatment planning in metastatic thyroid cancer (Abraham and Schöder, 2011).

2.2.14 Bladder

White-light cystoscopy (WLC) is the standard technique used for detecting and resecting bladder tumors. However, CIS (carcinoma in situ) might be missed and lead to recurrent tumors. Therefore, other modalities such as narrow-band imaging (NBI) cystoscopy and photodynamic diagnosis (PDD)/blue light cystoscopy (BLC) have been introduced. NBI is a noninvasive modality that relies on the longer wavelength of light that enable deeper penetration and visualization of detailed structure of bladder mucosa (Cheung et al., 2013). In PDD, a 5-aminolevulinic acid (5-ALA) dye or its hexyl ester hexaminolevulinate is infused into the bladder and absorbed by abnormal tissue, enabling photosensitization that emits a red color under blue reference light, while normal tissue appears blue. The technique is recommended during initial transurethral resection of bladder tumor (TURBT) and in patients with positive urine cytology but negative WLC results, for the assessment of tumor recurrences, and in the initial follow-up of patients with CIS or multifocal tumors (Witjes et al., 2010).

References

Abraham T, Schöder H. 2011. Thyroid cancer—Indications and opportunities for positron emission tomography/computed tomography imaging. *Semin Nucl Med* 41:121–138.

Aldrich JE. 2007. Basic physics of ultrasound imaging. *Crit Care Med* 35(5) (Suppl.):S131–S137.

Ali M, Magee D, Dasgupta U. 2008. Signal processing overview of ultrasound systems for medical imaging. Texas Instruments, White Paper SPRAB12, Texas, pp. 1–26. http://www.medimaging.jp/whitepaper/750.pdf

Bertholdo D, Watcharakorn A, Castillo M. 2013. Brain proton magnetic resonance spectroscopy: Introduction and overview. *Neuroimaging Clin N Am* 23(3):359–380. doi:10.1016/j.nic.2012.10.002. Epub 2013 Jan 20.

Bharwani N, Reznek RH, Rockall AG. 2011. Ovarian cancer management: The role of imaging and diagnostic challenges. *Eur J Radiol* 78:41–51.

Bolan PJ, Nelson MT, Yee D, Garwood M. 2005. Imaging in breast cancer: Magnetic resonance spectroscopy. *Breast Cancer Res* 7(4):149–152.

Brem RF, Floerke AC, Rapelyea JA, Teal C, Kelly T, Mathur V. 2008. Breast-specific gamma imaging as an adjunct imaging modality for the diagnosis of breast cancer. *Radiology* 247(3):651–657.

Brush J, Boyd K, Chappell F, Crawford F, Dozier M, Fenwick E, Glanville J et al. 2011. The value of FDG positron emission tomography/computerised tomography (PET/CT) in pre-operative staging of colorectal cancer: A systematic review and economic evaluation. *HTA* 15(35):19–130.

Bushberg JT, Seibert JA, Leidholdt EM, Boone JJM. 2012. *The Essential Physics of Medical Imaging* (3rd edn.). Lippincott Williams & Wilkins, Philadelphia, PA.

Chan V, Perlas A. 2011. Basics of ultrasound imaging. In *Atlas of Ultrasound-Guided Procedures in Interventional Pain Management*. Narouze, SN (ed.) pp. 13–19. Springer Science & Business Media, New York.

Chao F, Zhang H. 2012. PET/CT in the staging of the non-small-cell lung cancer. *J Biomed Biotechnol* 2012:783739. doi:10.1155/2012/783739. Epub March 7, 2012.

Chen P, Wang J, Hope K, Jin L, Dick J, Cameron R, Brandwein J, Minden M, Reilly RM. 2006. Nuclear localizing sequences promote nuclear translocation and enhance the radiotoxicity of the anti-CD33 monoclonal antibody HuM195 labeled with 111In in human myeloid leukemia cells. *J Nucl Med* 47:827–836.

Cherry SR. 2006. The 2006 Henry N. Wagner Lecture: Of mice and men (and positrons)—Advances in PET imaging technology. *J Nucl Med* 47:1735–1745.

Cheung G, Sahai A, Billia M, Dasgupta P, Khan MS. 2013. Recent advances in the diagnosis and treatment of bladder cancer. *BMC Med* 11:13. doi:10.1186/1741-7015-11-13.

Chi X, Huanga D, Zhaoa Z, Zhoua Z, Yinb Z, Gaoa J. 2012. Nanoprobes for in vitro diagnostics of cancer and infectious diseases. *Biomaterials* 33:189–206.

Czernin J, Benz MR, Allen-Auerbach MS. 2010. PET/CT imaging: The incremental value of assessing the glucose metabolic phenotype and the structure of cancers in a single examination. *Eur J Radiol* 73:470–480.

De Giorgi U, Aliberti C, Benea G, Conti M, Marangolo M. 2005. Effect of angiosonography to monitor response during imatinib treatment in patients with metastatic gastrointestinal stromal tumors. *Clin Cancer Res* 11:6171–6176.

Dove EL. 2004. Physics of medical imaging: An introduction. Biomedical Engineering, The University of Iowa, IA, pp. 1–51.

Evans CE, Mattock K, Humphries J, Saha P, Ahmad A, Waltham M, Patel A et al. 2011. Techniques of assessing hypoxia at the bench and bedside. *Angiogenesis* 14:119–124.

Fass L. 2008. Imaging and cancer: A review. *Mol Oncol* 2:115–152.

Fayed N, Olmos S, Morales H, Modrego PJ. 2006. Physical basis of magnetic resonance spectroscopy and its application to central nervous system diseases. *Am J Appl Sci* 3:1836–1845.

Figueiras RG, Padhani AR, Vilanova JC, Goh V, Martín CV. 2010. Functional imaging of tumors; Part 2. *Radiología* 52(3):208–220.

Gillies RJ, Morse DL. 2005. In vivo magnetic resonance spectroscopy in cancer. *Annu Rev Biomed Eng* 7:287–326.

Girish G, Finlay K, Fessell D, Pai D, Dong Q, Jamadar D. 2012a. Imaging review of skeletal tumors of the pelvis-malignant tumors and tumor mimics. *Scientific World J* 2012:Article ID 240281, 12. doi:10.1100/2012/240281.

Girish G, Finlay K, Morag Y, Brandon C, Jacobson J, Jamadar David. 2012b. Imaging review of skeletal tumors of the pelvis—Part I: Benign tumors of the pelvis. *Scientific World J* 2012:Article ID 290930, 10 doi:10.1100/2012/290930.

Gore JC, Manning HC, Quarles CC, Waddell KW, Yankeelov TE. 2011. Magnetic resonance in the era of molecular imaging of cancer. *Magn Reson Imaging* 29(2011):587–600.

Haberkorn U, Markert A, Eisenhut M, Mier W, Altmann A. 2011. Development of molecular techniques for imaging and treatment of tumors. *Q J Nucl Med Mol Imaging* 55:655–670.

Halter RJ, Hartov A, Paulsen KD. 2007. Experimental justification for using 3D conductivity reconstructions in electrical impedance tomography. *Physiol Meas* 28(7):S115–S127.

Hampton T. 2008. New studies contribute to ongoing quest for better breast cancer screening, care. *JAMA* 300(15):1749–1750.

Holloway CMB, Easson A, Escallon J, Leong WL, Quan ML, Reedjik M, Wright FC, McCready DR. 2010. Technology as a force for improved diagnosis and treatment of breast disease. *J Can Surg* 53(4):268–277.

Hornak JP. 2011. *The Basics of MRI.* Interactive Learning Software, Henietta, New York.

Ibusuki M, Yamamoto Y, Kawasoe T, Shiraishi S, Tomiquchi S, Yamashita Y, Honda Y, Iyama K, Iwase H. 2010. Potential advantage of preoperative three-dimensional mapping of sentinel nodes in breast cancer by a hybrid single photon emission CT (SPECT)/CT system. *Surg Oncol* 19(2):88–94.

Iglesias-García J, Lindkvist B, Lariño-Noia J, Domínguez-Muñoz JE. 2012. The role of endoscopic ultrasound (EUS) in relation to other imaging modalities in the differential diagnosis between mass forming chronic pancreatitis, autoimmune pancreatitis and ductal pancreatic adenocarcinoma. *Rev Esp Enferm Dig* (Madrid) 104(6):315–321.

James TL. 1998. Fundamentals of NMR, Indian Academy of Sciences, Chapter 1, pp. 1–31.

Juweid ME, Cheson BD. 2006. Positron emission tomography and assessment of cancer therapy. *N Engl J Med* 354:496–507.

Kalinyak JE, Schilling K, Berg WA, Narayanan D, Mayberry JP, Rai R, Dupree EB et al. 2011. PET-guided breast biopsy. *Breast J* 17(2):143–151.

Kalkmanna J, Zeileb M, Antochc G, Bergerd F, Diederiche S, Dinterf D, Finkf C, Jankag R, Stattaus J. 2012. Consensus report on the radiological management of patients with gastrointestinal stromal tumours (GIST): Recommendations of the German GIST Imaging Working Group. *Cancer Imaging* 12:126–135.

Karaosmanoğlu AD, Blake MA. 2012. Applications of PET-CT in patients with esophageal cancer. *Diagn Interv Radiol* 18:171–182.

Kenyon B, Kleinberg R, Straley C, Gubelin G, Morriss C. 1995. Nuclear magnetic resonance image technology for the 21st century. *Oilfield Review* 7(3):19–33.

Kircher MF, Hricak H, Larson SM. 2012. Molecular imaging for personalized cancer care. *Mol Oncol* 6:182–195.

Kobus T, Hambrock T, Hulsbergen-van de Kaa CA, Wright AJ, Barentsz JO, Heerschap A, Scheenen TWJ. 2011. In vivo assessment of prostate cancer aggressiveness using magnetic resonance spectroscopic imaging at 3 T with an endorectal coil. *Eur Urol* 60:1074–1080.

Koh DM, Brown G, Temple L, Raja A, Toomey P, Bett N, Norman AR, Husband JE. 2004. Rectal cancer: Mesorectal lymph nodes at MR imaging with USPIO versus histopathologic findings—Initial observations. *Radiology* 231:91–99.

Kundu S, Chopra S, Verma A, Mahantshetty U, Engineer R, Shrivastava SK. 2012. Functional magnetic resonance imaging in cervical cancer: Current evidence and future directions. *TCRT* 8(1):11–18.

Lardinois D, Weder W, Hany TF, Kamel EM, Korom S, Seifert B, von Schulthess GK, Steinhert HC. 2003. Staging of non-small-cell lung cancer with integrated positron emission tomography and computed tomography. *N Engl J Med* 348:2500–2507.

Lee S, Bae J, Lee A, Park J. 2011. Metastatic ovarian cancers. In *Text Book of Gynecological Oncology*. Ayhan A, Reed N, Gultekin M, Dursun P (eds.) pp. 9–13. Günes publishing, Germany.

Lestón JS, Dios PD. 2010. Diagnostic clinical aids in oral cancer. *Oral Oncol* 46:418–422.

Li M, Wua N, Liua Y, Zhenga R, Lianga Y, Zhanga W, Zhaoa P. 2012. Regional nodal staging with 18F-FDG PET–CT in non-small cell lung cancer: Additional diagnostic value of CT attenuation and dual-time-point imaging. *Eur J Radiol* 81:1886–1890.

Lin M, Jackson EF. 2012. Applications of imaging technology in radiation research. *Radiat Res* 177(4):387–397.

Lungu GF, Li ML, Xie X, Wang LV, Stoica G. 2007. In vivo imaging and characterization of hypoxia-induced neovascularization and tumor invasion. *Int J Oncol* 30(1):45–54.

Mallidi S, Luke GP, Emelianov S. 2011. Photoacoustic imaging in cancer detection, diagnosis, and treatment guidance. *Trends Biotechnol* 29(5):213–221.

Mankoff DA, Link JM, Linden HM, Sundararajan L, Krohn KA. 2008. Tumor receptor imaging. *J Nucl Med* 49(Suppl 2):149S–163S.

Mazzone P. 2012. Lung cancer screening: Examining the issues. *Cleveland Clinic J Med* 79:eS1–eS6.

McDonnell LA, Corthalsb GL, Willemsc SM, van Remoorterea A, van Zeijla RJM, Deeldera AM. 2010. Peptide and protein imaging mass spectrometry in cancer research. *J Proteomics* 73:1921–1944.

McQuade P, Rowland DJ, Lewis JS, Welch MJ. 2005. Positron-emitting isotopes produced on biomedical cyclotrons. *Curr Med. Chem* 12(7):807–818.

Mital M, Scott EP. 2007. Thermal detection of embedded tumors using infrared imaging. *J Biomech Eng* 129(1):33–39.

Moadel RM. 2011. Breast cancer imaging devices. *Semin Nucl Med* 41(3):229–241.

Morris P, Perkins A. 2012. Physics medicine 2; Diagnostic imaging. *Lancet* 379:1525–1533.

Mottram JC. 1936. Factor of importance in radiosensitivity of tumors. *Br J Radiol* 9:606.

Nagar H, Dobbs S, McClelland HR, Price J, McCluggage WG, Grey A. 2006. The diagnostic accuracy of magnetic resonance imaging in detecting cervical involvement in endometrial cancer. *Gynecol Oncol* 103:431–434.

Nannia C, Rubellob D, Castelluccia P, Farsada M, Franchia R, Rampinb L, Grossc MD, Al-Nahhasd A, Fantia S. 2006. 18F-FDG PET/CT fusion imaging in paediatric solid extracranial tumours. *Biomed Pharmacother* 60(9):593–606.

Nariai T, Tanaka Y, Wakimoto H, Aoyagi M, Tamaki M, Ishiwata K, Senda M et al. 2005. Usefulness of L-[methyl-11C]methionine-positron emission tomography as a biological monitoring tool in the treatment of glioma. *J Neurosurg* 103:498–507.

National Research Council (US) and Institute of Medicine (US) Committee on State of the Science of Nuclear Medicine. 6 Radiotracer and Radiopharmaceutical Chemistry. *Advancing Nuclear Medicine through Innovation*. National Academies Press (US); Washington, DC, 2007.

Nothacker M, Duda V, Hahn M, Warm M, Degenhardt F, Madjar H, Weinbrenner S, Albert U. 2009. Early detection of breast cancer: Benefits and risks of supplemental breast ultrasound in asymptomatic women with mammographically dense breast tissue. A systematic review. *BMC Cancer* 9:335–343.

Numata K, Luo W, Morimoto M, Fukuda H, Sato N, Tanaka K. 2011. Clinical usefulness of contrast-enhanced three-dimensional ultrasound imaging with sonazoid for hepatic tumor lesions, ultrasound imaging. Tanabe M (ed.), pp. 151–170, *In Tech,* Europe, China.

O'Connor MK, Phillips SW, Hruska CB, Rhodes DJ, Collins DA. 2007. Molecular breast imaging: Advantages and limitations of a scintimammographic technique in patients with small breast tumors. *Breast J* 13(1):3–11.

Pinker K, Stadlbauerc A, Bognerb W, Gruberb S, Helbich TH. 2012. Molecular imaging of cancer: MR spectroscopy and beyond. *Eur J Radiol* 81:566–577.

Pirotte B, Goldman S, Massager N, David P, Wikler D, Vandesteene A, Salmon I, Brotchi J, Levivier M. 2004. Comparison of 18F-FDG and 11C-methionine for PET-guided stereotactic brain biopsy of gliomas. *J Nucl Med* 45:1293–1298.

Prasad SN, Houserkovaa D. 2007. The role of various modalities in breast imaging. *Biomed Pap Med Fac Univ Palacky Olomouc Czech Repub* 151(2):209–218.

Rajendran JG, Hendrickson KR, Spence AM, Muzi M, Krohn KA, Mankoff DA. 2006. Hypoxia imaging-directed radiation treatment planning. *Eur J Nucl Med Mol Imaging* 33:44–53.

Raylman RR, Majewski S, Smith MF, Proffitt J, Hammond W, Srinivasan A, McKisson J et al. 2008. The positron emission mammography/tomography breast imaging and biopsy system (PEM/PET): Design, construction and phantom-based measurements. *Phys Med Biol* 53(3):637–653.

Rhodes DJ, O'Connor MK, Phillips SW et al. 2005. Molecular breast imaging: A new technique using technetium Tc 99m scintimammography to detect small tumors of the breast. *Mayo Clin Proc* 80(1):24–30.

Rinck P. 2012. *Magnetic Resonance in Medicine. The Basic Textbook of the European Magnetic Resonance Forum*. 6th edn. Electronic version 6.8; 5 July 2013. www.magnetic-resonance.org

Rosen JE, Chan L, Shieh DB, Gu FX. 2012. Iron oxide nanoparticles for targeted cancer imaging and diagnostics. *Nanomedicine: NBM* 8:275–290.

Schilling K, Narayanan D, Kalinyak JE, The J, Velasquez MV, Kahn S, Saady M, Mahal R, Chrystal L. 2011. Positron emission mammography in breast cancer presurgical planning: Comparisons with magnetic resonance imaging. *Eur J Nucl Med Mol Imaging* 38:23–36.

Schwab S, Uder M, Schuiz-Wendtland R, Bautz W, Janka R, Wenkel E. 2008. Direct MR galactography: Feasibility study. *Radiobiology* 249(1):54–61.

Seitz M, Shukla-Dave A, Bjartell A, Touijer K, Sciarra A, Bastian PJ, Stief C, Hricak H, Graser A. 2009. Functional magnetic resonance imaging in prostate cancer. *Eur Urol* 55(4):801–814.

Shammas A, Lim R, Charron M. 2009. Pediatric FDG PET/CT: Physiologic uptake, normal variants, and benign conditions. *Radiographics* 29:1467–1486.

Sharkey RM, Goldenberg DM. 2005. Perspectives on cancer therapy with radiolabeled monoclonal antibodies. *J Nucl Med* 46:115S–127S.

Shields AF. 2006. Positron emission tomography measurement of tumor metabolism and growth: Its expanding role in oncology. *Mol Imaging Biol* 8:141–150.

Shields AF, Grierson JR, Dohmen BM, Machulla HJ, Stayanoff JC, Lawhorn-Crews JM, Obradovich JE, Muzik O, Managner TJ. 1998. Imaging proliferation in vivo with [F-18] FLT and positron emission tomography. *Nat Med* 4:1334–1336.

Sinha S, Lucas-Quesada FA, Sinha U, DeBruhl N, Bassett LW. 2002. In vivo diffusion-weighted MRI of the breast: Potential for lesion characterization. *J Magn Reson Imaging* 15(6):693–704.

Slamon DJ, Leyland-Jones B, Shak S, Fuchs H, Paton V, Bajamonde A, Fleming T et al. 2001. Use of chemotherapy plus a monoclonal antibody against HER2 for metastatic breast cancer that overexpresses HER2. *N Engl J Med* 344(11):783–792.

Sugimoto K, Shiraishi J, Moriyasu F, Saito K, Doi K. 2009. Improved detection of hepatic metastases with contrast-enhanced low mechanical-index pulse inversion ultrasonography during the liver-specific phase of sonazoid: Observer performance study with JAFROC analysis. *Acad Radiol* 16(7):789–809.

Tafreshi NK, Kumar V, Morse DL, Gatenby RA. 2010. Molecular and functional imaging of breast cancer. *Cancer Control* 17(3):143–155.

Tanaka C, Fujii H, Ikeda T, Jinno H, Nakahara T, Suzuki T, Kitagawa Y et al. 2007. Stereoscopic scintigraphic imaging of breast cancer sentinel lymph nodes. *Breast Cancer* 14(1):92–99.

Ternier F, Houvenaeghel G, Lecrivain F, Brigand BL, Margain D, Brunelle S, Stefano DD. 2006. Computed tomography in suspected local breast cancer recurrence. *Breast Cancer Res Treat* 100(3):247–254.

Thomenius KE. 2006. Instrumentation design for ultrasound imaging. In *Biomedical Engineering and Design Handbook Vol. 2: Applications*. Myer, K (ed.) pp. 249–256. McGraw-Hill, New York.

Warning K, Hildebrandt MG, Kristensen B, Ewertz M. 2011. Utility of 18FDG-PET/CT in breast cancer diagnostics—A systematic review. *Dan Med Bull* 58(7):1–6.

Weber WA, Wieder H. 2006. Monitoring chemotherapy and radiotherapy of solid tumors. *Eur J Nucl Med Mol Imaging* 33:27–37.

Wieder HA, Beer AJ, Lordick K, Ott K, Fischer M, Rummeny J, Ziegler S et al. 2005. Comparison of changes in tumor metabolic activity and tumor size during chemotherapy of adenocarcinomas of the esophago-gastric junction. *J Nucl Med* 46:2029–2034.

Williams R, Hudson JM, Lloyd BA, Sureshkumar AR, Lueck G, Milot L, Atri M, Bjarnason GA, Burns PN. 2011. Dynamic microbubble contrast-enhanced US to measure tumor response to targeted therapy: A proposed clinical protocol with results from renal cell carcinoma patients receiving antiangiogenic therapy. *Radiology* 260:581–590.

Witjes JA, Redorta JP, Jacqmin D, Sofras F, Malmström PU, Riedl C, Jocham D et al. 2010. Hexaminolevulinate-guided fluorescence cystoscopy in the diagnosis and follow-up of patients with non-muscle-invasive bladder cancer: Review of the evidence and recommendations. *Eur Urol* 57:607–614.

Yamamoto A, Fukushima H, Okamura R, Nakamura Y, Morimoto T, Urata Y, Mukaihara S, Hayakawa K. 2006. Dynamic helical CT mammography of breast cancer. *Radiat Med* 24(1):35–40.

Zhi H, Ou B, Luo BM, Feng X, Wen YL, Yang HY. 2007. Comparison of ultrasound elastography, mammography, and sonography in the diagnosis of solid breast lesions. *J Ultrasound Med* 26(6):807–815.

3

Role of PET in Cancer Diagnosis

Silvia Taralli, Antonella Stefanelli, and Giorgio Treglia

CONTENTS

ABSTRACT During the last years, positron emission tomography (PET) has become an essential functional imaging tool in oncology clinical practice worldwide, with growing impact on cancer staging, restaging, therapy response assessment, and follow-up. The high diagnostic accuracy of PET imaging relies on its molecular nature. Using different radiotracers, PET is able to early detect functional and biochemical alterations that occur at the molecular and cellular levels in cancer tissue, such as alterations in metabolism, proliferation, and angiogenesis or peculiar biological features of cancer cells such as specific receptor expression or tumor hypoxia. This unique behavior of PET as molecular imaging is emerging as the basis for a new clinical approach that could integrate the patient-specific and disease-specific molecular information with selection of personalized therapies or identification of more accurate prognostic groups of patients. A better knowledge of the biological tumor changes at the molecular level is the essential basis for the development of new PET tracers targeting more and more specific cancer biomarkers. It is, doubtless, the future direction for research and it will allow PET to play a more relevant and leading role in the "personalized" management of oncologic patients.

3.1 PET: An Overview

In the 1970s and 1980s, positron emission tomography (PET) was initially used for research applications; only in the late 1990s, the use of PET expanded into clinical application, and particularly in oncology, also thanks to the FDA approval of fluorine-18-fluoro-deoxy-glucose (^{18}F-FDG), currently the most employed oncologic PET tracer for routine clinical use, and to the PET procedures reimbursement guaranteed by Medicare or any other payer worldwide. During the last years, PET has become an essential imaging tool in clinical oncology worldwide, with growing impact on cancer staging, restaging, therapy response assessment, and follow-up as well as on grading malignancy, prognostic evaluation, and radiation therapy planning (Townsend, 2008; Vallabhajosula, 2007; Zhu et al., 2011).

PET is a noninvasive functional imaging technique that, in many cases, allows to overcome the limits of computed tomography (CT) and magnetic resonance imaging (MRI), the main morphologic diagnostic tools traditionally involved in oncology. Indeed, conventional morphologic imaging provides detailed anatomical information and based its diagnostic power on the assessment of structural changes, abnormality in contrast enhancement or signal intensity, or on the absolute size or change in size of a lesion, but it can fail to detect cancer in normal-sized structures or to differentiate post-therapy changes from viable malignancy; moreover, it is subject to considerable inter- and intra-observer variation. Otherwise, the high diagnostic accuracy of PET imaging relies on its molecular nature: With an increasing number of different radiotracers, it is able to early detect (prior to the macroscopic anatomical signs evident on CT or MRI) the functional and biochemical alterations that occur at the molecular and cellular levels in cancer tissue, such as alterations in metabolism, proliferation, and angiogenesis or peculiar biological features of cancer cells such as specific receptor expression or tumor hypoxia. This unique behavior of PET as molecular imaging is emerging as the basis for a new clinical approach that could integrate the patient-specific and disease-specific molecular information with selection of personalized therapies or identification of more accurate prognostic groups of patients, to cite some of the many interesting PET applications (Berry and Cook, 2006; Chen and Chen, 2011; Vallabhajosula, 2007; Zhu et al., 2011).

3.2 Fundamentals of PET

The diagnostic ability of PET relies on two essential elements, one pertaining to technical field (the PET scanner) and the other more purely "metabolic" (the radiotracer).

3.2.1 PET Scanner

The intrinsic high accuracy of PET is due to the high sensitivity of the radionuclide and to the specific biocharacters of the different radiotracers. Radiotracers (molecules labeled with a radionuclide) behave like "molecular imaging probes" because they target a specific biological process and are biochemically indistinguishable from their natural counterparts. Once the positron-emitting radiotracer is administered to the patient, the radionuclide decays emitting a positron; after traveling a short distance within the body tissues (up to few millimeters), the positron may combine with an electron in the vicinity and subsequently annihilates; in each annihilation event, the mass of the two particles is converted into electromagnetic energy in the form of a pair of 511 keV photons that are simultaneously emitted in opposite trajectories; the resulting gamma rays are the signal detected by the PET system. The most common PET system surrounds the patient with a complete cylindrical gantry consisting of continuous ring of many 511 keV photon detectors; they detect and position millions of oppositely directed coincident photon pairs emitted within the system (so-called coincidence events). Detectors are the most important and expensive components of a PET system. They are constituted by inorganic scintillator crystals that absorb the 511 keV photon energy and generate flash of light; photomultiplier tubes then collect the light from the crystals and convert it to an electronic signal that brings spatial, energy, and time information of each single photon event. From the electronic signal, the source of the annihilation event is then localized as precisely as possible as a point in the body regions of the patient; finally, a whole-body spatial distribution of the radiotracer is reconstructed by computerized processes that use mathematical algorithms and it is converted in tomographic images. Overall, a PET system performance is related to several important parameters such as photon sensitivity, coincidence photon detection efficiency, and spatial, energy, coincidence time, and contrast resolutions that are essentially determined by the specific characteristic of the detectors. Particularly, spatial resolution (the system's ability to distinguish as separate two closely spaced positron sources) of the common PET scanners used in clinical practice is in the range of 5–7 mm (Chen and Chen, 2011; Levin, 2005; Vallabhajosula et al., 2011; Zhu et al., 2011).

In addition to documenting the presence or absence of radiotracer tissue uptake by a pure qualitative analysis of the images, it is possible also to perform a semiquantitative analysis: the standardized uptake value (SUV), derived from the ratio of tumor activity concentration to that in the remainder of the body, has become the widely known and used semiquantitative PET parameter. Although SUV is affected by several variables related to the acquisition protocol and to the patient's characteristics and is not completely comparable and reproducible, it is commonly used in clinical practice, especially to assess tumor response to treatment (Berry and Cook, 2006; Shreve et al., 1999).

Traditionally, PET and CT have been seen as complementary technologies, used sequentially in the management of oncologic patients. Soon, the large potential of the multimodality image fusion, with the simultaneous acquisition of both anatomic and functional information, was recognized and translated into the first combined PET/CT scanner, developed in 1998 and introduced into the clinical practice in 2001. It is composed of the two scanners aligned so that the patient can undergo imaging in the two gantries by just moving the one system table and allows the acquisition of PET and CT images coregistered in the same session, with a common CT scan performed from the base of the skull to thighs or pelvic floor. Combined PET/CT has quickly proven to be a great advance in cancer imaging and to be more accurate in staging and restaging than either PET or CT alone. It is well evident considering that, from 2001 to 2006, the sales of PET-only scanners was replaced entirely by sales of PET/CT and PET/CT was the fastest-growing imaging modality in 2004 with up to 1000 scanners installed worldwide only in that year. The most significant advantages are the use of the CT data (modified to allow for the difference in photon energy between CT and PET) for attenuation correction, with consequent improvement of image quality, better accuracy in quantification of functional parameters, and important reduction of PET scanning times (typically a combined whole-body PET/CT scan is now completed in 15–30 min); the availability of anatomic landmarks, useful for a better localization and classification of uptake sites with a consequent improvement of PET specificity when foci of physiologic or non-malignant uptake are recognized; and the limitation of spatial and temporal differences between the two sets of images (Berry and Cook, 2006; Hany et al., 2002; Townsend, 2008; Zhu et al., 2011).

With the increasing use of PET/CT, the radiation exposure to the patient has become an emerging concern issue. Radiation exposure from PET/CT is due to both the CT scan (external dose) and the injected PET radiotracer (internal dose); the total dose, as sum of the two radiation sources, depends on several factors such as the exposed body region, the CT-specific parameters of acquisition (different if a diagnostic CT or a low-dose CT is acquired), the technical features and sensitivity of CT and PET scanner, the biodistribution and the physical and biological half-life of the radiotracer, and the administered activity, which varies considerably among different centers. For a typical low-dose CT scan, as requested for attenuation correction and localization only, the whole-body effective dose is estimated to be 3 mSv or even lower; regarding PET, the average whole-body effective dose for a typical administered activity of 10 mCi is estimated to be 7 mSv and even lower if a patient with a low body mass index or a high-sensitivity scanner are considered (Townsend, 2008).

3.2.2 PET Radiotracers

The most common positron-emitting radionuclides used to label PET radiotracers, both for research and clinical applications, include ^{18}F, ^{11}C, ^{15}O, ^{13}N, and ^{68}Ga, isotopes of natural elements with different energy, half-life, synthesis protocol, availability, and cost. They are synthesized by a cyclotron, a particle accelerator, or created using a nuclear generator. ^{18}F continues to be considered an ideal radionuclide for developing PET radiotracers for routine clinical use, based on its favorable chemical and physical properties (Chen and Chen, 2011; Levin, 2005).

Since the 1970s, several hundreds of PET radiotracers have been developed and listed with potential clinical applications. While many of them are still subject of research and some are applied in clinical research settings, only few have been approved by FDA for routine clinical use. In oncology, ^{18}F-FDG remains the most widely used PET tracer. Moreover, considering that more than 90% of oncologic PET imaging is performed with ^{18}F-FDG, PET is often made synonymous to a ^{18}F-FDG study. However, in the last years, many alternative PET tracers have been proposed, tested, and evaluated in preclinical and clinical studies to characterize other aspects of tumor biology, searching for a more "tumor-specific" radiotracer (Vallabhajosula, 2007; Vallabhajosula et al., 2011; Zhu et al., 2011).

The most important among PET tracers are then briefly reported.

3.2.2.1 Glucose Metabolism

FDG is an analog of glucose, transported across cell membranes through specific glucose transporters (GLUT); in the cytosol it is enzymatically phosphorylated by the hexokinase to FDG-6-phosphate that is not a substrate for further enzymes of the glycolytic pathway; thus, it is trapped and accumulates into the cells in proportion to glucose metabolism. Cancer cells need critical factors for their growth such as oxygen, growth factors, and glucose. Increased glucose metabolism is one of the functional changes observed and firstly recognized in most of cancer types, necessary to generate the required energy to tumor growth. Tumor cells are known to have a high glycolytic rate because of increased expression of glucose transporters and glycolytic enzymes, and, particularly, the anaerobic consume of glucose provides a major energy source both in hypoxic conditions and also under aerobic conditions. This is the basis of the increased ^{18}F-FDG uptake in many tumors and of the wide oncologic use of ^{18}FDG-PET. ^{18}F-FDG PET imaging is generally performed at about 60 min after intravenous administration of the radiotracer; this time interval allows, on the one hand, the increasing ^{18}F-FDG uptake by avid tumor cells and, on the other, the concomitant decrease of the overall background tracer activity, with a better detection of pathological sites of uptake. Because serum glucose is competitive with ^{18}F-FDG, patients are required to fast for at least 4 h before the study. ^{18}F-FDG physiologically accumulates in normal glucose-dependent tissues, such as brain and myocardium, and is excreted in the urine, with physiological visualization of the urinary system from kidneys to bladder. Physiological ^{18}F-FDG uptake is present also in the liver, spleen, and bone marrow and, variably, in the digestive tract, thyroid gland, skeletal muscle, thymic tissue of children, breast tissue of premenopausal women, genital organs, and in the foci of active brown fat, especially in cold weather and in young or female patients. Moreover, several benign causes of ^{18}F-FDG uptake are reported, typically sites of inflammation or infection such as bone healing, degenerative or inflammatory arthritis, reactive enlarged lymph nodes, different manifestations of granulomatous disease like tuberculosis and sarcoidosis, sites of recent surgery or radiation therapy, and soft tissue infections. It is therefore evident that ^{18}F-FDG is not a target-specific tracer and, sometimes, it is difficult to distinguish if a high metabolic rate is due to cancer or other non-neoplastic etiologies characterized, similarly, by increased glucose metabolism. The knowledge of physiological sites or benign causes of ^{18}F-FDG uptake is essential to avoid diagnostic errors and false-positive interpretations. In addition, if on the one hand some malignant tumors such as prostate cancer, neuroendocrine tumors (NETs), hepatic tumors, and, generally, well-differentiated low-grade or hypocellular tumors do not exhibit a significantly increased ^{18}F-FDG uptake and, therefore, may be undetectable, on the other hand, ^{18}F-FDG is not useful for evaluating malignancy in tissues with physiological high glucose metabolism such as the central nervous system (CNS) (Berry and Cook, 2006; Chen and Chen, 2011; Shreve et al., 1999; Vallabhajosula, 2007; Zhu et al., 2011).

To date, ^{18}F-FDG PET/CT is largely used for different clinical indications (staging, restaging, or treatment response evaluation) and in several tumors such as lung cancer, lymphomas, head and neck tumors, breast cancer, gastrointestinal tumors, genitourinary cancers, melanoma, and sarcomas (Treglia et al., 2010) (Figure 3.1).

3.2.2.2 Amino Acid Metabolism

Tumor growth and development of many types of cancers require active protein synthesis and a consequent increased amino acid uptake. It is demonstrated that cancer cells show a significant increase in amino acid transporter expression for energy, protein synthesis, and cell division. Radiolabeled amino acids and their analogs are transported into the cells by the same transporter proteins and metabolized (if natural amino acid) or non-metabolized (if synthetic analog) similarly to their natural counterpart. ^{11}C-methionine (^{11}C-MET), ^{18}F-fluoro-tyrosine (^{18}F-TYR), ^{18}F-alphamethyl-tyrosine (^{18}F-FMT), ^{18}F-fluoroethyl-tyrosine (^{18}F-FET), and ^{18}F-fluoro-dihydroxyphenylalanine (^{18}F-DOPA) are the most studied and known. Particularly, while ^{11}C-MET and ^{18}F-FET have shown to be useful and valuable in clinical management of brain tumors, ^{18}F-DOPA has clinical utility not only for brain tumor imaging but also to evaluate NETs (Caroli et al., 2010; Vallabhajosula, 2007; Zhu et al., 2011).

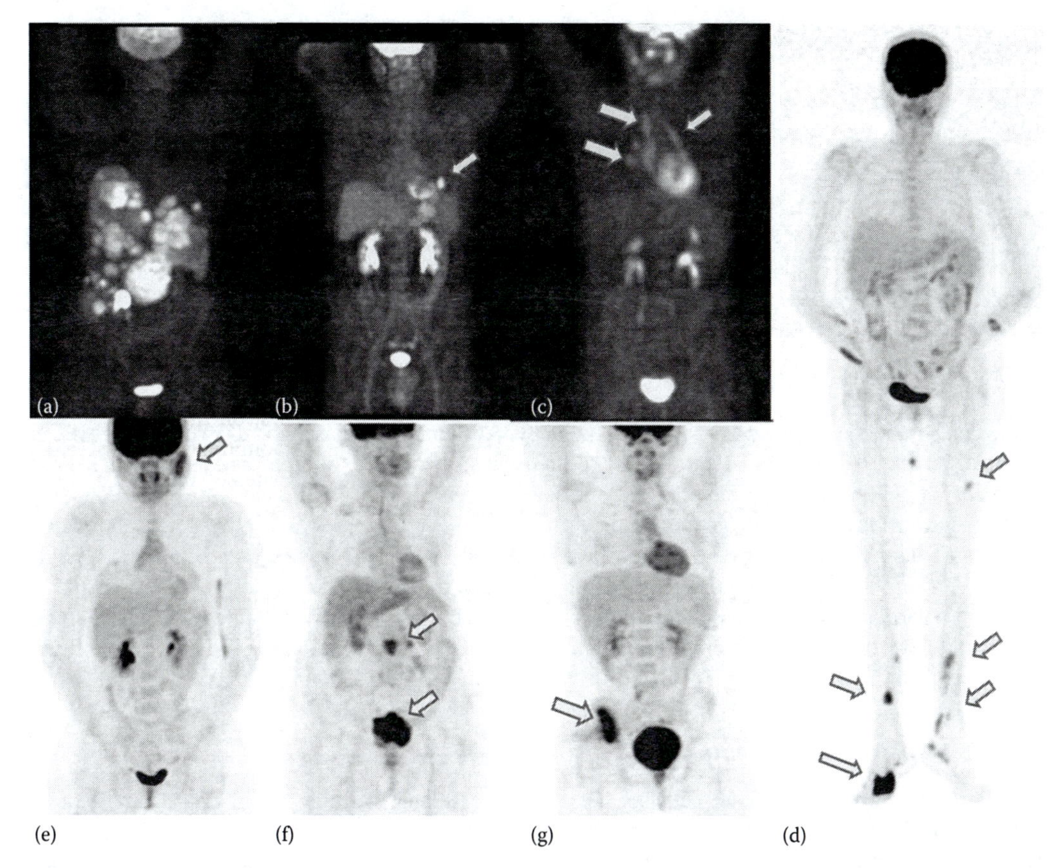

FIGURE 3.1 **(See color insert.)** ^{18}F-FDG PET scans showing (a) multiple liver metastases in a patient with colon cancer, (b) a solitary malignant pulmonary nodule, (c) multiple hypermetabolic mediastinal lymph node in a patient with lymphoma, (d) several cutaneous localizations in a patient with melanoma, (e) lymph nodal metastases in a patient with head and neck tumor, (f) an advanced endometrial cancer with lymph nodal metastases, and (g) a bone localization in a patient with osteosarcoma.

3.2.2.3 Membrane Lipid Synthesis

Phospholipids are essential components of all cell membranes. It is known that, for their proliferation and division, tumor cells show an increased demand for substrates of phospholipids synthesis. Choline is a major precursor for this biosynthetic pathway. Particularly, choline is transported in the cells by a specific transporter; within the cell it undergoes phosphorylation by the enzyme choline kinase and is further incorporated into phosphatidylcholine, a major constituent of membrane lipids. Malignant cells transformation and proliferation are associated with an increased choline kinase activity and consequent increased levels of phosphorylcholine. Radiolabeled choline analogs (^{11}C-choline and ^{18}F-choline) have been developed as marker of membrane metabolism and have a biodistribution very similar to that of natural choline, except for their very rapid urinary excretion. This aspect is a clear advantage for PET imaging because it translates in a low background activity in comparison to the most used ^{18}F-FDG. Radiolabeled choline is mainly involved in brain tumors and prostate cancer imaging (Figure 3.2) (Caroli et al., 2010; Vallabhajosula, 2007; Zhu et al., 2011).

3.2.2.4 Cell Proliferation

A major marker of cell proliferation is DNA synthesis. Tumor cells are characterized by an increased requirement of nucleotides as substrates for DNA synthesis and most of anticancer drugs are designed to just inhibit cell proliferation. Thymidine is the only nucleotide incorporated exclusively into DNA;

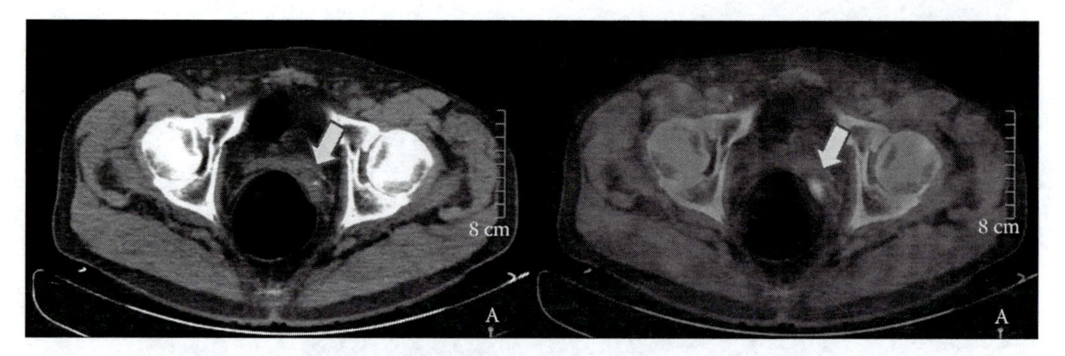

FIGURE 3.2 **(See color insert.)** ^{18}F-choline PET/CT showing a recurrence of prostate cancer (arrow).

in the cell, it undergoes phosphorylation by the enzyme thymidine kinase, which is overexpressed in cancer cells, and so incorporated into DNA. ^{11}C-thymidine first and ^{18}F-fluorothymidine (^{18}F-FLT) subsequently are the most known radiolabeled nucleotides developed for PET tumor imaging as specific markers of tumor cell proliferation rate. Particularly, ^{18}F-FLT is transported into cell and phosphorylated similar to thymidine, but only a really insignificant part is incorporated into DNA, the most part remaining metabolically trapped inside the cells. ^{18}F-FLT appears to demonstrate greater specificity than ^{18}F-FDG and a particular value in assessing tumor aggressiveness and monitoring therapy response. Lung cancer and CNS tumors are some of the many potential fields of application of ^{18}F-FLT (Caroli et al., 2010; Chen and Chen, 2011; Nanni et al., 2010; Vallabhajosula, 2007; Vallabhajosula et al., 2011).

3.2.2.5 Somatostatin Receptor

Several tumors, such as NETs, small cell lung cancer, and breast tumors, overexpress somatostatin receptors with different density and subtype prevalence. The subtype 2 (sst2) is the most expressed and bound by clinically used somatostatin analogs. Octreotide, a longer half-life and stable somatostatin analog, has been conjugated with various chelating agents and labeled with ^{68}Ga for PET imaging of somatostatin receptor-positive tumors. ^{68}Ga-DOTA-NOC, ^{68}Ga-DOTA-TOC, and ^{68}Ga-DOTA-TATE are the main PET somatostatin analogs employed in clinical trials, with the most relevant differences in the affinity to sst receptor subtypes. They seem useful not only as major diagnostic biomarkers of NETs but also for assessing somatostatin biodistribution in suitable candidates for radiometabolic therapy with ^{177}Lu- or ^{90}Y-labeled somatostatin analogs (Ambrosini et al., 2010; Caroli et al., 2010; Chen and Chen, 2011; Nanni et al., 2010) (Figure 3.3).

3.2.2.6 Hypoxia

A well-known consequence of the increasing tumor size during tumor progression is a deficiency in the amount of oxygen reaching all parts of the cancer mass by local vessels. The resulting hypoxia may be considered also as an adaptive response of the tumor and it has been established as one of the most important determinants of tumor progression and, especially, of therapy resistance, with evident prognostic implications. Particularly, poorly oxygenated cells are less sensitive to the cytotoxic effect of radiation therapy. ^{18}F-misonidazole (^{18}F-MISO), ^{18}F-arabino-furanosyl-nitroimidazole (^{18}F-FAZA), and ^{64}Cu-diacetyl-bis[N4-methylthiosemicarbazone] (^{64}Cu-ATSM) are the main studied hypoxic PET tracers. They bind selectively to hypoxic cells by electron reductions that occur in a poor-oxygen cellular environment and are metabolically trapped into the cell. Highlighting hypoxic areas of a tumor mass, they allow to perform a more effective overtreatment. Head and neck cancer and non-small cell lung cancer (NSCLC) are some of the fields of investigation of these radiotracers (Chen and Chen, 2011; Vallabhajosula, 2007; Vallabhajosula et al., 2011).

3.2.2.7 Angiogenesis

Neoangiogenesis is an essential mechanism developed by tumor mass during its progression to ensure adequate supply of growth factors and nutrients. It is the basis of tumor growth and metastatic spread and an

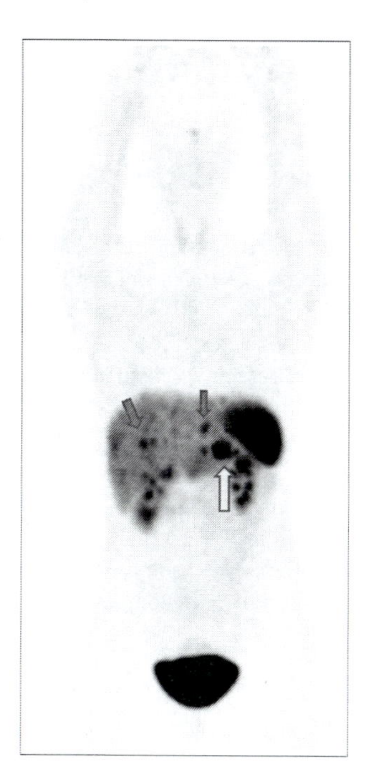

FIGURE 3.3 **(See color insert.)** Somatostatin receptor PET showing a NET of the pancreas (yellow arrow) with multiple liver metastases (blue arrows).

emerging target for cancer therapy and cancer imaging. Several PET radiotracers specific for the complex angiogenetic process have been developed and studied in clinical trials. Among these, the most investigated are the radiolabeled PET ligands for the vascular endothelial growth factor (VEGF) or the VEGF receptor, an important mediator of the angiogenic effects of VEGF, and for the $\alpha V\beta 3$ integrin, a cell adhesion receptor particularly involved in the angiogenetic process, expressed on the membrane of various tumor cells and upregulated in tumor angiogenesis (Chen and Chen, 2011; Nanni et al., 2010; Vallabhajosula et al., 2011).

3.2.2.8 Apoptosis

Apoptosis of cancer cells is a multistep programmed cell death process that could be induced by radiation therapy or chemotherapy. The apoptotic process is an interesting field of application of PET imaging because it could provide useful information to monitoring the anticancer therapy efficacy. Annexin-V is a protein with high and selective affinity for phosphatidylserine, a component of the cellular membrane that is expressed on the outer surface in cells undergoing apoptosis. The radiolabeled annexin-V (labeled with ^{18}F, ^{11}C, ^{124} I, ^{64}Cu, etc) is one of the most investigated probe targeting apoptosis (Chen and Chen, 2011; Nanni et al., 2010).

These are just some of the most promising PET tracers currently available. A better knowledge of the biological tumor changes at the molecular level is the essential basis for the development of new PET tracers targeting more and more specific cancer biomarkers. It is, doubtless, the future direction for research and it will allow PET to play a more relevant and leading role in the "personalized" management of oncologic patients (Chen and Chen, 2011; Zhu et al., 2011).

References

Ambrosini, V., Tomassetti, P., Franchi, R., and S. Fanti. 2010. Imaging of NETs with PET radiopharmaceuticals. *Q J Nucl Med Mol Imaging* 54:16–23.

Berry, J.D. and G.J.R. Cook. 2006. Positron emission tomography in oncology. *Br Med Bull* 79–80:171–186.

Caroli, P., Nanni, C., Rubello, D., Alavi, A., and S. Fanti. 2010. Non-FDG PET in the practice of oncology. *Indian J Cancer* 47:120–125.

Chen, K. and X. Chen. 2011. Positron emission tomography imaging of cancer biology: Current status and future prospects. *Semin Oncol* 38:70–86.

Hany, T.F., Steinert, H.C., Goerres, G.W., Buck, A., and G.K. von Schulthess. 2002. PET diagnostic accuracy: Improvement with in-line PET-CT system: Initial results. *Radiology* 225:575–581.

Levin, C.S. 2005. Primer on molecular imaging technology. *Eur J Nucl Med Mol Imaging* 32:S325–S345.

Nanni, C., Fantini, L., Nicolini, S., and S. Fanti. 2010. Non FDG PET. *Clin Radiol* 65:536–548.

Shreve, P.D., Anzai, Y., and R.L. Wahl. 1999. Pitfalls in oncologic diagnosis with FDG PET imaging: Physiologic and benign variants. *Radiographics* 19:61–77.

Townsend, D.W. 2008. Positron emission tomography/computed tomography. *Semin Nucl Med* 38:152–166.

Treglia, G., Cason, E., and G. Fagioli. 2010. Recent applications of nuclear medicine in diagnostics (first part). *Ital J Med* 4:84–91.

Vallabhajosula, S. 2007. ^{18}F-labeled positron emission tomographic radiopharmaceuticals in oncology: An overview of radiochemistry and mechanisms of tumor localization. *Semin Nucl Med* 37:400–419.

Vallabhajosula, S., Solnes, L., and B. Vallabhajosula. 2011. Broad overview of positron emission tomography radiopharmaceuticals and clinical applications: What is new? *Semin Nucl Med* 41:246–264.

Zhu, A., Lee, D., and H. Shim. 2011. Metabolic PET imaging in cancer detection and therapy response. *Semin Oncol* 38:55–69.

4

Innovative Tools for Early Detection of Cancer

Ali Tiss, Amal Hasan, Abdelkrim Khadir, Mohammed Dehbi, and Said Dermime

CONTENTS

ABSTRACT Early-stage detection of cancer is the key to provide a better outcome for therapeutic intervention. Most routine screening tools for cancer detection are largely based on examination of cell morphology, tissue histology, and measurement of serum markers, which lack sufficient sensitivity and/or specificity for early detection of cancer. Indeed, most secreted proteins studied as cancer screening biomarkers have low sensitivity and/or low specificity, and this could be due to the use of nonsensitive techniques or due the fact that several of these tumor markers are also produced by normal tissues. Altogether, these facts pinpoint to the urgent need for the discovery of innovative tools and novel tumor markers for cancer screening, diagnosis, and prognosis. Recently, scientists and clinicians have shifted to innovative techniques in order to identify and characterize biomarkers that drive the development and progression of cancer and to discover upstream genes/proteins, which could be useful to detect early-stage cancer, predict prognosis, and determine therapy efficacy or to be novel drug targets.

This chapter contains three sections that will discuss different but complementary innovative techniques that are being recently developed for the detection of early biomarkers in cancers. The first technique will focus on the use of reverse transcriptase polymerase chain reaction (RT-PCR) for the quantitation of the Wilms' tumor gene (WT1) mRNA (WT1 assay). The WT1 mRNA is a relatively new marker of several types of leukemia and myelodysplastic syndrome (MDS). This WT1 assay makes it possible to rapidly assess the effectiveness of treatment and to evaluate the degree of eradication of leukemic cells as well as the continuous assessment of the MDS progression and its evolution to overt acute myeloid leukemia. The second section will highlight the use of mass spectrometry (MS) technique as an important analytical tool in clinical proteomics, primarily in the disease-specific discovery, identification, and characterization of proteomic biomarkers and patterns. MS-based proteomics is increasingly being used in clinical validation and diagnostic method development. In this section, we will describe the current state of MS in clinical proteomics applied to early detection of cancer biomarkers with a focus on ovarian and breast cancers including both biomarker discovery and clinical diagnosis. In the last section, we will focus on the surface plasmon resonance (SPR) technique, which is primarily used to detect bimolecular interaction and has recently gained enormous interest and popularity for its versatility and high sensitivity especially when it is coupled to MS.

KEY WORDS: *qPCR, mass spectrometry, SPR, biomarker discovery, WT1.*

4.1 Real-Time PCR for the Detection of Wilms' Tumor Gene 1 in Cancer

4.1.1 Introduction

The Wilms' tumor gene 1 (WT1), located on chromosome 11p13, encodes a zinc finger transcription factor and activates or represses the transcription of various target genes, which are involved in important processes including the cell cycle, cell differentiation, cell proliferation, and apoptosis (Haber et al., 1991; Harrington et al., 1993; Hewitt et al., 1995; Scharnhorst et al., 2001). WT1 was initially described as a tumor suppressor gene (Call et al., 1990); however, it is now well accepted that WT1 has a profile more consistent with that of an oncogene. In this regard, the WT1 gene is highly expressed in most acute myeloid leukemia (AML) and acute lymphoid leukemia (ALL) (Bergmann et al., 1997; Brieger et al., 1994; Cilloni et al., 2002; Greiner et al., 2004; Inoue et al., 1994; Menssen et al., 1995, 1997; Miwa et al., 1992; Miyagi et al., 1993; Ogawa et al., 2003; Tamaki et al., 2003) and is also found in chronic myelogenous leukemia (CML) (Inoue et al., 1994). WT1 overexpression is considered as an adverse prognostic factor in AML (Bergmann et al., 1997; Miwa et al., 1992). Therefore, the WT1 mRNA is typically regarded as a tumor-specific marker for leukemic blast cells whereby a single leukemic cell (from 100,000 normal peripheral blood mononuclear cells [PBMCs]) can be detected by quantifying WT1 mRNA (Inoue et al., 1994). Importantly, the level of total WT1 expression can be used to monitor minimal residual disease (MRD) in AML and myelodysplastic syndrome (MDS) patients (Yang et al., 2007). In MDS (Tamaki et al., 1999) and CML (Inoue et al., 1994), WT1 mRNA expression levels increase with disease progression, and therefore, the WT1 assay is an essential tool in the detection of MRD in acute leukemia and MDS (Kletzel et al., 2002; Sugiyama, 2010). Furthermore, there are major differences in the expression of total WT1 between patient samples with distinct diagnosis; more specifically, in AML and MDS, total WT1 levels are different (among distinct "French–American–British" [FAB] subtypes) and show specific molecular aberrations (Barragan et al., 2004; Cilloni et al., 2002; Cilloni and Saglio, 2004; Kramarzova et al., 2012; Kreuzer et al., 2001; Lapillonne et al., 2006; Ostergaard et al., 2004; Rodrigues et al., 2007; Trka et al., 2002; Weisser et al., 2005). In addition, the WT1 gene is highly expressed in most types of solid tumors (Barbaux et al., 1997; Bickmore et al., 1992; Davies et al., 1998; Dechsukhum et al., 2000; Dumur et al., 2002; Gu et al., 2010; Hohenstein and Hastie, 2006; Ito et al., 2006; Mayo et al., 1999; Moorwood et al., 1999; Oji et al., 1999; Pelletier et al., 1991; Renshaw et al., 1997; Yang and Romaniuk, 2008), and the level of expression serves as a significant prognostic factor (Sugiyama, 2010). Indeed, overexpression of WT1 has been shown to be a poor prognostic factor in several solid tumors including ovarian (Netinatsunthorn et al., 2006), breast (Miyoshi et al., 2002), and hepatocellular carcinomas (HCCs) (Sera et al., 2008).

The precise relevance and contribution of WT1 to the malignant process remain to be elucidated. A number of aspects may contribute to the final outcome of WT1 pro- or antioncogenic effects; these include degradation of WT1 expression, discrepancy in the function of WT1 isoforms, interactions with other factors, and the status of the cell. A disturbed WT1 regulatory function may also lead to an alteration in the mesenchymal–epithelial balance, leading to malignant proliferation as well as nonmalignant diseases that are associated with the WT1 gene (Burwell et al., 2007; Scholz and Kirschner, 2011). Furthermore, given the prevalence of WT1 expression in a wide variety of malignancies and its limited physiological expression, the WT1 may be used as a potential immunotherapeutic target for vaccine development in various malignancies (reviewed in Ariyaratana and Loeb [2007]; Ellisen et al. [2001]; Scharnhorst et al. [2001]; Sugiyama [2001]; Virappane et al. [2008]; Wagner et al. [2003]; Yang et al. [2007].

4.1.2 WT1 Isoforms

At least 36 isoforms of the WT1 protein are produced from a single DNA template as a result of alternative splicing, alternative pre-mRNA splicing, mRNA editing, and alternative translation initiation (Bruening and Pelletier, 1996; Dallosso et al., 2004; Dutton et al., 2006; Florio et al., 2010; Haber et al., 1991; Hossain et al., 2006; Niksic et al., 2004; Scharnhorst et al., 2001; Sugiyama, 2001; Wagner et al., 2003). However, four major WT1 isoforms (WT1 variants A [EX5–/KTS–], B [EX5+/KTS–], C [EX5–/KTS+], and D [EX5+/KTS+]) are produced by an alternative splicing, and these vary in the presence or absence of the 17AA insert and KTS inserts (Bickmore et al., 1992; Davies et al., 1998; Ito et al., 2006; Mayo et al., 1999; Wang et al., 1995). In addition, studies have described an alternative WT1 transcript, namely, AWT1 (also known as short transcript, sWT1), which uses another first exon located in intron 1 of WT1 (exon 1a) but maintains WT1 exonic structure between exons 2 and 10 (Dallosso et al., 2004; Hossain et al., 2006). The alternative AWT1 transcript has been found to be overexpressed in leukemia samples (Hossain et al., 2006; Ishikawa et al., 2011). An N-terminally truncated transcript that lacks exons 1–5 has also been described, and it has been hypothesized that a cryptic promoter within WT1 intron 5 exists (Dechsukhum et al., 2000; Dumur et al., 2002). The 17AA (EX5) insert is located in the center of the protein and may function as a transcriptional activation domain. The KTS insert is located between the third and fourth zinc finger of the protein and alters the space between these fingers, which changes the DNA recognition site and thus decreases the DNA binding ability. The AWT1 transcript does not contain the repression domain (Figure 4.1) (Dallosso et al., 2004; Hossain et al., 2006; Moorwood et al., 1999; Renshaw et al., 1997; Scharnhorst et al., 2001; Sugiyama, 2001). The most prevalent isoforms are those that contain both splice inserts, and the least common transcripts are those that miss both inserts. The physiological ratio of A[–/–]: B[+/–]: C[–/+]: D[+/+] appears to be stable during the development of WT1 expressing tissues, and in the case of fetal kidney and Wilms' tumors, the ratio is 1.0:2.5:3.8:8.3 (Haber et al., 1991). In addition, defective splicing resulting in an altered ratio of WT1 KTS [+]/KTS[–] variants has been described in rare premalignant syndromes, such as Frasier syndrome and Denys–Drash syndrome (Barbaux et al., 1997; Hohenstein and Hastie, 2006; Pelletier et al., 1991; Yang and Romaniuk, 2008).

Various WT1 effects have been associated with particular WT1 isoforms (Bor et al., 2006; Burwell et al., 2007; Han et al., 2007; Ito et al., 2006; Jomgeow et al., 2006; Moriya et al., 2008; Morrison et al., 2006; Tatsumi et al., 2008). Previous methods used for the detection of WT1 isoforms, which include reverse transcriptase polymerase chain reaction (RT-PCR), GeneScan, and quantitative PCR (qPCR) of EX5 [+] and KTS[+] variants, have resulted in an approximate estimation of WT1 isoform levels. However, a more recent study has designed a real-time qPCR method that yields precise quantification of the four major WT1 variants, which enables the determination of the ratio of WT1 isoforms in childhood and adult AML and in MDS samples (Kramarzova et al., 2012). WT1 isoform expression patterns show significant differences among normal bone marrow (BM), AML, and MDS and between adult and children samples. However, the isoform expression patterns are more uniform in AML than in MDS. This reflects higher heterogeneity of MDS and its potential progression from BM harboring certain dysplastic

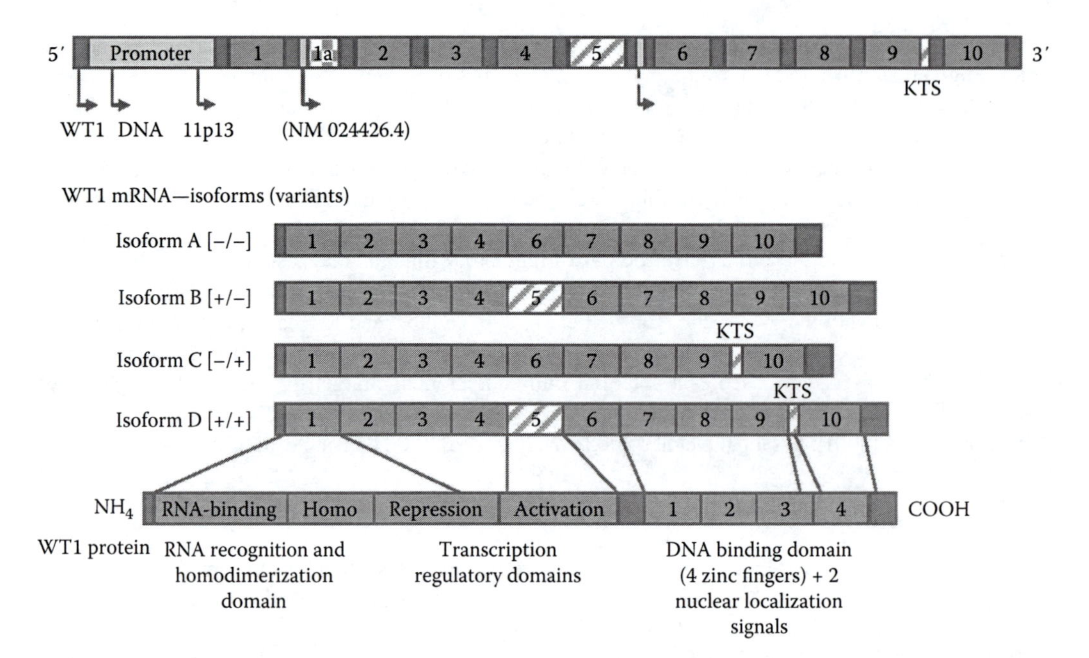

FIGURE 4.1 **(See color insert.)** Alternative splice sites are crosshatched. Blue arrows indicate alternative transcription initiation sites.

features to BM containing malignant cells. There are marked differences in the expression of total WT1, but not WT1 isoform ratios, among morphologically and cytogenetically defined subgroups of AML and MDS (Kramarzova et al., 2012). In this regard, AML has been associated with higher expression levels of EX5 [+] variants at both diagnosis and relapse (Gu et al., 2010; Renshaw et al., 1997; Siehl et al., 2004). Therefore, the use of sensitive and specific techniques for the detection, quantification, and monitoring of WT1 is essential.

4.1.3 Experimental Procedures

4.1.3.1 Sample Collection, Processing, and RNA Isolation

Peripheral blood or BM samples should be collected into sterile tubes with anticoagulant (ACD, K_2 or K_3EDTA) and immediately transported (at room temperature) to the lab. Mononuclear cells should be separated (within 4 h after collection) on a density gradient medium (Lymphoprep) as per manufacturers' instructions and stored at −80°C. In the case of solid tumors, biopsy samples should be obtained at the time of surgery and either used immediately or snap frozen in liquid nitrogen and stored at −80°C. For snap freezing, each piece of tissue may be cut into smaller aliquots to fit into plastic vials, with target weight being 0.1–0.2 g. The plastic vial can then be placed on a precision scale and the scale tarred (should read 0.0 with vial on it). The aliquot of tissue should then be placed into a vial and have the weight recorded. The Cryovial should then be held with long metal forceps and immersed approximately halfway down the height of the liquid nitrogen in a canister for at least 30 s. Cryovials may be either transferred to a dry ice cooler or kept in liquid nitrogen until transferred to a −80°C freezer (Ref.: http://www.cinj.org). For the isolation of RNA, an RNeasy Mini Kit (Qiagen) can be used as per manufacturers' instructions, and the concentration of RNA may be evaluated by spectrophotometry (NanoDrop or SPEC). Total RNA may be treated with DNaseI (Invitrogen) (Lehe et al., 2008).

4.1.3.2 Reverse Transcription PCR for WT1

RT-PCR for the detection of cDNA (starting from 1 μg of total RNA) can be performed according to the recommendations of the Europe Against Cancer (EAC) program (Beillard et al., 2003; Gabert et al., 2003), according to the BIOMED I™ protocol (Rossi et al., 2012), or as described previously (Lehe et al., 2008; Trka et al., 2002). In one of the described methods, 1 μg RNA in a total volume of 25 μL, oligo(dT) primers, Moloney murine leukemia virus reverse transcriptase (Invitrogen), and LightCycler FastStart DNA Master SYBR Green 1 Kit (Roche) were used for the quantification of WT1 mRNA expression (Lehe et al., 2008). Porphobilinogen deaminase (PBGD) was used as a housekeeping gene. The standard curve was generated using cDNA (2 μL) from K562 (Greiner et al., 2004; Lehe et al., 2008). The amplification was conducted in a total volume of 20 μL for 40 cycles/10 s at 95°C, 4 s/64°C, and 35 s/72°C. The forward primer TTCATCAAACAGGAGCCGAGC and the reverse primer GTGCGAGGGCGTGTGA were used for total WT1. For PBGD, the forward primer CATGTCTGGTAACGGCAATG and the reverse primer TCTTCTCCAGGGCATGTTCAA were used (Lehe et al., 2008). Alternatively, RT-PCR for total WT1 (starting from 1 mg of total RNA) can be performed using an iScript kit (Kramarzova et al., 2012). For the detection of the four main isoforms of WT1, a set of primers located on exon 5 (EX5+), exon 4/exon 6 boundary (EX5−), KTS (KTS+), and exon 9/exon 10 boundary (KTS−) can be used. Finally, PCR products can be analyzed either by electrophoresis on agarose gel or by capillary electrophoresis (Agilent 2100 Bioanalyzer) as described elsewhere (Kramarzova et al., 2012).

4.1.3.3 Real-Time qPCR for WT1

4.1.3.3.1 Plasmid Calibrators and qPCR for Total WT1

Using the TOPO TA Cloning Kit (Invitrogen), the WT1 sequence (obtained from the first round PCR) can be cloned into a PCR 2.1-TOPO vector and then transformed into a TOP10 *Escherichia coli* strain. The selected clones can be screened by PCR for the presence of the insert and then confirmed by sequencing. This should be followed by extraction of the plasmids, using the HiSpeed Plasmid Midi Kit (Qiagen), quantification by SPEC, and linearization with EcoRI (Invitrogen) restriction. The digested plasmid should then be serially diluted in a solution of Tris/EDTA/*E. coli* 16S and 23S rRNA (Roche), and a set of WT1 calibrators (with final concentrations of 10^6, 10^5, 10^4, 10^3, 10^2 and 10^1 copies/5 μL) should be prepared (Boublikova et al., 2006).

The expression of total WT1 can be quantified either by the use of a commercially available WT1 Kit (WT1 ProfileQuant) (Kramarzova et al., 2012) or as described previously (Boublikova et al., 2006): qPCR for the detection and quantification of total WT1 can be performed according to EAC protocols (Gabert et al., 2003). The Primer Express 2.0 software can be used to design primers and probes with the forward primer located on exon 6, the reverse primer on exon 7, and the 6FAM- and TAMRA-labeled probe on exon 6/7 boundary. For total WT1, the recommended primers and probes, reaction conditions, and parameters are listed in Table 4.1. The qPCR reaction can be performed either on an ABI PRISM 7700 Sequence Detection System (Applied Biosystems) or on an iCycler iQ (Bio-Rad). The detection of WT1 should be carried out in a triplicate reaction, while CG and calibrators for both WT1 and CG in duplicate. For WT1 and CG, the threshold should be set at the exponential phase (usually at 0.1) and the baseline set at 3–15 (baseline for B2M at 3–10).

4.1.3.3.2 Plasmid Calibrators and qPCR for Total WT1 and Its Main Isoforms

The products of RT-PCR can be cloned (with primers located on exon 4 and exon 10 of the WT1 gene) using the TOPO TA Cloning Kit as described previously (Boublikova et al., 2006). WT1 isoforms can also be identified by RT-PCR, and clones selected for bulk plasmid production. Sets of calibrators can be prepared for WT1 A, B, C, and D isoforms with final concentrations of 105, 104, 103, 102, and 101 copies per 5 mL. Notably, the detection of the four WT1 isoforms (A[EX5−/KTS−], B[+/−], C[−/+], and D[+/+]) by qPCR is associated with several difficulties; these are due to the length of the amplicon (B460 bases) and the high sequence homology between KTS[+] and KTS[−] variants (Kramarzova et al., 2012). A recent study has tested several approaches to overcome these difficulties and has established an optimal qPCR. The efficacy of the qPCR assays was further validated against the results of RT-PCR and GeneScan detection of WT1 isoforms (Kramarzova et al., 2012). Optimized primers and probe designs are shown in Figure 4.2 and Table 4.2, and the reaction conditions are summarized in Table 4.3. The qPCR reaction is performed on either the Applied Biosystems 7500 Fast Real-Time PCR System or

TABLE 4.1

qPCR Detection System for Total WT1

Reaction Primers and Probe

Primer	Probe Code	5′ Position	Size	Sequence 5′–3′
WT1-fwd	EX6	1253	21	TAC ACA CGC ACG GTG TCT TCA
WT1-rvs	EX7	1338	21	CTC AGA TGC CGA CCA TAC AAG
WT1-probe	EX6/7	1275	25	6FAM-AGG CAT TCA GGA TGT GCG ACG TGT G-TAMRA

Reaction Conditions

Reagent	Volume
cDNA	5 μL (10% of the RT mixture)
Fwd primer	300 nm
Rvs primer	300 nm
Probe	200 nm
2X TaqMan Universal Master Mix	12.5 μL
sdH_2O to total volume	25 μL

Reaction Incubation

Cycles/Temperature	Time
50°C	2 min
95°C	10 min
50 cycles of 95°C	15 s
60°C	60 s

Reaction Efficiency and Sensitivity

	Plasmid Calibrators	K-562 RNA
ΔRn	>1	>1
Standard curve slope	−3.45	−3.34
Standard curve intercept	39.4	21.7
Standard curve correlation coefficient	0.999	0.994
WT1/CG standard curve slope	0.055	0.075
Reproducible sensitivity	10 molecules	−5 log dilution

All positions correspond to WT1 mRNA variant D sequence, NM_024426.

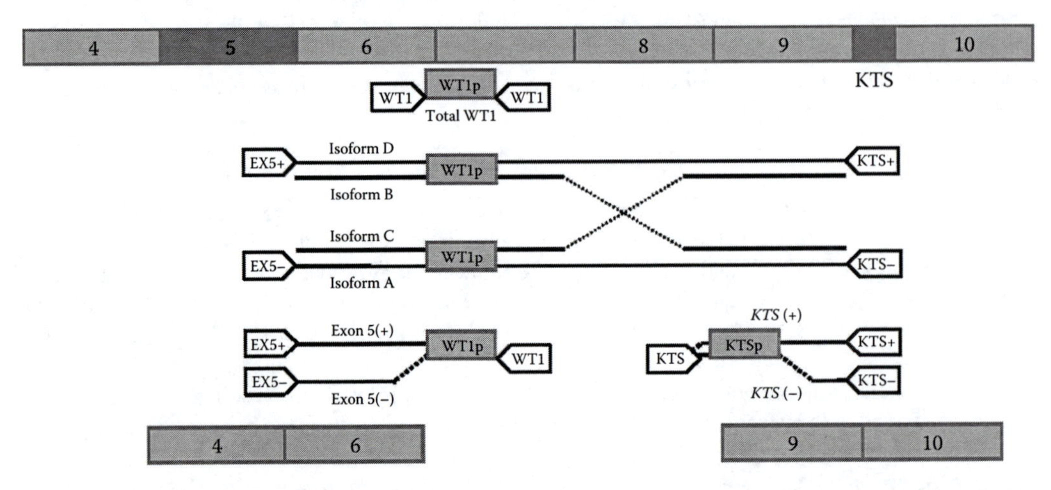

FIGURE 4.2 **(See color insert.)** qPCR detection systems for total WT1 and its four isoforms (primers are indicated by gray arrows and probes by black rectangles).

TABLE 4.2
qPCR Detection Systems for Total WT1 and Its Four Isoforms

Primer/Probe Code	5′ Position	Size	Sequence 5′–3′ and Exon Location
WT1-fwd	1257	21	TAC ACA CGCACG GTG TCT TCA ←— Exon 6 —→
WT1-rvs	1342	21	CTC AGA TGC CGA CCA TAC AAG ←— Exon 7 —→
WT1-probe	1279	25	6FAM-AGG CAT TCA GGA TGT GCG ACG TGT G-TAMRA ←— Exon 6 —→←— Exon 7 —→
KTS(com)-fwd	1501	24	GCT CAA AAG ACA CCA AAG GAG ACA ←— Exon 8 —→
KTS(−)-rvs	1639	22	GCT GAA GGG CTT TTC ACC TGT A ←— Exon 10 —→←— Exon 9 —→
KTS(+)-rvs	1638	25	CTGAAG GGC TTT TCA CTT GTT TTA C ←— Exon 10 —→←— KTS —→
KTS-probe	1562	24	6FAM-CGA AAG TTC TCC CGG TCC GAC CAC-TAMRA ←— Exon 9 —→
EX5(−)-fwd	1125	19	GAG CCA CCT TAA AGG GCC A ←— Exon 4 —→←— Exon 6 —→
EX5(+)-fwd	1171	20	ATG GAC AGA AGG GCA GAG CA ←— Exon 5 —→

TABLE 4.3
Reaction Conditions for the Detection of Total WT1 and Its Four Isoforms

qPCR Reaction Conditions for WT1 Isoforms and Total WT1		
Component	**WT1 Isoforms**	**Total WT1**
cDNA	5 μL (10% of RT mixture)	5 μL (10% of RT mixture)
fwd primer (15 μM)	1 μL (600 nM)	0.5 μL (300 nM)
rvs primer (15 μM)	1 μL (600 nM)	0.5 μL (300 nM)
Probe (5 μM)	1 μL (200 nM)	1 μL (200 nM)
dNTPs (10 mM)	2 μL (800 nM)	
$MgCl_2$ (25 mM)	2 μL (2 mM)	
PCR buffer 10X	2.5 μL	
ROX-5 or ROX-6 (10 μm)	0.1 μL (40 nM)	
Taq DNA polymerase (5 U/μL)	0.2 μL	
Universal master mix 2X		12.5 μL
sdH_2O to total volume	25 μL	25 μL
Incubation	**Temperature and Time**	
	50°C for 2 min	50°C for 2 min
	95°C for 10 min	95°C for 10 min
	10 cycles of touch-down:	50 cycles:
	95°C for 15 s	95°C for 15 s
	67°C–62.5°C for 60 s	60°C for 60 s
	40 cycles:	
	95°C for 15 s	
	62°C for 60 s	

LightCycler 480. ABL can be used as a control gene. The detection of the WT1 gene should be carried out in triplicate and the detection of ABL and calibrators in duplicate.

4.1.3.4 Result Interpretation of the qPCR

4.1.3.4.1 Result Interpretation of Total WT1

Samples should be considered positive if at least one of the triplicate or duplicate qPCR reactions is positive. The copy number of WT1, CG, and normalized WT1 (NCN, WT1/ABL, or WT1/100 B2M copies) can be calculated using the standard curve method. The standard curves can be created using plasmid DNA calibrators—ABL and B2M Control Gene Standards (Ipsogen) and WT1 plasmid calibrators. As a negative control, *E. coli* rRNA is recommended. The translocation of TEL-AML1 should be detected, quantified, and used for MRD monitoring according to BIOMED-1 and EAC recommendations (Beillard et al., 2003; van Dongen et al., 1999; Gabert et al., 2003).

4.1.3.4.2 Result Interpretation of WT1 Isoforms

Samples should be considered positive if at least one reaction of the replicate is positive and reported as negative if all reactions are negative (within the detection range) (Kramarzova et al., 2012). The plasmid standard curve can be used to calculate WT1 (total and isoform), ABL copy number, and WT1 normalized copy number (NCN¼WT1/ABL_104). The ratio of WT1 isoforms can be counted based on their proportion to the sum of all WT1 isoforms (Kramarzova et al., 2012). For the estimation of the ratios of A, B, C, and D isoforms, the ratios of the variants (EX5[+], EX5[−], KTS[+], and KTS[−]) can be multiplied by each other; for example, the ratio of EX5[−] can be multiplied with the ratio of KTS[−] to yield the ratio of isoform A, EX5[+] with KTS[−] for isoform B, EX5[−] with KTS[+] for isoform C, and EX5[+] with KTS[+] for isoform D (Siehl et al., 2004).

4.1.4 Challenges and Future Directions

The WT1 assay showed a good correlation of WT1 expression with the clinical course of the disease, and it can also correlate its expression with other follow-up markers that are assessed in parallel. Moreover, WT1 expression can reveal patients at high risk of treatment failure in the early phase of therapy, and that quantitative analysis of WT1 as postremission control can also enable early detection of imminent relapse.

The advantages of this method include sensitivity, specificity, reproducibility, and the yield of excellent correlation between the sum of isoforms and total WT1 (Kramarzova et al., 2012). However, the absolute numbers of detected copies of all isoforms are lower than total WT1 expression; this is likely to be due to the unequal performance of the qPCR detection systems for total WT1 and the isoforms (Kramarzova et al., 2012). Therefore, it is recommended that both EX5[−] and EX5[+], or KTS[−] and KTS[+], sites are always detected rather than deducing the values of EX5[−] or KTS[−] from total WT1 minus EX5[+] or KTS[+], respectively (Kramarzova et al., 2012). A certain minimum level of WT1 expression is required for a reliable evaluation of isoform ratios; otherwise WT1 isoform evaluation will be inaccurate. This assay limitation is especially important when comparing WT1 isoform ratios in leukemic cells expressing higher levels of total WT1 and normal BM with low total WT1 expression (Kramarzova et al., 2012).

There is ambiguity as to whether leukemic cells have been completely killed when complete remission is achieved in patients receiving conventional chemotherapy and/or BM transplantation. It may be able to treat leukemia patients with different clinical protocols based on the scope of MRD if we can monitor these patients for MRD. However, there is a limit of MRD detection: 1%–5% for morphologic techniques and 5%–10% for Southern blot technique and no more than 1% for fluorescence in situ hybridization; therefore, they are not currently practical for detection of MRD. On the other hand, flow cytometry has a sensitivity of 1 leukemic cell in 10^4, but this technique is valid only to leukemia with limited phenotypes. Moreover, although the PCR technique can detect leukemic cells at frequencies as low as 1 in 10^5–10^6 cells, it has been applied only to leukemia bearing tumor-specific DNA markers, which is useful for only 20%–30% of these leukemia patients. However, the detection of MRD RT-PCR WT1 assay is applicable to all leukemia patients, regardless of their type or the presence or absence of a tumor-specific marker.

Importantly, the WT1 assay can always be used for the detection of MRD even in cases in which chromosomal and DNA analyses of fresh leukemic cells were unsuccessful or could not be performed. Although basing treatment on the WT1 assay has not yet been demonstrated to be practically successful, this assay will be useful in the near future to individualize treatment protocols for all leukemia patients.

4.2 Mass Spectrometry-Based Proteomics for Detection of Cancer

4.2.1 Introduction

Genome sequencing and structure have received much attention in the last two decades and produced a wealth of information, including the full genome sequence. However, proteins are the workhorse biomolecules that functionally govern cellular processes, whereas genomics can provide only limited insight into the mechanisms of disease progress and malignancy. Accordingly, changes in levels or abundance of genes or their transcripts correlate poorly with protein abundance (Greenbaum et al., 2003; Vogel et al., 2010). Although the human genome contains about 22,000 protein-coding genes (Pertea and Salzberg, 2010), it is estimated that the human proteome comprises >500,000 proteins (Banks et al., 2000; Ewing and Green, 2000). In addition, alternative splicing and posttranslational modifications of proteins (e.g., phosphorylation, glycosylation, and proteolytic cleavage) further increase the diversity of the human proteome. Proteins are also very dynamic, compared to genes, due to proteins' varying localization, half-lives, and response to stimuli such as disease and treatment (Anderson and Anderson, 2002). This makes the proteome of a great interest to medical researchers. Thus, systematic large-scale study of the protein constituency of biological samples with a plethora of state-of-the-art techniques (proteomic studies) is thought to bridge between genomic information and functional proteins.

Proteomics is defined as the study of the structure and function of proteins in a cell or tissue at a specific time under certain predefined conditions and includes information on the way the proteins function and interact with each other inside cells. The possibility to systematically and simultaneously identify and quantify large number of proteins obviously positions proteomics on the forefront to track heterogeneous alterations in multiple pathways and mechanisms that drive the transformation of the malignant phenotype.

During the last decade, scientists and clinicians both shifted to proteomic strategies to identify and characterize proteins that drive the development and progress of malignancy, to discover protein biomarkers that could be useful to detect early-stage cancer, to predict prognosis, to determine therapy efficacy, or to be novel drug targets. Oncoproteomic profiling by comparing diseased samples (tumor tissue, biofluids) against healthy controls was greeted with much enthusiasm to meet the urgent need for new biomarkers to diagnose early stages of cancer as well as for prognostic needs to track disease progression and therapeutic response (Cox and Mann, 2007; Hanash et al., 2008).

Oncoproteomic approaches vary from basic biochemistry techniques up to the most complex and advanced microarray platforms containing thousands of proteins, peptides, or antibodies. In this part of the chapter, we will discuss and summarize mass spectrometry (MS)-based proteomic approaches and platforms used to study cancer biology. We will also discuss the benefits of proteomics, in particular novel biomarker discovery. Finally, we will discuss the limitations and challenges of current oncoproteomics and the available opportunities that will enhance our understanding of cancer biology to propel clinical proteomics in cancer research and applications.

4.2.2 Proteomic Approaches for Cancer Studies

Innovative proteomic technologies and strategies have been recently designed for protein fractionation, enrichment, identification, and quantitation to deeply investigate the oncoproteome using various human biospecimens including cell lines, tissue biopsies, blood components (serum, plasma, and mononuclear cells), urine, saliva, and cerebrospinal fluid. In addition, there is the need for high-throughput methods for biomarker validation and integration of the various platforms of oncogenomic and oncoproteomic data to fully comprehend cancer biology. These needs are being partially satisfied by the advancement

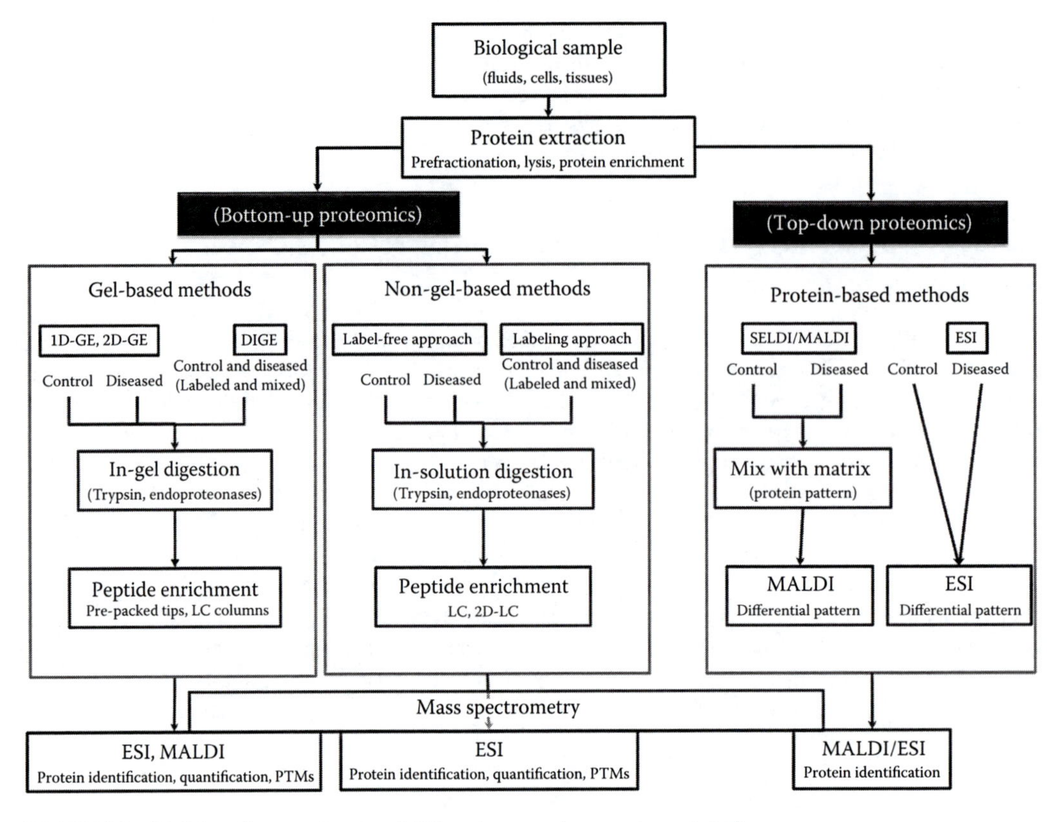

FIGURE 4.3 Workflow diagram of various MS-based proteomic strategies and platforms.

in sensitive MS technology and assisted by the growing array of gene and protein data available in compiled and curated databases (Baak et al., 2005). Figure 4.3 lists and compares some of the most common methods used in MS-based clinical proteomics applied to cancer. The analysis of proteins and peptides by MS is carried out using one of the two following strategies: The first is called a "top-down" approach referring to the determination of the protein sequence directly without breaking it a priori into pieces by enzymatic digestion. The second is the "bottom-up" approach, which refers to the reconstruction of the protein sequence from the sequences of the peptide fragments after proteolytic digestion, either by comparison with databases or derived from the analysis of their mass spectra.

As mentioned before, the discovery and clinical application of novel tumor markers for cancer screening, diagnosis, and prognosis are actually key focus areas of translational research in oncology. Accordingly, the main objectives of biomarker discovery are as follows: (1) presymptomatic diagnosis, including predisposition prediction, (2) stratification and assessment of progression of the disease, (3) following patient response to treatment, (4) predict and identify reoccurrences, and (5) identification of novel targets for therapeutic intervention. In line with these objectives, MS-based proteomics can be used either for biomarker discovery and validation or for clinical diagnosis and prognosis. Indeed, MS could be useful just for the early discovery steps, but it could be also used as an independent technique for validation of discovered biomarkers using other technologies or even as an endpoint clinical assay (summarized in Figure 4.4). Although conventional proteomics has become a key approach in biomarker discovery and validation, some of the most recent MS technologies have not yet been introduced to clinical application due to their low throughput, complexity, or high cost (Palmblad et al., 2009).

A mass spectrometer machine, the key element in this proteomic approach, consists of three main components: an ionization source, a mass analyzer, and an ion detector (Figure 4.5). The two most common ion sources used in proteomics are based on matrix-assisted laser desorption/ionization (MALDI) and electrospray ionization (ESI). The function of the ion source is to produce ions from the sample.

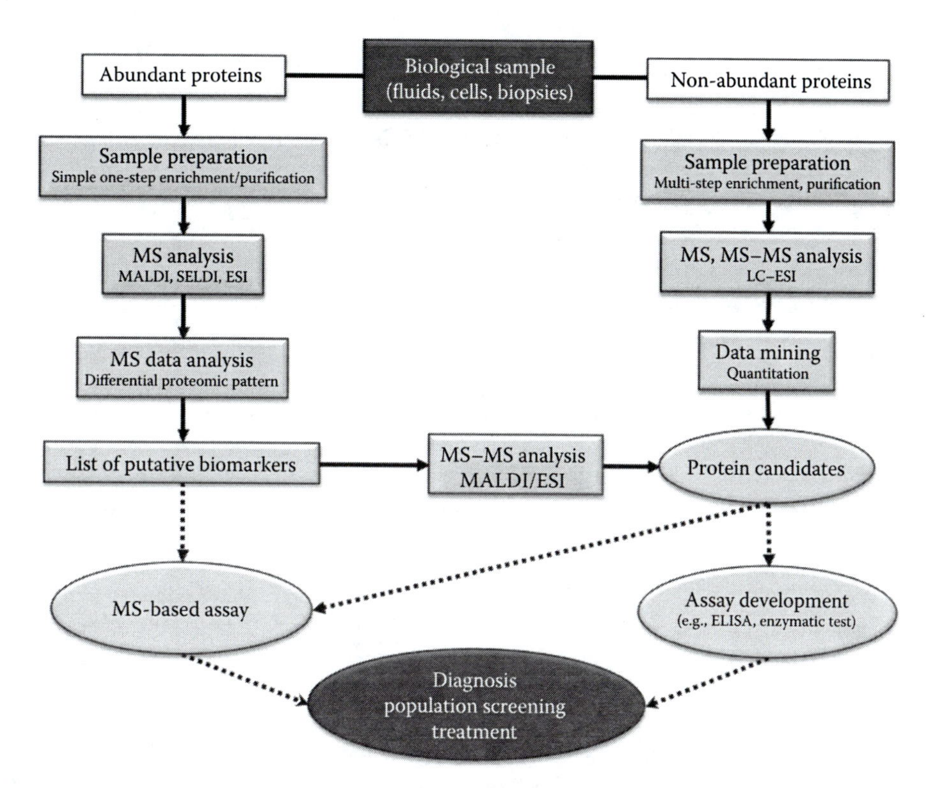

FIGURE 4.4 MS-based proteomic platforms used either as discovery/validation tool or as clinical assay.

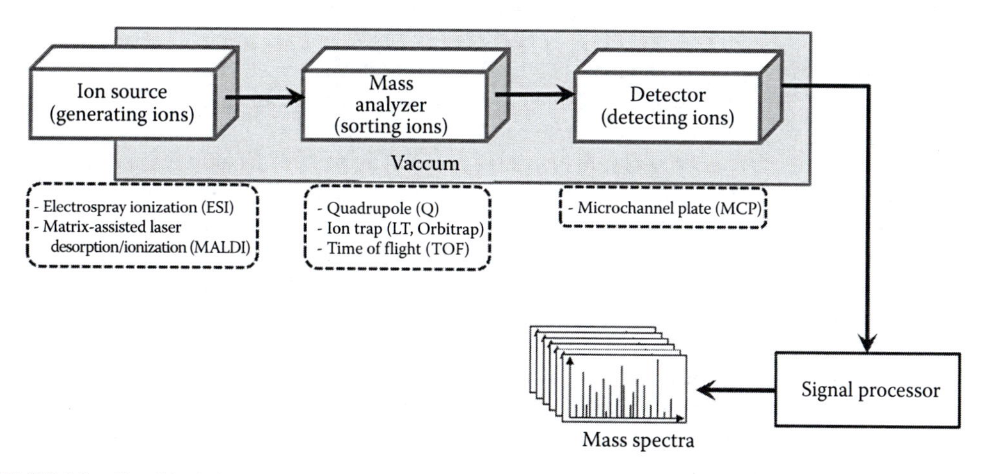

FIGURE 4.5 Simplified diagram and principles of mass spectrometer machine.

At this stage, peptides, proteins, and other molecules are converted to ions in the gas phase by the addition or loss of one or more protons in a so-called "soft" ionization technique that still maintains sample integrity. The function of the mass analyzer is to separate ions with different mass-to-charge ratios (m/z). The main ion analyzers used in proteomics are quadrupole (Q), time of flight (TOF), and ion traps. The amounts of different ions are finally measured by the detector that presents these as a mass spectrum or chart with a series of spiked peaks, each representing the charged protein or fragment ion present in a given sample (Figure 4.5).

The most commonly used techniques for the expression analysis of proteins are MALDI and surface-enhanced laser desorption/ionization (SELDI) combined with TOF-MS and ESI combined with liquid chromatography (LC)–(tandem) MS (LC–MS/MS). These techniques may also be combined with quantitative techniques such as isotope-coded affinity tags (ICATs), isobaric tags for relative and absolute quantification (iTRAQ), and stable isotope labeling by amino acids in cell culture (SILAC) (Gygi et al., 1999; Mann, 2006; Ong et al., 2002; Ross et al., 2004; Wiese et al., 2007). These MS techniques are particularly important for the analysis of low-molecular-weight (LMW) fraction of the proteome because, in this compartment of the proteome, the use of immunological assays such as enzyme-linked immunosorbent assay (ELISA) is limited owing to the difficulty in producing antibodies for LMW proteins, for example.

4.2.2.1 Biomarker Discovery

The present screening and diagnosis tools for cancer are mainly based on the examination of cell morphology and measurement of serum markers, such as carcinoembryonic antigen (CEA), prostate-specific antigen (PSA) for prostate cancer, CA-125 for ovarian cancer, and CA19-9 for colorectal and pancreatic cancer, which lack sufficient sensitivity and/or specificity for early detection (Tan et al., 2012). Indeed, most secreted proteins studied as cancer screening biomarkers have yielded too many false-negative results (failure to detect cancer in those who have it, a phenomenon known as low sensitivity) and/or too many false-positive results (indicate the presence of cancer in someone who does not have it, a phenomenon known as low specificity).

The poor sensitivity/specificity could be due to the fact that several of these tumor markers are also produced by nontumor tissues. For example, only 25%–30% of men referred for prostate biopsy on the basis of increased blood levels of PSA actually have prostate cancer as the level of PSA is also elevated in benign inflammatory diseases of the prostate (Parekh et al., 2007). Another example is the protein CA-125, which has been and still being used to screen for ovarian cancer, which has low sensitivity as blood levels of CA-125 are elevated in only 50%–60% of women who have early-stage ovarian cancer (Nossov et al., 2008). CA-125 also has low specificity since benign conditions, such as endometriosis and pregnancy, can elevate CA-125 levels (Bagan et al., 2008; Sarandakou et al., 2007). Alpha-fetoprotein (AFP) is the only clinical biomarker for the diagnosis of HCC, but it also has limited utility in early detection of HCC because about one-third of HCC patients have normal levels of serum AFP (Sun et al., 2008). The previously mentioned facts highlight the urgent, yet unmet, need for the discovery of novel tumor markers for cancer screening, diagnosis, and prognosis as well as fostering translational research in oncology to move from benchside to bedside.

Moreover, despite the recent discovery of many new potential markers with genomics and proteomics, only very few of these markers have been developed into clinical applications for cancer screening and patient monitoring. This is due to the long road from biomarker discovery to clinical diagnostics (Rifai et al., 2006). This long process from discovery to clinical application is exemplified in the development of OVA1, the first in vitro diagnostic multivariate index assay (IVDMIA) of proteomics biomarkers recently approved by the US FDA, to assess ovarian cancer risk in women diagnosed with ovarian tumor prior to a planned surgery (Zhang and Chan, 2010).

The following sections will provide a brief overview of two main approaches currently used in cancer proteomic research, which are protein identification and pattern recognition (Figure 4.6). We will mainly focus on oncoproteomic methodology using MALDI-MS, SELDI-MS, and LC–MS highlighting the introduction of these technologies in the area of cancer biomarker discovery and their introduction to the clinical application as well as the hurdles and challenges that need to be overcome. Both proteomic approaches require high-capacity computing and bioinformatic systems to process the enormous amount of data that are produced by proteomic studies. Furthermore, confidence in the identified biomarker signatures will require to be reproduced in different populations and by different laboratories, a process called validation.

4.2.2.1.1 Protein Identification

As compared to target-specific approaches such as Western blot and ELISA, the advent of discovery-based proteomics are better suited for discovery of novel diagnostic, prognostic, predictive biomarkers, and drug targets (Azad et al., 2006). Protein targets that are identified with proteomics could also be further characterized to understand their functional role in cancer biology. Protein identification approach is

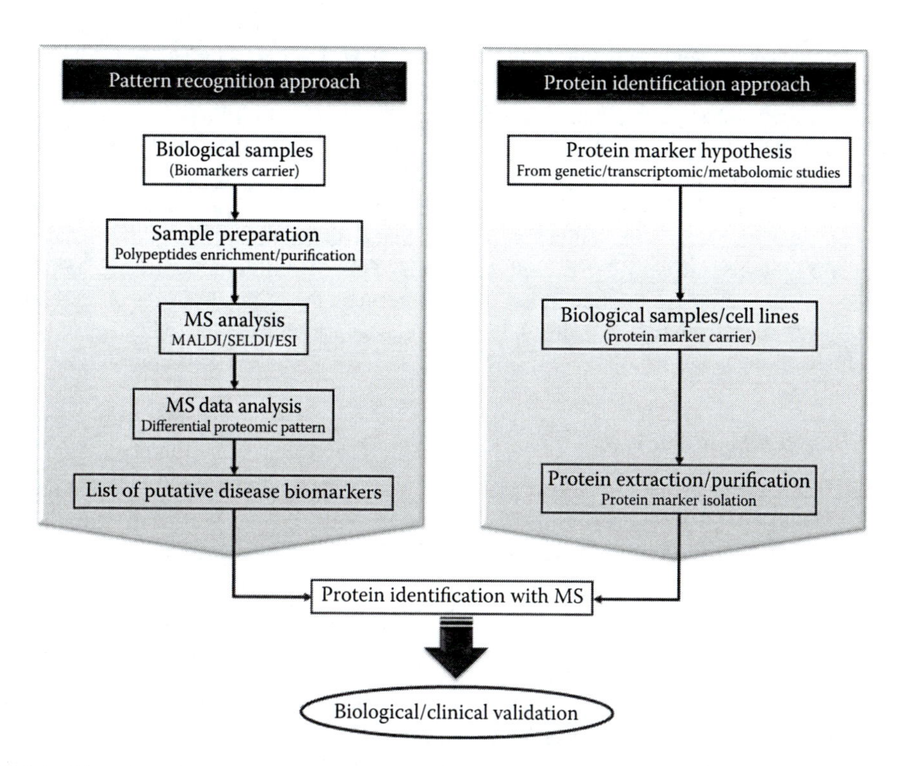

FIGURE 4.6 Biomarker discovery approaches based on MS.

a key step in the biomarker discovery and validation process rather than an independent discovery strategy (Figures 4.3 and 4.4). The identification of protein target will immediately facilitate its quantification and validation as well as evaluate its potential clinical value for further development (Tiss et al., 2010).

In practice, the identification of proteins using MS is a straightforward proteomic task even though some purification/enrichment steps might be needed. Those proteins could be generated from a differential expression panel between diseased and control subjects or just be selected as potential candidates from genetic, transcriptomic, and metabolomic studies (Figure 4.6). Another common strategy requiring protein identification is based on immunoprecipitation of protein complexes where there is an immediate need to identify the various partners of a given protein or DNA sequence. Indeed, cancer is often associated with differential expressions of several proteins in various signaling pathways that include large networks of protein complexes. Key signaling hubs of pathways involved in carcinogenesis are obviously potential molecular targets for therapeutics and inhibitor drugs against such proteins (Normanno et al., 2002; Zwick et al., 2002).

4.2.2.1.2 Pattern Recognition

Because of the heterogeneity of the cause and pathogenesis of cancer, multiple dysregulated proteins and cellular pathways are involved in the initiation and progression of cancer. In addition and as mentioned earlier, most proteins produced by tumor cells are not unique to cancer but also available in noncancerous cells. These proteins or fragments of proteins are often secreted into the bloodstream and other body fluids, such as urine and saliva (Kulasingam and Diamandis, 2008). Hence, a single biomarker is no longer thought to have sufficient sensitivity and/or specificity for population-based screenings. Instead, the discovery of biomarker panels called "protein signatures" that comprise several proteins would improve the detection of cancer patients and provide higher sensitivities and specificities (Jurisicova et al., 2008; Latterich et al., 2008; Paulovich et al., 2008; Wulfkuhle et al., 2004). In support to this vision, many recent proteomic studies have suggested that groups of proteins (protein signatures) are much more accurate tools for detecting cancer than individual proteins (Timms et al., 2011; Tiss et al., 2011; Villanueva et al., 2004, 2006, 2008). Several groups have screened for potential biomarker panels of ovarian, prostate, breast, bladder, pancreatic, and many other cancers with proteomics. For example, the OVA1 test, which was recently approved by the US FDA as clinical diagnostics for ovarian cancer, constitutes a panel of proteomic biomarkers (Zhang and Chan, 2010).

For pattern recognition, MS combined with some bioinformatic tools can be used to measure the mass and relative quantity of all proteins in a particular biological sample. MS machines can produce protein profiles (signatures) that can be compared between samples taken from patients with and without cancer even without the need to identify the individual proteins that produce the signatures. Independent identification of those proteins is usually carried out on MALDI-TOF-MS/MS or LC–MS/MS in the purpose of validation and also to reduce the likelihood that differences in protein signatures observed between biological samples taken from patients with and without cancer are actually due to bias related to sample collection and handling (Figure 4.6).

4.2.2.2 Clinical Diagnostics

After being essential in research, MS-based proteomic has found immediately its application in clinical analysis (Jellum et al., 1973; Lawson, 1975; Millington et al., 1990; Sweetman, 1996). Metabolite analysis is the most known clinical application of MS, which is now established in several countries in the neonatal screening programs for inborn errors of metabolism, in particular for phenylketonuria (Downing and Pollitt, 2008; Frazier et al., 2006; Wilcken et al., 2003).

MS is a powerful discovery tool, and most clinical applications of MS-based proteomics do not require MS to be physically available in the clinic. However, for prognosis, diagnosis, and monitoring disease progression, MS may very well be better employed on-site in the clinical setting or in local analytical laboratories (Palmblad et al., 2009). Nevertheless, MS has the potential to make the transition from a discovery tool (as largely used in conventional proteomics) to a clinical validation and diagnostic tool (Gramolini et al., 2008; Palmblad et al., 2009; Whiteaker et al., 2007). The wider introduction and use of MS-based proteomics at the bedside are foreseen for the very close future as the OVA1 test, for example, was recently approved by the US FDA as clinical diagnostics for ovarian cancer (Zhang and Chan, 2010).

4.2.3 Proteomic Platforms for Cancer Studies

4.2.3.1 SELDI-TOF

SELDI-MS uses a protein array chip (ProteinChip) with a functionalized surface that selectively binds subsets of proteins based on various physicochemical properties such as reverse phase, ion exchange, immobilized metal, or antibodies affinity. Organic matrix (a-cyano-4-hydroxycinnamic acid or sinapinic acid) is then added to the bound proteins on the chip surface as in MALDI, and in this way, the energy-absorbing matrix molecules co-crystallize with the proteins in the sample. The protein array chip is often coupled to TOF-MS and bioinformatics to derive proteome patterns for the samples analyzed (Petricoin and Liotta, 2004b). As other MS-based proteomic technologies, SELDI requires a low amount of samples (femtomole range), and it has real potential for clinical applications at the bedside to analyze samples for biomarker discovery (Petricoin and Liotta, 2004a,b; Wiesner, 2004). SELDI was widely used in researches related to signature detection of cancer proteome such as ovarian cancer (Kozak et al., 2005; Petricoin et al., 2002), prostate cancer (Malik et al., 2005; Petricoin et al., 2004; Stattin and Hakama, 2003), breast cancer (Becker et al., 2004; Lebrecht et al., 2009), lung cancer (Ueda et al., 2009), colon cancer (Albrethsen et al., 2005), and liver cancer (Orvisky et al., 2006).

The common applications of SELDI in cancer biomarker discovery were to find signature patterns correlated to healthy and diseased phenotypes. Indeed, several laboratories have applied SELDI-MS for the detection of various potential cancer biomarkers (Whelan et al., 2008). One of the first discovery studies carried out by Petricoin et al. (2002) generated a wide excitement in both the scientific community and the private sector, as their results were made into a commercially available diagnostic test (OvaCheck™, Correlogic, Inc., Germantown, MD).

Nevertheless, it became quickly obvious that SELDI-TOF-MS was insufficiently robust for biomarker discovery due to its inability to directly and accurately identify the proteins within proteome patterns, poor reproducibility between laboratories, and its relatively low mass resolution, which limited the use of SELDI-TOF-MS (Whelan et al., 2008). Furthermore, due to the high dynamic range of protein levels in serum and plasma, the ProteinChip array would be saturated with high-abundance proteins (Diamandis, 2004a,b), and thus, prefractionation steps were necessary to identify biomarkers present at low abundance. These limitations in SELDI-MS biomarker discovery were illustrated by its application in ovarian cancer screening, which was shortly later criticized for the lack of reproducibility, and the initial generated data were not validated in an independent test set (Baggerly et al., 2005; Diamandis, 2004b). Recently, the Lucid Proteomics System™, which combines SELDI from Bio-Rad (Hercules, CA) and MALDI-TOF/TOF-MS technologies from Bruker Daltonics (Billerica, MA), has however provided new hopes with top-down and bottom-up proteomic approaches for biomarker discovery on a single platform with improved spectra resolution and reproducibility (Jourdain et al., 2010). SELDI-MS technology can also, on the other hand, detect protein–protein, protein–DNA, and protein–metabolite interactions in complex biological samples to determine the biological functions of the proteins (Lehmann et al., 2005).

As an example of SELDI application in cancer relapse and prognosis, Cho et al. (2004) identified two isoforms of SAA protein as useful biomarkers to monitor relapse of nasopharyngeal carcinoma (NPC) by showing a large increase in SAA amounts in good correlation that relapse and a sharp fall with response to salvage chemotherapy. Further examination was conducted to identify other cancer targets that were associated with active disease or chemoresponse in NPC patients treated with two different drug combinations. Using MS/MS sequencing and immunoaffinity capture assay, two potential biomarkers were identified as a fragment of inter-a-trypsin inhibitor precursor and platelet factor-4 (Cho et al., 2007).

Direct-tissue proteomic analysis is on the other side a fast, highly sensitive, and reproducible application of SELDI-TOF-MS that opens the door to new perspectives in clinical proteomics. This high-throughput application allows proteomic analysis of tissue samples as a complement to other diagnostic methods. For example, Bouamrani and coworkers used SELDI to discriminate between glioblastomas and oligodendrogliomas that led to the identification of three potential cancer targets (Bouamrani et al., 2006).

4.2.3.2 MALDI-TOF

In MALDI, proteins or peptides are spotted onto a plate after being mixed with a large excess of a suitable organic matrix, absorbing energy at a specific wavelength of a pulsed laser. The dried mixture is then subjected to a laser pulse, which generates a plume of matrix and proteins converted into gas phase ions. The charged protein particles (ions) are accelerated into the vacuum flight tube of a TOF mass analyzer and travel through the tube until they impact the detector. The smaller ions have higher velocity and have a shorter flight time compared with the heavier ions. As the machine should be already calibrated using known polypeptide mixture, the relationship between the absolute mass of the ions and their TOF is used to determine the m/z ratio of the proteins or peptides (x-axis in mass spectra).

TOF analyzer can be operated either in linear or reflectron mode. In linear mode, the analyzer measures the TOF for ions flying from one end of the flight tube to the other. In reflectron mode however, when the ion reaches the end of the flight tube, a reflector will reflect them back toward a detector located near the MALDI ion source to lengthen the flight path. The reflectron mode helps in focusing ions with the same m/z value and in increasing the separation power/resolution of the mass spectrometer. Hence, protein or peptide ions are separated better and their masses are measured with more accuracy. The detector produces a response relative to the amount of each ion reaching it and converted to intensity with an arbitrary unit (y-axis in mass spectra). Thus, the mass spectrum is represented as a plot of m/z of ions against their respective intensity. In addition some MALDI instruments using a reflectron TOF analyzer have the ability to provide partial amino acid sequence data using its postsource decay (PSD) selection on ions with m/z values of up to 4 kDa, a feature not available with earlier SELDI-MS analyzers. This sequencing mode is, therefore, considered as an alternative approach to the more conventional MS/MS using ESI for protein sequencing (Spengler et al., 1992) with the advantage of being simple and having high sensitivity and higher tolerance to buffer and salt contaminants in comparison with ESI.

In a first approach, proteins are extracted from a biological sample, digested with a protease (e.g., trypsin) and then subjected to MALDI-TOF analysis to generate a list of m/z peaks known as peptide mass fingerprinting (PMF) specific to each protein. This approach has proven particularly useful in the discovery of biomarkers because of the technology's high sensitivity (down to attomol) and relatively wide dynamic range (3–4 orders of magnitude) added to the ability for high-throughput screening (Cramer, 2009). Alternatively, and as a second MALDI-MS-based approach, proteins/peptides can be separated, purified, and applied to target plates using high-throughput procedures (Figure 4.3). Then, specific patterns of proteins are generated from clinical samples such as serum and plasma that does not rely on protein identity, which can be used as a "diagnostic fingerprint" (Tiss et al., 2007; Veenstra et al., 2004; Villanueva et al., 2004, 2005).

Finally, MALDI-based technologies underpin high-throughput proteomic approaches that allow protein expression profiling of large sample sets with reasonable costs. MALDI-TOF platforms have been applied successfully to human cancer detection with reported high sensitivity and specificity using a variety of statistical pattern recognition and bioinformatic tools, for the early detection of cancers such as breast, ovarian, and lung cancer (for detailed reviews, see Bateson et al. [2011]; Gast et al. [2009]; Matharoo-Ball et al. [2007, 2008]; Mian et al. [2005]; Palmblad et al. [2009]).

4.2.3.3 1D and 2D Gels/MS

As mentioned before, complex biological specimens need most of the time a preliminary separation, enrichment, or fractionation of proteins before being analyzed by MS. Proteins from biological samples can be separated based on their size in a one-directional polyacrylamide gel electrophoresis (1D-PAGE), by applying an electric current to a gel matrix, where the smaller proteins move faster through the gel than the larger proteins. The gels can be stained and bands can be viewed. The proteins can then be visualized as spots after being stained, for example, using silver staining (Merril et al., 1979), Coomassie blue dye, fluorescent dyes (Patton, 2000), or radiolabels. It is usually performed for analytical purposes but may be used as a preparative technique before use of other methods such as MS for further characterization. This technique has however a major limitation as only few tens of proteins can be clearly separated at the same time and it cannot separate proteins of very similar size (e.g., protein isoforms).

An important development known as the "gold standard" method of 2D gel electrophoresis 2DE-PAGE, however, separates proteins using two different properties. In a first step, proteins are separated in a flat gel strip according to their isoelectric point (pI), that is, the specific point at which the net charge of the protein is zero. The proteins are then separated in a second experiment by placing the gel strip on top of a standard sodium dodecyl sulfate (SDS)-PAGE, which separates the proteins according their size.

The advantage of a 2DE-PAGE is its capability of separating many hundreds to few thousands proteins depending on the sample used, the gel size, and the sensitivity of the staining technique (Lopez, 1999). The main limitation in 2DE-PAGE, however, is the gel-to-gel variability, as the principle of the method relies on the comparison of the spot intensity within gels obtained from different samples or subjects. Another weakness of 2DE-PAGE is its low throughput as only being able to process at best two samples at a time, requiring relatively large amounts of sample and using a very laborious, time-consuming protocol and not suited to full automation. Furthermore, the limitation of 2DE-PAGE is the poor resolution of hydrophobic and membrane proteins and limited identification and quantification of proteins as these need to cut out the protein spots of the gel and digest them with proteases (e.g., trypsin). The generated peptides are then extracted from the gel slices and subjected to MS analysis to identify and quantify proteins of interest by submitting the MS or MS/MS profiles to the appropriate databases. The types of human cancers that have been investigated by this technique include lung, thyroid, colon, kidney, and bladder (Celis et al., 1996; Lin et al., 1995; Okuzawa et al., 1994; Sarto et al., 1997; Ward et al., 1990).

Gel-to-gel variations have been partially overcome with the development of new software packages but clearly enhanced by the development of the differential in-gel electrophoresis (2DE-DIGE) in 1997 by Unlu et al. (1997) that allows comparison of two or three protein samples simultaneously on the same gel. The method involves the covalent labeling of up to three different protein mixtures with different fluorescent dyes before 2D electrophoretic separation, which don't change migration properties of proteins in gels. Thus, the same proteins from different samples will migrate exactly to the same position on the same gel and allow the protein expression ratio (relative quantification) to be estimated on the same gel as the three used dyes will emit fluorescence at different wavelengths. The comparison between different gels also became possible by using internal standards to improve inter-gel variation.

As an example for cancer application using 2D-DIGE and MS, Dowling et al. (2007) identified several lung cancer-specific targets that may be useful for early detection of cancer, including apolipoprotein A-IV precursor, human complement component C3c, haptoglobin, serum amyloid A (SAA) protein precursor, Ras-related protein Rab-7b, alpha-2-HS glycoprotein, hemopexin precursor, proapolipoprotein, antithrombin III, and SP40. Other examples of using 2D-GE in clinical cancer research are illustrated by Bertucci et al. (2006), Galvao et al. (2011), and Gast et al. (2009).

4.2.3.4 LC-ESI-MS (/MS)

Liquid chromatography coupled with tandem mass spectrometry (LC–MS/MS) is used to identify proteins using database search tools such as Mascot, Phenyx, X!Tandem, or SEQUEST that allow quantification of all levels of proteins found in samples. The nano-LC method, widely implemented in proteomic studies, is a high-performance LC operating at high pressure (up to 1000 bars) used to separate components of a mixture by a variety of chemical interactions between the polypeptides and the chromatography column. It uses packed microcolumns with small internal diameter 75–150 μm and flow rates of 50–1000 nL/min and allows for a small sample amount and increase in sensitivity. An emergent strategy for "bottom-up" proteomics involves two or more dimensions of LC on the peptides from enzymatic protein digests coupled to ESI-MS, also called multidimensional protein identification technology (MudPIT) or "shotgun" proteomics (Delahunty and Yates, 2007; Liu et al., 2002; Motoyama et al., 2006; Palmblad et al., 2009). Multidimensional LC with orthogonal separation can be easily automated. It offers high reproducibility and works well for hydrophobic, acidic, basic, very small, very large, and low-abundance proteins, which are difficult to analyze by traditional separation techniques. In the multidimensional LC methods, the LC steps can be either on- or off-line with the subsequent MS or MS/MS analysis (Palmblad et al., 2009).

As compared to the off-line LC-MALDI, on-line LC-ESI generates more information in a given time and analysis time is often an important limiting factor in an experiment or study. It is also more suitable for relative quantification due to the ionization suppression issues linked to MALDI-MS.

On the other hand, the quantitative proteomics based on LC–MS/MS approaches has led to major development in the discovery of novel cancer biomarkers and potential therapeutic targets during the last decade. In "shotgun" quantitative proteomics, proteins are first labeled with stable isotopes, digested with proteases, and subsequently resolved generally with either 1D-LC or 2D-LC (Washburn et al., 2001) (Figure 4.3). The separated tryptic peptides are introduced into the mass spectrometer for identification. Quantitation typically involves ratio calculations from isotopically distinguishable peptides or tags at MS or MS/MS levels. The most used approach to perform quantitative proteomics is the differential stable isotope labeling (Gygi et al., 1999; Ong et al., 2002; Ross et al., 2004). In this approach, labeling is achieved by incorporating stable isotopes to biological samples (i.e., proteins or peptides) either by metabolic incorporation or by chemical tagging. Once introduced to the mass spectrometer, the mass shift due to labeling is easily detectable and quantifiable based on paired labeled versus native peptides or proteins. For example, ICAT-based quantitative proteomics has been used to identify potential biomarkers of pancreatic cancer (Chen et al., 2005), ovarian cancer (Stewart et al., 2006), and breast cancer (Kang et al., 2010) or in human myeloid leukemia (HL-60) cells (Han et al., 2001).

Approaches using isobaric tag for relative and absolute quantitation (iTRAQ) have been widely employed in cancer research, including search for cancer biomarkers and drug targets (Zieske, 2006). For example, in a head-and-neck squamous cell carcinoma biomarker discovery experiment, 4-plex iTRAQ was used to compare paired and nonpaired noncancerous samples with cancerous tissues (Ralhan et al., 2008). iTRAQ has also been applied to study cancer angiogenesis (Zhang et al., 2009), metastasis (Ho et al., 2009), epithelial–mesenchymal transition (Keshamouni et al., 2009), cancer therapy resistance (Li et al., 2010), and cancer secretome (Chenau et al., 2009).

Using metabolic labeling, in particular SILAC, coupled with 2D-LC–MS/MS in comprehensive proteomic analysis of MLL has discovered novel potential biomarkers and pharmacological targets for leukemia with MLL translocations (Yocum et al., 2006). SILAC was also employed to identify metastasis-associated proteins to understand cancer progression and predict prognosis, such as in patients with HCC, mammary, and melanoma cancers (Chen et al., 2008; Qiu and Wang, 2008; Xu et al., 2010). As metabolic labeling such as SILAC ethically is not allowed in humans due to issues linked to the incorporation of stable isotopes, SILAC quantification of human tumors was made possible by spiking the human samples with a mixture of SILAC-labeled cancer cell lines (Geiger et al., 2010). This approach is very promising for the isolation of new biomarkers linked to various forms of cancer as long as there are appropriate labeled cell lines that close reflecting the type of cancer.

As an alternative to isotope labeling, label-free quantification provides simple, low-cost measurements of cancerous proteomes (Zhang et al., 2006) (Figure 4.3). The straightforward method is a relative quantification based on peptides/proteins identified from spectra (spectral counting) with the assumption that precursor-ion intensities correlate with peptide abundance (Liu et al., 2004). Samples are analyzed in separate mass spectrometric analyses but using the same data acquisition protocol. Label-free quantification needs however good reproducibility between different MS runs. This approach has been used in a number of oncoproteomic analyses (Hu et al., 2009).

4.2.4 Challenges and Future Directions

The development of MS technologies has enabled generating huge amount of data characterizing the proteome of complex biological samples. Comparative analyses of samples from healthy and diseased persons became possible for the identification of highly specific biomarkers. In addition, the development of diagnostic platforms that offer the potential for highly multiplexed and sensitive analysis of the proteome is an advantage toward the development of new protein biomarkers. Nevertheless, the successful transition of proteomic technologies from research tools to integrated clinical diagnostic platforms still requires much development due to various limitations and challenges where some of them are technical and others are directly linked to the human physiology. In an attempt to evaluate the current situation of various MS-based proteomic platforms, we summarized in Table 4.4 the effectiveness of and usefulness of these platforms for biomarker discovery and/or clinical diagnosis.

4.2.4.1 Limitations and Challenges

The complex nature of the human proteome, the huge dynamic range of protein concentration, and the plethora of protein isoforms in human specimens added to the heterogeneity in diseases are major hurdles to overcome in proteomics (Schiess et al., 2009). Despite the development of standardized experimental protocols for enrichment, separation, and quantification of proteins, there is still a big gap in the expected reproducibility of proteomic analysis between different laboratories and samples mainly due to the alteration and degradation of protein samples during the collection, storage, and analysis steps. Therefore, stringent precautions are needed to maintain the integrity of proteins to ensure proteomic research results are accurate.

On the other hand, and regardless the tremendous progress in MS technologies, proteomic research is currently limited by the technologies and bioinformatic tools that are available for analyzing proteins. For example, mass spectrometers can accurately measure very small amounts of protein; however, proteins or peptides produced by cancer cells are often present in even smaller quantities, making their detection difficult. Both researchers and technologists are working to improve the sensitivity of MS to allow scientists to detect, identify, and quantify with confidence these rare cancer proteins.

Furthermore, the ultimate confirmation of the putative protein biomarkers or protein signatures shortlisted at the discovery levels will require their validation using independent assays as well as the reproduction of findings in different laboratories and additional populations of patients.

Most of previous proteomic studies were designed on a "snapshot" basis, where only a single time point from a given human sample was investigated, which most likely missed significant processes taking place over time. Therefore, it is now more relevant to look at serial time points, in particular for

TABLE 4.4
Throughput, Usefulness, and Cost-Effectiveness of Various MS-Based Proteomic Platforms

Technique	Protein Pattern	Identification (Protein/ Sample)	Quantification (Protein/ Sample)	Throughput (Sample per Day)	Information	Ease of Use	Cost-Effectiveness	
							Biomarker Discovery	Clinical Diagnosis
SELDI-MS	+++	–	–	>1000	+	+++	++	+++
MALDI-MS	+++	–	–	>1000	++	+++	++	+++
CE-MS	+	–	–	>100	+++	+	+	++
LC-MS	++	–	–	>20	+++	++	+	++
MALDI-MS/MS	–	>10	–	>100	++	++	++	++
LC-MS/MS	–	>100	>100	>10	+++	++	+++	+
2D-LC-MS/MS (MudPIT)	–	>1000	>500	<1	+++	+	+++	+
1D-GE—LC-MS/MS	–	>1000	>500	<1	+++	++	+++	+
2D-GE—MALDI-MS (/MS)	–	>200	>200	<1	+++	+	+++	+
LC-MS/MS (MRM)	–	–	>100	>20	+	+	+	+

screening and early detection of cancer (Timms et al., 2011; Tiss et al., 2011). This may help in getting access to the temporal and special dynamics of proteins as some of them may change in amounts or location within a short time.

4.2.4.2 Future Directions

Based on the large development during the last decade in proteomic strategies for biomarker discovery, some promising perspectives are foreseen including retuning some previous approaches, developing new ones, and combining proteomics with other omics approaches. Neither the so-called data-based strategy nor the hypothesis-based strategy was able to deliver the expected outcomes from proteomic studies, and the combination of both of them will definitely help in deciphering more secrets of disease-linked proteome and accelerating the path from the benchside to the bedside. MS-based oncoproteomics will most likely stay limited to the discovery and validation rather than clinical application area as the last is very stringent by all the legislations and approval procedures.

The direct-tissue analysis by MALDI imaging proteomic is a fast, sensitive, and reproducible approach that opens the door to new perspectives in clinical proteomics, and it may become a valuable alternative to immunohistochemistry (Caldwell and Caprioli, 2005; Chaurand et al., 2005; Reyzer and Caprioli, 2005). Combining known histological and pathophysiological data with molecular imaging data from the same tissue will, for instance, enhance the discovery of specific cancer cell biomarkers. Moreover, starting the biomarker mining at the disease-source tissue represents a straightforward approach to fish any new disease-specific proteins before trying to find it from the biofluids such as blood, urine, or saliva. Hence, this second step would be used for verification of the presence of these specific markers in the accessible body fluids in the aim of developing less invasive tests for cancer diagnosis or screening.

Another approach to overcome the complexity of the human proteome and the large dynamic range of proteins between different tissues or cellular compartments is to isolate profile-specific type of cells or cell organelles based on some preliminary biologically meaning hypotheses. On the other hand, the post-translational modifications in proteins make almost impossible to identify and quantify all isoforms of

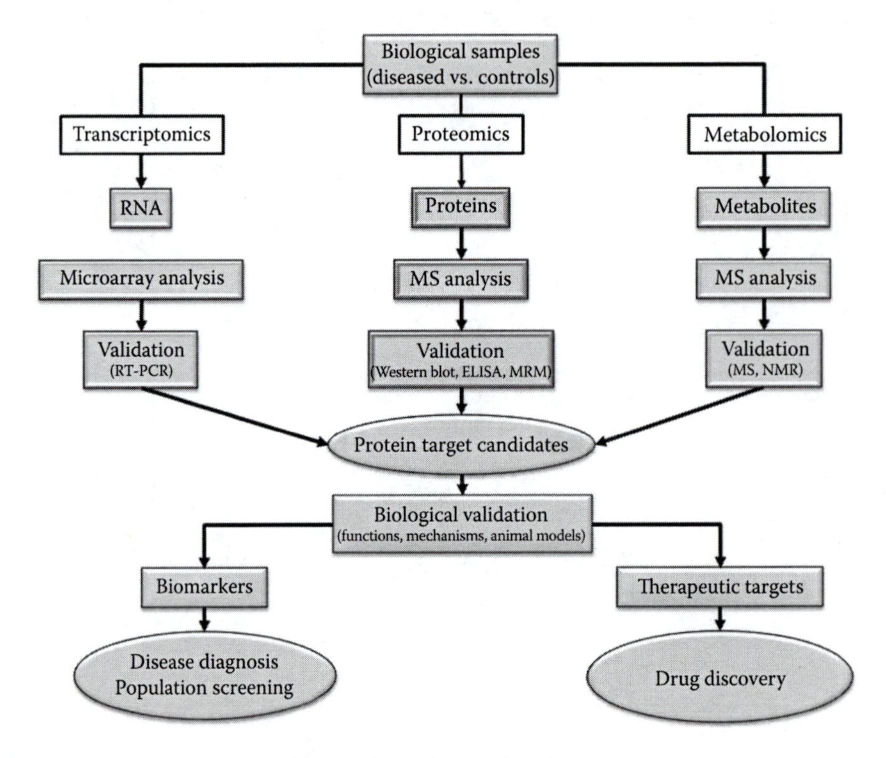

FIGURE 4.7 Omics integration and complementation as future approach.

the same protein in a single experiment. Thus, enrichment of specific and homogenous subproteome will increase the potential of discovered biomarkers. For example, the study of the kinome (the complement set of protein kinases) of human tissues associated with clinical outcome would clarify disease mechanisms, identify therapy targets, and develop predictive applications (Parikh and Peppelenbosch, 2010). The glycoproteome is also of particular interest because most traditional cancer biomarkers are glycoproteins and changes in patterns of glycosylation have been reported in cancer cells (Hung and Yu, 2010).

Strategies based on combining various gene and protein databases with robust bioinformatic tools for searching tissue-specific proteins might be also a good approach for a more targeted search for specific biomarkers. Besides, the selection of proteins likely to enter the circulation will prioritize candidates for further biological and clinical validation and thus will accelerate the transition from discovery to valuable clinical application.

Last but not least, the integration of the data generated from various omics approaches such as genomics, transcriptomics, proteomics, and metabolomic will help in making meaningful hypotheses and foster the discovery of real biomarkers by reducing the false-positive rates in the discovery and validation stages (see Figure 4.7 for a summary of the combined approaches). Obviously, this will dramatically reduce the research costs by putting scientists, clinicians, bioinformaticians, and technologists all together tightly collaborating to win the battle against cancer.

4.3 Surface Plasmon Resonance for Detection of Cancer

4.3.1 Introduction

Various analytical, biochemical, and molecular methods for cancer detection were developed and are currently used with success (Issaq et al., 2011). Surface plasmon resonance (SPR) or BiAcore is one of these approaches that emerged recently, and it is the subject of the section of this book chapter. Biosensors based on the optical phenomenon of SPR are among the most versatile techniques that are able to detect and measure biospecific interactions in real time using only small amounts of analytes with no chemical modification.

The ability to detect and quantify specific interactions from complex such as biological fluids or tissue lysates has led to a wide variety of proteomic applications for SPR biosensors. This ability has made coupling the SPR technique to downstream detection methods, in particular MS, a much sought after goal in proteomics. SPR-MS coupling enabled the combination of yet unmet need for biomarker fishing, identification, and quantification at the same time without the need for a deep fractionation of complex biological samples.

It is not within the scope of this chapter to describe in full details of the physics behind it, but we will briefly give an overview of the principle of SPR. A detailed description of SPR and its applications can be found in the literature (Day et al., 2002; Phillips and Cheng, 2007).

4.3.2 SPR Principles

SPR is an electron charge density wave phenomenon that was initially discovered in the late 1950s (Turbadar, 1959). After two decades of development and optimization, it was possible to apply it in life science to monitor various types of biomolecular interactions (Liedberg et al., 1983). For example, SPR detection systems have now been deployed in assays involving a wide range of biomolecular interaction such as protein–protein interaction, protein–nucleic acid interactions, antibodies, SNPs, sugars, narcotics, peptides, small molecules, and microRNAs. The principle of detection relies on the optical phenomenon of SPR, which is sensitive to the optical properties of the medium close to a metal surface. The phenomena of biosensing are based on measures of refractive index change occurring as molecules adsorb to or dissipate from a sensor surface during reaction (Huber and Mueller, 2006). BiAcore biosensors use this phenomenon for the detection of mass differences in a simple cell. A sensor chip carries a thin gold layer (50 nm) on a glass support. The chip is in direct contact with a flow cell (sample side) and a glass prism (detector side). A monochromatic, plane-polarized light beam at a wavelength of 760 nm is sent through the prism and is totally internally reflected at the interface. The generated evanescence field wave penetrates into the sample cell and allows the detection of refractive index properties to a distance of about 1 μm from the surface. The angle of minimum light intensity is detected using a 2D detector array.

Biomolecular interactions around the surface cause a change of the solute concentration and therefore of the refractive index of the medium, which can be detected as a change in the incidence light angle and converted into a response signal (Figure 4.8). The unit of the response signal is called resonance unit (RU) and represents a shift in the resonance angle of approximately 10^{-4} degree (Jonsson et al., 1991). The shift in resonance angle is monitored in real time and plotted in dependence of time generating a plot called sensorgram; the different stages of a binding event can be visualized and evaluated (Figure 4.8). With only buffer running through the flow system, the signal forms a stable baseline. Upon injection of the analyte solution, the sensorgram is dominated by the association phase, where analyte molecules bind to the target on the chip. However, bound molecules already start dissociating again during injection. After a certain injection time, a steady state is reached, where binding and dissociating molecules are in equilibrium. As soon as the injection is stopped, running buffer replaces the analyte cloud and only the pure dissociation phase is visible.

SPR biosensors are often referred as mass detectors because the mass of the molecules directly influences the refractive index. In the case of proteins, the correlation between sensor signal and mass increase was experimentally determined to be 1 RU = 1 pg/mm^2 (Stenberg et al., 1991). This correlation is practically constant for molecules with high protein and low lipid and carbohydrate content (Jonsson et al., 1991). This relationship stays applicable to other biomolecules such as nucleic acids, carbohydrates, lipids, or conjugate molecules even though possible minor deviations can exist. As a consequence, mass concentration can be detected with high sensitivity for nearly all molecules, regardless of their nature (Nagata and Handa, 2000). On the other side, sensitivity is dependent on the distance from the surface. Therefore, other changes around the interface like electrostatic attraction or conformational changes might also induce a shift of the incident light angle (Mannen et al., 2001).

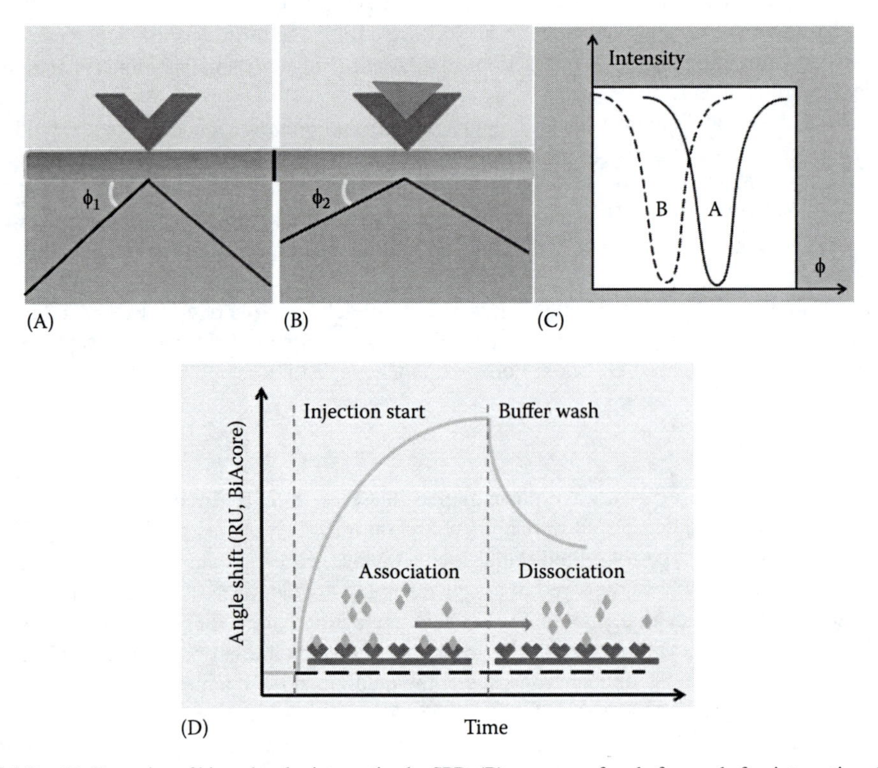

FIGURE 4.8 (A): Detection of biomolecular interaction by SPR, (B): sensor surface before and after interaction, (C): shift of light intensity dip upon interaction, and (D): schematic representation of a sensogram as the time course of binding events.

SPR/BiAcore biosensors gained enormous popularity in biomedical research and pharmaceutical industry due to their sensitivity, robustness, flexibility, and amenability to automation and throughput. One of the features of the technique is the possibility to obtain real-time data on the interaction of a ligand and its receptor allowing kinetic data to be determined. Moreover, compared to other technologies, the amount of material necessary to perform the experiments is less, labeling is not required, and variation in surface chemistries is possible, allowing various immobilization strategies and interaction experiments. Apart from the physicochemical information (Jacquemart et al., 2008; Karlsson, 1994), SPR also provides an accurate determination of the amount of ligand present on the sensor surface as there exists a linear relation between the quantity of a bound protein and the sensor response (Stigter et al., 2005). As an analytical method, SPR allows the quantification of a given analyte even at the picomolar range (Kikuchi et al., 2005; Yang et al., 2005). Recently, a major progress was made in SPR-based sensors, allowing the detection of small molecules (<300 Da) with high specificity, and this will have a significant impact on drug and metabolomic biomarker discovery.

4.3.3 Application of SPR in Cancer Biomarker Discovery

Several studies used SPR to detect biomarkers at clinically relevant concentrations highlighting the feasibility of using SPR in a clinical setting. These biomarkers can be identified from various specimens such as plasma, serum, saliva, and tissues. A summary of these efforts is illustrated in Table 4.5. Is it worth to mention that although SPR has been extensively used to monitor biomolecular interactions for many biological processes including measurement of biomolecules implicated in disease, its application to cancer biomarker discovery is so far limited and presents an opportunity to develop screening methods for diagnostic or for discovery of new targets if combined with other technology. A recent review documenting the applications of SPR-based biosensing approaches for biomarker discovery in different types of cancer was published recently (Reddy et al., 2012), and a list of various biomarkers of different cancers is illustrated in Table 4.6.

However, obtaining high sensitivity in complex biological samples under real physiological conditions remains one of the major challenges for bioanalytical applications with SPR biosensors. As the SPR response is based on the mass present at the sensor surface, there is no absolute certainty about the nature of the ligand interacting with the analyte particularly in interactions involving ligand with unknown analyte, or in the case of complex interactions involving more than two partners, "multicomponent assays" in addition to nonspecific adsorption to the surface of the chip and all of them are considered as inherent limitations of the SPR platform. Therefore, combining SPR with more sophisticated approaches that take into consideration these limitations is needed. As mentioned in Section 4.2 of this chapter, MS is one of the ideal technologies that could be easily integrated to SPR for identification of unknown targets regardless of the complexity of the interaction and sample.

TABLE 4.5

Summary of Biomarkers' Discovery Linked to Various Diseases Using SPR

Disease	Biomarker	Reference
Cardiovascular disease	B-type natriuretic peptide	Kurita et al. (2006)
	C-reactive protein	Hu et al. (2006)
Cystic fibrosis	W1282X mutation	Feriotto et al. (2001)
Inflammatory disease	Cystatin C	Lee et al. (2006)
Lyme borreliosis	Pathogen specific antibodies	Nagel et al. (2008)
Myocardial infarction	Cardiac troponin I	Masson et al. (2004, 2007)
	Myoglobin	Dutra et al. (2007)
Osteoporosis	N-telopeptide	Lung et al. (2003, 2004)
Type 2 diabetes	Retinol binding protein 4	Lee et al. (2008)
Viral meningitis	Beta2-microglobulin	Lee et al. (2006)

TABLE 4.6
Summary of Cancer Biomarkers' Discovery Using SPR

Type of Cancer	Biomarkers	References
Prostate	PSA	David et al. (2008); Kang et al. (2009); Krishnan et al. (2011)
	PSA-ACT complex	Cao et al. (2006); Jang et al. (2009); Malic et al. (2011)
	Haptoglobin	Kazuno et al. (2011)
Breast	BRCA1	Carrascosa et al. (2009)
	CA-15.3	Chang et al. (2010)
	LOX-12	Singh et al. (2011)
	CD24	Myung et al. (2010)
Colorectal	CEA autoantibody	Ladd et al. (2009a)
	CEA	Su et al. (2008)
	VEGF	Li et al. (2007)
	ALCAM/CD	Ladd et al. (2009b)
	Transgelin-2	Ladd et al., (2009b)
Oral	COX2	Kapoor et al. (2010)
	IL-8	Yang et al. (2005)
Pancreatic	AlCAM	Piliarik et al.; Vaisocherova et al. (2009)
	hCG	Vaisocherova et al. (2009)
Gastric	MG-7	Fang et al. (2010)
Hepatic	AFP	Teramura and Iwata (2007)
Lung	proGRP	Mie et al. (2012)
Ovarian	HE4	Yuan et al. (2012)
Other types	CA125	Suwansaard et al. (2009)
	TNFα	Law et al. (2009)

4.3.4 Integration of SPR with Mass Spectrometry

The combination of SPR with MS (SPR–MS) is a very powerful technique for pairing SPR interaction analysis or quantification with MS for target identification. As mentioned earlier, MS is most generally employed to provide supplementary information on the nature of isolated material. The ultimate goal of the SPR–MS is to recover the analytes captured on the SPR surface and subject them directly to MS identification. One of the advantages of this integrated approach is that it will provide complementary information about the affinity of the interaction occurring at the sensor surface as well as the quantification and identification of the isolated components. A summary of the main work done on biological matrices combing these two technologies is presented in Table 4.7. The surface commonly used for SPR sensor chips appear to be compatible with MALDI-TOF analysis. Two methods have been developed for integrating SPR–MS (Figure 4.9).

The first method called "on-chip MALDI-TOF-MS analysis" consists of using SPR and MS on the same sensor chip. The most important benefits of this approach are its ease of use and its sensitivity. The drawbacks of this method are the fact that sensors can only be used once and the necessity of manual intervention that hampers automation. To allow the identification of protein captured on-chip by MALDI-TOF-MS, a method consists of using carboxylated dextran (CM5) chip from BiAcore (Stigter et al., 2009). After several buffer washing steps, the chip is placed in an appropriate MALDI target after capture of analytes. A specially developed chip cutter is used for this purpose; it contains a circular heated cutterhead that excises the chip segment in a form that fits into the MALDI mass spectrometer target. The MALDI matrix applicator sprays a fine mist of matrix solution over the entire surface of the cutout chip. The sensor surface was connected to the target plate in order to create an electric field during MS analysis after which the matrix solution was applied allowing MALDI-TOF-MS analysis.

TABLE 4.7
Proteins Identified by Combined SPR–MS Methods

Ligand	Analyte	Matrix	Strategy	Reference
Antibody	Rat serum albumin	Plasma	On-chip MALD-TOF MS	Boireau et al. (2009)
Antibody	Cystatin, RBP, B2M, urinary protein 1	Plasma and urine	On-chip MALD-TOF MS	Natsume et al. (2002); Nedelkov and Nelson (2001a,b, 2003a,b); Nedelkov et al. (2003)
Antibody	A33 epithelial antigen	Cell extract	Elution-recovery MALD-TOF MS	Catimel et al. (2000)
Calmodulin binding protein	Calmodulin	Brain extract	Elution-recovery MALD-TOF MS	Zhukov et al. (2004)
p53	p53 binding proteins	Cell extract	Elution-recovery LC-ESI MS	Kikuchi et al. (2003)
Anti-TNFγ	Interferon-γ	Plasma (spiked)	Elution-recovery LC-ESI MS	Stigter et al. (2009)
Anti-β2-MG	B2M	Urine	Elution-recovery LC-ESI MS	Gilligan et al. (2002)

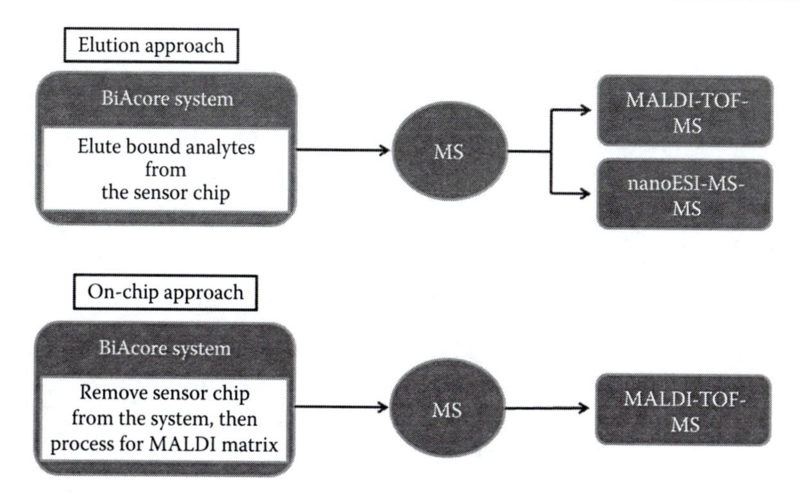

FIGURE 4.9 On-chip and elution SPR–MS approaches.

Although for these on-chip MS-approaches detection limits as low as 650 amol total protein originating from biological samples, such as serum or urine, have been reported (Stigter et al., 2009). These approaches described earlier allow very sensitive and accurate mass determination of the isolated protein and tandem MS information on peptide fragments obtained after proteolysis is required for the unambiguous identification of an isolated protein. A strategy to accomplish this using an on-chip SPR–MS approach was reported in a recent study (Boireau et al., 2009). The isolated protein was digested on-chip and subsequent MALDI-TOF-MS/MS allowed protein identification.

The second method called "elution SPR–MS" consists of eluting captured analyte from the sensor chip. An important feature of this strategy is the possibility of reusing the sensor, and for BiAcore 3000 series and T100/200 series, the technology is fully automated and therefore is the mostly used method for studies combining SPR with MS (Gilligan et al., 2002). A potential damage of the ligand might occur when kept in the buffer used for ligand desorption, and this may be considered as a drawback. The yield of microrecovery has been addressed in the design of the BiAcore systems by the introduction of air segments and reversal of the buffer flow to return the sample back through the flow cell for collection via the autosampler; this allows the recovery of a very small volume of sample (2 μL/cycle) (Situ et al., 2010). The recovery of hydrophobic proteins can be increased by the use of silica or C18-coated magnetic beads passed over the chip during the desorption process from the chip (Larsericsdotter et al., 2006). Tests have been performed with bovine serum albumin (BSA), a protein known for nonspecific binding to many

TABLE 4.8

Strengths and Weaknesses of qPCR, MS, and SPR Technologies in Cancer Biomarker Applications

Technique	Application	Information and Versatility	Ease of Use	Throughput (Sample per Day)	Quantification	Sensitivity	Specificity	Biomarker Discovery	Clinical Diagnosis	Cost-Effectiveness
qPCR	RNA, DNA	+	+++	>100	+++	+++	+++	+	+++	+++
MS-based proteomics	Proteins, metabolites	++	+	>1000	++	++	+	+++	+	+
SPR	DNA, RNA, proteins, metabolites	+++	++	>100	++	+++	++	++	+	+

materials, including those commonly used for fluidic systems. The silica particles increased the recovery of BSA from the chip twofold. This might be a useful approach when working with hydrophobic proteins showing high nonspecific binding. Although it is often a tedious procedure, microrecovery does allow tryptic digestion for protein identification. General protocols have been described by Borch and Roepstorff for binding, washing of the fluidic system, elution from the sensor chip, followed by tryptic digestion, and MS analysis including database searching of the peptide masses (Borch and Roepstorff, 2010).

4.3.5 Challenges and Future Directions

The feasibility of combining the affinity enrichment using SPR and identification by MS was demonstrated by different studies (Table 4.7). This is of major interest in proteomics and diagnosis applications. The combination of SPR and MS is indeed a strong asset because it allows the identification of the binding partners in complex mixtures.

Although the results obtained are promising, the coupling of SPR to MS still needs to be further optimized such as the capacity of the surface of the sensor chip, amount of bound target, sample loss, and carry-over during processing. One must also bear in mind that the capability of SPR to analyze binding kinetics of single known partners will be lost when analyzing complex mixtures of unknown proteins (e.g., human biofluids) due to the nonspecific adsorption on the sensor surface, and this is still considered as a big challenge. Moreover, improvements in the microfluidic systems and sensor surface of the SPR as well sensitivity of the MS are still required and will help in digging dipper into proteomics to isolate and characterize more disease-specific biomarkers available at very low amounts.

Finally, an attempt for benchmarking of the strengths and weaknesses of SPR and its usefulness in the cancer field as compared to the two previous technologies developed in this chapter (qPCR- and MS-based proteomics) is summarized in Table 4.8. Nevertheless, taking into account strengths and weaknesses as well as the possible hyphenation between these various platforms, we believe that integrative approaches will ensure comprehensive and accurate knowledge about biomarkers in cancer studies.

4.4 Considerations for Biological Samples

A tremendous progress has been recently achieved in both genomic and proteomic technologies, which enabled generating considerable amounts of data and knowledge about genes and proteins. Nevertheless, the successful transition of these technologies from research tools to integrated clinical diagnostic platforms is still hampered by some basic issues including those linked to the human physiology and biospecimen quality. Indeed, the complex nature and stability of the human clinical samples, due to the degradation of their quality and content linked to the presence of enzymes modifying DNA, RNA, and proteins, make the integrity of those samples a key to any analysis of their biomolecular content. The large dynamic range in gene expression and protein concentration is another hurdle to overcome before reaching the bedside applications.

For example, despite the development of standardized experimental protocols for enrichment, separation, and quantification of proteins, there is still big gap in the expected reproducibility of proteomic analysis between different laboratories mainly due to the alteration and degradation of protein samples during the collection, storage, and analysis steps (Diamandis, 2004b). Therefore, an extra effort was undertaken during the last few years to overcome the issues related to preanalytical (sample collection, handling, and storage) and analytical approaches to ensure reproducibility and avoid experimental bias. Consequently, many reports have been recently written about the potential confounding effects of preanalytical handling of specimens, and several groups have published recommendations addressing best practices for specimen handling with more stringent precautions to maintain the integrity of proteins and ensuring accuracy and reproducibility of proteomic results (ISBER, 2008; Leyland-Jones et al., 2008; Tiss et al., 2007; Villanueva et al., 2005).

On the other hand, specimen collection is often carried out in a clinical context and not under the control of the investigators studying disease markers; it is thus important to report as much information as possible about the way the biological samples were collected, handled, and preprocessed. It is also frequent that the sample analysis is performed after its storage for a certain period of time. Thus, it is important to report for how long and how the samples have been stored and processed before the marker analysis. Under these conditions, stringent criteria for acceptability of biospecimens to be used in marker investigation should be established prior to initiating any marker-based study to ensure high sample quality (Altman et al., 2012).

Furthermore, the adequacy of matching between cases and controls (gender, age, other morbidities, etc.) is a critical step in the experimental design to avoid systematic bias and reduce the false discovery rates and artifacts due to nonspecific disease-associated variations in biological samples.

Once all the optimal conditions for sample collection and handling are tuned, there is also the need to develop shared specimen resources to be used by independent research groups either for discovery or for validation of potential genomic or proteomic biomarkers. Cohort and time-serial samples collected before the onset of the cancer and appearance of diagnosed symptoms are on the other side particularly useful for discovering and validating biomarkers for early detection and follow-up of the disease.

Finally, combining good sample quality with optimized procedures for biospecimen analysis using advanced technology platforms aside with suitable bioinformatic tools for data processing might shorten the way from benchside to bedside by reducing the false-positive discovery and fostering real biomarkers to the validation and clinical trial stages.

References

Albrethsen, J., Bogebo, R., Gammeltoft, S., Olsen, J., Winther, B., and Raskov, H. (2005). Upregulated expression of human neutrophil peptides 1, 2 and 3 (HNP 1–3) in colon cancer serum and tumours: A biomarker study. *BMC Cancer* 5, 8.

Altman, D.G., McShane, L.M., Sauerbrei, W., and Taube, S.E. (2012). Reporting recommendations for tumor marker prognostic studies (REMARK): Explanation and elaboration. *BMC Med* 10, 51.

Anderson, N.L. and Anderson, N.G. (2002). The human plasma proteome: History, character, and diagnostic prospects. *Mol Cell Proteomics* 1, 845–867.

Ariyaratana, S. and Loeb, D.M. (2007). The role of the Wilms tumour gene (WT1) in normal and malignant haematopoiesis. *Expert Rev Mol Med* 9, 1–17.

Azad, N.S., Rasool, N., Annunziata, C.M., Minasian, L., Whiteley, G., and Kohn, E.C. (2006). Proteomics in clinical trials and practice: Present uses and future promise. *Mol Cell Proteomics* 5, 1819–1829.

Baak, J.P., Janssen, E.A., Soreide, K., and Heikkilae, R. (2005). Genomics and proteomics—The way forward. *Ann Oncol* 16(Suppl 2), ii30–ii44.

Bagan, P., Berna, P., Assouad, J., Hupertan, V., Le Pimpec Barthes, F., and Riquet, M. (2008). Value of cancer antigen 125 for diagnosis of pleural endometriosis in females with recurrent pneumothorax. *Eur Respir J* 31, 140–142.

Baggerly, K.A., Coombes, K.R., and Morris, J.S. (2005). Bias, randomization, and ovarian proteomic data: A reply to "producers and consumers". *Cancer Inform* 1, 9–14.

Banks, R.E., Dunn, M.J., Hochstrasser, D.F., Sanchez, J.C., Blackstock, W., Pappin, D.J., and Selby, P.J. (2000). Proteomics: New perspectives, new biomedical opportunities. *Lancet* 356, 1749–1756.

Barbaux, S., Niaudet, P., Gubler, M.C., Grunfeld, J.P., Jaubert, F., Kuttenn, F., Fekete, C.N. et al. (1997). Donor splice-site mutations in WT1 are responsible for Frasier syndrome. *Nat Genet* 17, 467–470.

Barragan, E., Cervera, J., Bolufer, P., Ballester, S., Martin, G., Fernandez, P., Collado, R., Sayas, M.J., and Sanz, M.A. (2004). Prognostic implications of Wilms' tumor gene (WT1) expression in patients with de novo acute myeloid leukemia. *Haematologica* 89, 926–933.

Bateson, H., Saleem, S., Loadman, P.M., and Sutton, C.W. (2011). Use of matrix-assisted laser desorption/ionisation mass spectrometry in cancer research. *J Pharmacol Toxicol Methods* 64, 197–206.

Becker, S., Cazares, L.H., Watson, P., Lynch, H., Semmes, O.J., Drake, R.R., and Laronga, C. (2004). Surfaced-enhanced laser desorption/ionization time-of-flight (SELDI-TOF) differentiation of serum protein profiles of BRCA-1 and sporadic breast cancer. *Ann Surg Oncol* 11, 907–914.

Beillard, E., Pallisgaard, N., van der Velden, V.H., Bi, W., Dee, R., van der Schoot, E., Delabesse, E. et al. (2003). Evaluation of candidate control genes for diagnosis and residual disease detection in leukemic patients using 'real-time' quantitative reverse-transcriptase polymerase chain reaction (RQ-PCR)—A Europe against cancer program. *Leukemia* 17, 2474–2486.

Bergmann, L., Miething, C., Maurer, U., Brieger, J., Karakas, T., Weidmann, E., and Hoelzer, D. (1997). High levels of Wilms' tumor gene (wt1) mRNA in acute myeloid leukemias are associated with a worse long-term outcome. *Blood* 90, 1217–1225.

Bertucci, F., Birnbaum, D., and Goncalves, A. (2006). Proteomics of breast cancer: Principles and potential clinical applications. *Mol Cell Proteomics* 5, 1772–1786.

Bickmore, W.A., Oghene, K., Little, M.H., Seawright, A., van Heyningen, V., and Hastie, N.D. (1992). Modulation of DNA binding specificity by alternative splicing of the Wilms tumor wt1 gene transcript. *Science* 257, 235–237.

Boireau, W., Rouleau, A., Lucchi, G., and Ducoroy, P. (2009). Revisited BIA-MS combination: Entire "on-a-chip" processing leading to the proteins identification at low femtomole to sub-femtomole levels. *Biosens Bioelectron* 24, 1121–1127.

Bor, Y.C., Swartz, J., Morrison, A., Rekosh, D., Ladomery, M., and Hammarskjold, M.L. (2006). The Wilms' tumor 1 (WT1) gene (+KTS isoform) functions with a CTE to enhance translation from an unspliced RNA with a retained intron. *Genes Dev* 20, 1597–1608.

Borch, J. and Roepstorff, P. (2010). SPR/MS: Recovery from sensorchips for protein identification by MALDI-TOF mass spectrometry. *Methods Mol Biol* 627, 269–281.

Bouamrani, A., Ternier, J., Ratel, D., Benabid, A.L., Issartel, J.P., Brambilla, E., and Berger, F. (2006). Direct-tissue SELDI-TOF mass spectrometry analysis: A new application for clinical proteomics. *Clin Chem* 52, 2103–2106.

Boublikova, L., Kalinova, M., Ryan, J., Quinn, F., O'Marcaigh, A., Smith, O., Browne, P. et al. (2006). Wilms' tumor gene 1 (WT1) expression in childhood acute lymphoblastic leukemia: A wide range of WT1 expression levels, its impact on prognosis and minimal residual disease monitoring. *Leukemia* 20, 254–263.

Brieger, J., Weidmann, E., Fenchel, K., Mitrou, P.S., Hoelzer, D., and Bergmann, L. (1994). The expression of the Wilms' tumor gene in acute myelocytic leukemias as a possible marker for leukemic blast cells. *Leukemia* 8, 2138–2143.

Bruening, W. and Pelletier, J. (1996). A non-AUG translational initiation event generates novel WT1 isoforms. *J Biol Chem* 271, 8646–8654.

Burwell, E.A., McCarty, G.P., Simpson, L.A., Thompson, K.A., and Loeb, D.M. (2007). Isoforms of Wilms' tumor suppressor gene (WT1) have distinct effects on mammary epithelial cells. *Oncogene* 26, 3423–3430.

Caldwell, R.L. and Caprioli, R.M. (2005). Tissue profiling by mass spectrometry: A review of methodology and applications. *Mol Cell Proteomics* 4, 394–401.

Call, K.M., Glaser, T., Ito, C.Y., Buckler, A.J., Pelletier, J., Haber, D.A., Rose, E.A. et al. (1990). Isolation and characterization of a zinc finger polypeptide gene at the human chromosome 11 Wilms' tumor locus. *Cell* 60, 509–520.

Celis, J.E., Ostergaard, M., Basse, B., Celis, A., Lauridsen, J.B., Ratz, G.P., Andersen, I. et al. (1996). Loss of adipocyte-type fatty acid binding protein and other protein biomarkers is associated with progression of human bladder transitional cell carcinomas. *Cancer Res* 56, 4782–4790.

Chang, C.C., Chiu, N.F., Lin, D.S., Chu-Su, Y., Liang, Y.H., and Lin, C.W. (2010). High-sensitivity detection of carbohydrate antigen 15-3 using a gold/zinc oxide thin film surface plasmon resonance-based biosensor. *Anal Chem* 82(4), 1207–1212.

Chaurand, P., Schwartz, S.A., Reyzer, M.L., and Caprioli, R.M. (2005). Imaging mass spectrometry: Principles and potentials. *Toxicol Pathol* 33, 92–101.

Chen, N., Sun, W., Deng, X., Hao, Y., Chen, X., Xing, B., Jia, W. et al. (2008). Quantitative proteome analysis of HCC cell lines with different metastatic potentials by SILAC. *Proteomics* 8, 5108–5118.

Chen, R., Yi, E.C., Donohoe, S., Pan, S., Eng, J., Cooke, K., Crispin, D.A. et al. (2005). Pancreatic cancer proteome: The proteins that underlie invasion, metastasis, and immunologic escape. *Gastroenterology* 129, 1187–1197.

Chenau, J., Michelland, S., de Fraipont, F., Josserand, V., Coll, J.L., Favrot, M.C., and Seve, M. (2009). The cell line secretome, a suitable tool for investigating proteins released in vivo by tumors: Application to the study of p53-modulated proteins secreted in lung cancer cells. *J Proteome Res* 8, 4579–4591.

Cho, W.C., Yip, T.T., Ngan, R.K., Podust, V.N., Yip, C., Yiu, H.H., Yip, V. et al. (2007). ProteinChip array profiling for identification of disease- and chemotherapy-associated biomarkers of nasopharyngeal carcinoma. *Clin Chem* 53, 241–250.

Cho, W.C., Yip, T.T., Yip, C., Yip, V., Thulasiraman, V., Ngan, R.K., Lau, W.H. et al. (2004). Identification of serum amyloid a protein as a potentially useful biomarker to monitor relapse of nasopharyngeal cancer by serum proteomic profiling. *Clin Cancer Res* 10, 43–52.

Cilloni, D., Gottardi, E., De Micheli, D., Serra, A., Volpe, G., Messa, F., Rege-Cambrin, G. et al. (2002). Quantitative assessment of WT1 expression by real time quantitative PCR may be a useful tool for monitoring minimal residual disease in acute leukemia patients. *Leukemia* 16, 2115–2121.

Cilloni, D. and Saglio, G. (2004). WT1 as a universal marker for minimal residual disease detection and quantification in myeloid leukemias and in myelodysplastic syndrome. *Acta Haematol* 112, 79–84.

Cox, J. and Mann, M. (2007). Is proteomics the new genomics? *Cell* 130, 395–398.

Cramer, R. (2009). MALDI MS. *Methods Mol Biol* 564, 85–103.

Dallosso, A.R., Hancock, A.L., Brown, K.W., Williams, A.C., Jackson, S., and Malik, K. (2004). Genomic imprinting at the WT1 gene involves a novel coding transcript (AWT1) that shows deregulation in Wilms' tumours. *Hum Mol Genet* 13, 405–415.

Davies, R.C., Calvio, C., Bratt, E., Larsson, S.H., Lamond, A.I., and Hastie, N.D. (1998). WT1 interacts with the splicing factor U2AF65 in an isoform-dependent manner and can be incorporated into spliceosomes. *Genes Dev* 12, 3217–3225.

Day, Y.S., Baird, C.L., Rich, R.L., and Myszka, D.G. (2002). Direct comparison of binding equilibrium, thermodynamic, and rate constants determined by surface- and solution-based biophysical methods. *Protein Sci* 11, 1017–1025.

Dechsukhum, C., Ware, J.L., Ferreira-Gonzalez, A., Wilkinson, D.S., and Garrett, C.T. (2000). Detection of a novel truncated WT1 transcript in human neoplasia. *Mol Diagn* 5, 117–128.

Delahunty, C.M. and Yates, J.R., 3rd (2007). MudPIT: Multidimensional protein identification technology. *Biotechniques* 43, 563, 565, 567 passim.

Diamandis, E.P. (2004a). Mass spectrometry as a diagnostic and a cancer biomarker discovery tool: Opportunities and potential limitations. *Mol Cell Proteomics* 3, 367–378.

Diamandis, E.P. (2004b). OvaCheck: Doubts voiced soon after publication. *Nature* 430, 611.

Dowling, P., O'Driscoll, L., Meleady, P., Henry, M., Roy, S., Ballot, J., Moriarty, M., Crown, J., and Clynes, M. (2007). 2-D difference gel electrophoresis of the lung squamous cell carcinoma versus normal sera demonstrates consistent alterations in the levels of ten specific proteins. *Electrophoresis* 28, 4302–4310.

Downing, M. and Pollitt, R. (2008). Newborn bloodspot screening in the UK—Past, present and future. *Ann Clin Biochem* 45, 11–17.

Dumur, C.I., Dechsukhum, C., Wilkinson, D.S., Garrett, C.T., Ware, J.L., and Ferreira-Gonzalez, A. (2002). Analytical validation of a real-time reverse transcription-polymerase chain reaction quantitation of different transcripts of the Wilms' tumor suppressor gene (WT1). *Anal Biochem* 309, 127–136.

Dutton, J.R., Lahiri, D., and Ward, A. (2006). Different isoforms of the Wilms' tumour protein WT1 have distinct patterns of distribution and trafficking within the nucleus. *Cell Prolif* 39, 519–535.

Ellisen, L.W., Carlesso, N., Cheng, T., Scadden, D.T., and Haber, D.A. (2001). The Wilms tumor suppressor WT1 directs stage-specific quiescence and differentiation of human hematopoietic progenitor cells. *Embo J* 20, 1897–1909.

Ewing, B. and Green, P. (2000). Analysis of expressed sequence tags indicates 35,000 human genes. *Nat Genet* 25, 232–234.

Florio, F., Cesaro, E., Montano, G., Izzo, P., Miles, C., and Costanzo, P. (2010). Biochemical and functional interaction between ZNF224 and ZNF255, two members of the Kruppel-like zinc-finger protein family and WT1 protein isoforms. *Hum Mol Genet* 19, 3544–3556.

Frazier, D.M., Millington, D.S., McCandless, S.E., Koeberl, D.D., Weavil, S.D., Chaing, S.H., and Muenzer, J. (2006). The tandem mass spectrometry newborn screening experience in North Carolina: 1997–2005. *J Inherit Metab Dis* 29, 76–85.

Gabert, J., Beillard, E., van der Velden, V.H., Bi, W., Grimwade, D., Pallisgaard, N., Barbany, G. et al. (2003). Standardization and quality control studies of 'real-time' quantitative reverse transcriptase polymerase chain reaction of fusion gene transcripts for residual disease detection in leukemia—A Europe Against Cancer program. *Leukemia* 17, 2318–2357.

Galvao, E.R., Martins, L.M., Ibiapina, J.O., Andrade, H.M., and Monte, S.J. (2011). Breast cancer proteomics: A review for clinicians. *J Cancer Res Clin Oncol* 137, 915–925.

Gast, M.C., Schellens, J.H., and Beijnen, J.H. (2009). Clinical proteomics in breast cancer: A review. *Breast Cancer Res Treat* 116, 17–29.

Geiger, T., Cox, J., Ostasiewicz, P., Wisniewski, J.R., and Mann, M. (2010). Super-SILAC mix for quantitative proteomics of human tumor tissue. *Nat Methods* 7, 383–385.

Gilligan, J.J., Schuck, P., and Yergey, A.L. (2002). Mass spectrometry after capture and small-volume elution of analyte from a surface plasmon resonance biosensor. *Anal Chem* 74, 2041–2047.

Gramolini, A.O., Peterman, S.M., and Kislinger, T. (2008). Mass spectrometry-based proteomics: A useful tool for biomarker discovery? *Clin Pharmacol Ther* 83, 758–760.

Greenbaum, D., Colangelo, C., Williams, K., and Gerstein, M. (2003). Comparing protein abundance and mRNA expression levels on a genomic scale. *Genome Biol* 4, 117.

Greiner, J., Ringhoffer, M., Taniguchi, M., Li, L., Schmitt, A., Shiku, H., Dohner, H., and Schmitt, M. (2004). mRNA expression of leukemia-associated antigens in patients with acute myeloid leukemia for the development of specific immunotherapies. *Int J Cancer* 108, 704–711.

Gu, W., Hu, S., Chen, Z., Qiu, G., Cen, J., He, B., He, J., and Wu, W. (2010). High expression of WT1 gene in acute myeloid leukemias with more predominant WT1+17AA isoforms at relapse. *Leuk Res* 34, 46–49.

Gygi, S.P., Rist, B., Gerber, S.A., Turecek, F., Gelb, M.H., and Aebersold, R. (1999). Quantitative analysis of complex protein mixtures using isotope-coded affinity tags. *Nat Biotechnol* 17, 994–999.

Haber, D.A., Sohn, R.L., Buckler, A.J., Pelletier, J., Call, K.M., and Housman, D.E. (1991). Alternative splicing and genomic structure of the Wilms tumor gene WT1. *Proc Natl Acad Sci USA* 88, 9618–9622.

Han, D.K., Eng, J., Zhou, H., and Aebersold, R. (2001). Quantitative profiling of differentiation-induced microsomal proteins using isotope-coded affinity tags and mass spectrometry. *Nat Biotechnol* 19, 946–951.

Han, Y., San-Marina, S., Yang, L., Khoury, H., and Minden, M.D. (2007). The zinc finger domain of Wilms' tumor 1 suppressor gene (WT1) behaves as a dominant negative, leading to abrogation of WT1 oncogenic potential in breast cancer cells. *Breast Cancer Res* 9, R43.

Hanash, S.M., Pitteri, S.J., and Faca, V.M. (2008). Mining the plasma proteome for cancer biomarkers. *Nature* 452, 571–579.

Harrington, M.A., Konicek, B., Song, A., Xia, X.L., Fredericks, W.J., and Rauscher, F.J., 3rd (1993). Inhibition of colony-stimulating factor-1 promoter activity by the product of the Wilms' tumor locus. *J Biol Chem* 268, 21271–21275.

Hewitt, S.M., Hamada, S., McDonnell, T.J., Rauscher, F.J., 3rd, and Saunders, G.F. (1995). Regulation of the proto-oncogenes bcl-2 and c-myc by the Wilms' tumor suppressor gene WT1. *Cancer Res* 55, 5386–5389.

Ho, J., Kong, J.W., Choong, L.Y., Loh, M.C., Toy, W., Chong, P.K., Wong, C.H. et al. (2009). Novel breast cancer metastasis-associated proteins. *J Proteome Res* 8, 583–594.

Hohenstein, P. and Hastie, N.D. (2006). The many facets of the Wilms' tumour gene, WT1. *Hum Mol Genet* 15(Spec No 2), R196–R201.

Hossain, A., Nixon, M., Kuo, M.T., and Saunders, G.F. (2006). N-terminally truncated WT1 protein with oncogenic properties overexpressed in leukemia. *J Biol Chem* 281, 28122–28130.

Hu, X., Zhang, Y., Zhang, A., Li, Y., Zhu, Z., Shao, Z., Zeng, R., and Xu, L.X. (2009). Comparative serum proteome analysis of human lymph node negative/positive invasive ductal carcinoma of the breast and benign breast disease controls via label-free semiquantitative shotgun technology. *OMICS* 13, 291–300.

Huber, W. and Mueller, F. (2006). Biomolecular interaction analysis in drug discovery using surface plasmon resonance technology. *Curr Pharm Des* 12, 3999–4021.

Hung, K.E. and Yu, K.H. (2010). Proteomic approaches to cancer biomarkers. *Gastroenterology* 138, 46–51 e41.

Inoue, K., Sugiyama, H., Ogawa, H., Nakagawa, M., Yamagami, T., Miwa, H., Kita, K. et al. (1994). WT1 as a new prognostic factor and a new marker for the detection of minimal residual disease in acute leukemia. *Blood* 84, 3071–3079.

ISBER (2008). International Society for Biological and Environmental Repositories, ISBER: 2008 Best practices for repositories: Collection, storage, retrieval and distribution of biological materials for research. *Cell Preserv Technol* 6, 5–58.

Ishikawa, Y., Kiyoi, H., and Naoe, T. (2011). Prevalence and clinical characteristics of N-terminally truncated WT1 expression in acute myeloid leukemia. *Leuk Res* 35, 685–688.

Issaq, H.J., Waybright, T.J., and Veenstra, T.D. (2011). Cancer biomarker discovery: Opportunities and pitfalls in analytical methods. *Electrophoresis* 32, 967–975.

Ito, K., Oji, Y., Tatsumi, N., Shimizu, S., Kanai, Y., Nakazawa, T., Asada, M. et al. (2006). Antiapoptotic function of 17AA(+)WT1 (Wilms' tumor gene) isoforms on the intrinsic apoptosis pathway. *Oncogene* 25, 4217–4229.

Jacquemart, R., Chavane, N., Durocher, Y., Hoemann, C., De Crescenzo, G., and Jolicoeur, M. (2008). At-line monitoring of bioreactor protein production by Surface Plasmon Resonance. *Biotechnol Bioeng* 100, 184–188.

Jellum, E., Stokke, O., and Eldjarn, L. (1973). Application of gas chromatography, mass spectrometry, and computer methods in clinical biochemistry. *Anal Chem* 46, 1099–1106.

Jomgeow, T., Oji, Y., Tsuji, N., Ikeda, Y., Ito, K., Tsuda, A., Nakazawa, T. et al. (2006). Wilms' tumor gene WT1 17AA(−)/KTS(−) isoform induces morphological changes and promotes cell migration and invasion in vitro. *Cancer Sci* 97, 259–270.

Jonsson, U., Fagerstam, L., Ivarsson, B., Johnsson, B., Karlsson, R., Lundh, K., Lofas, S. et al. (1991). Real-time biospecific interaction analysis using surface plasmon resonance and a sensor chip technology. *Biotechniques* 11, 620–627.

Jourdain, S., Bulman, A., and Dalmasso, E. (2010). The lucid proteomics system for top-down biomarker research. *Arch Physiol Biochem* 116, 158–162.

Jurisicova, A., Jurisica, I., and Kislinger, T. (2008). Advances in ovarian cancer proteomics: The quest for biomarkers and improved therapeutic interventions. *Expert Rev Proteomics* 5, 551–560.

Kang, U.B., Ahn, Y., Lee, J.W., Kim, Y.H., Kim, J., Yu, M.H., Noh, D.Y., and Lee, C. (2010). Differential profiling of breast cancer plasma proteome by isotope-coded affinity tagging method reveals biotinidase as a breast cancer biomarker. *BMC Cancer* 10, 114.

Kapoor, V., Singh, A.K., Dey, S., Sharma, S.C., and Das, S.N. (2010). Circulating cycloxygenase-2 in patients with tobacco-related intraoral squamous cell carcinoma and evaluation of its peptide inhibitors as potential antitumor agent. *J Cancer Res Clin Oncol* 136(12), 1795–1804.

Karlsson, R. (1994). Real-time competitive kinetic analysis of interactions between low-molecular-weight ligands in solution and surface-immobilized receptors. *Anal Biochem* 221, 142–151.

Kazuno, S., Fujimura, T., Arai, T., Ueno, T., Nagao, K., Fujime, M., and Murayama, K. (2011). Multi-sequential surface plasmon resonance analysis of haptoglobin-lectin complex in sera of patients with malignant and benign prostate diseases. *Anal Biochem* 419(2), 241–249.

Keshamouni, V.G., Jagtap, P., Michailidis, G., Strahler, J.R., Kuick, R., Reka, A.K., Papoulias, P. et al. (2009). Temporal quantitative proteomics by iTRAQ 2D-LC-MS/MS and corresponding mRNA expression analysis identify post-transcriptional modulation of actin-cytoskeleton regulators during TGF-beta-Induced epithelial-mesenchymal transition. *J Proteome Res* 8, 35–47.

Kikuchi, Y., Uno, S., Nanami, M., Yoshimura, Y., Iida, S., Fukushima, N., and Tsuchiya, M. (2005). Determination of concentration and binding affinity of antibody fragments by use of surface plasmon resonance. *J Biosci Bioeng* 100, 311–317.

Kletzel, M., Olzewski, M., Huang, W., and Chou, P.M. (2002). Utility of WT1 as a reliable tool for the detection of minimal residual disease in children with leukemia. *Pediatr Devel Pathol* 5, 269–275.

Kozak, K.R., Su, F., Whitelegge, J.P., Faull, K., Reddy, S., and Farias-Eisner, R. (2005). Characterization of serum biomarkers for detection of early stage ovarian cancer. *Proteomics* 5, 4589–4596.

Kramarzova, K., Stuchly, J., Willasch, A., Gruhn, B., Schwarz, J., Cermak, J., Machova-Polakova, K. et al. (2012). Real-time PCR quantification of major Wilms' tumor gene 1 (WT1) isoforms in acute myeloid leukemia, their characteristic expression patterns and possible functional consequences. *Leukemia* 26, 2086.

Kreuzer, K.A., Saborowski, A., Lupberger, J., Appelt, C., Na, I.K., le Coutre, P., and Schmidt, C.A. (2001). Fluorescent 5′-exonuclease assay for the absolute quantification of Wilms' tumour gene (WT1) mRNA: Implications for monitoring human leukaemias. *Br J Haematol* 114, 313–318.

Krishnan, S., Mani, V., Wasalathanthri, D., Kumar, C.V., and Rusling, J.F. (2011). Attomolar detection of a cancer biomarker protein in serum by surface plasmon resonance using superparamagnetic particle labels. *Angew Chem Int Ed Engl* 50(5), 1175–1178.

Kulasingam, V. and Diamandis, E.P. (2008). Strategies for discovering novel cancer biomarkers through utilization of emerging technologies. *Nat Clin Pract Oncol* 5, 588–599.

Lapillonne, H., Renneville, A., Auvrignon, A., Flamant, C., Blaise, A., Perot, C., Lai, J.L. et al. (2006). High WT1 expression after induction therapy predicts high risk of relapse and death in pediatric acute myeloid leukemia. *J Clin Oncol* 24, 1507–1515.

Larsericsdotter, H., Jansson, O., Zhukov, A., Areskoug, D., Oscarsson, S., and Buijs, J. (2006). Optimizing the surface plasmon resonance/mass spectrometry interface for functional proteomics applications: How to avoid and utilize nonspecific adsorption. *Proteomics* 6, 2355–2364.

Latterich, M., Abramovitz, M., and Leyland-Jones, B. (2008). Proteomics: New technologies and clinical applications. *Eur J Cancer* 44, 2737–2741.

Lawson, A.M. (1975). The scope of mass spectrometry in clinical chemistry. *Clin Chem* 21, 803–824.

Lebrecht, A., Boehm, D., Schmidt, M., Koelbl, H., and Grus, F.H. (2009). Surface-enhanced laser desorption/ionisation time-of-flight mass spectrometry to detect breast cancer markers in tears and serum. *Cancer Genomics Proteomics* 6, 75–83.

Lehe, C., Ghebeh, H., Al-Sulaiman, A., Al Qudaihi, G., Al-Hussein, K., Almohareb, F., Chaudhri, N. et al. (2008). The Wilms' tumor antigen is a novel target for human CD4+ regulatory T cells: Implications for immunotherapy. *Cancer Res* 68, 6350–6359.

Lehmann, R., Melle, C., Escher, N., and von Eggeling, F. (2005). Detection and identification of protein interactions of S100 proteins by ProteinChip technology. *J Proteome Res* 4, 1717–1721.

Leyland-Jones, B.R., Ambrosone, C.B., Bartlett, J., Ellis, M.J., Enos, R.A., Raji, A., Pins, M.R. et al. (2008). Recommendations for collection and handling of specimens from group breast cancer clinical trials. *J Clin Oncol* 26, 5638–5644.

Li, S.L., Ye, F., Cai, W.J., Hu, H.D., Hu, P., Ren, H., Zhu, F.F., and Zhang, D.Z. (2010). Quantitative proteome analysis of multidrug resistance in human ovarian cancer cell line. *J Cell Biochem* 109, 625–633.

Liedberg, B., Nylander, C., and Lundström, I. (1983). *Sensors Actuators* 4, 299–304.

Lin, J.D., Huang, C.C., Weng, H.F., Chen, S.C., and Jeng, L.B. (1995). Comparison of membrane proteins from benign and malignant human thyroid tissues by two-dimensional polyacrylamide gel electrophoresis. *J Chromatogr B Biomed Appl* 667, 153–160.

Liu, H., Lin, D., and Yates, J.R., 3rd (2002). Multidimensional separations for protein/peptide analysis in the post-genomic era. *Biotechniques* 32, 898, 900, 902 passim.

Liu, H., Sadygov, R.G., and Yates, J.R., 3rd (2004). A model for random sampling and estimation of relative protein abundance in shotgun proteomics. *Anal Chem* 76, 4193–4201.

Lopez, M.F. (1999). 2-D electrophoresis using carrier ampholytes in the first dimension (IEF). *Methods Mol Biol* 112, 111–127.

Malik, G., Ward, M.D., Gupta, S.K., Trosset, M.W., Grizzle, W.E., Adam, B.L., Diaz, J.I., and Semmes, O.J. (2005). Serum levels of an isoform of apolipoprotein A-II as a potential marker for prostate cancer. *Clin Cancer Res* 11, 1073–1085.

Mann, M. (2006). Functional and quantitative proteomics using SILAC. *Nat Rev Mol Cell Biol* 7, 952–958.

Mannen, T., Yamaguchi, S., Honda, J., Sugimoto, S., Kitayama, A., and Nagamune, T. (2001). Observation of charge state and conformational change in immobilized protein using surface plasmon resonance sensor. *Anal Biochem* 293, 185–193.

Matharoo-Ball, B., Miles, A.K., Creaser, C.S., Ball, G., and Rees, R. (2008). Serum biomarker profiling in cancer studies: A question of standardisation? *Vet Comp Oncol* 6, 224–247.

Matharoo-Ball, B., Ratcliffe, L., Lancashire, L., Ugurel, S., Miles, A.K., Weston, D.J., Rees, R. et al. (2007). Diagnostic biomarkers differentiating metastatic melanoma patients from healthy controls identified by an integrated MALDI-TOF mass spectrometry/bioinformatic approach. *Proteomics Clin Appl* 1, 605–620.

Mayo, M.W., Wang, C.Y., Drouin, S.S., Madrid, L.V., Marshall, A.F., Reed, J.C., Weissman, B.E., and Baldwin, A.S. (1999). WT1 modulates apoptosis by transcriptionally upregulating the bcl-2 proto-oncogene. *Embo J* 18, 3990–4003.

Menssen, H.D., Renkl, H.J., Rodeck, U., Kari, C., Schwartz, S., and Thiel, E. (1997). Detection by monoclonal antibodies of the Wilms' tumor (WT1) nuclear protein in patients with acute leukemia. *Int J Cancer* 70, 518–523.

Menssen, H.D., Renkl, H.J., Rodeck, U., Maurer, J., Notter, M., Schwartz, S., Reinhardt, R., and Thiel, E. (1995). Presence of Wilms' tumor gene (wt1) transcripts and the WT1 nuclear protein in the majority of human acute leukemias. *Leukemia* 9, 1060–1067.

Merril, C.R., Switzer, R.C., and Van Keuren, M.L. (1979). Trace polypeptides in cellular extracts and human body fluids detected by two-dimensional electrophoresis and a highly sensitive silver stain. *Proc Natl Acad Sci USA* 76, 4335–4339.

Mian, S., Ugurel, S., Parkinson, E., Schlenzka, I., Dryden, I., Lancashire, L., Ball, G. et al. (2005). Serum proteomic fingerprinting discriminates between clinical stages and predicts disease progression in melanoma patients. *J Clin Oncol* 23, 5088–5093.

Millington, D.S., Kodo, N., Norwood, D.L., and Roe, C.R. (1990). Tandem mass spectrometry: A new method for acylcarnitine profiling with potential for neonatal screening for inborn errors of metabolism. *J Inherit Metab Dis* 13, 321–324.

Miwa, H., Beran, M., and Saunders, G.F. (1992). Expression of the Wilms' tumor gene (WT1) in human leukemias. *Leukemia* 6, 405–409.

Miyagi, T., Ahuja, H., Kubota, T., Kubonishi, I., Koeffler, H.P., and Miyoshi, I. (1993). Expression of the candidate Wilm's tumor gene, WT1, in human leukemia cells. *Leukemia* 7, 970–977.

Miyoshi, Y., Ando, A., Egawa, C., Taguchi, T., Tamaki, Y., Tamaki, H., Sugiyama, H., and Noguchi, S. (2002). High expression of Wilms' tumor suppressor gene predicts poor prognosis in breast cancer patients. *Clin Cancer Res* 8, 1167–1171.

Moorwood, K., Salpekar, A., Ivins, S.M., Hall, J., Powlesland, R.M., Brown, K.W., and Malik, K. (1999). Transactivation of the WT1 antisense promoter is unique to the WT1[+/–] isoform. *FEBS Lett 456*, 131–136.

Moriya, S., Takiguchi, M., and Seki, N. (2008). Expression of the WT1 gene -KTS domain isoforms suppresses the invasive ability of human lung squamous cell carcinoma cells. *Int J Oncol* 32, 349–356.

Morrison, A.A., Venables, J.P., Dellaire, G., and Ladomery, M.R. (2006). The Wilms tumour suppressor protein WT1 (+KTS isoform) binds alpha-actinin 1 mRNA via its zinc-finger domain. *Biochem Cell Biol* 84, 789–798.

Motoyama, A., Venable, J.D., Ruse, C.I., and Yates, J.R., III (2006). Automated ultra-high-pressure multidimensional protein identification technology (UHP-MudPIT) for improved peptide identification of proteomic samples. *Anal Chem* 78, 5109–5118.

Myung, J.H., Launiere, C.A., Eddington, D.T., and Hong, S. (2010). Enhanced tumor cell isolation by a biomimetic combination of E-selectin and anti-EpCAM: implications for the effective separation of circulating tumor cells (CTCs). *Langmuir* 26(11), 8589–8596.

Nagata, K. and Handa, H. (2000). *Real-Time Analysis of Biomolecular Interactions: Applications of Biacore*, Tokyo, Japan: Springer-Verlag.

Netinatsunthorn, W., Hanprasertpong, J., Dechsukhum, C., Leetanaporn, R., and Geater, A. (2006). WT1 gene expression as a prognostic marker in advanced serous epithelial ovarian carcinoma: An immunohistochemical study. *BMC Cancer* 6, 90.

Niksic, M., Slight, J., Sanford, J.R., Caceres, J.F., and Hastie, N.D. (2004). The Wilms' tumour protein (WT1) shuttles between nucleus and cytoplasm and is present in functional polysomes. *Hum Mol Genet* 13, 463–471.

Normanno, N., Campiglio, M., De, L.A., Somenzi, G., Maiello, M., Ciardiello, F., Gianni, L., Salomon, D.S., and Menard, S. (2002). Cooperative inhibitory effect of ZD1839 (Iressa) in combination with trastuzumab (Herceptin) on human breast cancer cell growth. *Ann Oncol* 13, 65–72.

Nossov, V., Amneus, M., Su, F., Lang, J., Janco, J.M., Reddy, S.T., and Farias-Eisner, R. (2008). The early detection of ovarian cancer: From traditional methods to proteomics. Can we really do better than serum CA-125? *Am J Obstet Gynecol* 199, 215–223.

Ogawa, H., Tamaki, H., Ikegame, K., Soma, T., Kawakami, M., Tsuboi, A., Kim, E.H. et al. (2003). The usefulness of monitoring WT1 gene transcripts for the prediction and management of relapse following allogeneic stem cell transplantation in acute type leukemia. *Blood* 101, 1698–1704.

Oji, Y., Ogawa, H., Tamaki, H., Oka, Y., Tsuboi, A., Kim, E.H., Soma, T. et al. (1999). Expression of the Wilms' tumor gene WT1 in solid tumors and its involvement in tumor cell growth. *Jpn J Cancer Res* 90, 194–204.

Okuzawa, K., Franzen, B., Lindholm, J., Linder, S., Hirano, T., Bergman, T., Ebihara, Y., Kato, H., and Auer, G. (1994). Characterization of gene expression in clinical lung cancer materials by two-dimensional polyacrylamide gel electrophoresis. *Electrophoresis* 15, 382–390.

Ong, S.E., Blagoev, B., Kratchmarova, I., Kristensen, D.B., Steen, H., Pandey, A., and Mann, M. (2002). Stable isotope labeling by amino acids in cell culture, SILAC, as a simple and accurate approach to expression proteomics. *Mol Cell Proteomics* 1, 376–386.

Orvisky, E., Drake, S.K., Martin, B.M., Abdel-Hamid, M., Ressom, H.W., Varghese, R.S., An, Y. et al. (2006). Enrichment of low molecular weight fraction of serum for MS analysis of peptides associated with hepatocellular carcinoma. *Proteomics* 6, 2895–2902.

Ostergaard, M., Olesen, L.H., Hasle, H., Kjeldsen, E., and Hokland, P. (2004). WT1 gene expression: An excellent tool for monitoring minimal residual disease in 70% of acute myeloid leukaemia patients—Results from a single-centre study. *Br J Haematol* 125, 590–600.

Palmblad, M., Tiss, A., and Cramer, R. (2009). Mass spectrometry in clinical proteomics—From the present to the future. *Proteomics Clin Appl* 3, 6–17.

Parekh, D.J., Ankerst, D.P., Troyer, D., Srivastava, S., and Thompson, I.M. (2007). Biomarkers for prostate cancer detection. *J Urol* 178, 2252–2259.

Parikh, K. and Peppelenbosch, M.P. (2010). Kinome profiling of clinical cancer specimens. *Cancer Res* 70, 2575–2578.

Patton, W.F. (2000). A thousand points of light: The application of fluorescence detection technologies to two-dimensional gel electrophoresis and proteomics. *Electrophoresis* 21, 1123–1144.

Paulovich, A.G., Whiteaker, J.R., Hoofnagle, A.N., and Wang, P. (2008). The interface between biomarker discovery and clinical validation: The tar pit of the protein biomarker pipeline. *Proteomics Clin Appl* 2, 1386–1402.

Pelletier, J., Bruening, W., Kashtan, C.E., Mauer, S.M., Manivel, J.C., Striegel, J.E., Houghton, D.C. et al. (1991). Germline mutations in the Wilms' tumor suppressor gene are associated with abnormal urogenital development in Denys-Drash syndrome. *Cell* 67, 437–447.

Pertea, M. and Salzberg, S.L. (2010). Between a chicken and a grape: Estimating the number of human genes. *Genome Biol* 11, 206.

Petricoin, E.F., Ardekani, A.M., Hitt, B.A., Levine, P.J., Fusaro, V.A., Steinberg, S.M., Mills, G.B. et al. (2002). Use of proteomic patterns in serum to identify ovarian cancer. *Lancet* 359, 572–577.

Petricoin, E.F. and Liotta, L.A. (2004a). Clinical proteomics: Application at the bedside. *Contrib Nephrol* 141, 93–103.

Petricoin, E.F. and Liotta, L.A. (2004b). SELDI-TOF-based serum proteomic pattern diagnostics for early detection of cancer. *Curr Opin Biotechnol* 15, 24–30.

Petricoin, E.F., Ornstein, D.K., and Liotta, L.A. (2004). Clinical proteomics: Applications for prostate cancer biomarker discovery and detection. *Urol Oncol* 22, 322–328.

Phillips, K.S. and Cheng, Q. (2007). Recent advances in surface plasmon resonance based techniques for bioanalysis. *Anal Bioanal Chem* 387, 1831–1840.

Qiu, H. and Wang, Y. (2008). Quantitative analysis of surface plasma membrane proteins of primary and metastatic melanoma cells. *J Proteome Res* 7, 1904–1915.

Ralhan, R., Desouza, L.V., Matta, A., Chandra Tripathi, S., Ghanny, S., Datta Gupta, S., Bahadur, S., and Siu, K.W. (2008). Discovery and verification of head-and-neck cancer biomarkers by differential protein expression analysis using iTRAQ labeling, multidimensional liquid chromatography, and tandem mass spectrometry. *Mol Cell Proteomics* 7, 1162–1173.

Reddy, P.J., Sadhu, S., Ray, S., and Srivastava, S. (2012). Cancer biomarker detection by surface plasmon resonance biosensors. *Clin Lab Med* 32, 47–72.

Renshaw, J., King-Underwood, L., and Pritchard-Jones, K. (1997). Differential splicing of exon 5 of the Wilms tumour (WTI) gene. *Genes Chromosomes Cancer* 19, 256–266.

Reyzer, M.L. and Caprioli, R.M. (2005). MALDI mass spectrometry for direct tissue analysis: A new tool for biomarker discovery. *J Proteome Res* 4, 1138–1142.

Rifai, N., Gillette, M.A., and Carr, S.A. (2006). Protein biomarker discovery and validation: The long and uncertain path to clinical utility. *Nat Biotechnol* 24, 971–983.

Rodrigues, P.C., Oliveira, S.N., Viana, M.B., Matsuda, E.I., Nowill, A.E., Brandalise, S.R., and Yunes, J.A. (2007). Prognostic significance of WT1 gene expression in pediatric acute myeloid leukemia. *Pediatr Blood Cancer* 49, 133–138.

Ross, P.L., Huang, Y.N., Marchese, J.N., Williamson, B., Parker, K., Hattan, S., Khainovski, N. et al. (2004). Multiplexed protein quantitation in *Saccharomyces cerevisiae* using amine-reactive isobaric tagging reagents. *Mol Cell Proteomics* 3, 1154–1169.

Rossi, G., Minervini, M.M., Carella, A.M., de Waure, C., di Nardo, F., Melillo, L., D'Arena, G., Zini, G., and Cascavilla, N. (2012). Comparison between multiparameter flow cytometry and WT1-RNA quantification in monitoring minimal residual disease in acute myeloid leukemia without specific molecular targets. *Leuk Res* 36, 401–406.

Sarandakou, A., Protonotariou, E., and Rizos, D. (2007). Tumor markers in biological fluids associated with pregnancy. *Crit Rev Clin Lab Sci* 44, 151–178.

Sarto, C., Marocchi, A., Sanchez, J.C., Giannone, D., Frutiger, S., Golaz, O., Wilkins, M.R. et al. (1997). Renal cell carcinoma and normal kidney protein expression. *Electrophoresis* 18, 599–604.

Scharnhorst, V., van der Eb, A.J., and Jochemsen, A.G. (2001). WT1 proteins: Functions in growth and differentiation. *Gene* 273, 141–161.

Schiess, R., Wollscheid, B., and Aebersold, R. (2009). Targeted proteomic strategy for clinical biomarker discovery. *Mol Oncol* 3, 33–44.

Scholz, H. and Kirschner, K.M. (2011). Oxygen-dependent gene expression in development and cancer: Lessons learned from the Wilms' tumor gene, WT1. *Front Mol Neurosci* 4, 4.

Sera, T., Hiasa, Y., Mashiba, T., Tokumoto, Y., Hirooka, M., Konishi, I., Matsuura, B. et al. (2008). Wilms' tumour 1 gene expression is increased in hepatocellular carcinoma and associated with poor prognosis. *Eur J Cancer* 44, 600–608.

Siehl, J.M., Reinwald, M., Heufelder, K., Menssen, H.D., Keilholz, U., and Thiel, E. (2004). Expression of Wilms' tumor gene 1 at different stages of acute myeloid leukemia and analysis of its major splice variants. *Ann Hematol* 83, 745–750.

Singh, A.K., Kant, S., Parshad, R., Banerjee, N., and Dey, S. (2011). Evaluation of human LOX-12 as a serum marker for breast cancer. *Biochem Biophys Res Commun* 414(2), 304–308.

Situ, C., Buijs, J., Mooney, M.H., and Elliott, C.T. (2010). Advances in surface plasmon resonance biosensor technology towards high-throughput food-safety analysis. *Trends Anal Chem* 29, 1305–1315.

Spengler, B., Kirsch, D., Kaufmann, R., and Jaeger, E. (1992). Peptide sequencing by matrix-assisted laser-desorption mass spectrometry. *Rapid Commun Mass Spectrom* 6, 105–108.

Stattin, P. and Hakama, M. (2003). Correspondence re: B-L. Adam et al., Serum protein fingerprinting coupled with a pattern-matching algorithm distinguishes prostate cancer from benign prostate hyperplasia and healthy men. *Cancer Res*, 62, 3609–3614, 2002. *Cancer Res* 63, 2701; author reply 2701–2702.

Stenberg, E., Persson, B., Roos, H., and Urbaniczky, C. (1991). Quantitative determination of surface concentration of protein with surface plasmon resonance using radiolabeled proteins. *J Colloid Interf Sci* 143, 513–526.

Stewart, J.J., White, J.T., Yan, X., Collins, S., Drescher, C.W., Urban, N.D., Hood, L., and Lin, B. (2006). Proteins associated with Cisplatin resistance in ovarian cancer cells identified by quantitative proteomic technology and integrated with mRNA expression levels. *Mol Cell Proteomics* 5, 433–443.

Stigter, E.C., de Jong, G.J., and van Bennekom, W.P. (2005). An improved coating for the isolation and quantitation of interferon-gamma in spiked plasma using surface plasmon resonance (SPR). *Biosens Bioelectron* 21, 474–482.

Stigter, E.C., de Jong, G.J., and van Bennekom, W.P. (2009). Development of an on-line SPR-digestion-nanoLC-MS/MS system for the quantification and identification of interferon-gamma in plasma. *Biosens Bioelectron* 24, 2184–2190.

Sugiyama, H. (2001). Wilms' tumor gene WT1: Its oncogenic function and clinical application. *Int J Hematol* 73, 177–187.

Sugiyama, H. (2010). WT1 (Wilms' tumor gene 1): Biology and cancer immunotherapy. *Jpn J Clin Oncol* 40, 377–387.

Sun, Y., Mi, W., Cai, J., Ying, W., Liu, F., Lu, H., Qiao, Y. et al. (2008). Quantitative proteomic signature of liver cancer cells: Tissue transglutaminase 2 could be a novel protein candidate of human hepatocellular carcinoma. *J Proteome Res* 7, 3847–3859.

Sweetman, L. (1996). Newborn screening by tandem mass spectrometry (MS-MS). *Clin Chem* 42, 345–346.

Tamaki, H., Mishima, M., Kawakami, M., Tsuboi, A., Kim, E.H., Hosen, N., Ikegame, K. et al. (2003). Monitoring minimal residual disease in leukemia using real-time quantitative polymerase chain reaction for Wilms tumor gene (WT1). *Int J Hematol* 78, 349–356.

Tamaki, H., Ogawa, H., Ohyashiki, K., Ohyashiki, J.H., Iwama, H., Inoue, K., Soma, T. et al. (1999). The Wilms' tumor gene WT1 is a good marker for diagnosis of disease progression of myelodysplastic syndromes. *Leukemia* 13, 393–399.

Tan, H.T., Lee, Y.H., and Chung, M.C. (2012). Cancer proteomics. *Mass Spectrom Rev* 31, 583–605.

Tatsumi, N., Oji, Y., Tsuji, N., Tsuda, A., Higashio, M., Aoyagi, S., Fukuda, I. et al. (2008). Wilms' tumor gene WT1-shRNA as a potent apoptosis-inducing agent for solid tumors. *Int J Oncol* 32, 701–711.

Timms, J.F., Menon, U., Devetyarov, D., Tiss, A., Camuzeaux, S., McCurrie, K., Nouretdinov, I. et al. 2011. Early detection of ovarian cancer in samples pre-diagnosis using CA125 and MALDI-MS peaks. *Cancer Genomics Proteomics* 8, 289–305.

Tiss, A., Smith, C., Camuzeaux, S., Kabir, M., Gayther, S., Menon, U., Waterfield, M. et al. (2007). Serum peptide profiling using MALDI mass spectrometry: Avoiding the pitfalls of coated magnetic beads using well-established ZipTip technology. *Proteomics* 7, 77–89.

Tiss, A., Smith, C., Menon, U., Jacobs, I., Timms, J.F., and Cramer, R. (2010). A well-characterised peak identification list of MALDI MS profile peaks for human blood serum. *Proteomics* 10, 3388–3392.

Tiss, A., Timms, J.F., Smith, C., Devetyarov, D., Gentry-Maharaj, A., Camuzeaux, S., Burford, B. et al. 2011. Highly accurate detection of ovarian cancer using CA125 but limited improvement with serum matrix-assisted laser desorption/ionization time-of-flight mass spectrometry profiling. *Int J Gynecol Cancer* 20, 1518–1524.

Trka, J., Kalinova, M., Hrusak, O., Zuna, J., Krejci, O., Madzo, J., Sedlacek, P. et al. (2002). Real-time quantitative PCR detection of WT1 gene expression in children with AML: Prognostic significance, correlation with disease status and residual disease detection by flow cytometry. *Leukemia* 16, 1381–1389.

Turbadar, T. (1959). Complete absorption of light by thin metal films. *Proc Phys Soc Lond* 73, 40–44.

Ueda, K., Fukase, Y., Katagiri, T., Ishikawa, N., Irie, S., Sato, T.A., Ito, H. et al. (2009). Targeted serum glycoproteomics for the discovery of lung cancer-associated glycosylation disorders using lectin-coupled ProteinChip arrays. *Proteomics* 9, 2182–2192.

Unlu, M., Morgan, M.E., and Minden, J.S. (1997). Difference gel electrophoresis: A single gel method for detecting changes in protein extracts. *Electrophoresis* 18, 2071–2077.

van Dongen, J.J., Macintyre, E.A., Gabert, J.A., Delabesse, E., Rossi, V., Saglio, G., Gottardi, E. et al. (1999). Standardized RT-PCR analysis of fusion gene transcripts from chromosome aberrations in acute leukemia for detection of minimal residual disease. Report of the BIOMED-1 Concerted Action: Investigation of minimal residual disease in acute leukemia. *Leukemia* 13, 1901–1928.

Veenstra, T.D., Prieto, D.A., and Conrads, T.P. (2004). Proteomic patterns for early cancer detection. *Drug Discov Today* 9, 889–897.

Villanueva, J., Martorella, A.J., Lawlor, K., Philip, J., Fleisher, M., Robbins, R.J., and Tempst, P. (2006). Serum peptidome patterns that distinguish metastatic thyroid carcinoma from cancer-free controls are unbiased by gender and age. *Mol Cell Proteomics* 5, 1840–1852.

Villanueva, J., Nazarian, A., Lawlor, K., Yi, S.S., Robbins, R.J., and Tempst, P. (2008). A sequence-specific exopeptidase activity test (SSEAT) for "functional" biomarker discovery. *Mol Cell Proteomics* 7, 509–518.

Villanueva, J., Philip, J., Chaparro, C.A., Li, Y., Toledo-Crow, R., DeNoyer, L., Fleisher, M., Robbins, R.J., and Tempst, P. (2005). Correcting common errors in identifying cancer-specific serum peptide signatures. *J Proteome Res* 4, 1060–1072.

Villanueva, J., Philip, J., Entenberg, D., Chaparro, C.A., Tanwar, M.K., Holland, E.C., and Tempst, P. (2004). Serum peptide profiling by magnetic particle-assisted, automated sample processing and MALDI-TOF mass spectrometry. *Anal Chem* 76, 1560–1570.

Virappane, P., Gale, R., Hills, R., Kakkas, I., Summers, K., Stevens, J., Allen, C. et al. (2008). Mutation of the Wilms' tumor 1 gene is a poor prognostic factor associated with chemotherapy resistance in normal karyotype acute myeloid leukemia: The United Kingdom Medical Research Council Adult Leukaemia Working Party. *J Clin Oncol* 26, 5429–5435.

Vogel, C., Abreu Rde, S., Ko, D., Le, S.Y., Shapiro, B.A., Burns, S.C., Sandhu, D. et al. (2010). Sequence signatures and mRNA concentration can explain two-thirds of protein abundance variation in a human cell line. *Mol Syst Biol* 6, 400.

Wagner, K.D., Wagner, N., and Schedl, A. (2003). The complex life of WT1. *J Cell Sci* 116, 1653–1658.

Wang, Z.Y., Qiu, Q.Q., Huang, J., Gurrieri, M., and Deuel, T.F. (1995). Products of alternatively spliced transcripts of the Wilms' tumor suppressor gene, wt1, have altered DNA binding specificity and regulate transcription in different ways. *Oncogene* 10, 415–422.

Ward, L.D., Hong, J., Whitehead, R.H., and Simpson, R.J. (1990). Development of a database of amino acid sequences for human colon carcinoma proteins separated by two-dimensional polyacrylamide gel electrophoresis. *Electrophoresis* 11, 883–891.

Washburn, M.P., Wolters, D., and Yates, J.R., 3rd (2001). Large-scale analysis of the yeast proteome by multidimensional protein identification technology. *Nat Biotechnol* 19, 242–247.

Weisser, M., Kern, W., Rauhut, S., Schoch, C., Hiddemann, W., Haferlach, T., and Schnittger, S. (2005). Prognostic impact of RT-PCR-based quantification of WT1 gene expression during MRD monitoring of acute myeloid leukemia. *Leukemia* 19, 1416–1423.

Whelan, L.C., Power, K.A., McDowell, D.T., Kennedy, J., and Gallagher, W.M. (2008). Applications of SELDI-MS technology in oncology. *J Cell Mol Med* 12, 1535–1547.

Whiteaker, J.R., Zhang, H., Zhao, L., Wang, P., Kelly-Spratt, K.S., Ivey, R.G., Piening, B.D. et al. (2007). Integrated pipeline for mass spectrometry-based discovery and confirmation of biomarkers demonstrated in a mouse model of breast cancer. *J Proteome Res* 6, 3962–3975.

Wiese, S., Reidegeld, K.A., Meyer, H.E., and Warscheid, B. (2007). Protein labeling by iTRAQ: A new tool for quantitative mass spectrometry in proteome research. *Proteomics* 7, 340–350.

Wiesner, A. (2004). Detection of tumor markers with ProteinChip technology. *Curr Pharm Biotechnol* 5, 45–67.

Wilcken, B., Wiley, V., Hammond, J., and Carpenter, K. (2003). Screening newborns for inborn errors of metabolism by tandem mass spectrometry. *N Engl J Med* 348, 2304–2312.

Wulfkuhle, J., Espina, V., Liotta, L., and Petricoin, E. (2004). Genomic and proteomic technologies for individualisation and improvement of cancer treatment. *Eur J Cancer* 40, 2623–2632.

Xu, B.J., Yan, W., Jovanovic, B., An, A.Q., Cheng, N., Aakre, M.E., Yi, Y. et al. (2010). Quantitative analysis of the secretome of TGF-beta signaling-deficient mammary fibroblasts. *Proteomics* 10, 2458–2470.

Yang, C. and Romaniuk, P.J. (2008). The ratio of +/-KTS splice variants of the Wilms' tumour suppressor protein WT1 mRNA is determined by an intronic enhancer. *Biochem Cell Biol* 86, 312–321.

Yang, C.Y., Brooks, E., Li, Y., Denny, P., Ho, C.M., Qi, F., Shi, W. et al. (2005). Detection of picomolar levels of interleukin-8 in human saliva by SPR. *Lab Chip* 5, 1017–1023.

Yang, L., Han, Y., Suarez Saiz, F., and Minden, M.D. (2007). A tumor suppressor and oncogene: The WT1 story. *Leukemia* 21, 868–876.

Yocum, A.K., Busch, C.M., Felix, C.A., and Blair, I.A. (2006). Proteomics-based strategy to identify biomarkers and pharmacological targets in leukemias with t(4;11) translocations. *J Proteome Res* 5, 2743–2753.

Zhang, B., VerBerkmoes, N.C., Langston, M.A., Uberbacher, E., Hettich, R.L., and Samatova, N.F. (2006). Detecting differential and correlated protein expression in label-free shotgun proteomics. *J Proteome Res* 5, 2909–2918.

Zhang, J., Niu, D., Sui, J., Ching, C.B., and Chen, W.N. (2009). Protein profile in hepatitis B virus replicating rat primary hepatocytes and HepG2 cells by iTRAQ-coupled 2-D LC-MS/MS analysis: Insights on liver angiogenesis. *Proteomics* 9, 2836–2845.

Zhang, Z. and Chan, D.W. (2010). The road from discovery to clinical diagnostics: Lessons learned from the first FDA-cleared in vitro diagnostic multivariate index assay of proteomic biomarkers. *Cancer Epidemiol Biomarkers Prev* 19, 2995–2999.

Zieske, L.R. (2006). A perspective on the use of iTRAQ reagent technology for protein complex and profiling studies. *J Exp Bot* 57, 1501–1508.

Zwick, E., Bange, J., and Ullrich, A. (2002). Receptor tyrosine kinases as targets for anticancer drugs. *Trends Mol Med* 8, 17–23.

5

Noninvasive Nanodiagnostics for Cancer

Sandhiya Selvarajan, Melvin George, and Suresh Kumar

CONTENTS

ABSTRACT The most reliable factor in predicting cancer survival is the size of the tumor at the time of diagnosis. Hence, early diagnosis of cancer plays an important role in deciding the prognosis. The diagnostic methods available in the present scenario can detect tumors only when they contain a minimum of one billion cells. However, with the advances in the field of nanotechnology, it is possible to detect tumors 1000 times smaller than the usual detectable size as well as earlier than the current diagnostic methods available. Moreover, as nanoparticles can be designed to cross the biological barriers, they can also be used to detect tumors not accessible to conventional diagnostic methods. Inexpensive radio isotopes with short half-life can be combined with nanocarriers to target the specific tumor cells and to have a prolonged half-life.

The use of nanotechnology for clinical diagnostic purposes intended to meet the demands of increased sensitivity and earlier detection of disease is known as nanodiagnostics. The novel nanodiagnostic tools in early diagnosis of cancer include quantum dots (QDs), gold nanoparticles, and cantilevers (Arayne and Sultana 2006). These QDs are one of the most promising nanostructures for diagnostic applications, as they are semiconductor nanocrystals characterized by high photostability, single-wavelength excitation, and size-tunable emission. QDs and magnetic nanoparticles can be used for barcoding of specific analytes, while gold and magnetic nanoparticles are used as the key components of the bio-barcode assay, which has been proposed as a future alternative to the polymerase chain reaction (PCR). Magnetic nanoparticles can be used to capture circulating tumor cells in the bloodstream followed by rapid photoacoustic detection.

The increased demand for sensitivity requires a diagnostically significant interaction between analyte molecules and signal-generating particles, thus enabling detection of a single analyte molecule. Nanotechnology has enabled one-to-one interaction between analytes and signal-generating particles such as quantum dots in the size range of proteins and other biomolecules. Thus, nanotechnology has improved the early diagnosis of cancer, with the sensitive detection of multiple protein biomarkers using nanobiosensors. Nanoparticles used for targeted drug delivery in cancer facilitate the combination of both diagnostics and therapeutics known as theranostics. In addition, nanoparticles act as adjuncts to hyperthermia and photodynamic therapy. Thermosensitive liposomes (TSLs) loaded with MRI contrast agent have shown the release of MRI contrast agent gadolinium-loaded phosphatidylglyceroglycerol (Gd-TSL) in tumor-bearing mice at higher temperature. Thus, following intravenous injection of contrast agent loaded in TSL in tumor-bearing mice, the heated tumor tissue could be distinguished from unheated tumor tissue. This proves that apart from diagnosis, TSL could also be used to influence targeted drug therapy (Peller et al. 2008).

Furthermore, the applications of nanotechnology in surgical oncology include the use of nanoparticles to visualize tumor during surgery that aids proper removal and nanorobotics for remotely controlled diagnostics combined with therapeutics. Nanodiagnostics promise increased sensitivity, multiple capabilities, and reduced cost for many diagnostic applications as well as intracellular imaging. Further work is needed to fully optimize these diagnostic nanotechnologies for clinical laboratory setting and to address the potential health and environmental risks related to QDs. Hence, this chapter will discuss in detail the application of nanodiagnostics in the early detection of cancer.

KEY WORDS: *theranostics, quantum dots, paramagnetic nanoparticles, dendrimer, micelles.*

5.1 Introduction

Cancer, one of the most serious health threats worldwide, is on the rise over the last few decades. Early diagnosis of cancer offers the benefit of enhancing screening methods and the resultant reduction in morbidity and mortality owing to early intervention. However, early detection of cancer requires mandatory identification of the initial trace of disease-related biomarkers and molecular expression profile. Recent advances in medicine, life sciences, biotechnology, and nanotechnology offer the vista toward the early detection and diagnosis of cancer with the help of biomarkers like proteins, peptides, and molecular signatures. As tumor biomarkers appear earlier in the body well before the external appearance of the disease, lots of research is being undertaken for early cancer detection using molecular biology, proteomics, and nanotechnology (Bhati et al. 2012). Of these, nanotechnology is emerging as a promising tool in diagnosis and treatment of cancer.

Nanotechnology uses the knowledge of physics, chemistry, and biology to design nanoparticles and nanodevices of size 1–100 nm in at least one dimension. The application of nanotechnology in medicine for diagnosis and therapy is known as nanomedicine. The inherent properties of substances at nanoscale have been made use of in medicine to devise targeted, site-specific drugs, contrast agents, and drug carriers. As nanoparticles can be engineered into a multifunctional entity with the ability to target diseased area, carry contrast agents, and deliver therapeutic agents at the desired site, among the various specialties of medicine, oncology seems to reap the maximum benefit of nanotechnology.

Nanoparticles with large surface volume ratio and high surface reaction activity are one of the most useful drug carriers for delivering the drug at the desired site with least systemic toxicity. Nanoparticles used as drug carriers are divided into three generations with the first and second generation being single entity particles. Among the single entity molecules, the first generation nanovectors target the tumor site owing to their specific characteristic known as enhanced permeation and retention (EPR) effect. EPR phenomenon is attributed to the increased accumulation of drug at the tumor site as well as increased vascular permeability and the resultant retention due to lack of lymphatic drainage at the tumor site (Sandhiya et al. 2009). However, the second-generation nanovectors differ from their predecessors as they have distinct features like added targeting moieties, remove activation, and environmentally sensitive components. In contrast, third-generation nanovectors carry out multiple tasks using individual nanocomponents acting in a synergistic fashion. These nanocarriers can be used to carry both drug(s) and imaging agent(s) with application for both diagnosis and therapy. In addition, nanowires and cantilever arrays have shown promise in the detection of biomarkers. Thus, nanomedicine has immense potential for the overall diagnostic and therapeutic processes with the resultant enhanced quality of life in cancer. Hence, this chapter will discuss in detail the application of nanodiagnostics in the early detection of cancer.

5.2 Noninvasive Nanodiagnostics

The characteristics of nanoparticles have the potential to be used for medical imaging and diagnostic purposes. Iron oxide and colloidal gold nanoparticles are emerging as promising contrast agent for magnetic resonance imaging (MRI) and computed tomography (CT) imaging, respectively. Nevertheless optical imaging has been overwhelmed by the inability to provide valuable result in vivo imaging due to photobleaching. This could be overcome with the help of nanoparticles like quantum dots (QDs) with inherent ability to resist bleaching and tunable emission spectra. These advances will help in early detection of diseases owing to higher resolution of imaging agents used. Moreover, the enhanced understanding of disease progression and tumor location will help in the early detection of diseases. These advances in imaging and diagnosis play a major role in cancer as prognosis of the disease can be improved by initiating the therapy at the early stage of the disease.

Nanoparticles like QDs, nanoshells, and nanosomes have made the early detection of cancer more promising (Surendiran et al. 2009; Kateb et al. 2010; Ryvolova et al. 2012). Surface functionalization of nanocarriers with antibodies, aptamers, peptides, or small molecules that recognize either tumor-specific antigens (TSAs) or tumor-associated antigens (TAAs) in the tumor microenvironment can be used to enhance active tumor targeting. In addition to the drugs, nanomaterials can also be used to carry higher concentration of contrast agents in MRI, optical imaging, and photoacoustic imaging. Thus, nanocarriers carry the advantage of delivering higher concentration of the drug or contrast agents at the specific tumor site compared to the other conventional drug delivery systems (Ryvolova et al. 2012). The combination of diagnostics with therapeutics known as theranostics is emerging as an essential aspect of personalized medicine in cancer therapy (Fernandez-Fernandez et al. 2011). In the present scenario, theranostics have paved a novel approach toward personalized medicine with an increasing focus on the development of nano-imaging and drug delivery devices. The application of theranostics in medicine shows promise in the understanding of molecular mechanisms underlying the progression of diseases (Bae et al. 2011). Moreover, recently, substrate preparations for surface-enhanced laser desorption or ionization time of flight (SELDI-TOF) proteomic analysis protocols are being used for noninvasive and early cancer diagnosis (Gast et al. 2009). Nanodevices and nanoparticles have paved the way for developing novel imaging techniques for the early diagnosis of cancer.

5.2.1 Paramagnetic Nanoparticles

Magnetic nanoparticles derived with carbohydrate coatings such as dextran have shown properties well suited for the diagnostic purposes. The superparamagnetic iron oxide nanoparticles (SPIONs) have been shown to facilitate in vivo imaging with the help of magnetic resonance. The nanoparticle-based contrast agents developed are more potent than the conventional Gd-based contrast agents for MRI, and SPIONs are the first to be approved for this purpose. SPIONs have the capability of passively targeting and detecting changes in the reticuloendothelial system. One of the major advantages of SPIONs is their ability to integrate physiologically with the target organs as opposed to the usual heavy metal-based contrast agents in MRI. The iron oxide contrast agents have less systemic toxicity as they disintegrate in the body, initially get stored in the reticuloendothelial system followed by slow elimination over a period of 2–4 weeks. Animal dose escalation studies have demonstrated the lack of identifiable side effects with iron oxide up to a dose of 100 mg/kg of iron. This is well above the dose of iron oxide (<5 mg/kg) used in MRI. Similarly, studies in human beings has shown a rise in mean hemoglobin levels by 1.0 g/dL over a period of 35 days following intravenous administration of iron oxide nanoparticles coated with semisynthetic carbohydrates (Jain et al. 2008). In an in vivo study, use of an alpha(nu)beta3-targeted nanoparticle to detect neovascularity induced by implantation of the rabbit Vx-2 tumor using MRI showed the potential of this targeted molecular imaging agent to identify and characterize early angiogenesis induced by minute solid tumors. These findings suggest that alpha(nu)beta3-targeted nanoparticle can be used for diagnosis as well as assessment of the effectiveness of antitumor treatment during follow-up (Winter et al. 2003). Similarly paramagnetic nonionic vesicles known as niosomes along with polyethylene glycol (PEG) and glucose conjugates on their surface showed significant improvement in the targeting of tumors overexpressing glucose receptors as assessed by MRI scan in a xenograft model of human carcinoma (Luciani et al. 2004).

Dextran-coated SPIONs can be used as a platform for the synthesis of multifunctional imaging agents. Many nanoparticles having iron cores and carbohydrate coatings have been approved for use in humans. The loading of iron oxide inside nanoparticle results in hydrophobicity and hence merging iron oxide with drug inside the nanoparticle could result in suboptimal loading and particle instability. Nanoparticle coated with dextran is used to make iron oxide hydrophilic and facilitate the internalization of iron oxide into the particle. Dextran-coated nanoparticles influence iron oxide's ability to deliver both hydrophilic and hydrophobic drugs. However, the success of iron oxide–dextran core design depends on the loading of iron oxide into nanoparticle, stability of the outer shell of nanoparticle, and the final size of the nanoparticle (Erten et al. 2010). Similarly, monocrystalline iron oxide nanoparticles (MIONs) and cross-linked iron oxide nanoparticles (CLIOs) form amine groups that act as substrates for conjugation with targeting ligands in the tumor site (Huang et al. 2010). CLIO and their derivatives enhance the diagnostic imaging ability of magnetic resonance, optical, and positron emission tomography (PET) modalities. Moreover, CLIO provides a flexible stage for linking the targeting ligands resulting in specific cell toxicity with minimal systemic adverse effects (Tassa et al. 2011). In a study done to evaluate the tumor angiogenesis targeting ability of anti-$\alpha v\beta 3$ antibody guided magnetoliposomes revealed greater signal enhancement along the peripheral tumor. This study demonstrated the superparamagnetic properties of magnetoliposomes and their ability to localize in the neovasculature resulting in sensitive detection of tumor angiogenesis (Yan et al. 2013). In the present scenario, molecular imaging of angiogenesis is emerging as a promising approach in early tumor detection apart from playing a vital role in tumor biology-related research and discovery of drugs to prevent angiogenesis. In addition studies done to confirm the microvascular localization of rhodamine-labeled magnetic fluid-loaded liposomes in brain using real-time in vivo imaging have shown that these nanocarriers can be magnetically targeted toward selected areas of the brain through the microvasculature. This shows that liposomes have a promising role to play in the diagnosis as well as treatment of brain tumors (Rivière et al. 2007).

5.2.2 Polyethylene Glycol-Coated (PEGylated) Gold Nanoparticles

Gold-based nanomaterials have applications in diverse biomedical branches due to their unique surface chemistry and optical properties. The characteristic features of gold-based nanoparticles like size-tunable surface plasmon resonance, fluorescence, and easy surface functionalization have been widely used in the application of biosensors, cancer cell imaging, photothermal therapy (PTT), and drug delivery (Chatterjee et al. 2011). AuNP irradiated with near-infrared (NIR) light produce adequate heat to treat tumor tissue and this process strongly depends on the targeting ability of the AuNPs, size, and dosing strategy (Puvanakrishnan et al. 2012). Gold nanoshell-enabled PTT (NEPTT) uses thermal conversion of NIR light for the eradication of tumor cells (Nguyen et al. 2012). Thus, gold nanoparticles have been suggested as a novel radiosensitizer in radiotherapy due to their strong photoelectric absorption and acceleration of DNA strand breakage (Glazer and Curley 2010; Kim et al. 2013). However, studies have found that gold nanoparticle with a coating may reduce radiosensitization due to emission of lesser intensity of low-energy photoelectrons (Xiao et al. 2011).

PEG-coated (PEGylated) gold nanoparticles (AuNPs) are anticipated as drug carriers and diagnostic contrast agents. However, the impact of particle characteristics on the biodistribution and pharmacokinetics of PEGylated AuNPs is not clear. AuNPs coated with high-molecular-weight PEG were found to be more stable than AuNPs coated with low-molecular-weight PEG. The toxicity of PEG-coated gold nanoparticles is complex especially with 10 and 60 nm particles having more toxicity compared to that of 5 and 30 nm particles (Zhang et al. 2011). Silver nanoparticles (AgNPs) of diameter around 35 nm conjugated with nuclear and cytoplasmic targeting peptides incubated in HSC-3 and HaCat cancer cell lines demonstrated that DNA double-strand breaks and the resultant increase in apoptotic (sub G1) population occur at a lower concentration compared to gold nanoparticles (Austin et al. 2011). These differences between the metals due to the altered structure need to be explored in the diagnosis of cancer.

The recombinant antibody fragments like scFvs and Fabs attached to carbon nanotubes (CNTs), nanowires, cantilevers, and QDs can be used for enhancing the detection of biomarkers even at a lower concentration (pg/mL). Nanoshells with the help of sensing technologies like "surface-enhanced Raman scattering" or electrochemical detection have the potential to be effectively used in the detection of cancer biomarkers. In the coming days such devices may replace the conventional time-consuming diagnostic methods (Kierny et al. 2012).

Metal nanoparticles owing to their resonant light-absorbing and light-scattering properties provide a new and powerful tool for innovative diagnostic approaches. Gold nanoparticles conjugated to anti-epidermal growth factor receptor (EGFR) antibodies can be used to increase the energy threshold and selectivity of laser PTT through their plasmonic enhanced nonlinear optical processes. The potential of antibody-conjugated gold nanoparticles to target and illuminate cancer cells under a reflectance-based optical imaging system has proven their ability to discriminate between normal and tumor cells. In addition, the conjugation of gold nanoparticles with antibodies allows them to detect the expression of relevant biomarkers for molecular imaging (Kah et al. 2007).

5.2.3 Carbon Nanotubes

CNTs, a hexagonal configuration made of carbon, are hollow cylindrical nanostructure with characteristic electrical properties. They can be either single-walled CNTs (SWCNTs) or multiwalled CNTs (MWCNTs) with diameter ranging between 0.3 and 100 nm. CNTs can be used either as an electrode in an oxidation–reduction electrochemical reaction or as field effect transistor (FET) that recognizes the changes on the surface of the nanostructure. This property of CNT is used to detect antigen using immunosandwich assay. The recent studies using SWCNTs displayed high-density antibody attachment with increased sensitivity. SWCNTs have been found to be useful in detecting sentinel lymph nodes in breast cancer (Koo et al. 2012). SWCNTs owing to their physiochemical properties are widely used in drug delivery, imaging, and PTT (Ma et al. 2012). Similarly, it has been found that ultrasound signal of functionalized MWCNTs is more than that of graphene oxide and SWCNTs. MWCNTs have been found to be highly effective in imaging organs like the liver and heart. Moreover, MWCNT can also be used to detect lung cancer as shown in Table 5.1 (Guo et al. 2012).

TABLE 5.1

Nanodiagnostics and Their Potential Applications in Cancer Detection

Nanodiagnostics	Potential Applications
Gold nanoprobes	Detection and quantification of BCR-ABL mRNA-related changes associated with chronic myeloid leukemia (CML)
HER2-RQDs (HER2 monoclonal antibody-conjugated RNase A-associated CdTe QD cluster)	Detection of gastric cancer in animal models
CNT-FET	Detection of prostate cancer marker
MWCNT	Detection of lung cancer
Chitosan–CNTs-AuNPs nanocomposite film	Detection of carcinoembryonic antigen (CEA)
Multilayered nanoprobes made of magnetic nanoparticles and QDs	Used in multimodality tumor imaging
Microfluidic beads with QDs	Detection of AFP, a cancer biomarker in hepatocellular cancer, germ cell tumor, liver metastasis, etc.
QDs	In vivo imaging of sentinel lymph nodes in breast cancer
EGF-QDs	Detect level of EGFR expression in both cell lines and xenograft tumor
Thermally cross-linked SPIONs (TCL-SPIONs)	Early detection of prostate cancer

5.2.4 Quantum Dots

QDs are semiconducting fluorescent nanocrystals with diameters ranging between 1 and 10 nm. These nanoparticles with unique optical properties have strong resistance to photobleaching, size-dependent emission of wavelength, high molar extinction coefficient, etc. while possessing excellent quantum yield. QDs conjugated to antibodies, oligonucleotide, aptamer, etc., or coated with streptavidin can be used to target the tumor cells. QDs are neither water soluble nor biocompatible but various approaches like silanization and surface coating with water-soluble ligands are being investigated to improve their biocompatibility (Azzazy et al. 2006).

QDs are a heterogeneous group of fluorescent nanoparticles with unique optical and chemical properties. This characteristic feature makes them the most promising agent for biomedical applications in diagnosis, monitoring, as well as in understanding of the molecular pathology and heterogeneity of cancer. They are composed of a central core of heavy metal like cadmium and outer layer of zinc sulfide. Their distinct features include size- and composition-tunable emission from visible to infrared wavelengths, large absorption coefficients across a wide spectral range, and very high levels of brightness as well as photostability compared with organic dyes. These features make them fascinating fluorescent probes for bio-imaging applications including in situ cell or tissue labeling, live cell imaging, and in vivo imaging. However, in vivo imaging using QDs have many limitations like interferences from tissue autofluorescence and dearth of light available at deeper tissue sites (Xing et al. 2008).

QDs have unique optical and electronic properties such as size-tunable light emission, improved signal brightness, resistance against photobleaching, and simultaneous excitation of multiple fluorescence colors. These properties are most promising for improving the sensitivity of molecular imaging and quantitative cellular analysis by one- to twofolds. Recent advances have led to multifunctional nanoparticle probes that are highly bright and stable under complex in vivo conditions. A new structural design involves encapsulating luminescent QDs with amphiphilic block copolymers and linking the polymer coating to tumor-targeting ligands and drug delivery functionalities (Wang et al. 2011).

Polymer-encapsulated QDs have been found to be nontoxic to cells and small animals, but their long-term in vivo toxicity and degradation need to be studied carefully. Nonetheless, bioconjugated QDs have raised new possibilities for ultrasensitive and multiplexed imaging of molecular targets in living cells and animal models (Gao and Dave 2007). QDs attached to EGFR and conjugated with antigrowth factor antibody were found to be effective in detecting early biomarkers of cervical cancer as well as molecular changes occurring during the process of cancer development. Similarly, QDs attached to prostate gland-specific monoclonal antibody when injected in nude mice with prostate tumor were found to aggregate around the prostate tumor cells (Gao et al. 2004). Studies have found that the EGF-QDs can be a suitable imaging agent to find out the level of EGFR expression in both cell lines and xenograft tumors (Chopra 2009). QDs have shown excellent photostability during continuous illumination of cancerous cells and tissues that make them sensitive reporters for early detection of breast cancer markers like HER2 (Tabatabaei-Panah et al. 2013).

Recently, the technique of dissection and the biopsy of the sentinel lymph node in breast cancer that needs manipulation of radioactive products have been studied using QDs. Moreover, the possible anaphylactic reactions to the dye have been overcome by using QDs. This shows evidence toward the potential of QDs being used as fluorescent contrast agents for in vivo imaging of sentinel lymph nodes. This fluorescent imaging property of QDs can be used for effective and rapid detection of sentinel lymph nodes using very low doses of QDs with minimally invasive method (Robe et al. 2008).

Self-illuminating QDs, known as QD-BRET (bioluminescence resonance energy transfer) conjugates, are a new class of QDs that do not need external light for excitation. In this case, light emission relies on the BRET from the attached luciferase enzyme, which emits light upon the oxidation of its substrate. QD-BRET with combined advantages of QDs holds the promise for improved deep tissue in vivo imaging (Xing et al. 2008). Animal studies with self-illuminating QD conjugates have shown increased sensitivity in imaging techniques compared to existing QDs. However, currently the in vivo application of QD conjugates is minimal due to instability of the first generation of QD-BRET probes in the blood or serum. Moreover, the means of decline in bioluminescence activity of QD-BRET probes has not been found so far (So et al. 2006).

A study done to develop microfluidic beads-based immunosensor with the help of multienzyme-nanoparticle amplification and QDs labels for sensitive detection of α-fetoprotein (AFP), a cancer biomarker that showed a potential approach toward the early detection of disease-related biomolecules at the most minuscule level (Zhang et al. 2012). Recently cadmium-free, biocompatible QDs with long fluorescence lifetimes have been shown to be superior bio-imaging probes as they suppress cell autofluorescence and improve the signal–background ratio. Such biocompatible QDs may be used for designing safe fluorescence imaging probes for novel diagnostic devices to detect early malignancies especially in breast cancer (Mandal et al. 2013). Multilayered nanoprobes made of magnetic nanoparticles and QDs are studied for multimodality tumor imaging (Ma et al. 2012).

5.2.5 Dendrimers

Dendrimers are nano-sized core shell structures that can be used for both drug delivery and drug development. Polyvalent dendrimers have the ability to interact with multiple drug targets. Similarly dendrimers conjugated with folic acid have a promising approach toward targeted drug therapy as they can be used to recognize the tumors with overexpressed folate receptors (Choi et al. 2005). Dendrimers are polymers of well-defined spherical structures of 1–10 nm in the diameter. Studies done so far with poly-amidoamine (PAMAM) spherical dendrimers have proven their safety when given through intravenous route. In addition, the development of PEGylated biocompatible dendrimers provides the stage for dendrimer-based diagnostics and therapeutics (Cheng et al. 2011). Thus, dendrimers can be applied to a range of cancer treatment with improved safety and efficacy. Moreover, the applications of dendrimers in photodynamic therapy, boron neutron capture therapy, and gene therapy are being explored in cancer treatment. Apart from improving cancer therapy, dendrimers by integrating with advanced contrast agents can help to improve diagnosis of tumors using imaging techniques like MRI. This will facilitate the development of newer contrast agents targeted toward the diseased site (Baker, Jr. 2009).

5.2.6 Micelles

Micelles are lipid-based nanoparticles with biocompatibility and they have the capacity to carry high concentration of MRI contrast agent. They are target specific with the potential to be used in multiple imaging techniques (Straathof et al. 2011). Polymeric micelles are expanding as stimuli-responsive targeted therapies with the capability to release both diagnostic and therapeutic agents into tumor cells concurrently (Gao et al. 2013; Lin et al. 2013). Micelles tinted with PLZ4 have been found to have likely possibility of being developed as imaging and therapeutic agents used to selectively target bladder cancer cells in dog (Lin et al. 2013). SPIONs synthesized by loading hydrophobic SPIONs into micelles assembled from an amphiphilic block copolymer bearing folate has shown increased diagnostic efficiency and less toxicity (Hong et al. 2012). Micelles are flexible contrast agent and possess characteristic features for performing multiple imaging methods (Straathof et al. 2011).

5.2.7 Nano-Immunochemotherapy

Nanoparticles can be designed to diagnose disease at the cellular level or deliver drug at the tumor site. This could be achieved with the aid of disease-specific receptors on the surface of the tumor cells providing useful targets for nanoparticles. Various nanostructures with effective site targeting can be developed by combining a diverse selection of targeting, diagnostic, and therapeutic components. Incorporating immune target specificity to nanostructures introduces a new type of treatment modality, known as nano-immunochemotherapy for patients with cancer (Kateb et al. 2011).

The multistage nanovectors (MSVs) comprise several nanocomponents, each designed to cross one or more biological barriers (Godin et al. 2011). Administration of a single dose of MSVs loaded with neutral nanoliposomes containing small interfering RNA (siRNA) targeted against the EphA2 oncoprotein-enabled sustained EphA2 gene silencing for at least 21 days was found to reduce tumor burden in orthotopic mouse model of ovarian cancer (Godin et al. 2011). In addition MSVs include stage 1 mesoporous silicon particles (S1MPs) that are rationally designed and fabricated in a nonspherical geometry to enable superior blood margination and to increase cell surface adhesion. The main task of S1MPs is to efficiently transport nanoparticles that are loaded into their porous structure and to protect them during transport from the administration site to the disease lesion. Semiconductor fabrication techniques including photolithography and electrochemical etching allow for the exquisite control and precise reproducibility of S1MP physical characteristics such as geometry and porosity. Furthermore, S1MPs can be chemically modified with negatively/positively charged groups, PEG, polymers, fluorescent probes, contrast agents, and biologically active targeting moieties like antibodies, peptides, aptamers, and phage.

5.3 Conclusion

Nanomedicine takes advantage of the progress in the field of nanotechnology, medicine, chemistry, physics, and biology to create promising drug carriers that accumulate at the tumor site. Nanomedicine provides the potential to design devices that can accurately detect biomarkers for specific diseases rapidly at an initial stage. Moreover, nanotechnology offers the chance to analyze DNA, RNA, and proteins thus providing the opportunity for more accurate as well as rapid diagnostic methods at molecular level. The multifunctionality of nanoparticles gives an edge over the conventional diagnostic methods in early detection and diagnosis of tumors. Thus, nanotechnology is going to be one of the major tools in the future for early cancer detection and diagnosis.

Nanoparticles vary widely in size, chemical composition, surface charge, tissue affinity, and sensitivity. The concern about the exploration of social and ethical issues of nanotechnology has begun only a few years ago. The metabolism and excretion of these particles from the body will be the most important issue for medical applications of nanomaterials in future. Nanomedicine-related research has become dynamic owing to the prospective biomedical applications. However, as of now very little information is known regarding intracellular effects the nanoparticles in humans and other living organisms. The distinct physicochemical properties of nanoparticles may also be associated with the risk of health hazards both in humans and other living organisms. The toxic effects of nanoparticles depend on various factors like amount of exposure, accumulation in the body, systemic distribution, as well as elimination. Hence, the most challenging concern regarding the use of nanotechnology in medicine is the safety-related issues that need to be sorted out before the widespread use of nanoparticles for diagnostic and therapeutic purposes. This has to be supported with universal standard guidelines regarding the application of nanotechnology in various branches of medicine.

References

Arayne MS, Sultana N. 2006. Review: Nanoparticles in drug delivery for the treatment of cancer. *Pak J Pharm Sci* 19:258–268.

Austin LA, Kang B, Yen CW, El-Sayed MA. 2011. Nuclear targeted silver nanospheres perturb the cancer cell cycle differently than those of nanogold. *Bioconjug Chem* 22:2324–2331.

Azzazy HM, Mansour MM, Kazmierczak SC. 2006. Nanodiagnostics: A new frontier for clinical laboratory medicine. *Clin Chem* 52:1238–1246.

Bae KH, Chung HJ, Park TG. 2011. Nanomaterials for cancer therapy and imaging. *Mol Cells* 31:295–302.

Baker JR, Jr. 2009. Dendrimer-based nanoparticles for cancer therapy. *Hematol Am Soc Hematol Educ Prog* 2009:708–719.

Bhati A, Garg H, Gupta A, Chhabra H, Kumari A, Patel T. 2012. Omics of cancer. *Asian Pac J Cancer Prev* 13:4229–4233.

Chatterjee DK, Diagaradjane P, Krishnan S. 2011. Nanoparticle-mediated hyperthermia in cancer therapy. *Ther Deliv* 2:1001–1014.

Cheng Y, Zhao L, Li Y, Xu T. 2011. Design of biocompatible dendrimers for cancer diagnosis and therapy: Current status and future perspectives. *Chem Soc Rev* 40:2673–2703.

Choi Y, Thomas T, Kotlyar A, Islam MT, Baker JR, Jr. 2005. Synthesis and functional evaluation of DNA-assembled polyamidoamine dendrimer clusters for cancer cell-specific targeting. *Chem Biol* 12:35–43.

Chopra A. 2009. Epidermal growth factor conjugated to near-infrared fluorescent quantum dots. Molecular Imaging and Contrast Agent Database (MICAD) [Internet]. Bethesda (MD): National Center for Biotechnology Information; 2004–2013. February 02, 2009 (Updated February 25, 2009).

Erten A, Wrasidlo W, Scadeng M, Esener S, Hoffman RM, Bouvet M, Makale M. 2010. Magnetic resonance and fluorescence imaging of doxorubicin-loaded nanoparticles using a novel in vivo model. *Nanomedicine* 6:797–807.

Fernandez-Fernandez A, Manchanda R, McGoron AJ. 2011. Theranostic applications of nanomaterials in cancer: Drug delivery, image-guided therapy, and multifunctional platforms. *Appl Biochem Biotechnol* 165:1628–1651.

Gao GH, Cui Y, Lee DS. 2013. Environmental pH-sensitive polymeric micelles for cancer diagnosis and targeted therapy. *J Control Release* 169:180–184.

Gao X, Cui Y, Levenson RM, Chung LW, Nie S. 2004. In vivo cancer targeting and imaging with semiconductor quantum dots. *Nat Biotechnol* 22:969–976.

Gao X, Dave SR. 2007. Quantum dots for cancer molecular imaging. *Adv Exp Med Biol* 620:57–73.

Gast MC, Van Gils CH, Wessels LF, Harris N, Bonfrer JM, Rutgers EJ, Schellens JH, Beijnen JH. 2009. Serum protein profiling for diagnosis of breast cancer using SELDI-TOF MS. *Oncol Rep* 22:205–213.

Glazer ES, Curley SA. 2010. Radiofrequency field-induced thermal cytotoxicity in cancer cells treated with fluorescent nanoparticles. *Cancer* 116:3285–3293.

Godin B, Tasciotti E, Liu X, Serda RE, Ferrari M. 2011. Multistage nanovectors: From concept to novel imaging contrast agents and therapeutics. *Acc Chem Res* 44:979–989.

Guo NL, Wan YW, Denvir J, Porter DW, Pacurari M, Wolfarth MG, Castranova V, Qian Y. 2012. Multiwalled carbon nanotube-induced gene signatures in the mouse lung: Potential predictive value for human lung cancer risk and prognosis. *J Toxicol Environ Health A* 75:1129–1153.

Hong GB, Zhou JX, Yuan RX. 2012. Folate-targeted polymeric micelles loaded with ultrasmall superparamagnetic iron oxide: Combined small size and high MRI sensitivity. *Int J Nanomed* 7:2863–2872.

Huang FK, Chen WC, Lai SF, Liu CJ, Wang CL, Wang CH, Chen HH et al. 2010. Enhancement of irradiation effects on cancer cells by cross-linked dextran-coated iron oxide (CLIO) nanoparticles. *Phys Med Biol* 55:469–482.

Jain TK, Reddy MK, Morales MA, Leslie-Pelecky DL, Labhasetwar V. 2008. Biodistribution, clearance, and biocompatibility of iron oxide magnetic nanoparticles in rats. *Mol Pharm* 5:316–327.

Kah JC, Kho KW, Lee CG, James C, Sheppard R, Shen ZX, Soo KC, Olivo MC. 2007. Early diagnosis of oral cancer based on the surface plasmon resonance of gold nanoparticles. *Int J Nanomed* 2:785–798.

Kateb B, Chiu K, Black KL, Yamamoto V, Khalsa B, Ljubimova JY, Ding H et al. 2011. Nanoplatforms for constructing new approaches to cancer treatment, imaging, and drug delivery: What should be the policy? *Neuroimage* 54:S106–S124.

Kateb B, Yamamoto V, Alizadeh D, Zhang L, Manohara HM, Bronikowski MJ, Badie B. 2010. Multi-walled carbon nanotube (MWCNT) synthesis, preparation, labeling, and functionalization. *Methods Mol Biol* 651:307–317.

Kierny MR, Cunningham TD, Kay BK. 2012. Detection of biomarkers using recombinant antibodies coupled to nanostructured platforms. *Nano Rev* 3:17240. [Epub ahead of print]

Kim JH, Chung CH, Chung BH. 2013. Colorimetric detection of UV light-induced single-strand DNA breaks using gold nanoparticles. *Analyst* 138:783–786.

Koo J, Jeon M, Oh Y, Kang HW, Kim J, Kim C, Oh J. 2012. In vivo non-ionizing photoacoustic mapping of sentinel lymph nodes and bladders with ICG-enhanced carbon nanotubes. *Phys Med Biol* 57:7853–7862.

Lin TY, Li YP, Zhang H, Luo J, Goodwin N, Gao T, White Rde V et al. 2013. Tumor-targeting multifunctional micelles for imaging and chemotherapy of advanced bladder cancer. *Nanomedicine (London, U.K.)*. 8:1239–1251.

Luciani A, Olivier JC, Clement O, Siauve N, Brillet PY, Bessoud B, Gazeau F et al. 2004. Glucose-receptor MR imaging of tumors: Study in mice with PEGylated paramagnetic niosomes. *Radiology* 231:135–142.

Ma X, Zhang LH, Wang LR, Xue X, Sun JH, Wu Y, Zou G et al. 2012. Single-walled carbon nanotubes alter cytochrome c electron transfer and modulate mitochondrial function. *ACS Nano* 6(12):10486–10496.

Mandal G, Darragh M, Wang YA, Heyes CD. 2013. Cadmium-free quantum dots as time-gated bioimaging probes in highly-autofluorescent human breast cancer cells. *Chem Commun (Cambridge, U.K.)* 49:624–626.

Nguyen HT, Tran KK, Sun B, Shen H. 2012. Activation of inflammasomes by tumor cell death mediated by gold nanoshells. *Biomaterials* 33:2197–2205.

Peller M, Schwerdt A, Hossann M, Reinl HM, Wang T, Sourbron S, Ogris M, Lindner LH. 2008. MR characterization of mild hyperthermia-induced gadodiamide release from thermosensitive liposomes in solid tumors. *Invest Radiol* 43:877–892.

Puvanakrishnan P, Park J, Chatterjee D, Krishnan S, Tunnell JW. 2012. In vivo tumor targeting of gold nanoparticles: Effect of particle type and dosing strategy. *Int J Nanomed* 7:1251–1258.

Rivière C, Martina MS, Tomita Y, Wilhelm C, Tran Dinh A, Ménager C, Pinard E et al. 2007. Magnetic targeting of nanometric magnetic fluid loaded liposomes to specific brain intravascular areas: A dynamic imaging study in mice. *Radiology* 244:439–448.

Robe A, Pic E, Lassalle HP, Bezdetnaya L, Guillemin F, Marchal F. 2008. Quantum dots in axillary lymph node mapping: Biodistribution study in healthy mice. *BMC Cancer* 8:111–118.

Ryvolova M, Chomoucka J, Drbohlavova J, Kopel P, Babula P, Hynek D, Adam V et al. 2012. Modern micro and nanoparticle-based imaging techniques. *Sensors (Basel)* 12:14792–14820.

Sandhiya S, Dkhar SA, Surendiran A. 2009. Emerging trends of nanomedicine—An overview. *Fundam Clin Pharmacol* 23:263–269.

So MK, Xu C, Loening AM, Gambhir SS, Rao J. 2006. Self-illuminating quantum dot conjugates for in vivo imaging. *Nat Biotechnol* 24:339–343.

Straathof R, Strijkers GJ, Nicolay K. 2011. Target-specific paramagnetic and superparamagnetic micelles for molecular MR imaging. *Methods Mol Biol* 771:691–715.

Surendiran A, Sandhiya S, Pradhan SC, Adithan C. 2009. Novel applications of nanotechnology in medicine. *Indian J Med Res* 130:689–701.

Tabatabaei-Panah AS, Jeddi-Tehrani M, Ghods R, Akhondi MM, Mojtabavi N, Mahmoudi AR, Mirzadegan E et al. 2013. Accurate sensitivity of quantum dots for detection of HER2 expression in breast cancer cells and tissues. *J Fluoresc* 23:293–302.

Tassa C, Shaw SY, Weissleder R. 2011. Dextran-coated iron oxide nanoparticles: A versatile platform for targeted molecular imaging, molecular diagnostics, and therapy. *Acc Chem Res* 44:842–852.

Wang T, Sridhar R, Korotcov A, Ting AH, Francis K, Mitchell J, Wang PC. 2011. Synthesis of amphiphilic triblock copolymers as multidentate ligands for biocompatible coating of quantum dots. *Colloids Surf A Physicochem Eng Asp* 375:147–155.

Winter PM, Caruthers SD, Kassner A, Harris TD, Chinen LK, Allen JS, Lacy EK et al. 2003. Molecular imaging of angiogenesis in nascent Vx-2 rabbit tumors using a novel alpha(nu)beta3-targeted nanoparticle and 1.5 tesla magnetic resonance imaging. *Cancer Res* 63:5838–5843.

Xiao F, Zheng Y, Cloutier P, He Y, Hunting D, Sanche L. 2011. On the role of low-energy electrons in the radiosensitization of DNA by gold nanoparticles. *Nanotechnology* 22:465101.

Xing Y, So MK, Koh AL, Sinclair R, Rao J. 2008. Improved QD-BRET conjugates for detection and imaging. *Biochem Biophys Res Commun* 372:388–394.

Yan C, Wu Y, Feng J, Chen W, Liu X, Hao P, Yang R et al. 2013. Anti-αvβ3 antibody guided three-step pretargeting approach using magnetoliposomes for molecular magnetic resonance imaging of breast cancer angiogenesis. *Int J Nanomed* 8:245–255.

Zhang H, Liu L, Fu X, Zhu Z. 2012. Microfluidic beads-based immunosensor for sensitive detection of cancer biomarker proteins using multienzyme-nanoparticle amplification and quantum dots labels. *Biosens Bioelectron* 42:23–30.

Zhang XD, Wu D, Shen X, Liu PX, Yang N, Zhao B, Zhang H et al. 2011. Size-dependent in vivo toxicity of PEG-coated gold nanoparticles. *Int J Nanomed* 6:2071–2081.

6

Mitochondrial DNA in Early Cancer Diagnosis and Screening

Mukesh Verma, Neelesh Agarwal, and Mudit Verma

CONTENTS

ABSTRACT Biomarkers are used in cancer detection, diagnosis, and prognosis. In cancer, most genetic markers are based on nuclear DNA; mitochondrial DNA (mtDNA) has not been utilized very extensively. This article provides information about using mtDNA alterations as biomarkers to detect different tumor types at early stages of carcinogenesis. Mitochondria play an important role in cellular energy metabolism, free radical generation, and apoptosis. Alterations in respiratory activity and mtDNA alterations are an integral part of carcinogenesis. Mitochondria contain their own genome along with their own transcription, translation, and protein assembly machinery. Because mtDNA lacks introns, it does not have histones and is more susceptible to oxidative damage and other environmental insults. It has been suggested that most mutations and deletions will occur in coding sequences, and the subsequent accumulation of mutations may lead to tumor formation. Mitochondrial mutations have been reported in bladder, brain, breast, colon, cervical, esophageal, gastric, liver, lung, and prostate cancers. Some of these mutations occur quite early during cancer development and can be used in screening large populations to identify high-risk individuals. Mitochondrial DNA alteration can be detected in biospecimens collected non-invasively. The implications of using mitochondrial information in identifying populations that are at high risk of developing cancer are discussed.

KEY WORDS: *cancer, detection, diagnosis, epidemiology, haplogroups, mitochondria, prognosis, risk assessment, screening, survival, treatment.*

Abbreviations

miRNA	microRNA
mtDNA	mitochondrial DNA
ROS	reactive oxygen species
PSA	prostate specific antigen

6.1 Introduction

Genomic, proteomic, metabolomic, epigenomic, and imaging biomarkers are commonly used in cancer risk assessment, early diagnosis, prognosis, therapy, and follow-up survival (Yu, 2011). The advantages of using DNA biomarkers include their stability and the ability to conveniently isolate them from different cells (Chauhan et al., 2007). In epidemiologic studies, in which thousands of samples are analyzed, biomarkers should be assayed using high-throughput methods from conveniently stored samples and assays should not be expensive (Verma and Kumar, 2007; Verma et al., 2003). Proteomic biomarkers represent functional aspects of carcinogenesis and are more informative than genomic markers; because of the low stability of proteins, however, it is inconvenient to utilize proteomic biomarkers in epidemiologic studies (Verma et al., 2003, 2006). In retrospective studies, biomarkers are tested on samples that have been stored for several years; most proteomic biomarkers are degraded if they are not stored properly (Verma et al., 2004). Metabolomic markers are better than proteomic markers because the end products of the assay represent results of biology undergoing disease development. Furthermore, disease-associated metabolites are very stable and can be measured easily with high sensitivity and specificity in biofluids such as urine, blood, nipple aspirate, saliva, cerebrospinal fluid (CSF), and pancreatic juice. Epigenetic biomarkers represent functional aspects against the genomic background. Although DNA methylation, histone modification, microRNA (miRNA) expression, and chromatin modeling biomarkers are the major epigenetic biomarkers, only DNA methylation biomarkers are currently suitable for epidemiologic studies (Banerjee and Verma, 2009; Kumar and Verma, 2009; Verma et al., 2004, 2006). Imaging markers are excellent in most of the cases but are very expensive and time-consuming. Mitochondrial DNA (mtDNA) biomarkers may provide information that is complementary to the information gained from other biomarkers that are used for early cancer detection, diagnosis, prognosis, and survival (Greaves et al., 2009).

6.2 Why Mitochondrial DNA Markers?

Mitochondria are 0.002–0.008 nm long, membrane-bound, semiautonomous organelles that supply energy to the cell through the process known as oxidative phosphorylation (Parr et al., 2006; Valko et al., 2006). Mitochondria are susceptible to environmental insults. They do not have a well-developed repair system, and because of their proximity to the respiratory chain, damage to the mtDNA is greater than the damage to the nuclear genome (Radpour et al., 2009). The mutational rate of mtDNA is approximately 10-fold higher than that of nuclear DNA (nDNA) (Ebner et al., 2011). For a long time, mitochondria were considered to be simply the powerhouse of the cell that supplies energy in the form of adenosine triphosphate (ATP). Later, reactive oxygen species (ROS) and free radical-based damage to mitochondria were linked with different steps in carcinogenesis (Czarnecka et al., 2006, 2010; Ishikawa et al., 2008; Ralph et al., 2010). Along with other proteins, oncoproteins also are transported to mitochondria and initiate mitochondrial malignant transformation programs (Kulawiec et al., 2006; Verma et al., 2003; Yu, 2011).

Mitochondrial dysfunction is a hallmark of cancer cells (Ospelt and Gay, 2005). Mutations (both germ line and somatic) in mitochondria have been detected in different tumor types (Lievre et al., 2006). However, it is not clear whether the mitochondrial genomic status of human cells affects nuclear genome stability and whether proteins involved in intergenomic cross talk are involved in tumorigenesis. Somatic mitochondrial mutations are common in human cancers and can be used as a tool for early detection of cancer (Parr et al., 2006). Selected mutations and tumor types are discussed later. The majority of these somatic mutations are homoplasmic in nature, indicating that the mutant mtDNA becomes dominant in tumor cells. mtDNA copy numbers were found to be correlated with the advancement of liver cancer (Yin et al., 2004). It has been suggested that the extent of mtDNA mutations might be useful in determining cancer prognosis and/or response to certain therapies (Krishnan and Birch-Machin, 2006).

Mitochondria have been implicated in the carcinogenesis process because of their role in apoptosis and other aspects of tumor biology. mtDNA is present in high copy numbers per cell in cancer cells (Yu, 2011). The number of copies per cell varies between the normal and disease states. These copy numbers are determined based on nuclear hemoglobin gene copy numbers in the nuclear genome. The mtDNA codes for 13 polypeptides (involved in oxidative phosphorylation), 2 rRNAs, and 22 tRNAs. One noncoding region, the displacement region or D-region, also exists and contains the origins of replication. It is believed that the early mitochondrial genome derived from symbiotic bacteria in proto-eukaryotic cells could have contained other genes that were lost or integrated into the nDNA during evolution. Effect of environment, radiation, and genotoxic substances on the generation of heteroplasmic and homoplasmic mitochondria is shown in Figure 6.1. Effects of free oxygen radicals and oxidative stress and their contribution in alterations of mitochondrial and nuclear genomes are shown in Figure 6.2.

Two approaches are used to understand the utility of mtDNA in cancer epidemiology: one approach is to look for somatic mutations in mitochondria and the other approach is to look for disease-associated haplogroups. The inheritance pattern of mitochondria in patients with cancer has been studied by

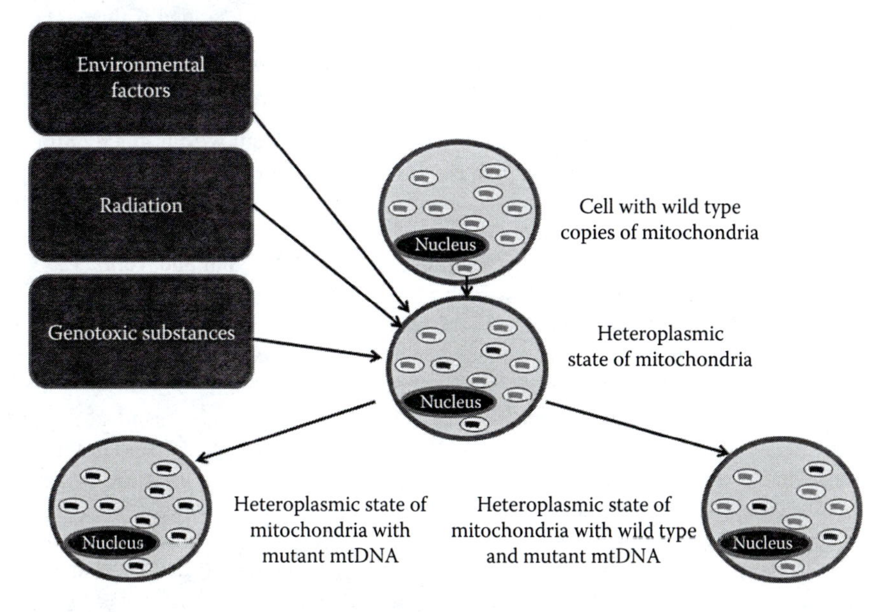

FIGURE 6.1 Effects of environment, radiation, and genotoxic substances on the generation of heteroplasmic and homoplasmic mitochondria.

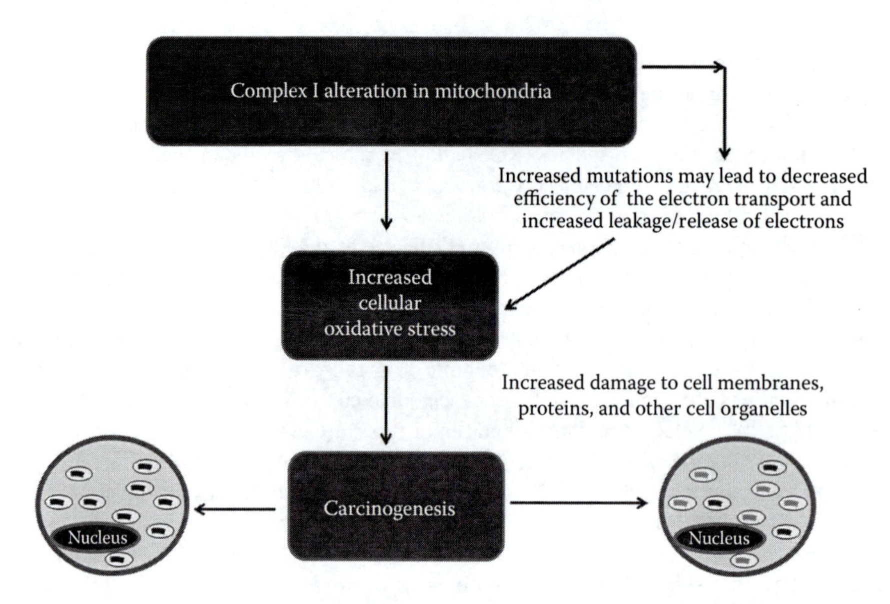

FIGURE 6.2 Alterations in mitochondrial and nuclear genomes due to oxidative stress and free radicals.

haplogroup analysis. Polymerase chain reaction of key polymorphic sites in the mitochondrial genome was performed in samples from cancer patients and normal individuals to determine if there is an association between mitochondrial genotype and cancer. Such an analysis has been accomplished in prostate and renal cancers.

mtDNA alterations are able to maintain genomic independence from the nucleus. However, as a consequence of protomitochondrial genes integrating into the nuclear genome throughout evolution, most mitochondrial proteins are encoded by nDNA and imported into the mitochondria. Quantification of the mitochondrial mutation load is easy to determine (Greaves et al., 2009).

6.3 Mitochondrial DNA in Different Cancers

Somatic mutations and germ line alterations in different tumor types are described in the following sections.

6.3.1 Bladder Cancer

According to data from the Surveillance, Epidemiology, and End Results (SEER) Program, in 2011, about 69,300 new bladder cancer cases were expected to be reported and about 15,000 people were expected to die as a result of this cancer (http://seer.cancer.gov/statfacts/html/urinb.html). Based on rates from 2006 to 2008, 2.41% of men and women born today will be diagnosed with cancer of the urinary bladder at some time during their lifetime. For analysis of mtDNA, human bladder cancer tissues were obtained by radical cystectomy and transurethral resection of bladder tumors (Chen et al., 2004; Dasgupta et al., 2008). Mutations were detected in the noncoding D-loop region and in different mtDNA genes. Deletions of variable lengths in mononucleotide repeats in the D-loop region, *ND2*, *ATPase 8*, and *COIII* genes also were observed. The repetitive sequences of mononucleotides within the mitochondria genome are known to be unstable and subject to deletions. The high incidence of mtDNA mutations in bladder cancer suggests that mtDNA and mitochondria could play an important role in the process of carcinogenesis and that mtDNA could be valuable as a marker for early bladder cancer diagnosis (Chen et al., 2004). In another study, urothelial carcinoma-specific mtDNA mutations were observed in 76% of patients (Yoo et al., 2010). Jakupciak et al. (2008) reported finding heteroplasmic mtDNA mutations in samples from bladder cancer patients. When mitochondrial genes ATPase6, CytB, ND1, and D310 were analyzed for bladder cancer-associated mutations in a population study, G8697A, G14905A, C15452A, and A15607G mutations were frequently observed (Guney et al., 2012).

6.3.2 Brain Cancer

SEER data estimated that there would be about 22,300 new cases and about 13,100 deaths from brain cancer in 2011. Mitochondrial pathways and energetics are critical in glioblastoma multiforme (Griguer and Oliva, 2011). Mutations in mtDNA also have been reported for glioblastoma (Krell et al., 2011). When the D-loop region of the mtDNA was analyzed to detect mutations in brain samples, 36% of the samples were found to contain mutations (Montanini et al., 2005). A follow-up study indicated that there was no correlation between these mutations and the aggressiveness of the disease. These mutations could be utilized for follow-up of the disease but not for diagnosis or prognosis (Montanini et al., 2005). In another study, CSF samples from medulloblastoma cases were analyzed to detect mtDNA mutations (Wong et al., 2003). A total of 18 mutations were detected in one-half of the samples analyzed (16); some of the mutations were found when treated samples were followed and the disease relapsed. This shows promise for future research using CSF in follow-up studies. Mutations also were reported in glioma (Montanini et al., 2005).

6.3.3 Breast Cancer

Breast cancer is the most prevalent cancer among women in the Western world. According to SEER data, in 2011, about 230,500 women were expected to be diagnosed with breast cancer and about 39,500 women were expected to die from breast cancer. Mutations and deletions have been reported in breast cancer by different groups of investigators (Canter et al., 2005; Gochhait et al., 2008; Singh et al., 2009; Tseng et al., 2011). Mutations in D310 region were reported during early development of breast cancer by Xu et al. (2012). Deletions ranged from 50 nucleotides to 4977 nucleotides (Radpour et al., 2009). The incidence of the 4977 base pair (bp) deletion and somatic mutations in the D-loop region were examined in breast cancer and adjacent tissues. Results indicated mutations in the D-loop region. Level of estrogen and survival data also were collected in this specific population in Taiwan. In another study, Zhu et al. reported several mutations in nipple aspirates collected from breast cancer patients (Zhu et al., 2005). In addition, an mtDNA G10398A polymorphism in breast cancer has been reported in African–American women (Canter et al., 2005; Darvishi et al., 2007). Two novel polymorphisms in the D-loop region were recently reported for breast cancer detection (Sultana et al., 2012).

6.3.4 Colon Cancer

Shimomura et al. (2011) reported mitochondrial mutations in traditional serrated adenomas of the colon. Other investigators also have reported mtDNA alterations in colorectal cancer (Czarnecka et al., 2006; Habano et al., 1999; Nooteboom et al., 2010). According to SEER data, in 2011, about 141,200 new cases were expected to be reported for colon cancer and about 49,400 deaths from colorectal cancer were expected. Colon cancer is divided into three histopathological categories: nonneoplastic polyps, neoplastic polyps (adenomatous polyps, adenomas), and cancers (Czarnecka et al., 2006). More than 95% of colon cancers are adenocarcinomas (Copeland et al., 2002). Vogelstein's group sequenced the mtDNA genome of 10 human cancer cell lines and found 12 different mutations in 7 of those 10 cell lines (Polyak et al., 1998). These mutations were localized in the protein-coding genes (*ND1*, *ND4L*, *ND5*, *COX subunit II* and *III*, *cytochrome b*) and in *rRNA* genes. This observation was confirmed by other investigators (Alonso et al., 1997; Copeland et al., 2002; Taylor et al., 2003). AT/GC transitions were observed in colon cancer samples by Alonso et al. (1997), and polycytidine tract mutations in the D-loop region and polyadenosine tract were observed by Habano et al. (1999). Although the D-loop region is only 1.12 kb long, numerous mutations are found in this region compared to the remaining mtDNA. The largest number of samples in which the D-loop region has been sequenced is 365, and the mutation rate was 38% (Czarnecka et al., 2006). A 3-year survival rate of 53% was observed in patients with mtDNA mutations, as opposed to a rate of 61% in patients without mutations. Thyagarajan et al. (2012) completed the first prospectively designed study in the Singapore Chinese Health Study and observed a U-shaped association between the relative mtDNA copy number and risk of colorectal cancer. Blood samples were used for this study from 422 colorectal cancer cases and 874 controls. Blood collection was from 168 prediagnosed cases and 254 postdiagnosed cases.

6.3.5 Endometrial Cancer

According to SEER data, in 2011, about 46,500 new cases of endometrial cancer were expected to be reported, and about 8,100 women were expected to die as a result of this cancer. Futyma et al. (2008) reported mtDNA4977 deletions in endometrial cancer. Somatic mutation, deletion, and microsatellite instability (MSI) were observed in a small (N = 50) endometrial cancer sample analysis. Mutations were located in the D-loop region and in the 12S and 16S *rRNA* genes; genomic instability was observed as a result of these mutations (Futyma et al., 2008; Liu et al., 2003). Mutational hot spot regions were located in the D-loop region and 12S *rRNA* genes. In a separate study, the *Cytb* gene region was found to be mutated when samples were collected from patients with gynecological malignancies as well as eight patients with benign gynecological tumors (Li et al., 2003). The malignant tumors were squamous cervical carcinomas, endometrial carcinomas, and epithelial ovarian cancers (EOCs); the benign tumors were ovarian epithelial tumors and uterine myomas. A mononucleotide repeat (D310) in mtDNA also has been identified as a mutational hot spot in cervical cancer (Parrella et al., 2003). Because individuals in these studies were not followed, it is not possible to say whether mtDNA is a marker of prognosis or how long the individuals survived.

6.3.6 Esophageal Cancer

According to SEER data, in 2011, about 17,000 new cases of esophageal cancer were expected to be reported, and about 14,700 people were expected to die from esophageal cancer. Somatic mutations of mtDNA have been reported to play an important role in the carcinogenesis of the esophagus and gastrointestinal tract (Gochhait et al., 2008; Tan et al., 2006). Samples of 82 esophageal cancers, 96 gastric cancers, and 138 colorectal cancers were examined to detect mtDNA mutations, and microsatellite assays were performed in the D310 mononucleotide repeat of mtDNA. The frequencies of mtDNA mutations were similar in esophageal, gastric, and colorectal cancers. No significant relationships were found between mtDNA mutations and patient age or sex, tumor location, depth of tumor invasion, and lymph node metastasis in each digestive tract cancer, which suggests that mtDNA mutations play a role in the development but not progression of each digestive tract cancer. The observations made in this study also suggest that the role of mtDNA mutations might be similar among the different digestive tract cancers. Another group of investigators reported frameshift mutations in the ND4L, ATP6 subunit, and *ND4* genes region and other mutations in the D-loop region (Tan et al., 2006).

6.3.7 Gastric Cancer

According to SEER data, in 2011, about 21,500 new cases of gastric cancer were expected to be reported, and about 10,300 people were expected to die from this disease. Gastric cancer is detected very late during disease development, and the 5-year survival rate is 10%–15%. Recently, Wei et al. (2011) reported finding a polymorphism in the D-loop region in gastric cancer. Somatic mutations in mtDNA have been detected in only 14% of gastric cancers (Hiyama et al., 2003; Hung et al., 2010; Kose et al., 2005). In another study, mutations in the *rRNA* gene of the mitochondria were found to be related to the development of gastric cancer (Hiyama et al., 2003). During the carcinogenesis process, heteroplasmic mtDNA was converted to homoplasmic DNA (Han et al., 2005). Mutations also have been reported in the D-loop region, and the number of mutations is higher in advanced stages of cancer compared to the early stages (Lee et al., 2005). ROS, apoptosis, and proliferation in the mutation group all were significantly higher than in the control group (Lee et al., 2005; Zhao et al., 2005). Shen et al. (2003) reported finding deletion of 4977 bp in gastric cancer. In another study, however, no correlation was observed between the presence of mutation in mtDNA and carcinogenesis (Martin et al., 2005). Validation of results from these two studies is needed to find a clear answer. *Helicobacter pylori* has been correlated with the development of gastric cancer, and Bax was found to be transported to mitochondria during this process (Ashktorab et al., 2004). No significant relationships were observed between mtDNA mutations and clinicopathological features such as patient age or sex, tumor location, depth of tumor invasion, and lymph node metastasis in gastric cancer.

6.3.8 Head and Neck Cancer

According to SEER data, in 2011, about 39,400 new cases of head and neck cancer were expected to be reported, and about 7,900 people were expected to die from this cancer. Parr's group observed mutations in mtDNA in head and neck cancer; some of these mutations were detected early in the carcinogenesis process (Parr et al., 2006). Head and neck cancer samples also were found to contain mutations in the D-loop region, although these mutations are not associated with the prognosis of head and neck cancer (Challen et al., 2011). These investigators suggested that mtDNA mutations in cancer might represent bystander genotoxic damage as a consequence of tumor development and progression. Mitochondrial mutations have been found in recurrent head and neck cancer tumors (Dasgupta et al., 2010).

6.3.9 Kidney Cancer

Samples from kidney cancer patients showed mitochondrial mutations in the D-loop region and in *rRNA* and *tRNA* genes (Meierhofer et al., 2006b; Nagy et al., 2002, 2003). Few groups have explored extensive mutation analysis in samples from kidney cancer patients (Sangkhathat et al., 2005). Germ line mitochondrial mutations in the succinate dehydrogenase gene were detected in kidney cancer samples (Housley et al., 2010). According to SEER data, in 2011, about 60,900 new cases were expected to be reported for kidney cancer, and about 13,100 people were expected to die from kidney cancer. Wada et al. (2006) reported mtDNA mutations and 8-hydroxy-2′ deoxyguanosine contents in the Japanese population in the United States.

6.3.10 Leukemia

According to SEER data, in 2011, about 44,600 new cases were expected to be reported for leukemia, and about 21,800 people were expected to die from this blood cancer. Meierhofer et al. (2006a) and Kwok et al. (2011) reported finding mtDNA mutations in leukemia. Most of the mutations were reported in the D-loop region in Kwok's study. Other groups also have reported mtDNA mutations in childhood leukemia (Sharawat et al., 2010). Previously somatic mtDNA mutations in isocitrate dehydrogenase 1 and 2 (IDH1 and IDH2) were reported in brain tumors and in a small proportion of acute myeloid leukemia (AML). This observational study led Chotirat et al. (2012) to conduct a large study with 230 newly diagnosed AML patients and evaluate the presence of mtDNA mutations in IDH1 and IDH2. About 19% of newly diagnosed patients had these mutations.

6.3.11 Liver Cancer

According to SEER data, in 2011, about 26,200 new cases of liver cancer were expected to be reported, and about 19,600 people were expected to die from this cancer. The mtDNA copy number was found to be correlated with advancement of liver cancer, but specific mutations in the D-loop region and specific deletions were not observed in liver cancer samples as compared to normal liver samples (Gwak et al., 2011; Lee et al., 2004; Wang et al., 2011; Wheelhouse et al., 2005; Yamada et al., 2006; Yin et al., 2004). A correlation was observed between tumor size and time of survival after the onset of disease. In another study, when a small number (n = 26) of samples from liver cancer patients who were undergoing interferon therapy after infection with the hepatitis C virus (HCV) was compared with biospecimens from liver cancer patients without HCV infection, the number of mutations in the mtDNA was found to be higher in the samples from the infected patients (Nishikawa et al., 2005). How the viral infection induces mtDNA mutation is not completely understood. A possible correlation between hepatitis B virus (HBV) infection and hepatocellular carcinoma (HCC) also was studied, and the number of mutations in the D-loop region was found to be higher in HBV-infected liver biopsy samples compared to age-matched normal tissues (Wheelhouse et al., 2005). In another study, fewer mtDNA mutations were observed compared to mutations in adjacent normal liver tissues (Tamori et al., 2004). Gwak et al. (2011) did not observe increased mutation rates in mtDNA or common 4977 bp deletion as a result of HBV infection or mutations in the HBV genome. Mitochondrial mutations also might indicate treatment outcomes in liver cancer (Wang et al., 2011).

6.3.12 Lung Cancer

Cigarette smoking in heavy smokers has been identified as a risk factor for lung cancer. ROS generated by cigarette smoke damage mtDNA. To compensate for the damage, cells produce a large number of mitochondrial copies. A case–control study (422 lung cancer patients and 504 controls) by Zheng et al. (2012) evaluated the role of mtDNA copy number and 822 bp deletions in cancer development. Multivariate logistic regression analysis indicated that haplogroups G and M7 might be risk factors for lung cancer, whereas haplogroups D and F were found to be related to individual lung cancer resistance. Lung cancer is a complex disease that has been divided into two categories: small-cell lung cancer (SCLC) and non-small-cell lung cancer (NSCLC). SCLC is further subtyped into small-cell, mixed small-cell/large-cell, and combined small-cell carcinoma. NSCLC is comprised of squamous cell carcinoma, adenocarcinoma, and large-cell carcinoma. D-loop mutations also have been reported in lung cancer patients (Dasgupta et al., 2012; Suzuki et al., 2003). In a high-throughput MitoChip assay, 18% of lung cancer samples had mutations in the mtDNA. Some of the mutations correlated with the stage of progression and prognosis in NSCLC (Matsuyama et al., 2003). In one report, most of the mtDNA lung cancer mutations that were investigated occurred randomly and were thought to have no impact on carcinogenesis, whereas the homoplasmic mutations might provide a potential diagnostic marker for lung cancer. Mutations in other regions also have been reported in lung cancer (Dai et al., 2006). According to SEER data, in 2011, about 221,100 new lung cancer cases were expected to be reported, and about 156,900 people were expected to die from lung cancer.

6.3.13 Oral Cancer

Each year in the United States, more than 21,000 men and 9,000 women are diagnosed with oral cancer. Oral cancer can develop in any part of the oral cavity (mouth and lips) or the part of the throat at the back of the mouth. Liu et al. (2012) reported mitochondrial mutations in the D-loop region of oral squamous carcinoma cells of 38 patients. This group also followed the effects of tobacco and betel chewing on the rate of mutations and correlated with overall survival. The focus of the mutation analysis was D-loop because this is a crucial site for replication and expression of mitochondrial genome as it holds the leading strand origin of replication and the main promoter for transcription of polycistronic message. Due to its triplet nature, this portion of the mtDNA is very variable and sensitive to external insults resulting in polymorphisms and mutations (Thyagarajan et al., 2012; Verma et al., 2003). The percentage of homoplasmic mutations in oral cancer was very high (68%) and 71% mutations were mononucleotide repeats located in the polycytidine stretch over 303nt of the mtDNA (Liu et al., 2012). Mitochondrial pathways are disturbed in oral cancer resulting in structure of genes (Lin et al., 2009).

6.3.14 Ovarian Cancer

According to SEER data, in 2011, about 22,000 new ovarian cancer cases were expected to be reported, and about 15,500 women were expected to die from this cancer. Histologically, three categories of ovarian cancer have been reported: ovarian epithelial cancer, sex cord–stromal tumors, and steroid cell tumors. The majority of tumors belong to the EOC category. Few reports have been published on mtDNA and ovarian cancer. In one study in which the D-loop region of 25 ovarian tumors was analyzed, 26 mutations were identified, resulting in a mutation rate of 32% (Shi et al., 2002). Another group screened several ovarian cancer samples to locate cancer-associated mutations but the mutations that were found had little clinical relevance (Bragoszewski et al., 2008). When multiple samples from the same patients were analyzed to detect mtDNA mutations, several mutations located in different regions of the genome were reported (Van Trappen et al., 2007). The 5-year survival rate for ovarian cancer is 25%.

6.3.15 Pancreatic Cancer

According to SEER data, in 2011, about 44,000 new pancreatic cancer cases were expected to be reported, and about 37,700 people were expected to die from this cancer. Pancreatic cancer mutations were identified in several genes, including *12S rRNA*, *16S rRNA*, *ND1*, *ND2*, *COXI*, *COXII*, *ATPase 6*, *COXIII*, *ND4*, *ND4L*, *ND5*, *ND6*, and *Cyt b*, as well as in the noncoding D-loop region (Jones et al., 2001). Analysis of other genes in the mtDNA molecule might demonstrate an even higher incidence of mtDNA somatic variants in patients (Kassauei et al., 2006). Germ line mtDNA variations exhibit associations with metabolism and outcome (Navaglia et al., 2006). In a recent epidemiologic study, haplogroup H contained the most mutations (Lam et al., 2012). This was a population-based, case–control study of 532 pancreatic cancer cases and 1701 controls that was conducted between 1994 and 2001 in the San Francisco Bay Area.

6.3.16 Prostate Cancer

Mitochondrial mutations have been reported in prostate cancer. For example, 6267G > A is a recurring mutation that introduces the Ala122Thr substitution in the mitochondrially encoded cytochrome c oxidase I (MT-CO1) (Gallardo et al., 2006; Petros et al., 2005). Most of the sequence variants were present in the D-loop region (52%), RNR2 (14%), and ND4 (13%) (Gomez-Zaera et al., 2006). Older age and a positive family history of prostate cancer are important risk factors (Jessie et al., 2001; Singh, 2006). Increased electron transport chain activity, increased oxygen consumption, and perhaps excess ROS production compared with normal prostate epithelial cells also might contribute to the development of prostate cancer (Feng et al., 2005; Schalken et al., 2005). Results from prostate-specific antigen (PSA) tests were compared with results from mtDNA alterations in prostate cancer samples, and the correlation between mutation rate and PSA level was observed (Kloss-Brandstätter et al., 2010). According to SEER data, about 240,900 new prostate cancer cases were expected to be reported in 2011, and about 33,700 men were expected to die from this cancer. Prostate cancer is the second most frequent cancer among men in the European Union and the most common cancer among men in the United States (Dakubo et al., 2006; Jeronimo et al., 2001).

6.3.17 Skin Cancer

According to SEER data, about 76,300 new skin cancer cases (excluding basal and squamous) were expected to be reported in 2011, and about 12,000 people were expected to die from this cancer. Multiple mtDNA deletions and tandem duplications have been reported in skin cancer (Hubbard et al., 2008; Krishnan and Birch-Machin, 2006; Mithani et al., 2008). These mutations have been used as biomarkers of photoaging in skin (Eshaghian et al., 2006; Krishnan and Birch-Machin, 2006). The most common deletions were 3715, 4977, and 6278 bp. Studies are being conducted in nonmelanoma skin cancer and photodamaged skin; it appears that more mutations are present in photodamaged skin. In another study, mtDNA instability in malignant melanoma of the skin was found to be restricted mostly to the nodular and metastatic stages (Poetsch et al., 2004). Induction of the common deletion was paralleled by a measurable decrease of oxygen consumption, mitochondrial membrane potential, and ATP content, as well as an increase of matrix metalloproteinase-1 (Berneburg et al., 2005). A high-throughput mitochondrial genome screening method also has been developed using multiplexed temperature gradient capillary electrophoresis (Girald-Rosa et al., 2005).

6.3.18 Thyroid Cancer

According to SEER data, in 2011, about 48,000 new thyroid cancer cases were expected to be reported, and about 1,700 people were expected to die from this cancer. Gasparre et al. (2007) demonstrated that disrupted mtDNA mutations can be markers of oncocytic phenotype in thyroid tumors. Other investigators have evaluated the presence of mtDNA mutations in thyroid cancer (Ding et al., 2010; Maximo et al., 2005; Tong et al., 2003). Witte et al. (2007) reported mtDNA mutations in differentiated thyroid cancer in older patients. Oncocytic tumors are proliferative lesions comprised of a high degree of mitochondrial hyperplasia that is frequent in the thyroid gland (Bonora et al., 2006). A literature survey did not show evidence of somatic mutations in mtDNA in other cancers such as leukemia and lymphoma.

6.4 Types of Samples Suitable for Isolating mtDNA and Mutation Analysis

A variety of clinical samples have been utilized to detect mtDNA mutations (Table 6.1). For example, tissues were used for thyroid cancer (Bonora et al., 2006; Maximo et al., 2005; Tong et al., 2003), nipple aspirate and paraffin-embedded specimens for breast cancer, urine for bladder cancer, buccal cells for head and neck cancer (Pai et al., 2006), CSF for medulloblastoma, and sputum for lung cancer (Pai et al., 2006). For epidemiologic studies in which thousands of samples are collected and analyzed, it is very important to determine which clinical samples should be collected. The procedure should be noninvasive and inexpensive. The characteristics of ideal biomarkers are shown in Figure 6.3.

TABLE 6.1

Patents in mtDNA Biomarkers in Cancer

Patent Application Reference	Inventor	Title	Remarks
US6649144	Zila, Inc., Phoenix, AZ	Methods for detecting and killing epithelial cells	A diagnostic method for detection of cancerous epithelial cells by selective marking of the mitochondria
US6605433	The Johns Hopkins University, Baltimore, MD	Mitochondria dosimeter	Determining mutation in D-loop region by PCR method Can be used for lung, head and neck, bladder, prostate, and pancreatic cancer detection
US8008008	Mitomics, Inc. Thunder Bay, Ontario, Canada	Mitochondrial mutations and rearrangements as a diagnostic tools for the detection of sun exposure, prostate cancer, and other cancers	Mutation detection in biological samples Deletion in regions covering genes encoding NADH dehydrogenase, tRNA histidine, tRNA serine2, and tRNA leucine 2

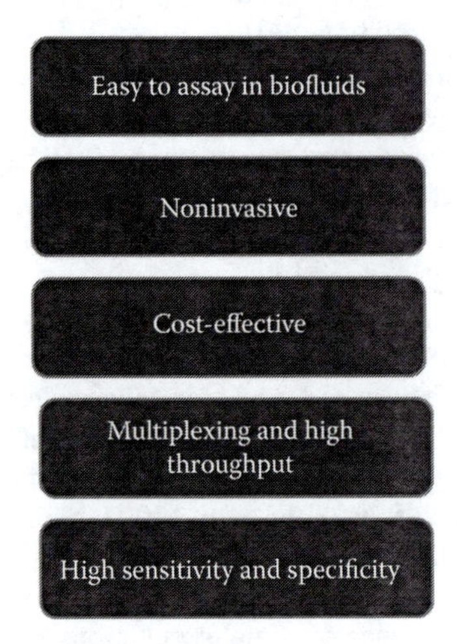

FIGURE 6.3 Characteristics of an ideal biomarker.

TABLE 6.2
Biospecimens Utilized for mtDNA Alterations in Cancer Detection

Biospecimens	References
Blood cells	Thyagarajan et al. (2012)
Buccal cells	Pai et al. (2006)
CSF	Wang et al. (2011)
Cervical swabs	Parrella et al. (2003)
Hair	Melton et al. (2012)
Nipple aspirate	Pai et al. (2006)
Paraffin-embedded specimens	Pai et al. (2006) and Xu et al. (2012)
Sputum	Pai et al. (2006)
Tissues	Bonora et al. (2006), Maximo et al. (2005), and Tong et al. (2003)
Urine	Pai et al. (2006)

6.5 Technological Advancements

Because of its small size, mtDNA is coprecipitated with nDNA and amplified using proper primers specific for mitochondria. However, microdissected samples have been used successfully to identify mtDNA mutations in clinical samples (Goebel et al., 2005). Pure populations of cells could be isolated from heterogeneous cells in the surgically isolated samples (Aldridge et al., 2003). The specificity of the mutational assays was 90%, whereas the sensitivity was 95% (Beck et al., 2010; Cai et al., 2011). Qiu et al. (2012) reported the sensitivity of the approach permitted detection of less than 5% mtDNA heteroplasmic levels. To understand the etiology of the disease and perform mitochondrial genotyping, a pure population of cells is needed. High-throughput microarray technologies (MitoChip) have been developed for somatic mutation detection (Kassauei et al., 2006; Maitra et al., 2004). Improved methods are needed to detect the integration of mtDNA in nDNA. Mitochondrial mutation detection assays have been patented (Table 6.2). Furukawa et al. (2012) developed MITO-Porter device that can be used to deliver chemicals and proteins in mitochondrial membrane to study the function of specific genes or study microenvironment inside the mitochondria. For complete genome of mitochondria, the term motogenome has been used (Meng et al., 2012).

6.6 Haplogroups in Mitochondria

Similar to nuclear genomic haplogroups, mitochondrial haplogroups have been reported (Darvishi et al., 2007; Ebner et al., 2011; Fang et al., 2010). mtDNA haplogroups have been used in characterizing admixed populations (Haber et al., 2012; Tofanelli et al., 2009). To understand the inheritance pattern of the mitochondrial genome in cancer, samples have been analyzed from different tissues (Darvishi et al., 2007). Haplogroup U, with an OR value of 1.95, also has been identified in prostate cancer samples. Inheritance of the U haplogroup is associated with a high risk of developing prostate cancer; about 20 million white individuals have this haplogroup. Thus far, nine mitochondrial haplogroups—H, I, J, K, T, U, V, W, and X—have been identified (Ebner et al., 2011; Li et al., 2011). The presence of a specific haplogroup predisposes an individual to a risk of prostate cancer. Haplogroup N contains the G10398A polymorphism, which is common in breast and esophageal cancer. Similar observations have been made for renal cancer. Haplotyping is performed by restriction analysis, whereas the whole mitochondrial genome is sequenced in mutation analysis.

6.7 Analytical and Clinical Validation of Mitochondrial Biomarkers

A number of biomarkers (SNPs, mutations, deletions, and copy number variances) have been reported by different investigators in different tumor types. However, results have not been verified or validated independently by other groups. As is true for other biomarkers, mitochondrial biomarkers should be validated: first by analytic techniques and then clinically. These processes are time-consuming and expensive but should be completed. Ideally, one national center should be created that can oversee the validation of biomarkers and coordinate all of the data generated from this research. The clinical implications of mitochondrial biomarker are shown in Figure 6.4. The implication of mitochondrial information in cancer epidemiology is summarized in Table 6.3. A few selected databases of mitochondrial information are presented in Table 6.4. The National Cancer Institute (NCI), National Institutes of Health, supports mitochondrial research in cancer etiology and cancer epidemiology where mtDNA biomarkers play a significant role. A few selected projects supported in this area are presented in Table 6.5. The Mitochondrial Medicine Society (http://mitosoc.org/blogs/about-us/) is an excellent resource for clinical application of mitochondrial-related information and getting updated about the criteria for mitochondrial biomarkers in different diseases and about other information related with mitochondrial diseases. The broad impact that Mitochondrial Medicine is now having on the biomedical sciences stems from the fact that traditional biomedical science has emphasized the tissue specificity of disease and the quantized genetics of Mendelian genes, while Mitochondrial Medicine also takes into account the systemic importance of energy and quantitative genetics of the mtDNA. Since the mitochondrial genome encompasses not only the energy genes of the mtDNA but also over 1500 nDNA genes that impact on mitochondrial structure and function, mitochondrial principles are providing new insights into the inheritance, development, and pathophysiology of a broad spectrum of clinical problems.

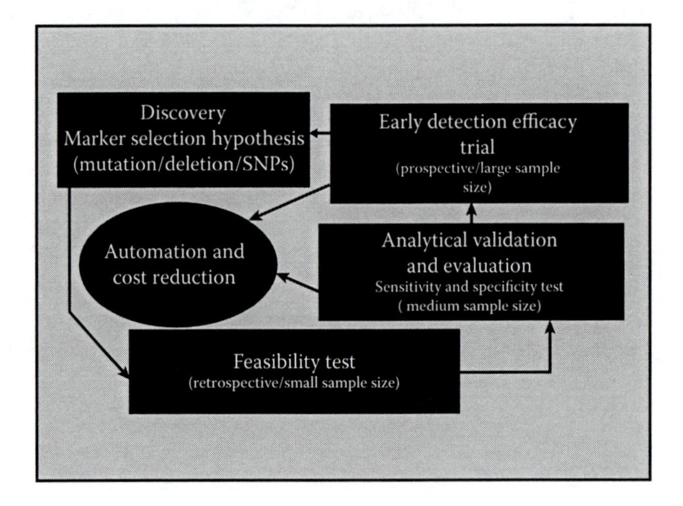

FIGURE 6.4 Clinical implication of mitochondrial markers.

TABLE 6.3

Implication of Mitochondrial Biomarker Information in Cancer Epidemiology

Implications
• Can we utilize mitochondrial haplogroup information to identify high-risk population?
• How can we utilize mitochondrial proteomic information to understand gene–gene and gene–environment studies and cancer etiology?
• Are different mitochondrial markers associated with development of cancer and are they mediated by specific nongenetic risk factors?
• Are mitochondrial markers useful for identification of high-risk groups before clinical onset of disease, and are they associated with recurrence of tumors?
• Can we utilize mitochondrial information to predict prognosis and better survival?

TABLE 6.4

Selected Databases for Mitochondrial Information

URLs of the Databases
• http://www.mitomap.org/MITOMAP
• http://mitowiki.research.chop.edu/MITOWIKI
• http://www.mtdb.igp.uu.se/
• http://www.smgf.org/pages/mtdatabase.jspx
• http://bioinfo.nist.gov/
• http://www.mrc-mbu.cam.ac.uk/faculty-and-research/mitominer

TABLE 6.5

Selected Projects Supported by the NCI, National Institutes of Health, in the Field of Cancer Epidemiology Where Mitochondrial Information Was Utilized

Subject of Projects Supported by NCI
Mitochondrial variants in metastatic breast cancer (CA173003)
An integrated study of mitochondrial pathways in colorectal cancer (oxidative stress and mutations) (CA172555)
mtDNA mutations in pancreatic cancer (CA133080)
Mitochondria as a novel biomarker of colorectal adenoma (CA167701)
Telomeric length, mitochondrial genome, oxidative stress, and breast cancer (CA155450)
mtDNA and ovarian cancer risk and survival (CA160669)
mtDNA copy number and skin cancer (CA165104)
The mitochondrial genome and ovarian cancer risk (CA149429)
mtDNA heteroplasmy and breast cancer risk (CA162131)
An association study of mtDNA variants and breast cancer risk (CA149435)

6.8 Concluding Remarks and Future Perspectives

Although problems still exist in the mtDNA field, mtDNA has potential to be used in the clinic, especially for risk assessment purposes. Areas requiring improvement include establishing a causative relationship between mitochondrial mutations and cancer development (an association with disease does not mean causation), identifying pathophysiological consequences of mtDNA alterations, validating already identified mtDNA mutation markers and polymorphisms in different populations, and assessing accidental amplification of nuclear mitochondrial pseudogenes (NUMTs) (Ospelt and Gay, 2005). Critical evaluation of mitochondrial primers is needed for high-quality results. Validating results in large numbers of population samples is recommended and has been adopted by a few investigators (Glazer et al., 2008). Correlating patient information (exposure history, lifestyle, BMI, alcohol consumption, smoking history, genetic background, and family history) with mitochondrial genetic alterations (copy number changes and mutations) should be accomplished before deriving any clinical inferences. No significant relationships have been identified between mtDNA mutations and clinicopathological features such as patient age or sex, tumor location, depth of tumor invasion, and lymph node metastasis in digestive tract cancers. Research in these directions is urgently needed. Some progress has been made in mitochondrial proteomics to identify new diagnostic and prognostic biomarkers of different tumor types (Bottoni et al., 2012).

The recent surge in mitochondrial research has been driven by the identification of mitochondria-associated diseases and the role of mitochondria in apoptosis. By virtue of their clonal nature and high copy numbers, mitochondrial mutations may provide a powerful molecular marker for the noninvasive detection of cancer. It has been suggested that the extent of mtDNA mutations might be useful in the prognosis of cancer outcome and/or response to certain therapies.

Although most cancer cells harbor somatic mutations in mtDNA, the question of whether such mutations contribute to the promotion of carcinomas remains unsolved. mtDNA mutations can initiate a cascade of events that leads to a continuous increase in the production of ROS (persistent oxidative stress), a condition that probably favors tumor development.

Mitochondria have been implicated in the process of carcinogenesis because of their vital role in energy production, nuclear–cytoplasmic signal integration, and control of metabolic pathways. Interestingly, at some point during neoplastic transformation, there is an increase in ROS, which damage the mitochondrial genome (Valko et al., 2006). This accelerates the somatic mutation rate of mtDNA. It has been proposed that these mutations may serve as an early indication of potential cancer development and may represent a means for tracking tumor progression.

The mechanisms responsible for the initiation and evolution of mtDNA mutations and their roles in the development of cancer, drug resistance, and disease progression are not completely understood. The mitochondrial genome is dependent upon the nuclear genome for transcription, translation, replication, and repair, but precise mechanisms for how the two genomes interact and integrate with each other are poorly understood. The relatively small size of the genome (16.5 kb) and the use of automated DNA sequencing make it possible to sequence the entire genome from clinical specimens in days.

The biggest challenge in this area is determining an accurate mtDNA copy number, because in some situations mtDNA becomes integrated into the nuclear genome at nonspecific sites. Another challenge is the simultaneous characterization of nuclear and mtDNA in cases and controls. Although this is technically possible, such studies have not yet been conducted within epidemiologic studies. Selection of sample is another problem. When mutations in blood DNA were compared with mutations in breast cancer tissues from the same patient, the mutations did not match. This suggests that blood might not be the appropriate biospecimen to use in such studies. Challenges exist in storing and mining data. There is general consensus that biology is transforming into an information science, and biomedical informatics is no longer an option but an integral component of all biomedical research. Traditional research methods must be complemented by comprehensive web and database searches for hypothesis generation. New computational methods and tools are constantly required to manage new types of data that often are unstructured, complex, massive, and nonintuitive. Peer-reviewed publications no longer provide the only source of fresh knowledge. Often, new discoveries are made by individuals who have the tools and skills to integrate and perform in-depth analyses of data from not only their own laboratories but, more importantly, from all accessible sources.

Replication of several studies mentioned in this chapter has not been completed. In epidemiology, replication of studies in different sets of participants with diverse exposure is very essential to reduce bias and confounding. Validation of findings also helps in identifying genetic variations that are influenced by environmental factors. Guidelines developed for proper reporting of observations and validation of biomarkers in molecular epidemiology should be followed.

Many challenges remain to be addressed before the use of information technology in everyday research is broadly accepted and adopted. These include the lack of user-friendly tools and training for bench biologists, especially in areas of emerging technologies, disengagement of tool builders and potential users, high overhead for data storage and dissemination, lack of common standards for data exchange, lack of computational infrastructure to accommodate new types of high-throughput data, and ineffective programs to attract computational scientists to the field of biology.

A coordination center (informatics forum) is needed that is responsible for (1) informing the research community about existing computational tools and resources, (2) disseminating technology from central institute supported tools, (3) gathering user feedback, and (4) identifying deficiencies in technology and critical needs through community consultation.

In summary, mtDNA information is promising and may lead to the identification of novel biomarkers for cancer detection, diagnosis, and follow-up of survival and treatment. It also might make it possible to identify populations that would be responsive to treatment.

Acknowledgment

I would like to thank to Joanne Brodsky of SCG, Inc., for reading the manuscript and providing suggestions.

References

Aldridge, B.A., Lim, S.D., Baumann, A.K., Hosseini, S., Buck, W., Almekinder, T.L., Sun, C.Q., and Petros, J.A. 2003. Automated sequencing of complete mitochondrial genomes from laser-capture microdissected samples. *Biotechniques* 35:606–607.

Alonso, A., Martin, P., Albarran, C., Aquilera, B., Garcia, O., Guzman, A., Oliva, H., and Sancho, M. 1997. Detection of somatic mutations in the mitochondrial DNA control region of colorectal and gastric tumors by heteroduplex and single-strand conformation analysis. *Electrophoresis* 18:682–685.

Ashktorab, H., Frank, S., Khaled, A.R., Durum, S.K., Kifle, B., and Smoot, D.T. 2004. Bax translocation and mitochondrial fragmentation induced by *Helicobacter pylori. Gut* 53:805–813.

Banerjee, H.N. and Verma, M. 2009. Epigenetic mechanisms in cancer. *Biomark. Med.* 3:397–410.

Beck, J., Urnovitz, H.B., Mitchell, W.M. et al. 2010. Next generation sequencing of serum circulating nucleic acids from patients with invasive ductal breast cancer reveals difference to healthy and nonmalignant control. *Mol. Can. Res.* 8:335–342.

Berneburg, M., Gremmel, T., Kürten, V. et al. 2005. Creatine supplementation normalizes mutagenesis of mitochondrial DNA as well as functional consequences. *J. Invest. Dermatol.* 125:213–220.

Bonora, E., Porcelli, A.M., Gasparre, G. et al. 2006. Defective oxidative phosphorylation in thyroid oncocytic carcinoma is associated with pathogenic mitochondrial DNA mutations affecting complexes I and III. *Cancer Res.* 66:6087–6096.

Bottoni, P., Giardina, B., Pontoglio, A. et al. 2012. Mitochondrial proteomic approaches for new potential diagnostic and prognostic biomarkers in cancer. *Adv. Exp. Med. Biol.* 942:423–440.

Bragoszewski, P., Kupryjanczyk, J., Bartnik, E., Rachinger, A., and Ostrowski, J. 2008. Limited clinical relevance of mitochondrial DNA mutation and gene expression analyses in ovarian cancer. *BMC Cancer* 8:292–296.

Cai, F.F., Kohler, C., Zhang, B. et al. 2011. Mutations of mitochondrial DNA as potential biomarkers in breast cancer. *Anticancer Res.* 31:4267–4271.

Canter, J.A., Kalianpur, A.R., Parl, F.F., and Millikan, R.C. 2005. Mitochondrial DNA G10398A polymorphism and invasive breast cancer in African American women. *Cancer Res.* 65:8028–8033.

Challen, C., Brown, H., Cai, C., Betts, G., Paterson, I., Sloan, P., West, C., Birch-Machin, M., and Robinson, M. 2011. Mitochondrial DNA mutations in head and neck cancer are infrequent and lack prognostic utility. *Br. J. Cancer* 104:1319–1324.

Chauhan, S.C., Kumar, D., Bell, M.C., Koch, M.D., and Verma, M. 2007. Molecular markers of miscellaneous primary and metastatic tumors of the uterine cervix. *Eur. J. Gynaecol. Oncol.* 28:5–14.

Chen, G.F., Chan, F.L., Hong, B.F., Chan, L.W., and Chan, P.S. 2004. Mitochondrial DNA mutations in chemical carcinogen-induced rat bladder and human bladder cancer. *Oncol. Rep.* 12:463–472.

Chotirat, S., Thongnoppakhun, W., Promsuwicha, O. et al. 2012. Molecular alterations of isocitrate dehydrogenase I and 2 (IDH1 and IDH2) metabolic genes and additional genetic mutations in newly diagnosed acute myeloid leukemia patients. *J. Hematol. Oncol.* 5:5–14.

Copeland, W.C., Wachsman, J.T., Johnson, F.M., and Penta, J.S. 2002. Mitochondrial DNA alterations in cancer. *Cancer Invest.* 20:557–569.

Czarnecka, A.M., Czarnecki, J.S., Kukwa, W., Cappello, F., Scińska, A., and Kukwa, A. 2010. Molecular oncology focus: Is carcinogenesis a "mitochondriopathy?" *J. Biomed. Sci.* 17:31–37.

Czarnecka, A.M., Golik, P., and Bartnik, E. 2006. Mitochondrial DNA mutations in human neoplasia. *J. Appl. Genet.* 47:67–78.

Dai, J.G., Xiao, Y.B., Min, J.X., Zhang, G.Q., Yao, K., and Zhou, R.J. 2006. Mitochondrial DNA 4977 BP deletion mutations in lung carcinoma. *Indian J. Cancer* 43:20–25.

Dakubo, G.D., Parr, R.L., Costello, L.C., Franklin, R.B., and Thayer, R.E. 2006. Altered metabolism and mitochondrial genome in prostate cancer. *J. Clin. Pathol.* 59:10–16.

Darvishi, K., Sharma, S., Bhat, A.K., Rai, E., and Bamezai, R.N. 2007. Mitochondrial DNA G10398A polymorphism imparts maternal Haplogroup N a risk for breast and esophageal cancer. *Cancer Lett.* 249:249–255.

Dasgupta, S., Hoque, M.O., Upadhyay, S., and Sidransky, D. 2008. Mitochondrial cytochrome B gene mutation promotes tumor growth in bladder cancer. *Cancer Res.* 68:700–706.

Dasgupta, S., Koch, R., Westra, W.H., Califano, J.A., Ha, P.K., Sidransky, D., and Koch, W.M. 2010. Mitochondrial mutation in normal margins and tumors of recurrent head and neck squamous cell carcinoma patients. *Cancer Prev. Res.* 3:205–1211.

Dasgupta, S., Soudry, E., Mukhopadhyay, N. et al. 2012. Mitochondrial DNA mutations in respiratory complex-I in never-smoker lung cancer patients contribute to lung cancer progression and associated with EGFR gene mutation. *J. Cell. Physiol.* 227:2451–2460.

Ding, Z., Ji, J., Chen, G., Fang, H., Yan, S., Shen, L., Wei, J., Yang, K., Lu, J., and Bai, Y. 2010. Analysis of mitochondrial DNA mutations in D-loop region in thyroid lesions. *Biochim. Biophys. Acta.* 1800:271–274.

Ebner, S., Lang, R., Mueller, E.E. et al. 2011. Mitochondrial haplogroups, control region polymorphisms and malignant melanoma: A study in middle European Caucasians. *PLoS One* 6:e27192.

Eshaghian, A., Vleugels, R.A., Canter, J.A., McDonald, M.A., Stasko, T., and Sligh, J.E. 2006. Mitochondrial DNA deletions serve as biomarkers of aging in the skin, but are typically absent in nonmelanoma skin cancers. *J. Invest. Dermatol.* 126:336–344.

Fang, H., Shen, L., Chen, T., He, J., Ding, Z., Wei, J., Qu, J., Chen, G., Lu, J., and Bai, Y. 2010. Cancer type-specific modulation of mitochondrial haplogroups in breast, colorectal and thyroid cancer. *BMC Cancer* 10:421–422.

Feng, T.H., Tsui, K.H., and Juang, H.H. 2005. Cholesterol modulation of the expression of mitochondrial aconitase in human prostatic carcinoma cells. *Chin. J. Physiol.* 48:93–100.

Furukawa, R., Yamada, Y., and Harashima, H. 2012. MITO-Porter; A cutting-edge technology for mitochondrial gene therapy. *Yakugaku Zasshi* 132:1389–1398.

Futyma, K., Putowski, L., Cybulski, M., Miotla, P., Rechberger, T., and Semczuk, A. 2008. The prevalence of mtDNA4977 deletion in primary human endometrial carcinomas and matched control samples. *Oncol. Rep.* 20:683–688.

Gallardo, M.E., Moreno-Loshuertos, R., Lopez, C., Casqueiro, M., Silva, J., Bonilla, F., Rodríguez de Córdoba, S., and Enríquez, J.A. 2006. m.6267G > A: A recurrent mutation in the human mitochondrial DNA that reduces cytochrome c oxidase activity and is associated with tumors. *Hum. Mutat.* 27:575–582.

Gasparre, G., Porcelli, A.M., Bonora, E. et al. 2007. Disruptive mitochondrial DNA mutations in complex I subunits are markers of oncocytic phenotype in thyroid tumors. *Proc. Natl. Acad. Sci. USA* 104:9001–9006.

Girald-Rosa, W., Vleugels, R.A., Musiek, A.C., and Sligh, J.E. 2005. High-throughput mitochondrial genome screening method for nonmelanoma skin cancer using multiplexed temperature gradient capillary electrophoresis. *Clin. Chem.* 51:305–311.

Glazer, C.A., Chang, S.S., Ha, P.K., and Califano, J.A. 2008. Applying the molecular biology and epigenetics of head and neck cancer in everyday clinical practice. *Oral Oncol.* 45:440–446.

Gochhait, S., Bhatt, A., Sharma, S., Singh, Y.P., Gupta, P., and Bamezai, R.N. 2008. Concomitant presence of mutations in mitochondrial genome and p 53 in cancer development—A study in north Indian sporadic breast and esophageal cancer patients. *Int. J. Cancer* 123:2580–2586.

Goebel, G., Zitt, M., and Muller, H.M. 2005. Circulating nucleic acids in plasma or serum (CNAPS) as prognostic and predictive markers in patients with solid neoplasias. *Dis. Markers* 21:105–120.

Gomez-Zaera, M., Abril, J., Gonzalez, L., Aguiló, F., Condom, E., Nadal, M., and Nunes, V. 2006. Identification of somatic and germline mitochondrial DNA sequence variants in prostate cancer patients. *Mutat. Res.* 595:42–51.

Greaves, L.C., Beadle, N.E., Taylor, G.A., Commane, D., Mathers, J.C., Khrapko, K., and Turnbull, D.M. 2009. Quantification of mitochondrial DNA mutation load. *Aging Cell* 8:566–572.

Griguer, C.E. and Oliva, C.R. 2011. Bioenergetics pathways and therapeutic resistance in gliomas: Emerging role of mitochondria. *Curr. Pharm. Des.* 17:2421–2427.

Guney, A.I., Ergec, D.S., Tavukcu, H.H. et al. 2012. Detection of mitochondrial mutations in nonmuscle invasive bladder cancer. *Genet. Test. Mol. Biomarkers* 16:672–678.

Gwak, G.Y., Lee, D.H., Moon, T.G., Choi, M.S., Lee, J.H., Koh, K.C., Paik, S.W., Joh, J.W., and Yoo, B.C. 2011. The correlation of hepatitis B virus pre-S mutation with mitochondrial D-loop mutations and common deletions in hepatocellular carcinoma. *Hepatogastroenterology* 58:522–528.

Habano, W., Sugai, T., Yoshida, T., and Nakamura, S. 1999. Mitochondrial gene mutation, but not large-scale deletion, is a feature of colorectal carcinomas with mitochondrial microsatellite instability. *Int. J. Cancer* 83:625–629.

Haber, M., Youhanna, S.C., Balanovsky, O. et al. 2012. mtDNA lineages reveal coronary artery disease-associated structures in the Lebanese population. *Ann. Hum. Genet.* 76:1–8.

Han, C.B., Ma, J.M., Xin, Y., Mao, X.Y., Zhao, Y.J., Wu, D.Y., Zhang, S.M., and Zhang, Y.K. 2005. Mutations of mitochondrial 12S rRNA in gastric carcinoma and their significance. *World J. Gastroenterol.* 11:31–35.

Hiyama, T., Tanaka, S., Shima, H. et al. 2003. Somatic mutation in mitochondrial DNA and nuclear microsatellite instability in gastric cancer. *Oncol. Rep.* 10:1837–1841.

Housley, S.L., Lindsay, R.S., Young, B., McConachie, M., Mechan, D., Baty, D., Christie, L., Rahilly, M., Qureshi, K., and Fleming, S. 2010. Renal carcinoma with giant mitochondria associated with germ-line mutation and somatic loss of the succinate dehydrogenase B gene. *Histopathology* 56:405–408.

Hubbard, K., Steinberg, M.L., Hill, H., and Orlow, I. 2008. Mitochondrial DNA deletions in skin from melanoma patients. *Ethn. Dis.* 18:S2-38–S2-43.

Hung, W.Y., Wu, C.W., Yin, P.H., Chang, C.J., Li, A.F., Chi, C.W., Wei, Y.H., and Lee, H.C. 2010. Somatic mutations in mitochondrial genome and their potential roles in the progression of human gastric cancer. *Biochim. Biophys. Acta.* 1800:264–270.

Ishikawa, K., Takenaga, K., Akimoto, M., Koshikawa, N., Yamaguchi, A., Imanishi, H., Nakada, K., Honma, Y., and Hayashi, J. 2008. ROS-generating mitochondrial DNA mutations can regulate tumor cell metastasis. *Science* 320:661–664.

Jakupciak, J.P., Maragh, S., Markowitz, M.E. et al. 2008. Performance of mitochondrial DNA mutations detecting early stage cancer. *BMC Cancer* 8:285–289.

Jeronimo, C., Nomoto, S., Caballero, O.L., Usadel, H., Henrique, R., Varzim, G., Oliveira, J., Lopes, C., Fliss, M.S., and Sidransky, D. 2001. Mitochondrial mutations in early stage prostate cancer and bodily fluids. *Oncogene* 20:5195–5198.

Jessie, B.C., Sun, C.Q., Irons, H.R., Marshall, F.F., Wallace, D.C., and Petros, J.A. 2001. Accumulation of mitochondrial DNA deletions in the malignant prostate of patients of different ages. *Exp. Gerontol.* 37:169–174.

Jones, J.B., Song, J.J., Hempen, P.M., Parmigiani, G., Hruban, R.H., and Kern, S.E. 2001. Detection of mitochondrial DNA mutations in pancreatic cancer offers a "mass"-ive advantage over detection of nuclear DNA mutations. *Cancer Res.* 61:1299–1304.

Kassauei, K., Habbe, N., Mullendore, M.E., Karikari, C.A., Maitra, A., and Feldmann, G. 2006. Mitochondrial DNA mutations in pancreatic cancer. *Int. J. Gastrointest. Cancer* 37:57–64.

Kloss-Brandstätter, A., Schäfer, G., Erhart, G., Hüttenhofer, A., Coassin, S., Seifarth, C., Summerer, M., Bektic, J., Klocker, H., and Kronenberg, F. 2010. Somatic mutations throughout the entire mitochondrial genome are associated with elevated PSA levels in prostate cancer patients. *Am. J. Hum. Genet.* 87:802–812.

Kose, K., Hiyama, T., Tanaka, S., Yoshihara, M., Yasui, W., and Chayama, K. 2005. Somatic mutations of mitochondrial DNA in digestive tract cancers. *J. Gastroenterol. Hepatol.* 20:1679–1684.

Krell, D., Assoku, M., Galloway, M., Mulholland, P., Tomlinson, I., and Bardella, C. 2011. Screen for IDH1, IDH2, IDH3, D2HGDH and L2HGDH mutations in glioblastoma. *PLoS One* 6:e19868.

Krishnan, K.J. and Birch-Machin, M.A. 2006. The incidence of both tandem duplications and the common deletion in mtDNA from three distinct categories of sun-exposed human skin and in prolonged culture of fibroblasts. *J. Invest. Dermatol.* 126:408–415.

Kulawiec, M., Arnouk, H., Desouki, M.M., Kazim, L., Still, I., and Singh, K.K. 2006. Proteomic analysis of mitochondria to nucleus retrograde response in human cancer. *Cancer Biol. Ther.* 5:967–975.

Kumar, D. and Verma, M. 2009. Methods in cancer epigenetics and epidemiology. *Methods Mol. Biol.* 471:273–288.

Kwok, C.S., Quah, T.C., Ariffin, H., Tay, S.K., and Yeoh, A.E. 2011. Mitochondrial D-loop polymorphisms and mitochondrial DNA content in childhood acute lymphoblastic leukemia. *J. Pediatr. Hematol. Oncol.* 33:e239–e244.

Lam, E.T., Bracci, P.M., Holly, E.A., Chu, C., Poon, A., Wan, E., White, K., Kwok, P.Y., Pawlikowska, L., and Tranah, G.J. 2012. Mitochondrial DNA sequence variation and risk of pancreatic cancer. *Cancer Res.* 72:686–695.

Lee, H.C., Li, S.H., Lin, J.C., Wu, C.C., Yeh, D.C., and Wei, Y.H. 2004. Somatic mutations in the D-loop and decrease in the copy number of mitochondrial DNA in human hepatocellular carcinoma. *Mutat. Res.* 547:71–78.

Lee, H.C., Yin, P.H., Lin, J.C., Wu, C.C., Chen, C.Y., Wu, C.W., Chi, C.W., Tam, T.N., and Wei, Y.H. 2005. Mitochondrial genome instability and mtDNA depletion in human cancers. *Ann. N. Y. Acad. Sci.* 1042:109–122.

Li, F.X., Ji, F.Y., Zheng, S.Z., Yao, W., Xiao, Z.L., and Qian, G.S. 2011. MtDNA haplogroups M7 and B in southwestern Han Chinese at risk for acute mountain sickness. *Mitochondrion* 11:553–558.

Li, H.X., Zhong, S., and Li, C.H. 2003. Study on the mitochondrion DNA mutation in tumor tissues of gynecologic oncology paticnts. *Zhonghua Fu Chan Ke Za Zhi* 38:290–293.

Lievre, A., Blons, H., Houllier, A.M., Laccourreye, O., Brasnu, D., Beaune, P., and Laurent-Puig, P. 2006. Clinicopathological significance of mitochondrial D-loop mutations in head and neck carcinoma. *Br. J. Cancer* 94:692–697.

Lin, S.Y., Lai, W.W., Ho, C.C. et al. 2009. Emodin induces apoptosis of human tongue squamous cancer SCC-4 cells through reactive oxygen species and mitochondrial dependent pathways. *Anticancer Res.* 29:327–335.

Liu, S.A., Jiang, R.S., Chen, F.J. et al. 2012. Somatic mutations in the D-loop of mitochondrial DNA in oral squamous cell carcinoma. *Eur. Arch. Otorhinolaryngol.* 269:1665–1670.

Liu, V.W., Yang, H.J., Wang, Y., Tsang, P.C., Cheung, A.N., Chiu, P.M., Ng, T.Y., Wong, L.C., Nagley, P., and Ngan, H.Y. 2003. High frequency of mitochondrial genome instability in human endometrial carcinomas. *Br. J. Cancer* 89:697–701.

Maitra, A., Cohen, Y., Gillespie, S.E. et al. 2004. The human MitoChip: A high-throughput sequencing microarray for mitochondrial mutation detection. *Genome Res.* 14:812–819.

Martin, R.C., Lan, Q., Hughes, K., Doll, M.A., Martini, B.D., Lissowska, J., Zatonski, W., Rothman, N., and Hein, D.W. 2005. No apparent association between genetic polymorphisms (−102 C>T) and (−9 T>C) in the human manganese superoxide dismutase gene and gastric cancer 1. *J. Surg. Res.* 124:92–97.

Matsuyama, W., Nakagawa, M., Wakimoto, J., Hirotsu, Y., Kawabata, M., and Osame, M. 2003. Mitochondrial DNA mutation correlates with stage progression and prognosis in non-small cell lung cancer. *Hum. Mutat.* 21:441–443.

Maximo, V., Lima, J., Soares, P., Botelho, T., Gomes, L., and Sobrinho-Simoes, M. 2005. Mitochondrial D-loop instability in thyroid tumours is not a marker of malignancy. *Mitochondrion* 5:333–340.

Meierhofer, D., Ebner, S., Mayr, J.A., Jones, N.D., Kofler, B., and Sperl, W. 2006a. Platelet transfusion can mimic somatic mtDNA mutations. *Leukemia* 20:362–363.

Meierhofer, D., Mayr, J.A., Fink, K., Schmeller, N., Kofler, B., and Sperl, W. 2006b. Mitochondrial DNA mutations in renal cell carcinomas revealed no general impact on energy metabolism. *Br. J. Cancer* 94:268–274.

Melton, T., Dimick, G., Higgins, B. et al. 2012. Mitochondrial DNA analysis of 114 hairs measuring less than 1 cm from a 19-year-old homicide. *Investig. Genet.* 3:12–13.

Meng, X., Shen, X., Zhao, N. et al. 2012. Mitogenomics reveals two subspecies in *Coelomactra antiquate* (Mollusca:Bivalvia). *Mitochondrial DNA* 24:102–104.

Mithani, S.K., Smith, I.M., Topalian, S.L., and Califano, J.A. 2008. Nonsynonymous somatic mitochondrial mutations occur in the majority of cutaneous melanomas. *Melanoma Res.* 18:214–219.

Montanini, L., Regna-Gladin, C., Eoli, M., Albarosa, R., Carrara, F., Zeviani, M., Bruzzone, M.G., Broggi, G., Boiardi, A., and Finocchiaro, G. 2005. Instability of mitochondrial DNA and MRI and clinical correlations in malignant gliomas. *J. Neurooncol.* 74:87–89.

Nagy, A., Wilhelm, M., and Kovacs, G. 2003. Mutations of mtDNA in renal cell tumours arising in end-stage renal disease. *J. Pathol.* 199:237–242.

Nagy, A., Wilhelm, M., Sükösd, F., Ljungberg, B., and Kovacs, G. 2002. Somatic mitochondrial DNA mutations in human chromophobe renal cell carcinomas. *Genes Chromosomes Cancer* 35:256–260.

Navaglia, F., Basso, D., Fogar, P. et al. 2006. Mitochondrial DNA D-loop in pancreatic cancer: Somatic mutations are epiphenomena while the germline 16519T variant worsens metabolism and outcome. *Am. J. Clin. Pathol.* 126:593–601.

Nishikawa, M., Nishiguchi, S., Kioka, K., Tamori, A., and Inoue, M. 2005. Interferon reduces somatic mutation of mitochondrial DNA in liver tissues from chronic viral hepatitis patients. *J. Viral Hepat.* 12:494–498.

Nooteboom, M., Johnson, R., Taylor, R.W., Wright, N.A., Lightowlers, R.N., Kirkwood, T.B., Mathers, J.C., Turnbull, D.M., and Greaves, L.C. 2010. Age-associated mitochondrial DNA mutations lead to small but significant changes in cell proliferation and apoptosis in human colonic crypts. *Aging Cell* 9:96–99.

Ospelt, C. and Gay, S. 2005. Somatic mutations in mitochondria: The chicken or the egg? *Arthritis Res. Ther.* 7:179–180.

Pai, C.Y., Hsieh, L.L., Lee, T.C., Yang, S.B., Linville, J., Chou, S.L., and Yang, C.H. 2006. Mitochondrial DNA sequence alterations observed between blood and buccal cells within the same individuals having betel quid (BQ)-chewing habit. *Forensic Sci. Int.* 156:124–130.

Parr, R.L., Dakubo, G.D., Thayer, R.E., McKenney, K., and Birch-Machin, M.A. 2006. Mitochondrial DNA as a potential tool for early cancer detection. *Hum. Genomics* 2:252–257.

Parrella, P., Seripa, D., Matera, M.G. et al. 2003. Mutations of the D310 mitochondrial mononucleotide repeat in primary tumors and cytological specimens. *Cancer Lett.* 190:73–77.

Petros, J.A., Baumann, A.K., Ruiz-Pesini, E. et al. 2005. mtDNA mutations increase tumorigenicity in prostate cancer. *Proc. Natl. Acad. Sci. USA* 102:719–724.

Poetsch, M., Dittberner, T., Petersmann, A., and Woenckhaus, C. 2004. Mitochondrial DNA instability in malignant melanoma of the skin is mostly restricted to nodular and metastatic stages. *Melanoma Res.* 14:501–508.

Polyak, K., Li, Y., Zhu, H., Lengauer, C., Willson, J.K., Markowitz, S.D., Trush, M.A., Kinzler, K.W., and Vogelstein, B. 1998. Somatic mutations of the mitochondrial genome in human colorectal tumors. *Nat. Genet.* 20:291–293.

Qiu, C., Kumar, S., Guo, J. et al. 2012. Mitochondrial single nucleotide polymorphism genotyping by matrix-assisted laser desorption/ionization time-of-flight mass spectrometry using cleavable biotinylated dideoxynucleotides. *Anal. Biochem.* 427:202–212.

Radpour, R., Fan, A.X., Kohler, C., Holzgreve, W., and Zhong, X.Y. 2009. Current understanding of mitochondrial DNA in breast cancer. *Breast J.* 15:505–509.

Ralph, S.J., Rodriguez-Enriquez, S., Neuzil, J., Saavedra, E., and Moreno-Sánchez, R. 2010. The causes of cancer revisited: "Mitochondrial malignancy" and ROS induced oncogenic transformation—Why mitochondria are targets for cancer therapy. *Mol. Aspects Med.* 31:145–170.

Sangkhathat, S., Kusafuka, T., Yoneda, A., Kuroda, S., Tanaka, Y., Sakai, N., and Fukuzawa, M. 2005. Renal cell carcinoma in a pediatric patient with an inherited mitochondrial mutation. *Pediatr. Surg. Int.* 21:745–748.

Schalken, J.A., Bergh, A., Bono, A. et al. 2005. Molecular prostate cancer pathology: Current issues and achievements. *Scand. J. Urol. Nephrol. Suppl.* 216:82–93.

Sharawat, S.K., Bakhshi, R., Vishnubhatla, S., and Bakhshi, S. 2010. Mitochondrial D-loop variations in paediatric acute myeloid leukaemia: A potential prognostic marker. *Br. J. Haematol.* 149:391–398.

Shen, H., Zhao, M., Dong, B., Tang, W., Xiao, B., Liu, J.Z., and Lu, Y.Y. 2003. Frequent 4 977 bp deletion of mitochondrial DNA in tumor cell lines, solid tumors and precancerous lesions of human stomach. *Zhonghua Yi Xue Za Zhi* 83:1484–1489.

Shi, H.H., Vincent, L., Hextan, N., and Yang, X.Y. 2002. Mutations in the D-loop region of mitochondrial DNA in ovarian tumors. *Zhongguo Yi Xue Ke Xue Yuan Xue Bao* 24:170–173.

Shimomura, T., Hiyama, T., Oka, S., Tanaka, S., Yoshihara, M., Shimamoto, F., and Chayama, K. 2011. Frequent somatic mutations of mitochondrial DNA in traditional serrated adenomas but not in sessile serrated adenomas of the colorectum. *J. Gastroenterol. Hepatol.* 26:1565–1569.

Singh, K.K. 2006. Mitochondria damage checkpoint, aging, and cancer. *Ann. N. Y. Acad. Sci.* 1067:182–190.

Singh, K.K., Ayyasamy, V., Owens, K.M., Koul, M.S., and Vujcic, M. 2009. Mutations in mitochondrial DNA polymerase-gamma promote breast tumorigenesis. *J. Hum. Genet.* 54:516–524.

Sultana, G.N., Rahman, A., Shahinuzzaman, A.D. et al. 2012. Mitochondrial DNA mutations—Candidate biomarkers for breast cancer diagnosis in Bangladesh. *Chin. J. Cancer.* 31:449–454.

Suzuki, M., Toyooka, S., Miyajima, K., Iizasa, T., Fujisawa, T., Bekele, N.B., and Gazdar, A.F. 2003. Alterations in the mitochondrial displacement loop in lung cancers. *Clin. Cancer Res.* 9:5636–5641.

Tamori, A., Nishiguchi, S., Nishikawa, M., Kubo, S., Koh, N., Hirohashi, K., Shiomi, S., and Inoue, M. 2004. Correlation between clinical characteristics and mitochondrial D-loop DNA mutations in hepatocellular carcinoma. *J. Gastroenterol.* 39:1063–1068.

Tan, D.J., Chang, J., Liu, L.L., Bai, R.K., Wang, Y.F., Yeh, K.T., and Wong, L.J. 2006. Significance of somatic mutations and content alteration of mitochondrial DNA in esophageal cancer. *BMC Cancer* 6:93–96.

Taylor, R.W., Barron, M.J., Borthwick, G.M. et al. 2003. Mitochondrial DNA mutations in human colonic crypt stem cells. *J. Clin. Invest.* 112:1351–1360.

Thyagarajan, B., Wang, R., Barcelo, H. et al. 2012. Mitochondrial copy number is associated with colorectal cancer risk. *Cancer Epi. Biom. Prev.* 21:1574–1581.

Tofanelli, S., Bertoncini, S., Castrì, L., Luiselli, D., Calafell, F., Donati, G., and Paoli, G. 2009. On the origins and admixture of Malagasy: New evidence from high-resolution analyses of paternal and maternal lineages. *Mol. Biol. Evol.* 26:2109–2124.

Tong, B.C., Ha, P.K., Dhir, K., Xing, M., Westra, W.H., Sidransky, D., and Califano, J.A. 2003. Mitochondrial DNA alterations in thyroid cancer. *J. Surg. Oncol.* 82:170–173.

Tseng, L.M., Yin, P.H., Yang, C.W., Tsai, Y.F., Hsu, C.Y., Chi, C.W., and Lee, H.C. 2011. Somatic mutations of the mitochondrial genome in human breast cancers. *Genes Chromosomes Cancer* 50:800–811.

Valko, M., Rhodes, C.J., Moncol, J., Izakovic, M., and Mazur, M. 2006. Free radicals, metals and antioxidants in oxidative stress-induced cancer. *Chem. Biol. Interact.* 160:1–40.

Van Trappen, P.O., Cullup, T., Troke, R., Swann, D., Shepherd, J.H., Jacobs, I.J., Gayther, S.A., and Mein, C.A. 2007. Somatic mitochondrial DNA mutations in primary and metastatic ovarian cancer. *Gynecol. Oncol.* 104:129–133.

Verma, M., Kagan, J., Sidransky, D., and Srivastava, S. 2003. Proteomic analysis of the cancer cell mitochondria. *Nat. Rev. Cancer* 3:789–795.

Verma, M. and Kumar, D. 2007. Application of mitochondrial genome information in cancer epidemiology. *Clin. Chim. Acta* 383:41–50.

Verma, M., Maruvada, P., and Srivastava, S. 2004. Epigenetics and cancer. *Crit. Rev. Clin. Lab. Sci.* 41:585–607.

Verma, M., Seminara, D., Arena, F.J., John, C., Iwamoto, K., and Hartmuller, V. 2006. Genetic and epigenetic biomarkers in cancer: Improving diagnosis, risk assessment, and disease stratification. *Mol. Diagn. Ther.* 10:1–15.

Wada, T., Tanji, N., Ozawa, A., Wang, J., Shimamoto, K., Sakayama, K., and Yokoyama, M. 2006. Mitochondrial DNA mutations and 8-hydroxy-2′-deoxyguanosine content in Japanese patients with urinary bladder and renal cancers. *Anticancer Res.* 26:3403–3408.

Wang, C., Zhang, F., Fan, H., Peng, L., Zhang, R., Liu, S., and Guo, Z. 2011. Sequence polymorphisms of mitochondrial D-loop and hepatocellular carcinoma outcome. *Biochem. Biophys. Res. Commun.* 406:493–496.

Wei, L., Zhao, Y., Guo, T.K., Li, P.Q., Wu, H., Xie, H.B., Ma, K.J., Gao, F., and Xie, X.D. 2011. Association of mtDNA D-loop polymorphisms with risk of gastric cancer in Chinese population. *Pathol. Oncol. Res.* 17:735–742.

Wheelhouse, N.M., Lai, P.B., Wigmore, S.J., Ross, J.A., and Harrison, D.J. 2005. Mitochondrial D-loop mutations and deletion profiles of cancerous and noncancerous liver tissue in hepatitis B virus-infected liver. *Br. J. Cancer* 92:1268–1272.

Witte, J., Lehmann, S., Wulfert, M., Yang, Q., and Röher, H.D. 2007. Mitochondrial DNA mutations in differentiated thyroid cancer with respect to the age factor. *World J. Surg.* 31:51–59.

Wong, L.J., Lueth, M., Li, X.N., Lau, C.C., and Vogel, H. 2003. Detection of mitochondrial DNA mutations in the tumor and cerebrospinal fluid of medulloblastoma patients. *Cancer Res.* 63:3866–3871.

Xu, C., Tran-Thann, D., Ma, C. et al. 2012. Mitochondrial D310 mutations in the early development of breast cancer. *Br. J. Cancer.* 106:1506–1511.

Yamada, S., Nomoto, S., Fujii, T., Kaneko, T., Takeda, S., Inoue, S., Kanazumi, N., and Nakao, A. 2006. Correlation between copy number of mitochondrial DNA and clinico-pathologic parameters of hepatocellular carcinoma. *Eur. J. Surg. Oncol.* 32:303–307.

Yin, P.H., Lee, H.C., Chau, G.Y., Wu, Y.T., Li, S.H., Lui, W.Y., Wei, Y.H., Liu, T.Y., and Chi, C.W. 2004. Alteration of the copy number and deletion of mitochondrial DNA in human hepatocellular carcinoma. *Br. J. Cancer* 90:2390–2396.

Yoo, J.H., Suh, B., Park, T.S., Shin, M.G., Choi, Y.D., Lee, C.H., and Choi, J.R. 2010. Analysis of fluorescence in situ hybridization, mtDNA quantification, and mtDNA sequence for the detection of early bladder cancer. *Genet. Cytogenet.* 198:107–117.

Yu, M. 2011. Generation, function and diagnostic value of mitochondrial copy number alterations in human cancers. *Life Sci.* 89:65–71.

Zhao, Y.B., Yang, H.Y., Zhang, X.W., and Chen, G.Y. 2005. Mutation in D-loop region of mitochondrial DNA in gastric cancer and its significance. *World J. Gastroenterol.* 11:3304–3306.

Zheng, S., Qian, P., Li, F. et al. 2012. Association of mitochondrial DNA variations with lung cancer risk in a Han Chinese population from southwestern China. *PLoS One* 7:e31322.

Zhu, W., Qin, W., Bradley, P., Wessel, A., Puckett, C.L., and Sauter, E.R. 2005. Mitochondrial DNA mutations in breast cancer tissue and in matched nipple aspirate fluid. *Carcinogenesis* 26:145–152.

7

Circulating miRNA Biomarkers in Various Solid Cancers

Martina Redova, Hana Mlcochova, and Ondrej Slaby

CONTENTS

ABSTRACT MicroRNAs (miRNAs) comprise an abundant class of endogenous, small noncoding RNAs, 18–25 nucleotides in length that posttranscriptionally regulate gene expression through binding to target mRNAs. Ability of miRNAs to inhibit translation of oncogenes and tumor suppressor genes implies their involvement in carcinogenesis. In the last decade, the number of evidences that miRNAs might contribute to the regulation of apoptosis, cellular proliferation, and differentiation is constantly growing. Specific miRNA expression signatures have been identified in a variety of human cancers. Recently, miRNAs' occurrence in the blood serum and plasma, where their levels are more stable, reproducible, and consistent among individuals of the same species, has been repeatedly observed. Circulating miRNAs have been successfully evaluated in various human cancers as promising novel noninvasive biomarkers of the early disease onset or its relapse. In this chapter, we describe the origin of circulating miRNAs, the principles of their immense stability, and proposed functions and comprehensively summarize studies focusing their significance in breast, colorectal, lung, and prostate cancer, proposing their potential application in clinical routine as relevant biomarkers.

KEY WORDS: *microRNA, body fluids, biomarkers, breast cancer, colorectal cancer, lung cancer, prostate cancer.*

7.1 miRNAs Are Relevant Cancer Biomarkers

MicroRNAs (miRNAs) are important regulators of gene expression that control both physiological and pathological processes, comprising an abundant class of endogenous, small noncoding RNAs. They are capable of either promoting mRNA degradation or attenuating protein translation. However, recently, it has been reported that several miRNAs could increase mRNA translation under some special cellular conditions (Vasudevan et al., 2007). miRNAs may serve as master regulators of many fundamental biological processes, such as embryogenesis, organ development, cellular differentiation, proliferation, and apoptosis, affecting such major biological systems as stemness, immunity, and cancer (Alvarez-Garcia and Miska, 2005, Carthew et al., 2009, Croce, 2009, Xiao and Rajewsky, 2009, Winter and Diedrichs, 2011). Bioinformatics and cloning studies have estimated that miRNAs may regulate up to 50% of all human genes and each miRNA can control hundreds of gene targets. Some miRNAs are expressed in a cell-specific, tissue-specific, and/or developmental stage-specific manner, while others are expressed ubiquitously (Calin and Croce, 2006). Moreover, the number of verified miRNAs is still growing—the latest version of miRBase (release 19.0, August 2012) has annotated over 1600 precursor and 2042 mature sequences in the human genome. Based on the annotations for the genomic position of miRNAs, which indicated that a vast majority of miRNAs is located in intergenic regions (>1 kb away from annotated or predicted genes), it has been postulated that most miRNA genes are transcribed as autonomous transcription units (Carthew et al., 2009).

Canonical biogenesis (Figure 7.1) of miRNAs follows three main steps: (1) transcription of primary transcript (pri-miRNA), generally driven by RNA polymerase II, followed by (2) its partial processing into a precursor miRNA (pre-miRNA) by the ribonuclease (RNase) Drosha in the nucleus, and (3) after nuclear transport using GTP-dependent transport protein Exportin 5, its final maturation into a miRNA duplex by the protein complex Dicer/TRBP in the cytoplasm (Beezhold et al., 2010, Siomi and Siomi, 2010). The leading strand from this duplex is finally incorporated into the RNA-induced silencing complex (RISC), which guides the complex into (1) the complementary 3′- or 5′-untranslated region (UTR) of the target mRNA, which control many aspects of mRNA metabolism, such as transport, localization, efficiency of translation and stability; (2) open reading frames; and (3) promoter regions (Lee et al., 2009, Krol et al., 2010). Recently, it has been shown that in some specific cases, both strands of the miRNA duplex are functional, which is contradictory to previous reports that the passenger strand is unwounded and degraded after incorporation of guide strand to the multiprotein RISC (Hu et al., 2009, Slaby and Sana, 2012).

Based on genome-wide miRNA expression profiling studies using high-throughput technologies, it has been repeatedly reported that miRNAs are commonly dysregulated in a wide range of human cancers, acting as either oncogenes or tumor suppressor genes, and actually, several miRNAs were observed to act as both oncogenes and tumor suppressors in various cancers and different cellular contexts (Hanahan and Wienberg, 2011). Different miRNA expression patterns in various malignancies may potentially serve as relevant biomarkers of cancer diagnosis, prognosis, and response to treatment. Moreover, if compared to mRNA, miRNAs are remarkably stable in routinely collected, formalin-fixed paraffin-embedded (FFPE) clinical tissues, as well as in fresh snap-frozen specimens (Li et al., 2007). Detecting miRNAs in the sera of various animal species (including human, mouse, rat, bovine, and horse) by stem-loop quantitative real-time polymerase chain reaction (qRT-PCR), it has been observed that levels of miRNAs in serum were reproducible and consistent among individuals of the same species (Chen et al., 2008).

An ideal tumor marker should be easily, reliably, and cost-effectively measured employing a minimally invasive assay with high analytical sensitivity and specificity. It is generally accepted that disease-related biomarkers, that is, antigens, enzymes, and lipid components, could be shed from the tissue or cells with ongoing disease and be present in blood. Among currently available blood-based biomarkers, carcinoembryonic antigen (CEA) (commonly used marker for colon cancer), cytokeratin 19 fragment (CYFRA21–1), alpha-fetoprotein (AFP) (associated marker for hepatocellular carcinoma), prostate-specific antigen (PSA), etc., holding a potential of analyzing tumors without involving a biopsy or a surgical procedure, could be mentioned (Huber et al., 1992, Schneider et al., 2000). Unfortunately, all these routinely used biomarkers express low sensitivities and specificities.

Circulating miRNAs, also known as cell-free miRNAs, represent a great promise as a new class of reliable minimally invasive cancer diagnostic, prognostic, and predictive. This potential could be

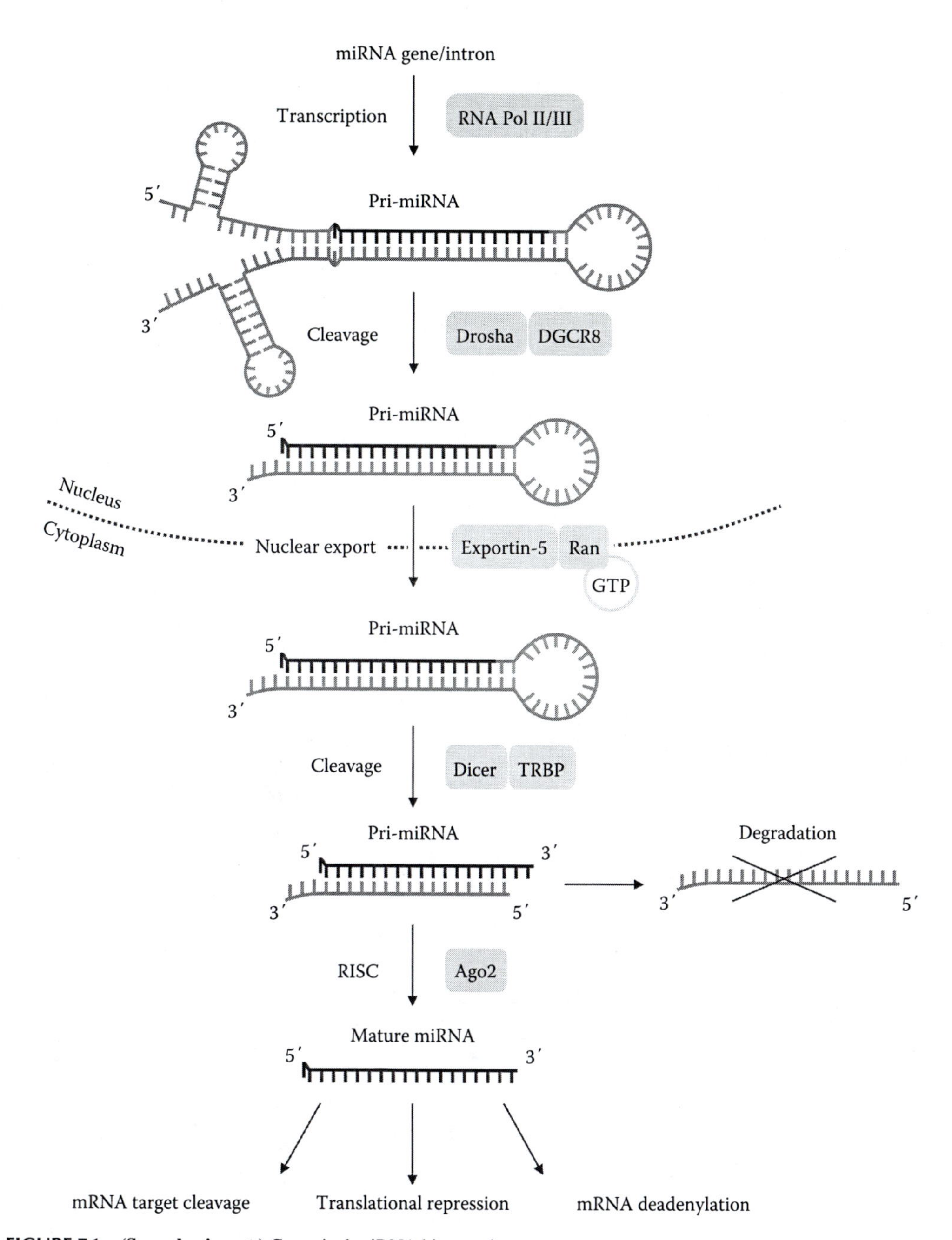

FIGURE 7.1 **(See color insert.)** Canonical miRNA biogenesis.

explained by the strikingly high stability of miRNAs in serum/plasma, association with disease state, and relative simplicity of sensitive and specific measurement. There are a number of studies focusing on the importance of circulating miRNAs in various human malignancies, including breast (Heneghan et al., 2010b), colorectal (Ng et al., 2009), lung (Mitchell et al., 2008), prostate (Bryant et al., 2012, Kelly et al., 2013), hepatocellular (Shigoka et al., 2010), gastric (Tsujiura et al., 2010, Valladares-Ayerbes et al., 2012), renal (Redova et al., 2012), and nasopharyngeal (Zeng et al., 2012) cancer. Furthermore, miRNAs have been described to be stable also in other body fluids such as urine, saliva, milk, and cell culture supernatants (Chen et al., 2008, Mitchell et al., 2008, Park et al., 2009). Studies focusing circulating miRNAs as potential biomarkers in various solid cancers are listed in Table 7.1.

TABLE 7.1

Studies Focusing Circulating miRNAs as Potential Biomarkers in Solid Cancer

Body Fluid	Study Design	Sample Size	miRNAs Examined	Technique	Normalization	Promising miRNAs	References
Breast cancer							
Serum	Tumor vs. normal	13 patients vs. 8 HC	3	qRT-PCR	18S rRNA	miR-155	Roth et al. (2010)
Whole blood	Tumor vs. normal	83 patients vs. 63 HC	7	qRT-PCR	miR-16	miR-195, let-7a	Heneghan et al. (2010a)
Plasma	Tumor vs. normal	20 patients vs. 20 HC in screening/ 25 patients vs. 25 HC in validation	31+18 in screening/2+2 in validation	Illumina microarray-based expression profiling/qRT-PCR	miR-16 in validation	miR-425*, miR-302b, let-7c	Zhao et al. (2010)
Serum	Tumor vs. normal	56 patients vs. 10 HC	4	qRT-PCR	miR-16	miR-125b	Schrauder et al. (2012)
Serum	Stages II–III locally advanced and inflammatory BC receiving neoadjuvant chemotherapy	42 patients in screening/26 patients in validation	800 in screening/8 in validation	Solexa deep sequencing/ qRT-PCR	miR-16 in validation	miR-375, miR-122	Wu et al. (2012)
Serum	Tumor vs. normal	89 patients vs. 29 HC	4	qRT-PCR	miR-16	miR-155, miR-34a, miR-10b	Roth et al. (2010)
Whole blood	Tumor vs. normal	48 patients vs. 57 HC in screening/ 24 patients vs. 24 HC in validation	2 in validation	Geniom biochip array/qRT-PCR	miR-16 in validation	miR-202	Schrauder et al. (2012)
Colorectal cancer							
Plasma	Tumor vs. normal/ correlation with tu. resection	5 CRC/healthy plasma + 5 CRC/adjacent normal tissue in screening; 25 patients vs. 25 HC in validation I; 90 CRC patients vs. 50 HC + 40 patients with other dg. in validation II	95 in screening/5 in validation I/2 in validation II	qRT-PCR array/ qRT-PCR	RNU6B	miR-17-3p, miR-92	Ng et al. (2009)
Plasma	Tumor vs. normal/ correlation with tu. resection and TNM stage	20 patients vs. 20 HC in screening; 80 CRC/ 37 advanced adenomas vs. 39 HC in validation	12 in screening/2 in validation	qRT-PCR	miR-16	miR-29, miR-92a	Huang et al. (2010)

Plasma	Tumor vs. normal/ correlation with tu. resection	30 CRC vs. 30 adjacent healthy tissue in screening; 16 CRC vs. 16 adjacent healthy tissue in validation I; 30 patients (plasma) vs. 30 HC in validation II; 20 patients (plasma) vs. 20 HC in validation III	4	qRT-PCR array/ qRT-PCR	RNU6B	miR-21, miR-31	Bandres et al. (2006)
Whole blood	Tumor vs. normal	63 patients vs. 45 HC	7	qRT-PCR	miR-425	miR-34a	Li et al. (2011)
Serum	Tumor vs. normal/ correlation with liver metastasis	38 metastatic sera vs. 36 nonmetastatic sera in screening; 20 CRC vs. 20 adjacent healthy tissue in validation	3	qRT-PCR	miR-16	miR-29a	Wang and Gu (2012)
Plasma	Tumor vs. normal/ correlation with distant metastasis	21 metastatic CRC tissue vs. 24 nonmetastatic CRC tissue in screening; 102 patients (plasma) vs. 156 HC in validation	3 in validation	qRT-PCR array/ qRT-PCR	cel-miR-39	miR-141	Cheng et al. (2011)
Plasma	Tumor vs. normal	103 patients vs. 37 HC	3	qRT-PCR	Serial dilutions	miR-221	Pu et al. (2010)
Lung cancer							
Serum	Tumor vs. normal	Pool in screening; 152 patients vs. 75 HC in validation	2 in validation	Solexa deep sequencing/ qRT-PCR	Total RNA	miR-25, miR-223	Chen et al. (2008)
Serum	Long vs. short survival (study on prognosis)	30 long survivals vs. 30 short survivals in screening; 120 patients in training set; 123 patients in testing set	4 in training and testing	Solexa deep sequencing/ qRT-PCR	Control healthy serum sample	miR-486, miR-30d, miR-1, miR-499	Hu et al. (2010)
Serum	Stages I–IV NSCLC	24 patients in stage I, 52 in stage II, 54 in stage III, 63 in stage IV	1	qRT-PCR	$2^{50\text{-Ct}}$	miR-125b	Yuxia et al. (2012)
Serum	Tumor vs. normal	21 NSCLC patients vs. 11 HC in screening; 97 NSCLC patients + 20 patients with benign lung disease vs. 30 HC in validation	2 in validation	Microarray profiling (microfluid biochips)/qRT-PCR	RNU6B, miR-1233	miR-361-3p, miR-625*	Roth et al. (2012)
Plasma	Tumor vs. normal	74 patients (different subtypes and stages) vs. 68 HC	6	qRT-PCR	Serial dilutions	miR-155, miR-197, miR-182	Zheng et al. (2011)

(continued)

TABLE 7.1 (continued)
Studies Focusing Circulating miRNAs as Potential Biomarkers in Solid Cancer

Body Fluid	Study Design	Sample Size	miRNAs Examined	Technique	Normalization	Promising miRNAs	References
Prostate cancer							
Plasma	Tumor vs. normal	25 patients vs. 25 HC	6	qRT-PCR	cel-miR-39, cel-miR-54, cel-miR-238	miR-141	Bryant et al. (2012)
Serum	Low vs. high grade; correlation with tu. progression	7 low grade vs. 14 high grade in screening; 45 patients in validation I; 71 patients in validation II	5 in validation I; 2 in validation II	qRT-PCR array/ qRT-PCR	cel-miR-39, cel-miR-54, cel-miR-238	miR-141, miR-375	Brase et al. (2011)
Serum	Tumor vs. normal	36 patients vs. 12 HC	96 in screening; 12 in validation	Multiplex qRT-PCR/ qRT-PCR	Subtracting the corresponding median for every sample and multiplex	miR-223, -874, -1207-5p, -24, 106a, -26b, -30c, -93, 1274a, 451	Moltzahn et al. (2011)

Note: HC, healthy controls; tu, tumor; qRT-PCR, quantitative reverse transcription polymerase chain reaction; dg, diagnosis; BC, breast cancer; CRC, colorectal cancer; NSCLC, non-small cell lung cancer.

7.1.1 Circulating miRNA Origin

Regarding the establishment of circulating miRNA-based novel cancer-relevant biomarker, it is of great importance to clarify the origin of such miRNAs (Figure 7.2) and their relationship with the disease onset. Lawrie et al. were the first who described miRNAs in circulation. They compared the levels of three cancer-associated miRNAs (miR-155, miR-210, and miR-21) in the serum of diffuse large B cell lymphoma (DLBCL) patients with those of healthy volunteers and described that DLBCL patients had generally higher levels of serum miRNAs than controls and, more interestingly, that high levels of miR-21 are associated with the longer relapse-free survival of these patients (Lawrie et al., 2008). Soon after that, Mitchell et al. demonstrated that plasma miRNAs, originating from human prostate cancer (PCa) xenografts, could be readily measured by miRNA cloning and TaqMan qRT-PCR (Mitchell et al., 2008).

Comparing the expression levels of miRNAs in various serum samples including serum from patients with lung cancer, colorectal cancer (CRC), and diabetes, Chen et al. observed significant differences

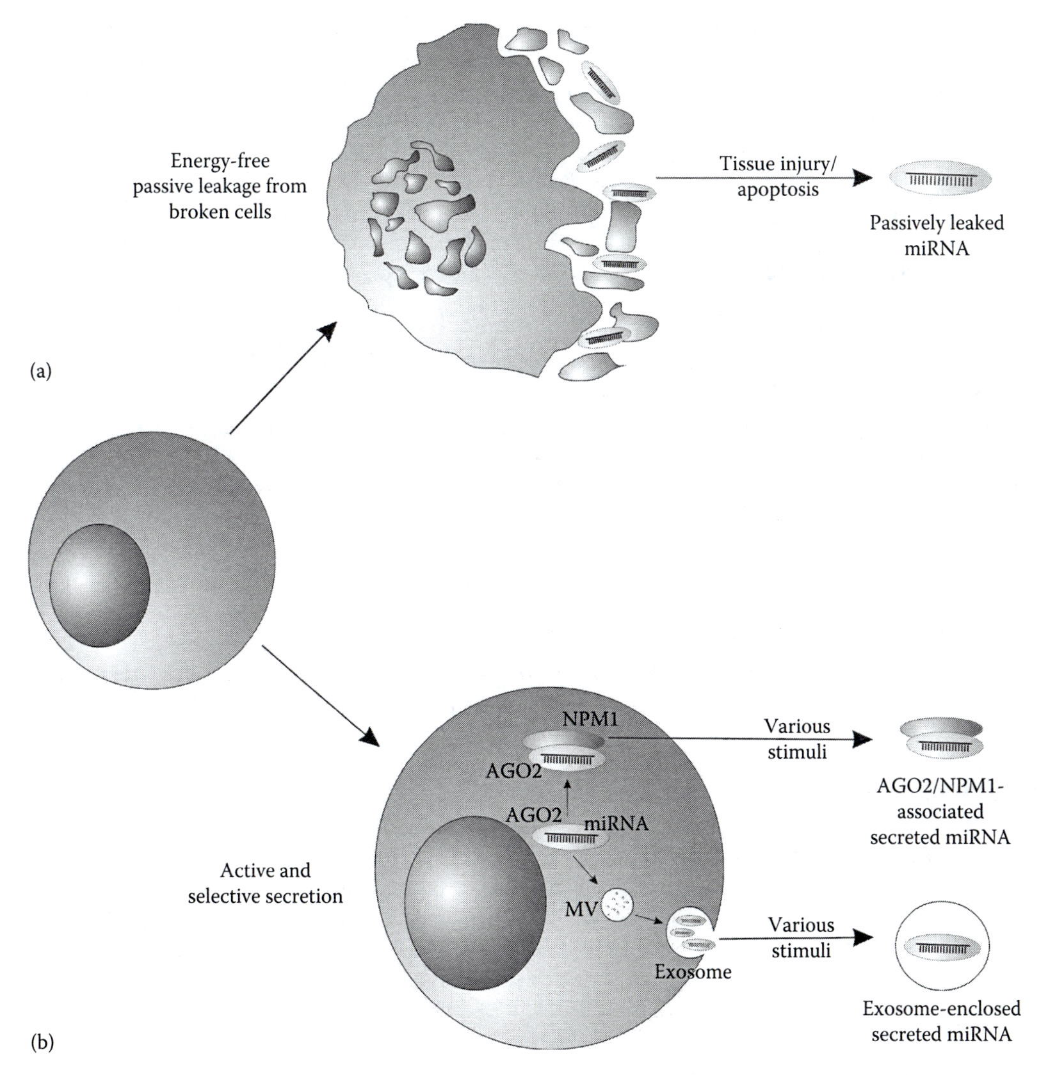

FIGURE 7.2 (See color insert.) Sources of circulating miRNAs: miRNAs may enter the circulation by (a) energy-free passive leakage from broken cells under conditions of tissue injury or apoptosis or by (b) active and selective secretion by cells as a response to various stimuli. This second pathway is ATP- and temperature-dependent and is similar to the release of certain hormones and cytokines. miRNAs could be released as MV-free nonmembrane-bound miRNAs associated with various multiprotein complexes or via cell-derived MVs (microparticles and exosomes).

between miRNAs in the serum and blood cells of cancer patients, and on the contrary, no differences between serum and blood cells of healthy individuals in their genome-wide expression profiling study employing Solexa sequencing (an ideal technical platform to analyze miRNAs). Based on these findings, they suggest that some specific serum miRNAs of cancer patients cannot be derived from circulating blood cells but likely from tumor cells or tissues associated with neoplastic transformation (Chen et al., 2008). However, Pritchard et al. enounced a cautionary note for miRNA-based cancer biomarker studies as they presented an evidence that blood cells are a major contributor to circulating miRNA and that perturbations in blood cell counts and hemolysis can alter plasma/serum miRNA biomarker levels by up to 50-fold (Pritchard et al., 2012).

Regarding the potential source of circulating miRNAs, there are major potential pathways hypothesized for miRNAs to enter the circulation. First, the energy-free passive leakage from broken cells, which is only a minor contributor to the process of circulating miRNAs generation, occurs predominantly under pathological circumstances such as tissue damage, cell apoptosis, tumor metastatic process, or chronic inflammation (Zen and Zhang, 2010). Confirming this pathway as a possible source of circulating miRNA, miR-208 was described as being exclusively expressed in the heart and was measured in the serum after myocardial injury (Ji et al., 2009). Second, active and selective secretion of miRNAs either as microvesicle (MV)-free miRNAs or via cell-derived MVs (Figure 7.2) as a response to various stimuli is ATP- and temperature-dependent and is similar to the release of certain hormones and cytokines (Han et al., 2009). Since there are a growing number of studies reporting that a significant portion of nuclease-resistant extracellular circulating miRNAs is floating outside exosomes or microparticles, the current model of circulating miRNAs encapsulated in membrane-bound vesicles should be revised. It has been confirmed that the vast majority (up to 90%) of circulating miRNAs is present in a non-membrane-bound form in association with Argonaute 2 (AGO2), the effector component of the miRISC, which directly binds different miRNAs and mediates messenger RNA (mRNA) repression in cells (Arroyo et al., 2011). The authors also hypothesized that vesicle-associated versus AGO2 complex-associated miRNAs originate from different cell types and reflect cell type-specific miRNA expression and/or release mechanisms and suggest that immunoaffinity enrichment of AGO2 complexes might be an effective strategy for improving sensitivity and miRNA biomarker performance. Moreover, Turchinovich et al. (2011) postulate that additional 96 kDa AGO proteins (AGO1, -3, -4) may also serve as miRNA carriers. Contradictory to the observation of extracellular circulating miRNAs floating outside the exosomes, Gallo et al. (2012) postulated that salivary miRNAs are predominantly enclosed in MVs, primarily exosomes.

miRNAs could be actively and selectively secreted into circulation also cell-derived membrane-bound MVs, microparticles, and exosomes. MVs have been detected in various body fluids such as blood, urine, malignant ascites, bronchoalveolar lavage fluid, synovial fluid, breast milk, and saliva, released under both physiological and pathological conditions from almost all cell types (Gutwein et al., 2005, Lodes et al., 2009). Exosomes, specialized membranous 50–90 nm vesicles that are exocytically released by many cell types (Fevrier and Raposo, 2004), arise from multivesicular bodies by a multistep and tightly controlled process of inward budding from the limiting membrane (Zomer et al., 2010). Circulating miRNAs could be carried also via larger membrane-bound particles that range in size to as large as 1 μm, produced by shedding of the plasma membrane (Lodes et al., 2009). Unfortunately the mechanisms that specifically direct miRNAs, or any RNA molecules, into multivesicular bodies and exosomes, are still unknown. It has been described by Gibbings et al. (2009) that miRNAs loading into exosomes is not a random event but is rather mediated by specific proteins involved in the miRNA network—the authors showed a presence of AGO2 protein and a significant enrichment of GW182 in purified monocyte-derived exosome-like vesicles, suggestive of the selective sorting of GW182 into exosomes. Further secretion of miRNAs was demonstrated to be triggered by the elevation of the cellular amount of ceramide, a bioactive sphingolipid, the synthesis of which is regulated by neutral sphingomyelinase (nSMase2).

7.1.2 Circulating miRNA Functions

Although the role of miRNAs released by tumors is not well established, among the proposed functions of circulating miRNAs, the role of exosomes in cell–cell communication including hematostasis, involvement in antigen presentation to T cells, and development of tolerance could be mentioned, although the exact mechanisms regarding circulating MV formation and miRNA incorporation are still unclear. Regarding the maintenance of homeostasis, the role of circulating miRNAs is supported by the observation that many of circulating miRNAs are derived from peripheral blood mononuclear cells (PBMCs) and other blood cells (Li et al., 2007, Hunter et al., 2008). For example, miR-223 is proposed to play a role in the regulation of differentiation of various blood cell lineages, as well as that of hematopoietic stem cells; miR-16 together with miR-24, detectable also in normal circulation, regulates lymphoid and red cell development. Circulating miRNAs were also proven to influence some metabolic pathways—for example, miR-486, confirmed to be differentially expressed between the plasma MVs and the PBMC, was predicted to regulate phenylalanine and cyanoamino acid metabolism, insulin receptor signaling, antigen presentation, and pentose phosphate pathway (Hunter et al., 2008). Moreover, cellular proliferation and immune and lymphatic system development could be modulated by miR-146a, which is highly expressed in the plasma MVs (Cameron et al., 2008). It has been recently reported that miR-150 secreted in MVs from human blood cells can modulate the expression of c-Myb, confirmed target of miR-150, through its uptake by HMEC-1 microvascular endothelial cells (Zhang et al., 2010). Furthermore, Zomer et al. (2010) described that miRNAs released in exosomes by Epstein–Barr virus (EBV)-infected cells can be taken up by peripheral PBMCs and, consequently, may suppress confirmed EBV target genes.

There are two relevant options based on which exosomes are believed to serve as transporters of genetic information, including miRNAs, to surrounding cells employed by tumor cells with a view to support tumor growth and progression. These are the findings that the quantity of tumor-derived exosomes in the peripheral circulation is highly correlated with different human cancers (Taylor and Gercel-Taylor, 2008, Krichevsky and Gabriely, 2009), and that the content of tumor cell-derived exosomes is correlated to the miRNA levels in primary tumor (Rabinowits et al., 2009). Recently, it has been reported by Fabbri et al. (2012) that tumor-secreted miRNAs (miR-21 and miR-29a) can regulate gene expression in the receiving cells also by different mechanisms than canonical binding to their target mRNAs. The authors described secreted miRNAs as key regulators of the tumor microenvironment by acting as paracrine agonists of Toll-like receptors (TLRs), that is, secreted miR-21 and miR-29a bind as ligands to different TLRs, murine TLR7, and human TLR8, in immune cells, triggering a TLR-mediated prometastatic inflammatory response that ultimately may lead to tumor growth and metastasis.

7.1.3 Circulating miRNA Stability

It is of great interest that circulating miRNAs are highly stable even in harsh conditions including RNase digestion, extreme temperature and pH (pH = 1 or 13), extended storage in frozen conditions, and repeated freeze–thaw cycles (Gilad et al., 2008, Mitchell et al., 2008).

One of the potential explanations of circulating miRNAs high stability deals with miRNA encapsulation in cell-derived lipid vesicles such as exosomes, microparticles (Hunter et al., 2008, Kosaka et al., 2010, Zhang et al., 2010), and apoptotic bodies (Zernecke et al., 2009). Recently, Arroyo et al. (2011) provided a novel model for the stability of non-vesicular circulating miRNAs based on AGO2–miRNA non-membrane-bound complexes localized in human circulation. Their proposed hypothesis of protection by a protein complex as a mechanism for circulating miRNAs stability in RNase-rich circulation was further supported by the observation of non-vesicle-associated miRNA-specific destabilization by proteinase K digestion of plasma. They also hypothesized that vesicle-associated versus AGO2 complex-associated miRNAs originate from different cell types and reflect cell type-specific miRNA expression and/or release mechanisms. It has been showed that also other miRNA-binding proteins, such as nucleophosmin 1 (NPM1), may be involved in the exportation, packaging, and protection of extracellular miRNAs (Wang et al., 2010).

Another explanation of circulating miRNAs stability in even harsh conditions in terms of resistance to RNase digestion takes into account the possibility of various modifications, including methylation (Yu et al., 2005), adenylation (Katoh et al., 2009), and uridylation (Jones et al., 2009). Recently, Katoh et al. described that mammalian miRNAs could be selectively stabilized by 3′ adenylation mediated by the cytoplasmic poly(A) polymerase GLD-2, but it is still unknown whether circulating miRNAs are either methylated or adenylated (Katoh et al., 2009).

7.1.4 Circulating miRNA Analysis

Although the circulating miRNAs in plasma, saliva, sputum, and urine seem to serve as excellent sources for noninvasive biomarkers, the RNA isolated from these body fluids is usually in relatively low concentrations. Majority of these samples do not pass through standard RNA quality criteria (A260:A230 and A260:A280 ratios) to be suitable for consequent molecular analysis. Despite the RNA samples isolated from previously mentioned sources not being considered pure enough through conventional quality assessment criteria, they still perform well in qRT-PCR.

Regardless, the technically challenging extraction due to the small amount of circulating miRNAs and the large amount of proteins, one of the most challenging issues that have to be addressed in association with circulating miRNA sample comparison is the quantification. Both high- and low-throughput techniques are extremely useful in circulating miRNA research, but microarray-based expression analysis is challenging since a large amount of RNA and preamplification step is required. On the contrary, qRT-PCR is the most widely performed and successful approach in terms of sensitivity and specificity due to its robustness and reproducibility (Chen et al., 2005). Of course, new armamentarium of circulating miRNAs analytical methods is emerging. For example, Lusi et al. (2009) were able to directly detect miRNAs in PCR- and label-free manner performing the miRNA detection through an electrochemical genosensor. This detection approach seems to be ultrasensitive since the detection limit is 0.1 pmol. As the first indications of disease-specific miRNA fingerprints in serum are emerging (Hu et al., 2010, Kozomara and Griffiths-Jones, 2011), the large-scale miRNA sequencing appears to be a very promising tool for further application of circulating miRNAs as noninvasive biomarkers for the diagnosis of various human cancers. Next-generation sequencing (NGS) platforms provide comprehensive and accurate measurements for transcripts as well as miRNAs, and furthermore, since the NGS approach is largely sequence independent, it does not rely on primers of probes specific to each miRNA design (Yang et al., 2011b). On the contrary, NGS remains expensive and labor-consuming, both in the sample preparation and in final data analysis.

A proper strategy of raw data normalization is a critical issue in quantification of circulating miRNAs since there is a lack of internal control for proper normalization. Regarding the quantification of circulating miRNA, literature-based tissue endogenous controls in the serum should be employed (Peltier and Latham, 2008), which is in contrast to tissue or cellular miRNAs, of which the expression levels of certain miRNAs can be normalized using U6 small nuclear ribonucleic acid (snRNA) or housekeeping miRNAs. In several studies, miR-16 consistently expressed in different human tissues and also detectable in serum was used (Lawrie et al., 2008, Huang et al., 2010, Redova et al., 2012). Another possible approach to standardization is normalizing the level of circulating miRNAs by the volume of serum/plasma sample. Currently, the spike-in normalization approach to control for technical variances during the purification process reported by Mitchell et al. is believed to be a gold standard for experimental miRNA data normalization (Mitchell et al., 2008). This approach is based on the use of exogenous synthetic nonhuman mature miRNA from *Caenorhabditis elegans* (cel-miR-39, -54, and -238) or plants as controls, which are spiked into the serum samples prior to RNA extraction (summarized in Kroh et al., 2010).

Also the presence of cellular contaminants such as platelets or erythrocytes and the imprecision introduced from the day-to-day setup of the RNA extraction and amplification procedures are critical to investigating the utility of miRNAs as circulating biomarkers and must considered before starting the study (Mitchell et al., 2008, Duttagupta et al., 2011, McDonald et al., 2011, Watson and Witwer, 2012).

7.1.5 Detection of miRNAs in Other Body Fluids

As it has been mentioned, membrane-bound MVs that could selectively and actively secrete miRNAs were detected also in other body fluids such as urine, malignant ascites, bronchoalveolar lavage fluid, synovial fluid, breast milk, and saliva (Gutwein et al., 2005, Lodes et al., 2009). Regarding the miRNA origin in other body fluids, it has been described that the urinary exosomes are delivered to the urinary space by fusion of its outer membrane with the apical plasma membrane of renal tubule epithelial cells. Exosomes have been shown to derive from every epithelial cell type facing the urinary space, from the podocyte to the transitional epithelium of the bladder (Zen and Zhang, 2010). Regarding the research of urine-based miRNAs as potential noninvasive biomarkers, Yun et al. (2012) validated the stability of miRNA in the supernatant of urine and conclude that even after seven cycles of freezing and thawing or 72 h long storage at room temperature, miRNA levels in the urine remained unchanged. RNA yield and concentration of saliva samples were observed to be stable over 48 h at room temperature (Patel et al., 2011). Concerning the urinary miRNA stability, urine samples contain lower levels of proteins than blood-based samples, which reduce the interference of proteins during the RNA isolation (Hanke et al., 2010).

Although the proper functions of tumor-released miRNAs are not well established, it is of note that miR-223, miR-16, and miR-24, functions of which were proposed as regulation of differentiation of various blood cell lineages, and regulation of lymphoid and red cell development, were abundantly expressed in saliva of healthy donors (Patel et al., 2011).

Regarding the challenging issues in circulating miRNA analysis, the detection of miRNAs in other body fluids is also complicated by the lack of suitable reference miRNA for data normalization. For the detection of urinary miRNAs, mostly small RNA U6 (RNU6B) and RNU48 were used as reference genes when voided urine was analyzed, but neither was regularly detected in urine supernatant, which contains mostly cell-free miRNAs originating in MVs (Wang et al., 2012a). In the study of Hanke et al. (2010), miR-152 was detected in all urine samples and used as an endogenous control.

7.2 miRNAs on Market

7.2.1 miRNAs' Relevant Patents

Regarding the miRNA exploitation, Thomas Tuschl's patents from Max Planck Society are pivotal in this field. Tuschl, a founder of Alnylam Pharmaceuticals, uncovered more than 100 naturally occurring miRNAs in mammalian cells. Some of these miRNAs could be pursued as drug targets. In 2001, Tuschl has licensed isolated nucleic acid consisting of 18–25 nucleotides having at least 90% identity or complementarity to mature sequence of miRNA-122 ("Tuschl I") and miRNA-21 ("Tuschl II"). While oligonucleotides complementary to miRNAs including miRNA-122a are taught by Tuschl, Esau et al. from Regulus Therapeutics have licensed (in 2003) methods for inhibiting miRNA-122 using oligonucleotides consisting of 17–25 linked nucleosides, wherein the oligo has at least 90% complementarity to a specified sequence and each nucleoside comprises a 2′-*O*-methoxyethyl sugar modification. Regarding methodology, Sarnow et al. from Stanford University have licensed methods of reducing hepatitis C virus (HCV) replication using antisense oligonucleotides complementary to miRNA-122 (in 2004), Horvitz et al. from Massachusetts Institute of Technology have licensed a method for identifying miRNA expression in a sample by contacting labeled miRNA to a microarray (in 2004), Li et al. from Stanford University have patented methods of raising T cell receptor signaling threshold and decreasing sensitivity of T cell to antigen by administering modified oligo of 12–25 nucleotides that is complementary to miRNA-181a (in 2006), and Safe et al. have licensed methods of inhibiting miR-27a in a breast cancer cell by delivering an antisense miR-27a oligonucleotide having a specific sequence and claim to the antisense molecule consisting of the specific sequence (in 2007) (McLeod et al., 2011). Other miRNA-related patents are listed in Table 7.2.

7.2.2 miRNAs and Market Players

The immense concern on miRNA research has raised the feedback of biotechnology companies. For example, the Santaris Pharma (www.santaris.com) is screening for disease-related miRNAs that might be feasible drug targets to inhibit and, having a broad experience in the creation of locked nucleic acid-based (LNA) antisense oligonucleotides that have drug-like properties, is designing and making miRNA antagonists for use in research and as possible diagnostic and therapeutic agents. Their flagship Miravirsen (SPC3649) is a novel LNA-Anti-miR™ oligonucleotide and a "first-in-class" specific inhibitor of miR-122. Miravirsen has the ability to inhibit a host factor needed for all subtypes of the HCV

TABLE 7.2

Relevant miRNA-Related US Patents

Patent No.	Inventor	Assignee	Title	Filed	Expire	Key Information
US 7,812,003	Safe SH		*Antisense miRNA and uses therefor*	August 1, 2008	October 12, 2010	Provides methods of treating a cancer using the antisense miRNA oligonucleotide. Also provides antisense miRNA-27a oligonucleotides usefulness in the methods described herein
US 8,349,568	Croce CM	The Ohio State University Research Foundation (Columbus, OH), Unites States, as represented by the Department of Health and Human Services (Washington, DC)	*Method of diagnosing poor survival prognosis colon cancer using let-7g*	November 14, 2011	January 8, 2013	Provides novel methods and compositions for the diagnosis and treatment of colon cancers
US 8,343,725	Croce CM	The Ohio State University Research Foundation (Columbus, OH), United States, as represented by the Secretary of the Department of Health and Human Services, National Institute of Health, Office of Technology Transfer (Washington, DC)	*Method of diagnosing poor survival prognosis colon cancer using miR-10a*	November 15, 2011	January 1, 2013	Provides diagnostics and prognostics for colon (including colon adenocarcinoma) cancer patients, wherein the methods related to measuring miR-10a levels can predict poor survival. The invention also provides methods of identifying inhibitors of tumorigenesis
US 8,338,106	Croce CM	The Ohio State University Research Foundation (Columbus, OH), United States, as represented by the Secretary of the Department of Health and Human Services, National Institute of Health, Office of Technology Transfer (Washington, DC)	*Method of diagnosing poor survival prognosis colon cancer using miR-29a*	November 15, 2011	December 25, 2012	Provides diagnostics and prognostics for colon (including colon adenocarcinoma) cancer patients, wherein the methods related to measuring miR-29a levels can predict poor survival
US 8,338,105	Croce CM	The Ohio State University Research Foundation (Columbus, OH), United States, as represented by the Secretary of the Department of Health and Human Services, National Institute of Health, Office of Technology Transfer (Washington, DC)	*Method of diagnosing poor survival prognosis colon cancer using miR-203*	November 15, 2011	December 25, 2012	Provides diagnostics and prognostics for colon (including colon adenocarcinoma) cancer patients, wherein the methods related to measuring miR-203 levels can predict poor survival

US 8,338.104	Croce CM	The Ohio State University Research Foundation (Columbus, OH), United States, as represented by the Secretary of the Department of Health and Human Services, National Institute of Health, Office of Technology Transfer (Washington, DC)	*Method of diagnosing poor survival prognosis colon cancer using miR-103-2*	November 15, 2011	December 25, 2012	Provides diagnostics and prognostics for colon (including colon adenocarcinoma) cancer patients, wherein the methods related to measuring miR-103-2 levels can predict poor survival
US 8,338,103	Croce CM	The Ohio State University Research Foundation (Columbus, OH), United States, as represented by the Secretary of the Department of Health and Human Services, National Institute of Health, Office of Technology Transfer (Washington, DC)	*Method of diagnosing poor survival prognosis colon cancer using miR-106a*	November 14, 2011	December 25, 2012	Provides diagnostics and prognostics for colon (including colon adenocarcinoma) cancer patients, wherein the methods related to measuring miR-106a levels can predict poor survival
US 8,338,102	Croce CM	The Ohio State University Research Foundation (Columbus, OH), United States, as represented by the Secretary of the Department of Health and Human Services, National Institute of Health, Office of Technology Transfer (Washington, DC)	*Method of diagnosing poor survival prognosis colon cancer using miR-181b*	November 14, 2011	December 25, 2012	Provides diagnostics and prognostics for colon (including colon adenocarcinoma) cancer patients, wherein the methods related to measuring miR-181b levels can predict poor survival
US 8,361,710	Croce CM	The Ohio State University Research Foundation (Columbus, OH), United States as represented by the Department of Health and Human Services (Washington, DC)	*miRNA-based methods and compositions for the diagnosis, prognosis and treatment of lung cancer using miR-21*	March 30, 2011	January 29, 2013	Provides novel methods and compositions for the diagnosis, prognosis, and treatment of lung cancer. The invention also provides methods of identifying anti-lung cancer agents

multiplication rather than attacking the virus itself, which lowers the risk of viral resistance and offers the advantage of broad genotype coverage. The company focused exclusively on miRNA is Rosetta Genomics (www.rosettagenomics.com) with its powerful bioinformatic platform enabling development of both diagnostic and therapeutic products for the detection and regulation of miRNAs. Furthermore, they are specialized on the technology related to cancer. Their portfolio comprise a molecular test that identifies the primary origin of tumors (miRview® mets[2]; 90% sensitivity and 99% specificity), a molecular test enabling accurate differentiation of lung primary tumors to the histological subtypes (miRview lung; 93.7% sensitivity and 97.9% specificity), additionally, the test differentiating squamous from non-squamous NSCLC (miRview squamous; 97% sensitivity and 91% specificity), the first single test that differentiates malignant pleural mesothelioma from carcinomas in the lung and pleura (miRview meso; 95% sensitivity and 96% specificity), and as a newcomer also a novel molecular test enabling proper differentiation of the four main histological types of primary kidney tumors (miRview kidney). Moreover, Rosetta Genomics has developed extraction protocols to isolate miRNAs from serum and other body fluids such as urine, saliva, amniotic, and follicular fluids. It is believed that circulating miRNA-based biomarkers could represent a crucial first step toward the development of highly sensitive miRNA-based tests that can be used for early detection, population screening, and developing noninvasive diagnostic tests, which can replace current surgical procedures. Moreover, such tests might be suitable for evaluating response to treatment or tumor reoccurrence.

7.3 Circulating miRNAs as Potential Biomarkers of Various Solid Cancers

Circulating miRNAs, considered as "extracellular communication RNAs," play an important role in various cellular processes, and escape from the proper regulatory network seems to be a common characteristic of several disease processes and malignant transformation. In this chapter we aimed to summarize the data related to the action of cellular miRNAs on the onset of various human cancers, including colorectal, lung, breast, and PCa. Up to date, there are tens of miRNAs reported as plasma or serum miRNA biomarkers of solid tumors. Detailed analysis of circulating miRNAs could potentially support the diagnosis of various cancers improvement and could predict outcome for cancer patients. Moreover, the profiling of alterations in circulating miRNAs that may signal a predisposition to cancer could also be a therapeutic target in these patients. Studied circulating miRNAs with diagnostic and prognostic potential are listed in Tables 7.3 and 7.4.

7.3.1 Colorectal Cancer

Colorectal cancer (CRC) is one of the leading causes of cancer-related death worldwide. A significant proportion of patients who develop CRC have no specific risk factor for the disease, and disease stage at diagnosis remains the best indicator of prognosis. Although several screening tests, including fecal occult blood testing (FOBT), colonoscopy, and stool DNA test, have been available for years, none of these methods has been established as a well-accepted screening tool due to their low adherence rates and low sensitivity and reproducibility (Huang et al., 2010). Also fecal immunochemical occult blood tests (FITs), which detect specifically human-specific globin, deal with unexceptionable limitations. For these reasons, the detection of early-stage cancer and precancerous lesions seems to be a key to reduce the mortality rate, and a promising approach for the identification of colorectal and other tumors is to assay stool or bodily fluids for molecular biomarkers that represent the spectrum of genetic and/or epigenetic alterations associated with cancer.

Among the set of circulating miRNAs relevant to CRC, miR-92a was the first potential noninvasive molecular marker for CRC detection. As reported by Ng et al., miR-92a reached 89% sensitivity and 70% specificity in plasma samples of CRC patients. miR-92a is a member of the miR-17–92 gene cluster, located on chromosome 13q13, and as an oncomir, this cluster promotes cell proliferation, suppresses apoptosis, induces angiogenesis, and accelerates tumor progression (Bandres et al., 2006, Ng et al., 2009, Li et al., 2011). Another study found significantly higher levels of miR-29a and miR-92a in plasma samples from patients with advanced CRC in comparison with healthy controls (Huang et al., 2010).

TABLE 7.3

Relevant Diagnostic miRNAs in Various Human Cancers

Diagnosis	miRNA	Source	Sensitivity, Specificity/ p-Value/AUC	Reference
Colorectal cancer	miR-92a	Plasma	89%, 70%	Ng et al. (2009)
	miR-29a + miR-92a	Plasma	83%, 85%	Huang et al. (2010)
	miR-21	Plasma	90%, 90%	Kanaan et al. (2012)
	miR-221	Plasma	86%, 41%	Pu et al. (2010)
	miR-21	Stool	$p < 0.05$	Link et al. (2010)
	miR-106a	Stool	$p < 0.05$	Link et al. (2010)
Lung cancer	miR-155 + miR-197 + miR-182	Plasma	82%, 87%	Zheng et al. (2011)
	miR-21 + miR-126 + miR-210 + miR-486-5p	Plasma	87%, 97%	Shen et al. (2011)
	miR-25, miR-223	Serum	$p < 0.0001$; $p < 0.0001$	Chen et al. (2008)
	34 miRNAs model	Serum	71%, 90%	Bianchi et al. (2012)
	miR-361-3p	Serum	AUC = 0.861	Roth et al. (2012)
	miR-625*	Serum	AUC = 0.770	Roth et al. (2012)
	miR-190b, miR-630, miR-942, miR-1284	Whole blood	91%, 100%	Patnaik et al. (2012)
	miR-155 + miR-197 + miR-182	Plasma	81.33%, 86.76%	Zheng et al. (2011)
	miR-125b	Serum	AUC = 0.786	Yuxia et al. (2012)
	miR-21, miR-143, miR-155, miR-210, miR-372	Sputum	83.3%, 100%	Roa et al. (2012)
	miR-21 + miR-486 + miR-375 + miR-200b	Sputum	80.6%, 91.7%	Yu et al. (2010)
	miR-205 + miR-210 + miR-708	Sputum	73%, 96%	Xing et al. (2010)
Breast cancer	Total RNA + miR-155	Serum	$p = 0.0001$	Roth et al. (2010)
	miR-10b, miR-34a, miR-155	Serum	$p = 0.005$; $p = 0.001$; $p = 0.008$	Roth et al. (2010)
	miR-195	Whole blood	88%, 91%	Heneghan et al. (2010b)
	miR-195 + let-7a + miR-155	Whole blood	94%; $p < 0.001$	Heneghan et al. (2010b)
	miR-193-3p	Whole blood	$p = 0.0001$	Schrauder et al. (2012)
	miR-425*, let-7c, let-7d*	Plasma	$p = 0.00328$; $p = 0.015$; $p = 0.03063$	Zhao et al. (2010)
Prostate cancer	miR-107, miR-574-3p	Urine	$p = 0.034$; $p = 0.034$	Bryant et al. (2012)
	miR-30c, miR-26b, miR-223, miR-24, miR-874, miR-1274a, miR-1207-5p, miR-93, miR-106a	Serum	$p = 0.01$; $p < 0.001$; $p < 0.001$; $p = 0.005$; $p < 0.001$; $p < 0.001$; $p < 0.001$; $p < 0.001$; $p < 0.001$	Moltzahn et al. (2011)
Gastric cancer	miR-221, miR-376c, miR-744	Serum	82.4%, 58.8%	Song et al. (2012)
	miR-17-5p, miR-21, miR-106a, miR-106b, let-7a	Plasma	$p = 0.05$; $p = 0.006$; $p = 0.008$; $p < 0.001$; $p = 0.002$	Tsujiura et al. (2010)
	miR-200c	Whole blood	65.4%, 100%	Valladares-Ayerbes et al. (2012)
	miR-223, miR-21, miR-218	Plasma	$p < 0.001$; $p < 0.001$; $p < 0.001$	Li et al. (2012)
Pancreatic cancer	miR-18a	Plasma	$p < 0.0001$	Morimura et al. (2011)
	miR-210	Plasma	$p < 0.00004$	Ho et al. (2010)

(continued)

TABLE 7.3 (continued)

Relevant Diagnostic miRNAs in Various Human Cancers

Diagnosis	miRNA	Source	Sensitivity, Specificity/ p-Value/AUC	Reference
	miR-21	Cyst fluid	p < 0.01; 76%, 80%	Ryu et al. (2011)
	miR-21 + miR-210 + miR-155 + miR-196a	Plasma	64%, 89%	Wang et al. (2009)
Oral cancer	miR-125a, miR-200a	Saliva	p < 0.05; p < 0.05	Park et al. (2009)
	miR-181a, miR-181b; miR-181a + miR-181b	Plasma	AUC = 0.84, AUC = 0.74; AUC = 0.89	Yang et al. (2011a)
	miR-333-3p, miR-29a, miR-223, miR-16, let-7b	Serum	80%, 80%; 76.7%, 76.9 0%; 60.0%, 96.2%; 93.3%, 61.5%; 80.0%, 80.8%	MacLellan et al. (2012)
Esophageal cancer	miR-21, miR-375	Plasma	p = 0.0649; p < 0.0001	Komatsu et al. (2011)
	miR-155	Plasma	AUC = 66%	Liu et al. (2012)
Liver cancer	miR-122	Serum	p < 0.001	Qi et al. (2011)
	miR-15b + miR-130b	Serum	98.2%, 91.5%	Liu et al. (2012)
	miR-885-5p	Serum	90.53%, 79.17%	Gui et al. (2011)
Thyroid cancer	let-7e + miR-151-5p + miR-222	Serum	86.8%, 79.5%	Yu et al. (2012a)
Kidney cancer	miR-10a + miR-30d	Urine	p < 0.01	Wang et al. (2012c)
	miR-378, miR-451, miR-378 + miR-451	Serum	p = 0.0003; p < 0.0001; 81%, 83%	Redova et al. (2012)
	miR-508-3p	Plasma	p < 0.01	Zhai et al. (2012)
	miR-1233	Serum	77.4%, 37.6%	Wulfken et al. (2011)
Ovarian cancer	miR-200a, miR-200b, miR-200c; miR-200b + miR-200c	Serum	p < 0.05; p = 0.05; p = 0.0005; AUC = 0.784	Kan et al. (2012)
	miR-21, miR-92, miR-93, miR-126, miR-29a	Serum	p < 0.01	Resnick et al. (2009)
Endometrial cancer	miR-155	Serum	p < 0.01	Tan et al. (2010)
	miR-9 + miR-1228, miR-9 + miR-92a	Plasma	AUC = 0.909; AUC = 0.913	Torres et al. (2012a)
	miR-199b, miR-99a, miR-199b + miR-99a	Plasma	AUC = 0.704, AUC = 0.810; 88%, 93%	Torres et al. (2012b)
Cervical cancer	miR-218	Serum	p < 0.001	Yu et al. (2012b)
Melanoma	miR-221	Serum	p < 0.0001	Kanemaru et al. (2010)
Rhabdomyosarcoma	miR-206	Serum	100%; 91.3%	Miyachi et al. (2010)

Note: AUC, area under curve.

Moreover, performed combined receiver operating characteristic (ROC) analyses of miR-29a and miR-92a yielded and increased AUC with 83% sensitivity and almost 85% specificity in discriminating CRC from healthy controls. Further, the authors demonstrated that both miR-29a and miR-92a could have significant diagnostic value even for advanced adenomas.

Another issue regarding CRC diagnostics and prognostication is discriminating metastatic and non-metastatic CRC patients. Wang and Gu proposed serum miR-29a as a promising novel marker for early detection of liver metastases in CRC patients (Wang and Gu, 2012). Another diagnostically valuable miRNA is miR-21 enabling discriminating CRC patients from controls with 90% specificity and sensitivity (Kanaan et al., 2012) or decreased miR-34a (Nugent et al., 2012). Concerning the prognostication of CRC patients, circulating plasma miR-141 may represent a novel biomarker that complements CEA in

TABLE 7.4

Relevant Prognostic and Predictive miRNAs in Various Human Cancers

Diagnosis	miRNA	Source	Sensitivity, Specificity/p-Value	References
Colorectal cancer	miR-29a	Serum	75%, 75% (liver meta)	Wang and Gu (2012)
	miR-141	Plasma	p = 0.004, resp. 0.002 (distant meta, poor prognosis; two cohorts)	Cheng et al. (2011)
	miR-221	Plasma	p = 0.043 (OS)	Pu et al. (2010)
Lung cancer	miR-155 + miR-197	Plasma	p < 0.001 (responsiveness)	Zheng et al. (2011)
	miR-486, miR-30d, miR-1, miR-499	Serum	p < 0.001 (OS)	Hu et al. (2010)
	miR-125b	Serum	p < 0.0001 (OS)	Yuxia et al. (2012)
Breast cancer	miR-155	Serum	p = 0.016 (hormone sensitive vs. insensitive)	Zhu et al. (2009)
	miR-141	Serum	p = 0.1 (PFS in M1); p = 0.06 (RFS in M0)	Roth et al. (2010)
	miR-122 + miR-375	Serum	80%, 100% (response to neoadj. therapy and relapse with metastatic disease)	Wu et al. (2012)
	miR-125b	Serum	p = 0.008 (responsiveness)	Wang et al. (2012b)
	miR-210	Plasma	p = 0.003 (lymph node meta)	Jung et al. (2012)
Prostate cancer	miR-141, miR-375	Serum	p = 0.034; p = 0.003 (recurrence)	Bryant et al. (2012)
	miR-20a, miR-21, miR-145, miR-221	Plasma	AUC = 0.824 (intermediate + high risk vs. low risk)	Shen et al. (2012)
	miR-451, miR-223, miR-24, miR-874, miR-1274a, miR-1207-5p, miR-93, miR-106a	Serum	p = 0.02; p = 0.002; p = 0.02; p = 0.003; p < 0.001; p < 0.001; p < 0.001; p < 0.001 (healthy vs. high risk)	Moltzahn et al. (2011)
Gastric cancer	miR-200c	Whole blood	p = 0.028 (OS); p = 0.028 (PFS)	Valladares-Ayerbes et al. (2012)
Oral cancer	miR-181	Plasma	p = 0.027 (poor survival)	Yang et al. (2011a)
Esophageal cancer	miR-21	Plasma	p = 0.0164 (recurrence)	Komatsu et al. (2011)
Liver cancer	miR-122, miR-21	Serum	p = 0.055, p = 0.051 (tumor size)	Qi et al. (2011)
Thyroid cancer	miR-151-5p, miR-222	Serum	p = 0.012, p = 0.001 (lymph node meta); p < 0.001 (tumor size - miR-151-5p)	Yu et al. (2012b)
Cervical cancer	miR-218	Serum	p < 0.001 (tumor stages and 2-year survival)	Yu et al. (2012a)
Melanoma	miR-221	Serum	p = 0.0257 (tumor thickness)	Kanemaru et al. (2010)

Note: OS, overall survival; PFS, progression-free survival; RFS, recurrence-free survival; meta, metastases.

detecting CRC with distant metastasis, as high expression levels of miR-141 in plasma were associated with poor prognosis (Cheng et al., 2011). Based on plasma samples of CRC patients and healthy controls, it has been shown that plasma level of miR-221 is a potential biomarker for differentiating CRC patients from controls. Furthermore, the study shows that elevated plasma miR-221 level may serve as a significant prognostic factor for poor overall survival in CRC patients (Pu et al., 2010).

Link et al. (2010) start their pilot study of fecal miRNAs as potential novel biomarkers for CRC screening from an option considering the increased number of exfoliated colonocytes shed in the colon from CRC patients; it is highly likely that the earliest detectable neoplastic changes in the expression pattern of specific miRNAs may be in feces rather than in blood (Nagasaka et al., 2009). Their observation of higher expression of miR-21 and miR-106a in stool samples from patients with colonic neoplasia (adenomas and/or CRC) compared to subjects with normal colonoscopy is in accordance with results of

Ahmed et al. (2009) who performed a study in which the expression of several miRNAs was analyzed in stool samples from CRC patients, inflammatory bowel disease patients, and healthy subjects. The authors summarize that miRNAs can be easily, effectively, and reproducibly extracted from freshly collected stools, as well as from FOBT kits, and that differential expression of miRNA in the stools of patients with colorectal neoplasia suggests that fecal miRNAs may provide a novel, promising, and non-invasive approach for the diagnosis of early colorectal neoplasia. Moreover, in another study performed by Schetter et al. (2008), the increased expression of miR-21 and miR-160a was also associated with poor survival and poor therapeutic outcome.

In conclusion, miRNAs circulating in various body fluids hold a great promise in CRC patients' management as they may be indicative of the presence of CRC. However, larger diagnostic studies are needed to evaluate potential use of miRNA expression in early detection and diagnosis of CRC.

7.3.2 Lung Cancer

Lung cancer remains the leading cause of cancer-related deaths worldwide, and unfortunately, the majority of patients are diagnosed at advanced stages with an overall survival rate of only 15% (Siegel et al., 2011). Major histological subtype, the non-small cell lung carcinoma (NSCLC), accounts for approximately 80%–85% of all cases of lung cancer. Although the availability of targeted agents has provided some clinical benefit, the prognosis for NSCLC remains poor, and furthermore, an extensive number of patients are insensitive to treatment, and cancer cells often develop drug resistance, leading to a relapse or worsening the prognosis (Martoni et al., 2005). Analyses of circulating miRNAs are thus of great interest as they may improve the NSCLC diagnostics and prognostication, and moreover, circulating miRNAs are believed to hold a potential to provide higher level of therapy individualization, such as monitoring therapy response and chemotherapy resistance.

Concerning the early detection of lung cancer, Zheng et al. described that levels of miR-155, miR-197, and miR-182 were significantly elevated in plasma of lung cancer patients in comparison to healthy controls ($p < 0.001$) (Zheng et al., 2011). They also reported that combination of these three plasma miRNAs further increases the discrimination power to almost 82% sensitivity and 87% specificity. Another set of circulating miRNAs (miR-21, miR-126, miR-210, and miR-486-5p) could discriminate NSCLC patients from cancer-free subjects with almost 87% sensitivity and 97% specificity (Shen et al., 2011). Regarding potential noninvasive diagnostic markers of NSCLC, elevated levels of circulating miR-25 and miR-223, previously shown to be involved in cancer development, could be mentioned (Chen et al., 2008). Recently, Bianchi et al. (2012) identified a serum miRNA diagnostic test to identify asymptomatic high-risk individuals with early-stage lung cancer with almost 80% accuracy. Their 34-miRNA model comprises, for example, the members of the let-seven family, which are often downregulated in lung cancer with diagnostic and prognostic value (Yanaihara et al., 2006); members of the miR-17–92 cluster, the first oncomir identified (He et al., 2005); miR-126 with its potential to inhibit cancer cell growth and metastasis in vitro and in vivo (Tavazoie et al., 2008); and miR-486, repeatedly reported to be downregulated in primary cancer and in the sera of NSCLC patients (Boeri et al., 2011, Shen et al., 2011). The authors postulate that the simplicity of the procedure (minimally invasive, requires <1 mL of serum) and its relatively low cost should encourage population compliance to large-scale screening programs, thus accelerating its application in the clinic as a "first line screening test" to identify those high-risk individuals who should undergo further testing, including by low-dose spiral computed tomography. Based on the study of expression levels of miR-361-3p and miR-625* in various cohorts of samples (NSCLC patients, benign disease, healthy individuals, large cell lung cancer (LCLC) patients, lung adenocarcinoma patients, non-/smoking patients), Roth et al. (2012) conclude that miR-361-3p and miR-625* might have a protective influence on the development of NSCLC, and the quantitative assessment of these miRs in blood serum might have diagnostic potential to detect NSCLC, in particular in smokers. Finally, Patnaik et al. (2012) studied miRNA expression profiles of whole blood in lung adenocarcinoma patients. They identified four miRNAs (miR-190b, miR-630, miR-942, and miR-1284) to be present in a majority of the classifiers that were generated in the cross-validation analyses to distinguish patients from healthy controls.

Regarding the potential of circulating miRNAs as relevant prognostic and predictive factors, Zheng et al. (2011) have shown that plasma levels of miR-155 and miR-197 were significantly elevated in metastatic patients and, together with miR-182, were decreased after chemotherapy in the majority of clinically responsive cancer patients. Moreover, employing Solexa sequencing, Hu et al. described 11 serum miRNAs to be significantly altered between longer-survival and shorter-survival groups, and expression levels of 4 miRNAs (miR-486, miR-30d, miR-1, miR-499) to be significantly associated with overall survival (Hu et al., 2010). The authors conclude that these four miRNAs may serve as an independent predictor of overall survival. Also miR-125b could be potential independent prognostic factor for survival of NSCLC patients as the cohort of patients with high miR-125b expression displayed a significantly poorer prognosis compared with patients with low expression (Yuxia et al., 2012).

Interestingly, Roa et al. (2012) have presented a novel approach for the early detection of NSCLC based on profiling of miRNAs in sputum. Employing a qRT-PCR and cluster analysis on an optimized miRNA profile consisting of five miRNAs (miR-21, miR-143, miR-155, miR-210, miR-372), they were able to accurately detect NSCLC patients with 83.3% sensitivity and 100% specificity. Regarding the early detection of lung adenocarcinoma, which is the most common type of lung cancer, Yu et al. (2010) described four miRNAs from sputum (miR-21, miR-486, miR-375, and miR-200b), combination of which produced the best prediction in distinguishing lung adenocarcinoma patients from normal subjects with 80.6% sensitivity and 91.7% specificity. Also the early detection of lung squamous cell carcinoma could be improved by the miRNA sputum markers as postulated by Xing et al. (2010) who observed that combination of sputum miR-205, miR-210, and miR-708 could exclusively distinguish lung squamous cell carcinoma patients from normal subjects with 73% sensitivity and 96% specificity.

To conclude, plasma, serum, and even sputum miRNAs might serve as next-generation biomarkers for early lung cancer detection and could potentially provide a noninvasive strategy for prognostication and predicting drug response.

7.3.3 Breast Cancer

Breast cancer is the second leading cause of cancer death in women worldwide with only lung cancer responsible for more female cancer-related deaths (Jemal et al., 2008). It is a heterogenous disease due to complicated etiology involving both genetic and environmental factors. This malignity comprises multiple entities associated with distinctive histological and biological features, clinical presentations, and behaviors and responses to therapy. Although the proposed sensitivity of mammography ranges between 67% and 95% and is strongly influenced by several factors, for example, age, breast density, and professional experience of the examiner (Kroh et al., 2010), it still remains the modality of choice for early breast cancer screening.

Regarding the breast cancer diagnostics, commercially available molecular diagnostic tests show great promise in enhancing the standard methods of assessing disease status and proper treatment for breast cancer patients. The MammaPrint test as a molecular diagnostic tool uses a 70-gene signature that has been shown to have independent prognostic value over clinicopathologic risk assessment in patients with node-negative breast cancer (Buyse et al., 2006). Although this test has been shown to have an extremely high correlation of prognostic prediction to tumor recurrence ($p < 0.0001$), there are still some unexceptionable limitations. This screening is recommended only to a very specific breast cancer patients subgroup; furthermore, the test requires a large amount of fresh sample that will be sent to the Agendia laboratory in Amsterdam in an RNA-stabilizing solution for analysis (Glas et al., 2006). Moreover, Oncotype DX, a 21-gene expression assay that uses qRT-PCR and microarray technologies, has the ability to predict a patient's risk of recurrence and benefit from chemotherapy (Harris et al., 2007, Wolff et al., 2007). Although these tests infer a great progression in breast cancer diagnostics and patients management, it is of great interest to search for a universal, reproducible, and effective test to predict therapeutic response and outcome.

It has been repeatedly reported that deregulation of miRNAs plays a crucial role in carcinogenesis of various types of cancer, including breast cancer, and that this aberrant expression of tissue miRNAs might be associated with clinical stage and clinicopathologic features, such as hormone receptor (HR) status, histological subtypes, metastatic potential, progression-free survival, and overall survival (Iorio et al., 2005, Blenkiron et al., 2007, Yan et al., 2008, Lowery et al., 2009, Svoboda et al., 2012).

As novel noninvasive biomarkers based on circulating miRNAs suitable for breast cancer are apparent, it is of note that a cellular selection mechanism for miRNA release may exist and that the extracellular and cellular miRNA profiles may differ, as indicated by Roth et al. (2010). Authors described that the bulk of miR-451 and miR-1246 produced by malignant mammary epithelial cells was released, while the majority of these miRNAs produced by nonmalignant mammary epithelial cells was retained. Concerning the proper early diagnostics, it has been demonstrated in the study of Roth et al. (2010) that the relative concentrations of total RNA and miR-155 in serum significantly discriminated M0-breast cancer patients from healthy controls ($p = 0.0001$) and that the miR-10b ($p = 0.005$), miR-34a ($p = 0.001$), and miR-155 ($p = 0.008$) expression levels could be used to discriminate between M1-breast cancer patients and healthy controls with significant correlation with the presence of overt metastases. The relative potential of miR-155 in discriminating among women with hormone-sensitive compared to women with hormone-insensitive breast cancer has been proposed (Zhu et al., 2009) (Table 7.1). Moreover, the higher expression levels of miR-10b were observed in breast cancer patients with estrogen receptor (ER)-negative disease (Heneghan et al., 2010a). Later on, Heneghan et al. (2010b) observed that elevated circulating miR-195 is breast cancer specific and could differentiate breast cancer from other cancers and from controls with a sensitivity of 88% at a specificity of 91%. Moreover, the combination of circulating levels of miR-195, let-7a, and miR-155 increased the sensitivity for differentiating breast cancer cases from controls to 94% ($p < 0.001$).

Another serum miRNA-based potential prognostic marker relevant in node-negative breast cancer patients is miR-141 (Roth et al., 2010). miR-202, reported by Schrauder et al. (2012) to be highly upregulated in early-stage breast cancer patients' blood samples, belongs to the let-7 family, known to be involved in self-renewal and tumorigenicity of breast cancer cells, and influences many cancer-relevant biological pathways. It has been confirmed that let-7e and miR-202 target the proto-oncogene MYCN in vitro. Furthermore, altered expression levels of circulating miR-425*, let-7c, let-7d*(Zhao et al., 2010), and miR-122 in combination with miR-375 (Wu et al., 2012) might have great potential to serve as novel, noninvasive biomarkers for early detection of breast cancer and possibly may allow optimized chemotherapy treatments and preventive anti-metastasis interventions in future clinical applications.

Regarding the prediction of chemoresistance in breast cancer patients, (1) miR-125b, exhibiting higher expression levels ($p = 0.008$) in nonresponsive patients who had higher percentage of proliferating cells and lower percentage of apoptotic cells in the corresponding surgical specimens obtained after neoadjuvant chemotherapy (Wang et al., 2012b); (2) miR-221, expression levels of which were described to be significantly associated with HR status; and (3) miR-210, circulating expression levels of which were associated with trastuzumab sensitivity, tumor presence, and lymph node metastases ($p = 0.003$), are of great interest in the field of searching a relevant noninvasive biomarker to predict and perhaps monitor response to breast cancer patients therapies (Jung et al., 2012).

7.3.4 Prostate Cancer

PCa is the second most common cancer and the sixth leading cause of cancer-related death among the men worldwide (Jemal et al., 2011). Actual diagnostics is based on the detection of the androgen-regulated serine protease, PSA, in serum. Although the expression of PSA is highly specific to prostate tissue, the routine use of PSA as diagnostic marker is limited by several issues: (1) elevated serum PSA levels are not specific only to PCa but could be associated also with benign prostatic hyperplasia (BPH) and prostatitis (Schroder et al., 2009); (2) PCa early detection using PSA and biopsy is associated with the critical problem of overdiagnosis and overtreatment of clinically significant PCa (Bastian et al., 2009). Although some molecules have been investigated as potential biomarkers for PCa, including KLK2, KLK11, PSMA, and PCA3, their benefit in clinical application still needs to be further validated (Sardana et al., 2008, Fradet, 2009, Ploussard and De La Taille, 2010).

Panel of circulating miRNAs that could serve as potential PCa biomarker enabling accurate discrimination of PCa from BPH and healthy controls has been identified by Chen et al., who employed the illumina microarray platform to describe the upregulated, let-7e, let-7c, and miR-30c, and downregulated, miR-622 and miR-1285. Moreover, further principal component analysis indicated component 1 extracted from expression data of the five miRNAs could differentiate PCa from BPH and healthy controls with high diagnosis performance, with an AUC of 0.924 and 0.860, respectively (Chen et al., 2012). Authors have proposed higher diagnostic value of the panel if combined with routinely used PSA. Concerning the diagnostic potential of circulating miRNAs in PCa early detection, miR-107 ($p = 0.034$) and miR-574-3p ($p = 0.034$), which were quantified at significantly higher concentrations in the urine of PCa patients compared with controls, were confirmed (Bryant et al., 2012). Authors conclude that the utilization of assays such as plasma and urine miR-107 measurement may potentially improve the accuracy of conventional PCa detection and case finding when combined with PSA level measurement, although this hypothesis requires formal testing in larger prospective studies. Specific serum miRNA signature identified by microfluidic-based multiplex qRT-PCR and consisting of both oncogenic and tumor-suppressive miRNAs (miR-223, -874, 1207-5p, -24, -106a, -26b, -30c, -93, -1274a, and -451) could participate on proper diagnostics of PCa patients and correlation with their prognosis (Moltzahn et al., 2011).

In PCa management, distinguishing the patients with varied aggressiveness is of great importance. miR-141 ($p = 0.034$) and miR-375 ($p = 0.003$), association of which with metastatic PCa was confirmed using serum-derived exosomes and MVs in a separate cohort of patients with recurrent or nonrecurrent disease following radical prostatectomy, may be potentially used to proper PCa staging (Bryant et al., 2012). Furthermore, a large-scale study investigating 667 different miRNAs in PCa patients showed that miR-375 and miR-141 were associated with advanced PCa (Brase et al., 2011). Hence, miR-375 might represent useful marker of micrometastases in order to aid appropriate selection of patients with organ-confined prostate cancer for invasive therapy such as radical prostatectomy. Additionally, miR-375, miR-378*, and miR-141 were observed as significantly overexpressed in serum from castration-resistant PCa patients compared with serum from low-risk localized patients, confirming their potential for monitoring cancer status (Nguyen et al., 2012). Based on previously mentioned studies, Shen et al. (2012) reported that combination of circulating miR-20a, miR-21, miR-145, and miR-221 expression levels may distinguish intermediate- or high-risk patients from those with low-risk score for aggressiveness. Moreover, the authors observed higher levels of serum miR-21 in both androgen-dependent PCa and hormone-refractory PCa and conclude that expression level of miR-20a and miR-21 are associated with clinicopathologic variables.

Conclusions of these studies confirm the potential of circulating miRNAs to serve as relevant novel noninvasive PCa biomarkers relevant for proper diagnostics and prognostication, but additional large prospective profiling studies, aiming at improving of clinical prediction of PCa prognosis, and enhancing the quality of PCa patients' life, are warranted.

7.4 Conclusion

Circulating miRNAs hold a great promise as a novel class of noninvasive cancer biomarkers due to their surprisingly high stability in plasma, association with disease states, and ease of sensitive measurement. However, there are still several limitations to the technology and study design, and important issues need to be addressed. Standardized and robust technologies have to be established aiming purification and reproducible detection of tumor-specific miRNAs in body fluids. Before translation of circulating miRNAs from bench to bedside, larger independent studies are required to establish a well-characterized panel of miRNAs specific to each tumor type, early or advanced cancer stage, response to treatment, patient outcome, and recurrence. These should be followed by larger prospective clinical trials validating the results obtained in retrospective exploratory cohorts. Afterward, efforts aiming at translating the validated findings into clinical routine must be increased.

Acknowledgment

This work was supported by grant IGA NT13549-4/2012 and NT13860 4/2012 of the Czech Ministry of Health, by Institutional Resources for Supporting the Research Organization provided by the Czech Ministry of Health in 2012 to Masaryk Memorial Cancer Institute and by the project "CEITEC–Central European Institute of Technology" (CZ.1.05/1.1.00/02.0068).

References

Ahmed, F.E., C.D. Jeffries, P.W. Vos et al. 2009. Diagnostic microRNA markers for screening sporadic human colon cancer and active ulcerative colitis in stool and tissue. *Cancer Genom Proteom* 6:281–295.

Alvarez-Garcia, I., and E.A. Miska. 2005. MicroRNA functions in animal development and human disease. *Development* 132:4653–4662.

Arroyo, J.D., J.R. Chevillet, E.M. Kroh et al. 2011. Argonaute2 complexes carry a population of circulating microRNAs independent of vesicles in human plasma. *Proc Natl Acad Sci USA* 108:5003–5008.

Bandres, E., E. Cubedo, X. Agirre et al. 2006. Identification by real-time PCR of 13 mature microRNAs differentially expressed in colorectal cancer and non-tumoral tissues. *Mol Cancer* 5:29.

Bastian, P.J., B.H. Carter, A. Bjartell et al. 2009. Insignificant prostate cancer and active surveillance: From definition to clinical implications. *Eur Urol* 55:1321–1330.

Beezhold, K.J., V. Castranova, and F. Chen. 2010. Microprocessor of microRNAs: Regulation and potential for therapeutic intervention. *Mol Cancer* 9:134.

Bianchi, F., F. Nicassio, G. Veronesi et al. 2012. Circulating microRNAs: Next-generation biomarkers for early lung cancer detection. *Ecancermedicalscience* 6:246.

Blenkiron, C., L.D. Goldstein, N.P. Thorne et al. 2007. MicroRNA expression profiling of human breast cancer identifies new markers of tumor subtype. *Genome Biol* 8:R214.

Boeri, M., C. Verri, D. Conte et al. 2011. MicroRNA signatures in tissues and plasma predict development and prognosis of computed tomography detected lung cancer. *Proc Natl Acad Sci USA* 108:3713–3718.

Brase, J.C., M. Johannes, T. Schlomm et al. 2011. Circulating miRNAs are correlated with tumor progression in prostate cancer. *Int J Cancer* 128:608–616.

Bryant, R.J., T. Pawlowski, J.W. Catto et al. 2012. Changes in circulating microRNA levels associated with prostate cancer. *Br J Cancer* 106:768–774.

Buyse, M., S. Loi, L. van 't Veer et al. 2006. Validation and clinical utility of a 70-gene prognostic signature for women with node-negative breast cancer. *J Natl Cancer Inst* 98:1183–1192.

Calin, G.A. and C.M. Croce. 2006. MicroRNA signatures in human cancers. *Nat Rev Cancer* 6:857–866.

Cameron, J.E., Q. Yin, C. Fewell et al. 2008. Epstein-Barr virus latent membrane protein 1 induces cellular microRNA miR-146a, a modulator of lymphocyte signaling pathways. *J Virol* 82:1946–1958.

Carthew, R.W. and E.J. Sontheimer. 2009. Origins and mechanisms of miRNAs and siRNAs. *Cell* 136:642–655.

Chen, C., D.A. Ridzon, A.J. Broomer et al. 2005. Real-time quantification of microRNAs by stem-loop RT-PCR. *Nucleic Acids Res* 33:e179.

Chen, X., Y. Ba, L. Ma et al. 2008. Characterization of microRNAs in serum: A novel class of biomarkers for diagnosis of cancer and other diseases. *Cell Res* 18:997–1006.

Chen, Z.H., G.L. Zhang, H.R. Li et al. 2012. A panel of five circulating microRNAs as potential biomarkers for prostate cancer. *Prostate* 72:1443–1452.

Cheng, H., L. Zhang, D.E. Cogdell et al. 2011. Circulating plasma MiR-141 is a novel biomarker for metastatic colon cancer and predicts poor prognosis. *PLoS One* 6:e17745.

Croce, C.M. 2009. Causes and consequences of microRNA dysregulation in cancer. *Nat Rev Genet* 10:704–714.

Duttagupta, R., R. Jiang, J. Gollub et al. 2011. Impact of cellular miRNAs on circulating miRNA biomarker signatures. *PLoS One* 6:e20769.

Fabbri, M., A. Paone, F. Calore et al. 2012. MicroRNAs bind to toll-like receptors to induce prometastatic inflammatory response. *Proc Natl Acad Sci USA* 109:E2110–E2116.

Fevrier, B. and G. Raposo. 2004. Exosomes: Endosomal-derived vesicles shipping extracellular messages. *Curr Opin Cell Biol* 16:415–421.

Fradet, Y. 2009. Biomarkers in prostate cancer diagnosis and prognosis: Beyond prostate-specific antigen. *Curr Opin Urol* 19:243–246.

Gallo, A., M. Tandon, I. Aleviyos et al. 2012. The majority of microRNAs detectable in serum and saliva is concentrated in exosomes. *PLoS One* 7:e30679.

Gibbings, D.J., C. Ciaudo, M. Erhardt et al. 2009. Multivesicular bodies associate with components of miRNA effector complexes and modulate miRNA activity. *Nat Cell Biol* 11:1143–1149.

Gilad, S., E. Meiri, Y. Yogev et al. 2008. Serum microRNAs are promising novel biomarkers. *PLoS One* 3:e3148.

Glas, A.M., A. Floore, L.J. Delahaye et al. 2006. Converting a breast cancer microarray signature into a high-throughput diagnostic test. *BMC Genomics* 7:278.

Gui, J., Y. Tian, X. Wen et al. 2011. Serum microRNA characterization identifies miR-885-5p as a potential marker for detecting liver pathologies. *Clin Sci (London, U.K.)* 120:183–193.

Gutwein, P., A. Stoeck, S. Riedle et al. 2005. Cleavage of L1 in exosomes and apoptotic membrane vesicles released from ovarian carcinoma cells. *Clin Cancer Res* 11:2492–2501.

Han, C., T. Chen, M. Yang et al. 2009. Human SCAMP5, a novel secretory carrier membrane protein, facilitates calcium-triggered cytokine secretion by interaction with SNARE machinery. *J Immunol* 182:2986–2996.

Hanahan, D. and R.A. Weinberg. 2011. Hallmarks of cancer: The next generation. *Cell* 144:646–674.

Hanke, M., K. Hoefig, H. Merz et al. 2010. A robust methodology to study urine microrna as tumor marker: Microrna-126 and microrna-182 are related to urinary bladder cancer. *Urol Oncol* 28:655–661.

Harris, L., H. Fritsche, R. Mennel et al. 2007. American society of clinical oncology 2007 update of recommendations for the use of tumor markers in breast cancer. *J Clin Oncol* 25:5287–5312.

He, L., J.M. Thomson, M.T. Hemann et al. 2005. A microRNA polycistron as a potential human oncogene. *Nature* 435:828–833.

Heneghan, H.M., M. Miller, A.J. Lowery et al. 2010a. Circulating microRNAs as novel minimally invasive biomarkers for breast cancer. *Ann Surg* 251:499–505.

Heneghan, H.M., N. Miller, R. Kelly et al. 2010b. Systemic miRNA-195 differentiates breast cancer from other malignancies and is a potential biomarker for detecting noninvasive and early stage disease. *Oncologist* 15:673–682.

Ho, A.S., X. Huang, H. Cao et al. 2010. Circulating miR-210 as a novel hypoxia marker in pancreatic cancer. *Transl Oncol* 3:109–113.

Hu, H.Y., Z. Yan, Y. Xu et al. 2009. Sequence features associated with microRNA strand selection in humans and flies. *BMC Genomics* 10:413.

Hu, Z., X. Chen, Y. Zhao et al. 2010. Serum microRNA signatures identified in a genome-wide serum microRNA expression profiling predict survival of non-small-cell lung cancer. *J Clin Oncol* 28:1721–1726.

Huang, Z., D. Huang, S. Ni et al. 2010. Plasma microRNAs are promising novel biomarkers for early detection of colorectal cancer. *Int J Cancer* 127:118–126.

Huber, K., J.C. Kirchheimer, D. Ermler et al. 1992. Determination of plasma urokinase-type plasminogen activator antigen in patients with primary liver cancer: Characterization as tumor-associated antigen and comparison with alpha-fetoprotein. *Cancer Res* 52:1717–1720.

Hunter, M.P., N. Ismail, X. Zhang et al. 2008. Detection of microRNA expression in human peripheral blood microvesicles. *PLoS One* 3:e3694.

Iorio, M.V., M. Ferracin, C.G. Liu et al. 2005. MicroRNA gene expression deregulation in human breast cancer. *Cancer Res* 65:7065–7070.

Jemal, A., F. Bray, M.M. Center et al. 2011. Global cancer statistics. *CA Cancer J Clin* 61:69–90.

Jemal, A., R. Siegel, E. Ward et al. 2008. Cancer statistics. *CA Cancer J Clin* 58:71–96.

Ji, X., R. Takahashi, Y. Hiura et al. 2009. Plasma miR-208 as a biomarker of myocardial injury. *Clin Chem* 55:1944–1949.

Jones, M.R., L.J. Quinton, M.T. Blahna et al. 2009. Zcchc11-dependent uridylation of microRNA directs cytokine expression. *Nat Cell Biol* 11:1157–1163.

Jung, E.J., L. Santarpia, J. Kim et al. 2012. Plasma microRNA 210 levels correlate with sensitivity to trastuzumab and tumor presence in breast cancer patients. *Cancer* 118:2603–2614.

Kan, C.W., M.A. Hahn, G.B. Gard et al. 2012. Elevated levels of circulating microRNA-200 family members correlate with serous epithelial ovarian cancer. *BMC Cancer* 12:627.

Kanaan, Z., S.N. Rai, M.R. Eichenberger et al. 2012. Plasma miR-21: A potential diagnostic marker of colorectal cancer. *Ann Surg* 256:544–551.

Kanemaru, H., S. Fukushima, J. Yamashita et al. 2011. The circulating microRNA-221 level in patients with malignant melanoma as a new tumor marker. *J Dermatol Sci* 61:187–193.

Katoh, T., Y. Sakaguchi, K. Miyauchi et al. 2009. Selective stabilization of mammalian microRNAs by 3′ adenylation mediated by the cytoplasmic poly(A) polymerase GLD-2. *Genes Dev* 23:433–438.

Kelly, B.D., N. Miller, N.A. Healy et al. 2013. A review of expression profiling of circulating microRNAs in men with prostate cancer. *BJU Int* 111:17–21.

Komatsu, S., D. Ichikawa, H. Takeshita et al. 2011. Circulating microRNAs in plasma of patients with oesophageal squamous cell carcinoma. *Br J Cancer* 105:104–111.

Kosaka, N., H. Iguchi, and T. Ochiya. 2010. Circulating microRNA in body fluid: A new potential biomarker for cancer diagnosis and prognosis. *Cancer Sci* 101:2087–2092.

Kozomara, A. and S. Griffiths-Jones. 2011. miRBase: Integrating microRNA annotation and deep-sequencing data. *Nucleic Acids Res* 39:(Database issue)D152–D157.

Krichevsky, A.M. and G. Gabriely. 2009. miR-21: A small multi-faceted RNA. *J Cell Mol Med* 13:39–53.

Kroh, E.M., R.K. Parkin, P.S. Mitchell et al. 2010. Analysis of circulating microRNA biomarkers in plasma and serum using quantitative reverse transcription-PCR (qRT-PCR). *Methods* 50:298–301.

Krol, J., I. Loedige, and W. Filipowicz. 2010. The widespread regulation of microRNA biogenesis, function and decay. *Nat Rev Genet* 11:597–610.

Lawrie, C.H., S. Gal, H.M. Dunlop et al. 2008. Detection of elevated levels of tumour-associated microRNAs in serum of patients with diffuse large B-cell lymphoma. *Br J Haematol* 141:672–675.

Lee, I., S.S. Ajay, J.I. Yook et al. 2009. New class of microRNA targets containing simultaneous 5′-UTR and 3′-UTR interaction sites. *Genome Res* 19:1175–1183.

Li, B., Y. Zhao, G. Guo et al. 2012. Plasma microRNAs, miR-223, miR-21 and miR-218, as novel potential biomarkers for gastric cancer detection. *PLoS One* 7:e41629.

Li, J., P. Smyth, R. Flavin et al. 2007. Comparison of miRNA expression patterns using total RNA extracted from matched samples of formalin-fixed paraffin-embedded (FFPE) cells and snap frozen cells. *BMC Biotechnol* 7:36.

Li, Y., H. Zhang, and Y. Chen. 2011. MicroRNA-mediated positive feedback loop and optimized bistable switch in a cancer network involving miR-17–92. *PLoS One* 6:e26302.

Link, A., F. Balaguer, Y. Shen et al. 2010. Fecal microRNAs as novel biomarkers for colon cancer screening. *Cancer Epidemiol Biomarkers Prev* 19:1766–1774.

Liu, A.M., T.J. Yao, W. Wang et al. 2012. Circulating miR-15b and miR-130b in serum as potential markers for detecting hepatocellular carcinoma: A retrospective cohort study. *BMJ Open* 2:e000825.

Lodes, M.J., M. Caraballo, D. Suciu et al. 2009. Detection of cancer with serum miRNAs on an oligonucleotide microarray. *PLoS One* 4:e6229.

Lowery, A.J., N. Miller, A. Devaney et al. 2009. MicroRNA signatures predict oestrogen receptor, progesterone receptor and HER2/neu receptor status in breast cancer. *Breast Cancer Res* 11:R27.

Lusi, E.A., M. Passamano, P. Guarascio et al. 2009. Innovative electrochemical approach for an early detection of microRNAs. *Anal Chem* 81:2819–2822.

MacLellan, S.A., J. Lawson, J. Baik et al. 2012. Differential expression of miRNAs in the serum of patients with high-risk oral lesions. *Cancer Med* 1:268–274.

Martoni, A., A. Marino, F. Sperandi et al. 2005. Multicentre randomised phase III study comparing the same dose and schedule of cisplatin plus the same schedule of vinorelbine or gemcitabine in advanced non-small cell lung cancer. *Eur J Cancer* 41:81–92.

McDonald, J.S., D. Milosevic, H.V. Reddi et al. 2011. Analysis of circulating microRNA: Preanalytical and analytical challenges. *Clin Chem* 57:833–840.

McLeod, B., M.L. Hayman, A.L. Purcell et al. 2011. The "real world" utility of miRNA patents: Lessons learned from expressed sequence tags. *Nat Biotechnol* 29:129–133.

Mitchell, P.S., R.K. Parkin, E.M. Kroh et al. 2008. Circulating microRNAs as stable blood-based markers for cancer detection. *Proc Natl Acad Sci USA* 105:10513–10518.

Miyachi, M., K. Tsuchiya, H. Yoshida et al. 2010. Circulating muscle-specific microRNA, miR-206, as a potential diagnostic marker for rhabdomyosarcoma. *Biochem Biophys Res Commun* 400:89–93.

Moltzahn, F., A.B. Olshen, L. Baehner et al. 2011. Microfluidic-based multiplex qRT-PCR identifies diagnostic and prognostic microRNA signatures in the sera of prostate cancer patients. *Cancer Res* 71:550–560.

Morimura, R., S. Komatsu, D. Ichikawa et al. 2011. Novel diagnostic value of circulating miR-18a in plasma of patients with pancreatic cancer. *Br J Cancer* 105:1733–1740.

Nagasaka, T., N. Tanaka, H.M. Cullings et al. 2009. Analysis of fecal DNA methylation to detect gastrointestinal neoplasia. *J Natl Cancer Inst* 101:1244–1258.

Ng, E.K., W.W. Chong, H. Jin et al. 2009. Differential expression of microRNAs in plasma of patients with colorectal cancer: A potential marker for colorectal cancer screening. *Gut* 58:1375–1381.

Nguyen, H.C., W. Xie, M. Yang et al. 2012. Expression differences of circulating microRNAs in metastatic castration resistant prostate cancer and low-risk, localized prostate cancer. *Prostate* doi: 10.1002/pros.22572.

Nugent, M., N. Miller, and M.J. Kerin. 2012. Circulating miR-34a levels are reduced in colorectal cancer. *J Surg Oncol* 106:947–952.

Park, N.J., H. Zhou, D. Elashoff et al. 2009. Salivary microRNA: Discovery, characterization, and clinical utility for oral cancer detection. *Clin Cancer Res* 15:5473–5477.

Patel, R.S., A. Jakymiw, B. Yao et al. 2011. High resolution of microRNA signatures in human whole saliva. *Arch Oral Biol* 56:1506–1513.

Patnaik, S.K., S. Yendamuri, E. Kannisto et al. 2012. MicroRNA expression profiles of whole blood in lung adenocarcinoma. *PLoS One* 7:e46045.

Peltier, H.J. and G.J. Latham. 2008. Normalization of microRNA expression levels in quantitative RT-PCR assays: Identification of suitable reference RNA targets in normal and cancerous human solid tissues. *RNA* 14:844–852.

Ploussard, G. and A. De La Taille. 2010. Urine biomarkers in prostate cancer. *Nat Rev Urol* 7:101–109.

Pritchard, C.C., E. Kroh, B. Wood et al. 2012. Blood cell origin of circulating microRNAs: A cautionary note for cancer biomarker studies. *Cancer Prev Res (Phila)* 5:492–497.

Pu, X.X., G.L. Huang, H.Q. Guo et al. 2010. Circulating miR-221 directly amplified from plasma is a potential diagnostic and prognostic marker of colorectal cancer and is correlated with p53 expression. *J Gastroenterol Hepatol* 25:1674–1680.

Qi, P., S. Cheng, H. Wang et al. 2011. Serum microRNAs as biomarkers for hepatocellular carcinoma in Chinese patients with chronic hepatitis B virus infection. *PLoS One* 6:e28486.

Rabinowits, G., C. Gercel-Taylor, J.M. Day et al. 2009. Exosomal microRNA: A diagnostic marker for lung cancer. *Clin Lung Cancer* 10:42–46.

Redova, M., A. Poprach, J. Nekvindova et al. 2012. Circulating miR-378 and miR-451 in serum are potential biomarkers for renal cell carcinoma. *J Transl Med* 10:55.

Resnick, K.E., H. Alder, J.P. Hagan et al. 2009. The detection of differentially expressed microRNAs from the serum of ovarian cancer patients using a novel real-time PCR platform. *Gynecol Oncol* 112:55–59.

Roa, W.H., J.O. Kim, R. Razzak et al. 2012. Sputum microRNA profiling: A novel approach for the early detection of non-small cell lung cancer. *Clin Invest Med* 35:E271.

Roth, C., B. Rack, V. Muller et al. 2010. Circulating microRNAs as blood-based markers for patients with primary and metastatic breast cancer. *Breast Cancer Res* 12:R90.

Roth, C., I. Stuckrath, K. Pantel et al. 2012. Low levels of cell-free circulating miR-361-3p and miR-625* as blood-based markers for discriminating malignant from benign lung tumors. *PLoS One* 7:e38248.

Ryu, J.K., H. Matthaei, M. dal Molin et al. 2011. Elevated microRNA miR-21 levels in pancreatic cyst fluid are predictive of mucinous precursor lesions of ductal adenocarcinoma. *Pancreatology* 11:343–350.

Sardana, G., B. Dowell, and E.P. Diamandis. 2008. Emerging biomarkers for the diagnosis and prognosis of prostate cancer. *Clin Chem* 54:1951–1960.

Schetter, A.J., S.Y. Leung, J.J. Sohn et al. 2008. MicroRNA expression profiles associated with prognosis and therapeutic outcome in colon adenocarcinoma. *JAMA* 299:425–436.

Schneider, J., H.G. Velcovsky, H. Morr et al. 2000. Comparison of the tumor markers tumor M2-PK, CEA, CYFRA 21-1, NSE and SCC in the diagnosis of lung cancer. *Anticancer Res* 20:5053–5058.

Schrauder, M.G., R. Strick, R. Schulz-Wendtland et al. 2012. Circulating micro-RNAs as potential blood-based markers for early stage breast cancer detection. *PLoS One* 7:e29770.

Schroder, F.H., J. Hugosson, M.J. Roobol et al. 2009. Screening and prostate-cancer mortality in a randomized European study. *N Engl J Med* 360:1320–1328.

Shen, J., G.W. Hruby, J.M. Mckiernan et al. 2012. Dysregulation of circulating microRNAs and prediction of aggressive prostate cancer. *Prostate* 72:1469–1477.

Shen, J., N.W. Todd, H. Zhang et al. 2011. Plasma microRNAs as potential biomarkers for non-small-cell lung cancer. *Lab Invest* 91:579–587.

Shigoka, M., A. Tsuchida, T. Matsudo et al. 2010. Deregulation of miR-92a expression is implicated in hepatocellular carcinoma development. *Pathol Int* 60:351–357.

Siegel, R., E. Ward, O. Brawley et al. 2011. Cancer statistics, 2011: The impact of eliminating socioeconomic and racial disparities on premature cancer deaths. *Cancer J Clin* 61:212–236.

Siomi, H. and M.C. Siomi. 2010. Posttranscriptional regulation of microRNA biogenesis in animals. *Mol Cell* 38:323–332.

Slaby, O. and J. Sana. 2012. MicroRNAs biogenesis, function and decay. In: *MicroRNAs in Solid Cancer: From Biomarkers to Therapeutic Targets* (ed.) O. Slaby, pp. 1–21. Nova Science Publishers, Hauppauge, NY.

Song, M., K. Pan, H. Su et al. 2012. Identification of serum microRNAs as novel non-invasive biomarkers for early detection of gastric cancer. *PLoS One* 7:e33608.

Svoboda, M., J. Sana, M. Redova et al. 2012. MiR-34b is associated with clinical outcome in triple-negative breast cancer patients. *Diagn Pathol* 7:31.

Tan, Z.Q., F.X. Liu, H.L. Tang et al. 2010. Expression and its clinical significance of hsa-miR-155 in serum of endometrial cancer. *Zhonghua Fu Chan Ke Za Zhi* 45:772–774.

Tavazoie, S.F., C. Alarcon, T. Oskarsson et al. 2008. Endogenous human microRNAs that suppress breast cancer metastasis. *Nature* 451:147–152.

Taylor, D.D. and C. Gercel-Taylor. 2008. MicroRNA signatures of tumor-derived exosomes as diagnostic biomarkers of ovarian cancer. *Gynecol Oncol* 110:13–21.

Torres, A., K. Torres, A. Pesci et al. 2012a. A Diagnostic and prognostic significance of miRNA signatures in tissues and plasma of endometrioid endometrial carcinoma patients. *Int J Cancer* 132:1633–1645.

Torres, A., K. Torres, A. Pesci et al. 2012b. Deregulation of miR-100, miR-99a and miR-199b in tissues and plasma coexists with increased expression of mTOR kinase in endometrioid endometrial carcinoma. *BMC Cancer* 12:369.

Tsujiura, M., D. Ichikawa, S. Komatsu et al. 2010. Circulating microRNAs in plasma of patients with gastric cancers. *Br J Cancer* 102:1174–1179.

Turchinovich, A., L. Weiz, A. Langheinz et al. 2011. Characterization of extracellular circulating microRNA. *Nucleic Acids Res* 39:7223–7233.

Valladares-Ayerbes, M., M. Reboredo, V. Medina-Villaamil et al. 2012. Circulating miR-200c as a diagnostic and prognostic biomarker for gastric cancer. *J Transl Med* 10:186.

Vasudevan, S., Y. Tong, and J.A. Steitz. 2007. Switching from repression to activation: MicroRNAs can up-regulate translation. *Science* 318:1931–1934.

Wang, G., E.S. Chan, B.C. Kwan et al. 2012a. Expression of micrornas in the urine of patients with bladder cancer. *Clin Genitourin Cancer* 10:106–113.

Wang, H., G. Tan, L. Dong et al. 2012b. Circulating miR-125b as a marker predicting chemoresistance in breast cancer. *PLoS One* 7:e34210.

Wang, J., J. Chen, P. Chang et al. 2009. MicroRNAs in plasma of pancreatic ductal adenocarcinoma patients as novel blood-based biomarkers of disease. *Cancer Prev Res (Philadelphia, PA)* 2:807–813.

Wang, K., S. Zhang, J. Weber et al. 2010. Export of microRNAs and microRNA-protective protein by mammalian cells. *Nucleic Acids Res* 38:7248–7259.

Wang, L.G. and J. Gu. 2012. Serum microRNA-29a is a promising novel marker for early detection of colorectal liver metastasis. *Cancer Epidemiol* 36:e61–e67.

Wang, N., Y. Zhou, L. Jiang et al. 2012c. Urinary microRNA-10a and microRNA-30d serve as novel, sensitive and specific biomarkers for kidney injury. *PLoS One* 7:e51140.

Watson, A.K. and K.W. Witwer. 2012. Do platform-specific factors explain microRNA profiling disparities? *Clin Chem* 58:472–474; author reply 474–475.

Winter, J. and S. Diederichs. 2011. MicroRNA biogenesis and cancer. *Methods Mol Biol* 676:3–22.

Wolff, A.C., M.E. Hammond, J.N. Schwartz et al. 2007. American Society of Clinical Oncology/College of American Pathologists guideline recommendations for human epidermal growth factor receptor 2 testing in breast cancer. *Arch Pathol Lab Med* 131:18.

Wu, X., G. Somlo, Y. Yu et al. 2012. De novo sequencing of circulating miRNAs identifies novel markers predicting clinical outcome of locally advanced breast cancer. *J Transl Med* 10:42.

Wulfken, L.M., R. Moritz, C. Ohlmann et al. 2011. MicroRNAs in renal cell carcinoma: Diagnostic implications of serum miR-1233 levels. *PLoS One* 6:e25787.

Xiao, C. and K. Rajewsky. 2009. MicroRNA control in the immune system: Basic principles. *Cell* 136:26–36.

Xing, L., N.W. Todd, L. Yu et al. 2010. Early detection of squamous cell lung cancer in sputum by a panel of microRNA markers. *Mod Pathol* 23:1157–1164.

Yan, L.X., X.F. Huang, Q. Shao et al. 2008. MicroRNA miR-21 overexpression in human breast cancer is associated with advanced clinical stage, lymph node metastasis and patient poor prognosis. *RNA* 14:2348–2360.

Yanaihara, N., N. Caplen, E. Bowman et al. 2006. Unique microRNA molecular profiles in lung cancer diagnosis and prognosis. *Cancer Cell* 9:189–198.

Yang, C.C., P.S. Hung, P.W. Wang et al. 2011a. miR-181 as a putative biomarker for lymph-node metastasis of oral squamous cell carcinoma. *J Oral Pathol Med* 40:397–404.

Yang, Q., J. Lu, S. Wang et al. 2011b. Application of next-generation sequencing technology to profile the circulating microRNAs in the serum of preeclampsia versus normal pregnant women. *Clin Chim Acta* 412:2167–2173.

Yu, B., Z. Yang, J. Li et al. 2005. Methylation as a crucial step in plant microRNA biogenesis. *Science* 307:932–935.

Yu, J., Y. Wang, R. Dong et al. 2012a. Circulating microRNA-218 was reduced in cervical cancer and correlated with tumor invasion. *J Cancer Res Clin Oncol* 138:671–674.

Yu, L., N.W. Todd, L. Xing et al. 2010. Early detection of lung adenocarcinoma in sputum by a panel of microRNA markers. *Int J Cancer* 127:2870–2878.

Yu, S., Y. Liu, J. Wang et al. 2012b. Circulating microRNA profiles as potential biomarkers for diagnosis of papillary thyroid carcinoma. *J Clin Endocrinol Metab* 97:2084–2092.

Yun, S.J., P. Jeong, W.T. Kim et al. 2012. Cell-free micrornas in urine as diagnostic and prognostic biomarkers of bladder cancer. *Int J Oncol* 41:1871–1878.

Yuxia, M., T. Zhennan, and Z. Wei. 2012. Circulating miR-125b is a novel biomarker for screening non-small-cell lung cancer and predicts poor prognosis. *J Cancer Res Clin Oncol* 138:2045–2050.

Zen, K. and C.Y. Zhang. 2010. Circulating microRNAs: A novel class of biomarkers to diagnose and monitor human cancers. *Med Res Rev* 32:326–348.

Zeng, X., J. Xiang, M. Wu et al. 2012. Circulating miR-17, miR-20a, miR-29c, and miR-223 combined as non-invasive biomarkers in nasopharyngeal carcinoma. *PLoS One* 7:e46367.

Zernecke, A., K. Bidzhekov, H. Noels et al. 2009. Delivery of microRNA-126 by apoptotic bodies induces CXCL12-dependent vascular protection. *Sci Signal* 2:ra81.

Zhai, Q., L. Zhou, C. Zhao et al. 2012. Identification of miR-508-3p and miR-509-3p that are associated with cell invasion and migration and involved in the apoptosis of renal cell carcinoma. *Biochem Biophys Res Commun* 419:621–626.

Zhang, Y., D. Liu, X. Chen et al. 2010. Secreted monocytic miR-150 enhances targeted endothelial cell migration. *Mol Cell* 39:133–144.

Zhao, H., J. Shen, L. Medico et al. 2010. A pilot study of circulating miRNAs as potential biomarkers of early stage breast cancer. *PLoS One* 5:e13735.

Zheng, D., S. Haddadin, Y. Wang et al. 2011. Plasma microRNAs as novel biomarkers for early detection of lung cancer. *Int J Clin Exp Pathol* 4:575–586.

Zhu, W., W. Qin, U. Atasoy et al. 2009. Circulating microRNAs in breast cancer and healthy subjects. *BMC Res Notes* 2:89.

Zomer, A., T. Vendrig, E.S. Hopmans et al. 2010. Exosomes: Fit to deliver small RNA. *Commun Integr Biol* 3:447–450.

8

Stem Cell Biomarkers in Early Diagnosis, Prognosis, and Therapy of Cancer

Dipali Dhawan and Harish Padh

CONTENTS

ABSTRACT Cancer stem cells (CSCs) have been categorized in a large number of hematopoietic cancers and solid tumors and are identified by virtue of the expression of cell surface markers. These CSCs have been isolated from the bulk tumor by the expression of cell surface proteins, like CD44, CD24, and CD133, and efflux of Hoechst dye or aldehyde dehydrogenase (ALDH) activity by flow cytometry and/or fluorescence-activated cell sorting (FACS). The identification of markers allows the prospective isolation of CSCs from whole tumor tissues, which would lead to the elucidation of important biological properties of CSCs and provide the possibility to target them. This chapter reviews the advances in this field of cancer stem cells in various cancer types.

8.1 Stem Cell Origin of Cancer

8.1.1 Theories of Cellular Origin of Cancer

There are two hypotheses regarding the origin of cancer stem cells (CSCs) (Figure 8.1): The first suggests that these cells are a result of the transformation of the normal stem cells, whereas the second one suggests that the differentiated cells undergo a transdifferentiation program to give rise to these stemlike cells.

It is postulated that if the CSCs arise from the normal stem cells, dedifferentiation would not be necessary for generating a tumor. Hence, the cancer cells would utilize the existing stem cell machinery to promote self-renewal. The stem cells have a longer life-span than those of mature cells. Many characteristics of the leukemia-initiating cells support the stem cell origin theory.

The other theory suggests that CSCs could arise from adult, differentiated cells that in some way are reprogrammed to become more stem cell-like. This means that a large number of cells in the tissue might have a tumorigenic potential and a small group out of those would initiate the tumor. However, it is still not fully understood what decides the selection of these cells that would eventually dedifferentiate.

8.1.2 CSCs

CSCs are a specific subset of transformed cells that are able to sustain primary tumor growth according to a hierarchical pattern. There is strong evidence in literature supporting the existence of such cells in many cancer types, although it may not be true for all cancer types and/or all stages. The normal stem cells have three main properties: (1) capability of self-renewal, (2) strict control on stem cell numbers, and (3) ability to divide and differentiate to generate all functional elements of that particular tissue (Bixby et al., 2002). However, the CSCs have no control on the cell numbers as compared to normal stem cells. CSCs form very small numbers in tumors and are said to be responsible for the growth of the tumor. A large number of cells are needed to generate a new tumor in an animal model; however, with

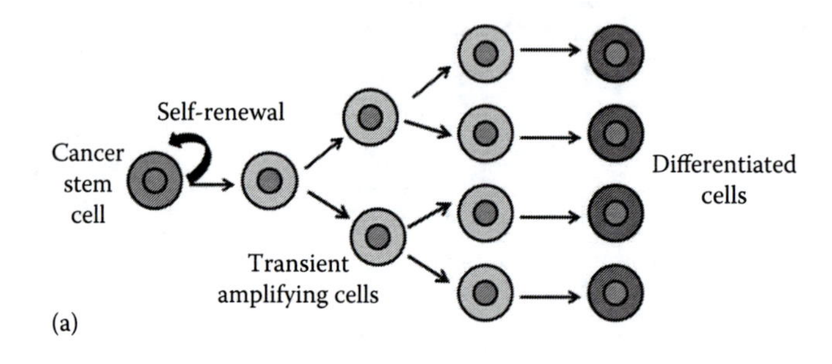

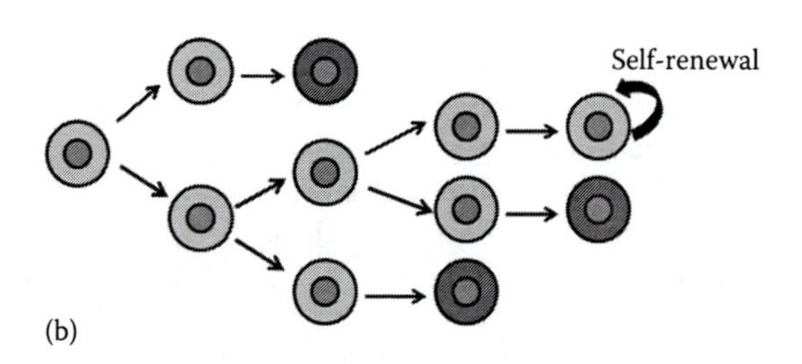

FIGURE 8.1 Theories for origin of cancer. (a) The CSC theory suggests that a clear hierarchy of cells exists within a tumor, whereas (b) the stochastic model suggests that tumor growth is a random process to which all cells can contribute equally.

the elucidation of CSCs, it may be explained that the higher numbers may be due to the probability of a higher number of CSCs being injected in the animal.

CSCs are considered a new concept; however, their presence was identified around 1971 almost 35 years back when they were called leukemic stem cells (Park et al., 1971). Now, CSCs have also been identified in solid tumors like breast, brain, and many others (Dick, 2003; Galderisi et al., 2006). The CSCs have the property of self-renewal and also give rise to other differentiated cells (Al-Hajj et al., 2003). These CSCs can be identified by the different markers expressed by these cells and are different in the cancers that have been studied (Table 8.1).

TABLE 8.1

Distribution of CSC Markers

Marker	Tumor Type
CD133	Brain (Cheng et al., 2009)
	Hepatic (Suetsugu et al., 2006)
	Prostate (Vander Griend et al., 2008)
	Pancreatic (Immervoll et al., 2008)
	Melanoma (Jaksch et al., 2008)
	Colon (Jaksch et al., 2008)
	Liver (Ding et al., 2009)
	Lung (Bertolini et al., 2009)
	Ovarian (Stewart et al., 2011)
CD44	Colon (Dalerba et al., 2007)
	Ovarian (Zhang et al., 2008)
	Head and neck (Prince et al., 2007)
	Breast (Al-Hajj et al., 2003)
	Prostate (Collins et al., 2005)
	Pancreatic (Li et al., 2007)
ALDH	Breast (Croker et al., 2009)
	Lung (Jiang et al., 2009)
	Head and neck (Visus et al., 2007)
	Colon (Huang et al., 2009)
	Liver (Ma et al., 2008)
	Pancreatic (Tomuleasa et al., 2011)
	Gastric (Zhi et al., 2011)
	Prostate (Hellsten et al., 2011)
ABCG2	Pancreatic (Lechner et al., 2002)
	Lung (Summer et al., 2003)
	Limbal epithelium (Watanabe et al., 2004)
	Brain (Islam et al., 2005)
	Prostate (Apati et al., 2008)
	Liver (Shi et al., 2008)
	Ovarian (Dou et al., 2011)
	Retinoblastoma (Seigel et al., 2005)
CD90	T-acute lymphoblastic leukemia (Yamazaki et al., 2009)
	Gliomas (He et al., 2012)
	Liver (Yang et al., 2008)
ABCB5	Melanoma (Gazzaniga et al., 2010)
Ep-CAM	Lung (Eramo et al., 2008)
	Colon (Ricci-Vitiani et al., 2007)

8.2 CSCs and Metastasis

8.2.1 Basics of Tumor Progression: Invasion and Metastasis

Invasion and metastasis leads to death in about 90% of tumors in humans (Sporn, 1996). The tumor cells acquire an ability to colonize in other organs of the body and form new tumors without any shortage of nutrients and space (Hanahan and Weinberg, 2000; Bergers and Benjamin, 2003; Fidler, 2003). Metastasis is accomplished after a long process involving the destruction of the basement membrane, invasion of cells into adjacent tissues, intravasation and survival in the bloodstream, extravasation into other distant organs, and in the end colonizing at these organs and forming new tumors.

Invasion is the preceding step of metastasis, which is highly complex and regulated. The invasion begins with changes in the cell adhesion properties of the tumor cells at the periphery that affects cell–cell contacts and the contact between cell and extracellular matrix. This leads to detachment of cells from the parent tumor mass, degradation of the extracellular matrix, and migration of the cells into distant organs via the bloodstream (Figure 8.2). There are a number of proteins involved in the invasion and metastasis process like cell adhesion proteins (Birchmeier and Behrens, 1994; Hood and Cheresh, 2002; Cavallaro and Christofori, 2004; Guo and Giancotti, 2004), extracellular matrix proteases (Lopez-Otin and Overall, 2002; Folgueras et al., 2004) playing significant roles.

The key player involved in cell–cell adhesion and their alteration during the invasion process is E-cadherin, which is a calcium-dependent adhesion protein of the cadherin family of proteins and is well studied in most of the cancers (Birchmeier and Behrens, 1994; Cavallaro and Christofori, 2004). Integrins are another group of essential players supporting the interactions between the cell and extracellular matrix; however, their role is not completely elucidated (Hood and Cheresh, 2002; Guo and Giancotti, 2004).

It has been demonstrated that stem cells and metastatic cancer cells have numerous properties in common that are vital to the metastatic process, which includes the prerequisite of a precise microenvironment (or "niche") to sustain growth and offer protection, the use of definite cellular pathways for migration, increased resistance to cell death, and an enhanced capacity for drug resistance (Croker and Allan, 2008). Metastatic sites for any specific cancer could represent those tissues that support the development of a well-matched CSC niche, from which CSCs could increase through normal or deregulated cellular signaling. Further, normal stem cells tend to be quiescent except if they are triggered to divide (Pardal et al., 2003).

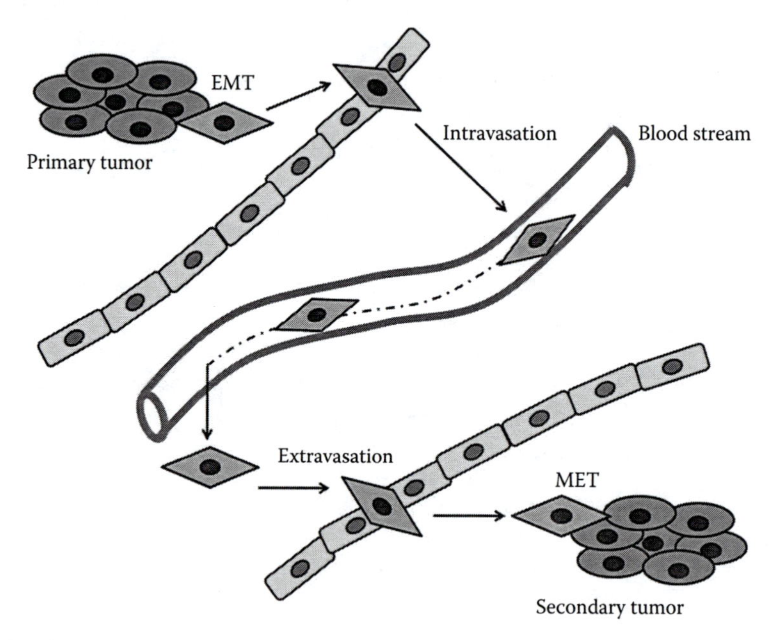

FIGURE 8.2 Invasion and metastasis.

8.2.2 Epithelial-to-Mesenchymal Transition in Cancer

The transformation of cells along with changes in cellular morphology is associated with an epithelial-to-mesenchymal transition (EMT) (Mani et al., 2008; Morel et al., 2008). The process involves the conversion of polarized, well-adhered epithelial cells into individual motile mesenchymal cells (Figure 8.2). The process of EMT is an essential event in early stages of embryonic development under the control of signaling molecules; however, its aberrant reactivation in cancer is considered an important factor in the dissociation of cells (Thiery et al., 2009) and further in imparting the cell properties of a stemlike cell (Mani et al., 2008; Morel et al., 2008; Vesuna et al., 2009). The EMT hence converts differentiated epithelial cells into CSCs and is also affected by the microenvironment. EMT is a reversible transdifferentiation process related with an intense genetic reprogramming and major consequent phenotypic alterations.

The association of tumor invasion with EMT has been well proven in cancer cell lines and animal models (Christofori and Semb, 1999; Thiery, 2002; Kang and Massague, 2004); however, the evidence for EMT occurrence in human tumors is very meager limiting its actual interpretation in relevance to human cancers (Tarin et al., 2005; Thompson et al., 2005; Christiansen and Rajasekaran, 2006). The major constraint for this is that EMT might not be easily identified in time and space in human cancers, probably because EMT may occur transiently at times and in less number of cells or even in isolated cells of tumor-invasive areas (Thiery, 2002; Kang and Massague, 2004; Peinado et al., 2004). However, it has been observed that the cell lines undergo stable EMT in response to external stimuli or expression of specific genes (Huber et al., 2005; Thiery and Sleeman, 2006).

A number of signaling pathways are involved in the EMT, and there is often a cross talk among the molecules of this pathway, which finally results in the cells converting from epithelial to mesenchymal. The major pathways involved include Hedgehog (Hh), Notch, Wnt, and TGF-β signaling pathways (Takebe et al., 2011a) (Figure 8.3).

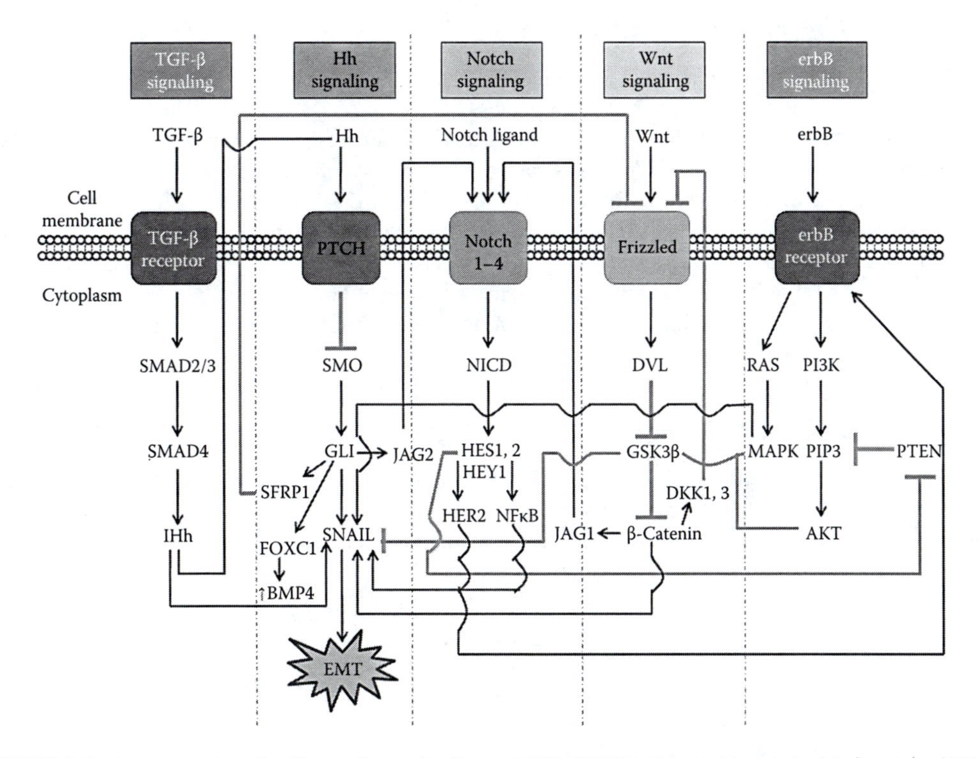

FIGURE 8.3 Interconnected signaling pathways leading to EMT. (SFRP1, Secreted frizzled-related protein; DKK1, Dickkopf homolog 1; NICD, Notch intracellular domain; DVL, Disheveled; R-SMAD, Receptor regulated SMAD; FOXC1, Forkhead box C1; JAG1, 2, Jagged 1, 2; PTCH, Patched; SMO, Smoothened; IHh, Indian Hedgehog; Hh, Hedgehog; PI3K, Phosphoinositide 3-kinase; HEY1, HES1 related; HES1, Hairy and enhancer of split 1; HER2, erbB2; BMP, Bone morphogenetic protein; MAPK, Mitogen-activated protein kinase). (Based on Takebe, N. et al., *Breast Cancer Res.*, 13, 211, 2011b.)

8.2.3 Evidence of Epithelial-to-Mesenchymal Transition in Clinical Cancer Samples

Metastasis is a highly complex process that involves several chronological steps like escape from the primary tumor (intravasation), survival within circulation, extravasation into a secondary site, and sustained growth in a distinct microenvironment (Woodhouse et al., 1997; Chambers et al., 2002; Pantel and Brakenhoff, 2004). About 0.02%–0.1% of the cancer cells that reach the circulation can only develop macrometastases (Weiss, 1990; MacDonald et al., 2002; Allan et al., 2006). CSCs can initiate and sustain secondary tumor growth as is evident from an experimental model (Li et al., 2007). There have been many studies that propose CSCs as a source of the metastatic increase (Wicha, 2006; Li et al., 2007; Goss et al., 2008; Visvader and Lindeman, 2008).

One example of full EMT in human cancer is the possibility that stromal components surrounding carcinoma cells like myofibroblasts might originate directly from tumoral cells. Also peritumoral stromal cells sometimes exhibit similar genetic alterations to those exhibited by the adjacent carcinoma cells, which suggests a common origin for both cell types (Moinfar et al., 2000; Wernert et al., 2000). However, such examples showing conversion of tumor cells into mesenchymal cells may not totally reflect the occurrence of EMT in human cancers. In case of cell lines, the ability to undergo EMT differs from cell line to cell line even with the exposure of the same external stimuli (Grunert et al., 2003; Peinado et al., 2003); hence, it means that complete EMT might not be easy to achieve, but partial EMT may be sufficient for some cell lines to have a migratory phenotype. Hence, researchers study the expression of mesenchymal markers and loss of epithelial markers as signs of partial EMT (Grunert et al., 2003).

8.3 CSCs in Various Cancer Types

8.3.1 Leukemia and Other Hematological Malignancies

8.3.1.1 Isolation and Identification of CSCs

Only about 0.1%–1.0% of acute myeloid leukemia (AML) cells can give rise to new tumors in severe combined immunodeficient (SCID) mice (Lapidot et al., 1994; Bonnet and Dick, 1997). Hence, with the scarce presence of leukemia stem cells (LSCs), it becomes difficult to isolate these cells from clinical blood samples, bone marrow, or leukemia cell lines. The LSCs can be isolated based on two methods: (1) by fluorescence-activated cell sorting using cell surface markers like CD9, CD33, CD44, CD90, CD96, CD110, and CD123 that are expressed in the different hematological diseases as mentioned in Table 8.2 and (2) by fluorescence-activated cell sorting based on the capacity of the side population (SP) cells to exclude the fluorescent dye Hoechst 33342. These cells have the ability to self-renew and also differentiate into other cell types.

These LSCs can be characterized on the basis of expression profiles of cell surface markers and by testing their functional characteristics.

8.3.1.2 LSCs in Metastasis

In case of hematopoietic stem cells (HSCs), two stem cells niches have been identified, the osteoblastic niche (Calvi et al., 2003; Zhang et al., 2003) and the vascular niche (Kiel et al., 2005), which regulates the number and function of normal tissue stem cells (Papayannopoulou and Scadden, 2008). This stem cell

TABLE 8.2

Cell Surface Markers for Hematological Disorders

Disorder	Cell Surface Markers
Acute B-lymphoblastic leukemia (B-ALL)	$CD9^+CD34^+CD10^-CD19^-$
Acute T-lymphoblastic leukemia (T-ALL)	$CD34^+CD4^-CD7^-CD19^-CD90^+CD110^+$
AML	$CD33^+CD34^+CD38^-CD44^+CD90^+CD96^+CD117^-CD123^+$
Chronic myeloid leukemia (CML)	$CD34^+CD38^-CD44^+$

Source: Deng, C.H. and Zhang, Q.P., *Chin. Med. J.*, 123, 954, 2010.

niche also plays an integral part in the functional regulation of LSCs. This niche supports the migration of the LSCs leading to metastasis (Hendrix et al., 2007; Wang et al., 2007). The niche required by metastatic tumor cells, like in the case of normal cells and CSCs, is known as the "metastatic niche." It has been observed that bone marrow-derived VEGFR1$^+$ hematopoietic cells can reside in tumor-specific premetastatic lesions thereby forming clusters of cells. By altering the local microenvironment, they cause the activation of integrins and chemokines, such as stroma cell-derived factor-1 (SDF-1). SDF-1 is known to promote cell attachment and further supports survival and growth of the tumor cells. The anti-VEGFR1 antibody treatment leads to the eradication of pre-metastatic clusters of cells and migration is prevented; hence, the metastasis of the tumor cells is averted (Kaplan et al., 2005).

8.3.2 Prostate Cancer

8.3.2.1 Isolation and Identification of CSCs

CSCs can be identified using cell surface markers, SP, and sphere formation. In case of prostate cancer cell lines, LAPC-9 xenograft tumors contained a detectable SP, but there was no detectable SP in DU 145, LNCaP, PC3, and PPC-1 cell lines (Patrawala et al., 2005). The tumorigenicity of SP cells of LAPC-9 was much more compared to non-SP cells, where less than 100 SP cells could give rise to tumors, while more than 300,000 non-SP cells were needed to induce a tumor. Patrawala and colleagues showed that SP cells are enriched for CSCs and contain the most primitive of stem cells along with more differentiated transit amplifying (TA) cells (Patrawala et al., 2005). Another approach for the identification and enrichment of CSCs is by culturing the nonadherent spheres. In case of prostate cancer-purified prostate, CSCs can grow as prostataspheres in culture (Patrawala et al., 2006; Hurt et al., 2008). There are a number of markers that are being studied for the isolation of prostate CSCs. The CD44$^+$ cells displayed significant properties of CSCs like long-term retention of BrdU indicating that the cells are relatively quiescent, initiation of tumors at low numbers, serial transplantation ability, and long-term maintenance in culture (Patrawala et al., 2006; Tang et al., 2007). Collins and colleagues have shown that in case of patient primary samples, the CD44$^+$CD133$^+$integrin-$\alpha 2\beta 1^{hi}$ cells were highly proliferative and more invasive than CD133$^-$ cells. In case of DU145 cell line, the CD44$^+$CD133$^+$integrin-$\alpha 2\beta 1^{hi}$ cells showed increased tumorigenicity, which confirmed another important property of CSCs (Wei et al., 2007). However, there are very few studies confirming the role of CD44$^+$CD133$^+$integrin-$\alpha 2\beta 1^{hi}$CD24$^-$ cells as prostatic CSCs; hence, more studies to confirm the same are warranted.

8.3.3 Breast Cancer

8.3.3.1 Isolation and Identification of CSCs

Al-Hajj and colleagues reported the discovery of CSCs in human breast tumors in 2003. A cellular population was characterized on the basis of cell surface markers CD44$^+$/CD24$^{-/low}$/ESA$^+$ markers and lineage$^-$ (lineage markers CD2, CD3, CD10, CD16, CD18, CD31, CD64, and CD140b) markers (Al-Hajj et al., 2003). Literature suggests that breast CSCs can also be isolated from patient samples after in vitro propagation (Ponti et al., 2005) as well as from breast cancer cell lines (Fillmore and Kuperwasser, 2008). The breast CSCs can form mammospheres in culture that can allow the propagation of mammary epithelial cells in an undifferentiated state by proliferation of cells in suspension as spheres (Dontu et al., 2003, 2004). It has been observed that the mammospheres from breast cancer cells are enriched in cells with CD44$^+$/CD24$^{-/low}$ phenotype, and further on injecting these cells into non-obese diabetic (NOD)/SCID mice, the cells retain their tumor-initiating capability. Interestingly, only a fraction of CD44$^+$/CD24$^{-/low}$ cells are able to form secondary mammospheres (Ponti et al., 2005).

Hence, the study of additional markers like aldehyde dehydrogenase (ALDH) has become inevitable. In mammalian cells ALDH1 is the predominant isoform and increased ALDH activity has been observed in human HSCs as well as in CSCs (Hess et al., 2004; Corti et al., 2006). The identification of breast CSCs is by ALDEFLUOR staining that involves an uncharged ALDH substrate, BODIPY-aminoacetaldehyde (BAAA). BAAA is taken up by live cells through passive diffusion and is converted to a negatively charged product BODIPY-aminoacetate (BAA$^-$) by the intracellular ALDH. BAA$^-$ is maintained inside cells expressing elevated levels of ALDH, leading them to fluoresce intensely (Christ et al., 2007). ALDH-expressing cells can hence be detected in the green fluorescence channel (520–540 nm) of a standard flow cytometer. The ALDH$^+$ breast tumor cells are able to generate tumors in NOD/SCID mice with characteristics resembling the parental tumor. Hence, the collection of ALDH$^+$ cells also contains the CSC population (Ginestier et al., 2007).

A number of new approaches have been tried recently to improve the efficiency of identification and isolation of breast CSCs (Cicalese et al., 2009; Pece et al., 2010; Sajithlal et al., 2010). PKH26 has been used to identify the proportion of stem cells in normal human mammary cells. The cell membrane is labeled with PKH26 and then mammary cells are cultured in suspension to form mammospheres. After 7–10 days only the slow cycling cells retain the PKH26 dye and can be sorted on the basis of its fluorescence. The cells with a high PKH26 intensity (PKH26^{hi}) are able to form secondary mammospheres, divide asymmetrically, express markers of pluripotency, and can reconstitute a normal mammary epithelium when transplanted into NOD/SCID mice. This indicates that this population is highly enriched in stem cells (Pece et al., 2010). Another method recently reported by Sajithlal and colleagues involved tagging the CSC pool from human cancer cell lines with green fluorescent protein (GFP) under the control of the Oct3/4 promoter. It was observed that in case of MCF-7 cells, only 1% population expressed GFP, and majority of those cells were CD44$^+$/CD24$^-$. The GFP$^+$ cells were sorted and maintained in culture. Surprisingly, the CD44$^+$/CD24$^-$/GFP$^+$ phenotype remained stable in these cells for over 1 year, suggesting that the incorporation of the promoter blocked the CSC differentiation. These cells were more tumorigenic (100–300 times) than the rest of the tumor cells (Sajithlal et al., 2010).

8.3.3.2 CSCs in Breast Tumor Metastasis

A pool of circulating tumor cells that express stem cell markers has been identified in metastatic breast cancer patients, and a high percentage of CD44$^+$/CD24$^-$ tumor cells has been observed in metastases (Balic et al., 2006; Aktas et al., 2009; Theodoropoulos et al., 2010). Also the expression of stem cell marker ALDH in samples of inflammatory breast cancer (IBC) correlates with the development of distant metastasis and decreased survival (Charafe-Jauffret et al., 2010). Several in vitro and in vivo studies have proved the ability of breast CSCs to invade and proliferate at the metastatic sites. Increased invasiveness and elevated expression levels of genes involved in invasion like IL-1α, IL-6, IL-8, CXCR4, MMP-1, and UPA have been observed in CSCs isolated from cancer cell lines (Sheridan et al., 2006). Similarly, ALDH$^+$ cells isolated from breast cancer cell lines were more invasive than ALDH$^-$ cells (Charafe-Jauffret et al., 2009; Crocker et al., 2009). Further, ALDH$^+$ cells, when injected intracardially to NOD/SCID mice, generated metastases at distant organs, while ALDH$^-$ cells generated only occasional metastases limited to lymph nodes (Charafe-Jauffret et al., 2009, 2010).

8.3.4 Lung Cancer

8.3.4.1 Identification and Isolation of CSCs

Carney and coworkers observed the presence of a clonogenic population of cells in human lung cancer in the early 1980s. They observed that specimens from small cell lung cancer (SCLC) and adenocarcinoma possessed a small subpopulation of cells that had the ability to form colonies on agar. Further when injected intracranially into athymic nude mice, these cells gave rise to cancers with features like the original specimen (Carney et al., 1982). SP cells have also been isolated in non-small cell lung cancer (NSCLC) and in clinical specimens of lung cancer cell lines. The SP cells when cultured in vitro showed a higher invasiveness and resulted in self-renewal as well as differentiation of the cells. The tumorigenicity of these cells was much higher, which was proved by their ability to generate new tumors in immunodeficient mice as compared to non-SP cells (Ho et al., 2007).

The marker CD177 (c-Kit) and its ligand were identified in the 1990s by Hibi and colleagues. This is a stem cell factor in pulmonary neuroendocrine tumors (Hibi et al., 1991) and is associated with poor prognosis in early stage lung adenocarcinoma and squamous cancer patients (Pelosi et al., 2004). However, other studies have contradictory results regarding the expression of c-Kit (Altundag et al., 2005; Dy et al., 2005; Gross et al., 2006). Another marker CD44 that is a universally expressed transmembrane cell surface adhesion glycoprotein has functions in cell–matrix and cell–cell interactions. It has been associated with poor prognosis and resistance to chemotherapy in a number of different cancers (Liu and Jiang, 2006). CD44 has been associated with increased metastasis, which supports its role as a supporter in the survival of disseminated cells (Desai et al., 2007). Increased levels of CD44 have been observed in both SCLC and NSCLC and have been observed to be associated with survival (Lee et al., 2005; Le et al., 2006). Further, a study analyzing SCLC and NSCLC tumors identified a subset of $CD133^+$ cells that produced lung tumor spheres that could differentiate and produce tumors in vivo (Eramo et al., 2008).

8.3.5 Gliomas

Gliomas are brain tumors with glial cell characteristics, composed of a heterogeneous mix of cells, including glioma stem cells. Gliomas include astrocytomas, oligodendrogliomas, ependymoma, and mixed gliomas. They account for 32% of all brain and central nervous system (CNS) tumors and 80% of all malignant brain and CNS tumors (CBTRUS, 2010).

8.3.5.1 Isolation and Identification of CSCs

There is extensive heterogeneity among gliomas; hence, it is likely that tumors from different patients originate from different stages of the adult neural hierarchy, which also explains the distinct molecular subclasses of gliomas (Phillips et al., 2006). The three properties that are considered essential for a cell to be universally accepted as a glioma stem cell include capability of the cells to self-renew, potential for high proliferation, and lastly capable of forming new tumors (Rich, 2008). Due to the higher heterogeneity, there is no single marker that is consistent for all patients, specific to glioma stem cells, and includes all glioma stem cells in a tissue. CD133, CD15, and A2B5 are the most commonly used markers to identify and isolate glioma stem cells. Though CD133 is the widely used marker, it has become clear from the various studies that individual gliomas are very heterogeneous and further tumors vary greatly from patient to patient (Phillips et al., 2006). However, presently there is no universally accepted collection of markers for isolation of a pure population of glioma stem cells (Gilbert and Ross, 2009).

8.3.6 Colorectal Cancer

8.3.6.1 Isolation and Identification of CSCs

Several studies have hinted toward the existence of colorectal CSCs (O'Brien et al., 2007; Ricci-Vitiani et al., 2007; Todaro et al., 2007). CD133 was the first surface marker used for purification of a CRC cell population, which further induced tumor formation in mice (O'Brien et al., 2007; Ricci-Vitiani et al., 2007; Todaro et al., 2007). This marker has been utilized for studying various other types of cancers. The function of the CD133 protein is obscure; however, it is considered to be involved in plasma membrane physiology since its expression is in membrane protrusions and it co-localizes with membrane cholesterol (Mizrak et al., 2008). Less than 100–3000 $CD133^+$ cells were able to initiate a new tumor whereas more than 10×10^5–6×10^6 $CD133^-$ cells failed to generate a new tumor (O'Brien et al., 2007; Ricci-Vitiani et al., 2007; Todaro et al., 2007). Hence, selection of $CD133^+$ cells fraction led to the enrichment of CSCs. Other markers like $CD44^+/ESA^{high}$ have also been observed to have CSC population (Dalerba et al., 2007) and have been summarized in Table 8.3. There is an overlap observed between the $CD133^+$ and $CD44^+/ESA^{high}$ populations, indicating that a combination of these markers may enrich the colon CSC population.

TABLE 8.3
Colon CSC Markers

Markers	Function	Percentage (%)
$CD44^+/ESA^{high}/CD166^+$	CD44; adhesion molecule, ESA; adhesion molecule, CD166 (ALCAM); adhesion molecule	0.2–38 (mean 11.8)
$CD133^+$	Unknown	0.2–20

8.4 Treatment Implications

Most contemporary cancer treatments have limited selectivity against the tumors. Hence, these methods must be used cautiously to limit adverse effects associated with treatment. It has also been observed that cancers that are treated with the current chemotherapy or radiotherapy tend to recur after some time and may arise at a new site. Hence, a more selective and targeted approach would help in the better eradication of the tumor. If the CSC hypothesis proves to be acceptable, then an approach can be aimed to selectively stop the tumor. Some studies have shown that the tumor aggressiveness may correlate with the proportion of CSCs within a corresponding tumor (Smalley and Ashworth, 2003; Bao et al., 2006; Diehn and Clarke, 2006). Evidence also supports that CSCs may be able to selectively resist many current therapies (Croker and Allan, 2008). There are several common drug-resistant genes that are overexpressed in normal stem cells and metastatic cancer cells. All these discoveries have led researchers to propose numerous strategies for treating cancer by aiming at molecules concerned with CSC renewal and proliferation pathways. Potential strategies include interfering with molecular pathways that augment drug resistance, aiming at proteins that may sensitize CSCs to radiation or preventing the CSCs' self-renewal capacity by modifying their cell differentiation potential (Croker and Allan, 2008). The researchers need to characterize the CSCs associated with a particular tumor type, recognize relevant molecules to target, develop effective agents, and test the agents in preclinical models, such as animals or cell lines.

8.5 Future Perspectives

The discovery of CSCs in some tumor types has ushered in a new era of cancer research. CSC science is a promising field that will eventually impact the understanding of cancer progression and may enable the identification of novel therapeutic strategies. However, a lot needs to be explored about these exceptional cells, which as of now have not been recognized in all types of cancer. Currently, evidence persists to rise to support a CSC hypothesis—that cancers are proliferate by a small number of tumor-initiating cells that demonstrate various stem cell-like properties. It is not clear if the hypothesis ultimately proves true in all cases; however, by understanding the similarities between cancer cells and stem cells, the molecular pathways that are triggered in carcinogenesis will be revealed. The characterization of these CSCs will probably play a major role in the development of novel targeted therapies designed to eradicate the most notorious tumor cells that may be resistant to current chemotherapy regimens, thereby providing scientists and clinicians with additional targets to ease the burden of cancer.

References

Aktas, B., Tewes, M., Fehm, T., Hauch, S., Kimmig, R., and Kasimir-Bauer, S. 2009. Stem cell and epithelial-mesenchymal transition markers are frequently overexpressed in circulating tumor cells of metastatic breast cancer patients. *Breast Cancer Res* 11:R46.

Al-Hajj, M., Wicha, M.S., Benito-Hernandez, A., Morrison, S.J., and Clarke, M.F. 2003. Prospective identification of tumorigenic breast cancer cells. *Proc Natl Acad Sci USA* 100:3983–3988.

Allan, A.L., Vantyghem, S.A., Tuck, A.B., and Chambers, A.F. 2006. Tumor dormancy and cancer stem cells: Implications for the biology and treatment of breast cancer metastasis. *Breast Dis* 26:87–98.

Altundag, O., Altundag, K., Boruban, C., Silay, Y.S., and Turen, S. 2005. Imatinib mesylate lacks activity in small cell lung carcinoma expressing c-kit protein: A phase II clinical trial. *Cancer* 104:2033–2034.

Apati, A., Orban, T.I., Varga, N. et al. 2008. High level functional expression of the ABCG2 multidrug transporter in undifferentiated human embryonic stem cells. *Biochim Biophys Acta Biomembr* 1778:2700–2709.

Balic, M., Lin, H., Young, L. et al. 2006. Most early disseminated cancer cells detected in bone marrow of breast cancer patients have a putative breast cancer stem cell phenotype. *Clin Cancer Res* 12:5615–5621.

Bao, S., Wu, Q., McLendon, R.E. et al. 2006. Glioma stem cells promote radio resistance by preferential activation of the DNA damage response. *Nature* 444:756–760.

Bergers, G. and Benjamin, L.E. 2003. Tumorigenesis and the angiogenic switch. *Nat Rev Cancer* 3:401–410.

Bertolini, G., Roz, L., Perego, P. et al. 2009. Highly tumorigenic lung cancer CD133$^+$ cells display stem-like features and are spared by cisplatin treatment. *Proc Natl Acad Sci USA* 106:16281–16286.

Birchmeier, W. and Behrens, J. 1994. Cadherin expression in carcinomas: Role in the formation of cell junctions and the prevention of invasiveness. *Biochim Biophys Acta* 1198:11–26.

Bixby, S., Kruger, G.M., Mosher, J.T., Joseph, N.M., and Morrison, S.J. 2002. Cell-intrinsic differences between stem cells from different regions of the peripheral nervous system regulate the generation of neural diversity. *Neuron* 35:643–656.

Bonnet, D. and Dick, J.E. 1997. Human acute myeloid leukemia is organized as a hierarchy that originates from a primitive hematopoietic cell. *Nat Med* 3:730–737.

Calvi, L.M., Adams, G.B., Weibrecht, K.W. et al. 2003. Osteoblastic cells regulate the hematopoietic stem cell niche. *Nature* 425:841–846.

Carney, D.N., Gazdar, A.F., Bunn, P.A. Jr, and Guccion, J.G. 1982. Demonstration of the stem cell nature of clonogenic tumor cells from lung cancer patients. *Stem Cells* 1:149–164.

Cavallaro, U. and Christofori, G. 2004. Cell adhesion and signalling by cadherins and Ig-CAMs in cancer. *Nat Rev Cancer* 4:118–132.

CBTRUS. 2010. *CBTRUS Statistical Report: Primary Brain and Central Nervous System Tumors Diagnosed in the United States in 2004–2006*. Hinsdale, IL: Central Brain Tumor Registry of the United States.

Chambers, A.F., Groom, A.C., and MacDonald, I.C. 2002. Dissemination and growth of cancer cells in metastatic sites. *Nat Rev Cancer* 2:563–572.

Charafe-Jauffret, E., Ginestier, C., and Iovino, F. 2009. Breast cancer cell lines contain functional cancer stem cells with metastatic capacity and a distinct molecular signature. *Cancer Res* 69:1302–1313.

Charafe-Jauffret, E., Ginestier, C., and Iovino, F. 2010. Aldehyde dehydrogenase 1-positive cancer stem cells mediate metastasis and poor clinical outcome in inflammatory breast cancer. *Clin Cancer Res* 16:45–55.

Cheng, J.X., Liu, B.L., and Zhang, X. 2009. How powerful is CD133 as a cancer stem cell marker in brain tumors? *Cancer Treat Rev* 35:403–408.

Christ, O., Lucke, K., Imren, S. et al. 2007. Improved purification of hematopoietic stem cells based on their elevated aldehyde dehydrogenase activity. *Haematologica* 92:1165–1172.

Christiansen, J.J. and Rajasekaran, A.K. 2006. Reassessing epithelial to mesenchymal transition as a prerequisite for carcinoma invasion and metastasis. *Cancer Res* 66:8319–8326.

Christofori, G. and Semb, H. 1999. The role of the cell-adhesion molecule E-cadherin as a tumor-suppressor gene. *Trends Biochem Sci* 24:73–76.

Cicalese, A., Bonizzi, G., Pasi, C.E. et al. 2009. The tumor suppressor p53 regulates polarity of self-renewing divisions in mammary stem cells. *Cell* 138:1083–1095.

Collins, A.T., Berry, P.A., Hyde, C., Stower, M.J., and Maitland, N.J. 2005. Prospective identification of tumorigenic prostate cancer stem cells. *Cancer Res* 65:10946–10951.

Corti, S., Locatelli, F., Papadimitriou, D. et al. 2006. Identification of a primitive brain-derived neural stem cell population based on aldehyde dehydrogenase activity. *Stem Cells* 24:975–985.

Croker, A.K. and Allan, A.L. 2008. Cancer stem cells: Implications for the progression and treatment of metastatic disease. *J Cell Mol Med* 12:374–390.

Croker, A.K., Goodale, D., Chu, J. et al. 2009. High aldehyde dehydrogenase and expression of cancer stem cell markers selects for breast cancer cells with enhanced malignant and metastatic ability. *J Cell Mol Med* 13:2236–2252.

Dalerba, P., Dylla, S.J., Park, I.K. et al. 2007. Phenotypic characterization of human colorectal cancer stem cells. *Proc Natl Acad Sci USA* 104:10158–10163.

Deng, C.H. and Zhang, Q.P. 2010. Leukemia stem cells in drug resistance and metastasis. *Chin Med J* 123:954–960.

Desai, B., Rogers, M.J., and Chellaiah, M.A. 2007. Mechanisms of osteopontin and CD44 as metastatic principles in prostate cancer cells. *Mol Cancer* 6:18.

Dick, J.E. 2003. Breast cancer stem cells revealed. *Proc Natl Acad Sci USA* 100:3547–3549.

Diehn, M. and Clarke, M.F. 2006. Cancer stem cells and radiotherapy: New insights into tumor radioresistance. *J Natl Cancer Inst* 98:1755–1757.

Ding, W., Mouzaki, M., You, H. et al. 2009. CD133$^+$ liver cancer stem cells from methionine adenosyl transferase 1A-deficient mice demonstrate resistance to transforming growth factor (TGF)-beta-induced apoptosis. *Hepatology* 49:1277–1286.

Dontu, G., Abdallah, W.M., Foley, J.M. et al. 2003. In vitro propagation and transcriptional profiling of human mammary stem/progenitor cells. *Genes Dev* 17:1253–1270.

Dontu, G., Jackson, K.W., McNicholas, E., Kawamura, M.J., Abdallah, W.M., and Wicha, M.S. 2004. Role of Notch signaling in cell-fate determination of human mammary stem/progenitor cells. *Breast Cancer Res* 6:R605–R615.

Dou, J., Jiang, C.L., Wang, J. et al. 2011. Using ABCG2-molecule-expressing side population cells to identify cancer stem-like cells in a human ovarian cell line. *Cell Biol Int* 35:227–234.

Dy, G.K., Miller, A.A., Mandrekar, S.J. et al. 2005. A phase II trial of imatinib (ST1571) in patients with c-kit expressing relapsed small-cell lung cancer: A CALGB and NCCTG study. *Ann Oncol* 16:1811–1816.

Eramo, A., Lotti, F., Sette, G. et al. 2008. Identification and expansion of the tumorigenic lung cancer stem cell population. *Cell Death Differ* 15:504–514.

Fidler, I.J. 2003. The pathogenesis of cancer metastasis: The 'seed and soil' hypothesis revisited. *Nat Rev Cancer* 3:453–458.

Fillmore, C.M. and Kuperwasser, C. 2008. Human breast cancer cell lines contain stem-like cells that self-renew, give rise to phenotypically diverse progeny and survive chemotherapy. *Breast Cancer Res* 10:R25.

Folgueras, A.R., Pendas, A.M., Sanchez, L.M., and Lopez-Otin, C. 2004. Matrix metalloproteinases in cancer: From new functions to improved inhibition strategies. *Int J Dev Biol* 48:411–424.

Galderisi, U., Cipollaro, M., and Giordano, A. 2006. Stem cells and brain cancer. *Cell Death Differ* 13:5–11.

Gazzaniga, P., Cigna, E., Panasiti, V. et al. 2010. CD133 and ABCB5 as stem cell markers on sentinel lymph node from melanoma patients. *Eur J Surg Oncol* 36:1211–1214.

Gilbert, C.A. and Ross, A.H. 2009. Cancer stem cells: Cell culture, markers, and targets for new therapies. *J Cell Biochem* 108:1031–1038.

Ginestier, C., Hur, M.H., Charafe-Jauffret, E. et al. 2007. ALDH1 is a marker of normal and malignant human mammary stem cells and a predictor of poor clinical outcome. *Cell Stem Cell* 1:555–567.

Goss, P., Allan, A.L., Rodenhiser, D.I., Foster, P.J., and Chambers, A.F. 2008. New clinical and experimental approaches for studying tumor dormancy: Does tumor dormancy offer a therapeutic target? *APMIS* 116:552–568.

Gross, D.J., Munter, G., Bitan, M. et al. 2006. The role of imatinib mesylate (Glivec) for treatment of patients with malignant endocrine tumors positive for c-kit or PDGF-R. *Endocr Relat Cancer* 13:535–540.

Grunert, S., Jechlinger, M., and Beug, H. 2003. Diverse cellular and molecular mechanisms contribute to epithelial plasticity and metastasis. *Nat Rev Mol Cell Biol* 4:657–665.

Guo, W. and Giancotti, F.G. 2004. Integrin signalling during tumor progression. *Nat Rev Mol Cell Biol* 5:816–826.

Hanahan, D. and Weinberg, R.A. 2000. The hallmarks of cancer. *Cell* 100:57–70.

He, J., Liu, Y., Zhu, T. et al. 2012. CD90 is identified as a marker for cancer stem cells in primary high-grade gliomas using tissue microarrays. *Mol Cell Proteomics* 11:M111.010744.

Hellsten, R., Johansson, M., Dahlman, A., Sterner, O., and Bjartell, A. 2011. Galiellalactone inhibits stem cell-like ALDH-positive prostate cancer cells. *PLoS One* 6:e22118.

Hendrix, M.J., Seftor, E.A., Seftor, R.E., Kasemeier-Kulesa, J., Kulesa, P.M., and Postovit, L.M. 2007. Reprogramming metastatic tumor cells with embryonic microenvironments. *Nat Rev Cancer* 7:246–255.

Hess, D.A., Meyerrose, T.E., Wirthlin, L. et al. 2004. Functional characterization of highly purified human hematopoietic repopulating cells isolated according to aldehyde dehydrogenase activity. *Blood* 104:1648–1655.

Hibi, K., Takahashi, T., Sekido Y. et al. 1991. Coexpression of the stem cell factor and the c-kit genes in small-cell lung cancer. *Oncogene* 6:2291–2296.

Ho, M.M., Ng, A.V., Lam, S., and Hung, J.Y. 2007. Side population in human lung cancer cell lines and tumors is enriched with stem-like cancer cells. *Cancer Res* 67:4827–4833.

Hood, J.D. and Cheresh, D.A. 2002. Role of integrins in cell invasion and migration. *Nat Rev Cancer* 2:91–100.

Huang, E.H., Hynes, M.J., Zhang, T. et al. 2009. Aldehyde dehydrogenase 1 is a marker for normal and malignant human colonic stem cells (SC) and tracks SC overpopulation during colon tumorigenesis. *Cancer Res* 69:3382–3389.

Huber, M.A., Kraut, N., and Beug, H. 2005. Molecular requirements for epithelial–mesenchymal transition during tumor progression. *Curr Opin Cell Biol* 17:548–558.

Hurt, E.M., Kawasaki, B.T., Klarmann, G.J., Thomas, S.B., and Farrar, W.L. 2008. CD44(+)CD24(−) prostate cells are early cancer progenitor/stem cells that provide a model for patients with poor prognosis. *Br J Cancer* 98:756–765.

Immervoll, H., Hoem, D., Sakariassen, P.O., Steffensen, O.J., and Molven, A. 2008. Expression of the "stem cell marker" CD133 in pancreas and pancreatic ductal adenocarcinomas. *BMC Cancer* 8:48.

Islam, M.O., Kanemura, Y., Tajria, J. et al. 2005. Functional expression of ABCG2 transporter in human neural stem/progenitor cells. *Neurosci Res* 52:75–82.

Jaksch, M., Munera, J., Bajpai, R., Terskikh, A., and Oshima, R.G. 2008. Cell cycle-dependent variation of a CD133 epitope in human embryonic stem cell, colon cancer, and melanoma cell lines. *Cancer Res* 68:7882–7886.

Jiang, F., Qiu, Q., Khanna, A. et al. 2009. Aldehyde dehydrogenase 1 is a tumor stem cell-associated marker in lung cancer. *Mol Cancer Res* 7:330–338.

Kang, Y. and Massague, J. 2004. Epithelial–mesenchymal transitions: Twist in development and metastasis. *Cell* 118:277–279.

Kaplan, R.N., Riba, R.D., Zacharoulis, S. et al. 2005. VEGFR1-positive hematopoietic bone marrow progenitors initiate the pre-metastatic niche. *Nature* 438:820–826.

Kiel, M.J., Yilmaz, O.H., Iwashita, T., Yilmaz, O.H., Terhorst, C., and Morrison, S.J. 2005. SLAM family receptors distinguish hematopoietic stem and progenitor cells and reveal endothelial niches for stem cells. *Cell* 121:1109–1121.

Lapidot, T., Sirard, C., Vormoor, J. et al. 1994. A cell initiating human acute myeloid leukaemia after transplantation into SCID mice. *Nature* 367:645–648.

Le, Q.T., Chen, E., Salim A. et al. 2006. An evaluation of tumor oxygenation and gene expression in patients with early stage non-small cell lung cancers. *Clin Cancer Res* 12:1507–1514.

Lechner, A., Leech, C.A., Abraham, E.J., Nolan, A.L., and Habener, J.F. 2002. Nestin-positive progenitor cells derived from adult human pancreatic islets of Langerhans contain side population (SP) cells defined by expression of the ABCG2 (BCRP1) ATP-binding cassette transporter. *Biochem Biophys Res Commun* 293:670–674.

Lee, L.N., Kuo, S.H., Lee, Y.C. et al. 2005. CD44 splicing pattern is associated with disease progression in pulmonary adenocarcinoma. *J Formos Med Assoc* 104:541–548.

Li, C.W., Heidt, D.G., Dalerba, P. et al. 2007. Identification of pancreatic cancer stem cells. *Cancer Res* 67:1030–1037.

Liu, J. and Jiang, G. 2006. CD44 and hematologic malignancies. *Cell Mol Immunol* 3:359–365.

Lopez-Otin, C. and Overall, C.M. 2002. Protease degradomics: A new challenge for proteomics. *Nat Rev Mol Cell Biol* 3:509–519.

Ma, S., Chan, K.W., Lee, T.K. et al. 2008. Aldehyde dehydrogenase discriminates the CD133 liver cancer stem cell populations. *Mol Cancer Res* 6:1146–1153.

MacDonald, I.C., Groom, A.C., and Chambers, A.F. 2002. Cancer spread and micrometastasis development: Quantitative approaches for in vivo models. *Bioessays* 24:885–893.

Mani, S.A., Guo, W., Liao, M.J. et al. 2008. The epithelial-mesenchymal transition generates cells with properties of stem cells. *Cell* 133:704–715.

Mizrak, D., Brittan, M., and Alison, M.R. 2008. CD133: Molecule of the moment. *J Pathol* 214:3–9.

Moinfar, F., Man, Y.G., Arnould, L., Bratthauer, G.L., Ratschek, M., and Tavassoli, F.A. 2000. Concurrent and independent genetic alterations in the stromal and epithelial cells of mammary carcinoma: Implications for tumorigenesis. *Cancer Res* 60:2562–2566.

Morel, A.P., Lievre, M., Thomas, C., Hinkal, G., Ansieau, S., and Puisieux, A. 2008. Generation of breast cancer stem cells through epithelial-mesenchymal transition. *PLoS One* 3:e2888.

O'Brien, C.A., Pollett, A., Gallinger, S., and Dick, J.E. 2007. A human colon cancer cell capable of initiating tumour growth in immunodeficient mice. *Nature* 445:106–110.

Pantel, K. and Brakenhoff, R.H. 2004. Dissecting the metastatic cascade. *Nat Rev Cancer* 4:448–456.

Papayannopoulou, T. and Scadden, D.T. 2008. Stem-cell ecology and stem cells in motion. *Blood* 111:3923–3930.

Pardal, R., Clarke, M.F., and Morrison, S.J. 2003. Applying the principles of stem-cell biology to cancer. *Nat Rev Cancer* 3:895–902.

Park, C.H., Bergsagel, D.E., and McCulloch, E.A. 1971. Mouse myeloma tumor stem cells: A primary cell culture assay. *J Natl Cancer Inst* 46:411–422.

Patrawala, L., Calhoun, T., Schneider-Broussard, R., Zhou, J., Claypool, K., and Tang, D.G. 2005. Side population is enriched in tumorigenic, stem-like cancer cells, whereas ABCG2$^+$ and ABCG2$^-$ cancer cells are similarly tumorigenic. *Cancer Res* 65:6207–6219.

Patrawala, L., Calhoun, T., Schneider-Broussard, R. et al. 2006. Highly purified CD44$^+$ prostate cancer cells from xenograft human tumors are enriched in tumorigenic and metastatic progenitor cells. *Oncogene* 25:1696–1708.

Pece, S., Tosoni, D., Confalonieri, S. et al. 2010. Biological and molecular heterogeneity of breast cancers correlates with their cancer stem cell content. *Cell* 140:62–73.

Peinado, H., Portillo, F., and Cano, A. 2004. Transcriptional regulation of cadherins during development and carcinogenesis. *Int J Dev Biol* 48:365–375.

Peinado, P., Quintanilla, M., and Cano, A. 2003. Transforming growth factor beta 1 induces Snail transcription factor in epithelial cell lines: Mechanisms for epithelial mesenchymal transitions. *J Biol Chem* 278:21113–21123.

Pelosi, G., Barisella, M., Pasini, F. et al. 2004. CD117 immunoreactivity in stage I adenocarcinoma and squamous cell carcinoma of the lung: Relevance to prognosis in a subset of adenocarcinoma patients. *Mod Pathol* 17:711–721.

Phillips, H.S., Kharbanda, S., Chen, R. et al. 2006. Molecular subclasses of high-grade glioma predict prognosis, delineate a pattern of disease progression, and resemble stages in neurogenesis. *Cancer Cell* 9:157–173.

Ponti, D., Costa, A., Zaffaroni, N. et al. 2005. Isolation and in vitro propagation of tumorigenic breast cancer cells with stem/progenitor cell properties. *Cancer Res* 6513:5506–5511.

Prince, M.E., Sivanandan, R., Kaczorowski, A. et al. 2007. Identification of a subpopulation of cells with cancer stem cell properties in head and neck squamous cell carcinoma. *PNAS* 104:973–978.

Ricci-Vitiani, L., Lombardi, D.G., Pilozzi, E. et al. 2007. Identification and expansion of human colon-cancer-initiating cells. *Nature* 445:111–115.

Rich, J.N. 2008. The implications of the cancer stem cell hypothesis for neuro-oncology and neurology. *Future Neurol* 3:265–273.

Sajithlal, G.B., Rothermund, K., Zhang, F. et al. 2010. Permanently blocked stem cells derived from breast cancer cell lines. *Stem Cells* 28:1008–1018.

Seigel, G.M., Campbell, L.M., Narayan, M., and Gonzalez-Fernandez, F. 2005. Cancer stem cell characteristics in retinoblastoma. *Mol Vis* 11:729–737.

Sheridan, C., Kishimoto, H., Fuchs, R.K. et al. 2006. CD44$^+$/CD24$^-$ breast cancer cells exhibit enhanced invasive properties: An early step necessary for metastasis. *Breast Cancer Res* 8:R59.

Shi, G.M., Xu, Y., Fan, J. et al. 2008. Identification of side population cells in human hepatocellular carcinoma cell lines with stepwise metastatic potentials. *J Cancer Res Clin Oncol* 134:1155–1163.

Smalley, M. and Ashworth, A. 2003. Stem cells and breast cancer: A field in transit. *Nat Rev Cancer* 3:832–844.

Sporn, M.B. 1996. The war on cancer. *Lancet* 347:1377–1381.

Stewart, J.M., Shaw, P.A., Gedye, C., Bernardini, M.Q., Neel, B.G., and Ailles, L.E. 2011. Phenotypic heterogeneity and instability of human ovarian tumor-initiating cells. *Proc Natl Acad Sci USA* 108:6468–6473.

Suetsugu, A., Nagaki, M., Aoki, H., Motohashi, T., Kunisada, T., and Moriwaki, H. 2006. Characterization of CD133$^+$ hepatocellular carcinoma cells as cancer stem/progenitor cells. *Biochem Biophys Res Commun* 351:820–824.

Summer, R., Kotton, D.N., Sun, X., Ma, B., Fitzsimmons, K., and Fine, A. 2003. Side population cells and Bcrp1 expression in lung. *Am J Physiol Lung Cell Mol Physiol* 285:L97–L104.

Takebe, N., Harris, P.J., Warren, R.Q., and Ivy, S.P. 2011a. Targeting cancer stem cells by inhibiting Wnt, Notch, and Hedgehog pathways. *Nat Rev Clin Oncol* 8:97–106.

Takebe, N., Warren, R.Q., and Ivy, S.P. 2011b. Breast cancer growth and metastasis: Interplay between cancer stem cells, embryonic signaling pathways and epithelial-to-mesenchymal transition. *Breast Cancer Res* 13:211.

Tang, D.G., Patrawala, L., Calhoun, T. et al. 2007. Prostate cancer stem/progenitor cells: Identification, characterization and implications. *Mol Carcinog* 46:1–14.

Tarin, D., Thompson, E.W., and Newgreen, D.F. 2005. The fallacy of epithelial mesenchymal transition in neoplasia. *Cancer Res* 65:5996–6001.

Theodoropoulos, P.A., Polioudaki, H., Agelaki, S. et al. 2010. Circulating tumor cells with a putative stem cell phenotype in peripheral blood of patients with breast cancer. *Cancer Lett* 288(1):99–106.

Thiery, J.P. 2002. Epithelial-mesenchymal transitions in tumor progression. *Nat Rev Cancer* 2:442–454.

Thiery, J.P., Acloque, H., Huang, R.Y., and Nieto, M.A. 2009. Epithelial–mesenchymal transitions in development and disease. *Cell* 139:871–890.

Thiery, J.P. and Sleeman, J.P. 2006. Complex networks orchestrate epithelial–mesenchymal transitions. *Nat Rev Mol Cell Biol* 7:131–142.

Thompson, E.W., Newgreen, D.F., and Tarin, D. 2005. Carcinoma invasion and metastasis: A role for epithelial–mesenchymal transition? *Cancer Res* 65:5991–5995.

Todaro, M., Perez Alea, M., Di Stefano, A.B. et al. 2007. Colon cancer stem cells dictate tumor growth and resist cell death by production of interleukin-4. *Cell Stem Cell* 1:389–402.

Tomuleasa, C., Mosteanu, O., Susman, S., and Cristea, V. 2011. ALDH as a tumor marker for pancreatic cancer. *J Gastrointestin Liver Dis* 20:443–444; author reply 444.

Vander Griend, D.J., Karthaus, W.L., Dalrymple, S., Meeker, A., DeMarzo, A.M., and Isaacs, J.T. 2008. The role of CD133 in normal human prostate stem cells and malignant cancer-initiating cells. *Cancer Res* 68:9703–9711.

Vesuna, F., Lisok, A., Kimble, B., and Raman, V. 2009. Twist modulates breast cancer stem cells by transcriptional regulation of CD24 expression. *Neoplasia* 11:1318–1328.

Visus, C., Ito, D., Amoscato, A. et al. 2007. Identification of human aldehyde dehydrogenase 1 family member A1 as a novel $CD8^+$ T cell-defined tumor antigen in squamous cell carcinoma of the head and neck. *Cancer Res* 67:10538–10545.

Visvader, J.E. and Lindeman, G.J. 2008. Cancer stem cells in solid tumours: Accumulating evidence and unresolved questions. *Nat Rev Cancer* 8:755–768.

Wang, W.G., Eddy, R., and Condeelis, J. 2007. The cofilin pathway in breast invasion and metastasis. *Nat Rev Cancer* 7:429–444.

Watanabe, K., Nishida, K., Yamato, M. et al. 2004. Human limbal epithelium contains side population cells expressing the ATP-binding cassette transporter ABCG2. *FEBS Lett* 565:6–10.

Wei, C., Guomin, W., Yujun, L., and Ruizhe, Q. 2007. Cancer stem-like cells in human prostate carcinoma cells DU145: The seeds of the cell line? *Cancer Biol Ther* 6:763–768.

Weiss, L. 1990. Metastatic inefficiency. *Adv Cancer Res* 54:159–211.

Wernert, N., Locherbach, C., Wellmann, A., Behrens, P., and Hugel, A. 2000. Presence of genetic alterations in microdissected stroma of human colon and breast cancers. *J Mol Med* 78:B30.

Wicha, M.S. 2006. Cancer stem cells and metastasis: Lethal seeds. *Clin Cancer Res* 12:5606–5607.

Woodhouse, E.C., Chuaqui, R.F., and Liotta, L.A. 1997. General mechanisms of metastasis. *Cancer* 80:1529–1537.

Yamazaki, H., Nishida, H., Iwata, S., Dang, N.H., and Morimoto, C. 2009. CD90 and CD110 correlate with cancer stem cell potentials in human T-acute lymphoblastic leukemia cells. *Biochem Biophys Res Commun* 383:172–177.

Yang, Z.F., Ho, D.W., Ng, M.N. et al. 2008. Significance of CD90(+) cancer stem cells in human liver cancer. *Cancer Cell* 13:153–166.

Zhang, J., Niu, C., Ye, L. et al. 2003. Identification of the hematopoietic stem cell niche and control of the niche size. *Nature* 425:836–841.

Zhang, S., Balch, C., Chan, M.W., Lai, H., Matei, D. et al. 2008. Identification and characterization of ovarian cancer-initiating cells from primary human tumors. *Cancer Res* 68:4311–4320.

Zhi, Q.M., Chen, X.H., Ji, J. et al. 2011. Salinomycin can effectively kill ALDH (high) stem-like cells on gastric cancer. *Biomed Pharmacother* 65:509–515.

9

Salivary Biomarkers in Early Diagnosis and Monitoring of Cancer

Saroj K. Basak and Eri S. Srivatsan

CONTENTS

ABSTRACT Cancer is responsible for millions of deaths all over the world. Unfortunately, most cancer-related symptoms appear at late stages of the disease that leaves few treatment options. It is possible to prevent all cancer-related deaths if the disease is detected early. Early detection of cancer can also help in better monitoring and treatment of the disease. Till recently, blood and urine from cancer patients have been the choice of diagnostic fluids not because of their ease of availability but because of the presence of cancer-specific antigens in these body fluids. Though saliva is easily available, the intrinsic problem has been the low concentration of tumor antigens that could not be detected efficiently by using conventional methods, such as polymerase chain reaction (PCR), reverse transcriptase PCR (RT-PCR), enzyme-linked immunosorbent assay (ELISA), and immunoblotting techniques. However, recent advancements and improvements in the detection technology and new proteomic and genomic technologies have greatly improved the detection of salivary biomarkers in human diseases. It has also been realized that no single biomarker can identify a disease or its stage accurately in a population. Thus, the focus is to identify panels of biomarkers that can be related to a specific disease and stage of the disease. The use of salivary biomarkers for cancer detection is now at the discovery phase where by applying new exciting technologies, a panel of biomarkers are being validated in cancer patients. Identification of cancer-specific biomarkers is enhanced by global profiling of proteins, DNA, mRNA, microRNA, and metabolites. Further, analysis of the salivary transcriptome (RNA) and proteome from cancer patients is applied to identify RNA and protein markers.

This chapter summarizes the various salivary cancer biomarkers that have been identified by the applications of recent methodologies and techniques in the analysis of salivary samples. The pace of discovery of salivary biomarkers for cancer has increased in recent times, and one hopes for its application in early cancer diagnosis and monitoring of cancer in the affected patients.

9.1 Saliva as a Diagnostic Material for Cancer

Every year cancer kills about 7.6 million people and 70% of the deaths occur in low- to middle-income countries (WHO Report, 2013). These deaths are due to cancer of the lung, oral, breast, cervical, stomach, colon, and liver. Detection and diagnosis of cancer at an early stage can save lives due to better cure rate and treatment. A good example of early detection and good prognosis is ovarian cancer where 5-year survival rate post diagnosis can reach 70%–93%, if the disease is detected at an early stage (stage I and II), but drops to 10%–37%, if diagnosed at late stage (stage III and IV) (Holschneider and Berek, 2000). Oral cancer (oral squamous cell carcinoma [OSCC]) has about 50% mortality rate within 5 years of diagnosis (Kantola et al., 2000; Myers et al., 2000), which has remained the same over the last 50 years (Ribeiro et al., 2000; Sparano et al., 2004). Early diagnosis could therefore improve the survival of these patients.

Unfortunately, the current predictors of cancer are not up to mark for the early detection and prevention of cancer. This is due to the limitation of sensitive diagnostic techniques that can detect specific markers at an early stage of cancer (Bretthauer et al., 2013). However, recent development of new powerful screening tests particularly in proteomic, genomic, and imaging technologies (Sadick et al., 2012) combined with bioinformatic techniques can play an important role in early detection of cancer (Metallo, 2012; Wang et al., 2013). Another important factor for early detection of cancer is the routine/regular checkups, and general public and clinicians are aware of the importance of the role of regular checkup and early detection of cancer and its role in prevention. However, most morbid symptoms appear at late phase of cancer. This is further complicated by the reluctance of general public to give blood for diagnostic purposes that requires trained personnel and collection centers. Saliva on the other hand can be collected easily from people and thus has advantages over other body fluids for the detection of diseases including cancer (Mandel, 1990; Haeckel and Hänecke, 1993; Wong et al., 2006a,b; O'Driscoll, 2007; Giannobile et al., 2011; Sharma et al., 2010).

Early detection of cancer can help in better management of cancer by successful monitoring of the progression of cancer (Rusling et al., 2010; Printz, 2012). For the development and discovery of salivary biomarkers of cancer, it is necessary to evaluate the saliva for changes in protein, DNA, mRNA, and other markers and just not test the existence of cancer blood markers in the saliva. The rapid accent of salivary diagnosis of diseases and health monitoring is helped by the development of technologies such as PCR, mass spectroscopy (MS), and nanotechnology. These technologies when applied for large-scale data collection for human diseases and human populations have created new scientific fields such as genomics, proteomics, metabolomics, peptidomics, transcriptomics, and bioinformatics (Lee and Wong, 2009). The science collectively known as "omics" has led to a vast knowledge database that is currently used for monitoring of diseases. Further, recent salivary proteomic and genomic data available in the literature have important information for diagnostic applications of cancer (Helmerhorst and Oppenheim, 2007; Denny et al., 2008; Farnaud et al., 2010; Ai et al., 2012).

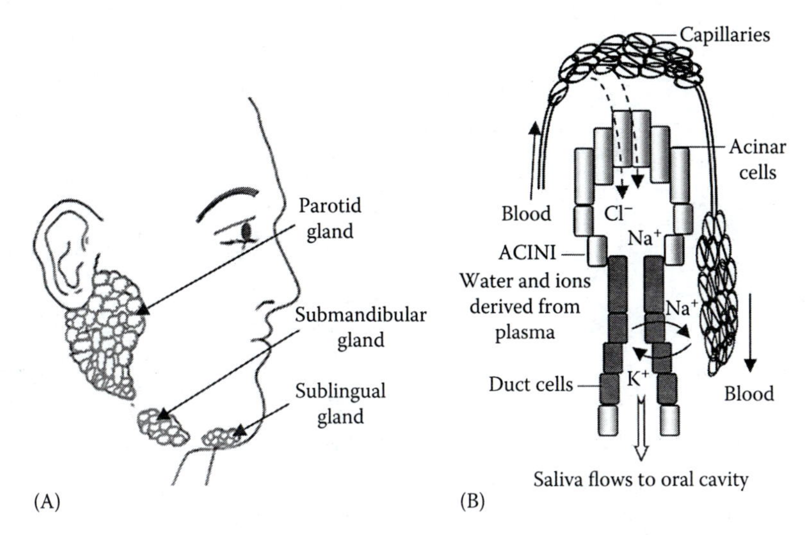

FIGURE 9.1 Salivary glands and saliva production. (A) Salivary glands: parotid, submandibular, and sublingual glands. (B) Biomarker transportation from serum to salivary gland acini. Biomarkers enter saliva through the space between cells by transcellular (passive intracellular diffusion and active transport) or paracellular routes (extracellular ultrafiltration). Acinar cells actively pump Na^+ into the duct. Duct cells pump Na^+ back into the blood. (Adapted from Pink, R. et al., *Biomed Pap Med Fac Univ Palacky Olomouc Czech Repub*, 153(2), 103, June 2009.)

9.2 Saliva as a Physiological Sample

Saliva is produced by three major salivary glands: the parotid, submandibular, and sublingual glands in association with minor glands including labial, buccal, lingual, and palatal tissue (Figure 9.1A). Saliva is a clear viscous and slightly acidic liquid (6.0–7.0 pH) that contains many biological compounds including cells of epithelial origin. In general, a healthy individual produces 1–1.5 L of saliva/day (Mandel, 1993; Humphrey and Williamson, 2001). Saliva plays an important role in human physiology as it helps in maintaining the healthy status of oral cavity including dental health. It also has a role in tasting of food and its digestion.

Since saliva is secreted from glands that are connected with the rest of the body by local vasculature that originates from carotid artery, it is a complex biological fluid that contains factors and compounds found in the blood as well as in the rest of the body tissues (Figure 9.1B) (Drobitch and Drobitch, 1992; Haeckel and et al., 1993, 1996; Jusko and Milsap, 1993; Forde et al., 2006). Thus, salivary factors such as proteins, genetic molecules (DNA/RNA), and biochemical compounds can serve as biomarkers that can represent the health status of an individual. In the last few years, scientific interest in using the salivary biomarkers for detection and monitoring of diseases has increased due to the development and availability of new methods and technologies (Lawrence, 2002; de Almeida et al., 2008; Yeh et al., 2010; Castagnola et al., 2011a,b; Pfaffe et al., 2011; Spielmann and Wong, 2011; Brinkmann et al., 2012; Shah et al., 2013).

9.3 Collection of Saliva

Saliva can be used as a diagnostic fluid primarily due to its ease of collection and noninvasive procedures. It can also be collected repeatedly at any location and can be obtained over long duration without any discomfort to the patient. Saliva can be collected from an individual as they are produced in general course over time or they can be collected by stimulating saliva production by chewing action such as chewing gum or rubber, to increase salivary flow. Stimulated saliva is generally collected from patients who have undergone radiation therapy of the oral region or have difficulty in producing saliva.

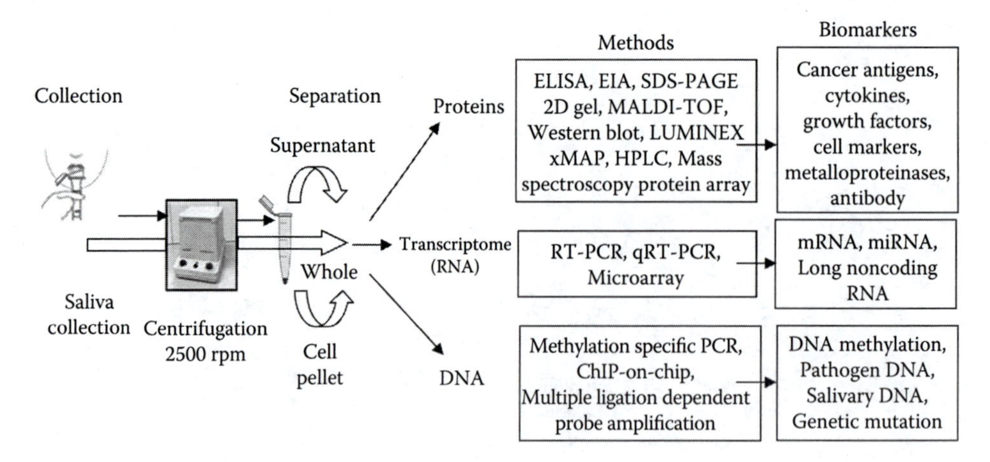

FIGURE 9.2 Saliva collection and processing. Saliva collected from patients is separated from cellular component by centrifugation. Supernatant, cell pellets, or total saliva can be procesed by different methods for detection of salivary protein, transcriptome, and DNA biomarkers.

Patients are advised to clean or rinse their mouth prior to collection of saliva that can be collected either by draining, spitting, or suction methods (Navazesh, 1993; Lee and Wong, 2009).

Though saliva is easily available, it has been reported that the method of preservation of saliva could affect the outcome of salivary diagnostic results indicating that there is a need for standardizing the collection method and storage. It has been reported that half-life of mRNA of β-actin in freshly collected saliva is only 12 min (Park et al., 2006a). However, the mRNA of saliva can be preserved up to 12 weeks at room temperature by using the reagent RNAprotect® saliva reagent (RPS, QIAGEN Inc., Valencia, CA) that can work better than other commercially available preservation reagents such as SUPERaseIn™ RNase inhibitor and RNALater® (Park et al., 2006b). Further studies have shown that RPS can also preserve DNA and protein. It has also been suggested that cell debris removal from saliva by centrifugation or filtration (5.0 μm syringe filter) helps in the preservation of salivary proteins (Jiang et al., 2009). Collection of saliva from xerostomia cancer patients due to oral surgery or radiation therapy is challenging, and this can be overcome by using Oragene® sponges that helps in the collection of sufficient amount of DNA/RNA for analysis (Matthews et al., 2013). Salivary RNAs are also being used recently for diagnosis of diseases including cancer (Martin et al., 2010). In the last few years, salivary RNA has also been used in the identification of dental health status of diabetic (Gomes et al., 2006; Nussbaumer et al., 2006) and in sleep-deprived patients (Seugnet et al., 2006). Salivary transcriptomes have been also used in the detection of oral cancer (Li et al., 2004; Zimmermann and Wong, 2008; Zimmermann et al., 2007; Lee et al., 2010; Markopoulos et al., 2010; Brinkmann et al., 2011; Zhang et al., 2012a), pancreatic cancer (Tang et al., 2010a), breast cancer (Zhang et al., 2010b), and Sjogren's syndrome (Hu et al., 2007b). Recently, it has been shown that direct salivary transcriptome analysis (DSTA) of salivary supernatant (cell-free supernatant) (Brinkmann and Wong, 2011) for RNA can be achieved after storage in ambient temperature without the need of mRNA isolation (Lee et al., 2011). Such improvement in salivary sample preparation has helped in the development of salivary-based diagnostic techniques for early stage detection of diseases including cancer (Figure 9.2).

9.4 Biomarkers of Saliva

Saliva, being a physiological fluid from the body, contains different molecules that can be used as biomarkers. Changes of salivary molecular markers during disease condition can be evaluated by comparing the molecular signature during healthy condition. Different markers such as DNA, RNA, or protein can act as indicators of the disease state. In addition to changes of such markers during pathological condition, abnormal genetic material or protein molecules can appear in saliva. Analysis of gene expression profiling of saliva can help in early detection of cancer (Westra and Califano, 2004; Adami and Adami, 2012). In addition to these molecules, saliva also contains enzymes, hormones, antibodies, growth factors, and antimicrobial constituents (Zelles et al., 1995; Rehak et al., 2000). Hormones such as cortisol are produced by adrenal glands in response to disease-related stress, and it can be detected in blood as well as in saliva. Recently, salivary cortisol levels have been measured in cancer patients and can be used as a cancer biomarker (Bernabé et al., 2012). Thus, saliva contains different biomarkers such as epigenetic, transcriptomes, microRNA (miRNA), protein, cytokines, pathogen-related biomarkers, exosomes, telomerase activity, microsatellite DNA, mitochondrial DNA (mtDNA), and metabolite/metabolomic biomarkers that are briefly discussed later.

9.4.1 Epigenetic Biomarkers

DNA methylation is an important regulator of gene transcription and it plays an important role in tumor development. Saliva can also be used for evaluating disease-related epigenetic changes such as DNA methylation (Markopoulou et al., 2012). This epigenetic modification of promoter methylation leads to repression of transcription and therefore inactivation of tumor suppressor genes. Genes involved in cell cycle, DNA repair, proliferation, and apoptosis are usually the targets of gene silencing by promoter methylation (Gonzalez-Ramirez et al., 2011). It is believed that there may be cancer-specific promoter methylation that could be helpful in cancer diagnosis. Thus, hypermethylation of the promoter regions is associated with suppression of gene function and is therefore considered a potential cancer biomarker. Some of the hypermethylated promoter regions of head and neck cancer are TIMP-3 (Rettori et al., 2013), RASSF1A, DAPK1, and p16 (Ovchinnikov et al., 2012) and DAPK, DCC, MINT-31, TIMP-3, p16, MGMT, CCNA1 (Carvalho et al., 2008, 2011), KIF1A, and EDNRB (Demokan et al., 2010) and for OSCC are HOXA9 and NID2 in OSCC (Guerrero-Preston et al., 2011).

9.4.2 Transcriptome-Based Markers

It has been shown recently that salivary transcriptomes (RNA molecules) that can be prepared from whole saliva or cell-free salivary can be used for detection of different cancers (Park et al., 2006a,b, 2007), including IL-8, SAT, IL-1β, OAZ1, H3F3A, DUSP, and S100P in OSCC (Li et al., 2004; Zimmerman et al., 2007; Park et al., 2009; Brinkmann and Wong, 2011; Brinkmann et al., 2011; Elashoff et al., 2012); ILL1RN, MAL, and MMP1 in head and neck squamous cell carcinoma (HNSCC) (Lallemant et al., 2009); CCN1, EGFR, FF19, FRS2, and GREB1 in lung cancer (Zhang et al., 2012a); S100A8, CSTA, GRM1, TPT1, GR1K1, H6PD, IGF2BP1, and MDM4 in breast cancer (Zhang et al., 2010b); KRAS, MBD3L2, ACRV1, and DPM1 in pancreatic cancer (Zhang et al., 2010a); and AGPAT1, B2M, BASP2, IER3, and IL-1β in ovarian cancer (Lee et al., 2012).

9.4.3 MicroRNA Biomarkers

miRNAs are short noncoding RNA molecules (19–24 nucleotides) and they bind to complementary sequence in 3′-untranslated region (3′-UTR) of mRNA, thus regulating protein expression/translation or degradation of mRNA (Lee et al., 1993; Lagos-Quintana et al., 2001; Lee and Ambros, 2001). One miRNA can bind to more than 100 different kinds of mRNA due to their imperfect complementary binding ability. Of the 708 human miRNAs detected in human (miRBase version 12.0), about 314 miRNAs have been detected in saliva (Liu et al., 2008; Park et al., 2009; Michael et al., 2010). miRNAs play important part in gene regulation; thus, they have important role in cell growth, differentiation, apoptosis, inflammation, stress response, invasion, metastasis, and immune response (Dalmay and Edwards, 2006; Kim et al., 2009; Garzon and Croce, 2011; Varol et al., 2011). Different cancers have different cell of origin and they also have different mechanism by which they become cancerous and they are regulated by different sets of miRNA. The cancer cells also show different miRNA expression patterns than its normal cell stage (Lu et al., 2005). Thus, miRNA profile of each cancer may depend on site of origin, its stage, and other factors. miRNAs in saliva have been recently used for diagnosis of diseases including cancer (Park et al., 2009; Brinkmann and Wong, 2011; Brinkmann et al., 2011; Liu et al., 2012a; Zen and Zhang, 2012; Yoshizawa and Wong, 2013).

In oral cancer it has been shown that miRNA regulates cell proliferation (Selcuklu et al., 2009), apoptosis (Wong et al., 2008), and drug resistance (Yu and Pestell, 2012) and they differ from their normal tissue counterpart (Kozaki et al., 2008) and fold/level of expression (Jiang et al., 2005). These data suggest that alteration in miRNA profile can be detected in saliva that bathe the cancerous tissue locally and it may be possible to detect the miRNA shed in saliva by different methods. miRNA can be shed directly from the local tumor microenvironment into saliva or in exosomes that protect their degradation (Valadi et al., 2007; Palanisamy et al., 2010). miRNA from distant tumor can also be detected in saliva as they are released in the blood and are transported to the local salivary glands where they are released in salivary acini and into the saliva.

Though many miRNAs have been identified and their role in different cancer has been validated, the process of detection and validation of miRNA in saliva has just started. It has been recently shown that in OSCC there is significant decrease of miR-125a and miR-200a (Park et al., 2009). It has also been shown that miR-31 is overexpressed in OSCC (Liu et al., 2010a).

In HNSCC promoter hypermethylation of miR-137 has been detected that is associated with gender and body mass index (BMI) (Langevin et al., 2010).

9.4.4 Protein Biomarkers

Saliva contains different proteins and several salivary cancer biomarkers have been detected for cancer diagnosis. Markers such as protein cancer markers CA-125 (Balan et al., 2012) and Cyfra 21–1 (Zhong et al., 2007), CA-50, CEA (He et al., 2009), IL-β, IL-6, IL-8 (St. John et al., 2004; Katakura et al., 2007; Korostoff et al., 2011), tetranectin protein (Arellano-Garcia et al., 2010), NNMT protein (Sartini et al., 2012), and cortisol (Bernabé et al., 2012) in OSCC; soluble CD44 (solCD44) (Franzmann et al., 2012), HA (Franzmann et al., 2003; Pereira et al., 2011), β-fibrin, S100, transferrin, and cofilin (Dowling et al., 2008) in HNSCC; CA15-3 and Her2/neu (Streckfus et al., 1999; Streckfus and Bigler, 2005) and VEGF (Brooks et al., 2008) in breast cancer; and alpha-fetoprotein (AFP) in hepatocellular carcinoma (You et al., 1993) are detected in primary tumor site and shed into the blood, which is also detected in the saliva of patients as biomarkers of cancer. Proteomics has revealed many protein biomarkers such as cystatin (Shintani et al., 2010), transferrin, ZNF510 (Jou et al., 2010, 2011) of OSCC. Similarly, proteomics has also revealed some biomarkers of lung cancer (Li et al., 2012; Xiao and Wong, 2012; Xiao et al., 2012) and gastric cancer (Wu et al., 2009).

9.4.5 Cytokine Biomarkers

During cancer progression and metastasis, cytokine and growth factors such as IL-8 (Yang et al., 2005; Kim et al., 2011), IL-6, IL-1β, TGF-β, and TNF-α (Brailo et al., 2012) are increased at tumor sites and in blood. These cytokines have also been used as biomarkers in saliva for the detection of OSCC (Yang et al., 2005; Brailo et al., 2012; Elashoff et al., 2012), tongue cancer (Korostoff et al., 2011), oral leukoplakia with dysplasia (Katakura et al., 2007; Tan et al., 2008; Sharma et al., 2011), and head and neck cancer (Demokan et al., 2010; Kim et al., 2011; Pereira et al., 2011).

9.4.6 Pathogen Biomarkers

Cancer can also be caused by pathogens such as viruses, bacteria, and parasites due to their persistent presence at the site of infection. Thus, the pathogen-specific antigens could be present in saliva, and direct detection of antigens or antibodies against such antigens has been evaluated for their use as salivary biomarkers of cancer. For example, cholangiocarcinoma is caused by *Opisthorchis viverrini* infection and detection of antibodies (IgG and IgA) to the bacterial antigens in the saliva is used for the diagnosis of the disease (Chaiyarit et al., 2011). Human papillomavirus (HPV) and Epstein–Barr virus (EBV) are also responsible for the development of oral cancer, head and neck cancer, and Kaposi's sarcoma, and the detection of viral RNA or DNA in the saliva has been used as cancer biomarkers in saliva (Zhao et al., 2005; Chuang et al., 2008; SahebJamee et al., 2009; Pow et al., 2011).

9.4.7 Exosome Biomarkers

Exosomes are small membrane-bound vesicles (40–100 nm) that are released by the cells. These membrane-bound vesicles originate from late endosomal state. They are found in different body fluids including plasma, amniotic fluid, urine, malignant fluid, ascites, and saliva. These exosomes contain proteins, mRNA, miRNA, and esRNA, and these can be used as a diagnostic marker of diseases (Marzesco et al., 2005; Palanisamy et al., 2010; Vlassov et al., 2012). Exosomes can be isolated from body fluids by differential centrifugation. Once isolated, the exosomes can be characterized by different methods such as immunoblot, ELISA, RT-PCR, and proteomics (Keller et al., 2011). Exosome-containing proteins and nucleic acid have been characterized in plasma of different diseases (e.g., cancer, neurodegenerative disorders, prion disease, cancers, type I and II diabetes), and progress is being achieved to correlate exosome-based biomarkers of saliva for cancer (Gonzalez-Begne et al., 2009).

9.4.8 Matrix Metalloproteinase Biomarkers

Matrix metalloproteinases (MMPs) are zinc-dependent endopeptidases that belong to the metzincin superfamily and cause degradation of the extracellular matrix and basement membrane and can play a major role in cancer development and progression (Stetler-Stevenson and Yu, 2001; Shpitzer et al., 2009; Shuman Moss et al., 2012). Recently, it has been shown that the MMP1 expression in saliva of *primary* OSCC is 200-fold higher than normal individuals. Similarly, in OSCC patients the MMP1 and MMP3 were 6.2 and 14.8 times higher, respectively, than controls, and the level goes up with higher-stage disease (Stott-Miller et al., 2011).

9.4.9 Telomerase Activity Biomarkers

Telomerase is a ribonuclease protein that inserts and elongates repeats ("TTAGGG" in all vertebrates) to the 3′ end of DNA strands by using a complementary intrinsic RNA strand as a template (Mocellin et al., 2013). In slow-growing cells or in senescence tissue, the telomerase activity is low and it is considered that to escape this and to become cancer cells, high telomerase activity is a prerequisite for the development of malignant cell. Tumor tissue (72%–100%) such as oral cancer, head and neck cancer, neuroblastoma, lung cancer, breast cancer, gastric cancer, prostate cancer, and other cancers expresses telomerase activity, whereas somatic tissue (except some blood and germ cells) does not express telomerase activity (Kim et al., 1994). Telomerase activity has been detected from oral rinses of HNSCC using PCR-based method with low positive rates (Califano et al., 1996; Sumida et al., 1998). Recently, the telomerase activity in OSCC patients has been assessed by telomerase PCR-ELISA method, and the results show that 75.0% of OSCC patients exhibit high telomerase activity and only 6.67% positive in control subjects, which was statistically significant ($p < 0.001$). However, no significant difference ($p < 0.05$) could be detected between early- and late-stage (lymph node metastasis) patients (Zhong et al., 2005).

9.4.10 Microsatellite Biomarkers

Microsatellites are repeat DNA sequences that are common and normal in genome. Any changes in the microsatellite DNA due to mutation in DNA repair genes results in longer or shorter microsatellite and is referred as microsatellite instability (MSI) (Okami et al., 2002). Molecular methods such as PCR can detect small number of cancer cells among normal cells. Using this technique, eight microsatellite markers were selected for analysis of MSI in tumor and saliva samples of oral and pharyngeal cancer patients. In this study only 22% had MSI in tumor samples; however, 80% of MSI positive sample had same/identical MSI in saliva (Okami et al., 2002). Similar technique when used in HNSCC patients with 23 microsatellite markers to assay DNA from patients produced much better detection results. MSI of at least one marker was detected in 86% of primary tumors. Identical alterations were also found in the saliva samples in 92% of those with markers (overall 79%). No MSI was detected in healthy control subjects (Spafford et al., 2001). Thus, MSI salivary biomarker detection can be a valuable technique for early detection of cancer.

9.4.11 Mitochondrial DNA Biomarkers

Human mtDNA mutations occur in cancer with high frequency. Analysis of bladder, head and neck, and lung tumors along with their paired salivary samples has indicated that mtDNA mutations could be detected in saliva at a much higher rate than p53 mutations. Since mtDNA mutations are clonal in nature and are in high copies, these molecular markers can be used as salivary diagnostic markers of cancer (Fliss et al., 2000; Mithani et al., 2007).

9.4.12 Metabolite/Metabolomic Biomarkers

Salivary biomarker detection of cancer patients by metabolomics has been developed in recent times. Metabolites in cancer patients have also been used for the detection and monitoring of cancer progression. Analysis of analyte tests (Tainsky et al., 2007) and salivary metabolites from cancer patients of oral (Wei et al., 2011), pancreatic, and breast cancers, periodontal disease patients, and healthy controls has revealed 57 metabolites that can help predict specific cancer types (Sugimoto et al., 2010).

9.5 Technological Advancement for Salivary-Based Diagnostics

Salivary diagnostics and biomarker detection are based on the presence of proteins and nucleic acids in the saliva. Saliva contains hundreds of major proteins and in addition contains peptides that can be used for the detection of diseases. One of the major problems in protein biomarker detection is the presence of low level of antigen in saliva that requires sample concentration for marker detection. However, new technologies such as molecular diagnostics and nanotechnology are being used to overcome this limitation of low concentration of markers in saliva (Baum et al., 2011; Genco, 2012).

Proteome (protein)-based technology has been used for detection of salivary biomarkers for some time. The common technologies applied for protein characterizations are 2D PAGE and mass spectrometry (MS). These proteins can be further subcharacterized by electrospray ionization (ES) and matrix-assisted laser desorption ionization (MALDI). These technologies can be coupled with mass analyzer such as quadruple time of flight (TOF) to improve the detection sensitivity, specificity, and efficiency (Denny et al., 2008). Proteins in saliva can also be detected by nano-biochip quantum dot bioconjugate labels (Jokerst et al., 2009) or optical detection by quantum dot composite nanoparticle (Lee et al., 2010).

One such technology known as surface plasmon resonance (SPR) system has been developed based on Au/ZnO technology that can detect tumor marker CA15-3 in human saliva at 2.5–20 U/mL. This higher sensitivity of detection can be used for measuring levels of CA15-3 in cancer patients without the need of concentrating the saliva (Liang et al., 2012). Other technologies such as single-step nanoplasmonic VEGF165 aptasensor (Cho et al., 2012) and electrochemical sensor for multiplex detection (Wei et al., 2009) have been used for detection of cancer markers. Cancer diagnostic immunoassay panel can be developed by surface-enhanced Raman scattering (SERS)-based technology (Granger et al., 2013). High-throughput antibody screening of clinical samples can be evaluated by layered peptide array technology (Gannot et al., 2005).

Other technologies have been developed for detection of posttranslational modification of proteins, where changes, such as phosphorylation, glycosylation, acetylation, and methylation, can change protein function. These posttranslational modifications may be common in cancer conditions and can be detected by different methods such as MALDI-MS and HPLC-ESI-MS/MS (Tao et al., 2005; Lee and Wong, 2009) and methylation enrichment pyrosequencing (Shaw et al., 2006). These techniques have been applied for salivary biomarker detection of OSCC (Yang et al., 2005; Shintani et al., 2010; Jou et al., 2011; Chitra et al., 2012), HNSCC (Dowling et al., 2008; Jarai et al., 2012; Matta et al., 2010), lung cancer (Li et al., 2012; Xiao et al., 2012), and gastric cancer (Wu et al., 2009) and for the detection of salivary metabolomics in various other cancers (Sugimoto et al., 2010).

Saliva also contains DNA and RNA and currently discovery of large number of transcripts by transcriptome analysis has opened up new avenues for biomarker detection in saliva (Li et al., 2004). The transcriptomic biomarker identification is usually done through microarray technology and is used for biomarker detection of several cancers including OSCC (Li et al., 2004; Zimmerman et al., 2007; Elashoff et al., 2012), HNSCC (Lallemant et al., 2009), lung cancer (Zhang et al., 2012a), pancreatic cancer (Zhang et al., 2010a), breast cancer (Zhang et al., 2010b), and ovarian cancer (Lee et al., 2012). Currently new methodologies are being developed for the refinement of these detection systems for use in salivary transcriptome analysis (Li et al., 2006; Hu et al., 2008). Methods have also been developed for quantitative detection of viral DNA (herpesvirus 8) in clinical specimens (Stamey et al., 2001).

9.6 Salivary Biomarkers of Cancer

Efforts to identify salivary biomarkers of cancer have been improved over the last decade due to availability of new technologies. Different salivary biomarkers of OSCC, HNSCC, and lung, breast, liver, and pancreatic cancer have been identified.

9.6.1 Oral Cancer

Oral cancer is the most common cancer that has been evaluated for salivary biomarkers because of its direct contact with saliva. OSCC is the most common cancer of the oral cavity and is the eighth most common cause of cancer death due to malignancy. The mortality and suffering from OSCC can be significantly reduced if OSCC can be detected early. Several groups have studied different biomarkers of oral cancer (Lingen, 2010; Shah et al., 2011) for early diagnosis by various methods and technologies that are listed in Table 9.1.

Saliva has been used for detection of OSCC cancer antigens CA-125, CA-50, and CEA by ELISA that measures proteins expressed in higher amounts than the normal controls. These studies indicate that OSCC-related antigens are shed into the oral cavity and are easier to detect such antigens in saliva than in the blood (Angelov et al., 1996; He et al., 2009; Balan et al., 2012). Other studies have studied the level of cytokines IL-6, IL-8, and TNF-α in the patient's saliva either alone or in combination with other cancer-associated markers. These studies indicate that it is possible to detect differential expression of cytokines in the saliva of patients by ELISA, RT-PCR, and quantitative RT-PCR (St John et al., 2004; Tan et al., 2008; Arellano-Garcia et al., 2010; Sharma et al., 2011; Brailo et al., 2012). New technology BiAcore SPR can even detect picomole levels of IL-8 in saliva (Yang et al., 2005). Other common cancer markers such as aldehyde dehydrogenase (ALDH) (Wroczynski et al., 2006; Giebułtowicz et al., 2008), salivary adenosine deaminase (SAD) (Rai et al., 2011), and reactive oxygen species (ROS) (Chitra et al., 2012) have been measured, and their higher expression in saliva shows promising results as biomarkers of OSCC.

Salivary proteomics has helped in the identification of oral cancer (Hu et al., 2007a, 2008).

DNA methylation studies have also been conducted in salivary samples using methylation-specific PCR and methylation array technology to identify genes specific for OSCC. Such studies have identified genes ECAD, TMEFF2, RARβ, and MGMT to be associated with DNA methylation in OSCC (Viet and Schmidt, 2008; Nagata et al., 2012).

Recently, salivary transcriptome analysis (cell-free supernatant or whole saliva) by quantitative RT-PCR and array technology along with ELISA have revealed the presence of diagnostic markers of OSCC such as mRNAs of IL-8, SAT, IL-1β, OAZ1, H3F3A, S110P and proteins IL-8, M2BP, and IL-1β (Brinkmann et al., 2011; Elashoff et al., 2012). Higher cytokine expression, IL-6, IL-1β, IL-8, TNF-α, VEGF (St John et al., 2004; Korostoff et al., 2011; Sharma et al., 2011; Brailo et al., 2012), that have previously been shown to be associated with cancer has also been detected in the saliva of OSCC patients.

The miRNAs detected in saliva of OSCC are miRNA125a, miRNA (Zen and Zhang, 2012; Yoshizawa and Wong, 2013), miRNA-200a (Park et al., 2009), and miR-31 (Liu et al., 2012a).

Saliva of OSCC patients has also been used for detection of cancer cells shed into the saliva. To detect these cells, microsatellite markers were selected and evaluated for MSI in the primary site and in salivary cells. Eighty percent of those patients that had MSI tested positive for identical MSI in saliva (El-Naggar et al., 2001; Okami et al., 2002). DNA specific to oral cancer (Chen and Lin, 2011) and exocyclic DNA adducts (Chen et al., 2011) have been also detected. Other markers that have been tested from OSCC patients and show promise are salivary cortisol (Bernabé et al., 2012), nicotinamide N-methyltransferase

TABLE 9.1

Salivary Biomarkers of Oral Squamous Cell Cancer

Biomarkers	Methods	Findings	References
Long noncoding RNAs (lncRNAs)	RT-PCR	Whole saliva contains detectable amount of some subsets of lncRNAs as potential markers.	Tang et al. (2013)
Cancer antigen 125 (CA-125)	ELISA	Noninvasive salivary CA-125 is significantly ($P < 0.001$) higher in OSCC patients than nontumor control samples. *Significant increase in the CA-125 level with higher of OSCC stages.*	Balan et al. (2012)
Amino acid profile	HPLC	Higher level of all amino acids in saliva of OSCC patients (well-differentiated OSCC and moderately differentiated OSCC) than nontumor individuals. These markers can serve as *diagnostic and prognostic markers.* All amino acid values except histidine and 5 threonine were significant ($P < 0.05$) than controls.	Reddy et al. (2012)
Cortisol (OSCC and oropharyngeal SCC)	ELISA	Significant higher level of salivary cortisol ($P < 0.01$) in OSCC than control saliva, oropharyngeal SCC, and advanced-stage OSCC had higher level ($P < 0.05$) than smokers and drinkers. Higher levels ($P < 0.05$) of cortisol in patients with advance-stage OSCC than initial clinical stage *help in diagnosis and prognosis.*	Bernabé et al. (2012)
Nicotinamide N-methyltransferase (NNMT)	Western blot	Upregulation of salivary NNMT protein in oral cancer and in unfavorable cases (N+) than that of favorable cases (N0).	Sartini et al. (2012)
RNA: IL-8, SAT, IL-1β, OAZ1, H3F3A, DUSP, and S100P	Quantitative PCR microarray analysis	Expression of all seven mRNAs and three protein markers was increased in OSCC versus controls. Can also be used for oral cancer detection. The ROC curve for prediction of OSCC status ranges from 0.74 to 0.86 across the cohorts.	Elashoff et al. (2012) Brinkmann et al. (2011)
Proteins: IL-8, M2BP, and IL-1β		Serbian OSCC patient population also displays similar markers, indicating multiethnic-based biomarkers of cancer. Four salivary mRNAs OAZ, SAT1, IL-8, and IL-1β can detect oral cancer with high efficiency. AUC = 0.86, sensitivity = 0.89, specificity = 0.78 for OSCC total.	Zimmerman et al. (2007) and Li et al. (2004)
Reactive oxygen species (RoS), proxidants, trace elements (Oral submucous fibrosis [OSMF])	Biochemical assays	Significant higher level of lipid peroxidase ($P < 0.001$), conjugate dienes ($P < 0.01$), hydroxy radicals ($P < 0.01$), superoxide dismutase ($P < 0.05$), copper ($P < 0.05$), calcium ($P < 0.01$), potassium ($P < 0.05$), iron ($P < 0.05$) and lower level of H_2O_2 ($P < 0.05$) and sodium ($P < 0.01$) in the saliva of OSMF patients. Treatment with α-tocopherol significantly alters the expression of markers.	Chitra et al. (2012)

Protein pattern comparison annexin 1 and peroxiredoxin 2 specific peptides	Electophoretic separation of bands, matrix-assisted laser-desorption ionization MALDI-time of flight (TOF)	Targeted MALDI-TOF MS analysis of unique peptides of putative saliva protein tumor biomarker could be used for high throughput screening of cancer.	Szanto et al. (2012)
ECAD, TMEFF2, RARβ, and MGMT	Methylation-specific PCR and microchip electrophoresis system	Methylation status of tumor-related genes were evaluated, detection was with 100% sensitivity and 87.5% specificity using combination of ECAD, TMEFF2, RARβ, MGMT; and 97.1% sensitivity and 91.7% specificity with ECAD, TMEFF2, and MGMT.	Nagata et al. (2012)
miR-31	RT-PCR	Salivary miR-31 is significantly increased in OSCC patients. This marker yielded a receiver operating characteristic curve area of 0.82 and an accuracy of 0.72. After excision of tumor, miR-31 level reduced significantly. *Detection and postoperative follow-up*.	Liu et al. (2012a)
Metalloproteinase (MMPs)	Affymetrix HG U133 Plus 2.0 Array (Affymetrix)	MMP1, MMP3, MMP10, and MMP12 were evaluated. MMP1 and MMP3 in saliva and primary tumor indicated robust diagnostic marker specificity for OSCC. (AUC% = 100; 95% CI: 100–100).	Stott-Miller et al. (2011)
Level of IL-1β, IL-6, and TNF-α	Commercial ELISA	Salivary IL-1β and IL-6 were significantly higher in oral cancer patients than controls ($P < 0.05$), no difference in salivary TNF-α level but serum TNF-α was low in cancer patients.	Brailo et al. (2012)
Promoter methylation of NID2, HOXA9, KIFIA, and EDNBR evaluated	HumanMethylation27 BeadChip, quantitative methylation specific PCR	NID2 (87% sensitivity, 21% specificity, and a 0.73 AUC) and HOXA9 (75% sensitivity, 53% specificity, and a 0.75 AUC) promoter hypermethylation can be used for early detection of OSCC. The HOXA9 and NID2 gene panel had 94% sensitivity, 97% specificity, and 0.97 AUC.	Guerrero-Preston et al. (2011)
Peptides, zinc finger proteins 510 (ZNF510)	ClinProt technique, MALDI-TOF MStechnology	ZNF510 peptide is present in 0% of healthy individuals versus 25% and 60% from OSCC patients with T1 + T2 and T3 + T4 stages respectively ($P < 0.001$).	Jou et al. (2011)
Protein profile: Transferin	2D-gel electrophoresis MALDI-TOF MS, Western blot, and ELISA	Increase in Transferin level strongly correlates with the size and stage of the tumor.	Jou et al. (2010)
Salivary biomarkers Cystatin SA_I	Surface-enhanced laser desorption/ionization time-of flight mass spectrometry: SELDI-TOF protein chip	Revealed 26 proteins with significantly different expression levels in the pre- and posttreatment samples. Truncated cystatin SA-I (loss of 3aa at the N terminus) was detected as primary biomarker of pre treatment saliva of OSCC. Significant difference in pre and posttreatment levels ($P < 0.05$).	Shintani et al. (2010)
micro-RNA	Quantitative RT-PCR	miRNA-125a and miR-200a are present in significantly ($P < 0.05$) lower level in OSCC.	Park et al. (2009)

(continued)

TABLE 9.1 (continued)

Salivary Biomarkers of Oral Squamous Cell Cancer

Biomarkers	Methods	Findings	References
Metastatic OSCC: Tetranectin protein	2-D gel electophoresis; liquid chromatography/tandem MS	Tetranectin is significantly underexpressed in serum and saliva of metastatic OSCC compared to primary OSCC.	Arellano-Garcia et al. (2010)
Salivary sialic acid, total protein, and total sugar	Ninhydrin reagent-Lowry method etc.	Salivary level of total protein, total sugar, protein-bound sialic acid, and free sialic acid is significantly higher in OSCC patient. $P < 0.001$ in all the results. Only sialic acid is significantly higher in well *differentiated SCC than moderately differentiated carcinoma* ($P < 0.001$).	Sanjay et al. (2008)
Protein biomarkers	Luminex xMAP single-plex ELISA	IL-8 and IL-1β are both high in OSCC subjects. Can be detected efficiently detected by multiplex assay.	Arellano-Garcia et al. (2008)
DNA methylation array analysis; pre- and postoperative samples	GoldenGate Methylation Array (Illumina), ELISA, CK-19 expression by RT-PCR and immunohistochemistry	Significant differences in pre- and postoperative saliva. Establishes gene classifier consisting of 41 gene loci from 34 genes that showed methylation in preoperative saliva and tissues but were not methylated in postoperative saliva or in normal subjects. Gene panels of 4–10 genes, sensitivity of 62%–77%, and specificity of 83%–100% for OSCC.	Viet and Schmidt (2008)
Cyfra 21-1		Cyfra 21-1, the soluble fragment of cytokeratin 19 (CK 19), correlates well with OSCC ($P = 0.009$). Higher in patient with tumor recurrence than without recurrence ($P = 0.023$). Great correlation between tissue CK19 protein expression and saliva Cyfra 21-1 concentration ($P = 0.051$).	Zhong et al. (2007)
IL-8	BiAcore surface plasmon resonance (SPR)	Sandwich assay was developed. Pre-concentrating saliva sample 10 fold prior to SPR analysis detects IL-8 levels in cancer patients.	Yang et al. (2005)
Telomerase activity	PCR-ELISA	75% positive in OSCC and 6.67% positive in normal controls ($P < 0.001$). Can be used as an adjuvant marker for OSCC.	Zhong et al. (2005)
IL-6 and IL-8	ELISA and qRT-PCR	IL-8 in saliva at higher concentration than normal ($P = 0.01$) and IL-6 in serum hold promise for OSCC biomarkers. Confirmed by mRNA and protein levels. For IL-8 in saliva, a threshold value of 600 pg/mL yields a sensitivity of 86% and a specificity of 97%.	St John et al. (2004)
TSCC (Tongue SCC): Long non-coding RNA	Quantitative RT-PCR	Whole saliva contained some lnRNAs.	Tang et al. (2013)
Cytokine protein levels IL-1β, IL-6, IL-8, TNF-α, and VEGF	ELISA	All five cytokines were elevated in endophytic TSCC (survival rate 10.4 months) in and only four except IL-8 were elevated in TSCC (survival rate 24 months). *Correlate with survival implies a prognostic benefit and future treatment targets.*	Korostoff et al. (2011)
TSCC: Adenosine deaminase (ADA)	Enzyme activity assay	Salivary ADA level was high in TSCC patient ($P < 0.001$). Levels significantly increased stage I to stage II of the disease ($P < 0.001$).	Rai et al. (2011)

Oral leukoplakia with dysplasia	Competitive enzyme linked immunosorbent assay	Tobacco use, elevation of IL-6 level in leukoplakia with coexisting periodontitis and in periodontitis patients, $P < 0.001$ when compared to normal controls. Within leukoplakia group IL-6 level increased with severity of dysplasia.	Sharma et al. (2011)
Premalignant: IL-6			
Oral malignant tumor: CA-50 and CEA	ELISA and immunoradiometric analysis	CEA and CA levels in saliva were more sensitive than in serum and higher in malignant tumors ($P < 0.001$) than in benign tumors and controls.	He et al. (2009)
ALDH	Fluorimetric method	Salivary ALDH3A1 activity higher in cancer patients.	Giebultowicz et al. (2008)
IL-8	Optical protein sensor	Confocal optics based sensor for IL-8 detection in oral cancer patient.	Tan et al. (2008)
IL-1β, IL-6, IL-8, and osteopontin	ELISA	Expression of cytokines was higher in oral cancer patients than controls. In particular IL-6 level was significant in cancer patients than controls.	Katakura et al. (2007)
Apoptosis cells detection	Detection of apoptotic epithelial cells	Detection of apoptotic cells in treated malignant patients (18.18 ± 12.65) was significantly higher than in healthy volunteers (6.99 ± 6.52), premalignant patients (4.43 ± 5.52), and untreated malignant patients (3.40 ± 5.14) ($P < 0.05$).	Cheng et al. (2004)
Oral and pharyngeal cancer: Cancer cells in saliva	Microsatellite analysis in tumor and saliva	Eight microsatellite markers selected to test for MSI. 22% had MSI in tumor samples and 80% of them tested identical MSI in saliva.	Okami et al. (2002) and El-Naggar et al. (2001)
		Forty nine patients had loss of hetrozygocity (LOH), markers: D3S1234, D9S156, and D17S799 identifies 72.2% with LOH in samples ($P < 0.001$), whereas combination of D3S1234, D9S156, D8S254 identifies 84.3% in saliva and 86% in tumor samples.	Nunes et al. (2000)
P53 autoantibodies IgA and IgG	ELISA, immunoprecipitation, competition assay	Sixty four percent of samples were positive tissue, 27% high level in saliva, matching saliva samples were positive.	Warnakulasuriya et al. (2000)
Oncofetal fibronectin (FN) isoform E-DA, ED-B, and OFFN	ELISA	No difference between OSCC and control group, would not be a test for OSCC.	Lyons and Cui (2000)
Lactate dehydrogenase LDH, alkaline, and acid phosphatase	Enzymatic assays	LDH, alkaline, and acid phosphatase were 1.5–6 times high in oral malignancies than in normal mucosa. Significant increase in alpha-amylase and acid phosphatase, tartrate inhibited fraction was detected in cancer patients (86%–96%).	Bassalyk et al. (1992)

(NNMT) (Sartini et al., 2012), annexin-1- and peroxiredoxin-2-specific peptides (Szanto et al., 2012), miR-31 (Liu et al., 2012a), salivary zinc finger protein ZNF510 (Jou et al., 2011), tetranectin protein (Arellano-Garcia et al., 2010), higher levels of salivary sialic acid, total protein and sugars (Sanjay et al., 2008), CK-19 (Zhong et al., 2007), and telomerase activity (Zhong et al., 2005).

It has been also shown that transferrin levels strongly correlate with the size and stage of tumors (Jou et al., 2010). Similarly, cytokine markers IL-1β, IL-6, TNF-α, and VEGF correlate with the survival of OSCC patients (Korostoff et al., 2011). These studies collectively indicate that salivary biomarkers of OSCC can be efficiently detected and used for early diagnosis and monitoring of cancer progression during and after treatment.

9.6.2 Head and Neck Cancer

HNSCC is the most common cancer of the oral cavity and is mainly caused by tobacco smoking, alcohol drinking, and HPV infection (Haddad and Shin, 2008; Leemans et al., 2011). Despite new treatment and improvement in detection and therapy methods, the 5-year survival rate is among the lowest of major cancers and relapses after therapy is common.

Similar to oral cancer previously discussed, the proximity of the head and neck cancer to salivary organs may help in the early detection of cancer. Thus, saliva of head and neck cancer patients is being extensively evaluated for early biomarker detection as indicated in Table 9.2.

Protein biomarkers expressed in saliva of HNSCC patients were evaluated by ELISA, 2D gel, western blot, and immunoprecipitation methods, and salivary IgA and IgG against p53 were detected in higher levels in HNSCC patients than control samples (Warnakulasuriya et al., 2000). Salivary hyaluronic acid (HA) and hyaluronidase levels are also increased in HNSCC patients (Franzmann et al., 2003). Analysis of salivary proteins by 3D DIGE MS has detected significantly higher levels of β fibrin, S100 calcium-binding protein, transferrin, and cofilin-1 and decreased levels of transthretin in HNSCC patients. (Dowling et al., 2008).

miR-137 promoter methylation has been detected in HNSCC where it is associated with gender and BMI (Langevin et al., 2010) and is also associated with poor survival of patients (Langevin et al., 2011).

It has been reported that CD44, a cancer stem cell marker, is also overexpressed in primary tumors of HNSCC (Tu et al., 2009; Zhang et al., 2012b). It is likely that this antigen is also shed into saliva and can serve as a biomarker for early detection of cancer. Recent studies have been able to detect solCD44 in oral rinse of HNSCC patients by ELISA (Pereira et al., 2011; Franzmann et al., 2012). It has also been suggested that when solCD44 level is low, then the detection sensitivity of HNSCC can be improved by including methylation status of the CD44 gene (Franzmann et al., 2005, 2007). Proteomics of salivary biomarkers by SDS PAGE and MALDI TOF/TOF mass spectrometric method has detected several biomarkers including annexin A1 and β- and γ-actin, cytokeratin 4 and 13, zinc finger protein, and p53 pathway proteins that can be used for the detection and monitoring of the disease progression during treatment (Drake et al., 2005; Jarai et al., 2012).

It has been reported that HNSCC tumor-specific p53 mutation can be detected in cancer patients (Boyle et al., 1994; Chai and Grandis, 2006; Koch et al., 1994). Genomic studies have revealed 11 genes that can predict HNSCC, and 2 of these genes, PMAIPI1and PTPN1, have been shown to identify HNSCC with 100% specificity (Sethi et al., 2009). Salivary transcriptome analysis has however revealed that of the three diagnostic markers (IL1RN, MAL, and MMP1) of the tumor, only MMP1 can serve as a biomarker of HNSCC (Lallemant et al., 2009). Extensive studies have also been done for identifying hypermethylation of genes that can be used as diagnostic markers from the saliva of HNSCC. These studies indicate that promoter methylation of RASSF1A, DAPK1, and p16 (Ovchinnikov et al., 2012); CCNA1, DAPK, DCC, MGMT, and TIMP-3 (Rettori et al., 2013); KIF1A and EDNRB (Demokan et al., 2010); and several other genes (Righini et al., 2007a,b, 2008; Sun et al., 2012a,b, 2008) can be used as biomarkers. Other studies have indicated that hypermethylation of at least one of the genes from the selective list (DAPK, DCC, MINT-31, TIMP-3, p16, MGMT, CCNA1) could predict HNSCC development and monitoring of tumor status in the salivary rinse could help in the treatment and surveillance of HNSCC (Carvalho et al., 2008, 2011). Recently, Rettori et al. (2013) have shown that in HNSCC, hypermethylation of promoter region of any of the five genes, CCNA1,

TABLE 9.2

Salivary Biomarkers of Head and Neck Squamous Cell Carcinoma

Biomarkers	Methods	Findings	References
Promoter hypermethylation of RASSF1A, DAPK1, and p16 genes	Methylation-specific polymerase chain reaction (MSP)	Noninvasive saliva, promoter methylation of genes is useful in early detection of HNSCC. The specificity of the MSP panel was 87% and the sensitivity 80% ($P < 0.0001$). For early stage HNSCC detection, the sensitivity was 94% and specificity 87%.	Ovchinnikov et al. (2012)
CCNA1, DAPK, DCC, MGMT, and TIMP-3	MSP	Five genes showed specificity (76%–84%) and sensitivity (20%–55%) and presence of hypermethylation in any of the genes showed *presence of tumors*. Hypermethylation of TIMP-3 after treatment indicated lower local recurrence-free survival ($P = 0.008$), indicating its value as a local independent *prognostic marker for survival*.	Rettori et al. (2013)
Genes: p16. CCNA1, DCC, TIMP-3, MGMT, DAPK, and MINT-31	Methylation-specific PCR	Strong correlation of gene hypermethylation. Salivary rinses collected with or without exfoliating brush offer reliable markers frequent methylation detected by rinse or eighth exfoliation of TIMP-3 (8.8% vs. 5.2%), CCNA1 (26.3% vs. 22.8%), DCC (33.3% vs. 29.8%) TIMP-3 (31.6% vs. 36.8%), p16 (8.8% vs. 5.2%), MGMT (29.8% vs. 38.6%), DAPK (14.0% vs. 19.2%), and MINT-31 (10.5% vs. 8.8%).	Sun et al. (2012a,b) Righini et al. (2007a,b, 2008)
Most abundant proteins: Annexin A1, β and γ-actin. Proteins in malignant cancer cytokeratin 4 and 13, ZFP 28, p53 pathway proteins	SDS page, MALDI TOF/TOF Mass spectrometric method	Proteomics can detect proteins related to HNSCC cancer and can be used for cancer diagnosis and follow-up treatment. Annexin 1, zinc finger protein 28, regulator G-protein 3, indoleamine 2,3-dioxygenase, OFD1 protein and CEP290.	Jarai et al. (2012)
Soluble CD44 (solCD44)	Protein assay, ELISA ELISA, methylation-specific PCR, Western blot	Oral rinse level of solCD44 and protein show promise for better detection of HNSCC. (odds ratio [OR] = 24.90; 95% confidence interval [CI], 9.04–68.57; area under the curve [AUC] = 0.786). It can be increase by combining solCD44 and protein level to AUC 0.796. solCD44 is elevated in cancer. In cases where low level of solCD44 is detected, sensitivity can be increased by including methylation status of the CD44 gene.	Franzmann et al. (2012) Franzmann et al. (2005, 2007)
TIMP-3 promoter hypermethylation	Methylation-specific quantitative RT-PCR	TIMP-3 promoter hypermethylation is a *predictor of local recurrence-free survival of* HNSCC (HR = 2.51; 95% CI: 1.10–5.68).	Sun et al. (2012a,b)
Hypermethylation of promoters of genes DAPK, DCC, MINT-31, TIMP-3, p16, MGMT, and CCNA1	Real-time quantitative methylation specific PCR (Q-MSP)	54.1% patient showed methylation of at least one of the selected genes. Local disease control ($P = 0.010$) and overall survival ($P = 0.015$) were significantly lower in patients with hypermethylation in salivary rinse. *This can help in treatment and surveillance of HNSCC*. Marker panels show improved detection, one panel with 35% sensitivity and 90% specificity and another panel with 85% sensitivity and 30% specificity.	Carvalho et al. (2011) Carvalho et al. (2008)
Sol CD44, IL-8, HA, and proteins	ELISA	A multivariate logistic model and significant improvement over univariate model, AUC of 0.853, sensitivity 75%–82.5%, and specificity 69.2%–82.1% depending on predictive probability cut points.	Pereira et al. (2011)
MicroRNA-137 promoter hypermethylation	Methylation-specific PCR	Only detected in 21.2% oral rinse from HNSCC patients and 3.0% from controls. Promoter methylation was associated with female gender and inversely associated with BMI.	Langevin et al. (2010, 2011)

(*continued*)

TABLE 9.2 (continued)

Salivary Biomarkers of Head and Neck Squamous Cell Carcinoma

Biomarkers	Methods	Findings	References
Promoter methylation of 10 genes evaluated: KIF1A, EDNRB, CDH4, TERT, CD44, NISCH, PAK3, VGF, MAL, and FKBP4	Bisulfate modification and quantitative methylation-specific PCR (Q-MSP)	Methylation of all genes were detected in normal salivary rinse, except CD44 no methylation was observed in normal or cancer salivary rinse. KIF1A and EDNRB were methylated in 38% and 67.6% respectively in patients (primary tissue 98% and 97% methylated) and may be potential biomarker for HNSCC.	Demokan et al. (2010)
Transcriptome analysis	qRT-PCR	IL1RN, MAL, and MMP1 were the most efficient diagnostic markers. Only MMP1 was detected in salivary rinse as biomarker with 100% specificity, sensitivity only 20%, thus technical improvement is needed.	Lallemant et al. (2009)
Salivary DNA 82 genes assayed	Multiplex ligation-dependent probe amplification	Eleven genes showed predictive ability to identify HNSCC by regression tree method. Identified two genes, PMAIP1 and PTPN1, that correctly identified 100% HNSCC. Validated by leave-one-out approach.	Sethi et al. (2009)
Salivary proteins	2D DIGE, mass spectrometry	Significant fold increased of β fibrin (+2.77), S100 calcium binding protein (+5.35), transferrin (+3.37), Ig constant region-γ (+3.28), cofilin-1 (+6.42), and significant decrease of transthyretin (−2.92) in HNSCC patients.	Dowling et al. (2008)
Salivary rinse mitochondrial mutation	MitoChip v2.0, array mitochondrial genome sequencing	Minor populations of mitochondrial DNA and disease-specific mitochondrial mutations can be detected in 76.9% of patients from HNSCC patient whose tumors carried mutation.	Mithani et al. (2007)
Cytotoxic effect on cell line	Chinese hamster cell line v79	Higher cytotoxic effect on cells correlating to high tobacco consumption and cancer patients ($P < 0.001$). 3.6-fold increased cancer risk in probands with cytotoxic saliva.	Bloching et al. (2007)
Hyaluronic acid (HA), Hyaluronidase (HAase)	ELISA, RT-PCR	Salivary HA (4.9-fold higher) and HAase (3.7-fold higher) levels are increased in cancer patients. The profile of HA species in HNSCC patients' and normal saliva are different. Depending on cutoff point and HNSCC site the sensitivity is 62%–70% and specificity 75%–88%.	Franzmann et al. (2003)
Primary and salivary cells	Microsatellite analysis in tumor and saliva	Twenty three informative MS markers evaluated. LOH or MSI was detected in 86% primary tumors, identical (92%) alterations found in saliva. None in controls.	Spafford et al. (2001) Nunes et al. (2000)
Primary and salivary cells	Microsatellite	Only 22% has MSI in tumor tissue, of then 80% MSI positive samples can be detected with identical MSI in saliva.	Okami et al. (2002)
Salivary cells: Promoter methylation	Methylation-specific PCR Genes p16 (CDKN2A), MGMT, DAP-K	Aberrant methylation of atleast one gene is detected in 56% primary tumors, and 65% of matched saliva, none of the saliva was positive from methylation negative tumors.	Rosas et al. (2001)
Salivary IgG and IgA against p53	ELISA, immunoprec-ipitation, competition assay	p53 antibodies were found only in serum and saliva of patients who showed p53 overexpression in their tumor tissues.	Warnakulasuriya et al. (2000)
Saliva p53 genetic mutation	PCR	Tumor specific p53 mutation were identified, salivary testing also reveal presence of mutations in preoperative samples (71%).	Boyle et al. (1994) and Koch et al. (1994)

DAPK, DCC, MGMT, and TIMP-3, could detect the presence of the tumor in oral cavity. It has also been shown that the promoter hypermethylation of TIMP-3 in salivary rinse can be used as a prognostic marker for recurrence-free survival in HNSCC patients.

Recently, in vitro bioassays have been developed to access the cytotoxicity effect of saliva of high tobacco- and alcohol-consuming cancer patients by using Chinese hamster cell line v79. It was found that normal control saliva does not induce such cytotoxicity. This assay shows that there is 3.6-fold higher increase of cancer risk in patients with cytotoxic saliva (Bloching et al., 2007). However, this study has not identified any specific factor/s in the saliva that is responsible for in vitro cytotoxic effect.

9.6.3 Lung Cancer

Lung cancer is the most common cause of cancer-related death for both men and women worldwide. About 1.4 million deaths are attributed to lung cancer (WHO, 2010). Lung cancer is usually detected at late stage due to late appearance of cancer-related symptoms. Early diagnosis will surely help in the diagnosis and early treatment of lung cancer that then can reduce mortality. Recent studies using proteomics and genomics have helped in the identification of biomarkers in the saliva of lung cancer patients as listed in Table 9.3. Cancer of the organs such as lung, breast, and liver though remotely located from oral cavity can also be detected in saliva with increased specificity and sensitivity through improved technology of proteomics and genomics (Hu et al., 2002; Bigler et al., 2009; Hassanein et al., 2012; Markopoulou et al., 2012).

No specific miRNA in the saliva has been reported for lung cancer. However, recent meta-analysis of human lung cancer miRNA expression profiling studies, where cancer tissue and normal tissues were compared, has revealed upregulation and downregulation of several miRNAs (Guan et al., 2012). The most reported four upregulated miRNAs were miR-210, miR-21, miR-31, and miR-182, and the two downregulated miRNAs were miR-126 and miR-145, and they were consistently reported for both squamous cell carcinoma and adenocarcinoma-based subgroup analysis. This study also reveals that the top two consistently reported lung cancer-related miRNAs were miR-210 and miR-21. These or related miRNAs in salivary samples of lung cancer patients may be potential diagnostic markers and need further testing.

Recently, microarray analysis of transcriptomes from saliva of lung cancer patients has identified five mRNAs (CCNI, EGFR, FF19, FRS2, GREB1) that can differentiate lung cancer patients from control subjects (Zhang et al., 2012a). Surface-enhanced Ramanspectroscopy (SER) analysis of salivary proteins and nucleic acids from lung cancer patients has revealed that most of the Raman peak intensities decrease when compared to nontumor controls (Li et al., 2012). Further, salivary proteome separation

TABLE 9.3

Salivary Biomarkers of Lung Cancer

Biomarkers	Methods	Findings	References
mRNA transcriptomics, CCNI, EGFR, FF19, FRS2, and GREB1	Affymetrix HG U133 Plus 2.0 Array (Affymetrix, Santa Clara, CA)	Five of the mRNA could differentiate lung cancer patient from normal controls, with AUC value of 0.925 with 93% sensitivity and 82.81% specificity.	Zhang et al. (2012a)
Proteins and nucleic acids	Surface-enhanced Ramanspectroscopy (SER)	Most of the Raman peak intensities decrease for lung cancer patients compared with that of normal people. The study resulted in accuracy, sensitivity, and specificity being 80%, 78%, and 83%, respectively.	Li et al. (2012)
Proteomics	2D difference gel electrophoresis with MS	16 candidate proteins identified by 2D difference gel electrophoresis and mass spectrometry. Patient and healthy control subject discriminatory power reach 88.5% sensitivity and 92.3% specificity with AUC = 0.90.	Xiao and Wong (2012) and Xiao et al. (2012)

TABLE 9.4
Salivary Biomarkers of Breast Cancer

Biomarkers	Methods	Findings	References
c-erbB-2 Her2/neu CA15-3	ELISA	Expression of c-erbB-2 correlate strongly with breast malignancy in women. Have practical use in initial detection and prognosis of the disease.	Streckfus et al. (1999, 2000a,b, 2001, 2005)
CA15-3 antigen level in serum and saliva	EIA	Salivary and serum level of CA15-3 was significantly higher ($P < 0.01$) in cancer patients than in normal controls. Higher in stage 2 than stage 1.	Agha-Hosseini et al. (2009)
Proteins: VEGF, EGF, and CEA	ELISA	Elevated levels of VEGF > EGF > CEA in cancer patients. The best prediction was combination of VEGF and EGF, sensitivity of 83%, specificity of 74%, and AUC of 84%.	Brooks et al. (2008)
Transcriptoms and proteomes	Affymetrix HG U133 Plus 2.0 Array, 2D-DIGE	Transcriptomic and proteomic profiling revealed significant variation in salivary molecular biomarkers between breast cancer patients and matched controls. Accuracy of 92% (83% sensitive, 97% specific). Eight salivary mRNA identified S100A8, CSTA, GRM1, TPT1, GRIK1, H6PD, IGF2BP1, and MDM4.	Zhang et al. (2010b)

and quantification by 2D gel electrophoresis and MS has identified 16 candidates that can be used as salivary biomarkers for the early detection of lung cancer (Xiao et al., 2012).

9.6.4 Breast Cancer

Breast cancer is the most common cancer in women worldwide and is responsible for 500,000 deaths a year and is the fifth largest cause of death due to cancer (WHO Media Center, 2013). Early detection and prevention of breast cancer can improve treatment efficacy and improve the life of patients (Chase, 2000a,b). Recent studies for salivary biomarkers of breast cancer are listed in Table 9.4.

Evaluation of breast cancer-specific antigens c-erbB-2/Her2/neu and CA15-3 by ELISA or EIA methods has revealed that antigens c-erB-2 (Streckfus et al., 1999, 2000a,b, 2001; Streckfus and Bigler, 2005) and CA15-3 (Agha-Hosseini et al., 2009) can be used as biomarkers for the detection of breast cancer. Beside the specific markers, higher levels of growth factors, VEGF and EGF, that are associated with tumor progression have been also detected in saliva of breast cancer patients (Brooks et al., 2008). In vitro studies have indicated that breast cancer exosome-like microvesicles can alter salivary gland cell-derived exosome-like microvesicles indicating that breast cancer cell may affect salivary glands to change their behavior (Lau and Wong, 2012). Recent studies of salivary transcriptomes and proteomes by microarray studies have identified eight mRNAs that are expressed significantly higher in the saliva of breast cancer patients than normal nontumor individuals (Zhang et al., 2010b). No salivary miRNA specific for detecting breast cancer has been defined yet. However, different miRNA upregulations or downregulations have been reported in breast cancer cells. The following miRNAs are downregulated such as let-7s and miR-30a/31/34a/125s/200s/203/205/206/342, or others are upregulated such as miR-10b/21/135a/155/221/222/224/373/520c in breast cancer cells that has role in breast cancer (Tang et al., 2012; Tu et al., 2012) and may be potential candidate as salivary diagnostic marker for breast cancer.

9.6.5 Gastric Cancer, Pancreatic Cancer, Liver Cancer, Ovarian Cancer, and Colon Cancer

Cancers of other organs such as gastric, pancreatic, liver, ovarian, and colon that have been evaluated for salivary biomarkers are shown in Table 9.5. Gastric cancer-related biomarkers are detected by protein fingerprinting of saliva by MALDI TOF/TOF mass spectrometric methods that has identified four

TABLE 9.5

Salivary Biomarkers of Gastric, Pancreatic, Liver, Ovarian, and Colon Cancers

Biomarkers	Methods	Findings	References
Gastric cancer: Protein fingerprint analysis	Proteomics MALDI TOF/TOF mass spectrometric method	Significant differences in mass to charge (M/Z) ratio of four proteins (1472.78, 2936.49, 6556.81, and 7081.17 Da) in patients than controls	Wu et al. (2009)
Pancreatic cancer: Transcriptomic biomarkers KRAS, MBD3L2, ACRV1, and DPM1	Affymetrix HG U133 Plus 2.0 Array, 2D-DIGE	Twelve mRNA were discovered and validated. Combination of 4 mRNA biomarkers KRAS, MBD3L2, ACRV1, and DPM1 could differentiate pancreatic cancer patients from non cancer individuals AUC = 0.971 with (0.0% sensitivity and 95.0% specificity.	Zhang et al. (2010a)
Hepatocellular carcinoma: AFP	Sandwich ELISA	Significant correlation between high serum and salivary levels in cancer patients; Salivary AFP (mean ± Sx: 3 552.6 ± 2 829.9 ng/L; normal controls mean ± 3.8 ng/L P < 0.001)	You et al. (1993)
Ovarian cancer: Serous papillary adenocarcinoma: Transcriptomes analysis	Affymetrix HG U133 Plus 2.0 Array Affy-metrix, Santa Clara, CA	Seven down-regulated mRNA biomarkers was validated by RT-qPCR (AGPAT1, B2M, BASP2, IER3, and IL-1β) and can be used with high sensitivity and specificity for detecting ovarian cancer. Sensitivity of 85.7%; Specificity of 91.4; AUC = 0.909	Lee et al. (2012)
Hereditary non-polyposis colon cancer: MSI of DNA	Small pool-polymerase chain reaction (SP-PCR)	Significant increase in saliva DNA from siblings with mismatch repair (MMR) mutation compared to normal controls (P < 0.001). Saliva testing is a viable alternative for identifying MSI in carriers with MMR gene mutations	Hu et al. (2011)
Colorectal cancer (CRC) TIMP-1	ELISA	A co-relationship was established with CRC patient and plasma level of TIMP-1, but not with salivary TIMP-1 level. Thus cannot substitute plasma TIMP-1 in detection of CRC	Holten-Andersen et al. (2012)

proteins of interest that show mass to charge differences in patients than control subjects (Wu et al., 2009). Salivary transcriptomes from pancreatic cancer patients (Hamada and Shimosegawa, 2011) analyzed by Affymetrix array technology and 2D difference gel electrophoresis (2D-DIGE) have identified combination of four mRNA biomarkers (KRAS, MBD3L2, ACRV1, DPM1) that can differentiate pancreatic cancer patients from noncancer individuals. High level of AFP in saliva of liver cancer patients has been detected (You et al., 1993). Recently, salivary biomarkers of ovarian cancer have been identified by transcriptome analysis and microarray technology and have detected seven downregulated mRNA biomarkers that can be used with high sensitivity and specificity for cancer detection (Lee et al., 2012). Comparison of salivary and plasma TIMP-1 levels has shown that the plasma levels but not the salivary levels correlate with diagnosis (Holten-Andersen, 2012).

In gastric cancer miRNAs are expressed in the tissues and many miRNAs are upregulated (35–40); about 3–4 are downregulated and many are correlated to prognosis.

Some of the miRNAs are released in the serum and can be used as diagnostic markers (miR-196a, miR-21, miR-17-5p, miR-106a, miR-106b, let-7a, miR-1, miR-20a, miR-27a, miR-34, miR-423-5p, miR-451, miR-486, miR-378, miR-223, miR-21, and miR-218). Detection of these gastric cancer-related miRNAs in saliva may help in early diagnosis and prognosis of gastric cancer. In pancreatic cancer several miRNAs have been suggested as useful as biomarker for pancreatic cancer detection (miR-21, miR-210, miR-155, miR-196a, miR-100a) (Fong and Winter, 2012; Winter et al., 2013). Similarly, several circulating miRNAs (miR-21, miR-122, and miR-223) are elevated in hepatocellular carcinoma; however, these miRNAs are also expressed in patients with chronic hepatitis (Xu et al., 2011). Combining these findings with other miRNAs expressed in hepatocellular carcinoma (miR-122, miR-21, and miR-34a) may provide specific biomarkers for detection of hepatic cancer (Xu et al., 2011). For ovarian cancer detection a serum-related predictive miRNA profile has been created where miR-200b + miR-200c can be used as diagnostic marker (Kan et al., 2012), and these can be evaluated for salivary diagnostic for ovarian cancer. In colon cancer the circulating miRNA, miR-141 (Cheng et al., 2011), miR-17-3p, and miR-92 (Ng et al., 2009) can be used as a diagnostic marker in serum that can also be evaluated for salivary diagnostic of colon cancer.

TABLE 9.6

Salivary Biomarkers for Causative Agent of Cancer

Biomarkers	Methods	Findings	References
Cholangiocarcinoma (CCA): Salivary IgA and IgG against crude *O. viverrini* antigens	ELISA	Significantly high salivary IgG ($P < 0.05$) and IgA in patients with liver fluke/*O. viverrini* and CCA. Levels of IgG correlates with burden of infection. *Can be used as a prognostic marker.*	Chaiyarit et al. (2011)
Nasopharngeal carcinoma (NPC): Salivary EBV DNA level	Real-time PCR	Primer and probes targeting the Bam HI-W region of the EBV genome. The EBV detection of pretreatment saliva was 80% and advanced stage *showed higher EBV DNA levels than patients with early stage*. Posttreatment EBV level was higher than pretreatment levels ($P < 0.01$).	Pow et al. (2011) Liu et al. (2012b)
OSCC: HPV detection HPV6, 11, 16, 18, 31, and 33	PCR	40.9% and 25% of patient and normal control respectively were positive for HPV. The study was *unable to support* the detection of HPV in saliva rinse as a diagnostic method for OSCC.	SahebJamee et al. (2009)
Kaposi's sarcoma: Human herpesvirus 8 (KSHV): Herpesvirus 8 (KSHV) Human herpesvirus 8 (HHV-8)	IFA, quantitative real time PCR in saliva and serum	KSHV blood, serum, and saliva viral load was comparable in all stages. The highest viral load was detected in saliva and decreased in stage II–IV compared to I–II patients. Higher KSHV lytic antibody (from serum) was detected as disease progressed from stage I–II to stage II–IV. KHSVA is associated with more rapid progressive disease. Antibody level and viral load together can be used for monitoring of disease progression. Oral HHV-8 shedding in seropositive patient independent of patient immune response.	Mancuso et al. (2008) Widmer et al. (2006) Casper et al. (2002) Ablashi et al. (2002); LaDuca et al. (1998); and Koelle et al. (1997)
OSCC and HIV patients: Comparison of salivary HPV in OSCC and HIV patient	L1 consensus PCR, restriction fragment length polymorphism (RFLP), DNA sequencing	HPV DNA was detected in 10.3% of oral cancer patients and 35.3% of HIV patients. A highly significant difference $P = 0.006$, odds ratio 4.753; 95% confidence interval (1.698–13.271). In both groups, the most common HPV type was high risk 16 (50% and 42.8% respectively).	Adamopoulou et al. (2008) Taylor et al. (2004)
HNSCC: Salivary HPV-16	E6 and E7 DNA copy number evaluated by PCR	Feasibility of posttreatment HPV DNA shed from persistent/recurrent HNSCC. Quantitative measurement of salivary HPV-16 DNA has promise for surveillance and early detection of recurrence. Recurrence: sensitivity 50%; no salivary HPV-16 DNA no recurrence: specificity = 100%. Using a cutoff of HPV-16 > 0.001 copies/cell in saliva rinse yield a sensitivity of 30.4% and specificity of 98.3% (Zhao et al., 2005). Methylation status of long control region (LCR) of E6 and E7, detection in saliva samples may have *diagnostic potential assessment of risk of high risk individuals.*	Chuang et al. (2008) Zhao et al. (2005) Park et al. (2011)

9.6.6 Biomarkers against Causative Agents of Cancer (Viruses, Bacteria, Parasite)

Some cancers are caused by pathogens such as viruses and bacteria. Attempts have been made to identify salivary biomarkers for early detection of these cancers by specifically looking for biomarkers against pathogens as shown in Table 9.6. Bacterial pathogens can cause OSCC and by DNA hybridization technique and checkerboard analysis, it has been shown that high salivary DNA count of *C. gingivalis*, *P. melaninogenica,* and *S. mitis* may be a diagnostic indicator of OSCC (Mager et al., 2005). Other studies have indicated significant higher levels of IgA and IgG against bacterial pathogen *O. viverrini* that can cause cancer (Chaiyarit et al., 2011); similarly, parasite-specific antibody can be detected in saliva of opisthorchiasis patients (Sawangsoda et al., 2012).

Oral and head and neck cancers are also caused by viruses such as HPV (Park et al., 2011), KSHV, and EBV (Saito et al., 1991; Frangou et al., 2005). New techniques have been developed to detect the viral load in the saliva of cancer patients by differential PCR techniques to improve sensitivity and specificity of detection (Widmer et al., 2006; Adamopoulou et al., 2008; Chuang et al., 2008; Mancuso et al., 2008, 2011; SahebJamee et al., 2009).

9.6.7 Other Cancer Biomarkers

Other cancer biomarkers such as mitochondrial DNA (Fliss et al., 2000) have been used for detection of cancer including lung, head and neck, and bladder cancer (Fliss et al., 2000; Mithani et al., 2007). Metabolomic markers have been used for detection of oral cancer, breast cancer, pancreatic cancer, and periodontal diseases (Sugimoto et al., 2010) and OSCC (Yan et al., 2008; Wei et al., 2011). Analysis of salivary microbiota DNA can also be used as salivary biomarker of OSCC with 80% sensitivity and 82% specificity (Mager et al., 2005) (Table 9.7).

TABLE 9.7

Other Cancer Biomarkers

Biomarkers	Methods	Findings	References
Metabolomics 57 principal metabolites (oral cancer, breast cancer, pancreatic cancer, and periodontal diseases)	Capillary electrophoresis time-of-flight mass spectrometry (CE–TOF–MS)	Identification of 57 principal metabolites that can be used to identify oral cancer, breast cancer, pancreatic cancer, and periodontal diseases. The AUCs were 0.865 for oral cancer, 0.973 for breast cancer, 0.993 for pancreatic cancer, and 0.969 for periodontal diseases to discriminate between disease and control subjects.	Sugimoto et al. (2010)
OSCC: Metabolomic approach, metabolic profile	HPLC/MS	Metabolic profiling can properly describe the pathologic characteristics of OSCC, oral lichen planus, and oral leukoplakia.	Yan et al. (2008)
Oral cancer: Metabolite: Y-aminobutyric acid, phenylalanine, valine, neicosanoic acid, and lactic acid	Ultra performance liquid chromatography, quadrupole/ TOF–MS	Valine, lactic acid, and phenylalanine in combination yield satisfactory accuracy of 0.89, sensitivity 86.5%, specificity of 82.4%, and positive predictive value of 81.6% in distinguishing OSCC from controls.	Wei et al. (2011)
Salivary microbiota DNA	Checkerboard DNA–DNA hybridization	Forty species tested, count of 3 (*C. gingivalis, P. melanogenica, S. mitis*) were elevated in saliva of OSCC ($P < 0.001$). Diagnostic sensitivity 80%, specificity 82% in the matched groups.	Mager et al. (2005)
Lung, HN, bladder, salivary, and primary tumors	Mutated mitochondrial DNA (mtDNA)	The mutated mtDNA was readily detected in paired bodily fluids from each type of cancer, was 19–200 times as about as mutated nuclear p53 DNA.	Fliss et al. (2000)

9.7 Cancer Biology and Salivary Biomarkers

Saliva from cancer patients can be used for the analysis of markers to understand the biology of cancer as well. It has been shown that treatment of cancer can alter the cytokine response of the tumor that can be monitored by evaluating salivary biomarkers (Korostoff et al., 2011). Despite aggressive treatment, the overall survival rate of HNSCC patients with advanced stage has remained poor, and 10%–40% of patients develop local or regional metastasis. Thus, other options of alternative cancer treatment strategies are being evaluated. Our studies have shown that "curcumin" could be used as an alternate therapy to suppress salivary cytokines in head and neck cancer patients (Kim et al., 2011). This study further shows that curcumin downregulates IKKβ kinase activity of salivary cells that results in the inhibition of cytokine expression in cancer patients. These results indicate that curcumin has a great promise to reduce cytokine response in head and neck cancer (Wilken et al., 2011).

Further, to access the effect of saliva of cancer patients on tumor cells, we have designed an in vitro assay. This assay can evaluate the plating efficiency of tumor cell lines when exposed to the saliva of cancer patients or normal individuals. Our preliminary studies have shown that saliva of normal individuals can significantly reduce the plating efficiency of tumor cell lines, whereas saliva of HNSCC cancer patients fails to efficiently reduce plating efficiency. Our studies have also indicated that inhibition of plating efficiency is due to the apoptosis of cancer cells by normal saliva. Currently, saliva collected from HNSCC cancer patients and control individuals is being evaluated to identify the factors responsible for such apoptotic effect on tumor cells that is missing in cancer patients (unpublished results). Such studies should lead to a better understanding of cancer biology in patients.

9.8 Commercial Entity and Availability of Salivary Diagnostic Kits

Salivary testing is a rapidly expanding field and many diagnostic tests are being developed for various diseases. Currently for laboratory and research use, several tests are available for periodontal pathogens. These include MyPerioPath, OralDNA Labs, and Brentwood, TN. There are also kits for accessing genetic predisposition to periodontal disease (MyPeriodID PST, OralDNA Labs) and kits to identify the presence of HPV (OraRisk HPV test and OralDNA Labs [Genco, 2012]) in salivary samples.

Some salivary test kits that have been approved by the Food and Drug Administration (FDA) are Oratect® HM15 oral fluid test screen PCP that detects drug abuse (Branan Medical Corporation), a kit that detects hormones (Hormonal Clarity Diagnostics™, Clarion, PA), and the kit OraQuick® that detects HIV antibody (OraSure Technologies, Inc., Bethlehem, PA). Currently no FDA-approved salivary diagnostic kits are available for cancer detection.

Patent search on the website "Patent Lens" (http://www.patentlens.net) with the words "Salivary detection cancer" in "title" search lists only 12 patents. For salivary detection of lung cancer, the following two patents are listed: patent nos. US 2011/0207622 A1 and WO 2011/100483 A1. Salivary detection of breast cancer lists eight patents: AU 2006/290222 A1, US 2007/0117123 A1, US 2011/0212851 A1, WO 2007/033367 A2, WO 2007/033367 A3R4, WO 2011/100472 A1, WO 2011/133770 A2, and WO 2011/133770 A3R4. Salivary detection of oral cancer lists two patents: US 2010/0210023 A1 (metabolic markers detection) and WO 2010/034037 A1. Whereas patent search in the same website for "cancer detection" in title search reveals 3061 results. These results indicate that the field of salivary biomarker detection and characterization for cancer is at the initiation stage, and new technology and biomarker detection tools can generate new patents for saliva as a diagnostic tool for cancer.

9.9 Future of Salivary Biomarkers of Cancer

Salivary diagnostics as a tool for detection of cancer were ignored for a long time due to limitation of sensitivity of assays. However, with the advent of new technologies and improvement in detection sensitivities, it is possible that early detection and prognosis of cancer can be monitored using salivary biomarkers (Poujol et al., 2006; Hu et al., 2007a). To reach this goal, more clinical evaluation of these technologies is required. Salivary biomarker detection technologies could then be extended for the detection of other diseases that have a limitation of blood collection and preservation. Thus, science of salivary biomarker detection has a bright future in human disease diagnostics.

Acknowledgments

This work is supported by grants from the Department of Medicine, UCLA, and the Robert W. Green Head and Neck Surgical Oncology Program at UCLA.

References

Ablashi DV, Chatlynne LG, Whitman JE Jr, Cesarman E. Spectrum of Kaposi's sarcoma-associated herpesvirus, or human herpesvirus 8, diseases. *Clin Microbiol Rev*. 2002 July;15(3):439–464. Review. PubMed PMID: 12097251; PubMed Central PMCID: PMC118087.

Adami GR, Adami AJ. Looking in the mouth for noninvasive gene expression-based methods to detect oral, oropharyngeal, and systemic cancer. *ISRN Oncol*. 2012;931301. doi: 10.5402/2012/931301. Epub September 24, 2012. PubMed PMID: 23050165; PubMed Central PMCID: PMC3462394.

Adamopoulou M, Vairaktaris E, Panis V, Nkenke E, Neukam FW, Yapijakis C. HPV detection rate in saliva may depend on the immune system efficiency. *In Vivo*. September–October 2008;22(5):599–602. PubMed PMID: 18853753.

Agha-Hosseini F, Mirzaii-Dizgah I, Rahimi A. Correlation of serum and salivary CA15-3 levels in patients with breast cancer. *Med Oral Patol Oral Cir Bucal*. October 1, 2009;14(10):e521–e524. PubMed PMID: 19680209.

Ai JY, Smith B, Wong DT. Bioinformatics advances in saliva diagnostics. *Int J Oral Sci*. June 2012;4(2):85–87. Review. PubMed PMID: 22699264; PubMed Central PMCID: PMC3412667.

Angelov A, Klissarova A, Dikranian K. Radioimmunological and immunohistochemical study of carcinoembryonic antigen in pleomorphic adenoma and mucoepidermoid carcinoma of the salivary glands. *Gen Diagn Pathol*. March 1996;141(3–4):229–234. PubMed PMID: 8705787.

Arellano-Garcia ME, Hu S, Wang J, Henson B, Zhou H, Chia D, Wong DT. Multiplexed immunobead-based assay for detection of oral cancer protein biomarkers in saliva. *Oral Dis*. November 2008;14(8):705–712. doi: 10.1111/j.1601-0825.2008.01488.x. PubMed PMID: 19193200; PubMed Central PMCID: PMC2675698.

Arellano-Garcia ME, Li R, Liu X, Xie Y, Yan X, Loo JA, Hu S. Identification of tetranectin as a potential biomarker for metastatic oral cancer. *Int J Mol Sci*. September 2, 2010;11(9):3106–3121. doi: 10.3390/ijms11093106. PubMed PMID: 20957082; PubMed Central PMCID: PMC2956083.

Balan JJ, Rao RS, Premalatha B, Patil S. Analysis of tumor marker CA 125 in saliva of normal and oral squamous cell carcinoma patients: A comparative study. *J Contemp Dent Pract*. September 1, 2012;13(5):671–675. PubMed PMID: 23250173.

Bassalyk LS, Gus'kova NK, Pashintseva LP, Liubimova NV. Enzyme and isoenzyme activity in patients with malignant tumors of the oral mucosa. *Vopr Onkol*. 1992;38(3):291–299. Russian. PubMed PMID: 1300720.

Baum BJ, Yates JR 3rd, Srivastava S, Wong DT, Melvin JE. Scientific frontiers: Emerging technologies for salivary diagnostics. *Adv Dent Res*. October 2011;23(4):360–368. doi: 10.1177/0022034511420433. PubMed PMID: 21917746; PubMed Central PMCID: PMC3172997.

Bernabé DG, Tamae AC, Miyahara GI, Sundefeld ML, Oliveira SP, Biasoli ÉR. Increased plasma and salivary cortisol levels in patients with oral cancer and their association with clinical stage. *J Clin Pathol*. October 2012;65(10):934–939. Epub June 25, 2012. PubMed PMID: 22734006.

Bigler LR, Streckfus CF, Dubinsky WP. Salivary biomarkers for the detection of malignant tumors that are remote from the oral cavity. *Clin Lab Med*. March 2009;29(1):71–85. doi: 10.1016/j.cll.2009.01.004. Review. PubMed PMID: 19389552.

Bloching MB, Barnes J, Aust W, Knipping S, Neumann K, Grummt T, Naim R. Saliva as a biomarker for head and neck squamous cell carcinoma: In vitro detection of cytotoxic effects by using the plating efficiency index. *Oncol Rep*. December 2007;18(6):1551–1556. PubMed PMID: 17982643.

Boyle JO, Mao L, Brennan JA, Koch WM, Eisele DW, Saunders JR, Sidransky D. Gene mutations in saliva as molecular markers for head and neck squamous cell carcinomas. *Am J Surg*. November 1994;168(5):429–432. PubMed PMID: 7977967.

Brailo V, Vucicevic-Boras V, Lukac J, Biocina-Lukenda D, Zilic-Alajbeg I, Milenovic A, Balija M. Salivary and serum interleukin 1 beta, interleukin 6 and tumor necrosis factor alpha in patients with leukoplakia and oral cancer. *Med Oral Patol Oral Cir Bucal*. January 1, 2012;17(1):e10–e15. PubMed PMID: 21743397; PubMed Central PMCID: PMC3448188.

Bretthauer M, Kalager M. Principles, effectiveness and caveats in screening for cancer. *Br J Surg*. January 2013;100(1):55–65. doi: 10.1002/bjs.8995. Review. PubMed PMID: 23212620.

Brinkmann O, Kastratovic DA, Dimitrijevic MV, Konstantinovic VS, Jelovac DB, Antic J, Nesic VS et al. Oral squamous cell carcinoma detection by salivary biomarkers in a Serbian population. *Oral Oncol*. January 2011;47(1):51–55. doi: 10.1016/j.oraloncology.2010.10.009. Epub November 24, 2010. PubMed PMID: 21109482; PubMed Central PMCID: PMC3032819.

Brinkmann O, Spielmann N, Wong DT. Salivary diagnostics: Moving to the next level. *Dent Today*. June 2012;31(6):54, 56–57; quiz 58–59. PubMed PMID: 22746063.

Brinkmann O, Wong DT. Salivary transcriptome biomarkers in oral squamous cell cancer detection. *Adv Clin Chem*. 2011;55:21–34. Review. PubMed PMID: 22126022.

Brooks MN, Wang J, Li Y, Zhang R, Elashoff D, Wong DT. Salivary protein factors are elevated in breast cancer patients. *Mol Med Report*. May–June 2008;1(3):375–378. PubMed PMID: 19844594; PubMed Central PMCID: PMC2763326.

Califano J, Ahrendt SA, Meininger G, Westra WH, Koch WM, Sidransky D. Detection of telomerase activity in oral rinses from head and neck squamous cell carcinoma patients. *Cancer Res*. December 15, 1996;56(24):5720–5722. PubMed PMID: 8971181.

Carvalho AL, Henrique R, Jeronimo C, Nayak CS, Reddy AN, Hoque MO, Chang S et al. Detection of promoter hypermethylation in salivary rinses as a biomarker for head and neck squamous cell carcinoma surveillance. *Clin Cancer Res*. July 15, 2011;17(14):4782–4789. doi: 10.1158/1078-0432.CCR-11-0324. Epub May 31, 2011. PubMed PMID: 21628494; PubMed Central PMCID: PMC3215270.

Carvalho AL, Jeronimo C, Kim MM, Henrique R, Zhang Z, Hoque MO, Chang S et al. Evaluation of promoter hypermethylation detection in body fluids as a screening/diagnosis tool for head and neck squamous cell carcinoma. *Clin Cancer Res*. January 1, 2008;14(1):97–107. doi: 10.1158/1078 0432.CCR-07-0722. PubMed PMID: 18172258.

Casper C, Krantz E, Taylor H, Dalessio J, Carrell D, Wald A, Corey L, Ashley R. Assessment of a combined testing strategy for detection of antibodies to human herpesvirus 8 (HHV-8) in persons with Kaposi's sarcoma, persons with asymptomatic HHV-8 infection, and persons at low risk for HHV-8 infection. *J Clin Microbiol*. October 2002;40(10):3822–3825. PubMed PMID: 12354890; PubMed Central PMCID: PMC130660.

Castagnola M, Cabras T, Vitali A, Sanna MT, Messana I. Biotechnological implications of the salivary proteome. *Trends Biotechnol*. August 2011a;29(8):409–418. doi: 10.1016/j.tibtech.2011.04. 002. Epub May 26, 2011a. Review. PubMed PMID:21620493.

Castagnola M, Picciotti PM, Messana I, Fanali C, Fiorita A, Cabras T, Calò L et al. Potential applications of human saliva as diagnostic fluid. *Acta Otorhinolaryngol Ital*. December 2011b;31(6):347–357. Review. PubMed PMID: 22323845; PubMed Central PMCID: PMC3272865.

Chai RL, Grandis JR. Advances in molecular diagnostics and therapeutics in head and neck cancer. *Curr Treat Options Oncol*. January 2006;7(1):3–11. Review. PubMed PMID: 16343364.

Chaiyarit P, Sithithaworn P, Thuwajit C, Yongvanit P. Detection of salivary antibodies to crude antigens of *Opisthorchis viverrini* in opisthorchiasis and cholangiocarcinoma patients. *Clin Oral Investig*. August 2011;15(4):477–483. doi: 10.1007/s00784-010-0421-y. Epub May 6, 2010. PubMed PMID: 20446100.

Chase WR. Salivary markers: Their role in breast cancer detection. *J Mich Dent Assoc*. February 2000a;82(2):12. PubMed PMID: 11323899.

Chase WR. Salivary markers: Their role in breast cancer detection. *J Okla Dent Assoc*. Summer 2000b; 91(1):10–11. PubMed PMID: 11314107.

Chen HJ, Lin WP. Quantitative analysis of multiple exocyclic DNA adducts in human salivary DNA by stable isotope dilution nanoflow liquid chromatography-nanospray ionization tandem mass spectrometry. *Anal Chem*. November 2011, 15;83(22):8543–8551. doi: 10.1021/ac201874d. Epub October 14, 2011. PubMed PMID: 21958347.

Chen J, Zhang J, Guo Y, Li J, Fu F, Yang HH, Chen G. An ultrasensitive electrochemical biosensor for detection of DNA species related to oral cancer based on nuclease-assisted target recycling and amplification of DNAzyme. *Chem Commun (Camb)*. July 28, 2011;47(28):8004–8006. doi: 10.1039/c1cc11929j. Epub June 14, 2011. PubMed PMID: 21670838.

Cheng B, Rhodus NL, Williams B, Griffin RJ. Detection of apoptotic cells in whole saliva of patients with oral premalignant and malignant lesions: A preliminary study. *Oral Surg Oral Med Oral Pathol Oral Radiol Endod*. April 2004;97(4):465–470. PubMed PMID: 15088030.

Cheng H, Zhang L, Cogdell DE, Zheng H, Schetter AJ, Nykter M, Harris CC, Chen K, Hamilton SR, Zhang W. Circulating plasma miR-141 is a novel biomarker for metastatic colon cancer and predicts poor prognosis. *PLoS One*. March 17, 2011;6(3):e17745. doi:10.1371/journal.pone. 0017745. PubMed PMID: 21445232; PubMed Central PMCID: PMC3060165.

Chitra S, Balasubramaniam M, Hazra J. Effect of α-tocopherol on salivary reactive oxygen species and trace elements in oral submucous fibrosis. *Ann Clin Biochem*. May 2012;49(Pt 3):262–265. doi: 10.1258/acb.2011.011050. Epub Feb 15, 2012. PubMed PMID: 22337705.

Cho H, Yeh EC, Sinha R, Laurence TA, Bearinger JP, Lee LP. Single-step nanoplasmonic VEGF165 aptasensor for early cancer diagnosis. *ACS Nano*. September 25, 2012;6(9):7607–7614. Epub Aug 21, 2012. PubMed PMID: 22880609; PubMed Central PMCID: PMC3458122.

Chuang AY, Chuang TC, Chang S, Zhou S, Begum S, Westra WH, Ha PK, Koch WM, Califano JA. Presence of HPV DNA in convalescent salivary rinses is an adverse prognostic marker in head and neck squamous cell carcinoma. *Oral Oncol*. October 2008;44(10):915–919. doi: 10.1016/j. oraloncology.2008.01.001. Epub March 7, 2008. PubMed PMID: 18329326; PubMed Central PMCID: PMC3215237.

Dalmay T, Edwards DR. MicroRNAs and the hallmarks of cancer. *Oncogene*. October 9, 2006;25(46): 6170–6175. Review. PubMed PMID: 17028596.

de Almeida Pdel V, Grégio AM, Machado MA, de Lima AA, Azevedo LR. Saliva composition and functions: A comprehensive review. *J Contemp Dent Pract*. March 1, 2008;9(3):72–80. Review. PubMed PMID: 18335122.

Demokan S, Chang X, Chuang A, Mydlarz WK, Kaur J, Huang P, Khan Z et al. KIF1A and EDNRB are differentially methylated in primary HNSCC and salivary rinses. *Int J Cancer*. November 15, 2010;127(10):2351–2359. doi: 10.1002/ijc.25248. PubMed PMID: 20162572; PubMed Central PMCID: PMC2946472.

Denny P, Hagen FK, Hardt M, Liao L, Yan W, Arellanno M, Bassilian S et al. The proteomes of human parotid and submandibular/sublingual gland salivas collected as the ductal secretions. *J Proteome Res*. May 2008;7(5):1994–2006. doi: 10.1021/pr700764j. Epub March 25, 2008. PubMed PMID: 18361515; PubMed Central PMCID: PMC2839126.

Dowling P, Wormald R, Meleady P, Henry M, Curran A, Clynes M. Analysis of the saliva proteome from patients with head and neck squamous cell carcinoma reveals differences in abundance levels of proteins associated with tumour progression and metastasis. *J Proteomics*. July 21, 2008;71(2):168–175. doi: 10.1016/j.jprot.2008.04.004. Epub May 1, 2008. PubMed PMID: 18617144.

Drake RR, Cazare LH, Semmes OJ, Wadsworth JT. Serum, salivary and tissue proteomics for discovery of biomarkers for head and neck cancers. *Expert Rev Mol Diagn*. January 2005;5(1):93–100. Review. PubMed PMID: 15723595.

Drobitch RK, Svensson CK. Therapeutic drug monitoring in saliva. An update. *Clin Pharmacokinet*. November 1992;23(5):365–379. Review. PubMed PMID: 1478004.

El-Naggar AK, Mao L, Staerkel G, Coombes MM, Tucker SL, Luna MA, Clayman GL, Lippman S, Goepfert H. Genetic heterogeneity in saliva from patients with oral squamous carcinomas: Implications in molecular diagnosis and screening. *J Mol Diagn*. November 2001;3(4):164–170. PubMed PMID: 11687600; PubMed Central PMCID: PMC1906964.

Elashoff D, Zhou H, Reiss J, Wang J, Xiao H, Henson B, Hu S et al. Prevalidation of salivary biomarkers for oral cancer detection. *Cancer Epidemiol Biomarkers Prev*. April 2012;21(4):664–672. doi: 10.1158/1055 9965.EPI-11-1093. Epub February 1, 2012. PubMed PMID: 22301830; PubMed Central PMCID: PMC3319329.

Farnaud SJ, Kosti O, Getting SJ, Renshaw D. Saliva: Physiology and diagnostic potential in health and disease. *Scientific World Journal*. March 16, 2010;10:434–456. doi: 10.1100/tsw.2010.38. Review. PubMed PMID: 20305986.

Fliss MS, Usadel H, Caballero OL, Wu L, Buta MR, Eleff SM, Jen J, Sidransky D. Facile detection of mitochondrial DNA mutations in tumors and bodily fluids. *Science*. March 17, 2000;287(5460):2017–2019. PubMed PMID: 10720328.

Fong ZV, Winter JM. Biomarkers in pancreatic cancer: Diagnostic, prognostic, and predictive. *Cancer J*. November–December 2012;18(6):530–538. doi: 10.1097/PPO.0b013e31827654ea. PubMed PMID: 23187839.

Forde MD, Koka S, Eckert SE, Carr AB, Wong DT. Systemic assessments utilizing saliva: Part 1 general considerations and current assessments. *Int J Prosthodont*. January–February 2006;19(1):43–52. Review. PubMed PMID: 16479760.

Frangou P, Buettner M, Niedobitek G. Epstein-Barr virus (EBV) infection in epithelial cells in vivo: Rare detection of EBV replication in tongue mucosa but not in salivary glands. *J Infect Dis*. January 15, 2005;191(2):238–342. Epub December 15, 2004. PubMed PMID: 15609234.

Franzmann EJ, Reategui EP, Carraway KL, Hamilton KL, Weed DT, Goodwin WJ. Salivary soluble CD44: A potential molecular marker for head and neck cancer. *Cancer Epidemiol Biomark Prev*. March 2005;14(3):735–739. PubMed PMID: 15767360.

Franzmann EJ, Reategui EP, Pedroso F, Pernas FG, Karakullukcu BM, Carraway KL, Hamilton K, Singal R, Goodwin WJ. Soluble CD44 is a potential marker for the early detection of head and neck cancer. *Cancer Epidemiol Biomark Prev*. July 2007;16(7):1348–1355. PubMed PMID: 17627000.

Franzmann EJ, Reategui EP, Pereira LH, Pedroso F, Joseph D, Allen GO, Hamilton K et al. Salivary protein and solCD44 levels as a potential screening tool for early detection of head and neck squamous cell carcinoma. *Head Neck*. May 2012;34(5):687–695. doi: 10.1002/hed.21810. Epub July 11, 2011. PubMed PMID: 22294418; PubMed Central PMCID: PMC3323768.

Franzmann EJ, Schroeder GL, Goodwin WJ, Weed DT, Fisher P, Lokeshwar VB. Expression of tumor markers hyaluronic acid and hyaluronidase (HYAL1) in head and neck tumors. *Int J Cancer*. September 1, 2003;106(3):438–445. PubMed PMID: 12845686.

Gannot G, Tangrea MA, Gillespie JW, Erickson HS, Wallis BS, Leakan RA, Knezevic V, Hartmann DP, Chuaqui RF, Emmert-Buck MR. Layered peptide arrays: High-throughput antibody screening of clinical samples. *J Mol Diagn*. October 2005;7(4):427–436. PubMed PMID: 16237212; PubMed Central PMCID: PMC1876163.

Garzon R, Croce CM. MicroRNAs and cancer: Introduction. *Semin Oncol*. December 2011;38(6):721–723. doi: 10.1053/j.seminoncol.2011.08.008. PubMed PMID: 22082757.

Genco RJ. Salivary diagnostic tests. *J Am Dent Assoc*. October 2012;143(10 Suppl):3S–5S. PubMed PMID: 23034835.

Giannobile WV, McDevitt JT, Niedbala RS, Malamud D. Translational and clinical applications of salivary diagnostics. *Adv Dent Res*. October 2011;23(4):375–380. doi: 10.1177/0022034511420434. PubMed PMID: 21917748; PubMed Central PMCID: PMC3172998.

Giebułtowicz J, Wroczyński P, Piekarczyk J, Wierzchowski J. Fluorimetric detection of aldehyde dehydrogenase activity in human tissues in diagnostic of cancers of oral cavity. *Acta Pol Pharm*. January–February 2008;65(1):81–84. PubMed PMID: 18536178.

Gomes MA, Rodrigues FH, Afonso-Cardoso SR, Buso AM, Silva AG, Favoreto S Jr, Souza MA. Levels of immunoglobulin A1 and messenger RNA for interferon gamma and tumor necrosis factor alpha in total saliva from patients with diabetes mellitus type 2 with chronic periodontal disease. *J Periodontal Res*. June 2006;41(3):177–183. PubMed PMID: 16677285.

Gonzalez-Begne M, Lu B, Han X, Hagen FK, Hand AR, Melvin JE, Yates JR. Proteomic analysis of human parotid gland exosomes by multidimensional protein identification technology (MudPIT). *J Proteome Res*. March 2009;8(3):1304–1314. doi: 10.1021/pr800658c. PubMed PMID: 19199708; PubMed Central PMCID: PMC2693447.

González-Ramírez I, García-Cuellar C, Sánchez-Pérez Y, Granados-García M. DNA methylation in oral squamous cell carcinoma: Molecular mechanisms and clinical implications. *Oral Dis*. November 2011;17(8):771–778. doi: 10.1111/j.1601-0825.2011.01833.x. Epub Jul 22, 2011. Review. PubMed PMID: 21781230.

Granger JH, Granger MC, Firpo MA, Mulvihill SJ, Porter MD. Toward development of a surface-enhanced Raman scattering (SERS)-based cancer diagnostic immunoassay panel. *Analyst*. January 2013;138(2):410–416. doi: 10.1039/c2an36128k. PubMed PMID: 23150876; PubMed Central PMCID: PMC3519366.

Guan P, Yin Z, Li X, Wu W, Zhou B. Meta-analysis of human lung cancer microRNA expression profiling studies comparing cancer tissues with normal tissues. *J Exp Clin Cancer Res*. June 6, 2012;31:54. doi: 10.1186/1756-9966-31-54. PubMed PMID: 22672859; PubMed Central PMCID: PMC3502083.

Guerrero-Preston R, Soudry E, Acero J, Orera M, Moreno-López L, Macía-Colón G, Jaffe A et al. NID2 and HOXA9 promoter hypermethylation as biomarkers for prevention and early detection in oral cavity squamous cell carcinoma tissues and saliva. *Cancer Prev Res (Phila)*. July 2011;4(7):1061–1072. doi: 10.1158/1940-6207.CAPR-11-0006. Epub May 10, 2011. PubMed PMID: 21558411; PubMed Central PMCID: PMC3131432.

Haddad RI, Shin DM. Recent advances in head and neck cancer. *N Engl J Med*. 2008;359:1143–1154.

Haeckel R, Hänecke P. The application of saliva, sweat and tear fluid for diagnostic purposes. *Ann Biol Clin (Paris)*. 1993;51(10–11):903–910. Review. PubMed PMID: 8210068.

Haeckel R, Hänecke P. Application of saliva for drug monitoring. An in vivo model for transmembrane transport. *Eur J Clin Chem Clin Biochem*. March 1996;34(3):171–191. Review. PubMed PMID: 8721405.

Hamada S, Shimosegawa T. Biomarkers of pancreatic cancer. *Pancreatology*. 2011;11 (Suppl 2):14–19. doi: 10.1159/000323479. Epub April 5, 2011. PubMed PMID: 21464582.

Hassanein M, Callison JC, Callaway-Lane C, Aldrich MC, Grogan EL, Massion PP. The state of molecular biomarkers for the early detection of lung cancer. *Cancer Prev Res (Phila)*. August 2012;5(8):992–1006. doi: 10.1158/1940-6207.CAPR-11-0441. Epub June 11, 2012. Review. PubMed PMID: 22689914.

He H, Chen G, Zhou L, Liu Y. A joint detection of CEA and CA-50 levels in saliva and serum of patients with tumors in oral region and salivary gland. *J Cancer Res Clin Oncol*. October 2009;135(10):1315–1321. doi: 10.1007/s00432-009-0572-x. Epub March 26, 2009. PubMed PMID: 19322585.

Helmerhorst EJ, Oppenheim FG. Saliva: A dynamic proteome. *J Dent Res*. August 2007;86(8):680–693. Review. PubMed PMID: 17652194.

Holschneider CH, Berek JS. Ovarian cancer: Epidemiology, biology, and prognostic factors. *Semin Surg Oncol*. July–August 2000;19(1):3–10. Review. PubMed PMID: 10883018.

Holten-Andersen L, Christensen IJ, Jensen SB, Reibel J, Laurberg S, Nauntofte B, Brünner N, Nielsen HJ. Saliva and plasma TIMP-1 in patients with colorectal cancer: A prospective study. *Scand J Gastroenterol*. October 2012;47(10):1234–1241. Epub August 8, 2012. PubMed PMID: 22871105.

Hu P, Lee CW, Xu JP, Simien C, Fan CL, Tam M, Ramagli L et al. Microsatellite instability in saliva from patients with hereditary non-polyposis colon cancer and siblings carrying germline mismatch repair gene mutations. *Ann Clin Lab Sci*. 2011 Fall;41(4):321–330. PubMed PMID: 22166501.

Hu S, Arellano M, Boontheung P, Wang J, Zhou H, Jiang J, Elashoff D, Wei R, Loo JA, Wong DT. Salivary proteomics for oral cancer biomarker discovery. *Clin Cancer Res*. October 1, 2008;14(19):6246–6252. doi: 10.1158/1078-0432.CCR-07-5037. PubMed PMID: 18829504; PubMed Central PMCID: PMC2877125.

Hu S, Loo JA, Wong DT. Human saliva proteome analysis. *Ann N Y Acad Sci*. March 2007a;1098:323–329. Review. PubMed PMID: 17435138.

Hu S, Wang J, Meijer J, Ieong S, Xie Y, Yu T, Zhou H et al. Salivary proteomic and genomic biomarkers for primary Sjögren's syndrome. *Arthritis Rheum*. November 2007b;56(11):3588–3600. PubMed PMID: 17968930; PubMed Central PMCID: PMC2856841.

Hu S, Yen Y, Ann D, Wong DT. Implications of salivary proteomics in drug discovery and development: A focus on cancer drug discovery. *Drug Discov Today*. November 2007c;12(21–22):911–916. Epub October 17, 2007. Review. PubMed PMID: 17993408.

Hu YC, Sidransky D, Ahrendt SA. Molecular detection approaches for smoking associated tumors. *Oncogene*. October 21, 2002;21(48):7289–7297. Review. PubMed PMID: 12379873.

Hu Z, Zimmermann BG, Zhou H, Wang J, Henson BS, Yu W, Elashoff D, Krupp G, Wong DT. Exon-level expression profiling: A comprehensive transcriptome analysis of oral fluids. *Clin Chem*. May 2008;54(5):824–832. doi: 10.1373/clinchem.2007.096164. Epub Mar 20, 2008. PubMed PMID: 18356245; PubMed Central PMCID: PMC2799536.

Humphrey SP, Williamson RT. A review of saliva: Normal composition, flow, and function. *J Prosthet Dent*. February 2001;85(2):162–169. Review. PubMed PMID: 11208206.

Jarai T, Maasz G, Burian A, Bona A, Jambor E, Gerlinger I, Mark L. Mass spectrometry-based salivary proteomics for the discovery of head and neck squamous cell carcinoma. *Pathol Oncol Res*. July 2012;18(3):623–628. doi: 10.1007/s12253-011-9486-4. Epub Feb 15, 2012. PubMed PMID: 22350791.

Jiang J, Lee EJ, Gusev Y, Schmittgen TD. Real-time expression profiling of microRNA precursors in human cancer cell lines. *Nucleic Acids Res*. September 28, 2005;33(17):5394–5403. Print 2005. PubMed PMID: 16192569; PubMed Central PMCID: PMC1236977.

Jiang J, Park NJ, Hu S, Wong DT. A universal pre-analytic solution for concurrent stabilization of salivary proteins, RNA and DNA at ambient temperature. *Arch Oral Biol*. March 2009;54(3):268–273. doi: 10.1016/j.archoralbio.2008.10.004. Epub Nov 28, 2008. PubMed PMID: 19047016; PubMed Central PMCID: PMC2674508.

Jokerst JV, Raamanathan A, Christodoulides N, Floriano PN, Pollard AA, Simmons GW, Wong J et al. Nano-bio-chips for high performance multiplexed protein detection: Determinations of cancer biomarkers in serum and saliva using quantum dot bioconjugate labels. *Biosens Bioelectron*. August 15, 2009;24(12):3622–3629. doi: 10.1016/j.bios.2009.05.026. Epub May 27, 2009. PubMed PMID: 19576756; PubMed Central PMCID: PMC2740498.

Jou YJ, Lin CD, Lai CH, Chen CH, Kao JY, Chen SY, Tsai MH, Huang SH, Lin CW. Proteomic identification of salivary transferrin as a biomarker for early detection of oral cancer. *Anal Chim Acta*. November 29, 2010;681(1–2):41–48. doi: 10.1016/j.aca.2010.09.030. Epub September 25, 2010. PubMed PMID: 21035601.

Jou YJ, Lin CD, Lai CH, Tang CH, Huang SH, Tsai MH, Chen SY, Kao JY, Lin CW. Salivary zinc finger protein 510 peptide as a novel biomarker for detection of oral squamous cell carcinoma in early stages. *Clin Chim Acta*. July 15, 2011;412(15–16):1357–1365. doi: 10.1016/j.cca. 2011.04.004. Epub April 8, 2011. PubMed PMID: 21497587.

Jusko WJ, Milsap RL. Pharmacokinetic principles of drug distribution in saliva. *Ann N Y Acad Sci*. September 20, 1993;694:36–47. Review. PubMed PMID: 8215084.

Kan CW, Hahn MA, Gard GB, Maidens J, Huh JY, Marsh DJ, Howell VM. Elevated levels of circulating microRNA-200 family members correlate with serous epithelial ovarian cancer. *BMC Cancer*. December 28, 2012;12:627. doi: 10.1186/1471-2407-12-627. PubMed PMID: 23272653; PubMed Central PMCID: PMC3542279.

Kantola S, Parikka M, Jokinen K, Hyrynkangs K, Soini Y, Alho OP, Salo T. Prognostic factors in tongue cancer—relative importance of demographic, clinical and histopathological factors. *Br J Cancer*. September 2000;83(5):614–619. PubMed PMID: 10944601; PubMed Central PMCID: PMC2363505.

Katakura A, Kamiyama I, Takano N, Shibahara T, Muramatsu T, Ishihara K, Takagi R, Shouno T. Comparison of salivary cytokine levels in oral cancer patients and healthy subjects. *Bull Tokyo Dent Coll*. November 2007;48(4):199–203. PubMed PMID: 18360107.

Keller S, Ridinger J, Rupp AK, Janssen JW, Altevogt P. Body fluid derived exosomes as a novel template for clinical diagnostics. *J Transl Med*. June 8, 2011;9:86. doi: 10.1186/1479-5876-9-86. PubMed PMID: 21651777; PubMed Central PMCID: PMC3118335.

Kim NW, Piatyszek MA, Prowse KR, Harley CB, West MD, Ho PL, Coviello GM, Wright WE, Weinrich SL, Shay JW. Specific association of human telomerase activity with immortal cells and cancer. *Science*. December 23, 1994;266(5193):2011–2015. PubMed PMID: 7605428.

Kim SG, Veena MS, Basak SK, Han E, Tajima T, Gjertson DW, Starr J et al. Curcumin treatment suppresses IKKβ kinase activity of salivary cells of patients with head and neck cancer: A pilot study. *Clin Cancer Res*. September 15, 2011;17(18):5953–5961. doi:10.1158/1078-0432.CCR-11-1272. Epub August 5, 2011. PubMed PMID: 21821700; PubMed Central PMCID: PMC3176971.

Kim VN, Han J, Siomi MC. Biogenesis of small RNAs in animals. *Nat Rev Mol Cell Biol*. February 2009;10(2):126–139. doi: 10.1038/nrm2632. Review. PubMed PMID: 19165215.

Koch WM, Boyle JO, Mao L, Hakim J, Hruban RH, Sidransky D. p53 gene mutations as markers of tumor spread in synchronous oral cancers. *Arch Otolaryngol Head Neck Surg*. September 1994;120(9):943–947. PubMed PMID: 8074821.

Koelle DM, Huang ML, Chandran B, Vieira J, Piepkorn M, Corey L. Frequent detection of Kaposi's sarcoma-associated herpesvirus (human herpesvirus 8) DNA in saliva of human immunodeficiency virus-infected men: Clinical and immunologic correlates. *J Infect Dis*. July 1997;176(1):94–102. PubMed PMID: 9207354.

Korostoff A, Reder L, Masood R, Sinha UK. The role of salivary cytokine biomarkers in tongue cancer invasion and mortality. *Oral Oncol*. April 2011;47(4):282–287. doi: 10.1016/j.oraloncology. 2011.02.006. PubMed PMID: 21397550.

Kozaki K, Imoto I, Mogi S, Omura K, Inazawa J. Exploration of tumor-suppressive microRNAs silenced by DNA hypermethylation in oral cancer. *Cancer Res*. April 1, 2008;68(7):2094–2105. doi: 10.1158/0008-5472.CAN-07-5194. PubMed PMID: 18381414.

LaDuca JR, Love JL, Abbott LZ, Dube S, Freidman-Kien AE, Poiesz BJ. Detection of human herpesvirus 8 DNA sequences in tissues and bodily fluids. *J Infect Dis*. December 1998;178(6):1610–1615. PubMed PMID: 9815212.

Lagos-Quintana M, Rauhut R, Lendeckel W, Tuschl T. Identification of novel genes coding for small expressed RNAs. *Science*. October 26, 2001;294(5543):853–858. PubMed PMID: 11679670.

Lallemant B, Evrard A, Combescure C, Chapuis H, Chambon G, Raynal C, Reynaud C et al. Clinical relevance of nine transcriptional molecular markers for the diagnosis of head and neck squamous cell carcinoma in tissue and saliva rinse. *BMC Cancer*. October 18, 2009;9:370. doi: 10.1186/1471-2407-9-370. PubMed PMID: 19835631; PubMed Central PMCID: PMC2767357.

Langevin SM, Stone RA, Bunker CH, Grandis JR, Sobol RW, Taioli E. MicroRNA-137 promoter methylation in oral rinses from patients with squamous cell carcinoma of the head and neck is associated with gender and body mass index. *Carcinogenesis*. May 2010;31(5):864–870. doi: 10.1093/carcin/bgq051. Epub Mar 2, 2010. PubMed PMID: 20197299; PubMed Central PMCID: PMC2864416.

Langevin SM, Stone RA, Bunker CH, Lyons-Weiler MA, LaFramboise WA, Kelly L, Seethala RR, Grandis JR, Sobol RW, Taioli E. MicroRNA-137 promoter methylation is associated with poorer overall survival in patients with squamous cell carcinoma of the head and neck. *Cancer*. April 1, 2011;117(7):1454–1462. doi: 10.1002/cncr.25689. Epub November 8, 2010. PubMed PMID: 21425146; PubMed Central PMCID: PMC3117118.

Lau CS, Wong DT. Breast cancer exosome-like microvesicles and salivary gland cells interplay alters salivary gland cell-derived exosome-like microvesicles in vitro. *PLoS One*. 2012;7(3):e33037. doi: 10.1371/journal.pone.0033037. Epub March 20, 2012. PubMed PMID: 22448232; PubMed Central PMCID: PMC3308964.

Lawrence HP. Salivary markers of systemic disease: Noninvasive diagnosis of disease and monitoring of general health. *J Can Dent Assoc*. March 2002;68(3):170–174. Review. PubMed PMID: 11911813.

Lee MH, Chen YC, Ho MH, Lin HY. Optical recognition of salivary proteins by use of molecularly imprinted poly(ethylene-co-vinyl alcohol)/quantum dot composite nanoparticles. *Anal Bioanal Chem*. June 2010;397(4):1457–1466. doi: 10.1007/s00216-010-3631-x. Epub March 28, 2010. PubMed PMID: 20349227.

Lee RC, Ambros V. An extensive class of small RNAs in *Caenorhabditis elegans*. *Science*. October 26, 2001;294(5543):862–864. PubMed PMID: 11679672.

Lee RC, Feinbaum RL, Ambros V. The *C. elegans* heterochronic gene lin-4 encodes small RNAs with antisense complementarity to lin-14. *Cell*. December 3, 1993;75(5):843–854. PubMed PMID: 8252621.

Lee YH, Kim JH, Zhou H, Kim BW, Wong DT. Salivary transcriptomic biomarkers for detection of ovarian cancer: For serous papillary adenocarcinoma. *J Mol Med (Berl)*. April 2012;90(4):427–434. doi: 10.1007/s00109-011-0829-0. Epub November 18, 2011. PubMed PMID: 22095100.

Lee YH, Wong DT. Saliva: An emerging biofluid for early detection of diseases. *Am J Dent*. August 2009;22(4):241–248. Review. PubMed PMID: 19824562; PubMed Central PMCID: PMC 2860957.

Lee YH, Zhou H, Reiss JK, Yan X, Zhang L, Chia D, Wong DT. Direct saliva transcriptome analysis. *Clin Chem*. September 2011;57(9):1295–1302. doi: 10.1373/clinchem.2010.159210. Epub July 26, 2011. PubMed PMID: 21791578.

Leemans CR, Braakhuis BJ, Brakenhoff RH. The molecular biology of head and neck cancer. *Nat Rev Cancer*. January 2011;11(1):9–22. doi: 10.1038/nrc2982. Epub December 16, 2010. Review. PubMed PMID: 21160525.

Li X, Yang T, Lin J. Spectral analysis of human saliva for detection of lung cancer using surface-enhanced Raman spectroscopy. *J Biomed Opt*. March 2012;17(3):037003. doi: 10.1117/1.JBO.17.3.037003. PubMed PMID: 22502575.

Li Y, Elashoff D, Oh M, Sinha U, St John MA, Zhou X, Abemayor E, Wong DT. Serum circulating human mRNA profiling and its utility for oral cancer detection. *J Clin Oncol*. April 10, 2006;24(11):1754–1760. Epub February 27, 2006. PubMed PMID: 16505414.

Li Y, St John MA, Zhou X, Kim Y, Sinha U, Jordan RC, Eisele D et al. Salivary transcriptome diagnostics for oral cancer detection. *Clin Cancer Res*. December 15, 2004;10(24):8442–8450. PubMed PMID: 15623624.

Liang YH, Chang CC, Chen CC, Chu-Su Y, Lin CW. Development of an Au/ZnO thin film surface plasmon resonance-based biosensor immunoassay for the detection of carbohydrate antigen 15-3 in human saliva. *Clin Biochem*. December 2012;45(18):1689–1693. doi: 10.1016/j. clinbiochem.2012.09.001. Epub September 12, 2012. PubMed PMID: 22981930.

Lingen MW. Screening for oral premalignancy and cancer: What platform and which biomarkers? *Cancer Prev Res (Phila).* September 2010;3(9):1056–1059. doi: 10.1158/1940-6207.CAPR-10-0173. Epub August 26, 2010. PubMed PMID: 20798207.

Liu CJ, Lin SC, Yang CC, Cheng HW, Chang KW. Exploiting salivary miR-31 as a clinical biomarker of oral squamous cell carcinoma. *Head Neck.* February 2012a;34(2):219–224. doi: 10.1002/hed.21713. Epub April 15, 2011. PubMed PMID:22083872.

Liu X, Fortin K, Mourelatos Z. MicroRNAs: Biogenesis and molecular functions. *Brain Pathol.* January 2008;18(1):113–121. doi: 10.1111/j.1750-3639.2007.00121.x. Review. PubMed PMID: 18226106.

Liu Y, Zhou ZT, He QB, Jiang WW. DAPK promoter hypermethylation in tissues and body fluids of oral precancer patients. *Med Oncol.* June 2012b;29(2):729–733. doi: 10.1007/s12032-011-9953-5. Epub April 24, 2011. PubMed PMID: 21516484.

Lu J, Getz G, Miska EA, Alvarez-Saavedra E, Lamb J, Peck D, Sweet-Cordero A et al. MicroRNA expression profiles classify human cancers. *Nature.* June 9, 2005;435(7043):834–838. PubMed PMID: 15944708.

Lyons AJ, Cui N. Salivary oncofoetal fibronectin and oral squamous cell carcinoma. *J Oral Pathol Med.* July 2000;29(6):267–270. PubMed PMID: 10890557.

Mager DL, Haffajee AD, Devlin PM, Norris CM, Posner MR, Goodson JM. The salivary microbiota as a diagnostic indicator of oral cancer: A descriptive, non-randomized study of cancer-free and oral squamous cell carcinoma subjects. *J Transl Med.* July 7, 2005;3:27. PubMed PMID: 15987522; PubMed Central PMCID: PMC1226180.

Mancuso R, Biffi R, Valli M, Bellinvia M, Tourlaki A, Ferrucci S, Brambilla L et al. HHV8 a subtype is associated with rapidly evolving classic Kaposi's sarcoma. *J Med Virol.* December 2008;80(12):2153–2160. doi: 10.1002/jmv.21322. Erratum in: *J Med Virol.* June 2009;81(6):1128. Athanasia, Tourlaki [corrected to Tourlaki, Athanasia]. PubMed PMID: 19040293; PubMed Central PMCID: PMC2596973.

Mancuso R, Brambilla L, Agostini S, Biffi R, Hernis A, Guerini FR, Agliardi C, Tourlaki A, Bellinvia M, Clerici M. Intrafamiliar transmission of Kaposi's sarcoma-associated herpesvirus and seronegative infection in family members of classic Kaposi's sarcoma patients. *J Gen Virol.* April 2011;92(Pt 4):744–751. doi: 10.1099/vir.0.027847-0. Epub January 7, 2011. PubMed PMID: 21216985.

Mandel ID. The diagnostic uses of saliva. *J Oral Pathol Med.* March 1990;19(3):119–125. Review. PubMed PMID: 2187975.

Mandel ID. Salivary diagnosis: Promises, promises. *Ann N Y Acad Sci.* September 20, 1993;694:1–10. Review. PubMed PMID: 8215047.

Markopoulos AK, Michailidou EZ, Tzimagiorgis G. Salivary markers for oral cancer detection. *Open Dent J.* 2010;4:172–178. doi: 10.2174/1874210601004010172. Epub August 27, 2010. PubMed PMID: 21673842; PubMed Central PMCID: PMC3111739.

Markopoulou S, Nikolaidis G, Liloglou T. DNA methylation biomarkers in biological fluids for early detection of respiratory tract cancer. *Clin Chem Lab Med.* October 1, 2012;50(10):1723–1731. doi: 10.1515/cclm-2012-0124. PubMed PMID: 23089700.

Martin KJ, Fournier MV, Reddy GP, Pardee AB. A need for basic research on fluid-based early detection biomarkers. *Cancer Res.* July 1, 2010;70(13):5203–5206. doi: 10.1158/0008-5472.CAN-10-0987. Epub June 29, 2010. Review. PubMed PMID: 20587531.

Marzesco AM, Janich P, Wilsch-Bräuninger M, Dubreuil V, Langenfeld K, Corbeil D, Huttner WB. Release of extracellular membrane particles carrying the stem cell marker prominin-1 (CD133) from neural progenitors and other epithelial cells. *J Cell Sci.* July 1, 2005;118(Pt 13):2849–2858. PubMed PMID: 15976444.

Matta A, Ralhan R, DeSouza LV, Siu KW. Mass spectrometry-based clinical proteomics: Head-and-neck cancer biomarkers and drug-targets discovery. *Mass Spectrom Rev.* November–December 2010;29(6):945–961. doi: 10.1002/mas.20296. Review. PubMed PMID: 20945361.

Matthews AM, Kaur H, Dodd M, D'Souza J, Liloglou T, Shaw RJ, Risk JM. Saliva collection methods for DNA biomarker analysis in oral cancer patients. *Br J Oral Maxillofac Surg.* July 2013;51(5):394–398.

Metallo CM. Expanding the reach of cancer metabolomics. *Cancer Prev Res (Phila).* December 2012;5(12):1337–1340. doi: 10.1158/1940-6207.CAPR-12-0433. Epub November 14, 2012. PubMed PMID: 23151806.

Michael A, Bajracharya SD, Yuen PS, Zhou H, Star RA, Illei GG, Alevizos I. Exosomes from human saliva as a source of microRNA biomarkers. *Oral Dis.* January 2010;16(1):34–38. doi: 10.1111/j.1601-0825.2009.01604.x. Epub July 15, 2009. PubMed PMID: 19627513; PubMed Central PMCID: PMC2844919.

Mithani SK, Smith IM, Zhou S, Gray A, Koch WM, Maitra A, Califano JA. Mitochondrial resequencing arrays detect tumor-specific mutations in salivary rinses of patients with head and neck cancer. *Clin Cancer Res*. December 15, 2007;13(24):7335–7340. PubMed PMID: 18094415.

Mocellin S, Pooley KA, Nitti D. Telomerase and the search for the end of cancer. *Trends Mol Med*. February 2013;19(2):125–133. doi: 10.1016/j.molmed.2012.11.006. Epub December 17, 2012. PubMed PMID: 23253475.

Myers JN, Elkins T, Roberts D, Byers RM. Squamous cell carcinoma of the tongue in young adults: Increasing incidence and factors that predict treatment outcomes. *Otolaryngol Head Neck Surg*. January 2000;122(1):44–51. PubMed PMID: 10629481.

Nagata S, Hamada T, Yamada N, Yokoyama S, Kitamoto S, Kanmura Y, Nomura M, Kamikawa Y, Yonezawa S, Sugihara K. Aberrant DNA methylation of tumor-related genes in oral rinse: A noninvasive method for detection of oral squamous cell carcinoma. *Cancer*. September 1, 2012;118(17):4298–4308. doi: 10.1002/cncr.27417. Epub Jan 17, 2012. PubMed PMID: 22252571.

Navazesh M. Methods for collecting saliva. *Ann N Y Acad Sci*. September 20, 1993;694:72–77. Review. PubMed PMID: 8215087.

Ng EK, Chong WW, Jin H, Lam EK, Shin VY, Yu J, Poon TC et al. Differential expression of microRNAs in plasma of patients with colorectal cancer: A potential marker for colorectal cancer screening. *Gut*. October 2009;58(10):1375–1381. doi: 10.1136/gut.2008.167817. Epub 2009 Feb 6. PubMed PMID: 19201770.

Nunes DN, Kowalski LP, Simpson AJ. Detection of oral and oropharyngeal cancer by microsatellite analysis in mouth washes and lesion brushings. *Oral Oncol*. November 2000;36(6):525–528. PubMed PMID: 11036246.

Nussbaumer C, Gharehbaghi-Schnell E, Korschineck I. Messenger RNA profiling: A novel method for body fluid identification by real-time PCR. *Forensic Sci Int*. March 10, 2006;157(2–3):181–186. Epub November 9, 2005. PubMed PMID: 16289614.

O'Driscoll L. Extracellular nucleic acids and their potential as diagnostic, prognostic and predictive biomarkers. *Anticancer Res*. May–June 2007;27(3A):1257–1265. Review. PubMed PMID: 17593617.

Okami K, Imate Y, Hashimoto Y, Kamada T, Takahashi M. Molecular detection of cancer cells in saliva from oral and pharyngeal cancer patients. *Tokai J Exp Clin Med*. September 2002;27(3):85–89. PubMed PMID: 12701646.

Ovchinnikov DA, Cooper MA, Pandit P, Coman WB, Cooper-White JJ, Keith P, Wolvetang EJ, Slowey PD, Punyadeera C. Tumor-suppressor gene promoter hypermethylation in saliva of head and neck cancer patients. *Transl Oncol*. October 2012;5(5):321–326. Epub October 1, 2012. PubMed PMID: 23066440; PubMed Central PMCID: PMC3468923.

Palanisamy V, Sharma S, Deshpande A, Zhou H, Gimzewski J, Wong DT. Nanostructural and transcriptomic analyses of human saliva derived exosomes. *PLoS One*. January 5, 2010;5(1):e8577. doi: 10.1371/journal.pone.0008577. PubMed PMID: 20052414; PubMed Central PMCID: PMC2797607.

Park IS, Chang X, Loyo M, Wu G, Chuang A, Kim MS, Chae YK et al. Characterization of the methylation patterns in human papillomavirus type 16 viral DNA in head and neck cancers. *Cancer Prev Res (Phila)*. February 2011;4(2):207–217. doi: 10.1158/1940–6207.CAPR-10-0147. PubMed PMID: 21292634; PubMed Central PMCID: PMC3079312.

Park NJ, Li Y, Yu T, Brinkman BM, Wong DT. Characterization of RNA in saliva. *Clin Chem*. June 2006a;52(6):988–994. Epub April 6, 2006. PubMed PMID: 16601067.

Park NJ, Yu T, Nabili V, Brinkman BM, Henry S, Wang J, Wong DT. RNAprotect saliva: An optimal room-temperature stabilization reagent for the salivary transcriptome. *Clin Chem*. December 2006b;52(12): 2303–2304. PubMed PMID: 17138851.

Park NJ, Zhou H, Elashoff D, Henson BS, Kastratovic DA, Abemayor E, Wong DT. Salivary microRNA: Discovery, characterization, and clinical utility for oral cancer detection. *Clin Cancer Res*. September 1, 2009;15(17):5473–5477. doi: 10.1158/1078-0432.CCR-09-0736. Epub August 25, 2009. PubMed PMID: 19706812; PubMed Central PMCID: PMC2752355.

Park NJ, Zhou X, Yu T, Brinkman BM, Zimmermann BG, Palanisamy V, Wong DT. Characterization of salivary RNA by cDNA library analysis. *Arch Oral Biol*. January 2007;52(1):30–35. Epub October 18, 2006. PubMed PMID: 17052683; PubMed Central PMCID: PMC2743855.

Pereira LH, Adebisi IN, Perez A, Wiebel M, Reis I, Duncan R, Goodwin WJ, Hu JJ, Lokeshwar VB, Franzmann EJ. Salivary markers and risk factor data: A multivariate modeling approach for head and neck squamous cell carcinoma detection. *Cancer Biomark*. 2011;10(5):241–249. PubMed PMID: 22699785.

Pfaffe T, Cooper-White J, Beyerlein P, Kostner K, Punyadeera C. Diagnostic potential of saliva: Current state and future applications. *Clin Chem*. May 2011;57(5):675–687. doi:10.1373/clinchem. 2010.153767. Epub March 7, 2011. Review. PubMed PMID: 21383043.

Pink R, Simek J, Vondrakova J, Faber E, Michl P, Pazdera J, Indrak K. Saliva as a diagnostic medium. *Biomed Pap Med Fac Univ Palacky Olomouc Czech Repub*. June 2009;153(2):103–110. PubMed PMID: 19771133.

Poujol S, Bressolle F, Duffour J, Abderrahim AG, Astre C, Ychou M, Pinguet F. Pharmacokinetics and pharmacodynamics of irinotecan and its metabolites from plasma and saliva data in patients with metastatic digestive cancer receiving Folfiri regimen. *Cancer Chemother Pharmacol*. September 2006;58(3): 292–305. Epub December 21, 2005. PubMed PMID: 16369821.

Pow EH, Law MY, Tsang PC, Perera RA, Kwong DL. Salivary Epstein-Barr virus DNA level in patients with nasopharyngeal carcinoma following radiotherapy. *Oral Oncol*. September 2011;47(9):879–882. doi: 10.1016/j.oraloncology.2011.06.507. Epub July 20, 2011. PubMed PMID: 21767975.

Printz C. Saliva yields clues to early cancer detection. *Cancer*. July 1, 2012;118(13):3224. doi: 10.1002/cncr.27700. PubMed PMID: 22711573. PubMed Central PMCID: PMC2674508.

Rai B, Kaur J, Jacobs R, Anand SC. Adenosine deaminase in saliva as a diagnostic marker of squamous cell carcinoma of tongue. *Clin Oral Investig*. June 2011;15(3):347–349. doi: 10.1007/s00784-010-0404-z. Epub April 9. PubMed PMID: 20379753.

Reddy I, Sherlin HJ, Ramani P, Premkumar P, Natesan A, Chandrasekar T. Amino acid profile of saliva from patients with oral squamous cell carcinoma using high performance liquid chromatography. *J Oral Sci*. September 2012;54(3):279–283. PubMed PMID: 23047040.

Rehak NN, Cecco SA, Csako G. Biochemical composition and electrolyte balance of "unstimulated" whole human saliva. *Clin Chem Lab Med*. April 2000;38(4):335–343. Erratum in: *Clin Chem Lab Med*. October 2000;38(10):1081. PubMed PMID: 10928655.

Rettori MM, de Carvalho AC, Bomfim Longo AL, de Oliveira CZ, Kowalski LP, Carvalho AL, Vettore AL. Prognostic significance of TIMP3 hypermethylation in post-treatment salivary rinse from head and neck squamous cell carcinoma patients. *Carcinogenesis*. January 2013;34(1):20–27. doi: 10.1093/carcin/bgs311. Epub October 5, 2012. PubMed PMID: 23042095.

Ribeiro KC, Kowalski LP, Latorre MR. Impact of comorbidity, symptoms, and patients' characteristics on the prognosis of oral carcinomas. *Arch Otolaryngol Head Neck Surg*. September 2000;126(9):1079–1085. PubMed PMID: 10979120.

Righini CA, de Fraipont F, Reyt E, Favrot MC. Aberrant methylation of tumor suppressor genes in head and neck squamous cell carcinoma: Is it clinically relevant? *Bull Cancer*. February 2007a;94(2):191–197. French. PubMed PMID: 17337388.

Righini CA, de Fraipont F, Timsit JF, Dassonville O, Milano G, Moro-Sibilot D. Study of aberrant methylation of TSG in saliva in case of upper-aerodigestive-tract cancer. *Rev Stomatol Chir Maxillofac*. September 2008;109(4):226–232. doi: 10.1016/j.stomax.2008.06.007. Epub August 29, 2008. French. PubMed PMID: 18760810.

Righini CA, de Fraipont F, Timsit JF, Faure C, Brambilla E, Reyt E, Favrot MC. Tumor-specific methylation in saliva: A promising biomarker for early detection of head and neck cancer recurrence. *Clin Cancer Res*. February 15, 2007b;13(4):1179–1185. PubMed PMID: 17317827.

Rosas SL, Koch W, da Costa Carvalho MG, Wu L, Califano J, Westra W, Jen J, Sidransky D. Promoter hypermethylation patterns of p16, O6-methylguanine-DNA-methyltransferase, and death-associated protein kinase in tumors and saliva of head and neck cancer patients. *Cancer Res*. February 1, 2001;61(3):939–942. PubMed PMID: 11221887.

Rusling JF, Kumar CV, Gutkind JS, Patel V. Measurement of biomarker proteins or point-of-care early detection and monitoring of cancer. *Analyst*. October 2010;135(10):2496–2511. doi: 10.1039/c0an00204f. Epub July 8, 2010. Review. PubMed PMID: 20614087; PubMed Central PMCID: PMC2997816.

Sadick M, Schoenberg SO, Hoermann K, Sadick H. Current oncologic concepts and emerging techniques for imaging of head and neck squamous cell cancer. *GMS Curr Top Otorhinolaryngol Head Neck Surg*. 2012;11:Doc08. doi: 10.3205/cto000090. Epub December 20, 2012. PubMed PMID: 23320060; PubMed Central PMCID: PMC3544205.

SahebJamee M, Boorghani M, Ghaffari SR, AtarbashiMoghadam F, Keyhani A. Human papillomavirus in saliva of patients with oral squamous cell carcinoma. *Med Oral Patol Oral Cir Bucal*. October 1, 2009;14(10):e525–e528. PubMed PMID: 19680210.

Saito I, Nishimura S, Kudo I, Fox RI, Moro I. Detection of Epstein-Barr virus and human herpes virus type 6 in saliva from patients with lymphoproliferative diseases by the polymerase chain reaction. *Arch Oral Biol.* 1991;36(11):779–784. PubMed PMID: 1662480.

Sanjay PR, Hallikeri K, Shivashankara AR. Evaluation of salivary sialic acid, total protein, and total sugar in oral cancer: A preliminary report. *Indian J Dent Res.* October–December 2008;19(4):288–291. PubMed PMID: 19075429.

Sartini D, Pozzi V, Renzi E, Morganti S, Rocchetti R, Rubini C, Santarelli A, Lo Muzio L, Emanuelli M. Analysis of tissue and salivary nicotinamide N-methyltransferase in oral squamous cell carcinoma: Basis for the development of a noninvasive diagnostic test for early-stage disease. *Biol Chem.* May 2012;393(6):505–511. doi: 10.1515/hsz-2012-0112. PubMed PMID: 22628313.

Sawangsoda P, Sithithaworn J, Tesana S, Pinlaor S, Boonmars T, Mairiang E, Yongvanit P, Duenngai K, Sithithaworn P. Diagnostic values of parasite-specific antibody detections in saliva and urine in comparison with serum in opisthorchiasis. *Parasitol Int.* March 2012;61(1):196–202. doi:10.1016/j.parint.2011.06.009. Epub June 17, 2011. PubMed PMID: 21704727.

Selcuklu SD, Donoghue MT, Spillane C. miR-21 as a key regulator of oncogenic processes. *Biochem Soc Trans.* August 2009;37(Pt 4):918–925. doi: 10.1042/BST0370918. Review. PubMed PMID: 19614619.

Sethi S, Benninger MS, Lu M, Havard S, Worsham MJ. Noninvasive molecular detection of head and neck squamous cell carcinoma: An exploratory analysis. *Diagn Mol Pathol.* June 2009;18(2):81–87. doi: 10.1097/PDM.0b013e3181804b82. PubMed PMID: 19430297; PubMed Central PMCID: PMC2693294.

Seugnet L, Boero J, Gottschalk L, Duntley SP, Shaw PJ. Identification of a biomarker for sleep drive in flies and humans. *Proc Natl Acad Sci USA.* December 26, 2006;103(52):19913–19918. Epub December 13, 2006. PubMed PMID: 17167051; PubMed Central PMCID: PMC1750902.

Shah FD, Begum R, Vajaria BN, Patel KR, Patel JB, Shukla SN, Patel PS. A review on salivary genomics and proteomics biomarkers in oral cancer. *Indian J Clin Biochem.* October 2011;26(4):326–334. Epub August 9, 2011. PubMed PMID: 23024467; PubMed Central PMCID: PMC3210231.

Sharma M, Bairy I, Pai K, Satyamoorthy K, Prasad S, Berkovitz B, Radhakrishnan R. Salivary IL-6 levels in oral leukoplakia with dysplasia and its clinical relevance to tobacco habits and periodontitis. *Clin Oral Investig.* October 2011;15(5):705–714. doi: 10.1007/s00784-010-0435-5. Epub June 19, 2010. PubMed PMID: 20563615.

Sharma S, Rasool HI, Palanisamy V, Mathisen C, Schmidt M, Wong DT, Gimzewski JK. Structural-mechanical characterization of nanoparticle exosomes in human saliva, using correlative AFM, FESEM, and force spectroscopy. *ACS Nano.* April 27, 2010;4(4):1921–1926. doi: 10.1021/nn901824n. PubMed PMID: 20218655; PubMed Central PMCID: PMC2866049.

Shaw RJ, Akufo-Tetteh EK, Risk JM, Field JK, Liloglou T. Methylation enrichment pyrosequencing: Combining the specificity of MSP with validation by pyrosequencing. *Nucleic Acids Res.* June 28, 2006;34(11):e78. PubMed PMID: 16807314; PubMed Central PMCID: PMC1904102.

Shintani S, Hamakawa H, Ueyama Y, Hatori M, Toyoshima T. Identification of a truncated cystatin SA-I as a saliva biomarker for oral squamous cell carcinoma using the SELDI ProteinChip platform. *Int J Oral Maxillofac Surg.* January 2010;39(1):68–74. doi: 10.1016/j.ijom. 2009.10.001. Epub November 5, 2009. PubMed PMID:19896329.

Shpitzer T, Hamzany Y, Bahar G, Feinmesser R, Savulescu D, Borovoi I, Gavish M, Nagler RM. Salivary analysis of oral cancer biomarkers. *Br J Cancer.* October 6, 2009;101(7):1194–1198. doi: 10.1038/sj.bjc.6605290. PubMed PMID: 19789535; PubMed Central PMCID: PMC2768098.

Shuman Moss LA, Jensen-Taubman S, Stetler-Stevenson WG. Matrix metalloproteinases: Changing roles in tumor progression and metastasis. *Am J Pathol.* December 2012;181(6):1895–1899. doi: 10.1016/j.ajpath.2012.08.044. Epub October 12, 2012. PubMed PMID: 23063657; PubMed Central PMCID: PMC3506216.

Spafford MF, Koch WM, Reed AL, Califano JA, Xu LH, Eisenberger CF, Yip L et al. Detection of head and neck squamous cell carcinoma among exfoliated oral mucosal cells by microsatellite analysis. *Clin Cancer Res.* March 2001;7(3):607–612. PubMed PMID: 11297256.

Sparano A, Weinstein G, Chalian A, Yodul M, Weber R. Multivariate predictors of occult neck metastasis in early oral tongue cancer. *Otolaryngol Head Neck Surg.* October 2004;131(4):472–476. PubMed PMID: 15467620.

Spielmann N, Wong DT. Saliva: Diagnostics and therapeutic perspectives. *Oral Dis.* May 2011;17(4):345–354. doi: 10.1111/j.1601-0825.2010.01773.x. Epub December 2, 2010. Review. PubMed PMID: 21122035; PubMed Central PMCID: PMC3056919.

St. John MA, Li Y, Zhou X, Denny P, Ho CM, Montemagno C, Shi W et al. Interleukin 6 and interleukin 8 as potential biomarkers for oral cavity and oropharyngeal squamous cell carcinoma. *Arch Otolaryngol Head Neck Surg*. August 2004;130(8):929–935. PubMed PMID: 15313862.

Stamey FR, Patel MM, Holloway BP, Pellett PE. Quantitative, fluorogenic probe PCR assay for detection of human herpesvirus 8 DNA in clinical specimens. *J Clin Microbiol*. October 2001;39(10):3537–3540. PubMed PMID: 11574569; PubMed Central PMCID: PMC88385.

Stetler-Stevenson WG, Yu AE. Proteases in invasion: Matrix metalloproteinases. *Semin Cancer Biol*. April 2001;11(2):143–152. Review. PubMed PMID: 11322833.

Stott-Miller M, Houck JR, Lohavanichbutr P, Méndez E, Upton MP, Futran ND, Schwartz SM, Chen C. Tumor and salivary matrix metalloproteinase levels are strong diagnostic markers of oral squamous cell carcinoma. *Cancer Epidemiol Biomark Prev*. December 2011;20(12):2628–2636. doi: 10.1158/1055-9965.EPI-11-0503. Epub September 29, 2011. PubMed PMID: 21960692; PubMed Central PMCID: PMC3237810.

Streckfus C, Bigler L. The use of soluble, salivary c-erbB-2 for the detection and post-operative follow-up of breast cancer in women: The results of a five-year translational research study. *Adv Dent Res*. June 2005;18(1):17–24. Review. PubMed PMID: 15998939.

Streckfus C, Bigler L, Dellinger T, Dai X, Cox WJ, McArthur A, Kingman A, Thigpen JT. Reliability assessment of soluble c-erbB-2 concentrations in the saliva of healthy women and men. *Oral Surg Oral Med Oral Pathol Oral Radiol Endod*. February 2001;91(2):174–179. PubMed PMID: 11174594.

Streckfus C, Bigler L, Dellinger T, Dai X, Kingman A, Thigpen JT. The presence of soluble c-erbB-2 in saliva and serum among women with breast carcinoma: A preliminary study. *Clin Cancer Res*. June 2000a;6(6):2363–2370. PubMed PMID: 10873088.

Streckfus C, Bigler L, Dellinger T, Pfeifer M, Rose A, Thigpen JT. CA 15-3 and c-erbB-2 presence in the saliva of women. *Clin Oral Investig*. September 1999;3(3):138–143. PubMed PMID: 10803125.

Streckfus C, Bigler L, Tucci M, Thigpen JT. A preliminary study of CA15-3, c-erbB-2, epidermal growth factor receptor, cathepsin-D, and p53 in saliva among women with breast carcinoma. *Cancer Invest*. 2000b;18(2):101–109. PubMed PMID: 10705871.

Sugimoto M, Wong DT, Hirayama A, Soga T, Tomita M. Capillary electrophoresis mass spectrometry-based saliva metabolomics identified oral, breast and pancreatic cancer-specific profiles. *Metabolomics*. March 2010;6(1):78–95. Epub September 10, 2009. PubMed PMID: 20300169; PubMed Central PMCID: PMC2818837.

Sumida T, Sogawa K, Hamakawa H, Sugita A, Tanioka H, Ueda N. Detection of telomerase activity in oral lesions. *J Oral Pathol Med*. March 1998;27(3):111–115. PubMed PMID: 9563802.

Sun W, Zaboli D, Liu Y, Arnaoutakis D, Khan T, Wang H, Koch W, Khan Z, Califano JA. Comparison of promoter hypermethylation pattern in salivary rinses collected with and without an exfoliating brush from patients with HNSCC. *PLoS One*. 2012a;7(3):e33642. doi: 10.1371/journal.pone.0033642. Epub Mar 16, 2012. PubMed PMID: 22438973; PubMed Central PMCID: PMC3306276.

Sun W, Zaboli D, Wang H, Liu Y, Arnaoutakis D, Khan T, Khan Z, Koch WM, Califano JA. Detection of TIMP3 promoter hypermethylation in salivary rinse as an independent predictor of local recurrence-free survival in head and neck cancer. *Clin Cancer Res*. February 15, 2012b;18(4):1082–1091. doi: 10.1158/1078-0432.CCR-11-2392. Epub Jan 6, 2012. PubMed PMID: 22228635; PubMed Central PMCID: PMC3288549.

Szanto I, Mark L, Bona A, Maasz G, Sandor B, Gelencser G, Turi Z, Gallyas F Jr. High-throughput screening of saliva for early detection of oral cancer: A pilot study. *Technol Cancer Res Treat*. April 2012;11(2):181–188. PubMed PMID: 22335413.

Tainsky MA, Chatterjee M, Levin NK, Draghici S, Abrams J. Multianalyte tests for the early detection of cancer: Speedbumps and barriers. *Biomark Insight*. July 10, 2007;2:261–267. PubMed PMID: 19662209; PubMed Central PMCID: PMC2717809.

Tan W, Sabet L, Li Y, Yu T, Klokkevold PR, Wong DT, Ho CM. Optical protein sensor for detecting cancer markers in saliva. *Biosens Bioelectron*. October 15, 2008;24(2):266–271. doi: 10.1016/j.bios.2008.03.037. Epub April 6, 2008. PubMed PMID: 18479906; PubMed Central PMCID: PMC2584973.

Tang H, Wu Z, Zhang J, Su B. Salivary lncRNA as a potential marker for oral squamous cell carcinoma diagnosis. *Mol Med Report*. March 2013;7(3):761–766.

Tang J, Ahmad A, Sarkar FH. The role of microRNAs in breast cancer migration, invasion and metastasis. *Int J Mol Sci*. October 18, 2012;13(10):13414–13437. doi: 10.3390/ijms131013414. PubMed PMID: 23202960; PubMed Central PMCID: PMC3497334.

Tao WA, Wollscheid B, O'Brien R, Eng JK, Li XJ, Bodenmiller B, Watts JD, Hood L, Aebersold R. Quantitative phosphoproteome analysis using a dendrimer conjugation chemistry and tandem mass spectrometry. *Nat Methods*. August 2005;2(8):591–598. PubMed PMID: 16094384.

Taylor MM, Chohan B, Lavreys L, Hassan W, Huang ML, Corey L, Ashley Morrow R et al. Shedding of human herpesvirus 8 in oral and genital secretions from HIV-1-seropositive and -seronegative Kenyan women. *J Infect Dis*. August 1, 2004;190(3):484–488. Epub July 7, 2004. PubMed PMID: 15243920.

Tu LC, Foltz G, Lin E, Hood L, Tian Q. Targeting stem cells-clinical implications for cancer therapy. *Curr Stem Cell Res Ther*. May 2009;4(2):147–153. Review. PubMed PMID: 19442199; PubMed Central PMCID: PMC3034385.

Tu Z, Li H, Ma Y, Tang B, Tian J, Akers W, Achilefu S, Gu Y. The enhanced antiproliferative response to combined treatment of trichostatin A with raloxifene in MCF-7 breast cancer cells and its relevance to estrogen receptor β expression. *Mol Cell Biochem*. July 2012;366(1–2):111–122. doi: 10.1007/s11010-012-1288-9. Epub April 4, 2012. PubMed PMID: 22476901.

Yu Z, Pestell RG. Small non-coding RNAs govern mammary gland tumorigenesis. *J Mammary Gland Biol Neoplasia*. March 2012;17(1):59–64. doi: 10.1007/s10911-012-9246-4. Epub March 1, 2012. Review. PubMed PMID: 22382486; PubMed Central PMCID: PMC3309138.

Valadi H, Ekström K, Bossios A, Sjöstrand M, Lee JJ, Lötvall JO. Exosome-mediated transfer of mRNAs and microRNAs is a novel mechanism of genetic exchange between cells. *Nat Cell Biol*. June 2007;9(6): 654–659. Epub May 7, 2007. PubMed PMID: 17486113.

Varol N, Konac E, Gurocak OS, Sozen S. The realm of microRNAs in cancers. *Mol Biol Rep*. February 2011;38(2):1079–1089. doi: 10.1007/s11033-010-0205-0. Epub June 20, 2010. Review. PubMed PMID: 20563858.

Viet CT, Schmidt BL. Methylation array analysis of preoperative and postoperative saliva DNA in oral cancer patients. *Cancer Epidemiol Biomark Prev*. December 2008;17(12):3603–3611. doi: 10.1158/1055-9965. EPI-08-0507. PubMed PMID: 19064577.

Vlassov AV, Magdaleno S, Setterquist R, Conrad R. Exosomes: Current knowledge of their composition, biological functions, and diagnostic and therapeutic potentials. *Biochim Biophys Acta*. July 2012;1820(7): 940–948. doi: 10.1016/j.bbagen.2012.03.017. Epub April 1, 2012. Review. PubMed PMID: 22503788.

Wang J, Peng W, Wu FX. Computational approaches to predicting essential proteins: A survey. *Proteomics Clin Appl*. January 2013;7(1–2):181–192. doi: 10.1002/prca.201200068. PubMed PMID: 23165920.

Warnakulasuriya S, Soussi T, Maher R, Johnson N, Tavassoli M. Expression of p53 in oral squamous cell carcinoma is associated with the presence of IgG and IgA p53 autoantibodies in sera and saliva of the patients. *J Pathol*. September 2000;192(1):52–57. PubMed PMID: 10951400.

Wei F, Patel P, Liao W, Chaudhry K, Zhang L, Arellano-Garcia M, Hu S et al. Electrochemical sensor for multiplex biomarkers detection. *Clin Cancer Res*. July 1, 2009;15(13):4446–4452. doi: 10.1158/1078-0432.CCR-09-0050. Epub June 9, 2009. PubMed PMID: 19509137; PubMed Central PMCID: PMC2799532.

Wei J, Xie G, Zhou Z, Shi P, Qiu Y, Zheng X, Chen T, Su M, Zhao A, Jia W. Salivary metabolite signatures of oral cancer and leukoplakia. *Int J Cancer*. November 1, 2011;129(9):2207–2217. doi: 10.1002/ijc.25881. Epub April 13, 2011. PubMed PMID: 21190195.

Westra WH, Califano J. Toward early oral cancer detection using gene expression profiling of saliva: A thoroughfare or dead end? *Clin Cancer Res*. December 15, 2004;10(24):8130–8131. PubMed PMID: 15623585.

WHO Media Center 2013: http://www.who.int/mediacentre/en/

WHO, International Agency for Research on Cancer 2010: http://globocan.iarc.fr

WHO Report 2013: http://www.who.int/cancer/en/

Widmer IC, Erb P, Grob H, Itin P, Baumann M, Stalder A, Weber R, Cathomas G. Human herpesvirus 8 oral shedding in HIV-infected men with and without Kaposi sarcoma. *J Acquir Immune Defic Syndr*. August 1, 2006;42(4):420–425. PubMed PMID: 16791117.

Wilken R, Veena MS, Wang MB, Srivatsan ES. Curcumin: A review of anti-cancer properties and therapeutic activity in head and neck squamous cell carcinoma. *Mol Cancer*. February 7, 2011;10:12. doi: 10.1186/1476-4598-10-12. Review. PubMed PMID: 21299897; PubMed Central PMCID: PMC3055228.

Winter JM, Yeo CJ, Brody JR. Diagnostic, prognostic, and predictive biomarkers in pancreatic cancer. *J Surg Oncol*. January 2013;107(1):15–22. doi: 10.1002/jso.23192. Epub June 21, 2012. Review. PubMed PMID: 22729569.

Wong DT. Salivary diagnostics for oral cancer. *J Calif Dent Assoc.* April 2006a;34(4):303–308. PubMed PMID: 16900988.

Wong DT. Towards a simple, saliva-based test for the detection of oral cancer 'oral fluid (saliva), which is the mirror of the body, is a perfect medium to be explored for health and disease surveillance'. *Expert Rev Mol Diagn.* May 2006b;6(3):267–272. PubMed PMID: 16706730.

Wong TS, Liu XB, Wong BY, Ng RW, Yuen AP, Wei WI. Mature miR-184 as potential oncogenic microRNA of squamous cell carcinoma of tongue. *Clin Cancer Res.* May 1, 2008;14(9):2588–2592. doi: 10.1158/1078-0432.CCR-07-0666. PubMed PMID: 18451220.

Wroczyński P, Giebułtowicz J, Piekarczyk J, Wierzchowski J. Fluorimetric detection of aldehyde dehydrogenase activity in human saliva in diagnostic of cancers of oral cavity. *Acta Pol Pharm.* September–October 2006;63(5):407–409. PubMed PMID: 17357596.

Wu ZZ, Wang JG, Zhang XL. Diagnostic model of saliva protein finger print analysis of patients with gastric cancer. *World J Gastroenterol.* February 21, 2009;15(7):865–870. PubMed PMID: 19230049; PubMed Central PMCID: PMC2653388.

Xiao H, Wong DT. Proteomic analysis of microvesicles in human saliva by gel electrophoresis with liquid chromatography-mass spectrometry. *Anal Chim Acta.* April 20, 2012;723:61–67. doi: 10.1016/j.aca.2012.02.018. Epub February 19, 2012. PubMed PMID: 22444574.

Xiao H, Zhang L, Zhou H, Lee JM, Garon EB, Wong DT. Proteomic analysis of human saliva from lung cancer patients using two-dimensional difference gel electrophoresis and mass spectrometry. *Mol Cell Proteomics.* February 2012;11(2):M111.012112. doi: 10.1074/mcp.M111. 012112. Epub November 17, 2011. PubMedPMID: 22096114; PubMed Central PMCID: PMC3277759.

Xu J, Wu C, Che X, Wang L, Yu D, Zhang T, Huang L, Li H, Tan W, Wang C, Lin D. Circulating microRNAs, miR-21, miR-122, and miR-223, in patients with hepatocellular carcinoma or chronic hepatitis. *Mol Carcinog.* February 2011;50(2):136–142. doi: 10.1002/mc.20712. Epub December 10, 2010. PubMed PMID: 21229610.

Yan SK, Wei BJ, Lin ZY, Yang Y, Zhou ZT, Zhang WD. A metabonomic approach to the diagnosis of oral squamous cell carcinoma, oral lichen planus and oral leukoplakia. *Oral Oncol.* May 2008;44(5):477–483. Epub October 23, 2007. PubMed PMID:17936673.

Yang CY, Brooks E, Li Y, Denny P, Ho CM, Qi F, Shi W et al. Detection of picomolar levels of interleukin-8 in human saliva by SPR. *Lab Chip.* October 2005;5(10):1017–1023. Epub August 18, 2005. PubMed PMID: 16175255.

Yeh CK, Christodoulides NJ, Floriano PN, Miller CS, Ebersole JL, Weigum SE, McDevitt J, Redding SW. Current development of saliva/oral fluid-based diagnostics. *Tex Dent J.* July 2010;127(7):651–661. Review. PubMed PMID: 20737986.

Yoshizawa JM, Wong DT. Salivary microRNAs and oral cancer detection. *Methods Mol Biol.* 2013;936: 313–324. PubMed PMID: 23007518.

You XY, Jiang J, Yin FZ. Preliminary observation on human saliva alpha-fetoprotein in patients with hepatocellular carcinoma. *Chin Med J (Engl).* March 1993;106(3):179–182. PubMed PMID: 7686840.

Yu ZW, Zhong LP, Ji T, Zhang P, Chen WT, Zhang CP. MicroRNAs contribute to the chemoresistance of cisplatin in tongue squamous cell carcinoma lines. *Oral Oncol.* April 2010;46(4):317–322. doi: 10.1016/j.oraloncology.2010.02.002. Epub March 9, 2010. PubMed PMID: 20219416.

Zen K, Zhang CY. Circulating microRNAs: A novel class of biomarkers to diagnose and monitor human cancers. *Med Res Rev.* March 2012;32(2):326–348.

Zelles T, Purushotham KR, Macauley SP, Oxford GE, Humphreys-Beher MG. Saliva and growth factors: The fountain of youth resides in us all. *J Dent Res.* December 1995;74(12):1826–1832. Review. PubMed PMID: 8600176.

Zhang L, Farrell JJ, Zhou H, Elashoff D, Akin D, Park NH, Chia D, Wong DT. Salivary transcriptomic biomarkers for detection of resectable pancreatic cancer. *Gastroenterology.* March 2010a;138(3):949–957. e1–e7. doi: 10.1053/j.gastro.2009.11.010. Epub November 18, 2009. PubMed PMID: 19931263; PubMed Central PMCID: PMC2831159.

Zhang L, Kirchhoff T, Yee CJ, Offit K. A rapid and reliable test for BRCA1 and BRCA2 founder mutation analysis in paraffin tissue using pyrosequencing. *J Mol Diagn.* May 2009;11(3):176–181. doi: 10.2353/jmoldx.2009.080137. Epub March 26, 2009. PubMed PMID: 19324993; PubMed Central PMCID: PMC2671333.

Zhang L, Xiao H, Karlan S, Zhou H, Gross J, Elashoff D, Akin D et al. Discovery and preclinical validation of salivary transcriptomic and proteomic biomarkers for the non-invasive detection of breast cancer. *PLoS One*. December 31, 2010b;5(12):e15573. doi: 10.1371/journal.pone.0015573. PubMed PMID: 21217834; PubMed Central PMCID: PMC3013113.

Zhang L, Xiao H, Zhou H, Santiago S, Lee JM, Garon EB, Yang J et al. Development of transcriptomic biomarker signature in human saliva to detect lung cancer. *Cell Mol Life Sci*. October 2012a;69(19):3341–3350. doi: 10.1007/s00018-012-1027-0. Epub June 12, 2012. PubMed PMID: 22689099.

Zhang Z, Filho MS, Nör JE. The biology of head and neck cancer stem cells. *Oral Oncol*. January 2012b;48(1):1–9. doi: 10.1016/j.oraloncology.2011.10.004. Epub November 8, 2011. Review. PubMed PMID: 22070916; PubMed Central PMCID: PMC3261238.

Zhao M, Rosenbaum E, Carvalho AL, Koch W, Jiang W, Sidransky D, Califano J. Feasibility of quantitative PCR-based saliva rinse screening of HPV for head and neck cancer. *Int J Cancer* November 20, 2005;117(4):605–610. PubMed PMID: 15929076.

Zhong LP, Chen GF, Xu ZF, Zhang X, Ping FY, Zhao SF. Detection of telomerase activity in saliva from oral squamous cell carcinoma patients. *Int J Oral Maxillofac Surg*. July 2005;34(5):566–570. Epub January 24, 2005. PubMed PMID: 16053879.

Zhong LP, Zhang CP, Zheng JW, Li J, Chen WT, Zhang ZY. Increased Cyfra 21-1 concentration in saliva from primary oral squamous cell carcinoma patients. *Arch Oral Biol*. November 2007;52(11):1079–1087. Epub July 5, 2007. PubMed PMID: 17612501.

Zimmermann BG, Park NJ, Wong DT. Genomic targets in saliva. *Ann N Y Acad Sci*. March 2007;1098:184–191. Review. PubMed PMID: 17435127; PubMed Central PMCID: PMC2910758.

Zimmermann BG, Wong DT. Salivary mRNA targets for cancer diagnostics. *Oral Oncol*. May 2008;44(5): 425–429. Epub December 3, 2007. PubMed PMID: 18061522; PubMed Central PMCID: PMC2408659.

Part II

Brain and Head and Neck Cancers

10

Biomarkers for Brain Gliomas

Yusuf Izci

CONTENTS

ABSTRACT Early detection of the brain gliomas is crucial for a successful management and satisfactory outcome. Different from the other tumors of human body that may produce specific proteins that are used as tumor markers, brain tumors do not release specific biomarkers into the blood circulation. The development of molecular techniques has opened up the potential of utilizing circulating nucleic acids as prospective tumor markers for brain tumors. Gliomas are one of the most commonly diagnosed adult primary tumors of the brain, and the most common types of gliomas are astrocytomas, oligodendrogliomas, and ependymomas. DNA fragments in human fluids may be potential biomarkers in patients with brain gliomas. Many studies exist for the use of brain tumor-derived circulating DNA as a diagnostic and research tool, and it is feasible to use the DNA fragments as noninvasive brain tumor marker. Methylated tumor-specific DNA is in use as a plasma biomarker in patients with glioma. For astrocytomas, the markers included promoter hypermethylation of both *MGMT* and *PTEN* and LOH of 10q. For oligodendroglial tumors, *MGMT* promoter methylation and LOH analysis of 10q, 1p, and 19q are potential biomarkers. None of these biomarkers have proven to be powerful enough to replace tissue diagnosis because their sensitivity and specificity for brain gliomas are limited and further studies are needed for noninvasive detection, follow-up, or prognostication of brain gliomas. In the near future, early and more accurate detection of such biomarkers make easy the follow-up and management of these tumors.

KEY WORDS: *biomarker, brain, glioma, methylation.*

10.1 Introduction

Gliomas are the most frequent type of primary brain tumors (Assem et al., 2012). These are the major parts of modern neurosurgical practice, and their treatments are always in debate despite many new technological improvements. Early diagnosis of the brain gliomas is critical for an early and appropriate management, as well as for a satisfactory outcome.

Gliomas arise from the glial cells, or supportive tissue, of the brain, and they account for approximately 77% of primary malignant brain tumors. Approximately 13,000 deaths and 18,000 new cases of primary malignant brain and central nervous system (CNS) tumors occur annually in the United States (Schwartzbaum et al., 2006). The available data of Central Brain Tumor Registry of the United States (CBTRUS) for a 10-year period from 1985 to 1994 showed a slight (0.9%) but statistically significant average annual percentage increase in incidence of brain tumors (Central Brain Tumor Registry of the United States, 2002). This increase may be related to improvements in radiological studies (computed tomography [CT] and magnetic resonance imaging [MRI]), increased availability of medical care systems and physicians, new approaches to the medical treatment of older patients, and changes in the classifications of brain tumors from benign to malignant (Australian Cancer Network Adult Brain Tumour Guidelines Working Party, 2009). The prognosis for patients with glioma is usually very poor (only approximately 2% of patients aged 65 years or older, and only 30% of those under the age of 45 years at glioblastoma diagnosis, survive for 2 years or more), and treatments to cure glioblastoma have yet to be devised (Schwartzbaum et al., 2006).

The type of glioma is determined by the cells that give rise to the tumor, and different types of gliomas were defined until today. Astrocytoma, oligodendroglioma, and ependymoma are the types of brain gliomas (Kleihues et al., 1993). Astrocytomas are the most common type, accounting for about half of all primary brain and spinal cord tumors. They develop from star-shaped glial cells called "astrocytes," which are the part of supportive tissue of the brain. They may occur in many regions of the CNS but most commonly in the cerebrum. They are more frequent in adults, particularly middle-aged male population. In children, most of these tumors are considered low grade, while in adults most are high-grade glioma or glioblastoma. There are different subtypes of astrocytomas, and these tumors are classified into several categories according to their appearance under a microscope. This classification is important because the appearance of an astrocytoma will often predict its behavior and, therefore, reflect the prognosis of the patient. These tumors are generally graded into one of three types: low-grade astrocytomas, anaplastic astrocytomas, and glioblastomas. Low-grade astrocytomas account for 10% of astrocytomas (Figure 10.1). These tumors are typically slow growing and may not require specific treatment at the time of diagnosis. Many patients with low-grade astrocytomas live for prolonged periods of time after the diagnosis. However, these tumors often advance into the higher grades and more rapidly growing forms

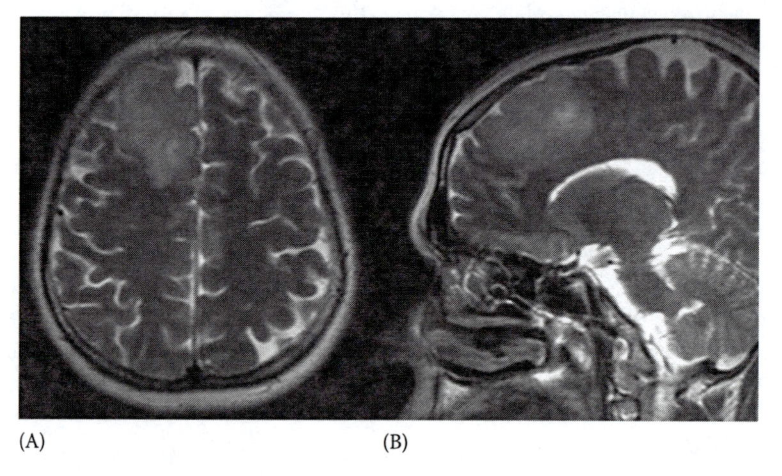

FIGURE 10.1 (A) T2-weighted axial and (B) T2-weighted sagittal MRI slices of the patient show left frontal hyperintense lesion. The diagnosis was grade II astrocytoma.

of brain gliomas. Anaplastic astrocytomas and glioblastomas are the most aggressive and, unfortunately, the most common types of astrocytoma. Glioblastomas are fast-growing astrocytomas that may contain many areas of necrotic tissue associated with tumor cells (Figure 10.2). In adults, glioblastoma occurs mostly in the cerebrum, especially in the frontal and temporal regions of the brain. The second type of gliomas is oligodendroglioma (Figure 10.3). They are thought to arise from the oligodendrocytes, which are the cells that wrap around nerve cells, produce myelin, and act as a form of electrical insulation for conducting the nerve impulses. Recent studies suggest that they may actually arise from progenitor cells, which are immature oligodendrocytes. These tumors also tend to occur in young adults and may contain calcium deposits that appear on brain scans as calcification. They tend to be slower growing than low-grade astrocytomas but have the potential to turn into more aggressive forms. The third type of brain

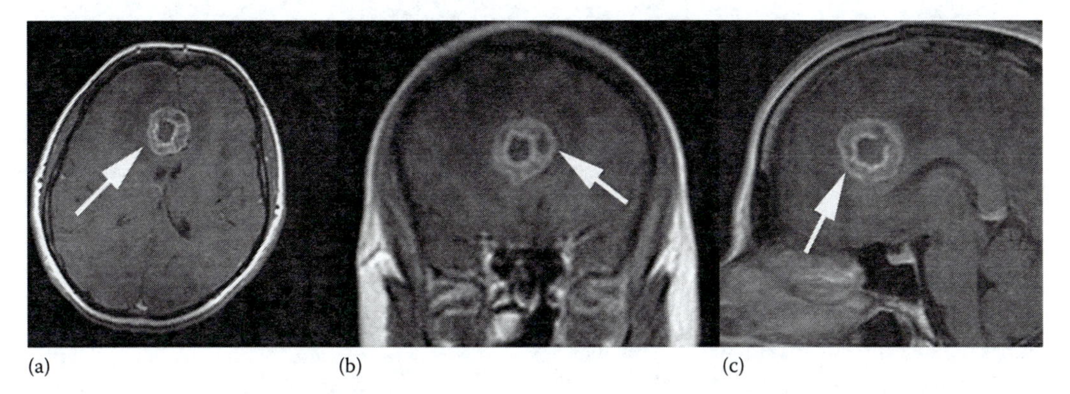

FIGURE 10.2 (a) T1-weighted axial, (b) T1-weighted coronal, and (c) T1-weighted sagittal MRI slices of the patient show frontal interhemispheric contrast-enhancing mass lesion. The diagnosis was glioblastoma.

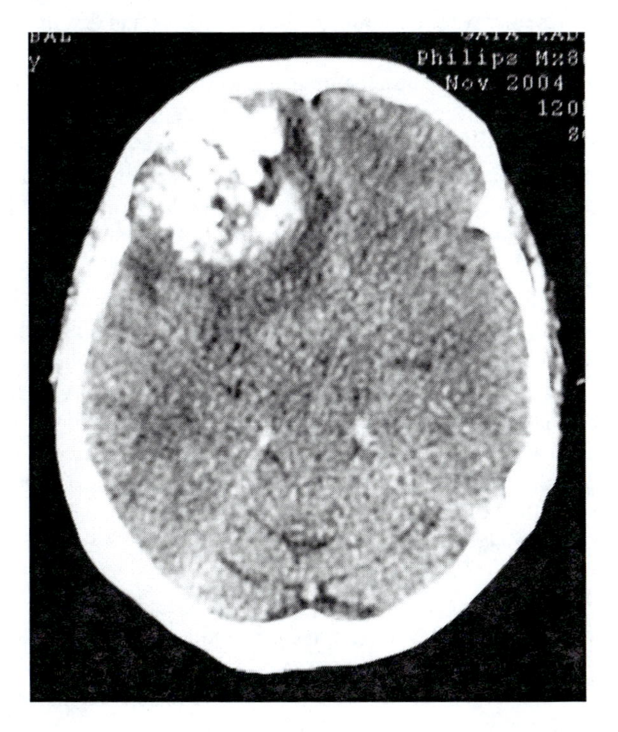

FIGURE 10.3 (See color insert.) The axial CT scan of a patient with left frontal calcified mass lesion. The diagnosis was oligodendroglioma.

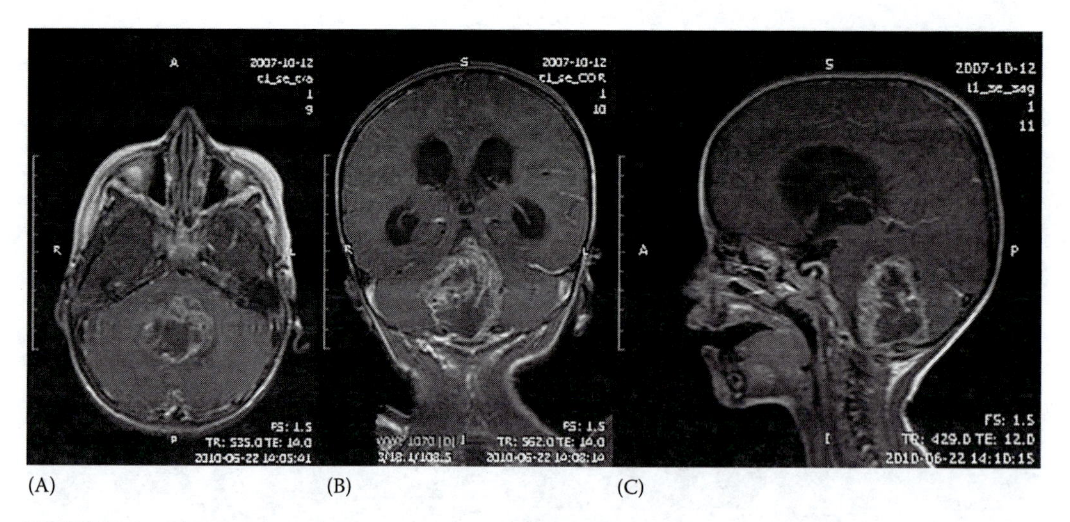

FIGURE 10.4 (A) T1-weighted axial, (B) T1-weighted coronal, and (C) T1-weighted sagittal MRI slices of a child patient show contrast-enhancing mass lesion in the posterior fossa and hydrocephalus. The diagnosis was ependymoma.

gliomas is ependymoma (Figure 10.4). This tumor arises from the ependymal cells lining the ventricles of the brain. It commonly affects children but may occur at any age. Ependymomas are also slow growing but may show aggressive behavior in many cases.

According to the World Health Organization (WHO) grading scale for tumors of the nervous system, lesions with no atypia/low proliferative activities are denoted as grade I, quite often curable upon surgical removal (Daumas-Duport et al., 1988). Once the lesion is infiltrative, it is designated as grade II, and tumors of this grade can progress to higher grades. Grade III are lesions with accelerated mitotic activity and nuclear atypia/anaplasia. Grade IV is the most malignant tumor grade with a fatal outcome. Grade IV tumors often present with infiltration into surrounding tissue, high mitotic activity, characteristic necrotic areas, and extensive microvascular proliferations (Kleihues and Cavenee, 1997). Diffuse astrocytomas grades II and III may progress to grade IV, which is then referred to as secondary glioblastoma. However, the majority of glioblastomas develop de novo, with no previous history, and are referred to as primary glioblastomas. The primary and secondary glioblastomas exhibit the same histopathological characteristics, even though they differ in both genetic changes and clinical history.

Unlike other cancers, brain gliomas grow in the confined and narrow space of the cranium. In order to grow, most cancers push healthy cells aside, but due to space constraints, gliomas must destroy normal brain tissue for growing and invasion (Sontheimer, 2008). To damage the normal brain structures, gliomas release large quantities of the neurotransmitter glutamate. Excess glutamate is toxic to neurons and causes seizures in up to 80% of people with gliomas (Ye and Sontheimer, 1999). So, brain gliomas are particularly damaging because they tend to quickly sprout and spread within the normal brain tissue.

Patients suspected with brain glioma need noninvasive preoperative evaluation of brain tumor grade for treatment planning and prediction of prognosis (Dean et al., 1990). Currently, the radiological studies such as CT, MRI, cerebral angiography, and skull x-ray; biochemical studies such as cerebrospinal fluid (CSF) examination; and histopathological techniques are in use for the diagnosis of brain gliomas (Table 10.1). But all of these studies do not provide early diagnosis for these tumors. So it is important to find some specific biomarkers associated with the development of gliomas for early and accurate diagnosis as well as treatment of brain gliomas. These biomarkers must have high specificity and sensitivity.

In the past decades, there have been considerable improvements on the characterization of brain tumors and gliomas. Information on the genomics and proteomics has increased; consequently the need for diagnostic biomarkers in gliomas has also increased (Furnari et al., 2007). Although studies on the molecular mechanisms and signaling pathways have provided more detailed knowledge on the initiation, maintenance, and progression of primary brain tumors, the prognosis for patients with malignant brain glioma is still very poor (Jung et al., 2011). Researchers have come closer to improving the prognosis

TABLE 10.1

Current Diagnostic Methods for Brain Gliomas

	Features			
Diagnostic Methods	**Specificity**	**Sensitivity**	**Advantages**	**Disadvantages**
1. CT (Goldman and Pirotte, 2011)	Low	Moderate	1. Easy available 2. Low cost	1. Radiation 2. Moderate sensitivity for gliomas
2. MRI (Upadhyay and Waldman, 2011)	Moderate	High	1. High sensitivity for gliomas 2. Nonradiation	1. High cost 2. Not easily available
3. Tissue sampling/biopsy	High	High	1. Accurate diagnosis	1. Invasive

by investigating the biology and behavior of gliomas in animals and humans. Studies are on the way to uncover the glioma's unique characteristics, including the mechanisms that help it survive and spread throughout the brain (Speert, 2008).

Brain gliomas show different histological characteristics, but they do not produce and release specific biomarkers into the human body fluids. There are currently no clinically approved serum markers for gliomas. Attempts to predict patient outcome have been limited by the heterogeneous clinical behavior of patients with glioma and by the different studies on the clinical, pathologic, and biological prognostic markers. The development of molecular techniques provides us new opportunity of utilizing circulating nucleic acids as prospective tumor markers for brain tumors. Today, circulating DNA fragments are potentially promising source of tumor-specific biomarkers in patients with brain gliomas. Numerous challenges exist for the possible use of brain tumor-derived circulating DNA as a diagnostic and research tool (Lavon et al., 2010). Initial discovery and worldwide studies of the epidermal growth factor (EGF) and transforming growth factor alpha (TGF-a), as well as the platelet-derived growth factor (PDGF) family, showed their presence in glioblastoma cell cultures and tissues. In addition, some experimental models were showed that brain gliomas may be induced by overexpression of PDGF-B in the brain (Terrile et al., 2010).

DNA fragments of different grade of gliomas can be detected in the circulation during the course of the brain tumor. It may be feasible to use these fragments as noninvasive brain tumor biomarker. Methylated tumor-specific DNA is in use as a plasma biomarker in patients with glioma (Weaver et al., 2006). For astrocytic tumors, the markers included promoter hypermethylation of both methylguanine-DNA methyltransferase (*MGMT*) and phosphatase and tensin homologue deleted on chromosome 10 (*PTEN*) and loss of heterozygosity (LOH) of 10q (Ohgaki, 2005). For oligodendroglial tumors, *MGMT* promoter methylation and LOH analysis of 10q, 1p, and 19q are potential biomarkers (Lavon et al., 2010). For ependymomas, Ki67 index is a reproducible and robust prognostic factor and can be considered a promising histopathological biomarker (Preusser et al., 2008). In addition, ependymoma relapses display a common gene expression signature, which is marked by the upregulation of kinetochore proteins and downregulation of metallothioneins (Peyre et al., 2010). In the future, the management and follow-up of brain gliomas will be easy and safe by the development of more sensitive and accurate biomarkers.

In this chapter, the epidemiology and characteristics of brain gliomas will be summarized firstly, then the biomarkers will be briefly defined, and lastly some of the important biomarkers for brain gliomas will be documented with the basic principles of genetic control of gene expression related to brain gliomas.

10.2 Treatment Strategies for Brain Gliomas

The treatment of brain gliomas is primarily surgery. Surgical resection is not only for treatment but also for accurate diagnosis of the tumor. The determination of the type of glioma is crucial for the further treatment protocol and the determination of patient's prognosis. Adjuvant methods are including radiotherapy and chemotherapy. The principal aims of surgical treatment are to establish the histological diagnosis, provide immediate palliation, reestablish the intracranial CSF dynamics and hemodynamics, enhance the effects of adjuvant therapies, decrease the tumor cells in the brain (cytoreduction), and extend the life of the patient. There are many operative approaches to the cerebral gliomas and the choice of approach depends on the location, size, and characteristics of the tumor. The clinical condition of the patient also affects the treatment protocol. The main goal of surgery is maximal tumor removal without deterioration of the neurological condition of the patient. The main target of the surgeon should be the glioma and surrounding gliotic tissue during the operation. Preservation of normal brain tissue is important to avoid additional neurological deficits after surgery. Recently, neuronavigation systems and intraoperative imaging techniques introduced in neurosurgery and operative treatment of brain glioma became more safe and effective by these new modalities (Schulz et al., 2012). Multimodality brain glioma management entails the simultaneous or sequential use of multiple therapeutic approaches that each produces a one to three log reduction in tumor cell count, the aim being to reduce the tumor burden to a level where it is again vulnerable to the host's defenses. To date, the adjuvant therapies are radiation therapy, chemotherapy, immunotherapy, and gene therapy (Candolfi et al., 2009). These therapies target the residual tumor cells into the brain tissue. The clinical outcomes of radiation and chemotherapies are not satisfactory for brain gliomas because of their side effects. High-grade gliomas are usually not responsive to these therapies, and surgical cytoreduction is the gold standard to increase the survival of the patient. Efforts to improve patients' immune response to tumor cells or "immunotherapy" are currently under investigation. Administration of interferon-, interleukin-2-, or lymphokine-activated killer cells revealed promising results in some trials (Jacobs et al., 1986). Numerous growth factors and their receptors have been identified, but their role in the control of cell proliferation and oncogenesis still remains unclear. The gene therapy strategies for brain gliomas are suicide gene therapy, genetic immunotherapy, and oncolytic virotherapy. The main target of gene therapy is the tumor cells, and the technique of this therapy is the use of genetically engineered viruses to destroy or modulate tumor cells within the brain while sparing the normal cells or tissue. Today, gene therapy has yielded encouraging results in preclinical animal models as well as promising safety profiles in phase I clinical trials but has failed to demonstrate significant therapeutic efficacy in phase III clinical trials (Tobias et al., 2013). Recent in vitro and in vivo studies have demonstrated the unique migratory capacity of neural and mesenchymal stem cells to target glioma. In the setting of glioblastoma therapy, mesenchymal stem cells are attractive because it is relatively easy to isolate them from patients, while neural stem cells have shown more specific migratory potential toward malignant gliomas (Auffinger et al., 2012). Nanomaterials are also under investigation in the treatment of brain gliomas. These materials can either act as drug carrier systems or induce glioma cytotoxicity directly. In addition, nanotechnology can be combined with other therapies, such as stem cell-based carriers, offering new concepts for treatment of brain gliomas (Roger et al., 2011).

Since the gliomas are histologically heterogeneous tumors with respect to cell cycle, antigen expression, and growth factor susceptibility, definitive treatment requires more prospective randomized studies on the molecular and genetic basis of such tumors.

10.3 Invasive and Noninvasive Biomarkers for Brain Gliomas

In medicine, a "biomarker" is a term often used to refer to a protein measured in the blood whose concentration reflects the presence or severity of some disease. Biomarkers may be specific cells, molecules, genes, gene products, enzymes, or hormones (Bhatt et al., 2010). Complex organ functions or general characteristic changes in biological structures can also serve as biomarkers. If a biomarker is used as an indicator of a particular disease, it is called as *diagnostic biomarker* (Kohn et al., 2007). If a biomarker is used to measure the progress of a disease or the effects of treatment, it is called as *prognostic biomarker*. These markers can be measured in CSF, blood, or tumor tissue in brain tumors.

Biomarkers have been used in preclinical research and clinical diagnosis for a considerable time. In molecular terms biomarker is the subset of markers that might be discovered using genomics, proteomics technologies, or imaging technologies. Today, gene-based biomarker is found to be an effective and acceptable marker in the scientific world (http://en.wikipedia.org/wiki/Biomarker_(medicine), accessed on September 22, 2012).

The validation of biomarkers can be difficult and require different levels of validation depending on their intended use (Febbo et al., 2011). If a biomarker is to be used to measure the success of a therapeutic intervention, the biomarker should reflect a direct effect of that intervention (Lee, 2009). Molecular and genetic biomarkers for brain gliomas are deeply analyzed in the next section of this chapter.

10.4 Invasive Molecular and Genetic Diagnostic Markers for Brain Gliomas

There is now overwhelming evidence that cancer is a genetic disease resulting from alterations in DNA. The diagnostic process starts with an appreciation of relevant clinical and radiological details. The precise histological diagnosis guides treatment and prognosis of the patient. The key point of accurate diagnosis is the knowledge molecular basis of the cancer by the laboratory techniques including nucleic acid hybridization and gene cloning.

Malignant gliomas arise in a unique environment where abundant vasculature, nutrients, and growth factors facilitate tumor proliferation and architectural scaffolding such as white matter tracts provide passage for invading cells to migrate to distant sites throughout the brain (De Groot and Sontheimer, 2011). These tumors are heterogeneous, diffuse, and highly infiltrating by nature.

The biomarkers for brain gliomas may be either invasive or noninvasive. The invasive markers are used during the histopathological analysis of tumor sample, which was obtained after surgery (Table 10.2). Conventional methods of neuropathology are now supplemented by the more sophisticated techniques of immunohistochemistry and molecular biology. Antigens with cell or tissue characteristics reveal information indicating the cellular origin of glioma, and these antigens act as tumor marker for gliomas. The antigenic determinants used most frequently to identify particular cell types are intermediate filaments, neuroectodermal markers, leukocytic or lymphoid antigens, epithelial cell markers, and vascular endothelial antigens. Intermediate filaments are glial fibrillary acidic protein (GFAP), neurofilaments, desmin, and vimentin. GFAP and vimentin are expressed in gliomas (Abaza et al., 1998). GFAP is nearly 100% sensitive as a marker of glial differentiation, but it is not a reliable marker for distinguishing astrocytomas from oligodendrogliomas, and it does not have prognostic significance in gliomas (Brat et al., 2008). There are also proliferation antigens indicating the level of malignancy in gliomas. Ki67 nuclear antigen is expressed in specific phases of cell cycle, and this antigen is a useful method for the detection of proliferating cells in gliomas (Preusser et al., 2008). Bromodeoxyuridine (BrdU) is a thymidine analogue, and it is also an indicator of proliferative potential of the tumor. BrdU incorporation was significantly elevated in glioma cells (Komohara et al., 2012). Monoclonal antibodies against DNA polymerase may be useful for the identification of proliferating cells (Brat et al., 2008). The advent of

TABLE 10.2

Current Molecular Biomarkers for Invasive (Tissue) Diagnosis of Brain Gliomas

	Features			
Invasive Molecular Biomarkers	**Specificity**	**Sensitivity**	**Advantages**	**Disadvantages**
1. GFAP (Brat et al., 2008)	Moderate	High	Easily available	Not for classification of gliomas
2. Ki67 (Preusser et al., 2008)	Low	High	Excellent marker for survival and tumor recurrence	Works only on frozen sections
3. Vimentin (Abaza et al., 1998)	Low	Moderate	Molecular structure is well characterized	Not specific for gliomas
4. Desmin (Abaza et al., 1998)	Low	Moderate	None	
5. S100 (Jung et al., 2011)	Low	High	Can also be detected in the blood and CSF	Not specific for gliomas, rise also in CNS injuries and neurodegenerative diseases

immunohistochemistry has contributed to the accuracy of diagnosis of gliomas. The immune markers may not only be used for the identification of tumor cell differentiation but also for the determination of proliferative activity of tumor.

A large number of genetic alterations have been described in brain gliomas, and several of them were found to be associated with the patient's survival (Bleeker et al., 2012). However, most of them are still lacking confirmation by an independent study, or the independent study has already demonstrated that the suggested prognostic or predictive value of this particular marker cannot be validated. Several genes, including tumor protein 53 (*TP53*), *PTEN*, cyclin-dependent kinase inhibitor 2A (*CDKN2A*), and *EGFR*, are altered in gliomas (Liu et al., 2011). LOH of chromosomes 1p and 19q is the most common genetic alteration in oligodendrogliomas. This specific alteration is detected in 40%–90% of oligodendrogliomas, and it can be easily detected by fluorescent in situ hybridization (FISH) or southern blotting in the laboratory. So, LOH of 1p/19q may be used as a diagnostic marker of oligodendrogliomas (Bell et al., 2011). *TP53* is the gene that encodes the important tumor suppressor protein, p53. p53 mutations are a hallmark of low-grade gliomas and consequently also occur in secondary glioblastoma that arise from lower-grade gliomas (Bell et al., 2011).

Currently, only two markers, MGMT promoter methylation and isocitrate dehydrogenase 1 (IDH1) mutations, are commonly accepted genetic biomarkers for patients with glioma (Riemenschneider et al., 2010). Today, MGMT is clinical application for the diagnosis of gliomas. The *TP53* mutation appears to be a relatively early event during the development of an astrocytoma, whereas the loss or mutation of *PTEN* and amplification of *EGFR* are characteristic of high-grade tumors.

In this section, some of the invasive biomarkers that are currently in use will be summarized and brief information about them will be given. This section also provides advantages, limitations, and evidence for use of these biomarkers in brain gliomas.

10.4.1 Glutamate

The glutamatergic system plays a key role in the proliferation, survival, and migration of gliomas. Glutamate is the main excitatory neurotransmitter in the CNS and is a highly abundant growth factor and motogen in the brain. It is a very good candidate for target role in the brain (De Groot and Sontheimer, 2011). Glioblastomas release glutamate to enhance their highly malignant behavior, and this imparts a survival advantage by promoting resistance to apoptosis and by promoting glioma proliferation and invasion. Multiple glutamate receptor subtypes have been shown to be expressed on glioma cell cultures and in primary glioblastoma specimens. In addition, glutamine synthetase expression can be used to distinguish astrocytic from oligodendroglial tumors and may play a role in the pathogenesis of astrocytomas (Zhuang et al., 2011). The multitude of effects of glutamate on glioma biology supports the rationale for pharmacological targeting of glutamate receptors and transporters. Several ongoing and recently completed clinical trials are exploring the therapeutic potential of interrupting glutamate-mediated brain tumor growth (De Groot and Sontheimer, 2011).

10.4.2 Vascular Endothelial Growth Factor

Immunohistochemistry and in situ hybridization studies showed high concentrations and upregulation of VEGF mRNA activity of angiogenic factors such as basic fibroblast growth factor (bFGF) and VEGF in glioblastoma (Brem et al., 1992; Plate and Risau, 1995). VEGF and bFGF levels of tumor extracts showed not only a significant correlation with microvessel density, which was higher in glioblastoma than in other gliomas (Takano et al., 1996), but also correlated with survival of patients with astrocytic tumors (Fukui et al., 2003) and indicated glioma grades (Takahashi et al., 1992). Angiogenic factors were also analyzed in CSF in relatively small patient groups of 15 and 27 patients (Peles et al., 2004). VEGF and bFGF levels in CSF correlated with the degree of tumor vascularity and were adversely associated with patient survival (Peles et al., 2004; Sampath et al., 2004).

Briefly, VEGF seems to be an invasive or noninvasive prognostic biomarker for brain glioma in the future if adequate investigations are performed for the detection of this biomarker in human body fluids. In addition, early detection of VEGF in the CSF may help to determine the vascularity of the glioma.

10.4.3 Platelet-Derived Growth Factor

PDGF is one of the growth factors that regulate the division and growth of human cells. Particularly, PDGF plays a role in the formation of blood vessel or angiogenesis (Hoeben et al., 2004). Discovered as a serum growth factor for fibroblasts, smooth muscle cells, and glial cells, the PDGF family has become one of the most extensively investigated growth factor groups (Heldin and Westermark, 1999; Andrae et al., 2008). The different isoforms of PDGF activate cellular response through receptors including PDGF receptor alpha (PDGFRa) and beta (PDGFRb). The in vitro studies showed that PDGFRa is produced by neurons and astrocytes and acts as a mitogen for oligodendrocyte progenitor cells (Nazarenko et al., 2012). Several experimental models have been created to induce gliomas in order to discover the functional role of PDGF in the development of brain tumors. The most important model is the development of glioma in mice by forced expression of PDGF (Nazarenko et al., 2012). Overexpression of PDGF in the brain usually leads to excessive production of oligodendrocyte progenitor cells and, if in a permissive setting, results in mainly oligodendroglioma-like tumors. It was also revealed that the upregulation of the PDGFRb on endothelial cells of vessels, which vascularize the tumor, is associated with malignant phenotype in human glial tumors (Plate et al., 1992). Overexpression or hyperactivity of PDGF ligands and receptors are frequent events in human gliomas of all grades, and their expression pattern in tumors suggests the presence of autocrine and paracrine stimulatory loops.

As a summary, the role of PDGFRa is consistent with the PDGFRa overexpression observed in human low-grade gliomas, whereas the role of PDGFRb was to promote the full-blown vascular proliferations that are characteristic of human glioblastomas. So, PDGFRa may be a noninvasive biomarker for low-grade glioma, but further studies are needed for the determination of specificity and sensitivity of this biomarker.

10.4.4 Methylguanine-DNA Methyltransferase

O6-MGMT is a protein that repairs the DNA and catalyzes the transfer of a methyl group from the O6-position of guanine to a cysteine at position 145. The gene encoding the *MGMT* has become one of the most investigated molecular markers in neurooncology since the first description of an association between *MGMT* promoter hypermethylation and response to alkylating drugs (Jung et al., 2011). The *MGMT* gene on 10q26 has 5 exons and a large CpG island of 763 bp with 98 CpG sites covering the first exon and large parts of the promoter. In normal brain the CpG sites are typically unmethylated. However, in tumors the cytosine in CpG sites often carries methyl groups, thereby increasing the affinity of methyl-CpG-binding proteins like methyl-CpG-binding protein 2 and methyl-CpG-binding domain protein 2 to the DNA. These proteins alter the chromatin structure and prevent binding of transcription factors, thereby silencing expression of MGMT (Nakagawachi et al., 2003).

The frequency of *MGMT* promoter hypermethylation in gliomas varies widely. In clinical studies, it has ranged from 35% to 73% in glioblastoma (Von Deimling et al., 2011). The alkylation of MGMT is a one way process that ends up with a degradation of MGMT (Olsson and Lindahl, 1980; Pegg et al., 1983; Gerson, 2004). Application of alkylating drugs like temozolomide causes, among other things, the binding of an alkyl group to the O6-position of guanine, thereby impairing DNA replication and triggering cell death. MGMT protein lessens the chemotherapeutical effect by repairing the desired DNA damage. A certain number of patients with a hypermethylated *MGMT* promoter in glioblastoma cells lack the corresponding DNA repair protein MGMT, and therefore, the cytotoxic effect of alkylating drugs becomes amplified. Thus, *MGMT* hypermethylation is a predictor for response to chemotherapy (Hegi et al., 2005). This widely accepted concept to understand the beneficial role of a hypermethylated *MGMT* promoter recently became challenged by the observation in patients with anaplastic gliomas, which showed that this alteration is associated with a better clinical course even if patients became treated by radiotherapy alone (Van den Bent et al., 2009a; Wick et al., 2009).

Since the first description of *MGMT* hypermethylation in glioblastoma (Esteller et al., 2000), various studies confirmed *MGMT* hypermethylation in glioblastoma and reported frequencies between 35% and 73% (Hegi et al., 2005; Herrlinger et al., 2006; Criniere et al., 2007; Wick et al., 2008; Van den Bent et al., 2009b; Brandes et al., 2009a,b; Clarke et al., 2009; Dunn et al., 2009; Prados et al., 2009; Weller et al., 2009; Zawlik et al., 2009; Weiler et al., 2010). This variation may be the result of different tumor sampling or differences in technical conditions (von Deimling et al., 2011). The predominant interest in *MGMT* promoter hypermethylation is based on the predictive role of this biomarker for temozolomide treatment. Glioblastoma patients with hypermethylated *MGMT* promoter exhibited survival rates of 49% after 2 years and 14% after 5 years when treated with concomitant and adjuvant temozolomide and radiotherapy. However, only 24% of glioblastoma patients with hypermethylated *MGMT* promoter survived after 2 years and 5% after 5 years when initially treated with radiotherapy only. Glioblastoma patients without hypermethylated *MGM* promoter demonstrated survival rates of 15% and 8% after 2 and 5 years while receiving radiochemotherapy, as well as 2% and 0% after 2 and 5 years when treated with radiotherapy alone (Hegi et al., 2005; Stupp et al., 2005, 2009). Many studies showed that *MGMT* promoter hypermethylation is one of the strongest prognostic factors for patients with newly diagnosed glioblastoma, and it is also pointed out that this alteration is a predictor for response to alkylating drugs (Esteller et al., 2000; Herrlinger et al., 2006; Gorlia et al., 2008; Brandes et al., 2009; Weller et al., 2009). Because of this important prognostic role in glioma, detection of *MGMT* promoter hypermethylation is currently required for every clinical trial, which is evaluating a new therapeutic agent or protocol for these tumors. Although in daily practice the determination of the MGMT promoter status might be helpful for management of patients who suffer from glioblastoma by neurooncologists, the lack of different therapeutic options for patients without hypermethylated MGMT promoter results in a similar therapy for both patient groups. So, determination of the MGMT status has no direct clinical implications or therapeutic influence (Jung et al., 2011).

10.4.5 Isocitrate Dehydrogenase 1

In a recent genome-wide analysis, somatic mutations at codon 132 of the isocitrate dehydrogenase 1 gene (*IDH1*) were identified in approximately 12% of glioblastomas (Labussiere et al., 2010). It was also suggested that *IDH1* mutations might occur after formation of a low-grade glioma and drive the progression of the tumor to a glioblastoma (Yan et al., 2009). Gliomas with *IDH* mutations were clinically and genetically distinct from gliomas with wild-type *IDH* genes. Notably, two types of gliomas of WHO grade II or III (astrocytomas and oligodendrogliomas) often carried *IDH* mutations, but not other genetic alterations that are detectable relatively early during the progression of gliomas (Hartmann et al., 2009; Ducray et al., 2009, 2011).

10.4.6 Glial Fibrillary Acidic Protein

GFAP is a member of the cytoskeletal protein family and is widely expressed in astroglial cells, in neural stem cells, and in astroglial tumors, such as astrocytoma and glioblastoma (Jacque et al., 1978; Hamaya et al., 1985; Abaza et al., 1998). The majority of astrocytomas express GFAP. However, glioblastoma tissues show a strong variability in GFAP expression ranging from <25% to 100% in others (Royds et al., 1986). GFAP has a relatively high molecular weight of 52 kDa (Yen et al., 1976), which limits its transit through the blood–brain barrier (BBB) under physiological conditions. However, under some clinical conditions such as head trauma, intracerebral hematoma, or brain ischemia, in which the BBB is disrupted, serum GFAP concentrations were elevated (Herrmann and Ehrenreich, 2003; Pelinka et al., 2004; Foerch et al., 2006). In addition, GFAP is present in the serum of patients with glioblastoma. In a study comparing GFAP serum levels of 50 glioblastoma patients with those of 31 astrocytoma grade II and III, 17 single brain metastases, and 50 healthy controls, serum GFAP levels of glioblastoma patients were significantly higher than those of patients with astrocytoma or with brain metastasis. Serum GFAP levels were correlated with the glioblastoma volume and tumor necrosis volume (Jung et al., 2007). As tumor necrosis is absent in low-grade glioma and present in glioblastoma, this might explain elevated GFAP serum levels in patients with voluminous glioblastoma. Interestingly, the product of GFAP expression in tissue samples and tumor necrosis, as a measure for necrotic GFAP positive cells in glioblastoma patients, was strongly correlated with GFAP serum levels, emphasizing the direct and/or indirect influence of these two factors on GFAP detectability in serum. In this study, an receiver operating characteristic (ROC) analysis cutoff point of 0.05 μg/L of serum GFAP afforded a sensitivity of 76% and a specificity of 100% for the differentiation of glioblastoma patients from nonglioblastoma tumor patients or healthy controls. The positive and negative predictive values were 1.0 and 0.89, respectively (Jung et al., 2007). Serum GFAP therefore appears to be a promising preoperative diagnostic biomarker for glioblastoma. Extending the scope to monitor clinical follow-up with serum GFAP is a different matter because elevated GFAP levels may also occur after head trauma, intracerebral hemorrhage, ischemic stroke, as well as in reactive gliosis (Herrmann and Ehrenreich, 2003; Pelinka et al., 2004; Foerch et al., 2006) as expected after cranial surgery. In addition, it is difficult to detect a recurrent glioblastoma with this marker, which is correlated with tumor volume. Moreover, there is no standardized GFAP-ELISA test for the early diagnosis of brain gliomas. So, the specificity and sensitivity of GFAP, as a noninvasive biomarker, are not high for brain glioma.

10.5 Noninvasive Molecular and Genetic Biomarkers for Brain Gliomas

Although some biomarkers for gliomas are detected in the blood or CSF (Table 10.3), there is no worldwide accepted biomarker in blood or CSF for detection, follow-up, or prognostication of brain gliomas (Von Deimling et al., 2011).

10.5.1 Biomarkers in the Blood

Because peripheral blood is readily accessible, research into tumor biomarkers is primarily aimed at serum. But the major problem of serum, as a main source of biomarkers, is the abundance of a few proteins, such as albumin, immunoglobulins, and acute-phase proteins, which comprise >90% of total serum protein and often prevent the discovery of the less abundant tumor markers. Brain gliomas usually disrupt the BBB, and thus, the bloodstream of these patients probably contains molecules, which not normally present with an intact BBB. Therefore, the search for serum markers has been mainly focused on proteins, many of which have been identified to directly correlate with tumor grade or better survival. Immunohistochemical analysis demonstrated that many of the protein biomarkers identified in peripheral blood specimens were expressed in malignant gliomas.

Staining levels for one of the biomarkers, macrophage inflammatory protein 1-α (MIP-1α), were found to correlate with WHO grade among invasive gliomas, and it was demonstrated that MIP-1α promotes human glioblastoma cell proliferation and migration (Xu et al., 2012).

Antitumor necrosis factor-induced apoptosis (ATIA) protein, which protects cells against apoptosis, is also highly expressed in glioblastoma and astrocytomas. ATIA may also be a potentially noninvasive diagnostic marker and therapeutic target in human gliomas (Choksi et al., 2011).

Cathepsin D is another indicator for glioma in the serum. It is an aspartyl protease enzyme involved in tissue remodeling and protein catabolism and is usually secreted by cancer cells. As the glioma grade rises, cathepsin D transcript levels determined by ELISA test would become significantly elevated (Fukuda et al., 2005). Similarly, GADD45 α (growth arrest and DNA damage-inducible protein) and follistatin-like 1 are upregulated in most primary and secondary glioblastomas (Reddy et al., 2008).

GFAP is the most promising noninvasive marker, and the expression of GFAP in patients with gliomas is highly elevated. However, GFAP levels are also elevated in other cerebral lesions. YKL-40 encodes a secreted protein with sequence similar to glycosyl hydrolases and is present in high levels in serum from patients with high-grade glioma (Iwamoto et al., 2011). Serum VEGF concentration is also significantly elevated in patients with high-grade gliomas. Many protein serum markers can be expressed or affected with other tumors, cerebral lesions, or brain trauma; therefore, the specificity of such markers will not be adequate for use of only one as a diagnostic protocol.

10.5.2 Biomarkers in CSF

CSF may be a source for noninvasive biomarkers, and many studies attempt to detect glioma biomarkers in the CSF, which is in contact with the tumor and may therefore contain higher levels of potential biomarkers than the serum (Baraniskin et al., 2012). In the last years, many biomarkers have been defined in the CSF of glioma patients, such as recoverin (protein A), S100 protein, neuron-specific enolase (NSE), and VEGF (Jung et al., 2011). However, these biomarkers could not be widespread used due to the limitation of repetition in CSF examinations (Liang and Shen, 2011). Moreover, exosomes are now becoming

TABLE 10.3

Current Molecular and Genetic Biomarkers for Noninvasive Diagnosis of Brain Gliomas

	Features			
Biomarkers	**Specificity**	**Sensitivity**	**Advantages**	**Disadvantages**
1. *Glutamate* (De Groot and Sontheimer, 2011)	Low	Low	Good prognostic factor	Not in clinical application
2. *GFAP* (Jung et al., 2007)	Moderate	High	Detectable in the blood	Not useful for classification of glioma
3. *ATIA* (Choksi et al., 2011)	Low	High for glioblastoma	None	Under investigation
4. *Cathepsin D* (Fukuda et al., 2005)	Low	High for aggressiveness of glioma		
5. *GADD45* α (Reddy et al., 2008)	Low	Moderate		
6. *YKL-40* (Iwamoto et al., 2011)	Low	Moderate		
7. *Ki67* (Preusser et al., 2008)	Low	High for glioblastoma	Shows cell proliferation in gliomas	None
8. *MIP-1α* (Xu et al., 2012)	Low	Moderate	None	Under investigation
9. *CDKN2A* (Liu et al., 2011)	Low	Low		
10. *IDH1* (Labussiere et al., 2010)	Low	High	1. Analysis is based on the morphologic identification of genetic alterations within tumor cell nuclei 2. Does not require microdissection of normal and tumor cells before analysis	1. Highly labor intensive 2. Automation has not yet reached for FISH technique
11. *MGMT* (Jung et al., 2011)	Moderate	High		
12. *VEGF* (Brem et al., 1992; Plate and Risau, 1995)	Low	Moderate		
13. *LOH of 10q* (Ohgaki, 2005)	Moderate	High		
14. *LOH 1p/19q* (Bell et al., 2011)	High for oligodendrogliomas	High for oligodendrogliomas		
15. *PDGF* (Heldin and Westermark, 1999; Andrae et al., 2008)	Low	Moderate for oligodendrogliomas		
16. *EGFR* (Liu et al., 2011)	Low	Moderate		

TABLE 10.3 (continued)

Current Molecular and Genetic Biomarkers for Noninvasive Diagnosis of Brain Gliomas

	Features			
Biomarkers	**Specificity**	**Sensitivity**	**Advantages**	**Disadvantages**
17. *miRNA-15b* (Baraniskin et al., 2012)	Low	High		
18. *PTEN* (Liu et al., 2011)	High	High		
19. *P53* (Bell et al., 2011)	Low	High		

Note: All of these markers are under investigation for serum or CSF analysis.

a hot spot to search for cancer biomarkers. They are 50–90 nm vesicle-like objects secreted by various mammalian cells. Tumor mutations in glioma can be detected in exosomes from serum, which is also facilitating a blood-based biomarker detection for solid tumors (Skog et al., 2008). Thus, tumor-derived exosomes may be used as a diagnostic biomarker and aid in therapeutic decisions for glioma patients.

10.5.3 Genetic Biomarkers

MicroRNAs (miRNAs) circulating in CSF may serve as novel biomarkers for the detection of glioma. Characteristic miRNA alterations (*miRNA-15a, miRNA-15b, miRNA-16, miRNA-19b, miRNA-21, miRNA-92, miRNA-106a, miRNA-155,* and *miRNA-204*) have been identified in gliomas (Baraniskin et al., 2012). Although there is no CSF biomarker in commercial use for brain gliomas, one study showed that the levels of *miRNA-15b,* as measured in quantitative reverse transcriptase-polymerase chain reaction (qRT-PCR) assays, were significantly increased in CSF samples from patients with glioma, compared with control subjects with miscellaneous neurological disorders or patients with primary CNS lymphoma or brain metastases (Baraniskin et al., 2012). Many other potential biomarkers are under investigation for diagnostic purposes in gliomas. Especially the biomarkers that are in use for the histopathological diagnosis may be used as noninvasive biomarkers for gliomas. DNA microarrays are often used to detect biomarkers of glioma tissue (Pope et al., 2008). Low- and high-grade astrocytomas and oligodendrogliomas have distinctive gene expression profiles and are clearly separable from each other and from normal brain tissue. Beyond the genomics, simultaneous screening for many tissue proteins to detect biomarkers can be done by 2D gel electrophoresis, mass spectrometry, or protein microarrays. New techniques detect posttranslational changes in proteins, which may markedly increase their diagnostic ability (Kalinina et al., 2011). Proteins, which are differentially expressed in low- and high-grade gliomas, are involved in cell division, cell migration, the cytoskeleton, stress response, and resistance to apoptosis. Serum or CSF mass spectra obtained from brain glioma patients are different from the corresponding spectra of control patients, raising the possibility of diagnosing brain tumors by testing body fluids. Proteomic studies have already generated a sizable number of candidate diagnostic and prognostic markers in human brain cancer. Before adapting discovered biomarkers to the clinic, it is necessary to address some of the significant challenges that still remain in the existing methodologies and technologies hindering an in-depth, nonbiased profiling of the human glioma proteome. In the near future, improved proteomic profiling is anticipated to bring about a merger of biology, engineering, and informatics, with a profound impact on glioma research and treatment (Kalinina et al., 2011).

10.6 Imaging Biomarkers for Gliomas

Radiological studies such as CT and MRI and physiological imaging using positron emission tomography (PET) and single-photon emission computed tomography (SPECT) scanning are the commonly used noninvasive methods for the diagnosis of brain tumors (Goldman and Pirotte, 2011). These methods have also played a pivotal role in defining landmarks used to manage primary brain tumors clinically (Fan, 2006). MRI using T1-weighted, T2-weighted, and gadolinium-enhanced sequences plays a central clinical role in diagnosis, characterization, surveillance, and therapeutic monitoring of gliomas (Upadhyay and Waldman, 2011). However, the differential diagnosis of brain tumors requires more sophisticated technique and knowledge. Magnetic resonance spectroscopy (MRS) provides information on tissue biochemistry that adds to anatomical information from MRI. Metabolites that can be identified on a standard MRS include *N*-acetyl aspartate (NAA), choline (Cho), creatine (Cr), myo-inositol (MI), and glutamate and glutamine compounds (Glu-n). NAA is a marker for neuronal density and viability. The NAA peak is assigned at 2.0 ppm and is the largest peak. The second largest peak is creatine. This peak is composed of resonances from Cr with contributions from creatine phosphate, gamma-aminobutyric acid, lysine, and glutathione. The peak is assigned at 3.03 ppm and serves as a marker for energy-dependent systems in the brain cells. The Cho peak is assigned at 3.2 ppm and contains contributions from glycerophosphocholine, phosphocholine, and phosphatidylcholine. It reflects the metabolism of cellular membrane turnover, and it is increased in all hypercellular lesions. In brain gliomas, MRS often indicates abnormalities in tissue that appears normal by conventional MRI. Specifically, an elevation in Cho with depression of NAA is a reliable indicator of glioma. In addition, the metabolite ratios of Cho/Cr, NAA/Cr, and MI/Cr and the presence of lipids and lactate are useful in grading of brain gliomas (Fan, 2006). Tumor progression can also be predicted using MRS by detecting metabolic abnormalities outside the MRI-defined treatment region. 18 Fludeoxyglucose positron emission tomography (^{18}F-FDG PET) has a potential role in providing prognostic information of brain gliomas. Amino acid tracers are promising in that they are more sensitive in imaging brain gliomas. With the development of targeted therapies, PET biomarkers might be used to select patients who are likely to respond to treatment, as well as to monitor treatment response (Chen, 2007). It was previously shown that SPECT is effective in differentiating viable glioma tissue from radiation necrosis and surrounding edema (Le Jeune et al., 2006). Moreover, higher tracer uptake on SPECT is associated with high-grade gliomas, decreased survival, and worse response to chemotherapy. However, the major limitation of SPECT images is the lack of objective and quantitative indexes during the interpretation (Deltuva et al., 2012). Advances in imaging techniques, including multivoxel MRS, tractography, functional MRI, and PET spectroscopy, are being used by neurosurgeons to target aggressive areas in brain gliomas and to help identify the real tumor borders, functional areas, and fiber tracts of the brain for a secure surgery (Brodbelt, 2011). Despite all of these noninvasive techniques, correct diagnosis of the gliomas cannot be achieved by the physicians. Today, tissue sampling by surgery seems the only method for the accurate diagnosis of brain gliomas.

10.7 Integrative "Omics"-Based Molecular Markers for Brain Gliomas

"Omics" is the term used to designate new biological sciences investigating a large group of molecules in biological samples. This term is in use since the mapping of the human genome (Idbaih, 2011). "Omics" is also used as a suffix in many words and refers to the study of "ome," defined as the whole set of something. The genome, for instance, is the sum total genetic information encoded in an organism. Similar definitions exist for proteome and metabolome and more recently the lipidome and glycome. Several emerging technologies have driven these new areas of research including DNA and protein microarrays and mass spectrometry. The field of bioinformatics has also developed to allow analysis of "omics" data and rapid data analysis, and information exchange is now possible by the help of the Internet (Petrik et al., 2006). "Omics" has enabled a better understanding of clinical and biological behavior of brain gliomas identifying new molecular abnormalities and relevant biomarkers (Idbaih, 2011). v-raf murine sarcoma viral oncogene homolog B1 (BRAF) gene abnormalities are diagnostic markers in low-grade astrocytomas. Translocation (1; 19) (q10; p10) is associated with oligodendrogliomas and showed better prognosis in these tumors (Idbaih, 2011). MGMT promoter methylation is predictive of response to chemotherapy in high-grade astrocytomas. Genetic and genomic disruptions of tyrosine kinase receptors, TP53 signaling pathways in the vast majority of cases, and several transcriptomic, epigenomic, and proteomic (such as EGFR and PDGFR) patterns with biological and/or clinical impacts have been discovered by the studies. Finally, "omics" have identified recurrent IDH1/IDH2 mutations with prognostic significance in gliomas and five single nucleotide polymorphisms associated with susceptibility to gliomas (Idbaih, 2011). So, the data generated by "omics" are huge and multidimensional. De Tayrac et al. (2009) introduced a data-mining approach, multiple factor analysis to combine multiple data sets and to add formalized knowledge. They illustrated this method with a glioma study performed with both comparative genomic hybridization array and expression microarray on the same tumor samples. Their results showed that both DNA copy number alteration and transcriptome data sets induce a good separation of the gliomas according to the WHO classification. The superimposition of the gene modules built since gene ontology (GO) annotation identifies regulatory mechanisms implicated in gliomagenesis. They also showed that this approach can handle a single data set with associated GO annotations and therefore be used as an exploratory tool in the case of classical single "omics" study (De Tayrac et al., 2009). As the results of "omics" studies on brain gliomas, the biomarkers that can be used in the histological classification and may serve as important prognostic and predictive markers are MGMT promoter methylation, IDH1 mutations, and codeletion of 1p/19q. BRAF gene fusion/mutations and EGFR amplification provide important clues diagnostically (Gupta and Salunke, 2012).

10.8 Conclusions

Although distinct progress has been achieved on the development of diagnostic marker for brain glioma, no established noninvasive biomarker exists because of its heterogeneous and complex structure.

However, there is a rapid expansion of our knowledge about the biology and genetics of brain gliomas and new promising molecular biomarkers has been developed. Some of them have shown diagnostic value, whereas others are useful for prognostic and predicting responses to treatments. For example, serum GFAP measurement seems to be most promising preoperative diagnostic marker for glioma (Jung et al., 2011). *MGMT* promoter hypermethylation has also been established as an important prognostic biomarker and has strong influence in every trial evaluating new therapeutic agents (Nagane, 2012). In addition, *IDH1* became one of the most important prognostic markers for diffusely infiltrating gliomas. Patients who exhibit IDH1 mutations have a better clinical course than the patients without these mutations. R132H is the most frequent mutational variant of IDH1, and it can be easily and reliably detected by immunohistochemistry. So, these markers might facilitate the diagnostic procedure and may influence the treatment of glioma (Jung et al., 2011). Beyond these biomarkers, the increasing number of antiangiogenic agents are currently investigated and developed by the clinical trials for gliomas. Furthermore, new biological concepts are emerging from the studies of stem cells, and new diagnostic techniques have been advanced from gene expression array and proteomic technologies that could revolutionize histopathology of gliomas. Better patient management and treatment strategy could only be achieved by the efforts to identify molecular markers for gliomas, which may predict the benefits of molecularly targeted treatments. In the future, beyond the molecular techniques, noninvasive MRI-based imaging and spectroscopy examinations may probably provide the identification of these biomarkers directly in the human brain.

References

Abaza, M.S., Shaban, F., Narayan, R.K., Atassi, M.Z. 1998. Human glioma associated intermediate filament proteins: Over-expression, co-localization and cross-reactivity. *Anticancer Res*. 18:1333–1340.

Andrae, J., Gallini, R., Betsholtz, C. 2008. Role of platelet-derived growth factors in physiology and medicine. *Genes Dev*. 22:1276–1312.

Assem, M., Sibenaller, Z., Agarwal, S., Al-Keilani, M.S., Alqudah, M.A., Ryken, T.C. 2012. Enhancing diagnosis, prognosis, and therapeutic outcome prediction of gliomas using genomics. *OMICS*. 16:113–122.

Auffinger, B., Thaci, B., Nigam, P., Rincon, E., Cheng, Y., Lesniak, M.S. 2012. New therapeutic approaches for malignant glioma: In search of the Rosetta stone. *F1000 Med Rep*. 4:18.

Australian Cancer Network Adult Brain Tumour Guidelines Working Party. 2009. *Clinical Practice Guidelines for the Management of Adult Gliomas: Astrocytomas and Oligodendrogliomas*. Cancer Council Australia, Australian Cancer Network and Clinical Oncological Society of Australia Inc., Sydney, New South Wales, Australia.

Baraniskin, A., Kuhnhenn, J., Schlegel, U., Maghnouj, A., Zöllner, H., Schmiegel, W., Hahn, S., Schroers, R. 2012. Identification of microRNAs in the cerebrospinal fluid as biomarker for the diagnosis of glioma. *Neuro Oncol*. 14:29–33.

Bell, E.H., Hadziahmetovic, M., Chakravarti, A. 2011. Evolvement of molecular biomarkers in targeted therapy of malignant gliomas. In: *Brain Tumors—Current and Emerging Therapeutic Strategies*. Abujamra AL (ed.). InTech Publication, New York, NY (accessed on September 27, 2012).

Bhatt, A.N., Mathur, R., Farooque, A., Verma, A., Dwarakanath, B.S. 2010. Cancer biomarkers—current perspectives. *Indian J Med Res*. 132:129–149.

Bleeker, F.E., Molenaar, R.J., Leenstra, S. 2012. Recent advances in the molecular understanding of glioblastoma. *J Neurooncol*. 108:11–27.

Brandes, A.A., Franceschi, E., Tosoni, A., Benevento, F., Scopece, L., Mazzocchi, V., Bacci, A. et al. 2009a. Temozolomide concomitant and adjuvant to radiotherapy in elderly patients with glioblastoma: Correlation with MGMT promoter methylation status. *Cancer*. 115:3512–3518.

Brandes, A.A., Tosoni, A., Franceschi, E., Sotti, G., Frezza, G., Amista, P., Morandi, L., Spagnolli, F., Ermani, M. 2009b. Recurrence pattern after temozolomide concomitant with and adjuvant to radiotherapy in newly diagnosed patients with glioblastoma: Correlation with MGMT promoter methylation status. *J Clin Oncol*. 27:1275–1279.

Brat, D.J., Prayson, R.A., Ryken, T.C., Olson, J.J. 2008. Diagnosis of malignant glioma: Role of neuropathology. *J Neurooncol*. 89:287–311.

Brem, S., Tsanaclis, A.M., Gately, S., Gross, J.L., Herblin, W.F. 1992. Immunolocalization of basic fibroblast growth factor to the microvasculature of human brain tumors. *Cancer*. 70:2673–2680.

Brodbelt, A. 2011. Clinical applications of imaging biomarkers. Part 2. The neurosurgeon's perspective. *Br J Radiol*. 84:Spec No 2:S205–S208.

Candolfi, M., Kroeger, K.M., Muhammad, A.K., Yagiz, K., Farrokhi, C., Pechnick, R.N., Lowenstein, P.R., Castro, M.G. 2009. Gene therapy for brain cancer: Combination therapies provide enhanced efficacy and safety. *Curr Gene Ther*. 9:409–421.

Central Brain Tumor Registry of the United States. Statistical Report: Primary Brain Tumors in the United States, 1995–1999. 2002. Published by the Central Brain Tumor Registry of the United States. pp. 20. http://www.CBTRUS.org

Chen, W. 2007. Clinical applications of PET in brain tumors. *J Nucl Med*. 48:1468–1481.

Choksi, S., Lin, Y., Pobezinskaya, Y., Chen, L., Park, C., Morgan, M., Li, T. et al. 2011. A HIF-1 target, ATIA, protects cells from apoptosis by modulating the mitochondrial thioredoxin, TRX2. *Mol Cell*. 42:597–609.

Clarke, J.L., Iwamoto, F.M., Sul, J., Panageas, K., Lassman, A.B., DeAngelis, L.M., Hormigo, A. et al. 2009. Randomized phase II trial of chemoradiotherapy followed by either dose-dense or metronomic temozolomide for newly diagnosed glioblastoma. *J Clin Oncol*. 27:3861–3867.

Criniere, E., Kaloshi, G., Laigle-Donadey, F., Lejeune, J., Auger, N., Benouaich-Amiel, A., Everhard, S. et al. 2007. MGMT prognostic impact on glioblastoma is dependent on therapeutic modalities. *J Neurooncol*. 83:173–179.

Daumas-Duport, C., Scheithauer, B., O'Fallon, J., Kelly, P. 1988. Grading of astrocytomas. A simple and reproducible method. *Cancer*. 62:2152–2165.

Dean, B.L., Drayer, B.P., Bird, C.R., Flom, R.A., Hodak, J.A., Coons, S.W., Carey, R.G. 1990. Gliomas: Classification with MR imaging. *Radiology*. 174:411–415.

De Groot, J., Sontheimer, H. 2011. Glutamate and the biology of gliomas. *Glia*. 59:1181–1189.

Deltuva, V.P., Jurkienė, N., Kulakienė, I., Bunevičius, A., Matukevičius, A., Tamašauskas, A. 2012. Introduction of novel semiquantitative evaluation of (99m)Tc-MIBI SPECT before and after treatment of glioma. *Medicina (Kaunas)*. 48:15–21.

De Tayrac, M., Lê, S., Aubry, M., Mosser, J., Husson, F. 2009. Simultaneous analysis of distinct Omics data sets with integration of biological knowledge: Multiple Factor Analysis approach. *BMC Genomics*. 10:32.

Ducray, F., El Hallani, S., Idbaih, A. 2009. Diagnostic and prognostic markers in gliomas. *Curr Opin Oncol*. 21:537–542.

Ducray, F., Idbaih, A., Wang, X.W., Cheneau, C., Labussiere, M., Sanson, M. 2011. Predictive and prognostic factors for gliomas. *Expert Rev Anticancer Ther*. 11:781–789.

Dunn, J., Baborie, A., Alam, F., Joyce, K., Moxham, M., Sibson, R., Crooks, D. et al. 2009. Extent of MGMT promoter methylation correlates with outcome in glioblastomas given temozolomide and radiotherapy. *Br J Cancer.* 101:124–131.

Etseller, M., Garcia-Foncillas, J., Andion, E., Goodman, S.N., Hidalgo, O.F., Vanaclocha, V., Baylin, S.B., Herman, J.G. 2000. Inactivation of the DNA-repair gene MGMT and the clinical response of gliomas to alkylating agents. *N Engl J Med.* 343:1350–1354.

Fan, G. 2006. Magnetic resonance spectroscopy and glioma. *Cancer Imaging.* 6:113–115.

Febbo, P.G., Ladanyi, M., Aldape, K.D., De Marzo, A.M., Hammond, M.E., Hayes, D.F., Iafrate, A.J. et al. 2011. NCCN Task Force report: Evaluating the clinical utility of tumor markers in oncology. *J Natl Compr Canc Netw.* 9(Suppl 5):S1–S32.

Foerch, C., Curdt, I., Yan, B., Dvorak, F., Hermans, M., Berkefeld, J., Raabe, A. et al. 2006. Serum glial fibrillary acidic protein as a biomarker for intracerebral haemorrhage in patients with acute stroke. *J Neurol Neurosurg Psychiatry.* 77:181–184.

Fukuda, M.E., Iwadate, Y., Machida, T., Hiwasa, T., Nimura, Y., Nagai, Y., Takiguchi, M. et al. 2005. Cathepsin D is a potential serum marker for poor prognosis in glioma patients. *Cancer Res.* 65:5190–5194.

Fukui, S., Nawashiro, H., Otani, N., Ooigawa, H., Nomura, N., Yano, A., Miyazawa, T. et al. 2003. Nuclear accumulation of basic fibroblast growth factor in human astrocytic tumors. *Cancer.* 97:3061–3067.

Furnari, F.B., Fenton, T., Bachoo, R.M., Mukasa, A., Stommel, J.M., Stegh, A., Hahn, W.C. et al. 2007. Malignant astrocytic glioma: Genetics, biology and paths to treatment. *Genes Dev.* 21:2683–2710.

Gerson, S.L. 2004. MGMT: Its role in cancer aetiology and cancer therapeutics. *Nat Rev Cancer.* 4:296–307.

Goldman, S., Pirotte, B.J. 2011. Brain tumors. *Methods Mol Biol.* 727:291–315.

Gorlia, T., van den Bent, M.J., Hegi, M.E., Mirimanoff, R.O., Weller, M., Cairncross, J.G., Eisenhauer, E. et al. 2008. Nomograms for predicting survival of patients with newly diagnosed glioblastoma: Prognostic factor analysis of EORTC and NCIC trial 26981-22981/CE.3. *Lancet Oncol.* 9:29–38.

Gupta, K., Salunke, P. 2012. Molecular markers of glioma: An update of recent progress and perspectives. *J Cancer Res Clin Oncol.* 138(12):1971–1981.

Hamaya, K., Doi, K., Tanaka, T., Nishimoto, A. 1985. The determination of glial fibrillary acidic protein for the diagnosis and histogenetic study of central nervous system tumors: A study of 152 cases. *Acta Med Okayama.* 39:453–462.

Hartmann, C., Meyer, J., Balss, J., Capper, D., Mueller, W., Christians, A., Felsberg, J. et al. 2009. Type and frequency of IDH1 and IDH2 mutations are related to astrocytic and oligodendroglial differentiation and age: A study of 1,010 diffuse gliomas. *Acta Neuropathol.* 118:469–474.

Hegi, M.E., Diserens, A.C., Gorlia, T., Hamou, M.F., de Tribolet, N., Weller, M., Kros, J.M. et al. 2005. MGMT gene silencing and benefit from temozolomide in glioblastoma. *N Engl J Med.* 352:997–1003.

Heldin, C.H., Westermark, B. 1999. Mechanism of action and in vivo role of platelet-derived growth factor. *Physiol Rev.* 79:1283–1316.

Herrlinger, U., Rieger, J., Koch, D., Loeser, S., Blaschke, B., Kortmann, R.D., Steinbach, J.P. et al. 2006. Phase II trial of lomustine plus temozolomide chemotherapy in addition to radiotherapy in newly diagnosed glioblastoma: UKT-03. *J Clin Oncol.* 24:4412–4417.

Herrmann, M., Ehrenreich, H. 2003. Brain derived proteins as markers of acute stroke: Their relation to pathophysiology, outcome prediction and neuroprotective drug monitoring. *Restor Neurol Neurosci.* 21:177–190.

Hoeben, A., Landuyt, B., Highley, M.S., Wildiers, H., Van Oosterom, A.T., De Bruijn, E.A. 2004. Vascular endothelial growth factor and angiogenesis. *Pharmacol Rev.* 56:549–580.

Idbaih, A. 2011. OMICS and biomarkers of glial tumors. *Rev Neurol (Paris).* 167:691–698.

Iwamoto, F.M., Hottinger, A.F., Karimi, S., Riedel, E., Dantis, J., Jahdi, M., Panageas, K.S. et al. 2011. Serum YKL-40 is a marker of prognosis and disease status in high-grade gliomas. *Neuro Oncol.* 13:1244–1251.

Jacobs, S.K., Wilson, D.J., Melin, G., Parham, C.W., Holcomb, B., Kornblith, P.L., Grimm, E.A. 1986. Interleukin-2 and lymphokine activated killer (LAK) cells in the treatment of malignant glioma: Clinical and experimental studies. *Neurol Res.* 8:81–87.

Jacque, C.M., Vinner, C., Kujas, M., Raoul, M., Racadot, J., Baumann, N.A. 1978. Determination of glial fibrillary acidic protein (GFAP) in human brain tumors. *J Neurol Sci.* 35:147–155.

Jung, C.S., Foerch, C., Schanzer, A., Heck, A., Plate, K.H., Seifert, V., Steinmetz, H., Raabe, A., Sitzer, M. 2007. Serum GFAP is a diagnostic marker for glioblastoma multiforme. *Brain.* 130:3336–3341.

Jung, C.S., Unterberg, A.W., Hartmann, C. 2011. Diagnostic markers for glioblastoma. *C Histol Histopathol.* 26:1327–1341.

Kalinina, J., Peng, J., Ritchie, J.C., Van Meir, E.G. 2011. Proteomics of gliomas: Initial biomarker discovery and evolution of technology. *Neuro Oncol.* 13:926–942.

Kleihues, P., Burger, P.C., Scheithauer, B.W. 1993. The new WHO classification of brain tumours. *Brain Pathol.* 3:255–268.

Kleihues, P., Cavenee, W.K. 1997. *Tumors of the Central Nervous System: Pathology and Genetics.* International Agency for Research on Cancer, Lyon, France.

Kohn, E.C., Azad, N., Annunziata, C., Dhamoon, A.S., Whiteley, G. 2007. Proteomics as a tool for biomarker discovery. *Dis Markers.* 23:411–417.

Komohara, Y., Horlad, H., Ohnishi, K., Fujiwara, Y., Bai, B., Nakagawa, T., Suzu, S. et al. 2012. Importance of direct macrophage-tumor cell interaction on progression of human glioma. *Cancer Sci.* 103(12):2165–2172.

Labussiere, M., Sanson, M., Idbaih, A., Delattre, J.Y. 2010. *IDH1* gene mutations: A new paradigm in glioma prognosis and therapy? *Oncologist.* 15:196–199.

Lavon, I., Refael, M., Zelikovitch, B., Shalom, E., Siegal, T. 2010. Serum DNA can define tumor-specific genetic and epigenetic markers in gliomas of various grades. *Neuro Oncol.* 12:173–180.

Lee, J.W. 2009. Method validation and application of protein biomarkers. Basic similarities and differences from biotherapeutics. *Bioanalysis.* 1:1461–1474.

Le Jeune, F.P., Dubois, F., Blond, S., Steinling, M. 2006. Sestamibi technetium-99m brain single-photon emission computed tomography to identify recurrent glioma in adults: 201 studies. *J Neurooncol.* 77:177–183.

Liang, S., Shen, G. 2011. Biomarkers of glioma. In: *Molecular Targets of CNS Tumors.* Garami M (ed.). InTech Publication, New York, NY, pp. 325–342.

Liu, W., Lv, G., Li, Y., Li, L., Wang, B. 2011. Downregulation of CDKN2A and suppression of cyclin D1 gene expressions in malignant gliomas. *J Exp Clin Cancer Res.* 30:76.

Nagane, M. 2012. Genetic alterations and biomarkers for glioma. *Brain Nerve.* 64:537–548.

Nakagawachi, T., Soejima, H., Urano, T., Zhao, W., Higashimoto, K., Satoh, Y., Matsukura, S. et al. 2003. Silencing effect of CpG island hypermethylation and histone modifications on O6-methylguanine-DNA methyltransferase (MGMT) gene expression in human cancer. *Oncogene.* 22:8835–8844.

Nazarenko, I., Hede, S.M., He, X., Hedrén, A., Thompson, J., Lindström, M.S., Nistér, M. 2012. PDGF and PDGF receptors in glioma. *Ups J Med Sci.* 117:99–112.

Ohgaki, H. 2005. Genetic pathways to glioblastomas. *Neuropathology.* 25:1–7.

Olsson, M., Lindahl, T. 1980. Repair of alkylated DNA in *Escherichia coli.* Methyl group transfer from O6-methylguanine to a protein cysteine residue. *J Biol Chem.* 255:10569–10571.

Pegg, A.E., Wiest, L., Foote, R.S., Mitra, S., Perry, W. 1983. Purification and properties of O6-methylguanine-DNA transmethylase from rat liver. *J Biol Chem.* 258:2327–2333.

Peles, E., Lidar, Z., Simon, A.J., Grossman, R., Nass, D., Ram, Z. 2004. Angiogenic factors in the cerebrospinal fluid of patients with astrocytic brain tumors. *Neurosurgery.* 55:562–567.

Pelinka, L.E., Kroepfl, A., Schmidhammer, R., Krenn, M., Buchinger, W., Redl, H., Raabe, A. 2004. Glial fibrillary acidic protein in serum after traumatic brain injury and multiple trauma. *J Trauma.* 57:1006–1012.

Petrik, V., Loosemore, A., Howe, F.A., Bell, B.A., Papadopoulos, M.C. 2006. OMICS and brain tumour biomarkers. *Br J Neurosurg.* 20:275–280.

Peyre, M., Commo, F., Dantas-Barbosa, C., Andreiuolo, F., Puget, S., Lacroix, L., Drusch, F. et al. 2010. Portrait of ependymoma recurrence in children: Biomarkers of tumor progression identified by dual-color microarray-based gene expression analysis. *PLoS One.* 5:e12932.

Plate, K.H., Breier, G., Farrell, C.L., Risau, W. 1992. Platelet-derived growth factor receptor-beta is induced during tumor development and upregulated during tumor progression in endothelial cells in human gliomas. *Lab Invest.* 67:529–534.

Plate, K.H., Risau, W. 1995. Angiogenesis in malignant gliomas. *Glia.* 15:339–347.

Pope, W.B., Chen, J.H., Dong, J., Carlson, M.R., Perlina, A., Cloughesy, T.F., Liau, L.M. et al. 2008. Relationship between gene expression and enhancement in glioblastoma multiforme: Exploratory DNA microarray analysis. *Radiology.* 249:268–277.

Prados, M.D., Chang, S.M., Butowski, N., DeBoer, R., Parvataneni, R., Carliner, H., Kabuubi, P. et al. 2009. Phase II study of erlotinib plus temozolomide during and after radiation therapy in patients with newly diagnosed glioblastoma multiforme or gliosarcoma. *J Clin Oncol.* 27:579–584.

Preusser, M., Heinzl, H., Gelpi, E., Höftberger, R., Fischer, I., Pipp, I., Milenkovic, I. et al. 2008. Ki67 index in intracranial ependymoma: A promising histopathological candidate biomarker. *Histopathology*. 53:39–47.

Reddy, S.P., Britto, R., Vinnakota, K., Aparna, H., Sreepathi, H.K., Thota, B., Kumari, A. et al. 2008. Novel glioblastoma markers with diagnostic and prognostic value identified through transcriptome analysis. *Clin Cancer Res*. 14:2978–2987.

Riemenschneider, M.J., Jeuken, J.W., Wesseling, P., Reifenberger, G. 2010. Molecular diagnostics of gliomas: State of the art. *Acta Neuropathol*. 120:567–584.

Roger, M., Clavreul, A., Venier-Julienne, M., Passirani, C., Montero-Menei, C., Menei, P. 2011. The potential of combinations of drug-loaded nanoparticle systems and adult stem cells for glioma therapy. *Biomaterials*. 32:2106–2116.

Royds, J.A., Ironside, J.W., Taylor, C.B., Graham, D.I., Timperley, W.R. 1986. An immunohistochemical study of glial and neuronal markers in primary neoplasms of the central nervous system. *Acta Neuropathol*. 70:320–326.

Sampath, P., Weaver, C.E., Sungarian, A., Cortez, S., Alderson, L., Stopa, E.G. 2004. Cerebrospinal fluid (vascular endothelial growth factor) and serologic (recoverin) tumor markers for malignant glioma. *Cancer Control*. 11:174–180.

Schulz, C., Waldeck, S., Mauer, U.M. 2012. Intraoperative image guidance in neurosurgery: Development, current indications, and future trends. *Radiol Res Pract*. 2012:197364.

Schwartzbaum, J.A., Fisher, J.L., Aldape, K.D., Wrensch, M. 2006. Epidemiology and molecular pathology of glioma. *Nat Clin Pract Neurol*. 2:494–503.

Skog, J., Würdinger, T., van Rijn, S., Meijer, D., Gainche, L., Sena-Esteves, M., Curry, W. Jr. et al. 2008. Glioblastoma microvesicles transport RNA and proteins that promote tumour growth and provide diagnostic biomarkers. *Nat Cell Biol*. 10:1470–1476.

Sontheimer, H. 2008. A role for glutamate in growth and invasion of primary brain tumors. *J Neurochem*. 105:287–295.

Speert, D. 2008. Glioma brain tumors. www.brainfacts.org/diseases-disorders/cancer/articles/2008/glioma-brain-tumors/ (accessed on January 20, 2013).

Stupp, R., Hegi, M.E., Mason, W.P., van den Bent, M.J., Taphoorn, M.J., Janzer, R.C., Ludwin, S.K. et al. 2009. Effects of radiotherapy with concomitant and adjuvant temozolomide versus radiotherapy alone on survival in glioblastoma in a randomised phase III study: 5-year analysis of the EORTC-NCIC trial. *Lancet Oncol*. 10:459–466.

Stupp, R., Mason, W.P., van den Bent, M.J., Weller, M., Fisher, B., Taphoorn, M.J., Belanger, K. et al. 2005. Radiotherapy plus concomitant and adjuvant temozolomide for glioblastoma. *N Engl J Med*. 352:987–996.

Takahashi, J.A., Fukumoto, M., Igarashi, K., Oda, Y., Kikuchi, H., Hatanaka, M. 1992. Correlation of basic fibroblast growth factor expression levels with the degree of malignancy and vascularity in human gliomas. *J Neurosurg*. 76:792–798.

Takano, S., Yoshii, Y., Kondo, S., Suzuki, H., Maruno, T., Shirai, S., Nose, T. 1996. Concentration of vascular endothelial growth factor in the serum and tumor tissue of brain tumor patients. *Cancer Res*. 56:2185–2190.

Terrile, M., Appolloni, I., Calzolari, F., Perris, R., Tutucci, E., Malatesta, P. 2010. PDGF-B-driven gliomagenesis can occur in the absence of the proteoglycan NG2. *BMC Cancer*. 10:550.

Tobias, A., Ahmed, A., Moon, K.S., Lesniak, M.S. 2013. The art of gene therapy for glioma: A review of the challenging road to the bedside. *J Neurol Neurosurg Psychiatry*. 84(2):213–222.

Upadhyay, N., Waldman, A.D. 2011. Conventional MRI evaluation of gliomas. *Br J Radiol*. 84(Spec No 2):S107–S111.

Van den Bent, M.J., Brandes, A.A., Rampling, R., Kouwenhoven, M.C., Kros, J.M., Carpentier, A.F., Clement, P.M. et al. 2009a. Randomized phase II trial of erlotinib versus temozolomide or carmustine in recurrent glioblastoma: EORTC brain tumor group study 26034. *J Clin Oncol*. 27:1268–1274.

Van den Bent, M.J., Dubbink, H.J., Sanson, M., van der Lee-Haarloo, C.R., Hegi, M., Jeuken, J.W., Ibdaih, A. et al. 2009b. MGMT promoter methylation is prognostic but not predictive for outcome to adjuvant PCV chemotherapy in anaplastic oligodendroglial tumors: A report from EORTC Brain Tumor Group Study 26951. *J Clin Oncol*. 27:5881–5886.

Von Deimling, A., Korshunov, A., Hartmann, C. 2011. The next generation of glioma biomarkers: MGMT methylation, BRAF fusions and IDH1 mutations. *Brain Pathol*. 21:74–87.

Weaver, K.D., Grossman, S.A., Herman, J.G. 2006. Methylated tumor-specific DNA as a plasma biomarker in patients with glioma. *Cancer Invest*. 24:35–40.

Weiler, M., Hartmann, C., Wiewrodt, D., Herrlinger, U., Gorlia, T., Bahr, O., Meyermann, R. et al. 2010. Chemoradiotherapy of newly diagnosed glioblastoma with intensified temozolomide. *Int J Radiat Oncol Biol Phys*. 77:670–676.

Weller, M., Felsberg, J., Hartmann, C., Berger, H., Steinbach, J.P., Schramm, J., Westphal, M. et al. 2009. Molecular predictors of progression-free and overall survival in patients with newly diagnosed glioblastoma: A prospective translational study of the German Glioma Network. *J Clin Oncol*. 27:5743–5750.

Wick, W., Hartmann, C., Engel, C., Stoffels, M., Felsberg, J., Stockhammer, F., Sabel, M.C. et al. 2009. NOA-04 randomized phase III trial of sequential radiochemotherapy of anaplastic glioma with procarbazine, lomustine, and vincristine or temozolomide. *J Clin Oncol*. 27:5874–5880.

Xu, B.J., An, Q.A., Srinivasa Gowda, S., Yan, W., Pierce, L.A., Abel, T.W., Rush, S.Z. et al. 2012. Identification of blood protein biomarkers that aid in the clinical assessment of patients with malignant glioma. *Int J Oncol*. 40:1995–2003.

Yan, H., Parsons, D.W., Jin, G., McLendon, R., Rasheed, B.A., Yuan, W., Kos, I. et al. 2009. IDH1 and IDH2 mutations in gliomas. *N Engl J Med*. 360:765–773.

Ye, Z., Sontheimer, H. 1999. Glioma cells release excitotoxic concentrations of glutamate. *Cancer Res*. 59:4383–4391.

Yen, S.H., Dahl, D., Schachner, M., Shelanski, M.L. 1976. Biochemistry of the filaments of brain. *Proc Natl Acad Sci USA*. 73:529–533.

Zawlik, I., Vaccarella, S., Kita, D., Mittelbronn, M., Franceschi, S., Ohgaki, H. 2009. Promoter methylation and polymorphisms of the MGMT gene in glioblastomas: A population-based study. *Neuroepidemiology*. 32:21–29.

Zhuang, Z., Qi, M., Li, J., Okamoto, H., Xu, D.S., Iyer, R.R., Lu, J. et al. 2011. Proteomic identification of glutamine synthetase as a differential marker for oligodendrogliomas and astrocytomas. *J Neurosurg*. 115:789–795.

11

Noninvasive Biomarkers in Head and Neck Squamous Cell Carcinoma

Anand Kumar, Mumtaz Ahmad Ansari, and Vivek Srivastava

CONTENTS

ABSTRACT The 5-year survival rates of head and neck squamous cell carcinomas (HNSCCs) have remained unchanged despite improved locoregional control and reduced treatment-related morbidity. This can be attributed to multiple factors like lack of suitable markers for screening, presentation of the disease at an advanced stage, failure of advanced lesions to respond to treatment, and variation in site-specific behavior of the tumor. The treatment of these cancers is most effective when the tumor burden is lowest and lymphatic spread is the least. The effective therapy for these tumors will depend on early diagnosis and intervention. Unfortunately, no strategy has yet proven to be consistent and effective with reference to its detection at an early stage. However, newer ongoing researches to detect various "biomarkers" that are biological factors within a tumor that affects the molecular process in tumor progression are in vogue. The present biomarkers for HNSCC include the *p53* gene and its protein; microsatellite regions throughout the genome; human papillomavirus; proteins and its metabolites involved in cellular proliferation, apoptosis, angiogenesis, genetic information, and their expression as DNA and RNA; intracellular adhesion molecules; epithelial growth factor receptor; and various measures of immune response to cancer. Biomarkers have potential clinical applications not only in early detection of primary disease but they are also helpful in detection of recurrent cancer as well as could be exploited in selecting molecular targets for possible diagnosis and therapy.

However, these tests need validation before these can be used in clinical practice.

11.1 Introduction

Cancers arising from the upper aerodigestive tract, mostly squamous cell carcinoma (SCC), are broadly classified as head and neck squamous cell carcinomas (HNSCCs). They account for nearly 500,000 new cases worldwide each year, constituting 5% of all malignancies and gradually increasing over the past few decades (Perez-Ordonez et al. 2006). Most HNSCCs arise in the oral cavity including oropharynx, hypopharynx, larynx, and trachea. Within the oral cavity, most tumors arise from the floor of the mouth, the ventrolateral tongue, or the soft palate, while the most common oropharyngeal site of involvement is the base of the tongue. The majority of laryngeal SCCs originate from the supraglottic and glottic regions. Tracheal SCCs are rare compared to laryngeal ones (Jemal et al. 2007).

The HNSCCs occur most frequently in the sixth and seventh decades and typically affect men (Ritchie et al. 2003). Over the last two decades, the incidence among women is on the rise because of increased prevalence of smoking (Barnes et al. 2005). The incidence is high in men for laryngeal, hypopharyngeal, and tracheal SCCs in Southern and Central Europe, some parts of South America, and among Blacks in the United States (Andl et al. 1998). The lowest rates are recorded in Southeast Asia and Central Africa. The disease is more common in urban than in rural areas. In the United States, incidence rates are twofold higher in Blacks compared to Whites (Barnes et al. 2005). In India also HNSCC is a major form of cancer, accounting for 23% of all cancer in males and 6% in females

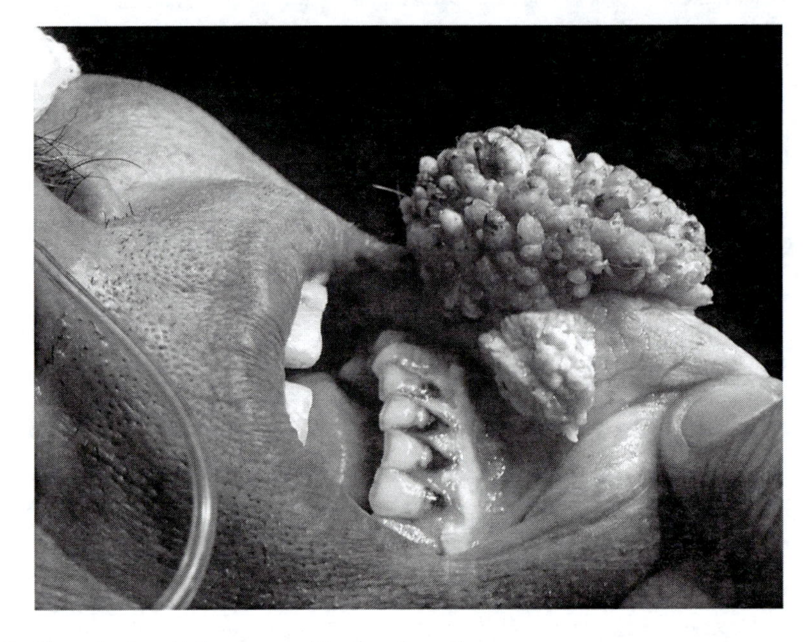

FIGURE 11.1 **(See color insert.)** Carcinoma arising from lower lip.

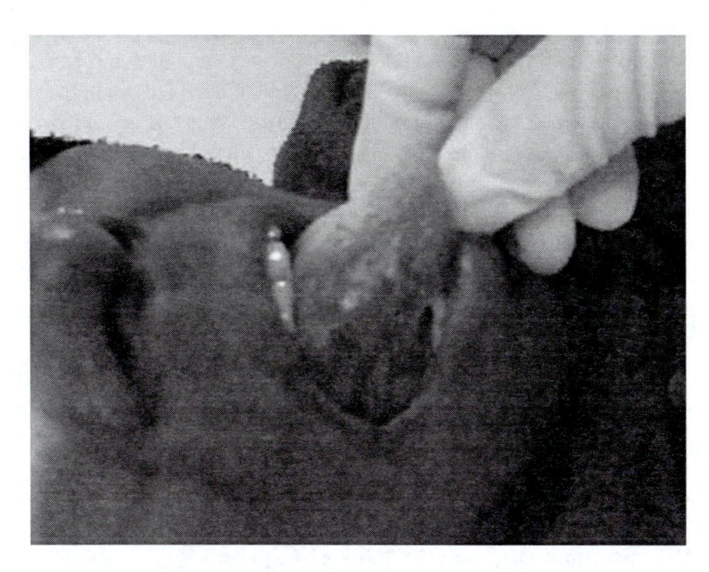

FIGURE 11.2 SCC arising from lateral border of tongue.

(Figures 11.1 and 11.2) (Belbin et al. 2008). The 5-year survival varies from 20% to 90% depending upon the anatomical site of origin and the clinical extent of disease at presentation (Jemal et al. 2007). Patients with early stage without nodal metastasis are treated with surgery and radiotherapy and have excellent 5-year survival rate. Unfortunately two-thirds of all patients present with advanced stage that is due to the fact that majority of HNSCCs arise de novo without preceding visible change in mucosa and also there is often delay in seeking consultation. Patients with advanced-stage tumor are treated by multimodality approach with chemoradiation and surgery that often leads to significant functional impairment in swallowing and speech, while their 5-year survival rate remains below 60% (Barnes et al. 2005, Jemal et al. 2007).

HNSCC is a preventable cancer owing to the established cause–effect relationship with consumption of tobacco and alcohol that play an important role in the etiopathogenesis of the disease. In the recent past there is an upsurge of human papillomavirus (HPV)-associated HNSCC especially in the tonsils and base of tongue region (Liang et al. 2012). The per capita consumption of cigarettes has increased by 2% over the last decade in India (Mehrotra et al. 2005) that corresponds to the increase in rate of HNSCC in the country. India has the dubious distinction of having the world's highest reported incidence of HNSCC in women (Rodrigo et al. 2005). The disproportionately higher prevalence of HNSCC in developing countries in relation to others may also be attributed to the use of tobacco in various forms (mainly smokeless tobacco), concomitant consumption of alcohol, and low socioeconomic condition related to poor hygiene, diet, or infections of viral origin (Bremmer et al. 2005) (Table 11.1).

TABLE 11.1

HNSCC Classification by World Health Organization, 2005

HNSCC Classification by World Health Organization, 2005
Conventional
Verrucous
Basaloid
Papillary
Spindle cell (sarcomatoid)
Acantholytic
Cuniculatum
Adenosquamous

Source: Barnes et al., 2005.

During the last decade a significant progress has been made in development of novel treatment for HNSCC. A successful treatment of the patients depends on early detection and correct therapy depending on the stage of disease. However, most cases of HNSCC are detected when the patient has become symptomatic of primary disease or when lymphatic metastasis has occurred and is clinically visible or palpable (Kreimer et al. 2005). Complains of pain, bleeding, ulceration, mass, otalgia, and dysphagia will usually direct the clinician to the primary lesion, which is typically at least stage II disease and often has associated cervical lymphadenopathy (Lipshutz et al. 1999). It has been reported that only 30% of HNSCC cases in the United States are diagnosed at an early clinical stage and two-thirds of patients present with advanced stage III or IV (Diamandis et al. 2004, Li et al. 2006). Despite improvements in current treatment including nonsurgical management and concomitant chemoradiation, less than 50% of the patients are cured and 15%–50% of patients develop locoregional recurrences (Ferlito et al. 2003, Takes 2004, Nagaraj et al. 2009). Such patients have poor prognosis with median survival of 6–10 months (van Wilgen et al. 2004). Further despite of intensive research, there are only a very few treatment options for those who experience recurrences. Chemotherapy with or without radiation remains the only effective option and is largely empirical with uncertain benefits (Hauswald et al. 2011).

11.2 Current Established Diagnostic Techniques

Early diagnosis and treatment is cornerstone of good outcome (Woolgar et al. 1995, Sciubba et al. 2001). Since the clinical examination has undetermined sensitivity and specificity, there is a need for more accurate diagnostic tools for early detection and determination of malignant potential of borderline and premalignant lesions. Currently available tools are shown in Table 11.2.

11.2.1 Biopsy and Histopathologic Examination

The prognostic value of histopathologic features related to a primary HNSCC tumor and the cervical lymph nodes has been extensively reviewed and is presently considered as the gold standard for diagnosis (Woolgar et al. 2006). Even histologic examination of a specimen is burdened with potential pitfalls and is subjective. Hence, the biopsy should be taken from the area likely to contain the greatest number of cellular changes suggestive of dysplasia. Vital staining may facilitate this. False-negative results are still occasionally possible and biopsies from leukoplakia and negative for dysplasia may harbor malignancy in up to 10% cases (Chiesa et al. 1986). Furthermore, pathologists have been shown to vary in their opinions, and even the same pathologist may offer a different opinion on different occasions if faced with exactly the same specimen specially in borderline malignant lesions (Figure 11.3) (Abbey et al. 1995; Karabulut et al. 1995; Fischer et al. 2004, 2005). Ideally a gold standard investigation should be unequivocal and should have the potential to reveal subtle epithelial molecular and/or DNA changes indicative of early carcinogenesis even where clinical lesions are not seen. This is the area where adjunct use of investigations like biomarker study could play an important role in eliciting changes undetectable on conventional hematoxylin- and eosin-stained sections.

11.2.2 Vital Staining

HNSCC is a cancer that is plagued with the presence of premalignant lesions and local tumor spread adjacent to location of primary tumor and is called as field change or field cancerization. It is seen in

TABLE 11.2

Diagnostic Tools in HNSCC

Diagnostic Tools in HNSCC
Biopsy and histopathologic examination
Vital staining
DNA ploidy (chromosomal polysomy)
Brush biopsy
Optical techniques

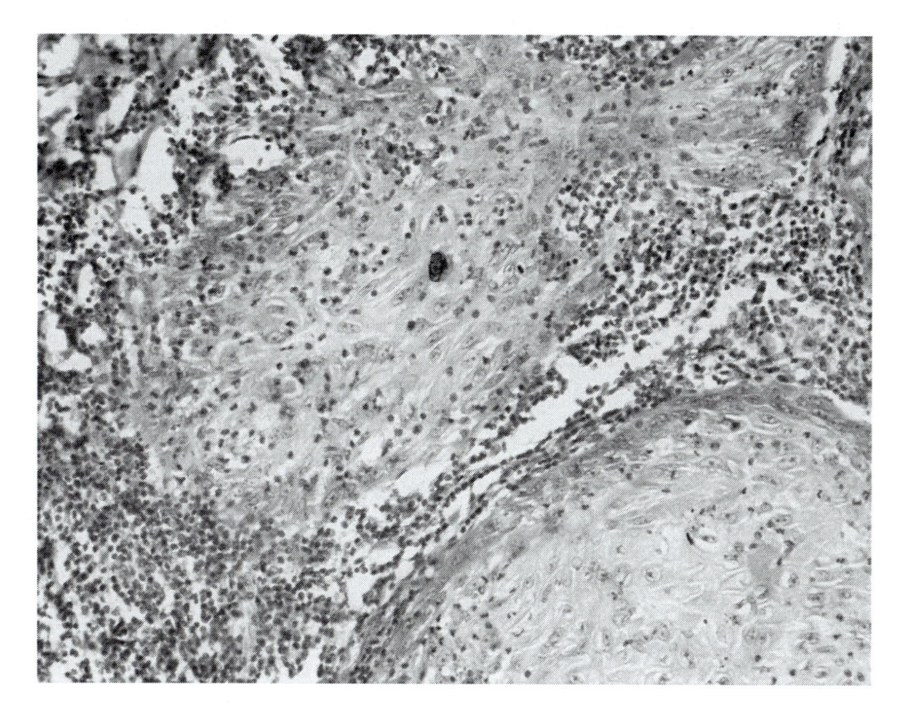

FIGURE 11.3 **(See color insert.)** Section under 20× magnification showing intact basal epithelial cells with variable shape and size with high nucleocytoplasmic ratio and hyperchromatic nuclei. There are dense mononuclear inflammatory infiltrates.

patients at high risk for HNSCC and is a major factor for tumor recurrence after surgical treatment. Adequate workup of HNSCC thus demands methods to highlight probable dysplastic areas prior to biopsy so that the diseased areas are not missed. Toluidine blue (TB), a basic metachromatic nuclear stain, is a simple and inexpensive diagnostic tool used to highlight abnormal areas of mucosa. In the high-risk population, TB has a higher sensitivity to detect carcinoma in situ (CIS) and invasive cancers when compared to a clinical oral examination (96.7% and 40%, respectively). False-positive staining is seen in 8%–10% of cases associated with keratotic lesions and the regenerating edges of ulcers and erosions. Various studies assessing TB have shown a sensitivity and specificity ranging from 93.5% to 97.8% and from 73.3% to 92.9%, respectively (Rosenberg et al. 1989, Mashberg et al. 1995).

11.2.3 DNA Ploidy in HNSCC

DNA ploidy is the measurement of nuclear DNA that provides a surrogate measure of gross chromosomal content. Multiple copies of DNA in excess of diploidy are termed polyploidy. If the chromosomes are not uniformly distributed to the daughter cells or if parts of chromosomes become detached, the chromosomal segregation during mitosis is termed aneuploidy and is commonly observed in many cancers (Hamidi et al. 2000, Diniz-Freitas et al. 2006). The methods of analyzing DNA content are flow cytometry and image analysis. The results from both the methods normally correlate well (Elsheikh et al. 1992). HNSCCs evolve from diploid squamous cells of the aerodigestive mucosa. At the time of diagnosis, about two-thirds of clinically diagnosed head and neck cancers are non-diploid, indicating that there must be an acquisition and accumulation of genetic material during tumor development. Therefore, measurement of DNA ploidy has been utilized to determine tumor's clinical behavior.

It has been demonstrated that in HNSCCs, the incidence of aneuploidy ranges from 29% to 80% (Sakr et al. 1989, Leemans et al. 1993, Wennerberg et al. 1998). Most studies have concluded that there is an association between a poor prognosis and aneuploid tumors (Stell et al. 1991, Milroy et al. 1997, Welkoborsky et al. 2000). There is no significant association for DNA ploidy in terms of locoregional recurrence or 2-year survival rate and mean DNA content of the tumor cells in node positive than in nonnegative tumors (Resnick et al. 1995, Welkoborsky et al. 2000). However, other studies could not validate this association between higher degree of aneuploidy and more aggressive behavior of tumor cell clones (Feinmesser et al. 1990). Ploidy may also play a role in determining response to radiotherapy and chemotherapy (Cooke et al. 1990). The drawbacks of ploidy study as a prognostic indicator are not only the intratumoral heterogeneity of the DNA content but also the fact that mere determination of ploidy may not be representative of existing chromosomal aberrations (El-Naggar et al. 1992). The comparative genomic hybridization (CGH) suggests that the aberrations that form the basis of aneuploidy are actually detectable in each and every HNSCC. Thus, aneuploidy is a frequent event suggesting that it is associated with early tumor development rather than advanced cancer progression and hence could not be consistently established as a prognostic marker.

Cytogenetic abnormalities including chromosomal disruptions have been shown to be a useful marker for the diagnosis and prognosis of various malignancies. The karyotypes of HNSCC are complex, often near triploid or tetraploid, and composed of multiple clonal numerical and structural chromosome abnormalities (Jin et al. 2000).

DNA aneuploidy being detectable in both nondysplastic and dysplastic lesions can be highly predictive for the subsequent development of cancer. Furthermore, tetraploidization is also detectable in preneoplasias. In multivariate analysis, DNA content was the only significant prognostic factor regarding progression toward cancer in contrast to the histological grade of dysplasia, sex, use of tobacco, size and location of lesions, and the presence of multiple lesions (Sudbo et al. 2001). Hence, the increase of DNA quantity by the induction of polyploid and then aneuploid karyotypes must be considered a very early event in HNSCC carcinogenesis. The quality of the DNA changes, that is, specific chromosomal imbalances, are then associated with different phenotypes of tumor progression.

11.2.4 Brush Biopsy

The brush biopsy uses a small nylon brush to gather cytology samples that are sent for computer scanning and analysis to identify and display individual cells. On identification of suspicious cells, a pathological examination of the sample is done that directs for a conventional incisional biopsy from clinically affected or suspicious site. The major drawback is the high false negativity and is of concern. The sensitivity, specificity, and positive and negative predictive values of brush biopsy in the diagnosis of premalignant

TABLE 11.3

Diagnostic Optical System
Laser-induced fluorescence spectroscopy
Light-induced fluorescence spectroscopy
Elastic-scattering spectroscopy
Raman spectroscopy
Photoacoustic imaging
Photon fluorescence
Orthogonal polarization spectral (OPS) imaging
Quantum dot optical coherence tomography (OCT)
Trimodal spectroscopy
Doppler OCT
Nuclear magnetic resonance spectroscopy
Chromoendoscopy
Narrow band imaging (NBI)
Immunophotodiagnostic techniques
Differential path length spectroscopy
2-Photon fluorescence
Second harmonic generation
Terahertz imaging

lesions are 71.4%, 32%, 44.1%, and 60%, respectively (Svirsky et al. 2002, Poate et al. 2004). Improved outcomes of brush biopsy may be obtained with the addition of molecular techniques. The diagnostic accuracy of brush biopsies in combination with DNA image cytometry showed an improved sensitivity of 97.8%, specificity of 100%, positive predictive value of 100%, and negative predictive value of 98.1% (Maraki et al. 2004). Besides DNA image cytometry, silver-stained nucleolar organizer region (AgNOR) analysis may be another useful adjunct. Remmerbach et al. (2003) used AgNOR and showed a sensitivity of 92.5%, specificity of 100%, positive predictive value of 100%, and negative predictive value of 84.6%.

11.2.5 Optical Systems

Interaction of light with tissues may highlight changes in tissue structure and metabolism. Optical spectroscopy systems to detect changes rely on the fact that the optical spectrum derived from a tissue will contain information about the histological and biochemical characteristics of the tissue. Such optical adjuncts may assist in identification of mucosal lesions including premalignant lesions and HNSCC, assist in biopsy site selection, and enhance visibility of surface texture and margins of lesions and may also assist in identification of cellular and molecular abnormalities not visible to the naked eye on routine examination. Some other potential diagnostic systems are listed in Table 11.3.

11.3 Biomarkers in HNSCC

With recent developments in gene sequencing, targeted therapies, and molecular diagnostics, cancer treatment is beginning to move from the traditional "trial-and-error" approach to more individualized approach, that is, giving the right drug at the right dose to the right patient. The required parameters for such effect are as follows:

- Detection of markers at an early stage of disease.
- Strong and independent prognostic markers that can reliably identify patients with indolent disease from those with aggressive forms.
- Patients with indolent disease may not need adjuvant chemotherapy, whereas those with aggressive disease are candidates for such treatment.
- Identification of markers that can prospectively predict response or resistance to specific therapy.
- Markers to identify patients who are likely to develop severe toxic effects.

Hence, the need of reliable biomarkers in HNSCC is being advocated. The use of biological markers in the body fluids for molecular detection of cancer has been the subject of an increasing number of translational studies with intent to improve overall screening accuracy and cost-effectiveness. Further, its use is being extended to identify premalignant and malignant tumor at an early stage and to prognosticate and predict therapeutic response to conventional treatment and also the treatment failure.

The study of biomarkers involves genetics, epigenetics, proteomics, RNA, and microRNA (miRNA) along with rapid development of high-throughput microarray technology and powerful bioinformatics that allow integration of complex data and molecular pathways involved in tumorigenesis.

11.3.1 Epigenetics

This is a stable inheritance of genetic information based on gene expression levels without changes in genetic code. The heritable modification of DNA occurs through several pathways including alteration in DNA methylation and histone modification. This alteration has been associated with cancer-specific gene expression differences in human malignancies and is known to occur early in tumorigenesis (Perez-Ordonez et al. 2006). As a novel mechanism of gene regulation, epigenetic control of tumor suppressor genes (TSGs) was quickly proposed as potentially important mechanism of carcinogenesis (Van Houten et al. 2004, Rodrigo et al. 2005, Belbin et al. 2008). Dysregulation of DNA methylation and associated gene expression changes in tumors and premalignant tissues makes DNA methylation profiling an attractive target for molecular studies. Since it is heritable but reversible, it also has great potential for identifying novel therapeutic targets (Bremmer et al. 2009). Studies of promoter methylation in primary tissues have revealed many TSGs in HNSCC that include *p16, Ch-6 (DIME-6), ATM, p15, TIMP-3, MGMT, RARB-2, DAP-K, E-cadherin, cyclin A-1, RASFIA, CDKN$_2$A, CDH-1,* and *DCC.* These genes function in pathways that control cell-cycle progression, apoptosis, cell to cell adhesion, DNA repair, and tumor invasion (Lipshutz et al. 1999, Ferlito et al. 2003, Diamandis et al. 2004, Rinaldo et al. 2004, Takes 2004, van Wilgen et al. 2004, Pentenero et al. 2005, Li et al. 2006, Suzuki et al. 2007, Alkureishi et al. 2008, Takes et al. 2008, Jung et al. 2009, Nagaraj et al. 2009). Hypermethylation profile gives us molecular ability to differentiate cancer for normal as well as specific cancer type (Becker et al. 2004, Yoshida et al. 2005). The use of different combinations of these genes allows improved detection of HNSCC in salivary rinse and serum (Cote et al. 1999). Evidence also supports a role for hypomethylation in tumor development (Shores et al. 2004; Elsheikh et al. 2005, 2006; Yamazaki et al. 2005). Upregulation of these genes has also shown to carry biological significance in tumor development and could be used for molecular detection. A challenge in study of epigenetic field is that epigenetic changes are tissue specific as compared to blood or other body fluid, but this can be exploited for detecting margin positivity during surgical excision (Goldenberg et al. 2004).

11.3.2 Proteomics

A number of tumor-associated proteins were frequently found to be altered in their expression in HNSCC, for example, stratifin, stathmin, heat shock protein 27, and superoxide dismutase 2 (SOD2) (Nieuwenhuis et al. 2003, Colnot et al. 2004, Ferris et al. 2005, Tsujimoto et al. 2007). Different proteins and its pattern identified in tissue and serum could be used to characterize the tumor and carry information about the carcinogenesis (Goda et al. 2009). Elevated SOD2 levels were also associated with lymph node metastasis and might provide predictive value for diagnosis of metastasis (Takes et al. 1997). Serum analysis by protein profiles used for molecular detection with reaction sensitivity and specificity of 80% and 100%, respectively (Chung et al. 2004, Roepman et al. 2005, Germani et al. 2009). Woolgar in 1999 reported development of a monofluid proteomic immunoassay to quantify total and load abundance protein isomers in nanoliter volumes, which promises to revolutionize the field of proteomics and potentially bring it one step closer for clinical diagnostic use. There are some drawbacks and limitation using proteomics to analyze valuable and limited clinical specimen. Once there is better understanding of the data produced by proteomic studies and the data is correlated with DNA and RNA expression profile and other known genetic alteration, the diagnosis, response to therapy, and recurrence might be detected by a simple blood test.

11.3.3 RNA and MicroRNA

RNA and miRNA are also being used for identification of altered gene expression in cancer. Nucleic acids can be isolated and detected in blood, urine, CSF and saliva using reverse transcription-10 chain reaction detection. This method can be used as biomarkers for cancer diagnosis (Simon et al. 2003, Michiels et al. 2005, Roepman et al. 2006). Microarray uncovered a large panel of human RNA signatures that exist in saliva and suggested that salivary transcriptome analysis could be useful in diagnostics and surveillance of oral cancer (Cromer et al. 2004). Differentially expressed mRNA transcripts between cancer and normal patients' salivary samples could be identified as potential biomarkers for cancer detection, for example, DUSPI, H$_3$F3A, OA21, S100P-SAT, IC8, and ILIB. Aberrantly expressed mRNA transcripts exhibited at least 3.5-fold elevations in cancer patients, and the combination of the biomarker panel yielded a sensitivity and specificity of 90% in distinguishing oral HNSCC from the control (O'Donnell et al. 2005). Nonetheless there is increasing evidence of aberrant expression of miRNA in HNSCC. While evaluating the expression pattern of 156 mature miRNA in HNSCC of the oral cavity, miRNA-133b was significantly reduced in tumor specimens when compared with paired normal epithelial samples, resulting in activation of a potential oncogene pyruvate kinase-type M2 (Schmalbach 2004). Using miRNA expression ratios, it was found that the miRNA-221/miRNA-375 seems to be predictive of HNSCC with sensitivity and specificity of 92% and 93%, respectively (Colella et al. 2008). The interactions of miRNA can be difficult to predict, and each one may have several hundreds to more than a thousand putative targets due to their relatively nonspecific binding to target mRNA. However, undoubtedly they play a major role in the regulation of gene expression and could potentially be utilized as molecular biomarker in tissues and body fluids (serum and saliva).

11.3.4 Human Papillomavirus Infection and HNSCC

HPV also plays an important role in unique subset of oropharyngeal HNSCC similar to cervical cancer (Wang et al. 2005, Akervall et al. 2006). HPV is present in 60% of patients with oropharyngeal HNSCC and confers a favorable prognosis in terms of recurrence and mortality. There are 13 known high-risk HPV types that can transform cells to cancer. Subtypes 6, 16, 18, 31, 33, and 35 have been identified to cause oropharyngeal HNSCC (Osman et al. 2002, Bradford et al. 2003, Foekens et al. 2006, Ganly et al. 2007). Regardless of study population, high-risk HPV 16 accounts for overwhelming majority (90%–95%) of HPV-positive tumor. HPV-positive HNSCC patients are usually nonsmoker and nondrinker and present at advanced stage. In a study of oropharyngeal cancer, nonsmokers were 15-fold more likely to be HPV positive than smokers (Bockmühl et al. 2000). Recently several clinical studies showed that HPV is an independent risk factor and does really modify the risk of HNSCCs associated with tobacco and alcohol exposure (Ashman et al. 2003). HPV-positive patients are five years younger than HPV-negative patients (Rodrigo et al. 2000, Wreesmann et al. 2004). Risk factors for seropositivity for HPV 16 viral capsid protein antibodies carry a 15-fold increased risk for HNSCC (Huang et al. 2002).

HPV status is also of prognostic value. HPV-positive patients have better response to chemoradiation than HPV-negative subset, better survival, and 60%–80% reduced risk of death (Rodrigo et al. 2009). They have much higher response, that is, 95% to chemoradiation as compared to HPV-negative patients whose response is 62% and who have higher 2-year survival rate (Gibcus et al. 2007). Considering its serological importance, the HPV positivity is labeled as valuable molecular biomarker (Brass et al. 1997).

In situ hybridization assay technique for determining the HPV DNA is presently the gold standard for clinical classification of HPV-positive tumor and is now commercially available (Singh et al. 2002). There are other tests like HPV 18, PNA and HPV 16 E6 and E7 seroactivity, and FISH (fluorescence in situ hybridization) and are currently being investigated. Similarly *Bcl 2* is also an important biomarker. Rocco et al. (2006) showed in their study that overexpressing *Bcl 2* had sixfold greater risk of treatment failure with chemoradiation (Eder et al. 2005, Kanao et al. 2005, Regala et al. 2005).

Immunohistochemical assessment of *Bcl 2* in pretreatment biopsies predicted response of oropharyngeal HNSCC to therapy and could prove to be another prognostic marker besides HPV as there was no correlation between HPV infection and *Bcl 2* status (Regala et al. 2005). More research is needed to determine correlation between HPV and *Bcl 2* statuses in predicting outcome in HNSCC.

11.3.5 Epidermal Growth Factor Receptor

Epidermal growth factor receptor (EGFR) is a tyrosine kinase receptor that belongs to Erb B family of cell receptor. This has many downstream signaling targets. When it gets activated, the receptor can signal via multiple pathways such as MAPK, AKt, RK, and JAB/sTAT. These pathways are related to cellular proliferation, apoptosis, invasion, angiogenesis, and metastasis. It is promising marker and has significant prognostic value for HNSCC. Understanding of its molecular biology has contributed in its targeted therapy. The adjacent tissue also shows overexpression and upregulation that signifies transition for dysplasia to HNSCC (Slebos et al. 2006, Singh 2008). EGFR is an important step in tumorigenesis and useful molecular marker since its elevated levels of expression confer poor survival (Smeets et al. 2009). In 2005 the continuous hyperfractionated accelerated radiotherapy (CHART) head and neck cancer phase III clinical trial demonstrated that overexpression of EGFR in pretreatment biopsies is a robust biomarker for improved response to radiotherapy and could serve as a predictive marker for therapeutic response (Sidransky et al. 1997). Follow-up studies showed that EGFR is also a potential therapeutic target for tyrosine kinase inhibitors as well as other anti-EGFR-targeted molecules (Boyle et al. 1994, Mao et al. 1994). Cetuximab is one of the best studied monoclonal antibodies directed against EGFR. A published phase III trial examined the effect of this drug in conjunction with radiotherapy in treatment of locoregionally advanced HNSCC. This study demonstrated an overall survival benefit (49 vs. 29 months) and increased duration of locoregional control (24.4 vs. 14.9 months) in the cetuximab plus radiotherapy alone versus the arm receiving only radiotherapy. This was the first randomized study showing a survival benefit with an EGFR-targeting agent in locally advanced HNSCC (Nawroz et al. 1996, Park et al. 1996).

11.3.6 Genetics and Loss of Heterozygosity

Loss of heterozygosity (LOH) is defined as the loss of a normal allele at a particular locus within a cell genome already harboring a deleterious mutation on the matching allele. LOH can arise via several pathways, including deletion, gene conversion, mitotic recombination, and chromosome loss. The latter event is sometimes followed by duplication of the remaining chromosome. Any of these events occurring at normal allele will leave the cell either hemizygous (one deleterious allele and one deleted allele) or homozygous for the deleterious allele. LOH is well known to play role in the inactivation of TSGs leading to the development of cancer. Several regions of chromosomal loss are commonly found in cancer. In HNSCC, one of the earliest and the most common of all genetic changes associated with tumorigenesis is the loss of chromosome region 9p21–22 that occurs at a frequency of 70% (van der Riet et al. 1994). Another example is the loss of chromosome region 3p (Nawroz et al. 1996). Thirty percent of benign hyperplastic lesions and the early precancerous lesions exhibited loss at either 9p21 or 3p (Nawroz et al. 1996). These studies indicate that LOH is a common event in both malignant and premalignant lesions. A retrospective study from M.D. Anderson in Houston showed that premalignant lesions demonstrating loss of chromosomes 9p21 and 3p14 more frequently progressed to HNSCC versus those patients without LOH at those loci (Mao et al. 1996). Another study done later similarly showed that patients with premalignant or benign leukoplakic lesions exhibiting losses of 3p and 9p had a 3.8-fold increased risk of progression to cancer. However, this study went on to demonstrate that additional chromosomal losses at 4q, 8p, 11q, or 17p had a 33-fold increased risk (Rosin et al. 2000). Another study screened premalignant lesions for LOH for several markers including 3p21, 8p21–23, 9p21, 13ql4.2, 17p13.1, and 18q21.1 and showed that having LOH in two or more of these regions carried a 73% probability of developing cancer in 5 years (Partridge et al. 1998) compared to those with fewer regions of loss. One of the most promising areas relating LOH to everyday practice is the ability to analyze premalignant and tumor margin tissue for regions of chromosomal loss, known to be associated with increased risk of progression to carcinoma. A few studies analyzing histologically normal margins have also shown that LOH within the field of cancerization may lead to tumor development (Tabor et al. 2001, 2004). Currently, LOH screening panels are not available commercially; however, commercial LOH testing is in the developmental phase and being used in screening and surveillance clinical trials for SCC of the upper aerodigestive tract. In the future, it is proposed that LOH testing will improve our ability to accurately diagnose and treat pre-microscopic disease and may be the only way to truly decrease the risk of recurrence in patients battling HNSCC.

There is relatively common pattern of DNA allelic loss during the progression from premalignant to malignant phenotype. Using simple polymerase chain reaction (PCR)-based molecular techniques, one can identify these losses of genetic material represented by complete deletion or loss of one allele. TSGs may be in the area of loss and thus would make the cell more susceptible to dysfunction that could further lead to cancer development especially if the same gene already contains a deleterious mutation on the matching allele.

11.4 Classification of Biomarkers

The classification of biomarkers are shown in Tables 11.4 and 11.5.

TABLE 11.4

Potential Biomarkers in Head and Neck Cancers

Major Classes	Member	Function
Cell-cycle regulation	*p16*^{INK4A}	A tumor suppressor gene regulating senescence and cell-cycle progression
	PT53	Suppressor gene regulating cell-cycle progression and cell survival
	PTEB	A tumor suppressor gene signaling pathways controlling cell proliferation and apoptosis
	Rb	A tumor suppressor gene regulating cell-cycle progression and apoptosis
	Cyclin D1	A proto-oncogene regulating cell-cycle progression
Signal transduction	EGFR	A transmembrane TK that acts as a central transducer of multiple signaling pathways
	VEGF	A transmembrane TK that promotes the proliferation, migration, and survival of endothelial cells during tumor growth
Extracellular matrix	Matrix metalloproteinases (MMPs)	A family of zinc-dependent proteolytic enzymes that degrade the basement membrane and other components of the extracellular matrix
Prostaglandin metabolism	Cox-2	A catalytic enzyme that decreases apoptosis, increases immunosuppression, and enhances the potential for tumor progression
Oncovirus	EBV	A causative agent for most nasopharyngeal carcinomas
	HPV	A causative agent for most oropharyngeal cancers

TABLE 11.5

Biomarkers for Early Detection of HNSCC with Sensitivity and Specificity

Reference	Specimen	Marker	Sensitivity (%)	Specificity (%)
Nunes et al. (2000)	Wash and brushing	Microsatellite instability (MSI)	84	100
Rosas et al. (2001)	Saliva	Methylation	65	96
Ranuncolo et al. (2002)	Plasma	MMP-9	81	80
Li et al. (2004)	Saliva	Transcriptomes	91	91
St. John et al. (2004)	Saliva and serum	IL-8 and IL-6	99	90
Lee et al. (2006)	Sputum	MAGE A1–A6	76	96
Linkov et al. (2007)	Serum	MMP, EGF, CK-19	84.5	98
Carvalho et al. (2008)	Serum	Methylation	65	72
Toyoshima (2008)	Tumor	CK-17 real-time quantitative PCR	94.6	—
Ries et al. (2008)	Tumor	MAGE A1–A6	85.5	100
Marcos et al. (2009)	Serum	MMP-13 and anti-*p53*	76	100
Park et al. (2009)	Saliva	miRNA	AUC 0.66	—

11.5 Methods of Assessment of Biomarkers

The various methods of assessment have been documented and currently practiced methods are as follows:

1. Autofluorescence
2. Western blot
3. Enzyme-linked immunosorbent assay (ELISA)
4. Immunohistochemistry (IHC)
5. 2D gel electrophoresis (2DGE) or 2D liquid chromatography (2DLC)

The criteria for using a particular technique should encompass the guidelines that the technology should be cost-effective, practical, and reproducible. ELISA and IHC are commonly employed methods to detect protein in body fluid and tissues, respectively. Recently, mass spectroscopy has been found to be an important method for detection of such proteins.

The various methods of assessment involve extracts from fresh frozen plasma, serum, for the assessment of autoantibodies. Fresh frozen plasma extraction (FFPE) is the most practical and simple since it provides enough archives of patients' sample, thereby permitting retrospective analysis as well. It preserves the morphological details within the cells because of cross-linking of intracellular proteins. The limitation has been the clinical validation for routine diagnosis (Table 11.6).

TABLE 11.6

Methods of Early Detection of Biomarkers

Sample	Method	Biomarker	Verification	Indication
FFPE	RPLC	Desmoglein 3	IHC	Carcinogenesis
		Cytokeratin 4		
		Cytokeratin 16		
		Desmoplakin		
		Vimentin		
	LCMS	Keratin 13	WB, IHC, RT-PCR	Epigenetically silenced gene
		Keratin 4		
		Annexin 1		
Tissue in HNSCC	2D DIGE	Keratin 4, 13	IHC	Premalignant tissue and second fluid tumor tissue
		Cornulin		
Tissue in HNSCC	CTRAQ/MDGC	S100-A7	IHC, WB, RT-PCR	HNSCC
Tissue in premalignant leukoplakia	iTRAQ	S100-A7	IHC, WB, RT-PCR	Epithelial dysplasia
Oral squamous cell carcinoma (OSCC) saliva	2DGE	S100-A9	ELISA	OSCC
	LC	Mac-2-binding protein	WB	
HNSCC saliva	2D DIGE	S100-A9	WB	Early detection
Tissue	IMAC 30 protein chip arrays	α-Defensin 1–3	IHC tissue microarray	Tumor relapse
Serum analysis	DIGF and iTRAQ	EGFR	ELISA, WB, IHC	Tissue and tumor invasion
Autoantibodies	2D-WB of OSCC and fibroblast cell lines	Sideroflexin 3	ELISA, IHC	Tumor burden

TABLE 11.7

Biomarkers according to Clinical Importance

Carcinogenesis Biomarkers	Tumor Progression Biomarkers	Tumor Relapse Biomarkers	Predictive Biomarkers
• Interleukin 8 and 6 • Melanoma-associated gene (MAGE) • MSI • MMPs • Cytokeratin 17 (CK-17) • miRNA • Actin and myosin	• Sideroflexin 3 • EGFR	• α-Defensins 1–3	• Keratin 13 • Keratin 4 • Annexin 1 • S100-A9 • Mac-2-binding protein

Common protein markers identified are S100-7, keratin 4, and keratin 13. S100-7 is upregulated, whereas keratins 4 and 7 are downregulated. S100-7 is a calcium-binding protein of S100 family, and its association is proven in dysregulation of keratinocyte differentiation and is considered as marker for invasion. Keratins 4 and 13 are present in supra-basal layer of the epithelium and have been shown to play important role in the premalignant conditions. These are found to be downregulated in epithelial tumors more so in HNSCC.

11.6 Role of Biomarkers in Clinical Setting

A biomarker is a biochemical, molecular, or genetic parameter that can be objectively measured and evaluated to discern the presence and progress of disease. With the onset of the molecular revolution and understanding of the molecular pathways, involved in tumor initiation and progression, the armament of potential biomarkers has been greatly expanded. Biomarkers were used primarily as prognostic indicators in the past, but today the role of biomarkers has been greatly expanded to address all aspects of patient care, from early cancer detection, to more accurate tumor staging, to the selection of those patients most likely to benefit from specific therapies, to posttreatment tumor surveillance (Table 11.7).

11.7 Identification of High-Risk Premalignant Lesions

Although premalignant lesions are at risk of progressing to overtly malignant lesions, assessment of histological parameters in such lesions may be subtle and overlapping with nonneoplastic reactive processes. Furthermore, there is considerable variation among pathologists in the recognition and grading of premalignant lesions. LOH at defined chromosomal loci may help in identifying the precursor lesions most likely to develop into HNSCCs. Several studies on oral dysplasias have shown that dual LOH at 3p and 9p can reliably distinguish those lesions that are likely to progress to invasive carcinoma from those that will not (Nawroz et al. 1996; Park et al. 2007, 2009).

11.8 Detection of HNSCC in Preclinical Stage (Screening)

Early cancer diagnosis using saliva as a substrate for biomarker assessment is one of the promising breakthrough in present time. Saliva has been used as a noninvasive, inexpensive, and readily accessible diagnostic substrate to assess diverse biomarkers including HPV status (Garber et al. 2004, Hu et al. 2008), promoter hypermethylation profile (van't Veer et al. 2002, Kallioniemi et al. 2004),

TP53 gene mutations (Ma et al. 2010), telomerase activity, and differential gene expression profiles (Tabor et al. 2001). For patients with HNSCCs the methylation profiles and HPV status of their tumors can be discerned from molecular genetic analysis of their oral washes. Despite the documented feasibility of saliva-based strategies, early-detection saliva assays have yet to prove their feasibility for broad population-based screening.

11.9 Tumor Localization

A significant subset of patients with HNSCC present with metastatic spread to cervical lymph nodes in the absence of a primary tumor by clinical, radiographic, endoscopic, and even histopathologic evaluation. Biomarkers can be used in pinpointing the primary site of tumor origin (Ramaswamy et al. 2003). In this regard the detection of certain oncogenic viruses that target specific regions of the upper aerodigestive tract can help in detection of primary lesion (Caldas et al. 2002). In effect, detection of a specific virus in the metastasis implicates the site of probable tumor origin. Most notably, detection of Epstein–Barr virus in a neck metastasis reliably points to tumor origin from the nasopharynx. Although this approach seems to be readily feasible for diagnostic laboratories with in situ hybridization facility, its far application is limited, as only few HNSCCs have been linked with tumorigenic virus. The application of this approach has been expanded with the recognition that HPV 16 is an important causative factor for HNSCCs arising from the oropharynx but not from nasopharyngeal sites; the study in individual cells aspirated from metastatic nodes can reliably point to the site of tumor origin as oropharynx (Caldas et al. 2002).

11.10 Tumor Extent, Including Its Relationship to Surgical Margins

Time-tested methods that rely on clinical inspection and microscopic examination to detect the extent of the neoplastic process have been frustratingly ineffective when it comes to cancer of the head and neck. Inexplicably, after excision, tumors can recur in microscopically free margins. The "field cancerization" effect leads to development of second tumor at different site and reappearance and progression of premalignant lesions that regress during chemoprevention once therapy is halted. Clearly, novel methods are required to permit better mapping of this elusive cancer spread. Assisted visualization of oral neoplasia in the intraoperative setting is being developed. Studies suggested staining the oral mucosa with the vital dye TB as a means of visualizing the subclinical disease. Abnormal staining of the oral mucosa has been shown to correlate with the presence of dysplasia, LOH, and increased cancer risk (van't Veer and Bernards et al. 2008). Studies on visual assessment of oral cavity luminescence under blue excitation light (400–460 nm) or following a chemical reaction (i.e., chemiluminescence) as a means of discrimination between normal and neoplasia mucosa have been done with encouraging results in detecting subclinical tumor extent (Reid et al. 2005, Dunkler et al. 2007). The changes in the metabolic activity of the surface epithelial cells induce spectral changes that impart tissue fluorescence signatures that are utilized for this purpose. At certain wavelengths, autofluorescence visualization of the oral mucosa provides a more complete topographical view of the neoplastic field, including its spatial relationship to surgical margins (Fakhry et al. 2006).

The traditional definition of a negative surgical margin now demands redefinition in light of the propensity of genetically damaged cells present in apparently normal-looking mucosa even on histologic examination to populate extended tracts of histologically normal oral mucosa. Indeed, the presence of genetically altered cells can be detected in histologically normal mucosal margins using a variety of strategies for detecting genetic alterations including *TP53* mutations (Lindel et al. 2001, D'Souza et al. 2007), LOH (Li et al. 2003), promoter hypermethylation (Mellin et al. 2000, Schwartz et al. 2001), and eIF4E proto-oncogene overexpression (Weinberger et al. 2006). Importantly, the presence of these genetically damaged cells has been shown to predict local tumor recurrence in patients who have undergone tumor resections with histologically clear margins. The biggest disadvantage of using biomarkers for detection of negative tumor margins is lack of retrieving instantaneous results unlike vital staining and autofluorescence. This limits its use intraoperatively; however, automation and streamlining of methodologies dramatically decrease turnaround times, even to the point that genetic analysis of surgical margins may become feasible in the intraoperative setting (Begum et al. 2003, Smeets et al. 2007, Chuang et al. 2008).

11.11 Detection of Micrometastasis

The incidence of occult subpathologic metastases in patients with HNSCC has a mean incidence of 15.2% (Rinaldo et al. 2004). In 2005, Yoshida et al. investigated immunohistochemically the presence of occult metastases in cervical lymph nodes from 24 patients with T2 N0 tongue cancer and found micrometastasis in 58% patients. The routine light microscopic histologic examination of neck dissection specimens fails to detect a portion of these occult nodal metastases. It is supported by the evidence that the recurrence rates of approximately 10% are reported in patients, who had histopathologically negative neck dissection but harboring occult metastasis (Becker et al. 2004). The observations merely indicate inaccurate staging in 10% patients. Further, the retrospective studies using the more sensitive and expensive techniques of complete sectioning and immune histochemistry of the lymph nodes have found that 8%–20% of patients with HNSCC have nodal metastases that were not identified by routine histopathologic examination (Rinaldo et al. 2004). In accordance, Cote et al. (1999) determined that the identification of regions of metastasis by hematoxylin and eosin (H&E) staining of negative lymph nodes on histologic examination required the analysis of up to 144 slides/patient, and therefore, it is not surprising that regions of metastasis within the lymph node are not detected on routine histopathologic examination. This emphasizes the need for serial microscopic sectioning of the nodes that might reveal micrometastases, but is impractical for routine use. Since the routine histology has significant chances of missing nodal metastasis, currently the molecular diagnostic techniques are being considered for its detection more effectively.

Several RNA-based markers were successfully used to detect lymph node metastasis in head and neck cancer. In 2005, Elsheikh et al. prospectively examined 48 patients with SCC of the oral cavity, with no palpable cervical lymph nodes who underwent an elective supraomohyoid neck dissection. The incidence of micrometastasis to lymph nodes was evaluated by pathological examination as well as by molecular analysis (CK20 mRNA expression). Of the 48 patients, 15 (31%) by pathological analysis and 22 (46%) by molecular analysis had lymph nodes positive for metastatic SCC. Using molecular analysis, 5 (10%) of the 48 patients had involvement of sublevel IIB lymph nodes, and the authors concluded that clinically uninvolved sublevel IIB lymph nodes can be left behind in elective supraomohyoid neck dissections in patients with SCC elsewhere in the oral cavity, but should be included whenever tongue is the primary site. The same authors prospectively investigated 31 patients with SCC of the larynx who underwent an elective lateral neck dissection (Elsheikh et al. 2006). The incidence of micrometastasis to lymph nodes in lateral neck dissection specimens was evaluated by nested reverse-transcription PCR (RT-PCR) for cytokeratin 19 (CK19) and cytokeratin 20 (CK20), as well as by pathological examination. Nested RT-PCR for CK19 and CK20 mRNA presented similar results to each other, but these results differed from those of routine pathological examination. Of the 31 patients, 6 (19%) by pathological analysis and 9 (29%) by molecular analysis had lymph nodes positive for metastatic SCC, and only 1 of the 31 patients had involvement of sublevel IIB lymph nodes. Other investigators used the detection of CK14 mRNA by RT-PCR as a marker of nodal metastases and found that CK14 RT-PCR is highly sensitive for detecting micrometastasis in lymph nodes that are negative by routine pathological examination, but with a relatively high false-positive (50%) rate (Shores et al. 2004). To avoid this problem, determination of *p53* mutations in lymph nodes using mutant allele-specific amplification (MASA) in 21 patients with HNSCC, 4 out of 10 pN0 (40%) were genetically positive, and 44 (9%) of the 476 lymph nodes diagnosed as negative by H&E staining were found to contain DNA with the same mutation as detected in the primary tumor (Yamazaki et al. 2005). In addition, they observed that patients with multiple or lower neck spread of micrometastases as detected by DNA assay have a poor prognosis. A potential problem in the use of DNA markers might be that DNA is an extremely stable molecule and tumor-derived DNA might find its way to the lymph nodes. This caused false-positive results when applied to the detection of minimal disease in histopathologically tumor-free surgical margins (Van Houten et al. 2004). In addition at the RNA level, HNSCC-associated antigens such as the E48 (hLy-6D) allow the detection of rare HNSCC cells in blood and bone marrow and also in lymph nodes and lymph node aspirates (Nieuwenhuis et al. 2003, Colnot et al. 2004).

A successful novel molecular diagnostic method for rapid evaluation of lymph node metastasis is one-step nucleic acid amplification (OSNA) (Tsujimoto et al. 2007). This intraoperative molecular diagnostic method can quantitatively measure CK19 mRNA expression. This assay consists of a sample preparation and rapid gene amplification by RT-LAMP (reverse-transcription loop-mediated isothermal amplification). The whole process takes only 30 min. Using quantitative reverse-transcription PCR (QRT-PCR), four markers have been identified that can discriminate between positive and benign nodes with accuracy greater than 97% (Ferris et al. 2005). These markers were PVA (pemphigus vulgaris antigen) (also known as desmoglein 3), SCCA1/2 (SCC antigen) (neutral and acidic forms), PTHrP (parathyroid hormone-related protein), and TACSTD1 (also known as EPCAM). Moreover, one of these markers, PVA, discriminated with 100% accuracy between positive and benign lymph nodes. A rapid QRT-PCR assay for PVA has been developed and incorporated into a completely automated RNA isolation and QRT-PCR instrument (the GeneXpert) for molecular diagnostic testing. This automated analysis is completed (from tissue to result) in about 30 min, thus demonstrating its feasibility in intraoperative staging of HNSCC sentinel lymph nodes. To develop a more efficient method for intraoperative genetic detection of lymph node metastasis in HNSCC, a total of 291 lymph nodes (59 patients) resected on SLN biopsy for cN0 HNSCC or neck dissection for cN1/2 HNSCC were diagnosed by OSNA method using GD-100 (Goda et al. 2009). It is speculated that because of high sensitivity and specificity, the OSNA assay could be used as a novel genetic detection tool of lymph node metastasis in HNSCC patients.

Apart from the time constraints, the major problem of all of these methods is that these do not easily fit in the routine logistics of the pathological examination of the dissection specimens. Most molecular methods work only reliably on fresh or frozen tissues and require direct sampling from the surgical specimen, are more sophisticated technically, and cannot be easily planned in daily practice. Alternatively, when methods would be suitable for analysis on formalin-fixed paraffin-embedded samples, then additional cuts of the block are required. These molecular methods seem, therefore, most suited for rapid and sensitive analysis of subgroups of lymph node, such as the sentinel lymph nodes.

11.12 Predictive Tests for Nodal Metastasis in Clinically N0 Patients

For decades, predictors for nodal metastasis have been sought, realizing that it would not be likely that a single marker could predict this event that is the result of very complex processes (Takes et al. 1997, 2008). Many patients with a clinically negative neck receive inappropriate treatment due to difficulties in preoperative detection of metastases in the cervical lymph nodes (Woolgar 1999, Robbins et al. 2002). However, numerous single markers have been studied that showed a significant correlation with nodal metastasis (Germani et al. 2009). However, no consistently relevant marker, validated in larger series, has been established till date. Recently, signatures have been identified for prediction of lymph node metastasis in patients with head and neck cancer based on the gene expression measurements in the primary tumor (Chung et al. 2004, Roepman et al. 2005). The potential clinical relevance of these signatures resides in the difficulties for currently diagnosing the absence of lymph node metastasis in patients with head and neck cancer. A large set of 825 genes have been identified that can be used for prediction of lymph node metastasis in clinically N0 patients, and based on this group of genes, multiple predictive signatures can be made with high-predictive accuracy (Michiels et al. 2005, Roepman et al. 2006).

11.13 Prognostication

Despite a bewildering large number of studies evaluating the prognostic significance of cell proliferation (e.g., *Ki67*, PCNA), *p53* immunohistochemical staining, apoptosis, aneuploidy, EGFR overexpression, and many other biomarkers, none has consistently proved reliable across multiple studies, and none is currently used in routine surgical practice.

The prognostic impact of currently used biomarkers is not altogether surprising, given the complexity of HNSCC tumorigenesis requiring the concerted actions of multiple genetic alterations and the differential impact of various gene-altering events. For example, about 50% of HNSCC harbors *TP53* gene mutations, but these mutations are highly divergent in their impact on *p53* protein structure, stability, DNA-binding properties, and clinical outcome, depending on where they occur. *TP53* mutational analysis is apparently a much more powerful prognostic indicator when clinical outcomes are measured against the specific type of *TP53* mutation (Zumbach et al. 2000). The *TP53* mutations that occur within the core domain completely blocking DNA binding have been correlated with accelerated tumor progression, reduced therapeutic responsiveness, and decreased patient survival compared to HNSCCs that harbor less disruptive *TP53* mutations.

The presence of HPV 16 is now recognized as a highly favorable prognostic indicator in HNSCC. When compared with HPV-negative to those with HPV-positive tumors, HPV-positive tumors have a lower risk of tumor progression and death (Gillison et al. 2006). A recent prospective multi-institutional study showed that when HNSCCs were uniformly treated with chemoradiation, HPV-positive tumor showed 73% lower risk of tumor progression and 64% lower risk of death when compared to HPV-negative patients (Capone et al. 2000). The mechanisms underlying these clinical differences may involve the combined effects of immune surveillance to viral-specific tumor antigens, an intact apoptotic response to radiation, and the absence of widespread genetic alterations (i.e., field cancerization).

11.14 Molecular-Targeted Therapy in HNSCC

Molecular-targeted therapies for HNSCC are rapidly becoming popular. A number of phase III trials in patients with advanced HNSCC are already underway especially with drugs targeting EGFR. Trial design now rests on the use of appropriate biomarkers to effectively identify those patients who will benefit from EGFR-targeted therapy. Confirmation of oncogenic HPV as an important causative agent in oropharyngeal cancer has opened the door for vaccine immunotherapy. Determination of HPV status will soon be a routine part of the pathologic evaluation of HNSCCs, at least for those cancers arising from the oropharynx.

11.14.1 Targeting the Epidermal Growth Factor Receptor Pathway

A growing understanding of the molecular genetic underpinning of HNSCC now permits the development of novel therapies that target specific components of the molecular genetic apparatus supporting tumor development and growth. A transmembrane tyrosine kinase receptor (EGFR) that acts as a central transducer of multiple signaling pathways is involved in tumor cell growth, angiogenesis, and invasion (Hynes et al. 2005). EGFR overexpression has been associated with a high local recurrence rate and poor survival in HNSCC (Rocco et al. 2006, Michaud et al. 2009). Although more than 90% of HNSCCs overexpress EGFR, only a small subset of HNSCCs demonstrate amplified copy numbers or mutational activation of the EGFR gene (Hynes et al. 2005). Instead, EGFR activation in HNSCC is driven in part by high expression of its ligands, resulting in the formation of powerful autocrine and paracrine loops. Binding of ligands to EGFR induces dimerization of EGFR, autophosphorylation of its intracellular kinase domain, and activation of multiple oncogenic pathways.

Targeted therapy has taken aim at different points along this signal transduction sequence in an effort to blockade EGFR function. Monoclonal antibodies (e.g., cetuximab) directed against the extracellular receptor domain seek to block ligand binding, prevent receptor dimerization, induce receptor degradation, and activate antitumoral immune responses. Tyrosine kinase inhibitors (e.g., erlotinib, gefitinib) are small molecules that interact with the cellular domain of EGFR to inhibit its phosphorylation function. EGFR gene silencing can be accomplished by various posttranscriptional strategies including the use of sequence-specific antisense oligodeoxynucleotides and small interfering RNAs (Rubin Grandis et al. 1998). Antisense oligodeoxynucleotides are antisense DNA strands that bind complementary EGFR mRNA and block protein synthesis. Small interfering RNAs are short double-stranded RNAs that bind a sequence-specific mRNA and trigger its destruction via the RNA interference pathway.

Despite the importance of overexpression in head and neck tumorigenesis, EGFR blockade as monotherapy has been only modestly successful in the treatment of patients with HNSCC (Rogers et al. 2005, Kalyankrishna et al. 2006). The limited success of monotherapy is not altogether surprising given the complexity and divergency of signaling pathways involved in tumor growth, invasion, and metastasis. Accordingly, current strategies seek to combine EGFR blockade with other traditional and nontraditional treatment modalities. Cetuximab used in combination with radiation therapy has recently been established as an effective regimen for improving locoregional control and survival in patients with locoregionally advanced HNSCC (Ishitoya et al. 1989, Ang et al. 2002). Additional trials suggest that cetuximab and other EGFR inhibitors may similarly enhance the effects of platinum-based chemotherapy (Maxwell et al. 1989, Kearsley et al. 1990, Grandis et al. 1993). Ongoing efforts to optimize EGFR blockade are combining agents with specific but no overlapping anti-EGFR activity, such as the combination of anti-EGFR monoclonal antibodies and tyrosine kinase inhibitor (Shin 1994). Another strategy involves the concomitant targeting of other signaling pathways that are independent of the EGFR pathways or that may intersect the EGFR pathway network. As one example, resistance to EGFR has been attributed, in part, to increased levels of vascular endothelial growth factor (VEGF). This in turn has generated interest in the use of dual inhibitors of both the EGFR and VEGF receptors (Grandis Rubin et al. 1998).

11.14.2 Newer Potential Targets for Therapy in HNSCC

Src kinases are involved in the regulation of a variety of normal cellular signal transduction pathways that influence cell proliferation and correlate with disease progression (Hofman et al. 2008). Src activation results in potentiation of EGFR-mediated tumor growth by stimulating FAK, STAT, and PI3K (Zhang et al. 2004). Recently published in vitro experiments show that Src family kinases are highly activated in cetuximab-resistant cells and enhance EGFR activation (Wheeler et al. 2009). Dual targeted treatment approaches directed at both EGFR and Src might therefore be a feasible strategy for overcoming or preventing acquired resistance to cetuximab. Dasatinib is a potent inhibitor of multiple oncogenic kinases including Src, cKIT, BCR-ABL, PDGFR, and ephrin A. Because of its ability to inhibit BCR-ABL, it was approved for treatment of chronic myeloid leukemia in 2006. Currently dasatinib is being evaluated in phase I clinical trials for solid tumors either alone or in combination with cetuximab (Johnson et al. 2005). Proteasomes are proteinases, which play a critical role in degradation of the proteins responsible for the control of cell growth. This has been documented through increased cytotoxic ability of bortezomib (a proteasome inhibitor) in EGF-stimulated HNSCCs cell lines (Wagenblast et al. 2008). Further, the bortezomib has demonstrated antitumor effects by induction of apoptosis and sensitization of malignant cells to conventional cytotoxic drugs in myeloma and lymphomas and was recently tested in phase II trials in HNSCC in combination with docetaxel or irinotecan (Chung et al. 2010). Preliminary results have shown 50% disease control rates in recurrent or metastasizing HNSCC patients with the use of low-dose bortezomib (Dudek et al. 2009). Phase III trials with optimized dosing schedules are needed to confirm these promising new treatment options, which were usually associated with acceptable toxicity.

11.15 Vaccine Strategies

The finding of HPV 16 in a distinct subset of HNSCCs provides a unique opportunity for the prevention and treatment of these cancers by vaccines, designed to induce appropriate HPV virus-specific immune response (Bentzen et al. 2005). The aim of a preventive vaccine is to prime the immune system so that it is able to induce high titers of neutralizing antibody upon exposure to a high-risk HPV to block cellular entry and prevent the development of an established infection. The ultimate prophylactic vaccine must (1) prime an antibody response that is specific for neutralizing epitopes on HPV, (2) induce an immune response that is long lasting, and (3) impede infection at the point of HPV contact, that is, the tonsillar crypts. A major breakthrough in preventive HPV vaccines came with the demonstration that the HPV capsid proteins can self-assemble resulting in high titers of neutralizing antibodies that inhibit the early stages of HPV cell binding and cell entry (Lin et al. 2003).

Therapeutic HPV vaccines aim to clear virally infected cells, inhibit progression of HPV-associated dysplasia, and eradicate established neoplasms. For established infections, utilization of T cell-mediated immunity against nonstructural viral antigens appears to be a more effective strategy in clearing infections and eradicating tumors. The HPV E6 and E7 proteins are ideal antigens for targeted immunotherapy. The reasons for this are as follows: (1) the E6 and E7 proteins are uniquely expressed by tumor cells but not by normal tissues, (2) HPV-associated carcinoma represents 20%–25% of all HNSCC and 60%–70% of HNSCCs arising in the oropharynx, (3) constitutive expression of E6 and E7 is requisite for maintenance of the tumor phenotype such that evasion of immune responses is not likely to occur by E6/E7 downregulation, and (4) these viral proteins are completely foreign and highly immunogenic.

A variety of HPV vaccines are under investigation including viral vector vaccines, bacterial vector vaccines, peptide/protein vaccines, DNA vaccines, and cell-based vaccines (Mackova et al. 2006). Preliminary data with an HPV DNA vaccine indicate that it is well tolerated in all patients. It is associated with minimal toxicity, and it generates significant levels of circulating HPV E7-specific immune cell postvaccination. Now that early-phase clinical trials have demonstrated the safety and feasibility of DNA-based HPV vaccines, efforts are now under way to enhance potency by optimizing delivery, frequency of immunizations, coadministration with adjuvant immune-enhancing agents, and two-staged delivery programs (i.e., prime–boost vaccines) (Califano et al. 1996, Karamouzis et al. 2007).

In June 2006, the US Food and Drug Administration approved the HPV vaccine Gardasil™ as an effective method of preventing cervical cancer and precancerous lesions due to HPV types 6, 11, 16, and 18. The Center for Disease Control recommends routine vaccination of girls and young women as a means of reducing cases of cervical cancer. The growing recognition of HPV-related HNSCCs in women and men underscores the reality that HPV-induced neoplasia is not gender specific (Devaraj et al. 2003). HPV-related malignancies of all types, including HNSCCs, are expected to retreat in the face of effective HPV prophylaxis. Accordingly, HPV vaccination will likely be recommended for all individuals, boys and girls alike, prior to onset of sexual activity. Clinical trials are already under way using HPV vaccines in the treatment of HPV-associated HNSCCs (Fiander et al. 2006). Based on animal models, HPV vaccines appear to be most effective for the eradication of low-volume disease (Badaracco et al. 2007). Accordingly, therapeutic vaccines may be most effective not as monotherapy, but as adjunctive therapy to clear residual microscopic disease following conventional surgical excision and/or radiation.

11.16 Patent Information on HNSCC Biomarkers

The available patent information on HNSCC biomarkers are shown in the following table.

Patent No	Filing Date	Inventor	Title	Comments/Assignee
US 7910293	March 28, 2008	Sinha, Uttam K. (United States), Los Angeles, CA (United States) Masood, Rizwan (United States), Los Angeles, CA (United States)	Development of prognostic markers from the saliva of head and neck cancer patients	Patent granted University of Southern California, Los Angeles, CA (United States)
US 8088591	May 14, 2007	Franzmann, Elizabeth J. (United States), Miami, FL (United States) Lokeshwar, Vinata B. (United States), Miami, FL (United States)	Biomarkers for detection and diagnosis of head and neck squamous cell carcinoma	Patent granted University of Miami, Miami, FL (United States)
US 2005/0214880 A1	March 28, 2005	Elizabeth J. Franzmann, Vinata B. Lokeshwar, Erika P. Reategui	Salivary soluble CD44: a molecular marker for head and neck cancer	Patent granted University of Miami, Miami, FL (United States)
WO 2011/095498 A1	February 2, 2011	DA Cruz, Luis A.G., 57 Nipigon Avenue Toronto, Ontario M2M 2V9 (CA) Franzmann, Elizabeth, Jane, 12701 SW 69th Avenue Miami, FL 33156 (United States)	A monoclonal antibody to CD44 for use in the treatment of head and neck squamous cell carcinoma	
AU 2007/249805 A1	May 14, 2007	Lokeshwar, Vinata B. Franzmann, Elizabeth J.	Biomarkers for detection and diagnosis of head and neck squamous cell carcinoma	
US 2009/0325201 A1	May 14, 2007	Franzmann, Elizabeth J. (United States), Miami, FL (United States) Lokeshwar, Vinata B. (United States), Miami, FL (United States)	Biomarkers for detection and diagnosis of head and neck squamous cell carcinoma	University of Miami, Miami, FL (United States)
US 2012/0115165 A1	December 13, 2011	Franzmann, Elizabeth J. (United States), Miami, FL (United States) Lokeshwar, Vinata B. (United States), Miami, FL (United States)	Biomarkers for detection and diagnosis of head and neck squamous cell carcinoma	University of Miami, Miami, FL (United States)
US 8088591	May 14, 2007	Franzmann, Elizabeth J. (United States), Miami, FL (United States) Lokeshwar, Vinata B. (United States), Miami, FL (United States)	Biomarkers for detection and diagnosis of head and neck squamous cell carcinoma	Patent granted University of Miami, Miami, FL (United States)
2007/133725 A1 591	May 14, 2007	Franzmann, Elizabeth J., 12701 SW 69th Avenue Miami, FL 33156 (United States) Lokeshwar, Vinata B., 12615 SW 112th Court Miami, FL 33176 (United States)	Biomarkers for detection and diagnosis of head and neck squamous cell carcinoma	
US 2011/0200556 A1	August 20, 2009	Gutkind, J. Silvio (United States), Potomac, MD (United States) Amornphimoltham, Panomwat (United States), Bethesda, MD (United States) Patel, Vyomesh (United States), Washington, DC (United States) Molinolo, Alfredo (United States), Rockville, MD (United States) Czerninski, Rakefet (Israel), Mevaseret Zion (Israel)	Chemoprevention of head and neck squamous cell carcinomas	The United States, as represented by the Secretary, Department of Health and Human Services, Bethesda, MD (United States)

(continued)

Patent No	Filing Date	Inventor	Title	Comments/Assignee
US 2009/ 0246761 A1	March 28, 2008	Sinha, Uttam K. (United States), Los Angeles, CA (United States) Masood, Rizwan (United States), Los Angeles, CA (United States)	Development of prognostic markers from the saliva of head and neck cancer patients	University of Southern California, Los Angeles, CA (United States)
US 7910293	March 28, 2008	Sinha, Uttam K. (United States), Los Angeles, CA (United States) Masood, Rizwan (United States), Los Angeles, CA (United States)	Development of prognostic markers from the saliva of head and neck cancer patients	Patent granted University of Southern California, Los Angeles, CA (United States)

11.17 Conclusion

Cancer and HNSCC in particular are the result of dysregulation of a complex system of molecular signaling pathways resulting from changes in DNA, RNA, and posttranscriptional molecules. Integration of information from several different "omics" is needed for understanding of the complex biology of cancer. Despite a substantial research effort over 25 years, very few prognostic markers and predictive assays have been established in routine clinical oncology specially in HNSCC like HPV, EGFR, LOH, and miRNA that have been of documented practical value. Large and multicentric collaborative networks with appropriately designed study are the need of the day for establishing the role of biomarkers in early detection and their therapeutic use in HNSCC. The most important initial ingredient will be large well-conducted validation studies that will provide definitive evidence on the diagnostic value of specific tests. After validation, a future could be envisaged in which classification systems and prognostic models contain molecular information enabling improved treatment choices and better outcomes.

References

Abbey LM, Kaugars GE, Gunsolley JC, Burns JC, Page DG, Svirsky JA, Eisenberg E, Krutchkoff DJ, and Cushing M. Intraexaminer and interexaminer reliability in the diagnosis of oral epithelial dysplasia. *Oral Surg Oral Med Oral Pathol* 1995;80:188–191.

Akervall J. Genomic screening of head and neck cancer and its implications for therapy planning. *Eur Arch Otorhinolaryngol* 2006;263:297–304.

Alkureishi LWT, Ross GL, and Shoaib T. Does tumor depth affect nodal upstaging in squamous cell carcinoma of the head and neck? *Laryngoscope* 2008;42(4):629–634. doi: 10.1097/MLG.0b013e31815e8bf0.

Andl T, Kahn T, Pfuhl A, Nicola T, Erber R, Conradt C et al. Etiological involvement of oncogenic human papillomavirus in tonsillar squamous cell carcinomas lacking retinoblastoma cell cycle control. *Cancer Res* 1998;58(1):5–13.

Ang KK, Berkey BA, Tu X, Zhang HZ, Katz R, Hammond EH et al. Impact of epidermal growth factor receptor expression on survival and pattern of relapse in patients with advanced head and neck carcinoma. *Cancer Res* December 15, 2002;62(24):7350–7356.

Ashman JN, Patmore HS, Condon LT, Cawkwell L, Stafford ND, and Greenman J. Prognostic value of genomic alterations in head and neck squamous cell carcinoma detected by comparative genomic hybridisation. *Br J Cancer* 2003;89:864–869.

Badaracco G and Venuti A. Human papillomavirus therapeutic vaccines in head and neck tumors. *Expert Rev Anticancer Ther* 2007;7:753–766.

Barnes L, Rogers S, Eveson JW, Reichart P, and Sidransky D. *Pathology and Genetics of Head and Neck Tumors.*World Health Organization Classification of Tumors. IARC Press, Lyon, 2005.

Becker MT, Shores CG, Yu KK, and Yarbrough WG. Molecular assay to detect metastatic head neck squamous cell carcinoma. *Arch Otolaryngol Head Neck Surg* 2004;130:21–27.

Begum S, Gillison ML, Ansari-Lari MA, Shah K, and Westra WH. Detection of human papillomavirus in cervical lymph nodes: A highly effective strategy for localizing site of tumor origin. *Clin Cancer Res* December 15, 2003;9(17):6469–6475.

Belbin TJ, Schlecht NF, Smith RV, Adrien LR, Kawachi N, Brandwein-Gensler M, Bergman A, Chen Q, Childs G, and Prystowsky MB. Site-specific molecular signatures predict aggressive disease in HNSCC. *Head Neck Pathol* 2008;2:243–256.

Bentzen SM, Atasoy BM, Daley FM, Dische S, Richman PI, Saunders MI et al. Epidermal growth factor receptor expression in pretreatment biopsies from head and neck squamous cell carcinoma as a predictive factor for a benefit from accelerated radiation therapy in a randomized controlled trial. *J Clin Oncol* August 20, 2005;23(24):5560–5567.

Bockmühl U, Schlüns K, Küchler I, Petersen S, and Petersen I. Genetic imbalances with impact on survival in head and neck cancer patients. *Am J Pathol* 2000;157:369–375.

Boyle JO, Mao L, Brennan JA, Koch WM, Eisele DW, Saunders JR, and Sidransky D. Gene mutations in saliva as molecular markers for head and neck squamous cell carcinomas. *Am J Surg* 1994;168:429–432.

Bradford CR, Zhu S, Ogawa H, Ogawa T, Ubell M, Narayan A, Johnson G, Wolf GT, Fisher SG, and Carey TE. P53 mutation correlates with cisplatin sensitivity in head and neck squamous cell carcinoma lines. *Head Neck* 2003;25:654–661.

Brass N, Heckel D, Sahin U, Pfreundschuh M, Sybrecht GW, and Meese E. Translation initiation factor eIF-4 gamma is encoded by an amplified gene and induces an immune response in squamous cell lung carcinoma. *Hum Mol Genet* 1997;6:33–39.

Bremmer JF, Graveland AP, Brink A, Braakhuis BJ, Kuik DJ, Leemans CR, Bloemena E, van der Waal I, and Brakenhoff RH. Screening for oral precancer with noninvasive genetic cytology. *Cancer Prev Res (Philadelphia, PA)* 2009;2:128–133.

Caldas C and Aparicio SA. The molecular outlook. *Nature* 2002;415:484–485.

Califano J, van der Riet P, Westra W, Nawroz H, Clayman G, Piantadosi S et al. Genetic progression model for head and neck cancer: Implications for field cancerization. *Cancer Res* June 1, 1996;56(11):2488–2489.

Capone RB, Pai SI, Koch WM, Gillison ML, Danish HN, Westra WH et al. Detection and quantitation of human papillomavirus (HPV) DNA in the sera of patients with HPV-associated head and neck squamous cell carcinoma. *Clin Cancer Res* November 2000;6(11):4171–4175.

Carvalho AL, Jeronimo C, Kim MM, Henrique R, Zhang Z, Hoque MO, Chang S et al. Evaluation of promoter hypermethylation detection in body fluids as a screening/diagnosis tool for head and neck squamous cell carcinoma. *Clin Cancer Res* 2008;14:97–107.

Chiesa F, Sala L, Costa L, Moglia D, Mauri M, Podrecca S, Andreola S, Marchesini R, Bandieramonte G, and Bartoli C. Excision of oral leukoplakias by CO_2 laser on an out-patient basis: A useful procedure for prevention and early detection of oral carcinomas. *Tumori* 1986;72:307–312.

Chuang AY, Chuang TC, Chang S, Zhou S, Begum S, Westra WH et al. Presence of HPV DNA in convalescent salivary rinses is an adverse prognostic marker in head and neck squamous cell carcinoma. *Oral Oncol* October 2008;44(10):915–919.

Chung CH, Aulino J, Muldowney NJ, Hatakeyama H, Baumann J, Burkey B, Netterville J et al. Nuclear factor-kappa B pathway and response in a phase II trial of bortezomib and docetaxel in patients with recurrent and/or metastatic head and neck squamous cell carcinoma. *Ann Oncol* April 2010;21(4):864–870.

Chung CH, Parker JS, Karaca G, Wu J, Funkhouser WK, Moore D, Butterfoss D et al. Molecular classification of head and neck squamous cell carcinomas using patterns of gene expression. *Cancer Cell* 2004;5:489–500.

Colella S, Richards KL, Bachinski LL, Baggerly KA, Tsavachidis S, Lang JC, Schuller DE, and Krahe R. Molecular signatures of metastasis in head and neck cancer. *Head Neck* 2008;30:1273–1283.

Colnot DR, Nieuwenhuis EJC, Kuik DJ, Leemans CR, Dijkstra J, Snow GB, Van Dongen GAMS, and Brakenhoff RH. Clinical significance of micrometastatic cells detected by E48 (Ly-6D) reverse transcriptase-polymerase chain reaction in bone marrow of head and neck cancer patients. *Clin Cancer Res* 2004;10:7827–7833.

Cooke LD, Cooke TG, Bootz F, Forster G, Helliwell TR, Spiller D, and Stell PM. Ploidy as a prognostic indicator in end stage squamous cell carcinoma of the head and neck region treated with cisplatinum. *Br J Cancer* May 1990;61(5):759–762.

Cote RJ, Peterson HF, Chaiwun B, Gelber RD, Goldhirsch A, Castiglione-Gertsch M, Gusterson B, and Neville AM. Role of immunohistochemical detection of lymph-node metastases in management of breast cancer. International Breast Cancer Study Group. *Lancet* 1999;354:896–900.

Cromer A, Carles A, Millon R, Ganguli G, Chalmel F, Lemaire F, Young J et al. Identification of genes associated with tumorigenesis and metastatic potential of hypopharyngeal cancer by microarray analysis. *Oncogene* 2004;23:2484–2498.

D'Souza G, Kreimer AR, Viscidi R, Pawlita M, Fakhry C, Koch WM et al. Case-control study of human papillomavirus and oropharyngeal cancer. *N Engl J Med* May 10, 2007;356(19):1944–1956.

Devaraj K, Gillison ML, and Wu TC. Development of HPV vaccines for HPV-associated head and neck squamous cell carcinoma. *Crit Rev Oral Biol Med* 2003;14:345–362.

Diamandis EP. Mass spectrometry as a diagnostic and a cancer biomarker discovery tool: Opportunities and potential limitations. *Mol Cell Proteomics* 2004;3:367–378.

Diniz-Freitas M, Garcia-Caballero T, Antunez-Lopez J, Gandara-Rey JM, and Garcia-Garcia A. Reduced E-cadherin expression is an indicator of unfavourable prognosis in oral squamous cell carcinoma. *Oral Oncol* 2006;42:190–200.

Dudek AZ, Lesniewski-Kmak K, Shehadeh NJ, Pandey ON, Franklin M, Kratzke RA, Greeno EW, and Kumar P. Phase I study of bortezomib and cetuximab in patients with solid tumours expressing epidermal growth factor receptor. *Br J Cancer* 2009;9:1379–1384.

Dunkler D, Michiels S, and Schemper M. Gene expression profiling: Does it add predictive accuracy to clinical characteristics in cancer prognosis? *Eur J Cancer* 2007;43:745–751.

Eder AM, Sui X, Rosen DG, Nolden LK, Cheng KW, Lahad JP, Kango-Singh M et al. Atypical PKCiota contributes to poor prognosis through loss of apical-basal polarity and cyclin E overexpression in ovarian cancer. *Proc Natl Acad Sci USA* 2005;102:12519–12524.

El-Naggar AK, Lopez-Varela V, Luna MA, Weber R, and Batsakis JG. Intratumoral DNA content heterogeneity in laryngeal squamous cell carcinoma. *Arch Otolaryngol Head Neck Surg* 1992;118:169–173.

Elsheikh MN, Mahfouz ME, and Elsheikh E. Level IIb lymph nodes metastasis in elective supraomohyoid neck dissection for oral cavity squamous cell carcinoma: A molecular-based study. *Laryngoscope* 2005;115:1636–1640.

Elsheikh MN, Mahfouz ME, Salim EI, and Elsheikh EA. Molecular assessment of neck dissections supports preserving level IIB lymph nodes in selective neck dissection for laryngeal squamous cell carcinoma with a clinically negative neck. *ORL J Otorhinolaryngol Relat Spec* 2006;68:177–184.

Elsheikh TM, Silverman JF, McCool JW, and Riley RS. Comparative DNA analysis of solid tumors by flow cytometric and image analyses of touch imprints and flow cell suspensions. *Am J Clin Pathol* 1992;98:296–304.

Fakhry C and Gillison ML. Clinical implications of human papillomavirus in head and neck cancers. *J Clin Oncol* June 10, 2006;24(17):2606–2611.

Feinmesser R, Freeman JL, and Noyek A. Flow cytometric analysis of DNA content in laryngeal cancer. *J Laryngol Otol* June 1990;104(6):485–487.

Ferlito A, Rinaldo A, Robbins KT, Leemans CR, Shah JP, Shaha AR, Andersen PE et al. Changing concepts in the surgical management of the cervical node metastasis. *Oral Oncol* 2003;39:429–435.

Ferris RL, Xi L, Raja S, Hunt JL, Wang J, Gooding WE, Kelly L, Ching J, Luketich JD, and Godfrey TE. Molecular staging of cervical lymph nodes in squamous cell carcinoma of the head and neck. *Cancer Res* 2005;65:2147–2156.

Fiander AN, Tristram AJ, Davidson EJ, Tomlinson AE, Man S et al. Prime-boost vaccination strategy in women with high-grade, noncervical anogenital intraepithelial neoplasia: Clinical results from a multicenter phase II trial. *Int J Gynecol Cancer* 2006;16:1075–1081.

Fischer DJ, Epstein JB, Morton TH, and Schwartz SM. Interobserver reliability in the histopathologic diagnosis of oral premalignant and malignant lesions. *J Oral Pathol Med* 2004;33:65–70.

Fischer DJ, Epstein JB, Morton TH, and Schwartz SM. Reliability of histologic diagnosis of clinically normal intraoral tissue adjacent to clinically suspicious lesions in former upper aerodigestive tract cancer patients. *Oral Oncol* 2005;41:489–496.

Foekens JA, Atkins D, Zhang Y, Sweep FC, Harbeck N, Paradiso A, Cufer T et al. Multicenter validation of a gene expression-based prognostic signature in lymph node-negative primary breast cancer. *J Clin Oncol* 2006;24:1665–1671.

Ganly I, Talbot S, Carlson D, Viale A, Maghami E, Osman I, Sherman E et al. Identification of angiogenesis/metastases genes predicting chemoradiotherapy response in patients with laryngopharyngeal carcinoma. *J Clin Oncol* 2007;25:1369–1376.

Garber K. Genomic medicine: Gene expression tests foretell breast cancer's future. *Science* 2004; 303:1754–1755.

Germani RM, Civantos FJ, Elgart G, Roberts B, and Franzmann EJ. Molecular markers of micrometastasis in oral cavity carcinomas. *Otolaryngol Head Neck Surg* 2009;141:52–58.

Gibcus JH, Menkema L, Mastik MF, Hermsen MA, de Bock GH, van Velthuysen ML, Takes RP et al. Amplicon mapping and expression profiling identify the Fas-associated death domain gene as a new driver in the 11q13.3 amplicon in laryngeal/pharyngeal cancer. *Clin Cancer Res* 2007;13:6257–6266.

Gillison ML. Human papillomavirus and prognosis of oropharyngeal squamous cell carcinoma: Implications for clinical research in head and neck cancers. *J Clin Oncol* December 20, 2006;24(36):5623–5625.

Goda H, Nakashiro K, Yoshimura T, Sumida T, Wakisaka H, Hato N, Hyodo M, and Hamakawa H. One-step nucleic acid amplification for detecting lymph node metastasis of head and neck cancer. *J Clin Oncol* 2009;27:15s.

Goldenberg D, Harden S, Masayesva BG, Ha P, Benoit N, Westra WH et al. Intraoperative molecular margin analysis in head and neck cancer. *Arch Otolaryngol Head Neck Surg* 2004;130(1):39–44.

Grandis JR, Melhem MF, Gooding WE, Day R, Holst VA, Wagener MM et al. Levels of TGF-alpha and EGFR protein in head and neck squamous cell carcinoma and patient survival. *J Natl Cancer Inst* June 3, 1998;90(11):824–832.

Grandis JR and Tweardy DJ. Elevated levels of transforming growth factor alpha and epidermal growth factor receptor messenger RNA are early markers of carcinogenesis in head and neck cancer. *Cancer Res* August 1, 1993;53(15):3579–3584.

Hamidi S, Salo T, Kainulainen T, Epstein J, Lerner K, and Larjava H. Expression of alpha(v)beta6 integrin in oral leukoplakia. *Br J Cancer* 2000;82:1433–1440.

Hauswald H, Simon C, Hecht S, Debus J, and Lindel K. Long-term outcome and patterns of failure in patients with advanced head and neck cancer. *Radiat Oncol* June 10, 2011;6:70.

Hofman P, Butori C, Havet K, Hofman V, Selva E, Guevara N, Santini J, and Van Obberghen-Schilling E. Prognostic significance of cortact in levels in head and neck squamous cell carcinoma: Comparison with epidermal growth factor receptor status. *Br J Cancer* March 11, 2008;98(5):956–964.

Hu S, Arellano M, Boontheung P, Wang J, Zhou H, Jiang J, Elashoff D, Wei R, Loo JA, and Wong DT. Salivary proteomics for oral cancer biomarker discovery. *Clin Cancer Res* 2008;14:6246–6252.

Huang X, Gollin SM, Raja S, and Godfrey TE. High-resolution mapping of the 11q13 amplicon and identification of a gene, TAOS1, that is amplified and overexpressed in oral cancer cells. *Proc Natl Acad Sci USA* 2002;99:11369–11374.

Hynes NE and Lane HA. ERBB receptors and cancer: The complexity of targeted inhibitors. *Nat Rev Cancer* May 2005;5(5):341–354.

Ishitoya J, Toriyama M, Oguchi N, Kitamura K, Ohshima M, Asano K et al. Gene amplification and overexpression of EGF receptor in squamous cell carcinomas of the head and neck. *Br J Cancer* April 1989;59(4):559–562.

Jemal A, Siegel R, Ward E, Murray T, Xu J, and Thun MJ. Cancer statistics. *CA Cancer J Clin* 2007;57(1): 43–66.

Jin C, Jin Y, Wennerberg J, Dictor M, and Mertens F. Nonrandom patterns of cytogenetic abnormalities in squamous cell carcinoma cell lines. *Genes Chromosomes Cancer* 2000;28:66–76.

Johnson FM, Saigal B, Talpaz M, and Donato NJ. Dasatinib (BMS-354825) tyrosine kinase inhibitor suppresses invasion and induces cell cycle arrest and apoptosis of head and neck squamous cell carcinoma and non-small cell lung cancer cells. *Clin Cancer Res* 2005;19(Pt 1):6924–6932.

Jung J, Cho NH, Kim J, Choi EC, Lee SY, Byeon HK, Park YM, Yang WS, and Kim SH. Significant invasion depth of early oral tongue cancer originated from the lateral border to predict regional metastases and prognosis. *Int J Oral Maxillofac Surg* 2009;38:653–660.

Kallioniemi O. Medicine: Profile of a tumour. *Nature* 2004;428:379–382.

Kalyankrishna S and Grandis JR. Epidermal growth factor receptor biology in head and neck cancer. *J Clin Oncol* June 10, 2006;24(17):2666–2672.

Kanao H, Enomoto T, Kimura T, Fujita M, Nakashima R, Ueda Y, Ueno Y et al. Overexpression of LAMP3/TSC403/DC-LAMP promotes metastasis in uterine cervical cancer. *Cancer Res* 2005;65:8640–8645.

Karabulut A, Reibel J, Therkildsen MH, Praetorius F, Nielsen HW, and Dabelsteen E. Observer variability in the histologic assessment of oral premalignant lesions. *J Oral Pathol Med* 1995;24:198–200.

Karamouzis MV, Grandis JR, and Argiris A. Therapies directed against epidermal growth factor receptor in aerodigestive carcinomas. *JAMA* July 4, 2007;298(1):70–82.

Kearsley JH, Furlong KL, Cooke RA, and Waters MJ. An immunohistochemical assessment of cellular proliferation markers in head and neck squamous cell cancers. *Br J Cancer* June 1990;61(6):821–827.

Kreimer AR, Clifford GM, Boyle P, and Franceschi S. Human papillomavirus types in head and neck squamous cell carcinomas worldwide: A systematic review. *Cancer Epidemiol Biomark Prev* 2005;14(2):467–475.

Lee KD, Lee HH, Joo HB, Lee HS, Yu TH, Chang HK, Jeon CH, and Park JW. Expression of MAGE A 1–6 mRNA in sputa of head and neck cancer patients—A preliminary report. *Anticancer Res* 2006;26:1513–1518.

Leemans CR, Tiwari R, Nauta JJ, van der Waal I, and Snow GB. Regional lymph node involvement and its significance in the development of distant metastases in head and neck carcinoma. *Cancer (Philadelphia, PA)* 1993;71:452–456.

Li W, Thompson CH, O'Brien CJ, McNeil EB, Scolyer RA, Cossart YE et al. Human papillomavirus positivity predicts favourable outcome for squamous carcinoma of the tonsil. *Int J Cancer* September 10, 2003;106(4):553–558.

Li Y, Elashoff D, Oh M, Sinha U, St John MA, Zhou X, Abemayor E, and Wong DT. Serum circulating human mRNA profiling and its utility for oral cancer detection. *J Clin Oncol* 2006;24:1754–1760.

Li Y, St. John MA, Zhou X, Kim Y, Sinha U, Jordan RC, Eisele D et al. Salivary transcriptome diagnostics for oral cancer detection. *Clin Cancer Res* 2004;10:8442–8450.

Liang C, Marsit CJ, McClean MD, Nelson HH, Christensen BC, Haddad RI, Clark JR et al. Biomarkers of HPV in head and neck squamous cell carcinoma. *Cancer Res* October 1, 2012;72(19):5004–5013.

Lin CT, Hung CF, Juang J, He L, Lin KY et al. Boosting with recombinant vaccinia increases HPV-16 E7-specificTcell precursor frequencies and antitumor effects of HPV-16 E7-expressing Sindbis virus replicon particles. *Mol Ther* 2003;8:559–566.

Lindel K, Beer KT, Laissue J, Greiner RH, and Aebersold DM. Human papillomavirus positive squamous cell carcinoma of the oropharynx: A radiosensitive subgroup of head and neck carcinoma. *Cancer* August 15, 2001;92(4):805–813.

Linkov F, Lisovich A, Yurkovetsky Z, Marrangoni A, Velikokhatnaya L, Nolen B, Winans M et al. Early detection of head and neck cancer: Development of a novel screening tool using multiplexed immunobead-based biomarker profiling. *Cancer Epidemiol Biomark Prev* 2007;16:102–107.

Lipshutz RJ, Fodor SP, Gingeras TR, and Lockhart DJ. High density synthetic oligonucleotide arrays. *Nat Genet* 1999;21(1 Suppl):20–24.

Ma XJ, Wang Z, Ryan PD, Isakoff SJ, Barmettler A, Fuller A, Muir B et al. Current potential and limitations of molecular diagnostic methods in head and neck cancer. *Eur Arch Otorhinolaryngol* 2010;267:851–860.

Mackova J, Stasikova J, Kutinova L, Masin J, Hainz P et al. Prime/boost immunotherapy of HPV16-induced tumors with E7 protein delivered by Bordetella adenylate cyclase and modified vaccinia virus Ankara. *Cancer Immunol Immunother* 2006;55:39–46.

Mao L, Lee DJ, Tockman MS, Erozan YS, Askin F, and Sidransky D. Microsatellite alterations as clonal markers for the detection of human cancer. *Proc Natl Acad Sci USA* 1994;91:9871–9875.

Mao L, Lee JS, Fan YH, Ro JY, Batsakis JG, Lippman S et al. Frequent microsatellite alterations at chromosomes 9p21 and 3p14 in oral premalignant lesions and their value in cancer risk assessment. *Nat Med* 1996;2(6):682–685.

Maraki D, Becker J, and Boecking A. Cytologic and DNA-cytometric very early diagnosis of oral cancer. *J Oral Pathol Med* 2004;33:398–404.

Marcos CA, Martinez DAK, de los Toyos JR, Dominguez Iglesias F, Hermsen M, Guervos MA, and Pendas JLL. The usefulness of new serum tumor markers in head and neck squamous cell carcinoma. *Otolaryngol Head Neck Surg* 2009;140:375–380.

Mashberg A and Samit A. Early diagnosis of asymptomatic oral and oropharyngeal squamous cancers. *CA Cancer J Clin* 1995;45:328–351.

Maxwell SA, Sacks PG, Gutterman JU, and Gallick GE. Epidermal growth factor receptor protein-tyrosine kinase activity in human cell lines established from squamous carcinomas of the head and neck. *Cancer Res* March 1, 1989;49(5):1130–1137.

Mehrotra R, Singh M, Gupta RK, Singh M, and Kapoor AK. Trends of prevalence and pathological spectrum of head and neck cancers in North India. *Indian J Cancer* 2005;42(2):89–93.

Mellin H, Friesland S, Lewensohn R, Dalianis T, and Munck-Wikland E. Human papillomavirus (HPV) DNA in tonsillar cancer: Clinical correlates, risk of relapse, and survival. *Int J Cancer* May 20, 2000;89(3):300–304.

Michaud WA, Nichols AC, Mroz EA, Faquin WC, Clark JR, Begum S et al. Bcl-2 blocks cisplatin-induced apoptosis and predicts poor outcome following chemoradiation treatment in advanced oropharyngeal squamous cell carcinoma. *Clin Cancer Res* March 1, 2009;15(5):1645–1654.

Michiels S, Koscielny S, and Hill C. Prediction of cancer outcome with microarrays: A multiple random validation strategy. *Lancet* 2005;365:488–492.

Milroy CM, Ferlito A, Devaney KO, and Rinaldo A. Role of DNA measurements of head and neck tumors. *Ann Otol Rhinol Laryngol* 1997;106:801–804.

Nagaraj NS. Evolving "omics" technologies for diagnostics of head and neck cancer. *Brief Funct Genomic Proteomic* 2009;8:49–59.

Nawroz H, Koch W, Anker P, Stroun M, and Sidransky D. Microsatellite alterations in serum DNA of head and neck cancer patients. *Natl Med* 1996;2:1035–1037.

Nieuwenhuis EJ, Jaspars LH, Castelijns JA, Bakker B, Wishaupt RG, Denkers F, Leemans CR, Snow GB, and Brakenhoff RH. Quantitative molecular detection of minimal residual head and neck cancer in lymph node aspirates. *Clin Cancer Res* 2003;9:755–761.

Nunes DN, Kowalski LP, and Simpson AJ. Detection of oral and oropharyngeal cancer by microsatellite analysis in mouth washes and lesion brushings. *Oral Oncol* 2000;36:525–528.

O'Donnell RK, Kupferman M, Wei SJ, Singhal S, Weber R, O'Malley B, Cheng Y et al. Gene expression signature predicts lymphatic metastasis in squamous cell carcinoma of the oral cavity. *Oncogene* 2005;24:1244–1251.

Osman I, Sherman E, Singh B, Venkatraman E, Zelefsky M, Bosl G, Scher H et al. Alteration of p53 pathway in squamous cell carcinoma of the head and neck: Impact on treatment outcome in patients treated with larynx preservation intent. *J Clin Oncol* 2002;20:2980–2987.

Park NJ, Zhou H, Elashoff D, Henson BS, Kastratovic DA, Abemayor E, and Wong DT. Salivary microRNA: Discovery, characterization, and clinical utility for oral cancer detection. *Clin Cancer Res* 2009;15:5473–5477.

Park NJ, Zhou X, Yu T, Brinkman BM, Zimmermann BG, Palanisamy V, and Wong DT. Characterization of salivary RNA by cDNA library analysis. *Arch Oral Biol* 2007;52:30–35.

Park OK, Schaefer TS, and Nathans D. In vitro activation of Stat3 by epidermal growth factor receptor kinase. *Proc Natl Acad Sci USA* 1996;93:13704–13708.

Partridge M, Emilion G, Pateromichelakis S, A'Hern R, Phillips E, and Langdon J. Allelic imbalance at chromosomal loci implicated in the pathogenesis of oral precancer, cumulative loss and its relationship with progression to cancer. *Oral Oncol* March 1998;34(2):77–83.

Pentenero M, Gandolfo S, and Carrozzo M. Importance of tumor thickness and depth of invasion in nodal involvement and prognosis of oral squamous cell carcinoma: A review of the literature. *Head Neck* 2005;27:1080–1091.

Perez-Ordonez B, Beauchemin M, and Jordan RCK. Molecular biology of squamous cell carcinoma of the head and neck. *J Clin Pathol* 2006;59:445–453.

Poate TW, Buchanan JA, Hodgson TA, Speight PM, Barrett AW, Moles DR, Scully C, and Porter SR. An audit of the efficacy of the oral brush biopsy technique in a specialist Oral Medicine unit. *Oral Oncol* 2004;40:829–834.

Ramaswamy S, Ross KN, Lander ES, and Golub TR. A molecular signature of metastasis in primary solid tumors. *Nat Genet* 2003;33:49–54.

Ranuncolo SM, Matos E, Loria D, Vilensky M, Rojo R, Bal de Kier Joffe E, and Ines Puricelli L. Circulating 92-kiloDalton matrix metalloproteinase (MMP-9) activity is enhanced in the euglobulin plasma fraction of head and neck squamous cell carcinoma. *Cancer* 2002;94:1483–1491.

Regala RP, Weems C, Jamieson L, Copland JA, Thompson EA, and Fields AP. Atypical protein kinase Ciota plays a critical role in human lung cancer cell growth and tumorigenicity. *J Biol Chem* 2005;280:31109–31115.

Reid JF, Lusa L, De Cecco L, Coradini D, Veneroni S, Daidone MG, Gariboldi M, and Pierotti MA. Limits of predictive models using microarray data for breast cancer clinical treatment outcome. *J Natl Cancer Inst* 2005;97:927–930.

Remmerbach TW, Weidenbach H, Muller C, Hemprich A, Pomjanski N, Buckstegge B, and Bocking A. Diagnostic value of nucleolar organizer regions (AgNORs) in brush biopsies of suspicious lesions of the oral cavity. *Anal Cell Pathol* 2003;25:139–146.

Resnick JM, Uhlman D, Niehans GA, Gapany M, Adams G, Knapp D, and Jaszcz W. Cervical lymph node status and survival in laryngeal carcinoma: Prognostic factors. *Ann Otol Rhinol Laryngol* 1995;104:685–694.

Ries J, Vairaktaris E, Mollaoglu N, Wiltfang J, Neukam FW, and Nkenke E. Expression of melanoma-associated antigens in oral squamous cell carcinoma. *J Oral Pathol Med* 2008;37:88–93.

Rinaldo A, Devaney KO, and Ferlito A. Immunohistochemical studies in the identification of lymph node micrometastases in patients with squamous cell carcinoma of the head and neck. *ORL J Otorhinolaryngol Relat Spec* 2004;66:38–41.

Ritchie JM, Smith EM, Summersgill KF, Hoffman HT, Wang D, Klussmann JP et al. Human papillomavirus infection as a prognostic factor in carcinomas of the oral cavity and oropharynx. *Int J Cancer* 2003;104(3):336.

Robbins KT, Clayman G, Levine PA, Medina J, Sessions R, Shaha A, Som P, Wolf GT, American Head and Neck Society, American Academy of Otolaryngology-Head and Neck Surgery. Neck dissection classification update: Revisions proposed by the American Head and Neck Society and the American Academy of Otolaryngology-Head and Neck Surgery. *Arch Otolaryngol Head Neck Surg* 2002;128:751–758.

Rocco JW, Leong CO, Kuperwasser N, DeYoung MP, and Ellisen LW. p63 mediates survival in squamous cell carcinoma by suppression of p73-dependent apoptosis. *Cancer Cell* January 2006;9(1):45–56.

Rodrigo JP, Ferlito A, Suárez C, Shaha AR, Silver CE, Devaney KO, Bradley PJ et al. New molecular diagnostic methods in head and neck cancer. *Head Neck* 2005;27:995–1003.

Rodrigo JP, García LA, Ramos S, Lazo PS, and Suárez C. EMS1 gene amplification correlates with poor prognosis in squamous cell carcinomas of the head and neck. *Clin Cancer Res* 2000;6:3177–3182.

Rodrigo JP, García-Carracedo D, García LA, Menéndez S, Allonca E, González MV, Fresno MF, Suárez C, and García-Pedrero JM. Distinctive clinicopathological associations of amplification of the cortactin gene at 11q13 in head and neck squamous cell carcinomas. *J Pathol* 2009;217:516–523.

Roepman P, Kemmeren P, Wessels LFA, Slootweg PJ, and Holstege FC. Multiple robust signatures for detecting lymph node metastasis in head and neck cancer. *Cancer Res* 2006;66:2361–2366.

Roepman P, Wessels LFA, Kettelarij N, Kemmeren P, Miles AJ, Lijnzaad P, Tilanus MGJ et al. An expression profile for diagnosis of lymph node metastases from primary head and neck squamous cell carcinomas. *Nat Genet* 2005;37:182–186.

Rogers SJ, Harrington KJ, Rhys-Evans P, Charoenrat PO, and Eccles SA. Biological significance of c-erbB family oncogenes in head and neck cancer. *Cancer Metastasis Rev* January 2005;24(1):47–69.

Rosas SL, Koch W, da Costa Carvalho MG, Wu L, Califano J, Westra W, Jen J, and Sidransky D. Promoter hypermethylation patterns of p16, O6-methylguanine-DNA-methyltransferase, and death-associated protein kinase in tumors and saliva of head and neck cancer patients. *Cancer Res* 2001;61:939–942.

Rosenberg D and Cretin S. Use of meta-analysis to evaluate tolonium chloride in oral cancer screening. *Oral Surg Oral Med Oral Pathol* 1989;67:621–627.

Rosin MP, Cheng X, Poh C, Lam WL, Huang Y, Lovas J et al. Use of allelic loss to predict malignant risk for low-grade oral epithelial dysplasia. *Clin Cancer Res* 2000;6(2):357–362.

Rubin Grandis J, Melhem MF, Gooding WE, Day R, Holst VA, Wagener MM et al. Levels of TGF-alpha and EGFR protein in head and neck squamous cell carcinoma and patient survival. *J Natl Cancer Inst* 1998;90(11):824–832.

Sakr W, Hussan M, Zarbo RJ, Ensley J, and Crissman JD. DNA quantitation and histologic characteristics of squamous cell carcinoma of the upper aerodigestive tract. *Arch Pathol Lab Med* 1989;113:1009–1014.

Schmalbach CE, Chepeha DB, Giordano TJ, Rubin MA, Teknos TN, Bradford CR, Wolf GT et al. Molecular profiling and the identification of genes associated with metastatic oral cavity/pharynx squamous cell carcinoma. *Arch Otolaryngol Head Neck Surg* 2004;130:295–302.

Schwartz SR, Yueh B, McDougall JK, Daling JR, and Schwartz SM. Human papillomavirus infection and survival in oral squamous cell cancer: A population-based study. *Otolaryngol Head Neck Surg* July 2001;125(1):1–9.

Sciubba JJ. Oral cancer. The importance of early diagnosis and treatment. *Am J Clin Dermatol* 2001;2:239–251.

Shin DM, Ro JY, Hong WK, and Hittelman WN. Dysregulation of epidermal growth factor receptor expression in premalignant lesions during head and neck tumorigenesis. *Cancer Res* June 15, 1994;54(12):3153–3159.

Shores CG, Yin X, Funkhouser W, and Yarbrough W. Clinical evaluation of a new molecular method for detection of micrometastases in head and neck squamous cell carcinoma. *Arch Otolaryngol Head Neck Surg* 2004;130:937–942.

Sidransky D. Nucleic acid-based methods for the detection of cancer. *Science* 1997;278:1054–1059.

Simon R, Radmacher MD, Dobbin K, and McShane LM. Pitfalls in the use of DNA microarray data for diagnostic and prognostic classification. *J Natl Cancer Inst* 2003;95:14–18.

Singh B and Pfister DG. Individualized treatment selection in patients with head and neck cancer: Do molecular markers meet the challenge? *J Clin Oncol* 2008;26:3114–3116.

Singh B, Reddy PG, Goberdhan A, Walsh C, Dao S, Ngai I, Chou TC et al. p53 regulates cell survival by inhibiting PIK3CA in squamous cell carcinomas. *Genes Dev* 2002;16:984–993.

Slebos RJ, Yi Y, Ely K, Carter J, Evjen A, Zhang X, Shyr Y et al. Gene expression differences associated with human papillomavirus status in head and neck squamous cell carcinoma. *Clin Cancer Res* 2006;12:701–709.

Smeets SJ, Brakenhoff RH, Ylstra B, van Wieringen WN, van de Wiel MA, Leemans CR, and Braakhuis BJM. Genetic classification of oral and oropharyngeal carcinomas identifies subgroups with a different prognosis. *Cell Oncol* 2009;31:291–300.

Smeets SJ, Hesselink AT, Speel EJ, Haesevoets A, Snijders PJ, Pawlita M et al. A novel algorithm for reliable detection of human papillomavirus in paraffin embedded head and neck cancer specimen. *Int J Cancer* December 1, 2007;121(11):2465–2472.

St. John MA, Li Y, Zhou X, Denny P, Ho CM, Montemagno C, Shi W et al. Interleukin-6 and interleukin-8 as potential biomarkers for oral cavity and oropharyngeal squamous cell carcinoma. *Arch Otolaryngol Head Neck Surg* 2004;130:929–935.

Stell PM. Ploidy in head and neck cancer: A review and meta-analysis. *Clin Otolaryngol* 1991;16:510–516.

Sudbo J, Ried T, Bryne M, Kildal W, Danielsen H, and Reith A. Abnormal DNA content predicts the occurrence of carcinomas in non-dysplastic oral white patches. *Oral Oncol* 2001;37:558–565.

Suzuki M, Suzuki T, Asai M, Ichimura K, Nibu K, Sugasawa M, and Kaga K. Clinicopathological factors related to cervical lymph node metastasis in a patient with carcinoma of the oral floor. *Acta Otolaryngol* 2007;Suppl 559:129–135. *Eur Arch Otorhinolaryngol* 2007;267:851–860.

Svirsky JA, Burns JC, Carpenter WM, Cohen DM, Bhattacharyya I, Fantasia JE, Lederman DA, Lynch DP, Sciubba JJ, and Zunt SL. Comparison of computer-assisted brush biopsy results with follow up scalpel biopsy and histology. *Gen Dent* 2002;50:500–503.

Tabor MP, Brakenhoff RH, Ruijter-Schippers HJ, Kummer JA, Leemans CR, and Braakhuis BJ. Genetically altered fields as origin of locally recurrent head and neck cancer: A retrospective study. *Clin Cancer Res* 2004;10(11):3607–3613.

Tabor MP, Brakenhoff RH, van Houten VM, Kummer JA, Snel MH, Snijders PJ et al. Persistence of genetically altered fields in head and neck cancer patients: Biological and clinical implications. *Clin Cancer Res* 2001;7(6):1523–1532.

Takes RP. Staging of the neck in patients with head and neck squamous cell cancer: Imaging techniques and biomarkers. *Oral Oncol* 2004;40:656–667.

Takes RP, Baatenburg de Jong RJ, Schuuring E, Hermans J, Vis AA, Litvinov SV, and van Krieken JHJM. Markers for assessment of nodal metastases in laryngeal carcinoma. *Arch Otolaryngol Head Neck Surg* 1997;123:412–419.

Takes RP, Rinaldo A, Rodrigo JP, Devaney KO, Fagan JJ, and Ferlito A. Can biomarkers play a role in the decision about treatment of the clinically negative neck in patients with head and neck cancer? *Head Neck* 2008;30:525–538.

Toyoshima T, Vairaktaris E, Nkenke E, Schlegel KA, Neukam FW, and Ries J. Cytokeratin-17 mRNA expression has potential for diagnostic marker of oral squamous cell carcinoma. *J Cancer Res Clin Oncol* 2008;134:515–521.

Tsujimoto M, Nakabayashi K, Yoshidome K, Kaneko T, Iwase T, Akiyama F, Kato Y et al. One-step nucleic acid amplification for intraoperative detection of lymph node metastasis in breast cancer patients. *Clin Cancer Res* 2007;13:4807–4816.

van der Riet P, Nawroz H, Hruban RH, Corio R, Tokino K, Koch W et al. Frequent loss of chromosome 9p21–22 early in head and neck cancer progression. *Cancer Res* 1994;54(5):1156–1158.

Van Houten VMM, Leemans CR, Kummer JA, Dijkstra J, Kuik DJ, Van den Brekel MWM, Snow GB, and Brakenhoff RH. Molecular diagnosis of surgical margins and survival of patients with head and neck cancer. *Clin Cancer Res* 2004;10:3614–3620.

van Wilgen CP, Dijkstra PU, van der Laan BF, Plukker JT, and Roodenburg JL. Shoulder complaints after nerve sparing neck dissections. *Int J Oral Maxillofac Surg* 2004;33:253–257.

van't Veer LJ and Bernards R. Enabling personalized cancer medicine through analysis of gene-expression patterns. *Nature* 2008;452:564–570.

van't Veer LJ, Dai H, van de Vijver MJ, He YD, Hart AA, Mao M, Peterse HL et al. Gene expression profiling predicts clinical outcome of breast cancer. *Nature* 2002;415:530–536.

Wagenblast J, Baghi M, Arnoldner C, Bisdas S, Gstöttner W, Ackermann H, May A, Knecht R, and Hambek M. Effect of bortezomib and cetuximab in EGF-stimulated HNSCC. *Anticancer Res* 2008;28(4B):2239–2243.

Wang Y, Klijn JG, Zhang Y, Sieuwerts AM, Look MP, Yang F, Talantov D et al. Gene-expression profiles to predict distant metastasis of lymph-node-negative primary breast cancer. *Lancet* 2005;365:671–679.

Weinberger PM, Yu Z, Haffty BG, Kowalski D, Harigopal M, Brandsma J et al. Molecular classification identifies a subset of human papillomavirus—Associated oropharyngeal cancers with favorable prognosis. *J Clin Oncol* February 10, 2006;24(5):736–747.

Welkoborsky HJ, Bernauer HS, Riazimand HS, Jacob R, Mann WJ, and Hinni ML. Patterns of chromosomal aberrations in metastasizing and nonmetastasizing squamous cell carcinomas of the oropharynx and hypopharynx. *Ann Otol Rhinol Laryngol* 2000;109:401–410.

Wennerberg J, Baldetorp B, and Wahlberg P. Distribution of non-diploid flow-cytometric DNA indices and their relation to the nodal metastasis in squamous cell carcinomas of the head and neck. *Invasion Metastasis* 1998;18:184–191.

Wheeler DL, Iida M, Kruser TJ, Nechrebecki MM, Dunn EF, Armstrong EA, Huang S, and Harari PM. Epidermal growth factor receptor cooperates with Src family kinases in acquired resistance to cetuximab. *Cancer Biol Ther* 2009;8:696–703.

Woolgar JA. Pathology of the N0 neck. *Br J Oral Maxillofac Surg* 1999;37:205–209.

Woolgar JA, Scott J, Vaughan ED, Brown JS, and West CR. Survival, metastasis and recurrence of oral cancer in relation to pathological features. *Am R Coll Surg Engl* 1995;77(5):325–331.

Woolgar JA. Histopathological prognosticators in oral and oropharyngeal squamous cell carcinoma. *Oral Oncol* 2006;42:229–239.

Wreesmann VB, Shi W, Thaler HT, Poluri A, Kraus DH, Pfister D, Shaha AR, Shah JP, Rao PH, and Singh B. Identification of novel prognosticators of outcome in squamous cell carcinoma of the head and neck. *J Clin Oncol* 2004;22:3965–3972.

Yamazaki Y, Chiba I, Hirai A, Satoh C, Sakakibara N, Notani K, Iizuka T, and Totsuka Y. Clinical value of genetically diagnosed lymph node micrometastasis for patients with oral squamous cell carcinoma. *Head Neck* 2005;27:676–681.

Yoshida K, Kashima K, Suenaga S, Nomi N, Shuto J, and Suzuki M. Immunohistochemical detection of cervical lymph node micrometastases from T2N0 tongue cancer. *Acta Otolaryngol* 2005;125:654–658.

Zhang Q, Thomas SM, Xi S, Smithgall TE, Siegfried JM, Kamens J, Gooding WE, and Grandis Jennifer R. SRC family kinases mediate epidermal growth factor receptor ligand cleavage, proliferation, and invasion of head and neck cancer cells. *Cancer Res* 2004;17:6166–6173.

Zumbach K, Hoffmann M, Kahn T, Bosch F, Gottschlich S, Gorogh T et al. Antibodies against oncoproteins E6 and E7 of human papillomavirus types 16 and 18 in patients with head-and-neck squamous-cell carcinoma. *Int J Cancer* March 15, 2000;85(6):815–818.

12

Biological Markers in Oral Squamous Cell Carcinoma

Mario Pérez-Sayáns García, Danielle Resende Camisasca, Abel García García, Simone de Queiroz Chaves Lourenço, and Anastasios Markopoulos

CONTENTS

ABSTRACT Oral squamous cell carcinomas (OSCCs) are the most frequent malignancy of the oral cavity, representing 90%–95% malignancies in the oral region. The development of OSCC is a multistep process requiring the accumulation of multiple genetic and epigenetic alterations, influenced by the patient's genetic predisposition and environmental factors. Cell-cycle regulation is crucial for tumorigenesis. This control in eukaryotic cells involves the sequential activation of cyclins, cyclin-dependent kinases (CDKs), and two great CDK inhibitors (CDK-Is): the INK4 family, comprised by inhibitors p16, p15, p18, and p19, and the Cip/Kip family, comprised by p27, p57, and p21. The inactivation of $p16^{INK4a}$ and $p21^{Waf1/CIP1}$ has been widely associated with this type of tumors. The OSCC is a characteristic locally aggressive tumor that presents large areas of tumoral necrosis, in which the levels of acidity and hypoxia are very high, causing low response to chemotherapy. Hypoxia-inducible factors (HIFs) include hypoxia-inducible factor 1 α (HIF-1α), hypoxia-inducible factor 1 β (HIF-1β), hypoxia-inducible factor 2 α (HIF-2α), and hypoxia-inducible factor 3 α (HIF-3α). HIF-1α overexpression has been associated with tumor cell growth and survival of these in head and neck tumors. Carbonic anhydrases (CAs), mainly CA-IX expression, have been thoroughly described in different tumors, including cervical carcinoma, lung, bladder, breast, esophagus, and colorectal cancers; however, this has not been so for head and neck carcinomas. Tumor development and progression are complex processes involving oncogenes, tumor suppressor genes, and tumoral microenvironment, through their contact with malignant cells, surrounding stromal cells (fibroblasts, endothelial cells, and inflammatory cells), and the extracellular matrix (ECM), formed by structural proteins (such as collagen and elastin), specialized proteins (such as fibrillin, fibronectin, and laminin), and proteoglycans. There are several proteases responsible for remodeling the ECM that enable dissemination and metastasis of tumor cells, such as serine proteases, cysteine cathepsins, and matrix metalloproteinases (MMPs). There is a group of specific and strong MMPs called endogenous tissue inhibitors of metalloproteinases (TIMPs), and although the expression of MMPs has been largely described in almost all the tumors of the body, the expression of TIMPs has been studied in a lesser degree. Altered mRNA transcripts are also a promising field for OSCC detection. Therefore, the goal of this chapter is to describe the expression of $p16^{INK4a}$; $p21^{Waf1/CIP1}$; HIFs; CA-IX; TIMPs; IL-8 and IL-1B; DUSP1; H3 histone, family 3A (H3F3A); ornithine decarboxylase antizyme 1 (OAZ1); S100 calcium binding protein P (S100P); and spermidine/spermine N1-acetyltransferasel (SAT1) in OSCC, determining their relation with clinical, histological, and prognostic factors regarding the different stages of the evolution of the tumors, looking for their detection through noninvasive techniques as exfoliative cytology.

KEY WORDS: *oral squamous cell carcinomas, exfoliative cytology, $p16^{INK4a}$, $p21^{Waf1/CIP1}$, hypoxia-inducible factor 1 α (HIF-1α), carbonic anhydrase IX, tissue inhibitors of metalloproteinases (TIMPs).*

12.1 Introduction

Oral squamous cell carcinomas (OSCCs) are the most frequent malignancy of the oral cavity, representing 90%–95% malignancies in the oral region. The development of OSCC is a multistep process requiring the accumulation of multiple genetic and epigenetic alterations, influenced by the patient's genetic predisposition and environmental factors. All these factors lead to a wide range of genetic and molecular alterations including inactivation of tumor suppressor genes and activation of oncogenes by deletions, specific mutations, promoter methylation, and gene amplification (Wood and Sawyer 1998, Perez-Sayans et al. 2009b).

Although biopsy is the only definitive diagnostic method for these sorts of lesions, other complementary diagnostic techniques, such as exfoliative cytology, have been proposed as faster and less invasive diagnostic alternatives. Exfoliative cytology provides sufficient epithelial cells for analysis (Navone et al. 2007, Perez-Sayans et al. 2009a). Classical applications of oral cytological evaluation, such as oral candidiasis, have been joined by others such as precancerous lesions and oral cancer (Acha et al. 2005, Mehrotra et al. 2006). The analytical methods for studying cytological samples are different and their results are variable. Although the development of molecular analysis techniques is currently attracting a growing interest in this technique, classical analysis, enhanced by liquid-based cytology, is still a suitable technique for the first screening of lesions of suspected malignancy (Diniz Freitas et al. 2004).

In liquid-based preparations, the samples and the samplings device are transported in a container with a liquid conservative. This permits immediate fixation of the cells; therefore, all the collected material can be used, thus obtaining preparations with abundant cells dispersed in a thin and homogeneous layer. Blood, inflammation, and mucus are reduced and distributed throughout the preparation increasing the quality of the sample for testing (Linder and Zahniser 1997, Nasuti et al. 2001). Compared with conventional smears, liquid-based preparations have considerably reduced the number of unsatisfactory or satisfactory, though limited, preparations due to the specimen's characteristics, thus reducing false negatives (Bishop et al. 1998).

The goal of this chapter is to describe the expression of $p16^{INK4a}$; $p21Waf1/CIP1^{Waf1/CIP1}$; hypoxia-inducible factors (HIFs); carbonic anhydrase IX (CA-IX); tissue inhibitors of metalloproteinases (TIMPs); interleukin-8 (IL-8); interleukin-1 beta (IL-1B); dual specificity protein phosphatase 1 (DUSP1); H3 histone, family 3A (H3F3A), ornithine decarboxylase antizyme 1 (OAZ1); S100 calcium binding protein P (S100P); and spermidine/spermine N1-acetyltransferase1 (SAT1) in OSCC, determining their relation with clinical, histological, and prognostic factors regarding the different stages of the evolution of the tumors and to analyze the possibility of their determination through noninvasive techniques, such as exfoliative cytology.

12.1.1 Types of Oral Cancers

Oral cancer comprises a variety of malignancies, with different origins and behaviors, such as salivary gland tumors, soft tissue and bone tumors, melanomas, odontogenic tumors, hematolymphoid tumors, and epithelial tumors (Barnes et al. 2005). However, squamous cell carcinoma (SCC) is the most frequent, remarking 90%–95% of all oral cancer cases and originates in the mucosal linings (Warnakulasuriya, 2009). Due to its high prevalence, this chapter will describe specifically OSCC.

OSCC remains one of the most difficult malignancies to control because of its high propensity for local invasion and cervical lymph node dissemination (de Vicente et al. 2007). The biological factors that underlie the locoregional and distant spreading of these neoplasms are not completely understood (Munoz-Guerra et al. 2005). The behavior of OSCC is difficult to predict solely using conventional clinical and histopathological parameters, and due to the location of the disease, the multimodal tumor therapy usually prescribed leads to a reduction in quality of life, making the psychosocial consequences of OSCC greater than other malignancies (Myoung et al. 2006, Dwivedi et al. 2012). For these reasons, despite advances in therapeutic strategies, the survival rate of OSCC patients is still poor (Carvalho et al. 2005, Jemal et al. 2011).

The development of OSCC is a multistep process requiring the accumulation of multiple genetic alterations, influenced by the patient's genetic predisposition as well as by environmental factors (Choi and Myers, 2008). It is not known what proportion of OSCC arises from precursor lesions (Figure 12.1a and b) and how many develop from apparently normal oral mucosa. However, studies have shown that between 16% and 62% of oral carcinomas are associated with leukoplakias when diagnosed (Bouquot et al. 2006).

Leukoplakia is a clinical term, and the presence or absence of dysplastic cells does not alter the clinical diagnosis; however, it has been suggested that leukoplakia should be redefined to be a combined clinical/histological term (Barnes et al. 2005, Bouquot et al. 2006). In the absence of validated molecular markers, histological grading of oral epithelial dysplasia remains the only determinant of potential malignant change (Figure 12.1). Severe epithelial dysplasia has an overall malignant transformation rate of approximately 16%, but studies have shown a wide range of transformation, varying from 7% to 50%. Other premalignant oral lesions are erythroplakia, verrucous leukoplakia, lichen planus, oral submucous fibrosis, and actinic cheilitis (Barnes et al. 2005).

Cancers of the oral cavity comprise tongue (C02.0, C02.1, C02.3, C02.2, C02.8, and C02.9), gingiva (C03.0, C03.1, and C03.9), floor of the mouth (C04.0), hard palate (C05.0, C05.8, C05.9), and buccal mucosa (C06.0, C06.1, C06.2, C02.8, C02.9) (WHO 1997, Edge et al. 2010). Nowadays, it is important to describe separately lip and oropharynx SCC, due to different etiology, pathogenesis, and prognosis (Camisasca et al. 2009, 2011, Lindenblatt et al. 2012). SCC can manifest itself on any mucosal surface but most commonly appears on lateral and ventral parts of the tongue, followed by the floor of the mouth (Figure 12.2a through c) (Neville and Day 2002, Camisasca et al. 2009).

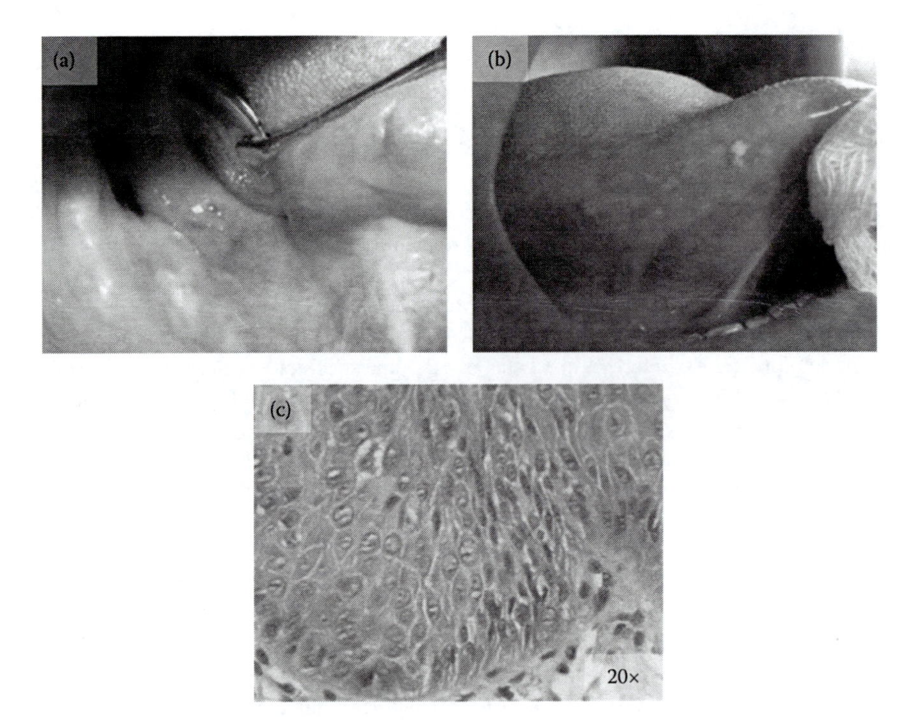

FIGURE 12.1 **(See color insert.)** Early diagnosis for OSCC relies on the detection of potentially malignant disorders and early-stage carcinomas. Discrete homogeneous oral leukoplakias are observed on the (a) floor of the mouth and (b) border of the tongue, which are high-risk areas for malignant transformation. (c) Dysplasia—as noted on routine hematoxylin and eosin histopathological analysis—is still the best available predictor of malignant transformation.

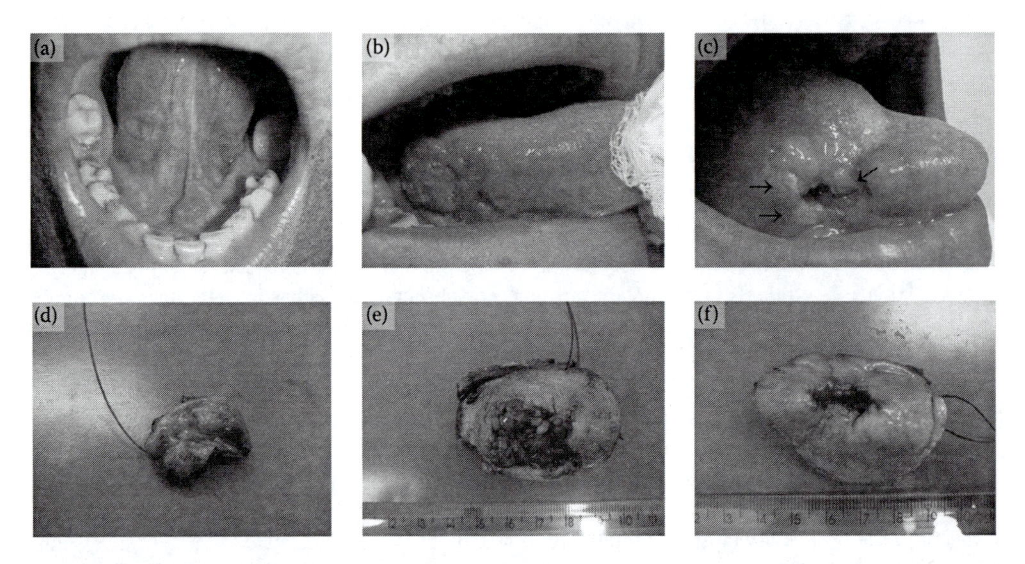

FIGURE 12.2 **(See color insert.)** Clinical aspect of stages I and II SCC and surgical specimens obtained after treatment: (a) Stage I SCC of the mouth floor. (b) Stage II SCC of the tongue. (c) Stage II SCC of the tongue with an adjacent area of leukoplakia (arrows). All patients were submitted to primary surgery followed by neck dissection, because tongue and floor of mouth SCC are predisposed to develop early cervical metastases. (d–f) Surgical specimens show about 1 cm free margins. Depending on histopathological analysis of the specimen and lymph node status, patients were referred to adjuvant radiation.

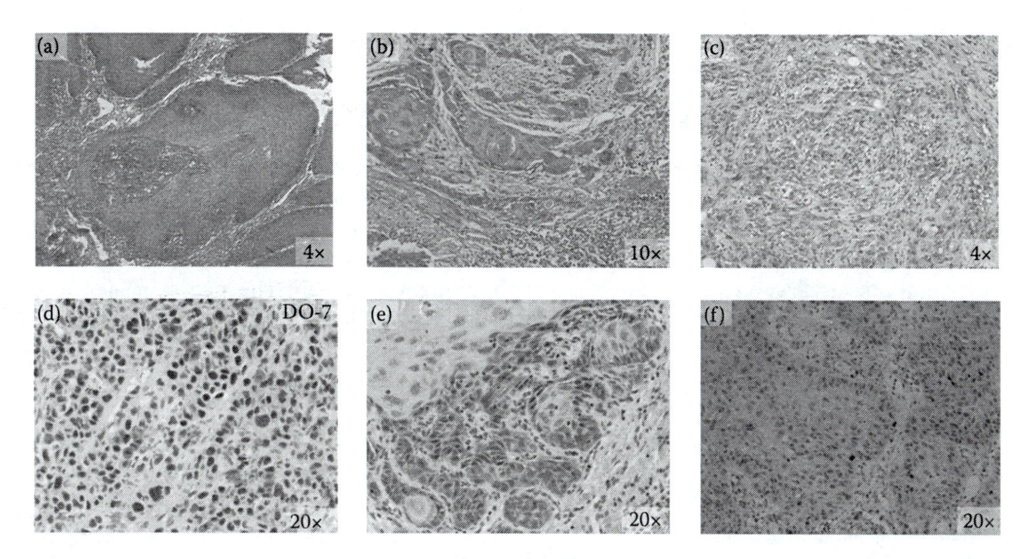

FIGURE 12.3 (See color insert.) OSCC histopathological grading and immunohistochemical staining. Usually OSCC is graded as (a) well, (b) moderately, and (c) poorly differentiated, according to keratinocyte resemblance with normal epithelium and as suggested by WHO guidelines. Immunohistochemistry is widely used in researches in an attempt to establish markers of malignant transformation, as well as prognostic markers. Clone DO-7 for p53 protein was extensively studied in leukoplakias and (d) OSCC. Bcl-2 protein, along with other family members, (e) shows prognostic value, and (f) p16 is used in association with HPV-16 to try to determine HPV activity in the tissue.

Tongue and floor of mouth SCCs are prone to develop cervical metastasis even in early clinical stages (Kligerman et al. 1994, Dias et al. 2001). OSCC is characterized by invasive and frequent perineural growth, a considerable rate of early recurrences, and frequent lymph node metastasis. Often these patients develop second primary cancers in the same or adjacent anatomical region. Nodal status appears to be the most important clinical prognostic indicator, once nodal metastases are associated with a high rate of regional recurrence and decreased survival (Barnes et al. 2005, Camisasca et al. 2011).

Other studies show that tumor differentiation (Figure 12.3a through c), treatment, and clinical stage can also be good prognostic indicators (Barnes et al. 2005, Lindenblatt et al. 2012). Histopathological subtypes of OSCC are verrucous carcinoma, spindle cell carcinoma, basaloid SCC, papillary SCC, carcinoma cuniculatum, acantholytic SCC, and adenosquamous carcinoma. The most frequent are the first three and verrucous carcinoma usually shows a much better prognosis than other carcinomas (Barnes et al. 2005, Pereira et al. 2007).

Even though lip and oral cavity are regions readily accessible to physical examination, most OSCC cases are still diagnosed in advanced stages (stages III and IV), in which the survival decreases significantly when compared to initial stage lesions (Carvalho et al. 2004, 2005). Besides that, patients with this type of cancer present high mortality and morbidity even if treated timely with the best available strategies, and this affects considerably their quality of life (Dwivedi et al. 2012). Usually the patient is put away from social contact, due either to the disease itself or to the disfiguring consequences of an extended surgery procedure. In this way, OSCC patients would benefit from screening strategies and biomarkers that could lead to higher figures of early diagnosis. Besides that, it is important to come up with technology or approaches that separate tumors with bad and good prognosis. Although it is not the most prevalent cancer all over the world, it is a public health concern in many countries (Warnakulasuriya 2009).

12.1.2 Epidemiology

Oral cancer is a serious and growing problem in many parts of the globe. Oral cancer accounts for 4% of all neoplastic diseases and it is increasing in incidence worldwide. The annual estimated incidence for 2008 was around 263,900 cases, and 128,000 deaths are caused from oral cavity cancer, of which two-thirds occurs in developing countries (Petersen et al. 2009, Jemal et al. 2011). The International Agency for Research on Cancer (IARC) estimates oral cancer to be among the 11 most frequent cancers in the world. However, broad differences in geographic distribution exist (Petersen et al. 2009).

The regional variation is such that in developing countries, the frequency of SCCs is much greater, accounting for up to 40% of all malignancies in the Indian subcontinent (Johnson 1997). Oral cancer is the most common cancer affecting men and the third one affecting women, after breast and cervix uteri tumors in India (Moore et al. 2000). Other geographic areas with high incidences are Europe, Australia, New Zealand, and Melanesia. Latin America and the Caribbean have intermediate incidence rates for oral cancer; however, intercountry rates in the region vary widely. The highest incidence rates occur in Pakistan, Brazil, India, and France (Warnakulasuriya 2009, de Camargo Cancela et al. 2010, Jemal et al. 2011).

12.1.2.1 Age Distribution

The incidence of oral cancer increases with age, although the pattern differs markedly in different countries and with different risk factors. In the West, 98% of cases concern patients over 40 years of age, with increasing incidence as age peaks in the sixth and seventh decades (Moore et al. 2000). In high-prevalence areas, many cases occur prior to the age of 35 years due to heavy abuse of various forms of oral smokeless tobacco (Llewellyn et al. 2004). There is an increasing incidence of oral cancer in young population (<40 years), but studies that investigated this group of patients showed contradictory results about risk factors involved and prognosis (Llewellyn et al., 2004, Garavello et al. 2007, Warnakulasuriya et al. 2007a, Kaminagakura et al. 2010).

12.1.2.2 Sex Distribution

Throughout the world, malignant neoplasms of the oral cavity rate as the eighth most common cancer in terms of incidence and as the 10th most common in terms of cancer mortality for men. In women, oral cancers ranked as the 13th in terms of incidence and mortality (de Camargo Cancela et al. 2010).

In industrialized countries, men are affected almost twice as often as women, probably due to their higher indulgence in risk factors such as alcohol and tobacco consumption. The incidence of oral cancer for women is, however, greater than or equal to that for men in high-prevalence areas such as India, where chewing and smoking are also common among women (Johnson 1997, de Camargo Cancela et al. 2010). Females still use less amounts of alcohol and cigarettes when compared to men (Kruse et al. 2011); however, studies have shown that changes in females' lifestyle in last decades have contributed for this variation in OSCC profile (Girod et al. 2009, Kruse et al. 2011).

12.1.2.3 Socioeconomic Status

Oral cancer is linked to social and economic status and deprivation, with the highest rates occurring in the most disadvantaged sections of the population. In developing countries, people are exposed to a wider range of risk factors, starting at younger ages (de Camargo Cancela et al. 2010). The association is particularly strong for men. An exception is the young group in which 25% are from professional classes (Llewellyn et al. 2004).

12.1.2.4 Survival

Oral cancer is particularly lethal, the crude 5-year survival rate being 30%–40%. Within the mouth, factors that influence survival are the site, the size of the lesion at the time of diagnosis, and the degree of differentiation (Figure 12.3a through c) (Carvalho et al. 2005). The best outcome is for the cancer of the lip, with an overall survival rate of up to 90% (Sargeran et al. 2009). Cancers that are detected at early stages (Figure 12.2) have a significantly better prognosis than those that are detected at advanced stages. The 5-year survival rate for patients with most cancer types is, on average, nearly 90% for patients who are diagnosed with stage I tumors and 10% or less for patients who are diagnosed with stage IV tumors

(Carvalho et al. 2004, 2005). Cancer survival tends to be poorer in developing countries, most likely because of a combination of a late stage at diagnosis and limited access to timely and standard treatment (Jemal et al. 2011).

12.1.2.5 Risk Factors

The main risk factor for oral cancer is exposure to exogenous carcinogens such as tobacco smoke and alcohol (Hashibe et al. 2009). Most patients diagnosed with OSCC are males who drink and smoke and show low socioeconomic status (Camisasca et al. 2011). However, close attention must be paid to certain groups that do not show this well-known and characteristic profile (Llewellyn et al. 2004, Dahlstrom et al. 2008, Girod et al. 2009). In general, sedentary lifestyle, ambiental risks, and alcohol and tobacco use predispose people to acquire diseases (Barnes et al. 2005, Danaei et al. 2005).

Different risk factors have specific effects on the incidence of oral cancer. Several studies have demonstrated that cigarette smoking is associated with a greater incidence of oral and pharyngeal cancer in a dose-dependent fashion (Blot et al. 1988). People who consume alcohol are three times more likely to develop oral cancer than nondrinkers. Many studies show that when alcohol is combined with tobacco use, the incidence of cancer is markedly increased (Blot et al. 1988, Lockhart et al. 1998, Rizzolo et al. 2007). Its consumption in populations suffering from malnutrition may also decrease immunity and hence promote oral cancer development (Leite and Koifman 1998). A person's cultural practices may increase risk, as well. The use of betel has been associated with OSCC (Rizzolo et al. 2007) and is widespread in South Asia, where they chew betel quid, a substance composed of the nut of the areca palm, betel pepper leaf, and quicklime (calcium hydroxide).

Human papillomaviruses (most frequently HPV-16) are implicated in the pathogenesis of OSCC; however, recent researches have shown that HPV-16 is involved in up to 70% of malignant tumors of the oropharynx (most commonly in palatine and tongue tonsils), mainly in those patients that do not drink alcohol or smoke (D'Souza et al. 2007, Syrjanen 2007). Dietary factors, such as a low intake of fruits and vegetables, may also be related to an increased cancer risk (Danaei et al. 2005). Finally, special attention could be given to sources of potential bias in population studies of gene–environment interaction, such as ethnicity. Beyond genetic predisposition, intracountry ethnic differences could be linked to specific risk factors such as socioeconomic status and access to health services, as well as diet, alcohol, and tobacco (Hashibe et al. 2009, Jemal et al. 2011).

12.1.3 Available Diagnoses

Early diagnosis aims at detecting carcinoma in situ and OSCC in its initial stages (Figure 12.2). Up to now, clinical screening is still the best tool to do it (Mehrotra and Gupta 2011). A previous step is detecting potentially malignant disorders (Figure 12.1) and apparently normal mucosa at risk to develop carcinoma and, besides and more importantly, identify the no return point, where the altered field (Braakhuis et al. 2003) will certainly become OSCC. In this sense, tissue, saliva, and serum or blood biomarkers would be useful, as well as optical tools that enhance visualization of the lesion.

Upon the detection of a clinically suspicious lesion, screening aids as toluidine blue and tissue fluorescence imaging are available. Toluidine blue staining is sensitive adjunct tool for identifying early OSCC and high-grade dysplasias (Mehrotra and Gupta 2011). Usually it is used to aid in the selection of the area for biopsy, and hence, it should not be viewed as a substitute for biopsy, and a negative test does not preclude the presence of dysplasia or even oral cancer. Nowadays, tissue fluorescence imaging (VELscope) (Huber 2012) is used with the same purpose as toluidine blue and should also be used to help identify lesions that may have been overlooked with a conventional oral examination. However, they should always be used with lesions clinically suspicious of malignancy; only a definitive test examining cells or tissue can determine the biologic behavior of a lesion.

Biopsy followed by histopathological analysis is still the gold standard of OSCC diagnosis (Figures 12.2 and 12.3). Attempts have been made to introduce cytopathological analysis as a routine method, similar to what is done for cervical cancer; however, cytological changes are not as well established for oral cancer as histological changes. Without a minimal invasiveness, it is not possible to access the deeper cell layers of the oral cavity with conventional exfoliative cytology. Brush biopsy appeared as a way to overcome this and should be able to analyze deeper cell layers; however, abnormal findings should be submitted to scalpel biopsy, retesting, or observation (Eisen and Frist 2005).

Clinically evident OSCCs do not pose a diagnostic problem. Diagnostic difficulties are faced with potentially malignant disorders and carcinoma in situ, in which the histopathological criteria for dysplasia (Figure 12.1) show low inter- and intraobserver agreement (Bouquot et al. 2006, Warnakulasuriya et al. 2007b). And besides, there is no direct association between the presence of severe epithelial dysplasia and malignant transformation to OSCC, since approximately 16% of these dysplasias develop into cancer. However, the best predictor for malignant transformations is still dysplasia (Bouquot et al. 2006).

Those OSCC that develop from an apparently normal mucosa would have early diagnosis enhanced by approaches investigating tissue, salivary, and serum/blood biomarkers (Szanto et al. 2012). Upon the detection of these altered fields, in which cancerization is probable, a biopsy could be performed to confirm the findings.

The investigation of phenotypic changes in OSCC cells may have a strategic prognostic value, and special attention has recently been focused on the use of potential molecular biomarkers as reliable predictors of tumor aggressiveness and to identify early molecular alterations present in potentially malignant disorders without dysplasia (Massano et al. 2006).

Advances in the understanding of cancer at the regulatory protein expression level have resulted in the identification of some prognostic tumor biomarkers, which can provide information complementary to that obtained from clinical examination and histopathological studies (Figure 12.3d through f). Tumor suppressor and apoptosis genes (p53, p63, blc-2 family, p21), cell proliferation markers (EGFR, ki-67, AKT1, cyclin D1), angiogenic markers (VEGF, podoplanin), and cell adhesion molecules and matrix degradation (caderina, catenina, CD44, matrix metalloproteinase [MMP]) have been studied as potential tools to predict the prognosis of patients with OSCC. In recent years, the number of molecular-based assays has increased, but histopathology remains the gold standard for most diagnostic and therapeutic decisions (Oliveira et al. 2011).

12.1.4 Treatment

The management of OSCC varies considerably: small cancers of the oral cavity are usually managed by surgery alone (Figure 12.2), whereas advanced oral cancers are usually treated with primary radical surgery followed by radiation or chemoradiation. Neck treatment is offered to patients who have a greater chance of having lymph node metastasis or who have neck involvement at the time of presentation (Kligerman et al. 1994, Jones 2012).

TNM classification system is used to evaluate the best possible predictors during clinical examination and to show the extent of the lesion before treatment. Three parameters are evaluated: T for size of the cancer lesion, N for lymph nodes status, and M for distant metastases. Image exams may be used to enhance clinical classification. If the patient is submitted to surgery and the surgical specimen is evaluated by pathologists, a pathological staging (pTNM) is assigned to the case. After that, the TNM is grouped in four stages. These stages are used to define the best treatment for the individual and to determine prognosis (Edge et al. 2010a,b).

Treatment is influenced by the stage of the disease and prognosis (Edge et al. 2010a), the need to spare the patient from mutilating surgery, the health of the patient, and the patient's desires. In general, wide surgical excision with or without lymph node dissection is the treatment of choice (Figure 12.2). Radiation alone tends to result in poor survival. On the other hand, prophylactic neck dissection to remove clinically negative nodes has been shown to increase survival (Kligerman et al. 1994, Dias et al. 2001). Patients undergoing neck dissection had the 5-year survival rate improved when compared to those who did not (Dias et al. 2001). Unfortunately, up to half of all cases with nodal involvement have disease that is too advanced for further therapy and can be treated only by supportive care. Furthermore, combination chemotherapy used adjunctively with surgery has not improved survival, although an aggressive regimen used recently with surgery showed an impressive overall survival rate of 85% (Hassel et al. 2012).

Regardless of the modality of treatment, patients face negative changes with reduced quality of life (Dwivedi et al. 2012). Moreover, an important issue for both patients and dentists is follow-up after treatment. Surgery may lead to the necessity for prostheses and/or obturators; speech and tongue mobility may then be compromised, making it difficult to perform an oral examination and dental treatment. Long-term fluoride treatment and close dental follow-up are also important components of postradiation management. Patients who continue to smoke after treatment are prone to develop second primary tumors, and advisement about this is crucial (Khuri et al. 2001).

12.2 p16^{INK4a} and p21$^{Waf1/CIP1}$ as Cell-Cycle Regulators in OSCC

Cell-cycle regulation is crucial for tumorigenesis. This control in eukaryotic cells involves the sequential activation of cyclins, cyclin-dependent kinases (CDKs), and two great CDK inhibitors (CDK-Is): the INK4 family, comprised by inhibitors p16, p15, p18, and p19, and the Cip/Kip family, comprised by p27, p57, and p21$^{Waf1/CIP1}$. These CDKIs block cell-cycle transition from G1 phase to S phase. The inactivation of p16^{INK4a} and p21$^{Waf1/CIP1}$ has been widely associated with these type of tumors (Serrano et al. 1993, Hunter and Pines 1994, Sherr 1994, Morgan 1995, Chen et al. 1999, Kapranos et al. 2001, Brennan et al. 2002) (Figure 12.4).

12.2.1 p16^{INK4a} Expression in OSCC

The decrease of p16^{INK4a} expression and its epigenetic silencing is associated with oral cancer and precancer, and its inactivation is believed to be an early and gradual event as the tumor stage and the grade of dysplasia advance in premalignant lesions, which is occasionally associated with certain clinical and pathological parameters or the expression of other cell-cycle regulatory proteins (Papadimitrakopoulou et al. 1997, Bradley et al. 2006, Uzawa et al. 2007, Vairaktaris et al. 2007, Angiero et al. 2008, Kresty et al. 2008, Schwarz et al. 2008, Takeshima et al. 2008).

The results of p16^{INK4a} expression in OSCC showed variable results between different research studies, showing both subexpression (Pande et al. 1998, Ai et al. 2003) and overexpression (Paradiso et al. 2004, Gologan et al. 2005). Alongside the immunohistochemical expression of p16^{INK4a}, some authors have tried to find a relationship between this expression and clinical and pathological parameters. Bova et al. considered that the loss of p16^{INK4a} expression is associated with a reduction in the 5-year disease-free survival and especially with the 5-year overall survival rate (Bova et al. 1999). These results were consistent with those reported by Jayasurya et al., who found a statistically significant association between p16^{INK4a} expression and the disease-free period (Jayasurya et al. 2005), and Pande et al., who linked the loss of p16^{INK4a} expression with tumor stage and progression (Pande et al. 1998). Karsai et al., in a study on 664 head and neck squamous cell carcinoma (HNSCC) cases by tissue microarray (the largest cohort study conducted on molecular biomarkers), found that the loss of p16^{INK4a} expression is related to a shorter survival, although the alteration in the expression pattern appears to be associated with early carcinogenic process (Karsai et al. 2007).

Suzuki et al. found that p16^{INK4a} expression is associated with greater sensitivity to chemotherapy (stage 2B and above in accordance with Ohboshi and Shimosato's criteria), while the reduction in expression is associated with a reduction in survival compared with normal or amplified gene expressions (Suzuki et al. 2006). Sailasree et al. observed that low levels or absence of p16^{INK4a} expression is associated with a lower initial response to treatment (Sailasree et al. 2008).

Other studies, however, found no relationship between p16^{INK4a} expression and clinical and pathological stages (Yakushiji et al. 2001), the mode of invasion of tumor cells described by Yamamoto et al. (Tokman et al. 2004), the survival (Muirhead et al. 2006), or recurrence rates (Gonzalez-Moles et al. 2007), suggesting a possible link between lack of protein expression and a reduction in the degree of keratinization and differentiation (Muirhead et al. 2006).

As we can see, the results are highly variable between different studies; the real applicability of determining p16^{INK4a} expression is controversial (Tanaka et al. 2001, Guo et al. 2007, Patel et al. 2007, Vekony et al. 2008). Thus, some studies show that p16^{INK4a} may be a clear potential marker in recognition of dysplasia in head and neck squamous mucosa (Gologan et al. 2005, Vairaktaris et al. 2007), for distinguishing branchial cleft cysts from cystic SCCs of the oropharynx (Pai et al. 2009). However, Buajeeb et al. state that p16^{INK4a} is not really a good marker for mucosal dysplasia or malignant transformation (Buajeeb et al. 2009).

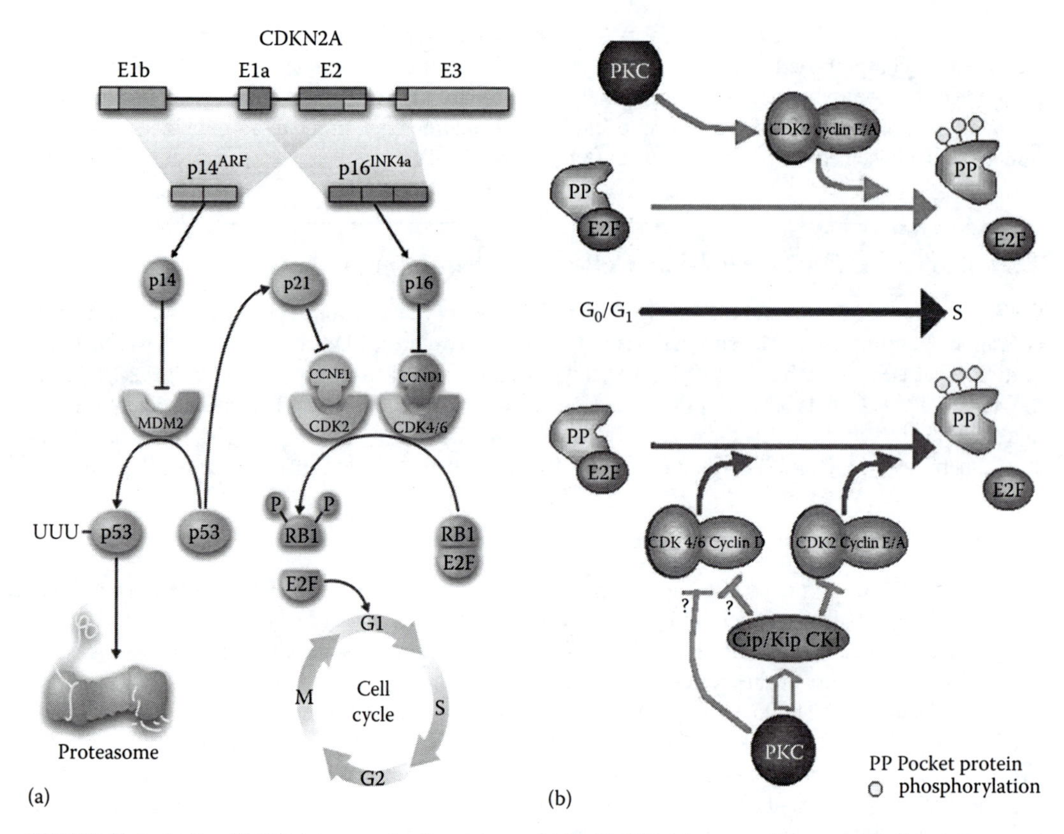

FIGURE 12.4 (a) The CDKN2A locus and cell-cycle control. The CDKN2A locus on chromosome 9p21 has an unusual structure because it encodes for two overlapping but very distinct proteins: p16^{INK4a} and p14^{ARF}. This is accomplished through selective use of an alternative first exon (exon E1a in p16^{INK4a} and exon E1b in p14^{ARF}). Although structurally very different, both protein products act as negative regulators of cell-cycle progression. The p16^{INK4a} protein inhibits the activation of CDK4 and CDK6 by cyclin D1 (CCND1), thereby preventing the subsequent phosphorylation of RB1. Underphosphorylated RB1 sequesters the transcription factor E2F and prevents it from inducing the progression from G1 to S phase of the cell cycle. The absence of functional p16^{INK4a}, therefore, leads to hyperphosphorylation of RB1 with resulting release of E2F and uninhibited cell-cycle progression. In contrast, p14^{ARF} regulates tumor protein 53 (p53) activity by inhibiting MDM2, a ubiquitin ligase that otherwise targets p53 for degradation by proteasome. High levels of p14^{ARF} stabilize p53, permitting it to induce p21$^{Waf1/CIP1}$, a cell-cycle inhibitor that blocks CDK2/cyclin E (CCNE1)-mediated phosphorylation of RB1. In the absence of functional p14^{ARF}, uncontrolled ubiquitination and degradation of p53 remove this important cell-cycle brake, leading ultimately to hyperphosphorylation of RB1 and cell-cycle progression. (From Sekulic, A. et al., *Mayo Clin. Proc. Mayo. Clin.*, 83(7), 825, 2008.) (b) Model of the molecular mechanisms underlying PKC-mediated regulation of G1–S progression. The upper portion of the figure (above the black arrow indicating G0/G1–S progression) shows the consequences of PKC activation in early G1, while the lower portion (below the arrow) depicts events resulting from PKC activation in mid-to-late G1 phase. (From Black, J.D., *Front. Biosci. J. Virt. Lib.*, 5, D406-23, 2000.)

12.2.2 Genetic and Epigenetic Alterations in p16^{INK4a} Expression Pattern

Gene silencing of p16^{INK4a}/CDKN2 and all other genes can be caused by physiological expression control mechanisms, as genetic or epigenetic alterations (homozygous deletion, methylation of the promoter region, or mutation). The final consequence of such alterations is gene silencing and the reduction or elimination of protein expression.

The frequency of genetic abnormalities of p16^{INK4a} in OSCCs is variable. Thus, Sailasree found that 62% of the cases have genetic abnormalities, deletion (33%), and methylation (29%). The deletion of p16^{INK4a} was associated with tumor aggressiveness (Sailasree et al. 2008). Shintani et al. observed homozygous deletion in 56.3% of the samples and three mutations, all in the second exon, and two of these were also methylated (Shintani et al. 2001). Tsai et al., in a group of 48 OSCCs, studied exons 1 and 2 of p16^{INK4a} by SSCP. They found 7 deletions (14.6%) and 5 mutations (10.4%); 26 specimens (54%) showed no expression of p16 protein, and 11 of them were due to genetic abnormalities (one of the mutations was nonsense) (Tsai et al. 2001). Ohta et al. described 20.5% of homozygous deletions (9 of 44 cases) and loss of heterozygosity at the locus 9p21$^{Waf1/CIP1}$ (encoding p16^{INK4a} and p14 proteins) in 68.8% (30 of 44 cases) (Ohta et al. 2009). Kim et al. described 11.76% mutations, associated concomitantly with LOH (Kim et al. 2000). Nakahara et al., in a sample population of 32 OSCCs, found 43.8% homozygous deletion in exon 1α and 34.4% in exon 2 (Nakahara et al. 2001).

Regarding the relationship between genetic abnormalities and clinical and pathological parameters, Tsai et al. found a high relationship between genetic alterations of p16^{INK4a} and regional metastasis (Tsai et al. 2001). Experimental studies in animals and cell lines also offer conflicting results regarding the frequency of genetic abnormalities, but nearly everyone agrees that methylation is a major cause of gene silencing of p16^{INK4a} (Akanuma et al. 1999, Cody et al. 1999, Lee et al. 2004, Ogawa et al. 2006, Hong et al. 2007, Li et al. 2008).

As far as epigenetic alterations are concerned, results are variable. According to Su et al., the frequency of methylation determined by Q-MSP in OSCC samples is 28.85%; they found no association between hypermethylation of p16^{INK4a} and low average age (<54 years), high-risk invasion of lymph nodes in young patients and distant metastases in older patients, and reduction of the disease-free interval (Su et al. 2010). Authors such as Sinha et al. found a statistically relevant relationship between p16^{INK4a} positivity in the surgical margins and tumor recurrence (Sinha et al. 2009).

Sailasree found a relationship between the hypermethylation pattern and increased tumor recurrence; this pattern also acts as an independent predictor agent for poor prognosis (Sailasree et al. 2008). Nakahara et al. found methylated p16^{INK4a} DNA in three of four patients with recurrences, suggesting that the MSP measurement may be a sensitive technique to detect recurrent OSCC (Nakahara et al. 2006), while Kato et al. found it in 27.27% (Kato et al. 2006). In fact, a study conducted by Zeidler et al. found a hypermethylation frequency of 9.7% (25 of 258) in 258 samples of smokers' normal oral mucosa without cancer, supporting the theory that p16^{INK4a} genetic silencing is an early event in carcinogenesis possibly conferring cell growth advantages (von Zeidler et al. 2004).

Cao et al. described similar results in a follow-up study of patients with dysplastic lesions. Of the 78 lesions, 22 evolved into OSCC (28.2%), and the relation with the p16^{INK4a} hypermethylation pattern was 43.8% of malignant lesions for methylated p16^{INK4a} and 17.4% for unmethylated p16^{INK4a} (Cao et al. 2009). A different perspective was shown by Hall et al., in which from 57% (8 of 14) patients suffering from malignant transformation of dysplastic lesions (≥3 years), 26% showed p16 methylation (Hall et al. 2008). Kresty et al. found 57.7% methylation in severe dysplastic lesions (Kresty et al. 2002).

12.2.3 p21$^{Waf1/CIP1}$ Expression in OSCC and Its Correlation with Clinical and Pathological Parameters

The results of p21$^{Waf1/CIP1}$ expression in OSCC showed mixed results in terms of positivity/negativity among different studies (from 53% to 96.6%) (Ralhan et al. 2000, Choi et al. 2003). Although all agree that expression of p21$^{Waf1/CIP1}$ is entirely nuclear, unlike other CDKIs such as p16, in which nuclear/cytoplasm location results are variable.

Regarding the relationship with clinicopathological parameters, the results are highly variable; thus, Fillies et al. (2007) accounted for a relationship between loss of p21$^{Waf1/CIP1}$ expression and a decrease in overall survival, and they also found an inverse correlation with tumor size. Tatemoto et al. (1998) found no association between p21$^{Waf1/CIP1}$ expression and tumor stage, mode of invasion of tumor cells, and the differentiation of the same. However, they found a correlation with the presence of metastases in lymph nodes. According to Kapranos et al. (2001), p21$^{Waf1/CIP1}$ shows positive expression in patients with HNSCC >65 years, in chemotherapy-responsive tumors and stage III patients with a higher overall survival rate. According to Xie et al. (2002), there is an inverse correlation between T classification and clinical stage, but not with N classification. Patients with p21$^{Waf1/CIP1}$ (+) tumors showed a greater disease-free interval than those patients with negative p21$^{Waf1/CIP1}$. The Hungarian group led by Nemes et al. (2005) found a correlation between the expression of p21$^{Waf1/CIP1}$ and T3 and T4 stage tumors, positive lymph node metastasis, cancer in advanced stages (III and IV), and tumors in the tongue and the retromolar trigone. Yen-Ping Kuo et al. (2002) reported a relationship between p21$^{Waf1/CIP1}$ (+) and a worst overall survival.

Other authors found no relationship between $p21^{Waf1/CIP1}$ expression and the clinical–pathological variables under study (Pande et al. 2002, Gonzalez-Moles et al. 2004). Osaki et al. (2000) found the same expression of $p21^{Waf1/CIP1}$ in both well-controlled tumors and lethal tumors; however, they found no correlation with treatment failure or metastatic sites. According to González-Moles et al. (2004), $p21^{Waf1/CIP1}$ expression is aberrant in all samples of nontumoral adjacent epithelium, and the absence of expression or decreased expression in tumors does not influence patient survival. Kuropkat et al. (2002) found no relation between survival or time and recurrence. Yook and Kim (1998) found no correlation with any of the clinicopathological parameters.

As mentioned earlier, $p21^{Waf1/CIP1}$ is regulated in two different ways: either through a p53-dependent pathway or through a p53-independent one, so it is very important to establish the relationship between these two proteins in OSCC. In fact, it seems that, although $p21^{Waf1/CIP1}$ expression is controlled in a p53-dependent manner, the coexpression of both in OSCC is not intrinsically related. The broad variety of molecules regulated by p53 result in a stricter control than $p21^{Waf1/CIP1}$ via p53 independence.

12.2.4 $p21^{Waf1/CIP1}$ Expression in Precancerous Lesions

Choi et al. (2003) described p21 expression in nondysplastic epithelium mainly in basal and suprabasal cells. In the dysplastic epithelium, p21 increases its expression as the degree of dysplasia increases. In OSCC, the expression is variable, especially in poorly differentiated tumor areas. They found no association whatsoever with any clinicopathological feature. Agarwal et al. (1998) found a rising percentage of p21 expression as hyperplasia is transformed into dysplasia, associated with differentiation and proliferative activity. Kudo et al. (1999) found that among 24 epithelial dysplasias, 23 (96%) were positive for p21, compared to 77% (36 of 47) of OSCC. Furthermore, 79% of these dysplasias were p53(−)/p21(+) compared with 25% of OSCC. Queiroz et al. (2010) found no statistically significant differences between p21 expression in normal oral epithelium, oral squamous papilloma, and OSCC. Chang et al. (2000) found a group of 53 verrucous leukoplakias, reporting p21 expression in 75% (40) of cases; 42% (22) developed OSCC in a period of 3½ years, 26% (14) were recurrent, and 32% (17) were free of disease. Aberrant p21 positivity was associated with 80% progression to OSCC compared with 32% of recurrences. On the other hand, Hogmo et al. (1998) found no relationship between p21 expression and risk assessment in terms of precancerous lesions.

Although it seems that the presence of HPV viral oncoproteins increases $p21^{Waf1/CIP1}$ levels, the small number of studies and the lack of statistically significant data of the same have forced us to disregard the hypothesis that HPV-infected lesions that present better prognosis are due to a $p21^{Waf1/CIP1}$-dependent control.

12.2.5 Genetic Alterations in $p21^{Waf1/CIP1}$ Expression Pattern

As regards to the genetic alterations of p21 in OSCC, Ralha et al. (2000) described polymorphism at codon 149 (A → G) in 11 of 30 premalignant lesions (37%) (7 hyperplastic lesions and 4 dysplastic lesions) and in 11 out of 30 OSCCs (37%), being statistically significant compared to the normal oral mucosa. It appears that this polymorphism is more common in precancerous lesions (10 of 11) and in OSCC (11 of 11) with weak p53 in lesions with mutated p53, suggesting that this polymorphism may affect the p53 pathway and play an important role in tumorigenesis.

The frequency of mutations (transitions and transversions) in exon 2 of p21, according to Ibrahim et al. (2002), ranges from 14% to 43% depending on the origin of tumors, being higher for Sudanese toombak-dipper tumors. In any case, the loss of 9p21 and its relationship with clinicopathological parameters can only be estimated in the context of the complex pattern of genomic imbalances that accompanies loss of chromosomes in the examined tumors (Gebhart et al. 2003).

12.2.6 Conclusions

We believe that differences in the expression of $p16^{INK4a}$ between the different working groups can be due to immunohistochemistry in addition to the populations' characteristics and specimens, which are at different stages and have widely varying degrees of differentiation. Likewise, we believe it is essential to standardize semiquantitative analysis methods to allow methodological unification of the different studies and thus enable performance of systematic reviews and meta-analyses. As we have seen, the role of $p21^{Waf1/CIP1}$ as cell-cycle regulator has been well described; however, in its relationship to OSCC, clinical and pathological variables of the tumors and HPV are not entirely clear. Thus, it would be very interesting to pursue further study of this protein, which may have a significant value in terms of diagnosis, prognosis, and therapy in this type of tumors.

12.3 HIFs and CA-IX as Regulators of the Hypoxia of the Microenvironment in OSCC

The SCC (OSCC) is a characteristic locally aggressive tumor that presents large areas of tumoral necrosis, in which the levels of acidity and hypoxia (which usually are related) are very high, causing low response to chemotherapy and providing basic resistance to anticancer drugs in these tumors (Moulder and Rockwell 1987, Perez-Sayans et al. 2009b, 2010). HIFs include hypoxia-inducible factor 1 α (HIF-1α), hypoxia-inducible factor 1 β (HIF-1β), hypoxia-inducible factor 2 α (HIF-2α), and hypoxia-inducible factor 3 α (HIF-3α) (Figure 12.5). HIF-1α overexpression has been associated with tumor cell growth and survival of these in cervical, breast, ovary, endometrium, stomach, and head and neck tumors (Ryan et al. 1998, Semenza 2000, Birner et al. 2001, Beasley et al. 2002, Makino et al. 2002, Schindl et al. 2002, Sivridis et al. 2002, Burri et al. 2003, Chen et al. 2005). CA-IX expression has been thoroughly described in different tumors, including cervical carcinoma (Brewer et al. 1996), lung (Giatromanolaki et al. 2001), bladder (Klatte et al. 2008), breast (Chia et al. 2001), esophagus (Turner et al. 1997), and colorectal cancers (Saarnio et al. 1998); however, this has not been so for head and neck carcinomas and, more specifically, in the case of OSCCs, which account for 95% of oral malignant neoplasms (Perez-Sayans et al. 2009b).

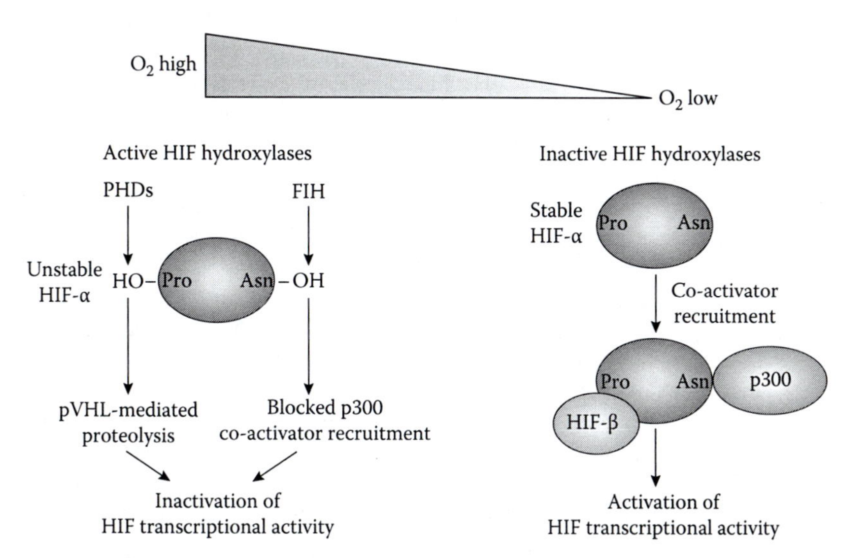

FIGURE 12.5 Dual regulation of HIF-α subunits by prolyl and asparaginyl hydroxylation. In the presence of oxygen, active HIF hydroxylases—that is, prolyl hydroxylase domains (PHDs) and factor inhibiting HIF (FIH)—downregulate and inactivate HIF-α subunits. PHDs hydroxylate a prolyl residue in the amino- and the carboxy-terminal oxygen-dependent degradation domains (NODDD and CODDD, respectively), which promotes von Hippel–Lindau tumor suppressor (pVHL)-dependent proteolysis and results in the destruction of HIF-α subunits. FIH, on the other hand, hydroxylates an asparaginyl residue in the carboxy-terminal activation domain (CAD), which blocks p300 co-activator recruitment and results in the inactivation of HIF-α-subunit transcriptional activity. In hypoxia, HIF hydroxylases are inactive, and these processes are suppressed, which allows the formation of a transcriptionally active complex. (From Schofield, C.J. and Ratcliffe, P.J., *Nat. Rev. Mol. Cell Biol.*, 5(5), 343, 2004.)

12.3.1 Effects of HIF Expression in OSCC Tumorigenesis and Its Relationship with Clinicopathological Parameters

In most tumors, HIF-1α overexpression is associated with increased mortality, but in HNSCCs, the results are controversial (Brennan et al. 2005, Koh et al. 2010, Majmundar et al. 2010, Lu and Kang 2010, Wong et al. 2010).

Uehara et al. (2009), using the computer-assisted measurement system by Wu et al. (1997), described the percentage of immunopositive HIF-1α (PHIA) in a sample population of 57 OSCC cases. They found statistically significant expression data in patients with poor prognosis (12.1%)/good prognosis (6.4%) and patients with lymph node metastases (11.7%)/patients free of metastases (7.5%).

Roh et al. (2009), analyzing the role of five hypoxia markers (HIF-1α, HIF-2α, CA-IX, GLUT-1, and EPOR), found that HIF-1α is significantly associated with disease-specific survival (DSS) in tongue carcinomas in stage T2, with a relative risk (RR) of 0.352, but not with other clinical and pathological parameters such as tumor thickness, involvement of lymph nodes, or the status of the resection margin. Liang et al. (2011) found in these tumors that HIF-1α overexpression is associated with a shorter disease-free survival, while HIF-2α did not show any correlation with overall survival or disease-free survival.

Lin et al. (2008), measuring the labeling indices (Lis) of HIF-1α nuclear expression (the proportion of immunopositive cells over the total number of cells), found, among the five groups of samples (normal oral mucosa; mild, moderate, and severe epithelial dysplasia; and OSCC), an increased expression of HIF-1α, with the highest levels appearing in the OSCC group (55% ± 23%). Differences with other groups were statistically significant. In normal oral mucosa, the expression is also positive (9% ± 6%); therefore, they concluded that this is an early event in oral carcinogenesis. These results are consistent with those described by Costa et al. (2001), who found that 14 of 15 lichen planus and 8 of 9 leukoplakias were negative for HIF-1α; however, 22 of 29 OSCCs were positive, particularly in well-differentiated cases, thus indicating an increased expression of this factor as the degree of dysplastic lesion advances.

Liu et al. (2008) found overexpression of HIF-1α in 69.64% of analyzed OSCCs and a positive correlation with the rate of tumor progression (tumor size, lymph node metastasis, histological differentiation, clinical stage, and the presence of tumor cell-lined vessels) and poorer survival. Eckert et al. (2010a) found a positive correlation between HIF-1α expression and tumor size, recurrences, and distant metastases.

Tilakaratne and Nissanka-Jayasuriya (2011) linked HIF-1α expression as an independent prognostic marker in OSCC and described a positive correlation between expression and tumor size (T1/T2 vs. T3/T4). HIF-1α-negative tumors, or those with a mild expression, had an 80% specific 5-year disease-free survival, compared to 49.4% for those with moderate or strong levels. The time of specific disease-free survival was 54 months for the first group and 38 months for the second. A recent study, carried out by Eckert et al. (2010b), which analyzed 82 patients with OSCC, attested that HIF-1α expression correlates with poor DSS. Patients with negative or low HIF-1α expression had a survival rate of 80%, which descended to only 33.6% in cases of moderate or strong expression. These results, however, were not confirmed by Beasley et al. (2002), who found that in HNSCC, both in cell lines and tissue samples, HIF-1α expression—in surgically treated patients—is associated with an improvement in disease-free survival and overall survival. According to Kyzas et al. (2005), in a retrospective study of 81 patients with HNSCC, HIF-1α expression had no impact on the prognosis of patients. These data support the hypothesis that tumor angiogenesis is closely related to, but not strictly dependent, hypoxic conditions of the tumors' microenvironment. Similarly, Fillies et al. (2005) associated HIF-1α expression in tumors of the floor of the mouth with improved 5-year survival rates and a greater disease-free period, regardless of the status of lymph nodes and tumor size. In node-negative tumors in stage T1/T2, the absence of HIF-1α was associated with a subgroup of high-risk patients.

12.3.2 HIF-1α as a Therapeutic Target in OSCC

As we described earlier, HIF-1α expression is associated with tumor progression and the resistance of tumor cells to radiotherapy (Aebersold et al. 2001) and chemotherapy (Unruh et al. 2003, Perez-Sayans et al. 2010). Yoshiba et al. (2009), in a study of OSCC cell lines exposed to 5-fluorouracil (5-Fu), found that hypoxia-sensitive cells develop resistance to 5-Fu under hypoxia. Sasabe et al. (2007) proved that treatment with cis-diamminedichloroplatinum, 5-Fu and γ-rays, causes an increase in the levels of HIF-1α. The inhibition of HIF-1α can enhance the results of these two therapeutic modalities, thus reducing the angiogenic effect, tumor growth, and spreading (Brennan et al. 2005).

Thus, Zhang et al. (2004) considered the possibility of inhibiting HIF-1α by siRNA (small interference of RNA) and antisense oligonucleotides. In this study, they showed that both siRNA and oligonucleotides induce apoptosis in OSCCs of the tongue through a caspase-dependent pathway. These same results have been found by Sasabe et al. (2007). Further studies are needed to corroborate the pro- or anticancer effect of HIF-1α expression under different conditions.

Novel molecules such as 17AAG, 2ME2, and NVP-AUY922 try to induce degradation to minimize the progression of tumors and enhance the effect of chemotherapy and radiotherapy (Isaacs et al. 2002, Mabjeesh et al. 2003, Okui et al. 2011). Other molecules such as trastuzumab, Celebrex, or imatinib are under research, although none of these specifically targets HIF-1α (Brennan et al. 2005).

12.3.3 CA-IX Expression in OSCC and Its Correlation with Clinical and Pathological Parameters CA-IX in Other HNSCCs

As we have established earlier, CA-IX expression is located in the plasma membrane, solely and exclusively in tumor cells; in some cases, tincture forms a continuous reticule that surrounds the contour of the cell, and in such cases, expression is strong; however, it tends to be diffuse in neoplasms, mainly in the center of tumor nests. The second pattern is similar, but membrane tincture is incomplete, weak, and limited to the periphery of the tumor (Choi et al. 2008, Roh et al. 2009, Eckert et al. 2011, Kondo et al. 2011, Oliveira 2011). The expression results for the different studies are summarized in Table 12.1.

As for the relationship with clinical and pathological parameters and especially with prognostic factors, the results are variable depending on the series of studied cases, as is the case of other markers of this type of tumors (Le 2007, Oliveira 2011). According to Choi et al. (2008), CA-IX expression is related to postsurgical recurrence and a worst average survival rate and is therefore considered as a good prognostic marker. For Kondo et al. (2011), CA-IX expression is positive in 98% of tumors, finding lower survival in patients with elevated CA-IX expression (≥50% of cells). Furthermore, patients with poorly

TABLE 12.1

CA-IX Immunohistochemical Expression in OSCC

Study	OSCC Cases	% (n) Positivity				% (n) Negativity	Quantification
Choi et al. (2008)	117	58.1% (68)				41.9% (49)	CA-IX (0) < 5%
		54 (1+)	14 (2+)				CA-IX (1+) 5%–20%
							CA-IX (2+) > 20%
Kondo et al. (2011)	107	98% (105)				2% (2)	CA-IX (–) < 10%
							CA-IX (+) ≥ 10%
Eckert et al. (2010b)	80	42.5% (34)				57.5% (46)	CA-IX (1) 1%–10%
							CA-IX (2) 11%–50%
		21 leve	11 mod.	2 intense			CA-IX (3) 51%–80%
							CA-IX (4) > 80%
Roh et al. (2009)	43	40.47%(26)				39.53% (17)	CA-IX (0) 0%
		7 (1+)	7 (2+)	10 (3+)	2 (4+)		CA-IX (1+) 1%–10%
							CA-IX (2+) 11%–50%
							CA-IX (3+) 51%–80%
							CA-IX (4+) 81%–100%
Kim et al. (2007)	60	CA-IX < 10%: 36.7% (22)					CA-IX < 10%
		CA-IX ≥ 10%: 63.3% (38)					CA-IX ≥ 10%

ND, not determined; Mod, moderate.

differentiated tumors, T4, lymph node metastasis, and stage IV with high CA-IX expression showed a worse outcome. For Kim et al. (2007), the percentage of positive cells ranges between 0% and 77.5%. In their series of OSCCs of the tongue, they found a relationship between high CA-IX (≥10%) expression and poorly differentiated tumors, with those located in the base of the tongue of smokers and patients who had been submitted to radiotherapy in contrast with those who had only undergone surgery.

In contrast, Roh et al. (2009) found that CA-IX levels were moderate to high in a sample of 43 OSCC patients, establishing a positive correlation only with tumor thickness, without affecting their overall survival nor the 5-year disease-free period. Eckert et al. (2010b) only found a greater expression of CA-IX in women, without relating such expression to prognostic factors.

12.3.4 CA-IX and Its Relationship with Angiogenesis and Resistance to Treatment

The relationship between CA and blood vessels has been described by several authors; thus, Koukourakis et al. (2001), in a series of 75 HNSCC cases that were treated with chemotherapy and radiotherapy, observed that CA-IX expression (26.6%, 20 of 75) takes place mainly in tumors with low vascularization (measured by microvascular density [MVD], positive for CD-31) and necrosis areas and is related to a poor overall response. These results were confirmed by Jonathan et al. (2006) and Beasley et al. (2001), the latter in three HNSCC cell lines and 79 specimens (31 OSCCs). The average CA-IX expression was 20% (0%–90%) and was induced by cell line hypoxia and was related to necrotic areas, high MVD (positive for CD-34), and advanced tumor staging; the average distance between blood vessels and the bottom line of the expression was 80 μm (40–140), thus confirming the results of Hoogsteen et al. (2005). A study of an HNSCC xenograft, conducted by Bhattacharya et al. (2004), confirmed the lack of microvessels in well-differentiated areas of the xenograft related to hypoxia and positive for CA-IX (detected by functional MRI), a limited use of chemotherapeutic drugs, and resistance to irinotecan therapy, thus confirming the hypothesis that hypoxia promoted the creation of resistant cell subpopulations. This same team tried to improve their results by adding tirapazamine (a chemotherapeutic drug with selective toxicity for hypoxic cells), but the results were not what they had expected, since it resulted in a reduction of blood vessels, thus reducing drug dosage in CA-IX-positive cells in hypoxic regions (Bhattacharya et al. 2008). These results were confirmed by Chintala et al. (2010), who studied the effect of Se-methylselenocysteine (molecule that increased the effect of irinotecan) in HNSCC cell lines and xenografts. They observed that, in cells and hypoxic areas, the combination of both drugs reduced HIF-1α levels, which, at the same time, transcriptionally regulated and lowered CA-IX levels. The hypothesis that CA-IX actively participates in chemoresistance has been confirmed by Zheng et al. (2010). In their research, they transformed an OSCC of the tongue cell line, which was moderately differentiated, into pingyangmycin (PYM) resistant (Tca8113/PYM) and cross-resistant to paclitaxel, Adriamycin, and mitomycin. It was confirmed that neither glycoprotein p (p-gp), nor multidrug resistance-associated protein 1, nor breast cancer resistance protein was involved in the acquired resistance. In order to verify the responsible factors, they analyzed cell lines by DNA microarray, PCA, and Western blot and found that the application of CA inhibitor, acetazolamide, and CA-IX silencing with oligonucleotides contributed to increase average pH in resistant cells, thus resulting in an increase of chemosensitivity to PYM, in addition to increasing activation of PYM-induced caspase 3. Currently, the possibility of using tumor-associated antigens (TAAs) such as G250/CA-IX for immunotherapy in HNSCC with up to 80% protein expression levels to produce a specific response of T $CD8^+$ cells is under study (Schmitt et al. 2009).

As regards to the role of CA-IX in radiotherapeutic treatments, Eriksen et al. (2007) tried to determine its role as a prognostic marker in a series of 320 HNSCCs undergoing radiotherapy treatments with concomitant nimorazole, a hypoxia-modifying drug. The research findings established that CA-IX is not related to any clinical, pathological, and prognostic (outcome and disease-free period) parameters; it was also proven useless as a marker for concomitant use of radiotherapy + nimorazole. As we have mentioned earlier, in the case of patients treated with ARCON vs. conventional surgery ± radiotherapy, the hypoxia and vascular density levels have no influence on treatment response (Kaanders et al. 2002). These same results were found by Jonathan et al. (2006) who reported that the relationship between CA-IX (expression >25% of tumor area) and the lack of locoregional control and freedom from distant metastasis and their relation with GLUT-3 disappears when tumors are treated with ARCON. According to Koukourakis et al. (2006), the joint expression of HIF-2α and CA-IX is responsible for poor continuous hyperfractionated accelerated radiotherapy (CHART) results, in contrast with conventional radiotherapy.

12.3.5 Conclusions

HIF functions are complex from a biological standpoint and even more from the pathological point of view. Hypoxia is a critical and decisive factor for malignancy and it appears to be controlled mainly by HIF-1α, in the case of OSCC. Furthermore, most studies relate their overexpression with increased tumor malignancy and therefore a worsening of survival rates, although results remain controversial. The number of molecules that control—and are controlled by—HIF is large and growing, hence the difficulty of establishing the correct molecular pattern of these tumors. However, results seem promising, including their inhibition as a potential therapeutic target. We believe that HIF, and especially HIF-1α, can be a suitable marker for diagnosis, prognosis, and therapy in OSCC, although further studies are needed.

It is clear that hypoxia in solid tumors is a decisive factor for the outcome of HNSCCs and especially OSCCs. However, despite the fact that the regulating endogenous markers have been perfectly described, the relevance of each one of them, especially CA-IX and their interrelations, has not been strongly confirmed. Probably this is due to the expression results in each of the different studies and their relationship with clinical and pathological parameters, as well as prognostic factors, which present great variability, resulting in a reduction of scientific evidences. These evidences, however, exist when relating hypoxia in solid tumors with chemoresistance and the failure of radiotherapy, both conventional and concomitant, in which CA-IX seems to play an important role. We consider that further studies of these tumors are needed to confirm the use of CA-IX as a prognostic marker and to evaluate its possible inhibition with minimal adverse effects, reducing the risk of metastasis and favoring the action of chemotherapeutic drugs and radiotherapy.

12.4 Tissue Inhibitors of Metalloproteinases as Metastasis Regulators in OSCC

Tumor development and progression are complex processes involving oncogenes, tumor suppressor genes, and tumoral microenvironment, through their contact with malignant cells, surrounding stromal cells (fibroblasts, endothelial cells, and inflammatory cells), and the extracellular matrix (ECM), formed by structural proteins (such as collagen and elastin), specialized proteins (such as fibrillin, fibronectin, and laminin), and proteoglycans (Stetler-Stevenson et al. 1993, Bhowmick et al. 2004). There are several proteases responsible for remodeling the ECM that enable dissemination and metastasis of tumor cells, such as serine proteases, cysteine cathepsins, and MMPs (Friedl and Wolf 2008, Hojilla et al. 2008). There is a group of specific and strong MMPs called endogenous tissue inhibitors of metalloproteinases (TIMPs), and although the expression of MMPs has been largely described in almost all the tumors of the body, the expression of TIMPs has been studied in a lesser degree and even less in the case of OSCCs (Poulsom et al. 1992, Khokha 1994, Imren et al. 1996, Thomas et al. 1999, Caterina et al. 2000, Hernandez-Barrantes et al. 2000, Okada 2000, Shiomi and Okada 2003, English et al. 2006).

12.4.1 Expression of TIMPs in OSCC

In regard to the immunohistochemical expression of mRNA and its relationship with different clinical, pathological, and prognostic parameters, the results vary from study to study. According to de Vicente et al. (2005), who performed a immunohistochemical analysis of 68 OSCC cases for TIMP-1 and TIMP-2, they found a positive expression of TIMP-1 in 45 cases (66.2%), all in tumoral tissue, and 19 (42.2%) of them also in the surrounding stroma. For TIMP-2, immunostaining was positive in 38 cases (56%) in tumors and 9 cases (13.2%) in stroma. The expression pattern was homogeneous, central, and irregular, and for TIMP-2, it was also in the invasive front of tumor nests. For Katayama et al. (2004), the expression of TIMP-2 is located mainly on the cell surface and in the cytoplasm of tumor cells, in addition to some endothelial cells and stromal fibroblasts surrounding tumoral cells; these data were also confirmed by Shimada et al. (2000). Following with the results obtained by de Vicente et al. (2005), the expression of TIMP-1 was not correlated with any of the clinicopathological parameters, whereas TIMP-2 was correlated with TNM staging, local recurrence, and worse survival rates. In a subsequent study, with the same study population (de Vicente et al. 2007), they found that positive immunostaining of MMP-7 correlated to TIMP-1 and TIMP-2 expressions. Similarly, TIMP-2 was related to MT1-MMP in the positive cases for lymph node affectation.

Singh et al. (2010) studied the expression of TIMPs in 75 OSCC patients, 50 healthy volunteers, and 42 coupled samples of normal mucosa adjacent to the tumor. Using different techniques, they found that plasma levels (determined by enzyme-linked immunosorbent assay [ELISA]) of TIMP-1 and TIMP-2 in OSCC were higher than the controls. As for mRNA levels determined by RT-PCR, the levels in tumor tissue were higher than in the adjacent normal mucosa. TIMP-1 was correlated with lymph node affectation and the degree of tumor differentiation, whereas TIMP-2 only correlated to lymph node affectation. On the other hand, Shimada et al. (2000) did not find a positive correlation between the expression of TIMP-1 and lymph node affectation.

Baker et al. (2006) determined the levels of TIMP-1 and TIMP-2 through ELISA (n = 38) and found higher average levels in tumor tissue (24.4 for TIMP-1 and 7.8 for TIMP-2) than in normal tissue (16.3 for TIMP-1 and 7.5 for TIMP-2), although such differences were not statistically significant. However, they found a relation with certain histological parameters, for example, TIMP-1 levels were higher in tumors that had not metastasized, and on the other hand, TIMP-2 showed higher levels in well-differentiated tumors than in poorly differentiated tumors. However, these results contrast with those of Schmalbach et al. (2004) who found an expression of TIMP-1 three times higher in metastatic tumors than in non-metastatic tumors. The same findings were included in the study by Shimada et al. (2000), who found statistically higher levels of TIMP-1 and not of TIMP-2 in tumor tissue, compared to normal tissue, although they found no relationship with clinical and pathological parameters.

In the research project by Kurahara et al. (1999), they analyzed the expression of TIMPs in 96 OSCC cases by immunohistochemistry, confirming the results of de Vicente et al. who affirmed that the expression is heterogeneous among the different cases, even showing individual variations depending on different areas. TIMP-1 was positive in 72 of 96 cases (75%), while TIMP-2 was positive in 84 (87.5%). TIMP-2 was expressed mainly in tumor cells and TIMP-1 in stromal cells. High levels of TIMP-1 (2+ and 3+) are related to cases with metastasis, which contrasts with those that show low or negative levels (0 and 1+). The expression of TIMP-1 was also related with lymph node affectation in a statistically significant way, while TIMP-2 was not. The increase of expression of TIMP-1 was related with the increase of expression of MMP-1, MMP-3, and MMP-9; TIMP-2 was not related with MMP-2 or MT1-MMP. However, for Katayama et al. (2004), the expression of TIMP-2 was related with the expression of MMP-2, but not with MMP-9 or MT1-MMP.

Katayama et al. (2004) studied the expression of TIMP-2 in 53 OSCC patients in initial stages (T1 or T2–N0–M0) conducting a follow-up routine for an average of 67 months. In regard to the prognosis, the patients that developed lymph node affectation and/or distant metastasis showed higher levels of TIMP-2 than those who did not develop metastasis. Intense expression of TIMP-2 was related with a worse and shorter average survival in contrast with patients showing negative or moderate expression, thus being an independent prognostic factor. On the other hand, in the case of TIMP-1, Ikebe et al. (1999) found that the group with lower levels had a higher risk of metastasis.

Gao et al. (2005) studied the expression of TIMP-2 in 40 OSCC cases and the adjacent mucosa at 2 and 5 cm, finding higher statistically significant levels in OSCCs (52.5%) than in normal mucosa at 2 cm (22.5%) and at 5 cm (25%). The expression of TIMP-2 was related to the degree of differentiation of tumor cells, lymph node status, and carcinoma staging, all of which are related to prognosis.

As per the genetic expression of TIMPs, the first analysis by in situ hybridization, around the year 1992, showed almost negligible levels in tumors and in healthy tissue (Gray et al. 1992). Subsequent studies, probably thanks to the improvement of molecular biology techniques, such as the one conducted by Birkedal-Hansen et al. (2000), found, in a coupled series of seven OSCCs and their adjacent healthy tissue, an expression of TIMP-1 reaching 100% in the tumor and adjacent tissue; TIMP-3, 85% in tumoral tissue and 43% in adjacent tissue; for the first time ever, they studied the expression of TIMP-4 in this type of tumors, without finding a positive expression in any of these cases. The expression of TIMP-3 showed statistically significant differences between both groups. Sutinen et al. (1998)

studied genetic and protein expression of TIMP-1, TIMP-2, and TIMP-3 in OSCC lesions and lymph node metastasis, epithelial dysplasia, lichen planus, and normal oral mucosa. The expression of mRNA TIMP-3 (in situ hybridization) was observed in stromal cells surrounding neoplastic islands in OSCCs and lymph nodes. mRNA TIMP-1 was only observed in some cases and TIMP-3 was practically negligible. The expression in the group of dysplastic lesions, lichen planus, and normal mucosa was mostly low. As per the protein expression (immunohistochemistry), the findings correlate exactly with the results obtained by in situ hybridization. Schmalbach et al. (2004) in a study by microarrays confirmed that the expression of TIMP-1 increases in metastatic tumors in a statistically significant manner.

Just like the measurements in tissue, the plasma levels of TIMPs can be used as prognostic markers. Thus, according to Pradhan-Palikhe et al. (2010), high blood levels of TIMP-1 are associated with a worse tumor prognosis, reducing survival of the OSCC case.

Improvements in the in vitro experimental models to study cell invasion in oral cancer (Duong et al. 2005) have allowed for studies on cell lines to confirm the hypothesis of clinical studies. Juarez et al. (1993) proved that the application of TIMP-2 on cell lines UM-SCC-1 and MDA-TU-138 substantially reduces in vitro invasion of these cells, via collagenase neutralization (since TIMPs do not have cytostatic effects on cells). Kinsenn et al. (2003), in the OSCC SAS cell line, found that the inhibiting effect against MMP-2 activation of TIMP-2 is dose-dependent, but this is not so in the case of TIMP-1. Moreover, Nii et al. (1996, 2000) found that TIMP-1 is expressed in nonmetastatic cell lines (SAT) but not in invasive or metastatic cell lines (HNOS). Kawamata et al. (1997) found that nonmetastatic cell lines (BHY) secrete TIMP-2; however, they barely found traces of TIMP-1, while metastatic cell lines (HM) secrete TIMP-1 but not TIMP-2. Trying to delve in the role of carcinogens in the expression of TIMPs, Lu et al. (2008) studied fibroblasts treated with areca nut extract and observed an increase in tumorigenesis of oral epithelial cells and a marked downregulation of TIMP-1 mRNA. Rosenthal et al. (2004), however, found no overexpression of TIMP-1, TIMP-2, or TIMP-3 in the fibroblasts related to HNSCC or in those related to normal stroma, thus confirming the results of Lu et al.

12.4.2 Exogenous TIMPs and Matrix Metalloproteinase Inhibitors in OSCC Antitumor Therapy

The development of matrix metalloproteinase inhibitor (MMI) has a key role in the field of academic and industrial research, since MMP blocking is complex, given its multifunctionality and participation in physiological and growth processes. There is a group of molecules, which we will call specific MMIs, since these have been specifically designed for the inhibition of MMPs, and a second group, which we call indirect MMIs, which are molecules designed for other purposes but with a spectrum of action that also includes inhibition of MMPs (Zucker et al. 2000, Sang et al. 2006). Currently, both small molecules (synthetic and natural) and endogenous macromolecules (especially TIMPs) have been used in anticancer therapy. TIMPs were initially considered for clinical therapy, and although they showed good activity in tumor-invasion models, metastasis and angiogenesis, their clinical use is limited since they are macromolecules and difficultly penetrate tissue barriers and are not susceptible to degradation by other enzymes (Bian et al. 1996, Ahonen et al. 2003). However, several natural and synthetic MMIs have been developed instead of TIMPs. Figure 12.6 shows those that have been accepted for use in cancer therapy clinical trials (Dorman et al. 2010, Devyand Dransfield 2011).

12.4.3 Conclusions

It seems that MMPs and their endogenous inhibitors (TIMPs) are essential for the regulation of ECM destruction, tumoral invasion, and metastasis. The expression of TIMPs in tumors is higher than in normal tissue, and although some discrepancies have been observed, it seems that an increase in these levels (especially TIMP-1), both in tumor and in plasma, is correlated with an increase in metastatic risk and regional lymph node affectation in cancer patients. Despite that some MMIs have shown encouraging results in certain tumor types, their use in OSCC has not been widely tested and there are very few clinical trials on this matter. Therefore, although MMIs provide some promising results, more studies are necessary to assess their effectiveness in anticancer treatments and especially in OSCC, for which research is still scarce.

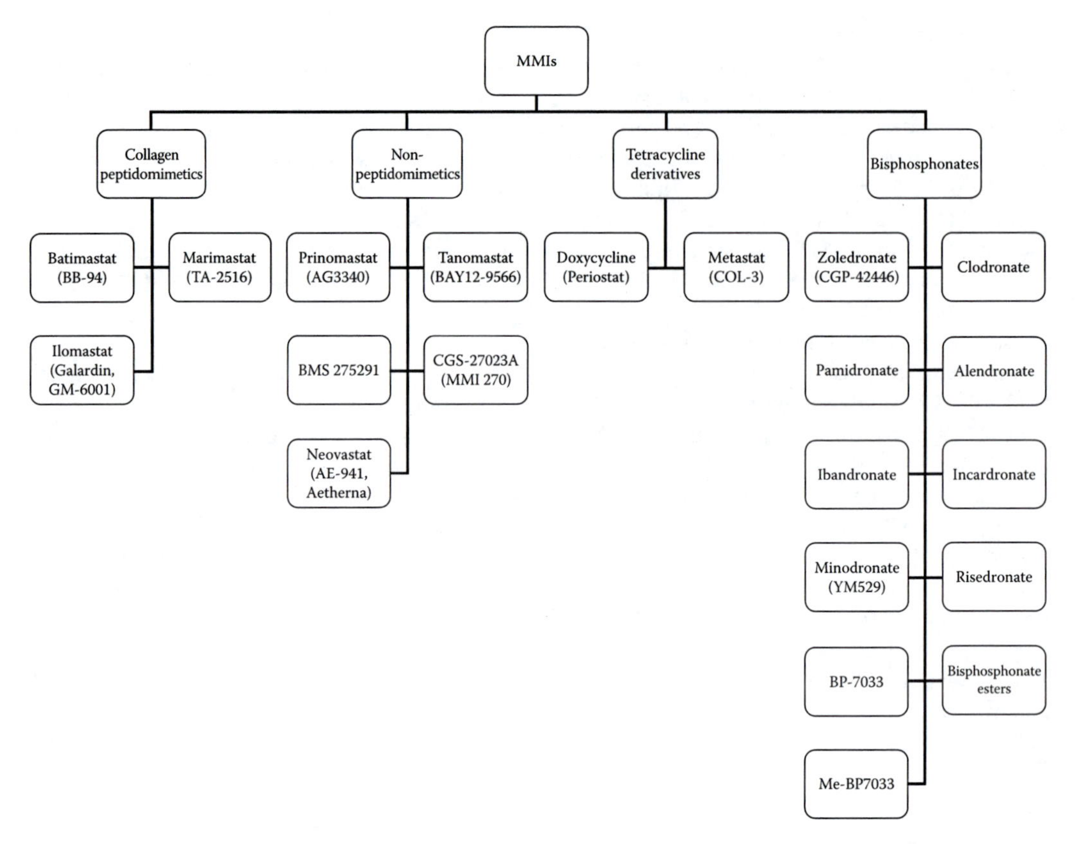

FIGURE 12.6 Natural and synthetic MMIs that have been developed and accepted for use in clinical trials for anticancer treatments.

Moreover, given the high invasive capacity of this type of tumors, patients could theoretically benefit from the progression-inhibiting effect and the metastatic destruction that is attributed to these compounds.

12.5 Altered mRNA Transcripts

RNA for years was thought to quickly degrade in saliva due to the various RNAses that saliva contains (Eichel et al. 1964). Despite the opposite reports (Kumar et al. 2006), cell-free RNA molecules seem to exist in saliva, both intact and fragmented (St. John et al. 2004). Various mRNA molecules, such as IL-1B, IL-8, DUSP1, H3F3A, OAZ1, S100P, and SAT, were found upregulated in the saliva of patients suffering from OSCC (Li et al. 2004, Zimmermann and Wong 2008, Wei et al. 2009).

Lately, microRNAs, small RNA molecules that seem to regulate transcription, were discovered existing in saliva of patients with OSCC (Hanson et al. 2009, Park et al. 2009, Michael et al. 2010).

A question that remains to be answered is the mechanism by which mRNA in saliva is protected by degradation. It has been proposed that salivary mRNA is contained in apoptotic bodies (Hasselmann et al. 2001, Ratajczak et al. 2006) or actively released in exosomes or microvesicles (Garcia et al. 2008, Skog et al. 2008, Al-Nedawi et al. 2009).

12.5.1 IL-8 and IL-1B

IL-8 is a cytokine produced by monocytes, T lymphocytes, neutrophils, endothelial and epithelial cells, and fibroblasts (Rollins 1997). IL-8 is one of the factors known to be involved in some types of cancer (Brennecke et al. 2005, Savage et al. 2004). It regulates humoral and immune responses. IL-8 is often associated with inflammation. IL-8 has been also involved in angiogenesis and neovascularization (Koch et al. 1992, Smith et al. 1994). In humans, IL-8 is encoded by the IL-8 gene (Modi et al. 1990). IL-8 gene expression is influenced by (-251A/T) polymorphism, which is found in the promoter region of the *IL-8* gene (Hull et al. 2006). IL-8 can be secreted by any cells with toll-like receptors. Usually, macrophages are the first cells that see an antigen and thus are the first cells to release IL-8 to recruit other cells.

IL-8 has been linked with cancer due to its angiogenic properties and its ability to induce cell proliferation and promote DNA damage through inhibition of DNA repair (Jaiswal et al. 2002, Moore 2002). It also has been proposed that higher levels of IL-8 may promote carcinogenesis not only by inducing cell proliferation and DNA damage but by upregulating gene transcription and activity of metalloproteinase-2 as well. Increased collagenase activity results in enhanced invasion of surrounding healthy tissues by tumor cells, increased angiogenesis, and, therefore, metastasis (Luca 1997). Interestingly, the suppression of IL-8 expression by synthesized positive inotropic agent vesnarinone inhibits both angiogenesis and tumorigenicity of human OSCC cells (Harada et al. 2005).

Elevated serum levels of IL-8 have been also observed in patients with ovarian and hepatocellular cancer (Al-Wabel et al. 1995, Watanabe et al. 2002). Significantly elevated salivary IL-8 levels were also found in OSCC patients. Several studies indeed have shown that IL-8 was elevated in the whole unstimulated saliva of subjects with OSCC and controls.

Interestingly, patients with metastatic melanoma who responded to chemotherapy show a significant decrease in the serum level for IL-8 (Brennecke et al. 2005, Brinkmann et al. 2011, Balija et al. 2005).

IL-1β is a cytokine protein that in humans is encoded by the IL-1B gene (Smirnova et al. 2003). This cytokine is produced by activated macrophages and is processed to its active form by caspase 1. IL-1β exerts various biological functions. Apart from regulating inflammatory response, this cytokine plays a significant role in the development of cancer. IL-1β acts as a potent promoter of tumorigenesis by enhancing the action of chemical carcinogens, which results in the proliferation of mutated cells and further accumulation of genetic damage (Dinarello 1996).

This proangiogenic, proinflammatory cytokine was found to be elevated in the saliva of oral leukoplakia or OSCC patients as compared to controls, thus suggesting its utility as indicator of malignant transformation from oral leukoplakia to OSCC (Rhodus et al. 2005).

Salivary IL-1β in a study was found to be high in OSCC patients. Interestingly in the same study, serum concentrations of IL-1β were below the level of detection (Brailo et al. 2012).

12.5.2 DUSP1

DUSP1 is a nuclear mitogen-activated protein kinase (MAPK) phosphatase. DUSP1 has the capability to inactivate MAPKs by dephosphorylating both phosphothreonine and phosphotyrosine residues located in the activation loop. It is also a transcriptional target of p53 that binds to the p53 binding site located in the second intron. Several factors, such as cellular and oxidative stress, DNA damaging factors, and hypoxia, can upregulate DUSP1 mRNA levels in a variety of cell types (Keyse and Emslie 1992, Franklin and Kraft 1997, Laderoute et al. 1999, Kristiansen et al. 2010).

DUSP1 is considered a negative regulator of cellular proliferation and regulator of cytokine biosynthesis in response to bacterial lipopolysaccharide (Huang et al. 2011). DUSP1 also plays a significant role in immune regulation and mediates the anti-inflammatory response to glucocorticoids (Hammer et al. 2005, Abraham et al. 2006, Chi et al. 2006, Zhao et al. 2006, Yu et al. 2011b). Several studies have also shown that DUSP1 significantly influences metabolic homeostasis and lipid metabolism (Wu et al. 2006, Flach et al. 2011). It also has been shown that DUSP1 protects the oral cavity against inflammation of bacterial etiology (Sartori et al. 2009, Yu et al. 2011a). During the last years, there is increasing evidence about the correlation of altered expression of DUSP1 and cancer. DUSP1 has been implicated as a mediator of tumor suppressor PTEN signaling pathway (Unoki and Nakamura 2001). It has been suggested that DUSP1 can act as tumor regulator according to the cancer type and stage (Patterson et al. 2009). The serum expression of DUSP1 has been shown to decrease in ovarian tumors, and a novel single-nucleotide polymorphism in the DUSP1 gene has been identified (Suzuki et al. 2001). In some human epithelial tumors, such as prostate, colon, and bladder cancer, an overexpression of DUSP1 was found only in the early phases of the disease. DUSP1 expression was also found to decrease in tumors with higher histological grade and metastasis (Loda et al. 1996). As for OSCC patients, several studies have shown that salivary DUSP1 expression is significantly increased compared with healthy individuals (Li et al. 2004, Lee et al. 2011).

12.5.3 H3 Histone, Family 3A

Histone genes are intronless genes that are transcribed into non-polyadenylated mRNAs. Histone H3.3 is a protein that is responsible for the structure of the chromosomal fiber in eukaryotes and has a DNA binding activity (Wells et al. 1987). H3F3A is commonly used as a proliferative marker and has been shown to be upregulated in prostate and colon cancer (Torelli 1987, Bettuzzi et al. 2000). Using standard procedures, it has been demonstrated that salivary H3F3A transcripts exhibit significantly different expression levels between normal and OSCC samples (Lee et al. 2011). Zimmermann and Wong (2008) have shown that H3F3A transcripts are elevated in the saliva of OSCC patients.

12.5.4 Ornithine Decarboxylase Antizyme 1

Ornithine decarboxylase catalyzes the conversion of ornithine to putrescine. Initially, it binds to and then destabilizes ornithine decarboxylase, which is finally degraded. It also inhibits cellular uptake of polyamines by inactivating the polyamine uptake transporter. It takes part in polyamine biosynthesis (Zimmermann and Wong 2008). It is encoded by the OAZ1 gene (Matsufuji et al. 1995).

OSCC patients have been found to have significant alterations of serum and salivary OAZ1 compared with healthy controls (Shpitzer et al. 2007). However, there are reports in the literature not validating OAZ1 as a single marker in the saliva of OSCC patients (Brinkmann et al. 2011).

12.5.5 S100 Calcium Binding Protein P

S100P is a 95 amino acid member of the S100 family of protein (Becker et al. 1992). It plays a role in protein binding and calcium ion binding. S100P expression is described in many different cancers and is associated with drug resistance, metastasis, and poor clinical outcome. S100P serum overexpression seems to be associated with prostate cancer. Recent studies have shown that serum differential expression of S100P is also associated with pancreatic carcinoma (Crnogorac-Jurcevic 2001, Logsdon 2003). In OSCC patients, the expression of S100P was associated with anoikis (a form of programmed cell death) resistance (Kupferman et al. 2007). S100P expression was measured in saliva of patients with OSCC and was found in increased levels (Li et al. 2004).

12.5.6 Spermidine/Spermine N1-Acetyltransferase1

SAT1 takes part in enzyme and transferase activity catalyzing the acetylation of polyamines. SAT1 allows a slight attenuation of the intracellular concentration of polyamines. It is also involved in the regulation of polyamine transport out of cells (Xiao et al. 1992). In several studies, SAT1 was found significantly elevated in serum and saliva of OSCC patients (Li et al. 2004, Brinkmann et al. 2011). Genes from SAT1 were able to discriminate and predict whether a saliva sample was from a patient with cancer or from a healthy subject, with a sensitivity and specificity of 91% (Wong 2006).

12.5.7 Conclusions

The utility of salivary transcriptome diagnostics is a promising field for OSCC detection. This novel diagnostic approach could be exploited to a robust and reproducible tool for early cancer detection.

References

Abraham, S.M., Lawrence, T., Kleiman, A., Warden, P., Medghalchi, M., Tuckermann, J., Saklatvala, J., and Clark, A.R. 2006. Antiinflammatory effects of dexamethasone are partly dependent on induction of dual specificity phosphatase 1. *The Journal of Experimental Medicine* 203(8), 1883–1889.

Acha, A., Ruesga, M.T., Rodriguez, M.J., Martinez de pancorbo, M.A., and Aguirre, J.M. 2005. Applications of the oral scraped (exfoliative) cytology in oral cancer and precancer. *Medicina Oral, Patologia Oral Y Cirugia Bucal* 10(2), 95–102.

Aebersold, D.M., Burri, P., Beer, K.T., Laissue, J., Djonov, V., Greiner, R.H., and Semenza, G.L. 2001. Expression of hypoxia-inducible factor-1alpha: A novel predictive and prognostic parameter in the radiotherapy of oropharyngeal cancer. *Cancer Research* 61(7), 2911–2916.

Agarwal, S., Mathur, M., Shukla, N.K., and Ralhan, R. 1998. Expression of cyclin dependent kinase inhibitor p21waf1/cip1 in premalignant and malignant oral lesions: Relationship with p53 status. *Oral Oncology* 34(5), 353–360.

Ahonen, M., Poukkula, M., Baker, A.H., Kashiwagi, M., Nagase, H., Eriksson, J.E., and Kahari, V.M. 2003. Tissue inhibitor of metalloproteinases-3 induces apoptosis in melanoma cells by stabilization of death receptors. *Oncogene* 22(14), 2121–2134.

Ai, L., Stephenson, K.K., Ling, W., Zuo, C., Mukunyadzi, P., Suen, J.Y., Hanna, E., and Fan, C.Y. 2003. The p16 (cdkn2a/ink4a) tumor-suppressor gene in head and neck squamous cell carcinoma: A promoter methylation and protein expression study in 100 cases. *Modern Pathology: An Official Journal of the United States and Canadian Academy of Pathology, inc* 16(9), 944–950.

Akanuma, D., Uzawa, N., Yoshida, M.A., Negishi, A., Amagasa, T., and Ikeuchi, T. 1999. Inactivation patterns of the p16 (ink4a) gene in oral squamous cell carcinoma cell lines. *Oral Oncology* 35(5), 476–483.

Al-Nedawi, K., Meehan, B., and Rak, J. 2009. Microvesicles: Messengers and mediators of tumor progression. *Cell Cycle* 8, 2014–2018.

Al-Wabel, A., Al-Knawy, B., and Raziuddin, S. 1995. Interleukin-8 and granulocyte-macrophage colony-stimulating factor secretion in hepatocellular carcinoma and viral chronic active hepatitis. *Clinical Immunology and Immunopathology* 74, 231–235.

Angiero, F., Berenzi, A., Benetti, A., Rossi, E., Del sordo, R., Sidoni, A., Stefani, M., and Dessy, E. 2008. Expression of p16, p53 and ki-67 proteins in the rogression of epithelial dysplasia of the oral cavity. *Anticancer Research* 28(5a), 2535–2539.

Baker, E.A., Leaper, D.J., Hayter, J.P., and Dickenson, A.J. 2006. The matrix metalloproteinase system in oral squamous cell carcinoma. *The British Journal of Oral & Maxillofacial Surgery* 44(6), 482–486.

Balija, M., Brennecke, S., Deichmann, M., Nacher, H., and Kurzen, H. 2005. Decline in angiogenic factors, such as interleukin-8, indicates response to chemotherapy of metastatic melanoma. *Melanoma Research* 15, 515–522.

Barnes, L., Eveson, J.W., Reichert, P., and Sidransky, D. 2005. *World Health Organization Classification of Tumours. Pathology and Genetics of Head and Neck Tumours*. Lyon, France: IARC Press.

Beasley, N.J., Leek, R., Alam, M., Turley, H., Cox, G.J., Gatter, K., Millard, P., Fuggle, S., and Harris, A.L. 2002. Hypoxia-inducible factors hif-1alpha and hif-2alpha in head and neck cancer: Relationship to tumor biology and treatment outcome in surgically resected patients. *Cancer Research* 62(9), 2493–2497.

Beasley, N.J., Wykoff, C.C., Watson, P.H., Leek, R. et al. 2001. Carbonic anhydrase ix, an endogenous hypoxia marker, expression in head and neck squamous cell carcinoma and its relationship to hypoxia, necrosis, and microvessel density. *Cancer Research* 61(13), 5262–5267.

Becker, T., Gerke, V., Kube, E., and Weber, K. 1992. S100P, a novel Ca(2+)-binding protein from human placenta. cDNA cloning, recombinant protein expression and Ca2+ binding properties. *European Journal of Biochemistry* 207(2), 541–547.

Bettuzzi, S., Davalli, P., Astancolle, S., Carani, C., Madeo, B., Tampieri, A., and Corti, A. 2000. Tumor progression is accompanied by significant changes in the levels of expression of polyamine metabolism regulatory genes and clusterin (sulfated glycoprotein 2) in human prostate cancer specimens. *Cancer Research* 60, 28–34.

Bhattacharya, A., Toth, K., Durrani, F.A., Cao, S., Slocum, H.K., Chintala, S., and Rustum, Y.M. 2008. Hypoxia-specific drug tirapazamine does not abrogate hypoxic tumor cells in combination therapy with irinotecan and methylselenocysteine in well-differentiated human head and neck squamous cell carcinoma a253 xenografts. *Neoplasia (New York)* 10(8), 857–865.

Bhattacharya, A., Toth, K., Mazurchuk, R., Spernyak, J.A. et al. 2004. Lack of microvessels in well-differentiated regions of human head and neck squamous cell carcinoma a253 associated with functional magnetic resonance imaging detectable hypoxia, limited drug delivery, and resistance to irinotecan therapy. *Clinical Cancer Research: An Official Journal of the American Association for Cancer Research* 10(23), 8005–8017.

Bhowmick, N.A., Neilson, E.G., and Moses, H.L. 2004. Stromal fibroblasts in cancer initiation and progression. *Nature* 432(7015), 332–337.

Bian, J., Wang, Y., Smith, M.R., Kim, H., Jacobs, C., Jackman, J., Kung, H.F., Colburn, N.H., and Sun, Y. 1996. Suppression of in vivo tumor growth and induction of suspension cell death by tissue inhibitor of metalloproteinases (timp)-3. *Carcinogenesis* 17(9), 1805–1811.

Birkedal-Hansen, B., Pavelic, Z.P., Gluckman, J.L., Stambrook, P., Li, Y.Q., and Stetler-Stevenson, W.G. 2000. Mmp and timp gene expression in head and neck squamous cell carcinomas and adjacent tissues. *Oral Diseases* 6(6), 376–382.

Birner, P., Schindl, M., Obermair, A., Breitenecker, G., and Oberhuber, G. 2001. Expression of hypoxia-inducible factor 1alpha in epithelial ovarian tumors: Its impact on prognosis and on response to chemotherapy. *Clinical Cancer Research: An Official Journal of the American Association for Cancer Research* 7(6), 1661–1668.

Bishop, J.W., Bigner, S.H., Colgan, T.J., Husain, M., Howell, L.P., Mcintosh, K.M., Taylor, D.A., and Sadeghi, M.H. 1998. Multicenter masked evaluation of autocyte prep thin layers with matched conventional smears. Including initial biopsy results. *Acta Cytologica* 42(1), 189–197.

Black, J.D. 2000. Protein kinase c-mediated regulation of the cell cycle. *Frontiers in Bioscience: A Journal and Virtual Library* 5, D406–D423.

Blot, W.J., McLaughlin, J.K. et al. 1988. Smoking and drinking in relation to oral and pharyngeal cancer. *Cancer Research* 48, 3282–3287.

Bouquot, J.E., Speight, P.M. et al. 2006. Epithelial dysplasia of the oral mucosa—Diagnostic problems and prognostic features. *Current Diagnostic Pathology* 12, 11–21.

Bova, R.J., Quinn, D.I., Nankervis, J.S., Cole, I.E., Sheridan, B.F., Jensen, M.J., Morgan, G.J., Hughes, C.J., and Sutherland, R.L. 1999. Cyclin d1 and p16ink4a expression predict reduced survival in carcinoma of the anterior tongue. *Clinical Cancer Research: An Official Journal of the American Association for Cancer Research* 5(10), 2810–2819.

Braakhuis, B.J., Tabor, M.P. et al. 2003. A genetic explanation of Slaughter's concept of field cancerization: Evidence and clinical implications. *Cancer Research* 63:1727–1730.

Bradley, K.T., Budnick, S.D., and Logani, S. 2006. Immunohistochemical detection of p16ink4a in dysplastic lesions of the oral cavity. *Modern Pathology: An Official Journal of the United States and Canadian Academy of Pathology, inc*. 19(10), 1310–1316.

Brailo, V., Vucicevic-Boras, V., Lukac, J., Biocina-Lukenda, D., Zilic-Alajbeg, I., and Milenovic, A. 2012. Salivary and serum interleukin 1 beta, interleukin 6 and tumor necrosis factor alpha in patients with leukoplakia and oral cancer. *Medicina Oral Patologia Oral y Cirugia Bucal* January 1, 17(1), e10–e15.

Brennan, P.A., Mackenzie, N., and Quintero, M. 2005. Hypoxia-inducible factor 1alpha in oral cancer. *Journal of Oral Pathology & Medicine: Official Publication of the International Association of Oral Pathologists and the American Academy of Oral Pathology* 34(7), 385–389.

Brennan, P.A., Palacios-Callender, M., Umar, T., Tant, S., and Langdon, J.D. 2002. Expression of type 2 nitric oxide synthase and p21 in oral squamous cell carcinoma. *International Journal of Oral and Maxillofacial Surgery* 31(2), 200–205.

Brennecke, S., Deichmann, M., Naeher, H., and Kurzen, H. 2005. Decline in angiogenic factors, such as interleukin-8, indicates response to chemotherapy of metastatic melanoma. *Melanoma Research* 15(6), 515–522.

Brewer, C.A., Liao, S.Y., Wilczynski, S.P., Pastorekova, S., Pastorek, J., Zavada, J., Kurosaki, T. et al. 1996. A study of biomarkers in cervical carcinoma and clinical correlation of the novel biomarker MN. *Gynecologic Oncology* 63(3), 337–344.

Brinkmann, O., Kastratovic, D.A., Dimitrijevic, M.V., Konstantinovic, V.S., Jelovac, D.B., Antic, J., Nesic V.S. et al. 2011. Oral squamous cell carcinoma detection by salivary biomarkers in a Serbian population. *Oral Oncology* 47(1), 51–55.

Buajeeb, W., Poomsawat, S., Punyasingh, J., and Sanguansin, S. 2009. Expression of p16 in oral cancer and premalignant lesions. *Journal of Oral Pathology & Medicine: Official Publication of the International Association of Oral Pathologists and the American Academy of Oral Pathology* 38(1), 104–108.

Burri, P., Djonov, V., Aebersold, D.M., Lindel, K., Studer, U., Altermatt, H.J., Mazzucchelli, L., Greiner, R.H., and Gruber, G. 2003. Significant correlation of hypoxia-inducible factor-1alpha with treatment outcome in cervical cancer treated with radical radiotherapy. *International Journal of Radiation Oncology, Biology, Physics* 56(2), 494–501.

Camisasca, D.R., Honorato, J. et al. 2009. Expression of Bcl-2 family proteins and associated clinicopathologic factors predict survival outcome in patients with oral squamous cell carcinoma. *Oral Oncology* 45, 225–233.

Camisasca, D.R., Silami, M.A. et al. 2011. Oral squamous cell carcinoma: Clinicopathological features in patients with and without recurrence. *Journal of Oto-Rhino-Laryngology and Its Related Specialties* 73, 170–176.

Cao, J., Zhou, J., Gao, Y., Gu, L., Meng, H., Liu, H., and Deng, D. 2009. Methylation of p16 cpg island associated with malignant progression of oral epithelial dysplasia: A prospective cohort study. *Clinical Cancer Research: An Official Journal of the American Association for Cancer Research* 15(16), 5178–5183.

Carvalho, A.L., Ikeda, M.K. et al. 2004. Trends of oral and oropharyngeal cancer survival over five decades in 3267 patients treated in a single institution. *Oral Oncology* 40, 71–76.

Carvalho, A.L., Nishimoto, I.N. et al. 2005. Trends in incidence and prognosis for head and neck cancer in the United States: A site-specific analysis of the SEER database. *International Journal of Cancer* 114, 806–816.

Caterina, J.J., Yamada, S., Caterina, N.C., Longenecker, G., Holmback, K., Shi, J., Yermovsky, A.E., Engler, J.A., and Birkedal-hansen, H. 2000. Inactivating mutation of the mouse tissue inhibitor of metalloproteinases-2(timp-2) gene alters prommp-2 activation. *The Journal of Biological Chemistry* 275(34), 26416–26422.

Chang, K.W., Lin, S.C., Kwan, P.C., and Wong, Y.K. 2000. Association of aberrant p53 and p21(waf1) immunoreactivity with the outcome of oral verrucous leukoplakia in Taiwan. *Journal of Oral Pathology & Medicine: Official Publication of the International Association of Oral Pathologists and the American Academy of Oral Pathology* 29(2), 56–62.

Chen, Q., Luo, G., Li, B., and Samaranayake, L.P. 1999. Expression of p16 and cdk4 in oral premalignant lesions and oral squamous cell carcinomas: A semi-quantitative immunohistochemical study. *Journal of Oral Pathology & Medicine: Official Publication of the International Association of Oral Pathologists and the American Academy of Oral Pathology* 28(4), 158–164.

Chen, W.T., Huang, C.J., Wu, M.T., Yang, S.F., Su, Y.C., and Chai, C.Y. 2005. Hypoxia-inducible factor-1alpha is associated with risk of aggressive behavior and tumor angiogenesis in gastrointestinal stromal tumor. *Japanese Journal of Clinical Oncology* 35(4), 207–213.

Chi, H., Barry, S.P., Roth, R.J., Wu, J.J., Jones, E.A., Bennett, A.M., and Flavell, R.A. 2006. Dynamic regulation of pro- and anti-inflammatory cytokines by MAPK phosphatase 1 (MKP-1) in innate immune responses. *Proceedings of the National Academy of Sciences of the USA* 103(7), 2274–2279.

Chia, S.K., Wykoff, C.C., Watson, P.H., Han, C., Leek, R.D., Pastorek, J., Gatter, K.C., Ratcliffe, P., and Harris, A.L. 2001. Prognostic significance of a novel hypoxia-regulated marker, carbonic anhydrase ix, in invasive breast carcinoma. *Journal of Clinical Oncology: Official Journal of the American Society of Clinical Oncology* 19(16), 3660–3668.

Chintala, S., Toth, K., Cao, S., Durrani, F.A., Vaughan, M.M., Jensen, R.L., and Rustum, Y.M. 2010. Se-methylselenocysteine sensitizes hypoxic tumor cells to irinotecan by targeting hypoxia-inducible factor 1alpha. *Cancer Chemotherapy and Pharmacology* 66(5), 899–911.

Choi, H.R., Tucker, S.A., Huang, Z., Gillenwater, A.M., Luna, M.A., Batsakis, J.G., and El-Naggar, A.K. 2003. Differential expressions of cyclin-dependent kinase inhibitors (p27 and p21) and their relation to p53 and ki-67 in oral squamous tumorigenesis. *International Journal of Oncology* 22(2), 409–414.

Choi, S. and Myers, J.N. 2008. Molecular pathogenesis of oral squamous cell carcinoma: Implications for therapy. *Journal of Dental Research* 87:14–32.

Choi, S.W., Kim, J.Y., Park, J.Y., Cha, I.H., Kim, J., and Lee, S. 2008. Expression of carbonic anhydrase ix is associated with postoperative recurrence and poor prognosis in surgically treated oral squamous cell carcinoma. *Human Pathology* 39(9), 1317–1322.

Cody, D.T., II, Huang, Y., Darby, C.J., Johnson, G.K., and Domann, F.E. 1999. Differential DNA methylation of the p16 ink4a/cdkn2a promoter in human oral cancer cells and normal human oral keratinocytes. *Oral Oncology* 35(5), 516–522.

Costa, A., Coradini, D., Carrassi, A., Erdas, R., Sardella, A., and Daidone, M.G. 2001. Re: Levels of hypoxia-inducible factor-1alpha during breast carcinogenesis. *Journal of the National Cancer Institute* 93(15), 1175–1177.

Crnogorac-Jurcevic, T., Missiaglia, E., Blaveri, E., Gangeswaranm, R., Jones, M., Terris, B., Costello, E., Neoptolemos, J.P., and Lemoine, N.R. 2003. Molecular alterations in pancreatic carcinoma: Expression profiling shows that dysregulated expression of S100 genes is highly prevalent. *Journal of Pathology* 201, 63–74.

Dahlstrom, K.R., Little, J.A. et al. 2008. Squamous cell carcinoma of the head and neck in never smoker-never drinkers: A descriptive epidemiologic study. *Head & Neck* 30, 75–84.

Danaei, G., Vander Hoorn, S. et al. 2005. Causes of cancer in the world: Comparative risk assessment of nine behavioural and environmental risk factors. *Lancet* 366, 1784–1793.

de Camargo Cancela, M., Voti, L. et al. 2010. Oral cavity cancer in developed and in developing countries: Population-based incidence. *Head & Neck* 32, 357–367.

de Vicente, J.C., Fresno, M.F., Villalain, L., Vega, J.A., and Lopez arranz, J.S. 2005. Immunoexpression and prognostic significance of timp-1 and -2 in oral squamous cell carcinoma. *Oral Oncology* 41(6), 568–579.

de Vicente, J.C., Lequerica-Fernandez, P. et al. 2007a. Expression of MMP-7 and MT1-MMP in oral squamous cell carcinoma as predictive indicator for tumor invasion and prognosis. *Journal of Oral Pathology & Medicine* 36, 415–424.

Devy, L. and Dransfield, D.T. 2011. New strategies for the next generation of matrix-metalloproteinase inhibitors: Selectively targeting membrane-anchored mmps with therapeutic antibodies. *Biochemistry Research International* 2011, 191670.

Dias, F.L., Kligerman, J. et al. 2001. Elective neck dissection versus observation in stage I squamous cell carcinomas of the tongue and floor of the mouth. *Otolaryngology Head and Neck Surgery* 125, 23–29.

Dinarello, C.A. 1996. Biologic basis for interleukin-1 in disease. *Blood* 87, 2095–2147.

Diniz Freitas, M., García García, A., Crespo Abelleira, A., Martins Carneiro, J.L., and Gándara Rey, J.M. 2004. Applications of exfoliative cytology in the diagnosis of oral cancer. *Medicina Oral, Patología Oral y Cirugía Bucal (ed.impresa)* 9, 355–361.

Dorman, G., Cseh, S., Hajdu, I., Barna, L., Konya, D., Kupai, K., Kovacs, L., and Ferdinandy, P. 2010. Matrix metalloproteinase inhibitors: A critical appraisal of design principles and proposed therapeutic utility. *Drugs* 70(8), 949–964.

D'Souza, G., Kreimer, A.R. et al. 2007. Case-control study of human papillomavirus and oropharyngeal cancer. *The New England Journal of Medicine* 356, 1944–1956.

Duong, H.S., Le, A.D., Zhang, Q., and Messadi, D.V. 2005. A novel 3-dimensional culture system as an in vitro model for studying oral cancer cell invasion. *International Journal of Experimental Pathology* 86(6), 365–374.

Dwivedi, R.C., St. Rose, S. et al. 2012. Evaluation of factors affecting post-treatment quality of life in oral and oropharyngeal cancer patients primarily treated with curative surgery: An exploratory study. *European Archives of Otorhinolaryngol* 269, 591–599.

Eckert, A.W., Lautner, M.H., Schutze, A., Bolte, K., Bache, M., Kappler, M., Schubert, J., Taubert, H., and Bilkenroth, U. 2010a. Co-expression of hif1alpha and caix is associated with poor prognosis in oral squamous cell carcinoma patients. *Journal of Oral Pathology & Medicine: Official Publication of the International Association of Oral Pathologists and the American Academy of Oral Pathology* 39(4), 313–317.

Eckert, A.W., Lautner, M.H., Schutze, A., Taubert, H., Schubert, J., and Bilkenroth, U. 2011. Coexpression of hypoxia-inducible factor-1alpha and glucose transporter-1 is associated with poor prognosis in oral squamous cell carcinoma patients. *Histopathology* 58(7), 1136–1147.

Eckert, A.W., Schutze, A., Lautner, M.H., Taubert, H., Schubert, J.M., and Bilkenroth, U. 2010b. Hif-1alpha is a prognostic marker in oral squamous cell carcinomas. *The International Journal of Biological Markers* 25(2), 87–92.

Edge, S., Byrd, D. et al. 2010. *AJCC Cancer Staging Manual*. New York: Springer.

Edge, S.B. and Compton, C.C. 2010. The American Joint Committee on Cancer: The 7th edition of the AJCC cancer staging manual and the future of TNM. *Annals of Surgical Oncology* 17, 1471–1474.

Eichel, H.J., Conger, N., and Chernick, W.S. 1964. Acid and alkaline ribonucleases of human parotid, submaxillary, and whole saliva. *Archives of Biochemistry and Biophysics* 107, 197–208.

Eisen, D. and Frist, S. 2005. The relevance of the high positive predictive value of the oral brush biopsy. *Oral Oncology* 41, 753–755; author reply 756.

English, J.L., Kassiri, Z., Koskivirta, I., Atkinson, S.J., Di Grappa, M., Soloway, P.D., Nagase, H. et al. 2006. Individual timp deficiencies differentially impact pro-mmp-2 activation. *The Journal of Biological Chemistry* 281(15), 10337–10346.

Eriksen, J.G., Overgaard, J., and Danish Head and Neck Cancer Study Group (DAHANCA). 2007. Lack of prognostic and predictive value of CA-IX in radiotherapy of squamous cell carcinoma of the head and neck with known modifiable hypoxia: An evaluation of the dahanca 5 study. *Radiotherapy and Oncology: Journal of the European Society for Therapeutic Radiology and Oncology* 83(3), 383–388.

Fillies, T., Werkmeister, R., Van diest, P.J., Brandt, B., Joos, U., and Buerger, H. 2005. Hif1-alpha overexpression indicates a good prognosis in early stage squamous cell carcinomas of the oral floor. *BMC Cancer* 5, 84.

Fillies, T., Woltering, M., Brandt, B., Van diest, J.P., Werkmeister, R., Joos, U., and Buerger, H. 2007. Cell cycle regulating proteins p21 and p27 in prognosis of oral squamous cell carcinomas. *Oncology Reports* 17(2), 355–359.

Flach, R.J., Qin, H., Zhang, L., and Bennett, A.M. 2011. Loss of mitogen-activated protein kinase phosphatase-1 protects from hepatic steatosis by repression of cell death-inducing DNA fragmentation factor A (DFFA)-like effector C (CIDEC)/fat-specific protein 27. *The Journal of Biological Chemistry* 286(25), 22195–22202.

Franklin, C.C. and Kraft, A.S. 1997. Conditional expression of the mitogen-activated protein kinase (MAPK) phosphatase MKP-1 preferentially inhibits p38 MAPK and stress-activated protein kinase in U937 cells. *The Journal of Biological Chemistry* 272(27), 16917–16923.

Friedl, P. and Wolf, K. 2008. Tube travel: The role of proteases in individual and collective cancer cell invasion. *Cancer Research* 68(18), 7247–7249.

Gao, Z.B., Duan, Y.Q., Zhang, L., Chen, D.W., and Ding, P.T. 2005. Expression of matrix metalloproteinase 2 and its tissue inhibitor in oral squamous cell carcinoma. *International Journal of Molecular Medicine* 16(4), 599–603.

Garavello, W., Spreafico, R. et al. 2007. Oral tongue cancer in young patients: A matched analysis. *Oral Oncology* 43, 894–897.

García, J.M., García, V., Peña, C., Domínguez, G., Silva, J., Diaz, R., Espinosa, P. et al. 2008. Extracellular plasma RNA from colon cancer patients is confined in a vesicle-like structure and is mRNA-enriched. *RNA* 14, 1424–1432.

Gebhart, E., Liehr, T., Wolff, E., Wiltfang, J., Koscielny, S., and Ries, J. 2003. Loss of 9p21 is embedded in a complex but consistent pattern of genomic imbalances in oral squamous cell carcinomas. *Cytogenetic and Genome Research* 101(2), 106–112.

Giatromanolaki, A., Koukourakis, M.I., Sivridis, E., Pastorek, J., Wykoff, C.C., Gatter, K.C., and Harris, A.L. 2001. Expression of hypoxia-inducible carbonic anhydrase-9 relates to angiogenic pathways and independently to poor outcome in non-small cell lung cancer. *Cancer Research* 61(21), 7992–7998.

Girod, A., Mosseri, V. et al. 2009. Women and squamous cell carcinomas of the oral cavity and oropharynx: Is there something new? *Journal of Oral and Maxillofacial Surgery* 67, 1914–1920.

Gologan, O., Barnes, E.L., and Hunt, J.L. 2005. Potential diagnostic use of p16ink4a, a new marker that correlates with dysplasia in oral squamoproliferative lesions. *The American Journal of Surgical Pathology* 29(6), 792–796.

Gonzalez-Moles, M.A., Gil-Montoya, J.A., Ruiz-Avila, I., Esteban, F., Delgado-Rodriguez, M., and Bascones-Martinez, A. 2007. Prognostic significance of p21waf1/cip1, p16ink4a and cd44s in tongue cancer. *Oncology Reports* 18(2), 389–396.

Gonzalez-Moles, M.A., Ruiz-Avila, I., Martinez, J.A., Gil-Montoya, J.A., Esteban, F., Gonzalez-Moles, S., Bravo-Perez, M., and Bascones, A. 2004. P21waf1/cip1 protein and tongue cancer prognosis. *Anticancer Research* 24(5b), 3225–3231.

Gray, S.T., Wilkins, R.J., and Yun, K. 1992. Interstitial collagenase gene expression in oral squamous cell carcinoma. *The American Journal of Pathology* 141(2), 301–306.

Guo, X.L., Sun, S.Z., Wang, W.X., Wei, F.C., Yu, H.B., and Ma, B.L. 2007. Alterations of p16ink4a tumour suppressor gene in mucoepidermoid carcinoma of the salivary glands. *International Journal of Oral and Maxillofacial Surgery* 36(4), 350–353.

Hall, G.L., Shaw, R.J., Field, E.A., Rogers, S.N., Sutton, D.N., Woolgar, J.A., Lowe, D. et al. 2008. P16 promoter methylation is a potential predictor of malignant transformation in oral epithelial dysplasia. *Cancer Epidemiology, Biomarkers & Prevention: A Publication of the American Association for Cancer Research, Cosponsored by the American Society of Preventive Oncology* 17(8), 2174–2179.

Hammer, M., Mages, J., Dietrich, H., Schmitz, F., Striebel, F., Murray, P.J., Wagner, H., and Lang, R. 2005. Control of dual-specificity phosphatase-1 expression in activated macrophages by IL-10. *European Journal of Immunology* 35(10), 2991–3001.

Hanson, E.K., Lubenow, H., and Ballantyne, J. 2009. Identification of forensically relevant body fluids using a panel of differentially expressed microRNAs. *Analytical Biochemistry* 387, 303–314.

Harada, K., Supriatno, Yoshida, H., and Sato, M. 2005. Vesnarinone inhibits angiogenesis and tumorigenicity of human oral squamous cell carcinoma cells by suppressing the expression of vascular endothelial growth factor and interleukin-8. *International Journal of Oncology* 27, 1489–1497.

Hashibe, M., Brennan, P. et al. 2009. Interaction between tobacco and alcohol use and the risk of head and neck cancer: Pooled analysis in the International Head and Neck Cancer Epidemiology Consortium. *Cancer Epidemiology Biomarkers & Prevention* 18, 541–550.

Hassel, A.J., Danner, D. et al. 2012. Oral health-related quality of life and depression/anxiety in long-term recurrence-free patients after treatment for advanced oral squamous cell cancer. *Journal of Cranio-Maxillofacial Surgery* 40, e99–e102.

Hasselmann, D., Rappl, G., Tilgen, W., and Reinhold, U. 2001. Extracellular tyrosinase mRNA within apoptotic bodies is protected from degradation in human serum. *Clinical Chemistry* 47, 1488–1489.

Hernandez-Barrantes, S., Toth, M., Bernardo, M.M., Yurkova, M., Gervasi, D.C., Raz, Y., Sang, Q.A., and Fridman, R. 2000. Binding of active (57 kda) membrane type 1-matrix metalloproteinase (mt1-mmp) to tissue inhibitor of metalloproteinase (timp)-2 regulates mt1-mmp processing and pro-mmp-2 activation. *The Journal of Biological Chemistry* 275(16), 12080–12089.

Hogmo, A., Lindskog, S., Lindholm, J., Kuylenstierna, R., Auer, G., and Munck-Wikland, E. 1998. Preneoplastic oral lesions: The clinical value of image cytometry DNA analysis, p53 and p21/waf1 expression. *Anticancer Research* 18(5b), 3645–3650.

Hojilla, C.V., Wood, G.A., and Khokha, R. 2008. Inflammation and breast cancer: Metalloproteinases as common effectors of inflammation and extracellular matrix breakdown in breast cancer. *Breast Cancer Research: BCR* 10(2), 205.

Hong, Y., Yang, L., Li, C., Xia, H., Rhodus, N.L., and Cheng, B. 2007. Frequent mutation of p16(cdkn2a) exon 1 during rat tongue carcinogenesis induced by 4-nitroquinoline-1-oxide. *Molecular Carcinogenesis* 46(2), 85–90.

Hoogsteen, I.J., Marres, H.A., Wijffels, K.I., Rijken, P.F., Peters, J.P., Van den hoogen, F.J., Oosterwijk, E., Van der kogel, A.J., and Kaanders, J.H. 2005. Colocalization of carbonic anhydrase 9 expression and cell proliferation in human head and neck squamous cell carcinoma. *Clinical Cancer Research: An Official Journal of the American Association for Cancer Research* 11(1), 97–106.

Huang, G., Wang, Y., Shi, L.Z., Kanneganti, T.D., and Chi, H. 2011. Signaling by the phosphatase MKP-1 in dendritic cells imprints distinct effector and regulatory T cell fates. *Immunity* 35(1), 45–58.

Huber, M.A. 2012. Adjunctive diagnostic aids in oral cancer screening: An update. *Texas Dental Journal* 129, 471–480.

Hull, J., Thomson, A., and Kwiatkowski, D. 2006. Association of respiratory syncytial virus bronchiolitis with the interleukin 8 gene region in UK families. *Thorax* 55, 1023–1027.

Hunter, T. and Pines, J. 1994. Cyclins and cancer. II: Cyclin d and cdk inhibitors come of age. *Cell* 79(4), 573–582.

Ibrahim, S.O., Lillehaug, J.R., Dolphine, O., Johnson, N.W., Warnakulasuriya, K.A., and Vasstrand, E.N. 2002. Mutations of the cell cycle arrest gene p21waf1, but not the metastasis-inducing gene s100a4, are frequent in oral squamous cell carcinomas from sudanese toombak dippers and non-snuff-dippers from the sudan, scandinavia, USA and UK. *Anticancer Research* 22(3), 1445–1451.

Ikebe, T., Shinohara, M., Takeuchi, H., Beppu, M., Kurahara, S., Nakamura, S., and Shirasuna, K. 1999. Gelatinolytic activity of matrix metalloproteinase in tumor tissues correlates with the invasiveness of oral cancer. *Clinical and Experimental Metastasis* 17(4), 315–323.

Imren, S., Kohn, D.B., Shimada, H., Blavier, L., and Declerck, Y.A. 1996. Overexpression of tissue inhibitor of metalloproteinases-2 retroviral-mediated gene transfer in vivo inhibits tumor growth and invasion. *Cancer Research* 56(13), 2891–2895.

Isaacs, J.S., Jung, Y.J., Mimnaugh, E.G., Martinez, A., Cuttitta, F., and Neckers, L.M. 2002. Hsp90 regulates a von hippel lindau-independent hypoxia-inducible factor-1 alpha-degradative pathway. *The Journal of Biological Chemistry* 277(33), 29936–29944.

Jaiswal, M., LaRusso, N.F., Burgart, L.J., and Gores, G.J. 2002. Inflammatory cytokines induce DNA damage and inhibit DNA repair in cholangiocarcinoma cells by a nitric oxide-dependent mechanism. *Cancer Research* 60, 184–190.

Jayasurya, R., Sathyan, K.M., Lakshminarayanan, K., Abraham, T., Nalinakumari, K.R., Abraham, E.K., Nair, M.K., and Kannan, S. 2005. Phenotypic alterations in Rb pathway have more prognostic influence than p53 pathway proteins in oral carcinoma. *Modern Pathology: An Official Journal of the United States and Canadian Academy of Pathology, inc* 18(8), 1056–1066.

Jemal, A., Bray, F. et al. 2011. Global cancer statistics. *CA: A Cancer Journal of Clinicans* 61, 69–90.

Johnson, N. 1997. Oral cancer—A worldwide problem. *FDI World* 6, 19–21.

Jonathan, R.A., Wijffels, K.I., Peeters, W., De Wilde, P.C., Marres, H.A., Merkx, M.A., Oosterwijk, E., Van der kogel, A.J., and Kaanders, J.H. 2006. The prognostic value of endogenous hypoxia-related markers for head and neck squamous cell carcinomas treated with arcon. *Radiotherapy and Oncology: Journal of the European Society for Therapeutic Radiology and Oncology* 79(3), 288–297.

Jones, D.L. 2012. Oral cancer: Diagnosis, treatment, and management of sequela. *Texas Dental Journal* 129, 459.

Juarez, J., Clayman, G., Nakajima, M., Tanabe, K.K., Saya, H., Nicolson, G.L., and Boyd, D. 1993. Role and regulation of expression of 92-kda type-iv collagenase (mmp-9) in 2 invasive squamous-cell-carcinoma cell lines of the oral cavity. *International Journal of Cancer. Journal International du Cancer* 55(1), 10–18.

Kaanders, J.H., Wijffels, K.I., Marres, H.A., Ljungkvist, A.S., Pop, L.A., Van den hoogen, F.J., De Wilde, P.C. et al. 2002. Pimonidazole binding and tumor vascularity predict for treatment outcome in head and neck cancer. *Cancer Research* 62(23), 7066–7074.

Kaminagakura, E., Vartanian, J.G. et al. 2010. Case-control study on prognostic factors in oral squamous cell carcinoma in young patients. *Head & Neck* 32, 1460–1466.

Kapranos, N., Stathopoulos, G.P., Manolopoulos, L., Kokka, E., Papadimitriou, C., Bibas, A., Yiotakis, J., and Adamopoulos, G. 2001. P53, p21 and p27 protein expression in head and neck cancer and their prognostic value. *Anticancer Research* 21(1b), 521–528.

Karsai, S., Abel, U., Roesch-Ely, M., Affolter, A., Hofele, C., Joos, S., Plinkert, P.K., and Bosch, F.X. 2007. Comparison of p16(ink4a) expression with p53 alterations in head and neck cancer by tissue microarray analysis. *The Journal of Pathology* 211(3), 314–322.

Katayama, A., Bandoh, N., Kishibe, K., Takahara, M., Ogino, T., Nonaka, S., and Harabuchi, Y. 2004. Expressions of matrix metalloproteinases in early-stage oral squamous cell carcinoma as predictive indicators for tumor metastases and prognosis. *Clinical Cancer Research: An Official Journal of the American Association for Cancer Research* 10(2), 634–640.

Kato, K., Hara, A., Kuno, T., Mori, H., Yamashita, T., Toida, M., and Shibata, T. 2006. Aberrant promoter hypermethylation of p16 and mgmt genes in oral squamous cell carcinomas and the surrounding normal mucosa. *Journal of Cancer Research and Clinical Oncology* 132(11), 735–743.

Kawamata, H., Nakashiro, K., Uchida, D., Harada, K., Yoshida, H., and Sato, M. 1997. Possible contribution of active mmp2 to lymph-node metastasis and secreted cathepsin l to bone invasion of newly established human oral-squamous-cancer cell lines. *International Journal of Cancer. Journal International du Cancer* 70(1), 120–127.

Keyse, S.M. and Emslie, E.A. 1992. Oxidative stress and heat shock induce a human gene encoding a protein-tyrosine phosphatase. *Nature* 359(6396), 644–647.

Khokha, R. 1994. Suppression of the tumorigenic and metastatic abilities of murine b16-f10 melanoma cells in vivo by the overexpression of the tissue inhibitor of the metalloproteinases-1. *Journal of the National Cancer Institute* 86(4), 299–304.

Khuri, F.R., Kim, E.S. et al. 2001. The impact of smoking status, disease stage, and index tumor site on second primary tumor incidence and tumor recurrence in the head and neck retinoid chemoprevention trial. *Cancer Epidemiol Biomarkers & Prevention* 10, 823–829.

Kim, H.S., Chung, W.B., Hong, S.H., Kim, J.A., Na, S.Y., Jang, H.J., Sohn, Y.K., and Kim, J.W. 2000. Inactivation of p16ink4a in primary tumors and cell lines of head and neck squamous cell carcinoma. *Molecules and Cells* 10(5), 557–565.

Kim, S.J., Shin, H.J., Jung, K.Y., Baek, S.K., Shin, B.K., Choi, J., Kim, B.S. et al. 2007. Prognostic value of carbonic anhydrase ix and ki-67 expression in squamous cell carcinoma of the tongue. *Japanese Journal of Clinical Oncology* 37(11), 812–819.

Kinsenn, H., Sato, H., Furukawa, M., and Yoshizaki, T. 2003. Modulation of cell growth and matrix metalloproteinase-2 activation of oral squamous cell carcinoma as a function of culture condition with type i collagen. *Acta Otolaryngologica* 123(8), 987–993.

Klatte, T., Belldegrun, A.S., and Pantuck, A.J. 2008. The role of carbonic anhydrase ix as a molecular marker for transitional cell carcinoma of the bladder. *BJU International* 101(Suppl 4), 45–48.

Kligerman, J., Lima, R.A. et al. 1994. Supraomohyoid neck dissection in the treatment of T1/T2 squamous cell carcinoma of oral cavity. *The American Journal of Surgery* 168, 391–394.

Koch, A.E., Polverini, P.J., Kunkel, S.L., Harlow, L.A., DiPietro, L.A., Elner, S.G. et al. 1992. Interleukin-8 as a macrophage-derived mediator of angiogenesis. *Science* 258, 1798.

Koh, M.Y., Spivak-Kroizman, T.R., and Powis, G. 2010. Hif-1alpha and cancer therapy. *Recent Results in Cancer Research. fortschritte der krebsforschung. progres dans les recherches sur le cancer* 180, 15–34.

Kondo, Y., Yoshikawa, K., Omura, Y., Shinohara, A., Kazaoka, Y., Sano, J., Mizuno, Y., Yokoi, T., and Yamada, S. 2011. Clinicopathological significance of carbonic anhydrase 9, glucose transporter-1, ki-67 and p53 expression in oral squamous cell carcinoma. *Oncology Reports* 25(5), 1227–1233.

Koukourakis, M.I., Bentzen, S.M., Giatromanolaki, A., Wilson, G.D., Daley, F.M., Saunders, M.I., Dische, S., Sivridis, E., and Harris, A.L. 2006. Endogenous markers of two separate hypoxia response pathways (hypoxia inducible factor 2 alpha and carbonic anhydrase 9) are associated with radiotherapy failure in head and neck cancer patients recruited in the chart randomized trial. *Journal of Clinical Oncology: Official Journal of the American Society of Clinical Oncology* 24(5), 727–735.

Koukourakis, M.I., Giatromanolaki, A., Sivridis, E., Simopoulos, K., Pastorek, J., Wykoff, C.C., Gatter, K.C., and Harris, A.L. 2001. Hypoxia-regulated carbonic anhydrase-9 (ca9) relates to poor vascularization and resistance of squamous cell head and neck cancer to chemoradiotherapy. *Clinical Cancer Research: An Official Journal of the American Association for Cancer Research* 7(11), 3399–3403.

Kresty, L.A., Mallery, S.R., Knobloch, T.J., Li, J., Lloyd, M., Casto, B.C., and Weghorst, C.M. 2008. Frequent alterations of p16ink4a and p14arf in oral proliferative verrucous leukoplakia. *Cancer Epidemiology, Biomarkers & Prevention: A Publication of the American Association for Cancer Research, Cosponsored by the American Society of Preventive Oncology* 17(11), 3179–3187.

Kresty, L.A., Mallery, S.R., Knobloch, T.J., Song, H., Lloyd, M., Casto, B.C., and Weghorst, C.M. 2002. Alterations of p16(ink4a) and p14(arf) in patients with severe oral epithelial dysplasia. *Cancer Research* 62(18), 5295–5300.

Kristiansen, M., Hughes, R., Patel, P., Jacques, T.S., Clark, A.R., and Ham, J. 2010. Mkp1 is a c-Jun target gene that antagonizes JNK-dependent apoptosis in sympathetic neurons. *The Journal of Neuroscience* 30(32), 10820–10832.

Kruse, A.L., Bredell, M. et al. 2011. Oral cancer in men and women: Are there differences? *Journal of Oral and Maxillofacial Surgery* 15, 51–55.

Kudo, Y., Takata, T., Ogawa, I., Sato, S., and Nikai, H. 1999. Expression of p53 and p21cip1/waf1 proteins in oral epithelial dysplasias and squamous cell carcinomas. *Oncology Reports* 6(3), 539–545.

Kumar, S.V., Hurteau, G.J., and Spivack, S.D. 2006. Validity of messenger RNA expression analyses of human saliva. *Clinical Cancer Research* 12, 5033–5039.

Kupferman, M.E., Patel, V., Sriuranpong, V., Amornphimoltham, P., Jasser, S.A., Mandal, M., and Zhou, G. 2007. Molecular analysis of anoikis resistance in oral cavity squamous cell carcinoma. *Oral Oncology* 43(5), 440–454.

Kurahara, S., Shinohara, M., Ikebe, T., Nakamura, S., Beppu, M., Hiraki, A., Takeuchi, H., and Shirasuna, K. 1999. Expression of mmps, mt-mmp, and timps in squamous cell carcinoma of the oral cavity: Correlations with tumor invasion and metastasis. *Head & Neck* 21(7), 627–638.

Kuropkat, C., Venkatesan, T.K., Caldarelli, D.D., Panje, W.R., Hutchinson, J., Preisler, H.D., Coon, J.S., and Werner, J.A. 2002. Abnormalities of molecular regulators of proliferation and apoptosis in carcinoma of the oral cavity and oropharynx. *Auris, Nasus, Larynx* 29(2), 165–174.

Kyzas, P.A., Stefanou, D., Batistatou, A., and Agnantis, N.J. 2005. Hypoxia-induced tumor angiogenic pathway in head and neck cancer: An in vivo study. *Cancer Letters* 225(2), 297–304.

Laderoute, K.R., Mendonca, H.L., Calaoagan, J.M., Knapp, A.M., Giaccia, A.J., and Stork, P.J. 1999. A candidate MKP for the inactivation of hypoxia-inducible stress-activated protein kinase/c-Jun N-terminal protein kinase activity. *The Journal of Biological Chemistry* 274(18), 12890–12897.

Le, Q.T. 2007. Identifying and targeting hypoxia in head and neck cancer: A brief overview of current approaches. *International Journal of Radiation Oncology, Biology, Physics* 69(2 suppl), S56–S58.

Lee, J.K., Kim, M.J., Hong, S.P., and Hong, S.D. 2004. Inactivation patterns of p16/ink4a in oral squamous cell carcinomas. *Experimental & Molecular Medicine* 36(2), 165–171.

Lee, Y.H., Zhou, H., Reiss, J.K., Yan, X., Zhang, L., Chia, D., and Wong, D.T. 2011. Direct saliva transcriptome analysis. *Clinical Chemistry* 57(9), 1295–1302, doi:10.1373/clinchem.2010.159210.

Leite, I.C. and Koifman, S. 1998. Survival analysis in a sample of oral cancer patients at a reference hospital in Rio de Janeiro, Brazil. *Oral Oncology* 34, 347–352.

Li, J., Warner, B., Casto, B.C., Knobloch, T.J., and Weghorst, C.M. 2008. Tumor suppressor p16(ink4a)/cdkn2a alterations in 7, 12-dimethylbenz(a)anthracene (dmba)-induced hamster cheek pouch tumors. *Molecular Carcinogenesis* 47(10), 733–738.

Li, Y., St. John, M.A.R., Zhou, X., Kim, Y., Sinha, U., Jordan, R.C.K., Eisele, D. et al. 2004. Salivary transcriptome diagnostics for oral cancer detection. *Clinical Cancer Research* December 15, 10, 8442. doi: 10.1158/1078–0432.CCR-04–1167.

Liang, X., Zheng, M., Jiang, J., Zhu, G., Yang, J., and Tang, Y. 2011. Hypoxia-inducible factor-1 alpha, in association with twist2 and snip1, is a critical prognostic factor in patients with tongue squamous cell carcinoma. *Oral Oncology* 47(2), 92–97.

Lin, P.Y., Yu, C.H., Wang, J.T., Chen, H.H., Cheng, S.J., Kuo, M.Y., and Chiang, C.P. 2008. Expression of hypoxia-inducible factor-1 alpha is significantly associated with the progression and prognosis of oral squamous cell carcinomas in Taiwan. *Journal of Oral Pathology & Medicine: Official Publication of the International Association of Oral Pathologists and the American Academy of Oral Pathology* 37(1), 18–25.

Lindenblatt R.C., Martinez, G.L. et al. 2012. Oral squamous cell carcinoma grading systems—Analysis of the best survival predictor. *Journal of Oral Pathology & Medicine* 41, 34–39.

Linder, J. and Zahniser, D. 1997. The thinprep pap test. A review of clinical studies. *Acta Cytologica* 41(1), 30–38.

Liu, S.Y., Chang, L.C., Pan, L.F., Hung, Y.J., Lee, C.H., and Shieh, Y.S. 2008. Clinicopathologic significance of tumor cell-lined vessel and microenvironment in oral squamous cell carcinoma. *Oral Oncology* 44(3), 277–285.

Llewellyn, C.D., Johnson, N.W. et al. 2004. Risk factors for oral cancer in newly diagnosed patients aged 45 years and younger: A case-control study in Southern England. *Journal of Oral Pathology & Medicine* 33, 525–532.

Llewellyn, C.D., Linklater, K. et al. 2004. An analysis of risk factors for oral cancer in young people: A case-control study. *Oral Oncology* 40, 304–313.

Lockhart, P.B., Norris, C.M. Jr. et al. 1998. Dental factors in the genesis of squamous cell carcinoma of the oral cavity. *Oral Oncology* 34, 133–139.

Loda, M., Capodieci, P., Mishra, R., Yao, H., Corless, C., Grigioni, W., Wang, Y., Magi-Galluzzi, C., and Stork, P.J. 1996. Expression of mitogen-activated protein kinase phosphase-1 in the early phases of human epithelial carcinogenesis. *American Journal of Pathology* 149, 1553–1564.

Logsdon, C.D., Simeone, D.M., Binkley, C., Arumugam, T., Greenson, J.K., Giordano, T.J., Misek, D.E., Kuick, R., and Hanash, S. 2003. Molecular profiling of pancreatic adenocarcinoma and chronic pancreatitis identifies multiple genes differentially regulated in pancreatic cancer. *Cancer Research* 63, 2649–2657.

Lu, H.H., Liu, C.J., Liu, T.Y., Kao, S.Y., Lin, S.C., and Chang, K.W. 2008. Areca-treated fibroblasts enhance tumorigenesis of oral epithelial cells. *Journal of Dental Research* 87(11), 1069–1074.

Lu, X. and Kang, Y. 2010. Hypoxia and hypoxia-inducible factors: Master regulators of metastasis. *Clinical Cancer Research: An Official Journal of the American Association for Cancer Research* 16(24), 5928–5935.

Luca, M., Huang, S., Gershenwald, J.E., Singh, R.K., Reich, R., Bar-Eli, M. et al. 1997. Expression of interleukin-8 by human melanoma cells up-regulates MMP-2 activity and increases tumor growth and metastasis. *American Journal of Pathology* 151, 1105–1113.

Mabjeesh, N.J., Escuin, D., Lavallee, T.M., Pribluda, V.S. et al. 2003. 2me2 inhibits tumor growth and angiogenesis by disrupting microtubules and dysregulating hif. *Cancer Cell* 3(4), 363–375.

Majmundar, A.J., Wong, W.J., and Simon, M.C. 2010. Hypoxia-inducible factors and the response to hypoxic stress. *Molecular Cell* 40(2), 294–309.

Makino, Y., Kanopka, A., Wilson, W.J., Tanaka, H., and Poellinger, L. 2002. Inhibitory pas domain protein (ipas) is a hypoxia-inducible splicing variant of the hypoxia-inducible factor-3alpha locus. *The Journal of Biological Chemistry*, 277(36), 32405–32408.

Markovic, S.Z., Martinovic, Z.R., Akina, D., Spielmanna, N., Zhoua, H., and Wonga, D.T. 2011. Oral squamous cell carcinoma detection by salivary biomarkers in a serbian population. *Oral Oncology* 47(1), 51–55

Massano, J., Regateiro, F.S. et al. 2006. Oral squamous cell carcinoma: Review of prognostic and predictive factors. *Oral Surgery Oral Medicine Oral Pathology Oral Radiology and Endodontology.* 102, 67–76.

Matsufuji, S., Matsufuji, T., Miyazaki, Y., Murakami, Y., Atkins, J.F., Gesteland, R.F., and Hayashi, S. 1995. Autoregulatory frameshifting in decoding mammalian ornithine decarboxylase antizyme. *Cell* 80(1), 51–60.

Mehrotra, R. and Gupta, D.K. 2011. Exciting new advances in oral cancer diagnosis: Avenues to early detection. *Head & Neck Oncology* 3, 33.

Mehrotra, R., Gupta, A., Singh, M., and Ibrahim, R. 2006. Application of cytology and molecular biology in diagnosing premalignant or malignant oral lesions. *Molecular Cancer* 5, 11.

Michael, A., Bajracharya, S.D., Yuen, P.S., Zhou, H., Star, R.A., Illei, G.G., and Alevizos, I. 2010. Exosomes from human saliva as a source of microRNA biomarkers. *Oral Dis* 16, 34–38.

Modi, W.S., Dean, M., Seuanez, H.N., Mukaida, N., Matsushima, K., and O'Brien, S.J. 1990. Monocyte-derived neutrophil chemotactic factor (MDNCF/IL-8) resides in a gene cluster along with several other members of the platelet factor 4 gene superfamily. *Human Genetics* 84(2), 185–187.

Moore, M.A. 2002. Cytokine and chemokine networks influencing stem cell proliferation, differentiation and marrow homing. *Journal of Cellular Biochemistry* 38, 29–38.

Moore, S.R., Johnson, N.W. et al. 2000. The epidemiology of mouth cancer: A review of global incidence. *Oral Diseases* 6, 65–74.

Morgan, D.O. 1995. Principles of cdk regulation. *Nature* 374(6518), 131–134.

Moulder, J.E. and Rockwell, S. 1987. Tumor hypoxia: Its impact on cancer therapy. *Cancer Metastasis Reviews* 5(4), 313–341.

Muirhead, D.M., Hoffman, H.T., and Robinson, R.A. 2006. Correlation of clinicopathological features with immunohistochemical expression of cell cycle regulatory proteins p16 and retinoblastoma: Distinct association with keratinisation and differentiation in oral cavity squamous cell carcinoma. *Journal of Clinical Pathology* 59(7), 711–715.

Munoz-Guerra, M.F., Marazuela, E.G. et al. 2005. P-cadherin expression reduced in squamous cell carcinoma of the oral cavity: An indicator of poor prognosis. *Cancer* 103, 960–969.

Myoung, H., Kim, M.J. et al. 2006. Correlation of proliferative markers (Ki-67 and PCNA) with survival and lymph node metastasis in oral squamous cell carcinoma: A clinical and histopathological analysis of 113 patients. *International Journal of Oral and Maxillofacial Surgery* 35, 1005–1010.

Nakahara, Y., Shintani, S., Mihara, M., Hino, S., and Hamakawa, H. 2006. Detection of p16 promoter methylation in the serum of oral cancer patients. *International Journal of Oral and Maxillofacial Surgery* 35(4), 362–365.

Nakahara, Y., Shintani, S., Mihara, M., Ueyama, Y., and Matsumura, T. 2001. High frequency of homozygous deletion and methalation of p16(ink4a) gene in oral squamous cell carcinomas. *Cancer Letters* 163(2), 221–228.

Nasuti, J.F., Tam, D., and Gupta, P.K. 2001. Diagnostic value of liquid-based (thinprep) preparations in nongynecologic cases. *Diagnostic Cytopathology* 24(2), 137–141.

Navone, R., Burlo, P., Pich, A., Pentenero, M., Broccoletti, R., Marsico, A., and Gandolfo, S. 2007. The impact of liquid-based oral cytology on the diagnosis of oral squamous dysplasia and carcinoma. *Cytopathology: Official Journal of the British Society for Clinical Cytology* 18(6), 356–360.

Nemes, J.A., Nemes, Z., and Marton, I.J. 2005. p21waf1/cip1 expression is a marker of poor prognosis in oral squamous cell carcinoma. *Journal of Oral Pathology & Medicine: Official Publication of the International Association of Oral Pathologists and the American Academy of Oral Pathology* 34(5), 274–279.

Neville, B.W. and Day, T.A. 2002. Oral cancer and precancerous lesions. *CA: A Cancer Journal of Clinicans* 52, 195–215.

Nii, M., Kayada, Y., Yoshiga, K., Takada, K., Okamoto, T., and Yanagihara, K. 2000. Suppression of metastasis by tissue inhibitor of metalloproteinase-1 in a newly established human oral squamous cell carcinoma cell line. *International Journal of Oncology* 16(1), 119–124.

Nii, M., Kayada, Y., Yoshiga, K., Takada, K., and Yanagihara, K. 1996. Expression of type iv collagen-degrading metalloproteinases and tissue inhibitors of metalloproteinases in newly established human oral malignant tumor lines. *Japanese Journal of Clinical Oncology* 26(3), 117–123.

Ogawa, K., Tanuma, J., Hirano, M., Hirayama, Y., Semba, I., Shisa, H., and Kitano, M. 2006. Selective loss of resistant alleles at p15ink4b and p16ink4a genes in chemically-induced rat tongue cancers. *Oral Oncology* 42(7), 710–717.

Ohta, S., Uemura, H., Matsui, Y., Ishiguro, H., Fujinami, K., Kondo, K., Miyamoto, H. et al. 2009. Alterations of p16 and p14arf genes and their 9p21 locus in oral squamous cell carcinoma. *Oral Surgery, Oral Medicine, Oral Pathology, Oral Radiology, and Endodontics* 107(1), 81–91.

Okada, Y. 2000. Tumor cell-matrix interaction: Pericellular matrix degradation and metastasis. *Verhandlungen der deutschen gesellschaft fur pathologie* 84, 33–42.

Okui, T., Shimo, T., Hassan, N.M., Fukazawa, T., Kurio, N., Takaoka, M., Naomoto, Y., and Sasaki, A. 2011. Antitumor effect of novel hsp90 inhibitor nvp-auy922 against oral squamous cell carcinoma. *Anticancer Research* 31(4), 1197–1204.

Oliveira, L.R. and Ribeiro-Silva, A. 2011. Prognostic significance of immunohistochemical biomarkers in oral squamous cell carcinoma. *The International Journal of Oral & Maxillofacial Surgery* 40, 298–307.

Osaki, T., Kimura, T., Tatemoto, Y., Dapeng, L., Yoneda, K., and Yamamoto, T. 2000. Diffuse mode of tumor cell invasion and expression of mutant p53 protein but not of p21 protein are correlated with treatment failure in oral carcinomas and their metastatic foci. *Oncology* 59(1), 36–43.

Pai, R.K., Erickson, J., Pourmand, N., and Kong, C.S. 2009. p16(ink4a) immunohistochemical staining may be helpful in distinguishing branchial cleft cysts from cystic squamous cell carcinomas originating in the oropharynx. *Cancer Cytopathology* 117(2), 108–119.

Pande, P., Mathur, M., Shukla, N.K., and Ralhan, R. 1998. prb and p16 protein alterations in human oral tumorigenesis. *Oral Oncology* 34(5), 396–403.

Pande, P., Soni, S., Kaur, J., Agarwal, S., Mathur, M., Shukla, N.K., and Ralhan, R. 2002. Prognostic factors in betel and tobacco related oral cancer. *Oral Oncology* 38(5), 491–499.

Papadimitrakopoulou, V., Izzo, J., Lippman, S.M., Lee, J.S., Fan, Y.H., Clayman, G., Ro, J.Y. et al. 1997. Frequent inactivation of p16ink4a in oral premalignant lesions. *Oncogene* 14(15), 1799–1803.

Paradiso, A., Ranieri, G., Stea, B., Zito, A., Zehbe, I., Tommasino, M., Grammatica, L., and De Lena, M. 2004. Altered p16ink4a and fhit expression in carcinogenesis and progression of human oral cancer. *International Journal of Oncology* 24(2), 249–255.

Park, N.J., Zhou, H., Elashoff, D., Henson, B.S., Kastratovic, D.A., Abemayor, E., and Wong, D.T. 2009. Salivary microRNA: Discovery, characterization, and clinical utility for oral cancer detection. *Clinical Cancer Research* 15, 5473–5477.

Patel, R.S., Rose, B., Bawdon, H., Hong, A., Lee, C.S., Fredericks, S., Gao, K., and O'Brien, C.J. 2007. Cyclin d1 and p16 expression in pleomorphic adenoma and carcinoma ex pleomorphic adenoma of the parotid gland. *Histopathology* 51(5), 691–696.

Patterson, K.I., Brummer, T., O'Brien, P.M., and Daly, R.J. 2009. Dual-specificity phosphatases: Critical regulators with diverse cellular targets. *Biochemical Journal* 418, 475–489.

Pereira, M.C., Oliveira, D.T. et al. 2007. Histologic subtypes of oral squamous cell carcinoma: Prognostic relevance. *Journal of Canadian Dental Association* 73, 339–344.

Perez-Sayans, M., Somoza-Martin, J., Barros-Angueira, F., Reboiras-Lopez, M., Gandara-Vila, P., Rey, J.G., and Garcia-Garcia, A. 2009a. Exfoliative cytology for diagnosing oral cancer. *Biotechnic & Histochemistry: Official Publication of the Biological Stain Commission* 85(3), 177–187.

Perez-Sayans, M., Somoza-Martin, J.M., Barros-Angueira, F., Diz, P.G., Rey, J.M., and Garcia-Garcia, A. 2010. Multidrug resistance in oral squamous cell carcinoma: The role of vacuolar atpases. *Cancer Letters* 295, 135–143.

Perez-Sayans, M., Somoza-Martin, J.M., Barros-Angueira, F., Reboiras-Lopez, M.D., Gandara Rey, J.M., and Garcia-Garcia, A. 2009b. Genetic and molecular alterations associated with oral squamous cell cancer (review). *Oncology Reports* 22(6), 1277–1282.

Petersen, P.E. et al. 2009. Oral cancer prevention and control—The approach of the World Health Organization. *Oral Oncology* 45, 454–460.

Poulsom, R., Pignatelli, M., Stetler-Stevenson, W.G., Liotta, L.A., Wright, P.A., Jeffery, R.E., Longcroft, J.M., Rogers, L., and Stamp, G.W. 1992. Stromal expression of 72 kda type iv collagenase (mmp-2) and timp-2 mrnas in colorectal neoplasia. *The American Journal of Pathology* 141(2), 389–396.

Pradhan-Palikhe, P., Vesterinen, T., Tarkkanen, J., Leivo, I., Sorsa, T., Salo, T., and Mattila, P.S. 2010. Plasma level of tissue inhibitor of matrix metalloproteinase-1 but not that of matrix metalloproteinase-8 predicts survival in head and neck squamous cell cancer. *Oral Oncology* 46(7), 514–518.

Queiroz, A.B., Focchi, G., Dobo, C., Gomes, T.S., Ribeiro, D.A., and Oshima, C.T. 2010. Expression of p27, p21(waf/cip1), and p16(ink4a) in normal oral epithelium, oral squamous papilloma, and oral squamous cell carcinoma. *Anticancer Research* 30(7), 2799–2803.

Ralhan, R., Agarwal, S., Mathur, M., Wasylyk, B., and Srivastava, A. 2000. Association between polymorphism in p21(waf1/cip1) cyclin-dependent kinase inhibitor gene and human oral cancer. *Clinical Cancer Research: An Official Journal of the American Association for Cancer Research* 6(6), 2440–2447.

Ratajczak, J., Wysoczynski, M., Hayek, F., Janowska-Wieczorek, A., and Ratajczak, M.Z. 2006. Membrane-derived microvesicles: Important and underappreciated mediators of cell-to-cell communication. *Leukemia* 20(9), 1487–1495.

Rhodus, N.L., Ho, V., Miller, C.S., Myers, S., and Ondrey, F. 2005. NF-kB dependent cytokine levels in saliva of patients with oral preneoplastic lesions and oral squamous cell carcinoma. *Cancer Detection and Prevention* 29(1), 42–45.

Rizzolo, D., Hanifin, C. et al. 2007. Oral cancer: How to find this hidden killer in 2 minutes. *JAAPA* 20, 42–47.

Roh, J.L., Cho, K.J., Kwon, G.Y., Ryu, C.H., Chang, H.W., Choi, S.H., Nam, S.Y., and Kim, S.Y. 2009. The prognostic value of hypoxia markers in t2-staged oral tongue cancer. *Oral Oncology* 45(1), 63–68.

Rollins, B.J. 1997. Chemokines. *Blood* 90, 909–928.

Rosenthal, E.L., Mccrory, A., Talbert, M., Carroll, W., Magnuson, J.S., and Peters, G.E. 2004. Expression of proteolytic enzymes in head and neck cancer-associated fibroblasts. *Archives of Otolaryngology—Head & Neck Surgery* 130(8), 943–947.

Ryan, H.E., Lo, J., and Johnson, R.S. 1998. Hif-1 alpha is required for solid tumor formation and embryonic vascularization. *The EMBO Journal* 17(11), 3005–3015.

Saarnio, J., Parkkila, S., Parkkila, A.K., Haukipuro, K., Pastorekova, S., Pastorek, J., Kairaluoma, M.I., and Karttunen, T.J. 1998. Immuno histo chemical study of colorectal tumors for expression of a novel transmembrane carbonic anhydrase, mn/ca ix, with potential value as a marker of cell proliferation. *The American Journal of Pathology* 153(1), 279–285.

Sailasree, R., Abhilash, A., Sathyan, K.M., Nalinakumari, K.R., Thomas, S., and Kannan, S. 2008. Differential roles of p16ink4a and p14arf genes in prognosis of oral carcinoma. *Cancer Epidemiology, Biomarkers & Prevention: A Publication of the American Association for Cancer Research, Cosponsored by the American Society of Preventive Oncology* 17(2), 414–420.

Sang, Q.X., Jin, Y., Newcomer, R.G., Monroe, S.C., Fang, X., Hurst, D.R., Lee, S., Cao, Q., and Schwartz, M.A. 2006. Matrix metalloproteinase inhibitors as prospective agents for the prevention and treatment of cardiovascular and neoplastic diseases. *Current Topics in Medicinal Chemistry* 6(4), 289–316.

Sargeran, K., Murtomaa, H. et al. 2009. Survival after lip cancer diagnosis. *Journal of Craniofacial Surgery* 20, 248–252.

Sartori, R., Li, F., Kirkwood, K.L. 2009. MAP kinase phosphatase-1 protects against inflammatory bone loss. *Journal of Dental Research* 88(12), 1125–1130.

Sasabe, E., Zhou, X., Li, D., Oku, N., Yamamoto, T., and Osaki, T. 2007. The involvement of hypoxia-inducible factor-1alpha in the susceptibility to gamma-rays and chemotherapeutic drugs of oral squamous cell carcinoma cells. *International Journal of Cancer. Journal International du Cancer* 120(2), 268–277.

Savage, S.A., Abnet, C.C., Mark, S.D., Qiao, Y.L., Dong, Z.W., Dawsey, S.M. et al. 2004. Variants of the IL8 and IL8RB genes and risk for gastric cardia adenocarcinoma and esophageal squamous cell carcinoma. *Cancer Epidemiology, Biomarkers & Prevention* 13, 2251–2257.

Schindl, M., Schoppmann, S.F., Samonigg, H., Hausmaninger, H., Kwasny, W., Gnant, M., Jakesz, R. et al. 2002. Overexpression of hypoxia-inducible factor 1alpha is associated with an unfavorable prognosis in lymph node-positive breast cancer. *Clinical Cancer Research: An Official Journal of the American Association for Cancer Research* 8(6), 1831–1837.

Schmalbach, C.E., Chepeha, D.B., Giordano, T.J., Rubin, M.A., Teknos, T.N., Bradford, C.R., Wolf, G.T. et al. 2004. Molecular profiling and the identification of genes associated with metastatic oral cavity/pharynx squamous cell carcinoma. *Archives of Otolaryngology—Head & Neck Surgery* 130(3), 295–302.

Schmitt, A., Barth, T.F., Beyer, E., Borchert, F., Rojewski, M., Chen, J., Guillaume, P. et al. 2009. The tumor antigens rhamm and g250/caix are expressed in head and neck squamous cell carcinomas and elicit specific cd8 + t cell responses. *International Journal of Oncology* 34(3), 629–639.

Schofield, C.J. and Ratcliffe, P.J. 2004. Oxygen sensing by hif hydroxylases. *Nature Reviews. Molecular Cell Biology* 5(5), 343–354.

Schwarz, S., Bier, J., Driemel, O., Reichert, T.E., Hauke, S., Hartmann, A., and Brockhoff, G. 2008. Losses of 3p14 and 9p21 as shown by fluorescence in situ hybridization are early events in tumorigenesis of oral squamous cell carcinoma and already occur in simple keratosis. *Cytometry. Part A: The Journal of the International Society for Analytical Cytology* 73(4), 305–311.

Sekulic, A., Haluska, P., Jr., Miller, A.J., Genebriera de Lamo, J., Ejadi, S., Pulido, J.S., Salomao, D.R. et al. 2008. Malignant melanoma in the 21st century: The emerging molecular landscape. *Mayo Clinic Proceedings. Mayo Clinic* 83(7), 825–846.

Semenza, G.L. 2000. Hif-1 and human disease: One highly involved factor. *Genes & Development* 14(16), 1983–1991.

Serrano, M., Hannon, G.J., and Beach, D. 1993. A new regulatory motif in cell-cycle control causing specific inhibition of cyclin d/cdk 4. *Nature* 366(6456), 704–707.

Sherr, C.J. 1994. G1 phase progression: Cycling on cue. *Cell* 79(4), 551–555.

Shimada, T., Nakamura, H., Yamashita, K., Kawata, R., Murakami, Y., Fujimoto, N., Sato, H., Seiki, M., and Okada, Y. 2000. Enhanced production and activation of progelatinase a mediated by membrane-type 1 matrix metalloproteinase in human oral squamous cell carcinomas: Implications for lymph node metastasis. *Clinical & Experimental Metastasis* 18(2), 179–188.

Shintani, S., Nakahara, Y., Mihara, M., Ueyama, Y., and Matsumura, T. 2001. Inactivation of the p14(arf), p15(ink4b) and p16(ink4a) genes is a frequent event in human oral squamous cell carcinomas. *Oral Oncology* 37(6), 498–504.

Shiomi, T. and Okada, Y. 2003. Mt1-mmp and mmp-7 in invasion and metastasis of human cancers. *Cancer Metastasis Reviews* 22(2–3), 145–152.

Shpitzer, T., Bahar, G., Feinmesser, R., and Nagler, R.M. 2007. A comprehensive salivary analysis for oral cancer diagnosis. *Journal of Cancer Research and Clinical Oncology* 133, 613–617.

Singh, R.D., Haridas, N., Patel, J.B., Shah, F.D., Shukla, S.N., Shah, P.M., and Patel, P.S. 2010. Matrix metalloproteinases and their inhibitors: Correlation with invasion and metastasis in oral cancer. *Indian Journal of Clinical Biochemistry* 25(3), 250–259.

Sinha, P., Bahadur, S., Thakar, A., Matta, A., Macha, M., Ralhan, R., and Gupta, S.D. 2009. Significance of promoter hypermethylation of p16 gene for margin assessment in carcinoma tongue. *Head & Neck* 31(11), 1423–1430.

Sivridis, E., Giatromanolaki, A., Gatter, K.C., Harris, A.L., Koukourakis, M.I., and Tumor and Angiogenesis Research Group, 2002. Association of hypoxia-inducible factors 1alpha and 2alpha with activated angiogenic pathways and prognosis in patients with endometrial carcinoma. *Cancer* 95(5), 1055–1063.

Skog, J., Würdinger, T., van Rijn, S., Meijer, D.H., Gainche, L., Sena-Esteves, M., Curry, W.T. Jr. et al. 2008. Glioblastoma microvesicles transport RNA and proteins that promote tumour growth and provide diagnostic biomarkers. *Nature Cell Biology* 10, 1470–1476.

Smirnova, M.G., Kiselev, S.L., Gnuchev, N.V. et al. 2003. Role of the pro-inflammatory cytokines tumor necrosis factor-alpha, interleukin-1 beta, interleukin-6 and interleukin-8 in the pathogenesis of the otitis media with effusion. *European Cytokine Network* 13(2), 161–172.

Smith, D.R., Polverini, P.J., Kunkel, S.L., Orringer, M.B., Whyte, R.I., Burdick, M.D. et al 1994. Inhibition of interleukin-8 attenuates angiogenesis in bronchogenic carcinoma. *Journal of Experimental Medicine* 179, 1409–1415.

St John, M.A., Li, Y., Zhou, X., Denny, P., Ho, C.M., Montemagno, C., Shi, W. et al. 2004. Interleukin 6 and interleukin 8 as potential biomarkers for oral cavity and oropharyngeal squamous cell carcinoma. *Archives of Otolaryngology—Head & Neck Surgery* 130(8), 929–935.

Stetler-Stevenson, W.G., Aznavoorian, S., and Liotta, L.A. 1993. Tumor cell interactions with the extracellular matrix during invasion and metastasis. *Annual Review of Cell Biology* 9, 541–573.

Su, P.F., Huang, W.L., Wu, H.T., Wu, C.H., Liu, T.Y., and Kao, S.Y. 2010. p16(ink4a) promoter hypermethylation is associated with invasiveness and prognosis of oral squamous cell carcinoma in an age-dependent manner. *Oral Oncology* 46(10), 734–739.

Sutinen, M., Kainulainen, T., Hurskainen, T., Vesterlund, E., Alexander, J.P., Overall, C.M., Sorsa, T., and Salo, T. 1998. Expression of matrix metalloproteinases (mmp-1 and -2) and their inhibitors (timp-1, -2 and -3) in oral lichen planus, dysplasia, squamous cell carcinoma and lymph node metastasis. *British Journal of Cancer* 77(12), 2239–2245.

Suzuki, C., Unoki, M., and Nakamura, Y. 2001. Identification and allelic frequencies of novel single-nucleotide polymorphisms in the DUSP1 and BTG1 genes. *Journal of Human Genetics* 46, 155–157.

Suzuki, H., Sugimura, H., and Hashimoto, K. 2006. p16ink4a in oral squamous cell carcinomas—A correlation with biological behaviors: Immunohistochemical and fish analysis. *Journal of Oral and Maxillofacial Surgery: Official Journal of the American Association of Oral and Maxillofacial Surgeons* 64(11), 1617–1623.

Syrjanen, S. 2007. Human papillomaviruses in head and neck carcinomas. *The New England Journal of Medicine* 356, 1993–1995.

Szanto, I., Mark, L. et al. 2012. High-throughput screening of saliva for early detection of oral cancer: A pilot study. *Technology in Cancer Research and Treatment* 11, 181–188.

Takeshima, M., Saitoh, M., Kusano, K., Nagayasu, H., Kurashige, Y., Malsantha, M., Arakawa, T. et al. 2008. High frequency of hypermethylation of p14, p15 and p16 in oral pre-cancerous lesions associated with betel-quid chewing in Sri Lanka. *Journal of Oral Pathology & Medicine: Official Publication of the International Association of Oral Pathologists and the American Academy of Oral Pathology* 37(8), 475–479.

Tanaka, N., Odajima, T., Mimura, M., Ogi, K., Dehari, H., Kimijima, Y., and Kohama, G. 2001. Expression of rb, prb2/p130, p53, and p16 proteins in malignant melanoma of oral mucosa. *Oral Oncology* 37(3), 308–314.

Tatemoto, Y., Osaki, T., Yoneda, K., Yamamoto, T., Ueta, E., and Kimura, T. 1998. Expression of p53 and p21 proteins in oral squamous cell carcinoma: Correlation with lymph node metastasis and response to chemoradiotherapy. *Pathology, Research and Practice* 194(12), 821–830.

Thomas, G.T., Lewis, M.P., and Speight, P.M. 1999. Matrix metalloproteinases and oral cancer. *Oral Oncology* 35(3), 227–233.

Tilakaratne, W.M. and Nissanka-Jayasuriya, E.H. 2011. Value of hif-1alpha as an independent prognostic indicator in oral squamous cell carcinoma. *Expert Review of Molecular Diagnostics* 11(2), 145–147.

Tokman, B., Gultekin, S.E., Sezer, C., and Alpar, R. 2004. The expression of p53, p16 proteins and prevalence of apoptosis in oral squamous cell carcinoma. Correlation with mode of invasion grading system. *Saudi Medical Journal* 25(12), 1922–1930.

Torelli, G., Venturelli, D., Colo, A., Zanni, C., Selleri, L., Moretti, L., Calabretta, B., and Torelli, U. 1987. Expression of c-myb protooncogene and other cell cycle-related genes in normal and neoplastic human colonic mucosa. *Cancer Research* 47, 5266–5269.

Tsai, C.H., Yang, C.C., Chou, L.S., and Chou, M.Y. 2001. The correlation between alteration of p16 gene and clinical status in oral squamous cell carcinoma. *Journal of Oral Pathology & Medicine* 30(9), 527–531.

Turner, J.R., Odze, R.D., Crum, C.P., and Resnick, M.B. 1997. Mn antigen expression in normal, preneoplastic, and neoplastic esophagus: A clinicopathological study of a new cancer-associated biomarker. *Human Pathology* 28(6), 740–744.

Uehara, M., Sano, K., Ikeda, H., Nonaka, M., and Asahina, I. 2009. Hypoxia-inducible factor 1 alpha in oral squamous cell carcinoma and its relation to prognosis. *Oral Oncology* 45(3), 241–246.

Unoki, M. and Nakamura, Y. 2001. Growth-suppressive effects of BPOZ and EGR2, two genes involved in the PTEN signaling pathway. *Oncogene* 20, 4457–4465.

Unruh, A., Ressel, A., Mohamed, H.G., Johnson, R.S., Nadrowitz, R., Richter, E., Katschinski, D.M., and Wenger, R.H. 2003. The hypoxia-inducible factor-1 alpha is a negative factor for tumor therapy. *Oncogene* 22(21), 3213–3220.

Uzawa, N., Sonoda, I., Myo, K., Takahashi, K., Miyamoto, R., and Amagasa, T. 2007. Fluorescence in situ hybridization for detecting genomic alterations of cyclin d1 and p16 in oral squamous cell carcinomas. *Cancer* 110(10), 2230–2239.

Vairaktaris, E., Yapijakis, C., Psyrri, A., Spyridonidou, S. et al. 2007. Loss of tumour suppressor p16 expression in initial stages of oral oncogenesis. *Anticancer Research* 27(2), 979–984.

Vekony, H., Roser, K., Loning, T., Raaphorst, F.M., Leemans, C.R., Van der Waal, I., and Bloemena, E. 2008. Deregulated expression of p16ink4a and p53 pathway members in benign and malignant myoepithelial tumours of the salivary glands. *Histopathology* 53(6), 658–666.

Von Zeidler, S.V., Miracca, E.C., Nagai, M.A., and Birman, E.G. 2004. Hypermethylation of the p16 gene in normal oral mucosa of smokers. *International Journal of Molecular Medicine* 14(5), 807–811.

Warnakulasuriya, S. 2009. Global epidemiology of oral and oropharyngeal cancer. *Oral Oncology* 45:309–316.

Warnakulasuriya, S., Johnson, N.W. et al. 2007a. Nomenclature and classification of potentially malignant disorders of the oral mucosa. *Journal of Oral Pathology & Medicine* 36, 575–580.

Warnakulasuriya, S., Mak, V. et al. 2007b. Oral cancer survival in young people in South East England. *Oral Oncology* 43, 982–986.

Watanabe, H., Iwase, M., Ohashi, M., and Nagumo, M. 2002. Role of interleukin-8 secreted from human oral squamous cell carcinoma cell lines. *Oral Oncology* 38, 670–679.

Wei, F., Patel, P., Liao, W., Chaudhry, K., Zhang, L., Garcia, M.A., Hu, S. et al. 2009. Electrochemical sensor for multiplex biomarkers detection. *Clinical Cancer Research* 15, 4446–4452.

Wells, D., Hoffman, D., and Kedes, L. 1987. Unusual structure, evolutionary conservation of non-coding sequences and numerous pseudogenes characterize the human H3.3 histone multigene family. *Nucleic Acids Research* 15(7), 2871–2889.

Wong, D.T. 2006. Salivary diagnostics powered by nanotechnologies, proteomics and genomics. *JADA* 137, 313–321.

Wood, N.K. and Sawyer, D.R. 1998. Cáncer oral. En Wood NK, Goaz PW, eds. Diagnóstico diferencial de las lesiones orales y maxilofaciales. Harcourt Brace: Barcelona, pp. 587–595.

World Health Organization. 1997. ICD-10. *International Statistical Classification of Diseases and Related Health Problems*. Geneva, Switzerland: World Health Organization.

Wu, J.J., Roth, R.J., Anderson, E.J., Hong, E.G. et al. 2006. Mice lacking MAP kinase phosphatase-1 have enhanced MAP kinase activity and resistance to diet-induced obesity. *Cell Metabolism* 4(1), 61–73.

Wu, L.C., D'Amelio, F., Fox, R.A., Polyakov, I., and Daunton, N.G. 1997. Light microscopic image analysis system to quantify immunoreactive terminal area apposed to nerve cells. *Journal of Neuroscience Methods* 74(1), 89–96.

Xiao, L., Celano, P., Mank, A.R., Griffin, C., Jabs, E.W., Hawkins, A.L., and Casero, R.A., Jr. 2011. Structure of the human spermidine/spermine N1-acetyltransferase gene (exon/intron gene organization and localization to Xp22.1). *Biochemical and Biophysical Research Communications* 187(3), 1493–1502.

Xie, X., Clausen, O.P., and Boysen, M. 2002. Prognostic significance of p21waf1/cip1 expression in tongue squamous cell carcinomas. *Archives of Otolaryngology—Head & Neck Surgery* 128(8), 897–902.

Yakushiji, T., Noma, H., Shibahara, T., Arai, K., Yamamoto, N., Tanaka, C., Uzawa, K., and Tanzawa, H. 2001. Analysis of a role for p16/cdkn2 expression and methylation patterns in human oral squamous cell carcinoma. *The Bulletin of Tokyo Dental College* 42(3), 159–168.

Yen-Ping Kuo, M., Huang, J.S., Kok, S.H., Kuo, Y.S., and Chiang, C.P. 2002. Prognostic role of p21waf1 expression in areca quid chewing and smoking-associated oral squamous cell carcinoma in Taiwan. *Journal of Oral Pathology & Medicine: Official Publication of the International Association of Oral Pathologists and the American Academy of Oral Pathology* 31(1), 16–22.

Yook, J.I. and Kim, J. 1998. Expression of p21waf1/cip1 is unrelated to p53 tumour suppressor gene status in oral squamous cell carcinomas. *Oral Oncology* 34(3), 198–203.

Yoshiba, S., Ito, D., Nagumo, T., Shirota, T., Hatori, M., and Shintani, S., 2009. Hypoxia induces resistance to 5-fluorouracil in oral cancer cells via g(1) phase cell cycle arrest. *Oral Oncology* 45(2), 109–115.

Yu, H., Li, Q., Herbert, B., Zinna, R., Martin, K., Junior, C.R., and Kirkwood, K.L. 2011a. Anti-inflammatory effect of MAPK phosphatase-1 local gene transfer in inflammatory bone loss. *Gene Therapy* 18(4), 344–353.

Yu, H., Sun, Y., Haycraft, C., Palanisamy, V., and Kirkwood, K.L. 2011b. MKP-1 regulates cytokine mRNA stability through selectively modulation subcellular translocation of AUF1. *Cytokine* 56(2), 245–255.

Zhang, Q., Zhang, Z.F., Rao, J.Y., Sato, J.D., Brown, J., Messadi, D.V., and Le, A.D. 2004. Treatment with sirna and antisense oligonucleotides targeted to hif-1alpha induced apoptosis in human tongue squamous cell carcinomas. *International Journal of Cancer. Journal International Du Cancer* 111(6), 849–857.

Zhao, Q., Wang, X., Nelin, L.D., Yao, Y., Matta, R., Manson, M.E., Baliga, R.S. et al. 2006. MAP kinase phosphatase 1 control innate immune responses and suppresses endotoxic shock. *Journal of Experimental Medicine* 203(1), 131–140.

Zheng, G., Zhou, M., Ou, X., Peng, B., Yu, Y., Kong, F., Ouyang, Y., and He, Z. 2010. Identification of carbonic anhydrase 9 as a contributor to pingyangmycin-induced drug resistance in human tongue cancer cells. *The FEBS Journal* 277(21), 4506–4518.

Zimmermann, B.G. and Wong, D.T. 2008. Salivary mRNA targets for cancer diagnostics. *Oral Oncology* 44(5), 425–429.

Zucker, S., Cao, J., and Chen, W.T. 2000. Critical appraisal of the use of matrix metalloproteinase inhibitors in cancer treatment. *Oncogene* 19(56), 6642–6650.

Part III

Gastrointestinal Cancers

13

Biomarkers for Gastric Cancer and the Related Premalignant Conditions

Marcis Leja, Jan Bornschein, Juozas Kupcinskas, and Peter Malfertheiner

CONTENTS

ABSTRACT Although gastric cancer is declining in incidence when estimated in standardized ratio statistics, it will still remain an important health-care problem during the coming decades. Currently, most of cancer cases outside Japan are diagnosed at advanced stages when radical management is substantially less effective. Infection with *Helicobacter pylori* bacteria is related to the majority of cases. Atrophy, intestinal metaplasia, and dysplasia are well-characterized precursors of the cancer. Currently, the only method available to diagnose exactly these lesions is upper endoscopy with an appropriate biopsy work-up. Biomarkers for noninvasive detection of early gastric cancer and/or the precursors would be of substantial importance to decrease the cancer-related mortality, in particular in the developing part of the world.

This chapter discusses the available gastric cancer screening programs and the potential existing methods, including modalities of endoscopy and tests for identification of the precursors (e.g., pepsinogen tests) as well as the limitations of these methods. The role of host genetic factors, including polymorphisms of proinflammatory cytokines, is addressed; the potential role of miRNAs and epigenetics is discussed. The rare entity of hereditary gastric cancer linked to *CDH1* gene mutation as well as the host genetic factors being related to increased cancer risk is also discussed. Insight is given into the new developments in the field, including the detection of specific cancer autoantibodies and volatile organic components in the exhaled breath.

13.1 Introduction

Despite the strongly declining incidence in developed Western countries, gastric cancer remains still a major burden for health systems worldwide socioeconomically and individually for the patients suffering from this disease (Parkin, 2006). Taken into consideration the predicted growth of the world population and increasing average life expectancies in many countries, the absolute number of gastric cancer cases is likely to be stable or even increases despite declining incidence (Parkin et al., 2005). Almost one million cases are newly diagnosed each year, and about 740,000 deaths are caused by this disease resulting in 8% of all cancer cases and 10% of all cancer-related deaths annually (Jemal et al., 2011). There is a regional variation of the incidence rates by the factor 10, with highest rates in East Asia, Eastern Europe, and parts of Central and Southern America and lowest rates in Southern Asia, North and East Africa, Australia, and North America (Bertuccio et al., 2009; Jemal et al., 2011). More than 70% of gastric cancers occur in developing countries due to lesser hygienic standards and higher *Helicobacter pylori* (*H. pylori*) prevalence rates (Jemal et al., 2011).

However, there has been a marked decrease of gastric cancer for several decades (Devesa et al., 1998; Schmassmann et al., 2009), most likely as a result of the significant reduction of various risk factors achieved by changes in food preservation (cooling and freezing instead of salting, smoking, and fermentation) and a decreasing prevalence of *H. pylori* by birth cohort (Forman and Burley, 2006). The underlying cause for the steadily decreasing incidence of *H. pylori* is most likely the reduced transmission in childhood due to better hygiene and less crowding as well as health education and adequate eradication therapies.

In contrast to a decline in the incidence of distal gastric cancer, there has been an increase of adenocarcinomas at the esophagogastric junction including gastric cardia cancer (Blot and McLaughlin, 1999; Crane et al., 2007). This trend is mainly documented for male Caucasians of advanced age in North America and Europe, but regional differences have to be taken into account (Devesa et al., 1998; Botterweck et al., 2000). In Asia, distal gastric cancer still remains the main entity.

At the time of diagnosis of gastric cancer, there is usually only a short period of symptoms such as unintentional weight loss, anemia, epigastric pain, nausea and vomiting, or dyspeptic symptoms. Forty percent of patients don't complain about any dyspeptic symptoms at all (Schmidt et al., 2005). Therefore, in the majority of cases, diagnosis is made at an advanced stage when only limited treatment options can be offered. Even though there has been minor improvement in the clinical management of gastric cancer, the 5-year survival rate is <30% in most countries and reported mortality rates mirror the incidence of gastric cancer adequately. Therefore, tools to diagnose the disease early are of critical importance.

13.2 Infection-Related Cancer

Infection with *H. pylori* is the major risk factor for the development of gastric cancer, and medical intervention represents the best option for the prevention of the disease (Malfertheiner et al., 2005). In 1994, the World Health Organization (WHO) classified *H. pylori* as class I carcinogen based mainly on epidemiological evidence for its role in gastric carcinogenesis (IARC Working Group on the Evaluation of Carcinogenic Risks to Humans, 1994), which has been reinforced in the more recent WHO contribution by the IARC (IARC, 2011). The majority of gastric cancer cases are related to *H. pylori* infection; globally 660,000 cases annually are caused by the infection (de Martel et al., 2012).

The first substantial evidence was obtained from animal studies on Mongolian gerbils, where *H. pylori* represents a complete carcinogen that is capable of inducing gastric adenocarcinomas without the influence of any cocarcinogens (Honda et al., 1998; Watanabe et al., 1998). However, the multifactorial etiology of gastric cancer was underlined, when supplementation of the animals with nitrosamines leads to higher rates of cancer incidence and a more rapid carcinogenesis (Shimizu et al., 1999; Maruta et al., 2000).

Numerous studies attempted to assess the attributable risk of *H. pylori* infection for gastric carcinogenesis in humans. A meta-analysis from Asia analyzed 19 studies with approximately 2500 gastric cancer patients and almost 4000 matched controls resulting in an odds ratio (OR) of 1.92 (95% CI, 1.32–2.78) for the development of noncardia gastric cancer in *H. pylori*-positive patients (Huang et al., 1998), which was in concordance with a previous similar analysis (Eslick, 1999).

In 2003, the *Helicobacter and Cancer Collaborative Group* combined data from the available case–control studies nested with prospective cohorts to assess more reliably the relative risk for gastric cancer. The evaluation of the data from 12 studies including 1228 patients demonstrated a clear association of *H. pylori* infection to noncardia gastric cancer (OR 3.0; 95% CI, 2.3–3.8) (Helicobacter and Cancer Collaborative Group, 2001). This association was even stronger when blood samples for *H. pylori* serology were obtained 10 years or longer before cancer diagnosis (OR 5.9; 95% CI, 3.4–10.3) (Helicobacter and Cancer Collaborative Group, 2001). A possible explanation is the loss of *H. pylori* colonization in the presence of atrophic gastritis and intestinal metaplasia, so that gastric cancer patients have already a loss of anti-*H. pylori* antibodies at the time of disease manifestation. In fact, in patients with early gastric cancer, the prevalence of *H. pylori* antibodies is much higher compared to individuals with advanced gastric cancer resulting in a different attributable risk (Huang et al., 1998). Further relevance is given by the time of serum sampling. The associated OR for gastric cancer development in case of *H. pylori* infection is significantly higher if serum samples are taken within 90 days after gastrectomy for the cure of the tumor (Brenner et al., 2004).

Several studies have shown that the risk of gastric cancer is further influenced by the presence of bacterial virulence factors like the cytotoxin-associated antigen A (CagA). A meta-analysis by Huang and colleagues revealed a further 1.64-fold increase of gastric cancer risk for CagA-positive strains compared to CagA-negative ones (16 studies, n = 5054) (Huang et al., 2003). Ekström reported an increase of the *H. pylori*-attributable OR for noncardia cancer from 2.2 to 21.0 if the CagA status was coevaluated by immunoblot analysis (Ekstrom et al., 2001). In this analysis, up to 91% of gastric cancer cases in the studied population were attributable to *H. pylori* infection.

While most studies claim that *H. pylori* is only related to distal gastric cancer, there is accumulating data that there is a high prevalence of the infection also in patients with proximally located adenocarcinomas if correct allocation of the primary tumor is performed and adenocarcinomas of the distal esophagus are strictly excluded (Bornschein et al., 2010). Finally, the risk for gastric carcinogenesis by *H. pylori* infection is equal in intestinal- and diffuse-type gastric cancer (Hansen et al., 2007; Bornschein et al., 2010).

The eradication of *H. pylori* has the potential to prevent gastric cancer. In 6695 patients included from various studies, *H. pylori* eradication significantly reduced gastric cancer risk (relative risk 0.65 [95% CI, 0.43–0.98]). Overall, 56 of 3307 (1.7%) of untreated (control) participants developed gastric cancer compared with 37 of 3388 (1.1%) treated patients (Fuccio et al., 2009).

The effect of *H. pylori* eradication on gastric cancer prevention was nearly exclusively studied in high-incidence regions in Asia. In an observational study from Japan, gastric cancer developed only in patients infected with *H. pylori*, but not in uninfected individuals (Uemura et al., 2001). In total, 1526 patients with dyspeptic symptoms were followed up for 7.8 years after endoscopic examination. Thirty-six of the *H. pylori*-positive patients (2.9%) developed gastric cancer, but in no case (0%), gastric malignancy was detected among the *H. pylori*-negative patients (Uemura et al., 2001).

The only prospective, randomized, placebo-controlled, population-based study to demonstrate primary gastric cancer prevention by the eradication of *H. pylori* has been performed in China (Wong et al., 2004). In total, 1630 healthy individuals were recruited for randomization on either *H. pylori* eradication or placebo treatment. In the period of 7.5-year follow-up, there have been 18 new cases of gastric cancer, 7 in the eradication group and 11 in the placebo group. Subgroup analysis revealed that all patients who developed gastric cancer presented with preneoplastic mucosal conditions (gastric atrophy, intestinal metaplasia) at baseline, whereas no case of gastric cancer was diagnosed without baseline mucosal changes ($p = 0.02$) (Wong et al., 2004). Thus, the major challenge is the detection and treatment of the *H. pylori* infection before mucosal changes have been developed that can no longer be stopped in the progression toward gastric cancer.

The individual risk for a stepwise development of gastric cancer from chronic active gastritis via premalignant lesions is still thought to be related to environmental influences combined with certain host susceptibility conditions since only about 1.0% of *H. pylori*-infected patients develop gastric cancer (Kuipers, 1999; Peek et al., 2002).

13.3 Classifications

The WHO and Laurén classifications are the most widely used histopathology-based classifications.

The *WHO classification* (Bosman et al., 2010) distinguishes five main types of gastric adenocarcinoma (tubular; papillary; mucinous; poorly cohesive, including signet-ring cell type; and mixed) and rare entities. Rare variants account for approximately 5% of all the gastric cancers and include adenosquamous carcinoma, squamous cell carcinoma, hepatoid adenocarcinoma, carcinoma with lymphoid stroma, choriocarcinoma, carcinosarcoma, parietal cell carcinoma, malignant rhabdoid tumor, mucoepidermoid carcinoma, Paneth cell carcinoma, undifferentiated carcinoma, mixed adenoneuroendocrine carcinomas, endodermal sinus tumor, embryonal carcinoma, pure gastric yolk sac tumor, and oncocytic adenocarcinoma. The WHO classification does not take in account histogenesis and differentiation.

The traditionally used *Laurén classification* is proposed back in 1965 (Laurén, 1965) distinguishing intestinal- (glandular epithelium composed of absorptive cells and goblet cells) and diffuse-type (poorly differentiated small cells in a dissociated noncohesive growth pattern) gastric adenocarcinomas. Tumors containing approximately equal quantities of intestinal and diffuse components are classified as mixed carcinomas, but those that are too undifferentiated to fit into either category are considered indeterminate. Laurén classification is still in use for either clinical or epidemiological purposes due to differences in patient populations, results of the management, and outcome; additionally to morphological also biological differences between these cancer types are considered responsible for the aforementioned (Lee et al., 2001).

Intestinal-type cancers are differentiated or moderately differentiated, sometimes with poorly differentiated tumor at the advancing margin, while diffuse-type cancers consist of poorly cohesive cells diffusely infiltrating the gastric wall with little or no gland formation; diffuse-type tumors resemble signet-ring cell cancers in the WHO classification.

Early gastric cancer is an invasive carcinoma limited to the mucosa or the mucosa and submucosa regardless of nodular status (Bosman et al., 2010).

The recent *TNM classification* (Edge et al., 2009) has introduced a change in the definition of cancer localization. The previously used terms of "cardia cancer" and "cancer of the esophagogastric junction" are discouraged since if the epicenter of the tumor is within 5 cm of esophagogastric junction and extends into the distal esophagus, it should be classified as esophageal carcinoma according to the TNM classification.

13.4 Screening and the Related Public Health Implications

13.4.1 Current Screening Programs

Currently, Japan and South Korea are the only countries having ongoing nationwide organized gastric cancer screening programs. In Japan, the screening program was launched in 1960, and still up for today, the only recommended screening method is photofluorography (Hamashima et al., 2008). In parallel to photofluorography, upper endoscopy is used as a screening tool in Korea (Choi et al., 2011). Kazakhstan has also decided to screen for upper digestive cancer with upper endoscopy; still the system is not well set up and the program is not yet launched.

A number of regional opportunistic screening activities that have been conducted should be more considered pilot studies (Leung et al., 2008). In Matsu island, a small island in Taiwan with high gastric cancer incidence, *H. pylori* screening with subsequent eradication in positive individuals has been conducted (Lee et al., 2012). A number of regional serological pepsinogen screening activities have been conducted in Japan (Miki, 2006). Another initiative of biomarker screening (*GastroPanel*) is ongoing in the North Italy.

13.4.2 Cost Implications

Endoscopic screening approach can only be cost-effective in moderate- to high-risk populations (Dan et al., 2006; Tashiro et al., 2006). In a decision model for the United States evaluating the cost-effectiveness of yearly endoscopy for a period of 10 years after a new diagnosis of intestinal metaplasia in the stomach, a cohort of 10,000 American patients was compared to no surveillance (Hassan et al., 2010). With an estimated gastric cancer incidence of 1.8% per year, 556 and 3738 endoscopies were needed to detect one case of gastric cancer and to prevent one cancer-related death, respectively. The incremental cost-effectiveness ratio (ICER) of endoscopic surveillance compared to nonsurveillance was US $72,519 per life year gained. Other estimations show a much higher ICER of US $544,500 per quality adjusted life year (QALY) if patients with intestinal metaplasia were followed consequently by upper gastrointestinal endoscopy, so that a recommendation for surveillance was only given for patients with epithelial dysplasia (Yeh et al., 2010). A practical approach from a logistic point of view is to combine screening for upper gastrointestinal malignancies with the screening colonoscopy for colorectal cancer prevention. One-time screening at the age of 50 years would result in US $115,664 per QALY (Gupta et al., 2011). The prevalence rates for gastric cancer have to rise by 337% to generate an ICER of less than US $50,000.

Another option would be a preventive approach not to screen for neoplastic or preneoplastic lesions itself but for the main risk factor, that is, infection with *H. pylori*. Taking into account the expenses for prior diagnostic procedures and the costs for antibiotic treatment, the cost-effectiveness of a "screen-and-eradicate" schedule for the prevention of gastric cancer is low (Malfertheiner et al., 2005). The estimations from the United States suggest the costs for *H. pylori* screening and treatment between €6,300 and €25,000 per life year saved (Parsonnet et al., 1996; Sonnenberg and Inadomi, 1998), and the data from the United Kingdom come up with a maximum cost of €8,500 if a positive effect on dyspeptic symptoms and peptic ulcer disease is included (Mason and Axon, 2002). However, calculation from Asia reveals that a single lifetime screening for the infection at the age of 20 years could reduce lifetime gastric cancer risk in men by 14.5% and in women by 26.6% costing less than US $1500 per life year saved compared to no screening (Yeh et al., 2009). Estimations for an older age seem less cost-effective, and additionally different costs for each modality of *H. pylori* screening have to be taken into account (Xie et al., 2008).

An effective vaccine against *H. pylori* would eliminate the necessity of screening and furthermore lead to an improvement of cost-effectiveness in the fight against gastric cancer. A prediction model estimates that a 10-year vaccination program would cause a decrease of *H. pylori* prevalence in the United States down to 0.07% by the end of the twenty-first century (Rupnow et al., 2001). This would have an effect not only on gastric cancer but on all *H. pylori*-related diseases. Vaccination of infants appears to be the most effective approach (Rupnow et al., 2009). However, it has to be considered that there is a latency of decades before the beneficial effect of this investment becomes obvious.

13.5 Invasive and Noninvasive Markers: Advantages and Disadvantages

The upper endoscopy being an invasive method with detailed analysis of visible lesions and proper biopsy sampling from gastric mucosa still represents the best and most effective screening modality; this includes also chromoendoscopy and newer developments in the visualization modalities. However, the method is not applicable for population screening in major part of the world with average and low risk, both because of the cost-efficacy issues and causing a discomfort for the individuals.

Traditionally, photofluorography has been used as the screening method of choice in Asia but not other parts of the world; multiple images are recorded and analyzed in detail during each investigation within the Japanese program. Although case–control studies have demonstrated 40%–60% decrease in mortality from gastric cancer, the results from prospective series are less convincing (Leung et al., 2008). Therefore, this is unlikely that the method will be introduced for organized gastric cancer screening elsewhere.

Noninvasive markers, discussed in detail later, are aiming to detect either parameter characteristic for gastric cancer (early detection) or premalignant conditions increasing the risk of the disease (atrophy, intestinal metaplasia, dysplasia); if those are identified, the group of patients at an increased risk may be subjected to surveillance programs.

13.6 Invasive Markers for High Risk of Gastric Cancer

13.6.1 New Imaging Techniques

Since there are no appropriate blood-based diagnostic tests for gastric cancer, upper gastrointestinal endoscopy with biopsy sampling for histopathological evaluation remains the gold standard for the determination of a definite diagnosis. Furthermore, a major focus on the endoscopic approach is not only to detect gastric cancer in its advanced stage but to identify early neoplastic lesions and to characterize preneoplastic conditions like intestinal metaplasia and atrophic gastritis as well as their extent. The diagnostic yield of traditional white light endoscopy can be enhanced by chromoendoscopic techniques (e.g., staining with methylene blue) (Peitz and Malfertheiner, 2002).

Technical advances that allow virtual chromoendoscopy by the use of optical filter systems have replaced the classical application of intraluminal dye (Uedo et al., 2011). The combination with optical magnification of the surface pattern of the gastric mucosa further increases the diagnostic accuracy. One major system is narrowband imaging (NBI) with special wavelength filters for red-colored structures like blood vessels or inflamed areas. The detection of even early neoplastic lesions in the stomach is dramatically increased compared to traditional white light endoscopy resulting in sensitivity and specificity above 90% in almost all trials (Kato et al., 2010; Ezoe et al., 2011; Zhang et al., 2011; Maki et al., 2012). Also, preneoplastic conditions can be classified more precisely and the number of lesions detected is clearly increased, so that this approach is of further benefit in surveillance of patients at high risk for gastric cancer development (Capelle et al., 2010b; Ang et al., 2012; Dutta et al., 2012).

The evaluation of the microvascular pattern as well as of the superficial structures allows the differentiation of small elevated lesions between adenomatous and cancerous tissue formations with higher accuracy, sensitivity, and specificity for NBI compared to white light endoscopy (Nakamura, 2010; Maki et al., 2012).

A challenge in diagnostic endoscopy is the correct assessment of small depressed lesions in the gastric mucosa. In a multicenter, prospective, randomized, controlled trial, depressed lesions with and lateral extent <10 mm have been assessed with white light endoscopy and magnified NBI (including crossover after white light). Again, accuracy, sensitivity, and specificity were higher with NBI (Ezoe et al., 2011). However, the highest diagnostic yield was gained, when both modalities were combined (accuracy 96.6%, sensitivity 95.0%, and specificity 96.8%).

By evaluation of surface and microvessel structure, it has even been possible to distinguish between Sm1 (cancers with intramucosal and minute submucosal invasion <500 μm in depth) and Sm2 (deeper submucosal invasion ≥500 μm in depth) early gastric cancer, with "nonstructure," "scattery vessels," and "multicaliber vessels" being an examiner-independent indicator for Sm2 (Kobara et al., 2012).

There are also criteria concerning the degree of differentiation of a neoplastic lesion, with differentiated early gastric cancer showing typically fine-network pattern or intralobular loop pattern 1, whereas undifferentiated lesions show more often corkscrew pattern or intralobular loop pattern 2 (Yokoyama et al., 2010).

During the past years, there has been strong effort to develop a general classification system for NBI-documented characteristics mainly focusing on the surface appearance including the gastric pit pattern, the microvascular structure, as well as the color and shape of the respective lesion (Pimentel-Nunes et al., 2012). The diagnostic quality of these patterns were satisfying although interobserver variation was still high (Kaise et al., 2009; Zhang et al., 2011). Compared with adenomas, carcinomas present at bigger size, depressed morphology, red color, and positive findings in surface and vessel structure (Tsuji et al., 2012). The efforts go on not only to develop a universal system for the differentiation of malignant from nonmalignant tissue but also to include preneoplastic conditions as well as different patterns of gastritis (Pimentel-Nunes et al., 2012).

A similar approach, but technically different systems, represents the flexible spectral imaging color enhancement (FICE) endoscopy, which offers more than just one optical filter in different digital channels, which can be easily switched during the investigation. Each mucosal structure can be assessed best by certain channels resulting in high interobserver agreement (Jung et al., 2011). Besides the accurate assessment of surface and microvessel patterns, the high contrast enhancement allows a better definition of the lateral demarcation line of gastric lesions compared with other approaches, especially for depressed lesions (Osawa et al., 2012a,b) (see Figure 13.1 for illustrations). The diagnostic yield can even be increased when additional intraluminal staining with, for example, indigo carmine is performed (Dohi et al., 2012).

The most recent technique is confocal laser endoscopy (CLE). Using these highly advanced endoscopes, an in vivo real-time assessment of the histopathological alterations present in the gastric mucosa is enabled. The first classifications of the related pit patterns have been developed on surgical specimens from gastric cancer patients and then validated in healthy volunteers (Zhang et al., 2008). The in vivo differentiation between physiological tissues from different regions of the stomach was possible as well as to distinguish between intestinal metaplasia, glandular atrophy, and neoplastic lesions (Zhang et al., 2008). This high-end magnification technique allows the detection of goblet cells and of a respective brush border in an absorptive intestinalized epithelium in case of intestinal metaplasia with a sensitivity around 90% and a specificity even higher and an acceptable interobserver agreement (Guo et al., 2008;

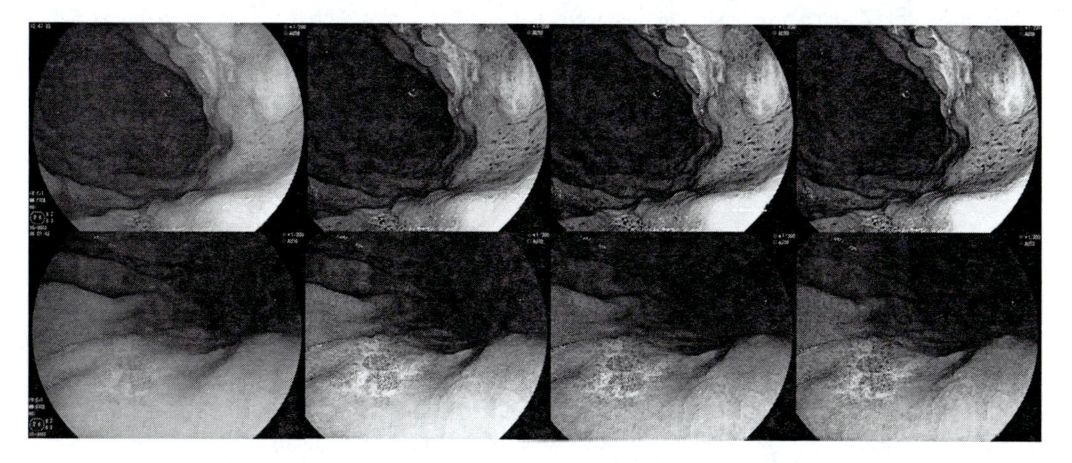

FIGURE 13.1 (See color insert.) FICE imaging: Endoscopic image of a gastric cancer (top line) as well as a focal area with intestinal metaplasia in high-resolution white light endoscopy (left panels) and in different filter channels of an FICE device.

Banno et al., 2010). However, it must be stated that for all CLE findings, the diagnostic accuracy and detection rate are significantly higher for experienced compared to inexperienced examiners since the investigation is time-consuming and demands high concentration and patience (Lim et al., 2011). In experienced hands—or better with experienced eyes—the diagnostic accuracy for the discrimination of cancerous lesions or even high-grade intraepithelial neoplasia (IEN) can be as high as 98.8% and by this comparable to classical histopathological evaluation (Li et al., 2010, 2011). This approach has further value in the assessment of resection margins after endoscopic treatment of early gastric cancer being even superior to biopsy sampling and histopathological assessment (Jeon et al., 2011; Ji et al., 2011).

In summary, there is an exciting technology development in the field; still so far at least in the Western world, this does not allow to replace routine standard biopsy work-up and use only targeted biopsies from suspected areas of visually identified lesions instead (Dinis-Ribeiro et al., 2012). However, by adopting the experience from Asia and being able to standardize this in other parts of the world, the situation might be changing.

13.6.2 Histopathology of Gastritis (The Sydney System)

The Sydney classification of gastritis with its updates is still the most widely used system for characterizing the status of gastric mucosa either for research or practice; this is combining topographic, morphological, and etiological information. The initial Sydney classification was first accepted in 1990 during the World Congress of Gastroenterology (Price and Misiewicz, 1991; Sipponen et al., 1991); in 1994, modifications were brought in during the Workshop on Histopathology and Gastritis in Houston (Dixon et al., 1996). The analysis of five biopsies—two from the antral part, one from the angulus, and two—from corpus is required to characterize gastritis in the absence of any visually detectable lesions. In addition to atrophy and intestinal metaplasia, each graded according to visual analogue scale, the classification requires also the reporting on the presence of *H. pylori*, active and chronic inflammation.

13.6.3 New Proposals for Scoring Gastritis (OLGA and OLGIM)

OLGA and OLGIM staging systems for gastric premalignant lesions are aimed to simplify the clinical approach while using the same biopsy work-up as for the Sydney system (i.e., five biopsies). The abbreviation OLGA stands for operative link on gastritis assessment, while OLGIM emphasizes the importance of intestinal metaplasia.

The initially proposed OLGA system is based on pooling the atrophy stages in each of parts of the stomach into a simple OLGA stage ranging from "0" to "4" (Rugge and Genta, 2005). This stage by itself does not allow to judge the topography of the lesion revealed (in particular for the lower stages), but it still could be linked to the prognosis and management issues since most of the cancer cases are expected to develop from stages III and IV (Rugge et al., 2010). In addition, such stage distribution is convenient also for research purpose (Daugule et al., 2011).

By considering that interobserver agreement is better for intestinal metaplasia than atrophy, the OLGIM system is using the same approach but staging intestinal metaplasia instead of atrophy (Capelle et al., 2010a).

13.6.4 Other Potential Markers

13.6.4.1 SPEM Metaplasia

During the past decade, another metaplastic alteration has been identified as a putative preneoplastic condition for gastric cancer development, the so-called spasmolytic polypeptide-expressing metaplasia (SPEM) (Nomura et al., 2004). SPEM is markedly characterized by an induction of the gene expression of the spasmolytic polypeptide, which has been identified as the trefoil factor 2 (TFF2) (Hoffmann, 2012). In surgical specimens from patients who had undergone gastrectomy in case of early gastric cancer, there was positive evidence of SPEM in the tumor surrounding mucosa if the tumor was located in the gastric body or at the body–antrum junction (Halldorsdottir et al., 2003). In three quarters of the cases, there was also SPEM in the body mucosa distant from the tumor. Furthermore, TFF2 could be detected already in 76% of dysplastic cells. In samples from a control cohort with gastritis and without neoplastic lesions, 82% of patients who developed gastric cancer during follow-up were positive for SPEM compared to 37% in case of no malignant transformation (Halldorsdottir et al., 2003). The same has been shown for the mucosa of patients with remnant adenocarcinoma after limited resection for gastric cancer (Yamaguchi et al., 2002).

It has been hypothesized by animal experiments that the metaplastic cells derive possibly from gastric chief cells or alternatively develop by the activation of basal crypt progenitor cells (Nozaki et al., 2008). However, recent data have shown that the leucine-rich repeat containing G-protein-coupled receptor 5 (Lgr5)-positive gastric stem cells are not the origin of SPEM (Nam et al., 2011). Signaling leading to the induction of these metaplastic changes seems to involve PGE2-related pathways and even the Wnt-signaling cascade (Oshima and Oshima, 2010).

13.6.4.2 Subtyping of Mucins and Intestinal Metaplasia

Intestinal metaplasia of the gastric mucosa is regarded as a premalignant condition and can be characterized by the differential expressions of certain mucins (MUC). There is a physiological expression of MUC5AC in the superficial epithelium and the upper part of the gastric pits, as well as MUC6 in the lower parts of the gastric glands (Babu et al., 2006). Further, gastric-type mucins are MUC1 and the human gastric mucin (HGM). MUC2 expression characterizes intestinal epithelium and is present in IM, mainly expressed by goblet cells (Babu et al., 2006). The induction of the intestinal transcription factor CDX2 leads to an upregulation of MUC2 gene expression, which is mostly accompanied by a downregulation of the gastric transcription factor SOX2 mirrored by decreased MUC5AC secretion (Tsukamoto et al., 2004; Kim et al., 2006).

These processes can be a response to *H. pylori*-induced chronic inflammation since the degree of the lymphocellular infiltration is concordant with the intramucosal level of MUC2 expression (Mejias-Luque et al., 2010). The proinflammatory cytokines *TNF*α and *IL1*β can induce MUC2 gene expression in gastric cancer cell lines (Mejias-Luque et al., 2010). In contrast, both gastric-type mucins, MUC5AC, MUC6, and MUC1 are significantly lower expressed in the gastric body of *H. pylori*-positive patients with increasing levels after eradication therapy (Wang and Fang, 2006; Kang et al., 2008a). Lower expression is maintained in case of the mucosal transformation toward atrophic changes, dysplasia, and gastric cancer. On the other hand, the gastric mucosal mucin profile can coregulate the expression of *H. pylori* virulence factors. The coculture of gastric epithelial cells with *H. pylori* under addition of specific mucins leads to an altered cytokine response and differential expression of BabA, CagA, and other *H. pylori*-related factors (Skoog et al., 2012).

According to the mucin expression profile, intestinal metaplasia in the stomach can be classified into a gastric, an intestinal, and a gastrointestinal (mixed) phenotype (Shiroshita et al., 2004; Wakatsuki et al., 2008). The mucin phenotype can even be distinguished by certain macroscopic criteria that can be assessed by magnifying NBI endoscopy (Kobayashi et al., 2011). The mucin phenotype can alter in relation to the status of *H. pylori* infection. Intestinal metaplasia after eradication of *H. pylori* is more often of the gastric predominant type, whereas in noneradicated patients, the intestinal type is more present with the latter being associated with a less favorable prognosis (Baldus et al., 2002; Wakatsuki et al., 2008; Yamamoto et al., 2011).

Atypical mucins like MUC13 are also upregulated in gastric cancer, mainly in adenocarcinomas of the intestinal type (Shimamura et al., 2005; Maher et al., 2011). MUC13 can also be detected in 90% of IM.

Interestingly, the phenotype of present intestinal metaplasia has not to be related to the histological type of an adenocarcinoma, although intestinal-type cancer shows more often a gastric mucin profile (Barresi et al., 2006; Ilhan et al., 2010). Despite positive associations of the mucin phenotype with Laurén type, differentiation of gastric cancer, and location of the primary tumor, there are still conflicting results that lack of a positive correlation of mucin expression with clinicopathological parameters (Tajima et al., 2006; Han et al., 2009; Lee et al., 2009; Oz Puyan et al., 2011; Xue et al., 2011). Similar are the data for MUC1. MUC1 expression in the tumor center correlates with advanced TNM stage and lymph node involvement, and the expression at the invasion front of the cancer is even an independent predictor for worse prognosis in multivariate analysis (Retterspitz et al., 2010). MUC1 expression is lost during dedifferentiation of gastric tumors, and most studies confirm a positive association to also distant metastases, accompanied in most cases also by a decrease of MUC5AC gene expression (Kocer et al., 2004; Ilhan et al., 2010). Especially in the aggressive mucinous-type gastric adenocarcinoma, there is a loss of gastric mucins and an increasing MUC2 transcription (Choi et al., 2009; Ilhan et al., 2010).

A recent genome-wide association study (GWAS) revealed single-nucleotide polymorphisms (SNPs) of the MUC1 promoter to be involved in differential regulation of this mucin and therefore to be related to gastric carcinogenesis, mainly of the diffuse type (Saeki et al., 2011). SNPs in the MUC1 gene have already been earlier reported to be related to gastric cancer, whereas SNPs for MUC5AC have only a minor impact (Jia et al., 2010). In contrast, polymorphisms of the MUC2 gene are associated with decreased risk of progression of premalignant alterations of the gastric mucosa and are interfering with the probability of regression after *H. pylori* eradication therapy (Marin et al., 2012). The effect can better be estimated when certain haplotype combinations are evaluated (Marin et al., 2012). MUC2 gene expression can also be epigenetically regulated by hypermethylation of its promoter region (Mesquita et al., 2003).

Unfortunately, the assessment of mucin phenotype and the expression profile remains a domain of histopathological analyses of biopsies or surgical specimens. Only in a minor proportion of gastric cancer patients, mucins can be detected in the peripheral blood as an indicator for an induced expression, and surrogates like anti-MUC1 IgG in the peripheral blood are not constantly present, having therefore no value for clinical practice (Klaamas et al., 2007; Dardaei et al., 2011).

13.7 Cancer Molecular Typing Implications: HER 2 Typing

In the era of individualized targeted therapy of malignant neoplasias, there has been a recent breakthrough for the treatment of gastric cancer when the results of the ToGA trial have been published, a prospective, randomized, placebo-controlled phase III trial on almost 600 patients with cancer of the stomach or at the esophagogastric junction (Bang et al., 2010). In these patients, trastuzumab, a monoclonal antibody against HER2, has been administered in combination with standard cisplatin/5-fluorouracil-based systemic chemotherapy in patients with positive expression of the HER2 molecule. The mean overall survival of patients receiving the trastuzumab combination has been 13.8 months compared to 11.1 months in the placebo group. Since this difference was not statistically significant, the major impact of the study was given, when a subgroup analysis revealed that in patients with strong expression of HER2 (IHC 3+ or IHC 2+/FISH+), survival was as high as 17.9 months being highly significant compared to the placebo group (Bang et al., 2010). A cost-effectiveness analysis indicated that indeed only treatment of these patients with highly positive HER2 status was reasonable in these clearly HER2-positive patients (Shiroiwa et al., 2011).

HER2 can be detected in 10.1%–20.6% of patients with gastric adenocarcinoma with higher positivity in intestinal-type tumors and in patients with distant metastases (Bang et al., 2010; Jones et al., 2011; Chua and Merrett, 2012; Gomez-Martin et al., 2012; Janjigian et al., 2012; Kataoka et al., 2012). Results concerning HER2 expression as prognostic indicator are still conflicting with studies showing partly poorer and partly improved survival for HER2-positive patients (Yan et al., 2010; Jones et al., 2011; Gomez-Martin et al., 2012). A systematic review on 42 publications including 12,749 patients reported in 71% of the trials an association of positive HER2 status with poor survival, serosal invasion, positive lymph node status, higher degree of distant metastases, and more advanced stage of the disease (Shitara et al., 2012). In another comprehensive review, 35 studies assessing survival were evaluated of which 20 could not demonstrate a difference in survival and 2 reported longer and 13 shorter survival in HER2-positive patients. The overall 5-year survival was 42% vs. 52% in favor of HER2-negative patients. However, the introduction of trastuzumab-based treatment regimens results in a clear survival advantage of HER2-positive patients (Yan et al., 2010).

HER2 expression is increasing with severity of mucosal alterations from lowest in low-grade IEN to highest in adenocarcinoma of the stomach, even showing further increase with dedifferentiation of the neoplastic lesions (Jorgensen and Hersom, 2012). Since there is high intratumor heterogeneity, there is an ongoing debate whether biopsy sampling during endoscopy is adequate for assessment of HER2 status and if tissue from metastatic sites (e.g., liver) can be used for the estimation of the primary. As of today, it can be stated that there is high concordance between HER2 expression in the primary tumor and distant metastases as well as affected lymph nodes (Bozzetti et al., 2011; Fassan et al., 2012; Janjigian et al., 2012). Despite the known tumor heterogeneity, there was also no significant difference in the diagnostic quality if tissue from surgical resection specimens or endoscopic biopsies were used (Janjigian et al., 2012; Pagni et al., 2012).

Since molecular testing and quantification of a positive test result have such a significant value for the treatment decision, there is ongoing debate on the best test method that should be applied as well as semiquantitative scoring systems. Fluorescence in situ hybridization (FISH) is superior to classical immunohistochemical staining (IHC) although it is more complicated and more expensive (Pirrelli et al., 2012). Another option is dual-color silver chromogenic ISH (CISH/SISH) that reveals even more precise test results and a higher detection rate than FISH (Gomez-Martin et al., 2012; Kataoka et al., 2012; Pirrelli et al., 2012). Even tissue microarrays have been discussed to enhance the diagnostic yield (Jones et al., 2011).

13.8 Current Knowledge on Noninvasive Marker Approaches

13.8.1 Noninvasive Tests for Atrophy

The serological analysis of conventional tumor markers for the diagnosis and follow-up of gastric cancer is of little clinical usefulness. CEA, CA19-9, and CA72-4 in the serum have an exceedingly low sensitivity (CEA, 16.4%–28.6%; CA19-9, 16.0%–41.0%; CA72-4, 18.6%–32.6%) (Kodera et al., 1996; Tocchi et al., 1998; Marrelli et al., 1999; Ishigami et al., 2001; Ucar et al., 2008). However, each of these markers is an independent risk factor for poor survival and high recurrence rates after curative resection in multivariate analyses (Kodera et al., 1996; Tachibana et al., 1998; Ishigami et al., 2001; Ucar et al., 2008). Controversial results exist on the association of each marker with clinicopathological characteristics. High serum levels of CEA might be associated with a higher risk for hepatic metastases, but there is also positive correlation of high CEA serum levels with serosal involvement and positive lymph node status (Kodera et al., 1996; Tachibana et al., 1998; Marrelli et al., 1999; Duraker and Celik, 2001; Ishigami et al., 2001; Ucar et al., 2008). However, serum markers for gastric cancer are currently not used in clinical practice. Even the design of multitumor marker chip arrays for serological assessment is costly and of limited advantage for clinical practice.

In the absence of reliable biomarkers for the detection of gastric cancer, a screening program would include the evaluation of surrogate markers that correlate with the presence of premalignant and malignant lesions. Glandular atrophy in the gastric body can be regarded as premalignant condition (Kamada et al., 2005), and the risk for gastric carcinogenesis correlates with the degree of baseline atrophy (Take et al., 2007).

13.8.1.1 Pepsinogens

Pepsinogens are proenzymes of pepsin, and their serum or plasma levels may indirectly reflect the function of the stomach secretion. Pepsinogen I (PgI) is exclusively produced by the chief and mucous neck cells of the corpus, while pepsinogen II (PgII) by these as well as cardiac, pyloric, and Brunner gland cells (di Mario and Cavallaro, 2008). Although only minor proportion (about 1%) of the secreted pepsinogens reaches the bloodstream, pepsinogen levels detected in blood constituents allow to judge the function of the stomach.

Pepsinogen levels are decreased if atrophy in the corpus of the stomach occurs, while an increase is observed during inflammation. To eliminate the possibility of false normal results at the occasion when both atrophy and *H. pylori*-caused inflammation coexist, the ratio between PgI and PgII (PgI/II) is considered a more reliable marker than PgI alone (Borch et al., 1989; Miki, 2006, 2011). A positive CagA status can be an independent influencing factor (Bornschein et al., 2012). Pepsinogen testing in opportunistic screening for gastric cancer and associated premalignant lesions has been used mainly in Japan for decades (Dinis-Ribeiro et al., 2004). However, in 2006, the results of a comprehensive meta-analysis on the available data of more than 40 studies including about 300,000 individuals indicated that tests on serum pepsinogens are not appropriate for gastric cancer screening itself but are useful to identify individuals at high risk to develop gastric cancer who would need further diagnostic work-up (Miki, 2006).

The diagnostic cutoff values for PgI and the PgI/II varied in former studies (Brenner et al., 2007). This should be mentioned that different test systems and methods have been traditionally used in the studies conducted in Asia and Europe; although there is a relatively good correlation between the obtained results, the absolute values differ; therefore, the results in absolute values cannot be translated between the different studies unless identical test systems are used (Miki and Fujishiro, 2009). Therefore, the current guidelines emphasize the need for regionally validated test systems (Malfertheiner et al., 2012).

Decreased pepsinogen levels revealed the best diagnostic reliability resulting in a sensitivity of 66.7%–84.6% and a specificity of 73.5%–87.1% for the detection of atrophic gastritis (Hattori et al., 1995; Kitahara et al., 1999; Kikuchi et al., 2006; Leja et al., 2009). However, other studies with similar cutoff values documented significantly lower sensitivity for gastric cancer screening (36.8%–62.3%) (Kang et al., 2008b; Yanaoka et al., 2008; Mizuno et al., 2009).

A large cohort study in a population from Portugal demonstrated the feasibility of pepsinogen testing approach in a Western population (Lomba-Viana et al., 2012). The authors followed a total of 13,118 individuals for five years; 446 individuals (3.4%) had decreased pepsinogen levels. From these, 274 were undergoing upper gastrointestinal endoscopy; 6 cancer cases were detected representing 1 cancer per 2200 tests or 1 incident case per 74 positive tests. However, three other cancer cases were detected in those with a negative pepsinogen test result (Lomba-Viana et al., 2012).

This method is not free of any challenge. In a Japanese study on an aging agricultural population with a high incidence of gastric cancer, there was also a high prevalence of gastric mucosal atrophy and *H. pylori* infection. Therefore, the number of subjects identified for further endoscopic examinations is too high in such populations to justify the "serological prescreening" (Shimoyama et al., 2012). Similar results have been reported from Latvia; therefore, setting of the right cutoff value for the particular territory is of importance (Leja et al., 2012).

An interesting question is if there are confounding factors given the gastric cancer characteristics that can modulate outcome of the pepsinogen test (Bornschein et al., 2012). The identification of these modifiers could be included in a further stratified analysis in order to improve the diagnostic value for gastric cancer screening. However, neither Laurén type nor tumor localization or tumor stage has an influence on the serum values for PgI, PgII, and PgI/II (Kwak et al., 2010; Bornschein et al., 2012). Only for the PgI/II, a significant difference between intestinal- and diffuse-type carcinomas is documented in some studies, which is related to the higher incidence of intestinal metaplasia and glandular atrophy in case of intestinal-type cancers (Boussioutas et al., 2003; Bornschein et al., 2010). Serum analysis of PgI, PgII, and gastrin-17 (G-17) can yield information about the distribution of intestinal metaplasia and atrophy in the stomach (Cao et al., 2007), but the location of a gastric adenocarcinoma has no significant influence on the results of these serological tests (Bornschein et al., 2012).

The Japanese investigators have suggested the combination of pepsinogen and *H. pylori* antibody detection to stratify the gastric cancer risk (Watabe et al., 2005; Miki, 2011), that is, ABC(D) method. According to the results of the serum test, individuals are classified in group A with a normal pepsinogen level and a negative *H. pylori* test, group B with a normal pepsinogen level and a positive *H. pylori* test, group C with a decreased pepsinogen level and a positive *H. pylori* test, and group D with a decreased pepsinogen level and a negative *H. pylori* test. Hazard ratios (HRs) for gastric cancer incidence if compared with group A were 1.1 (95% CI, 0.4–3.4), 6.0 (95% CI, 2.4–14.5), and 8.2 (3.2–21.5) for groups B, C, and D, respectively (Watabe, 2005). By this stratification, the individual risk assessment can be optimized and endoscopic surveillance individually tailored (Miki et al., 2009; Kudo et al., 2011). However, when using the approach, this is essential to consider the *H. pylori* eradication in the past; otherwise, patients with atrophy after successful *H. pylori* eradication therapy will be incorrectly placed in a higher-risk group than initially (i.e., moved from group "C" to group "D").

13.8.1.2 Gastrin-17

An additional marker has been suggested lately to characterize atrophy in the antral part of the stomach—amidated gastrin-17 (G-17)—since it is secreted exclusively by the G cells in this part of the organ (Sipponen et al., 2002; Vaananen et al., 2003; Agreus et al., 2012).

Within recent years, the importance of gastrin for an intact mucosal homeostasis in the stomach has been recognized and its complex role in gastric carcinogenesis has been revealed, including the gastrin-induced mediation of proliferation, angiogenesis, and tissue invasion (Watson et al., 2006). Animal models have shown that constitutive high expression leads to the development of gastric cancer in 100%, with a more rapid progression in animals that have been additionally infected by *Helicobacter felis* (Wang et al., 2000).

Konturek and colleagues suggested in 1999 for the first time a putative autocrine mechanism of stimulation of gastric cancer progression with gastric cancer cells expressing both gastrin and its receptor (Konturek et al., 1999). Median gastrin levels were higher in gastric cancer patients compared to controls, both concerning plasma and luminal levels. The positive expression of gastrin and its receptor is associated with better differentiation and intestinal-type gastric cancer (Hur et al., 2006).

Theoretically, there could be an additional gain of adding G-17 to the pepsinogen biomarker panel mainly because of two reasons: (1) A high G-17 at the presence of decreased pepsinogens would confirm the presence of atrophy in the corpus and (2) a low G-17 could be indicative for atrophy in the antral part of the stomach.

G-17 levels in the circulation are increased after food intake; therefore, the measurements of G-17 following a provocation with a protein-rich meal are considered the best indicator of antral G-cells functioning (Sipponen et al., 2003; Vaananen et al., 2003). However, the use of a provocation test is impractical and inconvenient in screening settings; therefore, fasting G-17 are being used in many studies instead (di Mario and Cavallaro, 2008).

In addition to diet, amidated G-17 levels in circulation are sensitive to other physiological stimuli, including drug intake (e.g., proton pump inhibitors) (Agreus et al., 2012). This diminishes the value of the test for detecting atrophy in the antral part of the stomach to the sensitivity levels far below the acceptable for a screening test (15.8% at fast and 36.8% after the stimulation) (Leja et al., 2011). No difference in G-17 levels was found also between proximally and distally localized gastric cancer (Hansen et al., 2007; Bornschein et al., 2012). Therefore, currently, there does not seem to be an important gain from investigating this parameter.

13.8.1.3 Other Markers: Ghrelin, Antiparietal Cell Antibodies

Ghrelin is a gastric hormone involved in the regulation of hunger and satiety. Ghrelin-positive cells can physiologically be detected in all parts of the stomach, but it is mainly distributed in the proximal parts, that is, the fundus and the proximal corpus region (Tanaka-Shintani and Watanabe, 2005; Kim et al., 2012). There is an inverse correlation of ghrelin expression with the degree of inflammation present in the stomach (Takiguchi et al., 2012). However, the number of ghrelin-positive cells as well as the ghrelin levels in the serum is decreasing with progression of preneoplastic and neoplastic alterations of the gastric mucosa (Mottershead et al., 2007; Zub-Pokrowiecka et al., 2010). Ghrelin is significantly lower in case of atrophic gastritis compared to early stages of *H. pylori*-induced gastric inflammation. In gastric cancer tissue, there is almost no expression of ghrelin. Low baseline concentrations of ghrelin in the serum are associated with a higher risk for gastric cancer (OR 1.75; 95% CI, 1.49–2.01) (Murphy et al., 2011).

The presence of antibodies against gastric parietal cells (APCAs) being the target for α- and β-subunits of proton pump has been also suggested as markers for atrophy in the stomach mucosa (di Mario and Cavallaro, 2008). APCA is considered a marker of autoimmune gastritis, and the presence of APCA correlates to the atrophy in the corpus part of the stomach (Lo et al., 2005); they may precede clinical manifestations of corpus gastritis as pernicious anemia (Betterle et al., 1988). However, in a majority of gastric cancer patients, APCA levels remain normal even in the presence of decreased pepsinogens (Ito et al., 2002; Sugiu et al., 2006).

13.8.2 *Helicobacter pylori* Subtyping

The malignant potential of each *H. pylori* strain is defined by certain bacterial virulence factors. The cytotoxin-associated antigen pathogenicity island (CagPAI) type IV secretion system that can induce a more severe inflammatory response and can increase the risk for gastric carcinogenesis is best investigated (Blaser et al., 1995; Parsonnet et al., 1997; Enroth et al., 2000). This type IV secretion system is a prerequisite for translocation of pathogenetic virulence factors (e.g., the CagA protein) of *H. pylori* into the epithelial cell (Backert et al., 2000; Odenbreit et al., 2000). CagA is rapidly phosphorylated by host Src kinases and has subsequently the potential to change intracellular signal transduction and to disrupt epithelial cell junctions (Stein et al., 2002; Saadat et al., 2007). The injected CagA leads to activation of the Ras–mitogen-activated protein kinase (MAPK) pathway, involving the Ras-dependent kinases ERK-1 and ERK-2 with further transactivation of host-related pathways (Higashi et al., 2002; Tsutsumi et al., 2003; Hatakeyama, 2004). The CagA-dependent activation of the Ras–Erk cascade increases also IL-8 release and consequent NF-κB activation responsible for the invasion of neutrophil granulocytes into the gastric mucosa (Brandt et al., 2005). NF-κB-related carcinogenesis is enhanced by *H. pylori*-associated release of tumor necrosis factor-α-inducing protein (*Tip*-α) inducing high expression of *TNF*-α with further involvement of IL-8- and COX-2-dependent pathways (Kim et al., 2001; Kuzuhara et al., 2007). The interaction of CagA with the e-cadherin/β-catenin system can lead to a direct transactivation of CDX1 and by this to metaplastic changes in the mucosa (Avidan et al., 2002).

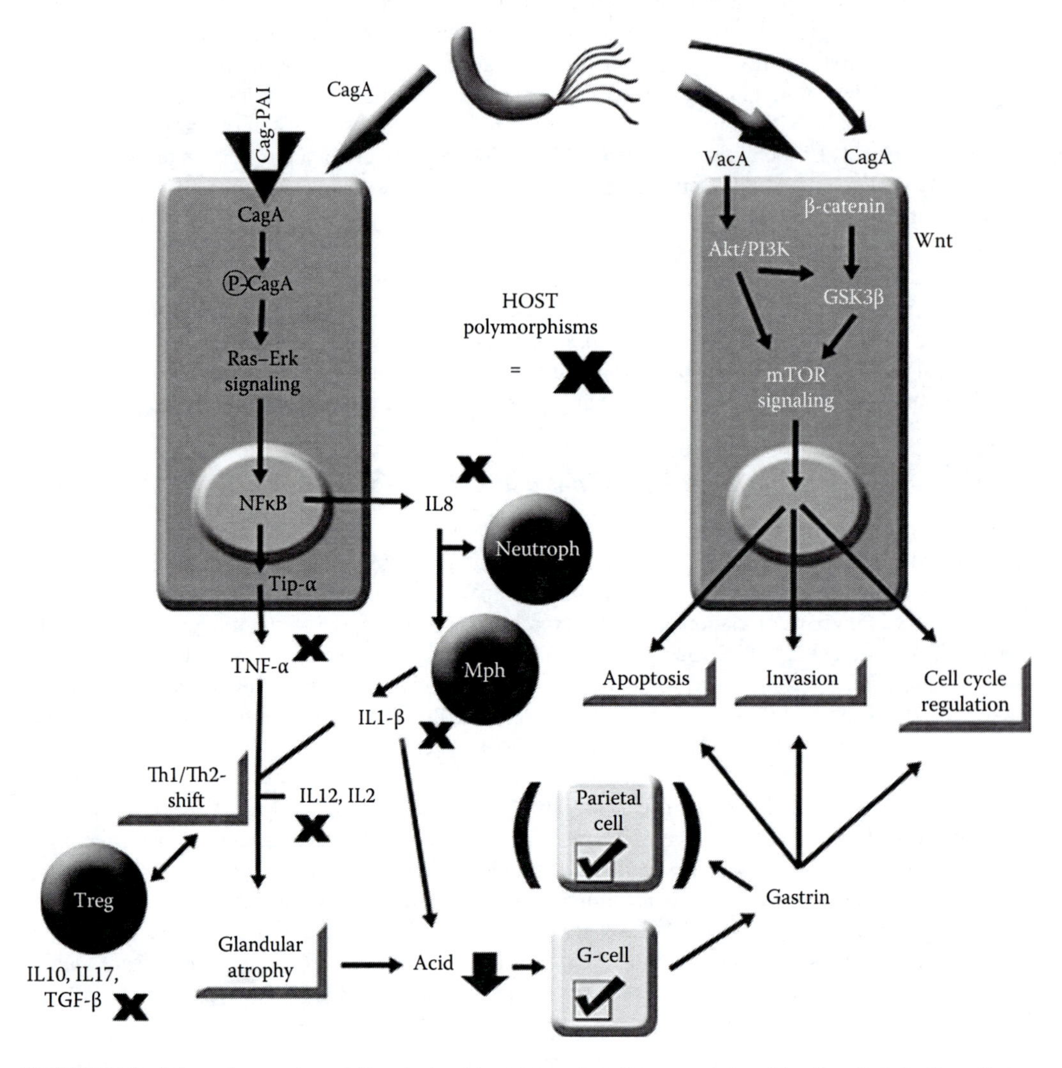

FIGURE 13.2 Schematic overview of *H. pylori* and host interaction: Processes induced by *H. pylori* virulence factors including the influence of host susceptibility factors. (From Bornschein, J. and Malfertheiner, P., *Langenbecks Arch. Surg.*, 396(6), 729, 2011.)

The genetic diversity of the Helicobacter plays an important role in *H. pylori*-driven carcinogenesis. CagA is phosphorylated at certain glutamate–isoleucine–tyrosine–alanine (EPIYA) motifs. Due to variations in the surrounding amino acid sequence, four distinct EPIYA motifs are described (EPIYA-A, EPIYA-B, EPIYA-C, EPIYA-D), which further influence the CagA-induced immune response as well as the related risk for gastric diseases (Higashi et al., 2005; Naito et al., 2006; Mueller et al., 2012). The prevalence of these motifs varies by region (Xia et al., 2009; Zhang et al., 2012). Especially C-terminal repeat of EPIYA-C motifs is associated with an increasing risk for gastric cancer development resulting in an OR of 7.3 in case of one EPIYA-C segment and up to 51-fold increased risk in case of two or more segments (Basso et al., 2008; Quiroga et al., 2010; Batista et al., 2011; Ferreira et al., 2012b).

A similar diversity has been identified for the vacuolating cytotoxin A (VacA). VacA has an inhibitory effect on GSK3β (glycogen synthase kinase 3-β)-regulated signaling pathways by phosphorylation through an Akt/PI3K (phosphatidylinositol-3-kinase)-mediated pathway, leading to a β-catenin release and, furthermore, modulation of apoptosis and cell cycle regulation (Manente et al., 2008; Nakayama et al., 2009). Due to variations in its gene structure, it can be stratified by variants of the signaling (s), the middle (m), and the intermediate (i) region showing also regional differences in its distribution (Uchida et al., 2009; Wroblewski et al., 2010). After the first identification of s1/m1-strains showing a higher attributable risk for gastric cancer development, more recently, also i1-strains have been demonstrated to be associated with not only dysplastic but also malignant invasive tissue formation (Basso et al., 2008; Douraghi et al., 2009; Breurec et al., 2012). Recent data suggested a strong interaction between VacA and CagA genotypes (Jang et al., 2010; Jones et al., 2011; Ferreira et al., 2012a).

The outer-membrane protein BabA is expressed by 40%–95% of the *H. pylori* strains, in dependency of the geographic region (Prinz et al., 2003). Patients infected with a BabA-positive strain show a higher density of bacterial colonization in the stomach and have an enhanced inflammation due to increased IL-8 levels (Rad et al., 2002). *H. pylori* strains expressing all three genes (*CagA*, *VacA*, *BabA*) are associated with the highest risk for developing gastric cancer (Gerhard et al., 1999) (see Figure 13.2 for schematic overview of *H. pylori* and host interaction).

13.9 Host Genetics

13.9.1 Hereditary Gastric Cancer and CDH1 Mutations

Hereditary genetic alterations account for about 5% of all gastric cancer cases with the majority of these being adenocarcinomas of the diffuse type by Laurén (Barber et al., 2006). The International Gastric Cancer Linkage Consortium (IGCLC) suggested criteria for the diagnosis and identification of hereditary diffuse gastric carcinomas (HDGCs). At diagnosis, two conditions must be fulfilled: (1) any family with two documented cases of diffuse-type gastric adenocarcinoma in first- or second-degree relatives, with one case diagnosed under the age of 50, and (2) three or more documented cases of diffuse-type gastric cancer in first- or second-degree relatives of any age (Park et al., 2000). These criteria facilitate the identification of affected families and enable the targeted search for genes responsible for gastric carcinogenesis.

In 2010, the IGCLC guidelines were updated (Fitzgerald et al., 2010), and the following indications for genetic testing were proposed: (1) two gastric cancer cases in the family, at least one of them being diffuse gastric carcinoma below the age of 50; (2) three confirmed diffuse-type cancers in first- or second-degree relatives irrespective the age of onset; (3) diffuse gastric cancer at the age below 40; and (4) personal or family history of diffuse gastric cancer and lobular breast cancer with the onset of one of them below the age of 50.

In 30%–50% of HDGC, a causative germ-line mutation of *CDH1*, the *e-cadherin* gene, can be identified. *CDH1* is a transmembrane glycoprotein involved in cell-to-cell adhesion. The loss of function of this gene is believed to contribute to carcinogenesis by stimulating proliferation and invasion (Semb and Christofori, 1998). Germ-line mutations of the *CDH1* gene are located on chromosome 16 and were first described in 1998 by Guilford et al. (1998). Alterations in *CDH1* gene include deletion, insertion, splice site and nonsense and missense variants (Guilford et al., 2010). A single-nucleotide substitution in the donor splice consensus sequence of exon 7 leads to a truncated gene product. A malfunction of the e-cadherin/β-catenin-complex frees β-catenin from the cell membrane and provides a higher cytoplasmatic pool, activating the Wnt-signaling pathway that plays a major role in gastric carcinogenesis (Park et al., 2000). This and β-catenin-related activation of T-cell factor (TCF)-dependent transcription induce signaling cascades like mTOR-related pathways leading to the induction of target genes like cyclins and matrix metalloproteinases (MMPs) that are relevant for the initiation of invasive gastric cancer (Kolligs et al., 2002).

The *CDH1* mutation is of the recessive type with one allele being altered and the other subsequently being inactivated in the gastric tissue either by hypermethylation, somatic mutation and loss of heterozygosity (LOH), intragenic deletion, or specific polymorphisms. More than 30 mutations are responsible for at least 30% of HDGC cases with a penetrance of 75%–80% (Pharoah et al., 2001). The estimated lifetime risk for developing gastric cancer for individuals bearing *CDH1* gene mutations is 40%–70% for men and 60%–80% for women (Corso et al., 2012). However, alterations of the *CDH1* gene are reported not only for hereditary gastric cancer; hypermethylation of the *CDH1*-promoter can be detected in 40%–80% of all primary gastric cancers (Graziano et al., 2003). Female patients that carry this mutation have additionally an increased risk (20%–30%) for developing lobular breast cancer (Cisco and Norton, 2008).

CDH1 genetic testing is indicated in individuals with family history of hereditary gastric cancer and can be used as the basis for making decisions on early radical gastric cancer prevention (Barber et al., 2006). The results of endoscopic surveillance of these patients are unsatisfying. Thus, *CDH1* gene mutation carriers should be offered the option of prophylactic gastrectomy (Fitzgerald et al., 2010). The debate is still controversial if prophylactic gastrectomy is a reasonable intervention for all carriers of *CDH1* germ-line mutations. Huntsman and colleagues performed the operation on five asymptomatic carriers of the specific mutation who presented with a positive family history of gastric cancer. All of the five resected specimens revealed early gastric cancer, in three cases of multifocal location (Huntsman et al., 2001). Others reported similar results evaluating larger cohorts of *CDH1* mutation-positive families with the detection of gastric cancer in 76.5%–83.3% of the patients after gastrectomy (Huntsman et al., 2001; Suriano et al., 2005; Lynch et al., 2008). This approach, however, is applied only in a small number of expertise centers. This genetic screening method, however, can be beneficial to a very small subgroup of hereditary diffuse-type gastric cancer patients that constitute only up to 5% of total gastric cancer cases.

13.9.2 Cytokine Polymorphisms

Genotyping costs have been dramatically reduced over the last decade due to pronounced advances in technology. Therefore, gene polymorphisms, including SNPs, emerged as attractive biomarkers for the identification of individuals with increased risk of developing different malignancies. The activation of proinflammatory pathways is the predominant carcinogenesis model of gastric cancer development, which has been demonstrated both in human studies and animal models (Watanabe et al., 1998; Fuccio et al., 2009). The postulated hypothesis suggests that subjects with a proinflammatory genetic profile are more vulnerable to *H. pylori* infection and gastric cancer development. Therefore, the role of proinflammatory and anti-inflammatory cytokines has been a core interest of different gastric cancer research groups.

In the year 2000, El-Omar and colleagues published an intriguing study in *Nature* journal reporting a significant association between proinflammatory interleukin-1B gene (*IL1B*) polymorphism and increased risk of *H. pylori*-induced gastric cancer (El Omar et al., 2000). Many associations between polymorphisms of the genes encoding cytokines and the risk of gastric cancer have been reported since then. The polymorphisms of the genes encoding cytokines *IL1B*, *IL1RN*, *IL2*, *IL6*, *IL8*, *IL10*, and many others have been studied extensively (Hishida et al., 2010). Different studies, however, reported partially conflicting results and conclusions drawn by the researchers are limited by small sample sizes, as well as anatomical, ethnical, and histological bias present among individual gastric cancer patients. Although initial studies have implicated a significant effect of certain cytokine gene alterations for the risk of gastric cancer development, data from more recent studies have shown opposite or null associations (El Omar et al., 2000; Kupcinskas et al., 2010). Polymorphisms of *IL1B* and interleukin-1 receptor antagonist gene (*IL1RN*) are the most famous cytokine-related gene alterations analyzed in the context of gastric cancer development risks. There are several meta-analyses in PubMed database pooling the data of smaller *IL1B* and *IL1RN* SNPs studies among gastric cancer patients (Camargo et al., 2006; Kamangar et al., 2006;

Peleteiro et al., 2010). Although the conclusions of separate meta-analyses vary in between, the overall impact of *IL1B* and *IL1RN* genetic alterations for gastric cancer development appears to be mild if any and slightly more relevant in subjects of Asian ethnicity. Low ORs present in these meta-analyses question the applicability of these genetic alterations as potential screening biomarkers. To date, none of the cytokine gene polymorphisms can be used in daily clinical practice for stratification of risk of gastric adenocarcinoma in an individual patient due to the lack of association strength (Malfertheiner et al., 2012). Further research, including GWASs, in the field is desirable, which may reveal new interesting gene susceptibility loci.

13.10 Emerging Areas of Biomarker Research

13.10.1 miRNAs and miRNA Coding Gene Polymorphisms

Gastric cancer is a complex disease, which is hypothesized to result from interaction of *H. pylori* infection, environmental, nutritional, and host factors. The interaction between different risk factors for gastric cancer is given in Figure 13.3.

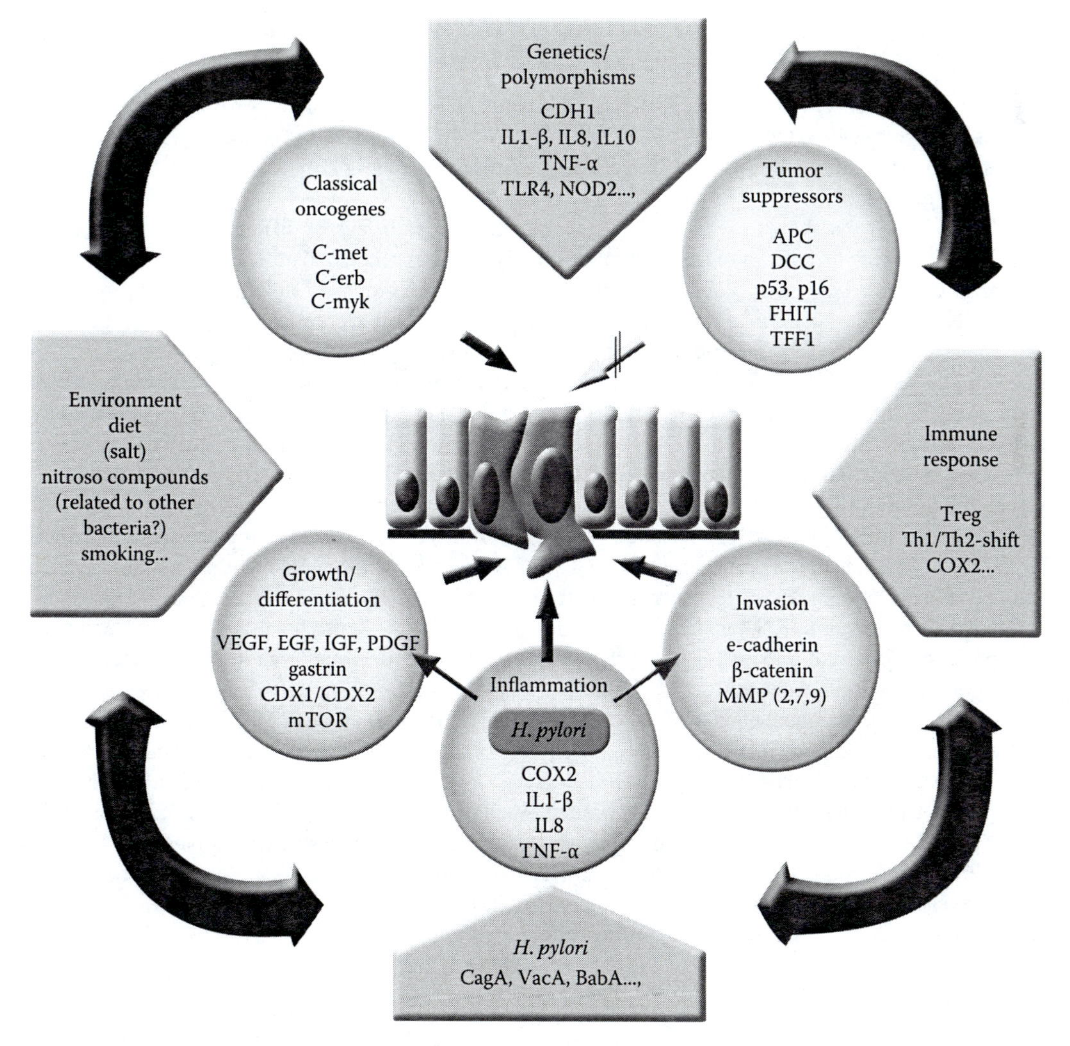

FIGURE 13.3 Gastric cancer risk factors: environmental and host-related factors as well as molecular changes related to gastric carcinogenesis. (Modified from Bornschein, J. et al., *Expert Opin. Med. Diagn.*, 3(5), 585, 2009.)

TABLE 13.1

List of Deregulated miRNAs in Gastric Adenocarcinoma

Downregulated miRNAs			Upregulated miRNAs	
let-7 family	miR-139	miR-377	miR-9	miR-196a/b
miR-9	miR-141	miR-429	miR-15/16	miR-199a
miR-15/16	miR-148a	miR-433	miR-21	miR-200 family
miR-10b	miR-148b	miR-449	miR-23a	miR-212
miR-29 family	miR-152	miR-451	miR-25-106b family	miR-214
miR-34	miR-155	miR-486	miR-27	miR-215
miR-34b	miR-181b	miR-497	miR-34b	miR-221–222 cluster
miR-43c	miR-181c	miR-512-5p	miR-103	miR-223
miR-101	miR-204	miR-622	miR-107	miR-320
miR-124a-1/3	miR-212	miR-652	miR-126	miR-372
miR-125a	miR-218		miR-130b	miR-379
miR-126	miR-331-3p		miR-146a	miR-421
miR-129-2	miR-335		miR-150	miR-429
miR-137	miR-375		miR-181c	miR-650

Source: Adapted from Link, A. et al., *Dig. Dis.*, 30(3), 255, 2012.

A recent discovery of microRNAs (miRNAs) has changed our perception of posttranscriptional gene expression regulation (Wightman et al., 1993). miRNAs are small ~22 bp noncoding RNAs, which have exceptional stability in different tissues. This feature makes miRNAs a very attractive target in biomarker research field.

miRNAs have been shown to participate in carcinogenesis pathways of different malignancies (Lu et al., 2005). A growing number of research groups outline the importance of miRNAs in different stages of gastric cancer development, including early steps of *H. pylori*-induced inflammation and atrophic gastritis (Link et al., 2012). miRNA profiling studies have revealed a promising miRNA deregulation pattern in stomach mucosa of gastric cancer patients. The most frequently reported deregulated miRNAs in gastric cancer include mir-19, mir-21, mir-25–106 family, mir-155, mir-181 family, and many others (Volinia et al., 2006; Ueda et al., 2010). The list of deregulated miRNAs in gastric cancer determined by different profiling studies is presented in Table 13.1. Furthermore, the importance of miRNAs has been shown in a growing number of functional studies, which identified direct miRNA target genes that function as either tumor suppressor or oncogenes (Link et al., 2012). The majority of the target genes affected by deregulated miRNAs in gastric adenocarcinoma are linked with cell cycle and apoptosis. Verified targets for miRNAs in gastric cancer include *BCL2*, *VEZT*, *p53*, *SOX2*, *KRAS*, and other numerous genes that play a major role in carcinogenesis pathways (Link et al., 2012).

Genetic alterations of miRNA genes may alter miRNA processing, induce functional changes, and alter susceptibility to different diseases. SNPs of the genes encoding miRNA may lead to loss of function and interaction with new target genes. Current bioinformatics projects offer online databases for miRNA-related SNPs and their potential interaction with target sites (miRanda, TargetScan, etc.). There are a growing number of studies examining the role of miRNA-related polymorphisms with respect to gastric cancer risk. The most explored in this field are rs2910164 (pre-miR-146a G > C) and rs11614913 (miR-196a2 C > T); however, the reported data are partially conflicting and limited by small sample sizes (Okubo et al., 2010; Zeng et al., 2010). The significance of these alterations remains poorly investigated in gastric cancer patients.

Current evidence suggests important role of miRNAs in gastric cancer pathogenesis. Further research in the field is required to determine potential applications of miRNA in daily clinical practice for diagnostic, prognostic, or even therapeutical purposes in gastric cancer patients.

13.10.2 Epigenetics

The epigenetic regulation of transcription has been studied extensively in different fields, underlying the significance of this process. Two patterns including global hypomethylation and promoter hypermethylation are common features in different malignancies. The first feature is linked with genomic instability and tumor formation, while the second is important for inactivation of tumor-suppressor genes and may affect important pathways of cell cycle regulation or proliferation. When a CpG island present in the promoter region of a gene is methylated, gene expression is downregulated (Gigek et al., 2012).

Aberrant methylation of CpG islands in promoter regions is a common event in gastric cancer. Therefore, the methylation of CpG islands has been studied in a large set of important genes related to gastric carcinogenesis (Miyamoto and Ushijima, 2005; Nobili et al., 2011). The pattern of aberrant methylation of CpG islands has potential to become a marker, which can be used to predict responses to chemotherapy and survival. A series of individual methylated genes has been related to prognosis in gastric cancer. The methylation of common tumor-suppressor genes, including *CDH1* (Huang et al., 2012), *CDX1* (Rau et al., 2012), *FOXD3* (Cheng et al., 2012), *RUNX3* (Lu et al., 2012), *SOX9* (Sun et al., 2012), *NDGR2* (Chang et al., 2012), *TPEF* (Ivanauskas et al., 2008), and many other genes, has been linked with gastric cancer development. A new player of carcinogenesis process—miRNAs—has also been shown to be deregulated by epigenetic changes in gastric cancer (Suzuki et al., 2010; Craig et al., 2011; Pavicic et al., 2011).

Advances in technologies over the last years allowed the identification of global methylation patterns in human malignancies, rather than looking at separate gene status. The methylation array analysis comparing three metastatic lymph nodes and three primary gastric cancer tissue samples without metastatic lymph node metastasis found a hypermethylation region, which could predict the presence of lymph node metastasis with a sensitivity of 43% and specificity of 85%. Additionally, the hypermethylation of the region was associated with a poor survival rate among gastric cancer patients. The results of the present study indicated that the methylation status of the region was a promising candidate marker to detect the presence of metastasis and may reflect the malignant potential of gastric cancers (Shigematsu et al., 2012). A study by Balassiano et al. found that global demethylation of tumor cell genomes occurs in gastric cancer, and their findings are consistent with the data that abnormal hypermethylation of specific genes (*ALDH2, MTHFR*) occurs concomitantly with genome-wide hypomethylation (Balassiano et al., 2011).

Current evidence suggests that epigenetic regulation of tumor-suppressor genes is an important mechanism in the development of gastric cancer. The definite role of methylation status detection for diagnostic, prognostic, or treatment benefits has yet to be established in the clinical setting.

13.10.3 Cancer Autoantibodies

Autoantibodies against tumor-associated antigens have been identified in several cancer types (Tureci et al., 1997; Preuss et al., 2002); because of their specificity and stability in the sera, they represent attractive targets for the development of noninvasive serological tests for the diagnosis or early detection of cancer (Zayakin et al., 2013). At the same time, the frequency of antibodies against particular tumor-associated antigens is rather low, typically ranging 1%–15%; therefore, an approach of panel testing has frequently been used to explore cancer-specific antibodies (Zayakin et al., 2013).

Recently, such an antibody search panel testing has been conducted in gastric cancer. A 45-autoantibody signature was found to discriminate gastric cancer from healthy controls with 59% sensitivity and 90% specificity (Zayakin et al., 2013).

13.10.4 Circulating Cancer Cells

The identification of circulating tumor cells (CTCs) has been related to the presence of a systemic disease and appearance of peripheral metastasis (Liotta et al., 1974). The detection of CTCs is suggested useful for estimating the prognosis and for monitoring the disease in several cancer types, including breast, lung, prostate, skin, colon, and gastrointestinal cancers (Kim et al., 2011; Krebs et al., 2011; Ito et al., 2012).

The larger number of CTCs has been found in metastatic gastric cancer than nonmetastatic disease ($p = 0.016$); the identification of two or more CTCs is an indicator for more advanced stage as well as peritoneal dissemination of gastric cancer (Hiraiwa et al., 2008).

In a recent study using a telomerase-specific viral agent to detect CTCs in peripheral blood of gastric cancer patients with different stages of the disease, a significant relationship between the number of CTCs and the prognosis of the disease was revealed.

However, not all the CTCs might have equal metastatic potential since the relapse of the early-stage disease was not identified even in the presence of CTCs (Ito et al., 2012).

The authors have suggested that the detection of CRCs might have a role for choosing an appropriate treatment approach, for example, neoadjuvant chemotherapy in patients with increased CRC count because of otherwise poor prognosis of the disease (Ito et al., 2012).

13.10.5 Volatile Organic Compounds in Exhaled Breath

A recent pilot study performed in patients from China suggests the possibility of highly sensitive, cross-reactive, and nanomaterial-based gas sensor use to identify and separate volatile marker patterns between gastric cancer patients and those with benign gastric conditions (Xu et al., 2013); with this approach, 89% sensitivity, 90% specificity, and 90% accuracy were achieved. Certain volatile organic compounds were found to be different in exhaled air between the groups when the analysis with gas chromatography combined to mass spectrometry was performed. The concentrations of 2-propenenitrile and 1-methoxy-2-propanol were very significantly elevated ($p = 0.0004$) in the breath of the gastric cancer patients, as compared to the patients with less severe gastric conditions without ulceration. The concentrations of tetrachlorobutyl acetate were significantly elevated in gastric cancer patients, as compared to the patients with gastric ulcers. Furthermore, the nonmalignant subpopulations (i.e., gastric ulcer and less severe gastric conditions) showed different concentration profiles, either elevated or reduced, for eight other volatile components from the families of alcohol ethers, aldehydes, esters, ketones, and alkenes (Xu et al., 2013). However, these results have to be treated as preliminary data; studies to demonstrate the reproducibility of the results in other populations have to be conducted.

13.11 Strategies and Future Perspective

Although the incidence of gastric cancer is globally declining in standardized ratio figures, the disease will still remain a major health-care issue during the decades to come; therefore, the identification of individuals at risk and finding the disease at early stage is going to remain a challenge during this period in major parts of the global population.

The Asia-Pacific guidelines encourage *H. pylori* screening and eradication in high-risk regions (Fock et al., 2009), but the implementation of these recommendations is still being discussed. European guidelines recommend to explore the screen-and-treat strategy for *H. pylori* in communities with a significant burden of gastric cancer (Malfertheiner et al., 2012). However, such strategy is highly controversial due to expected high incidence of undesirable events (adverse effects of drugs, increased resistance of microorganisms toward widely used antibiotics, etc.) even if cost-effective. The use of this strategy is likely to result in substantial overtreatment and may not be feasible to the entire population (Forman and Pisani, 2008). Vaccination would be an optimal solution but will not be available in the near future.

The recent guidelines on the management of precancerous conditions and lesions in the stomach (MAPS) (Dinis-Ribeiro et al., 2012) and the Maastricht IV guidelines (Malfertheiner et al., 2012) emphasize the importance of targeting the individuals at increased risk for gastric cancer development from the general population to enable the follow-up of this group.

Biomarker testing with pepsinogens for identifying individuals at increased risk for cancer development is considered also by the guidelines in the East and West (Fock et al., 2009; Dinis-Ribeiro et al., 2012; Malfertheiner et al., 2012). Although at the moment there is not any more effective screening tool for atrophy, the applicability of these tests in organized cancer screening programs still has to be studied. The sensitivity might not be high enough, in particular, when diffuse-type cancer risk is considered.

Therefore, additional research is required in respect to biomarker screening applications for gastric cancer; in addition, new screening tests are also required.

13.12 Commercially Available Markers and the Key Market Players

As mentioned earlier, there is no single ideal noninvasive gastric cancer screening marker ready to be applied in organized screening programs. However, many of the clinical tests discussed are in routine use.

A number of pepsinogen detection test kits are being used in Japan; the lists of the manufacturers are given in comprehensive reviews (Miki, 2006; Kim and Jung, 2010). Most of the Asian studies have been performed by using the test system from Eiken Chemical Co., Ltd., Tokyo; currently, the manufacturer has its latex-agglutination tests CE marked.

In Europe, mainly the ELISA method is used for pepsinogen (also for G-17) testing. The commercially available test panel *GastroPanel* (Biohit, Plc., Helsinki, Finland) is including several separate test kits, that is, for the detection of (1) PgI, (2) PgII, (3) G-17, and (4) *H. pylori* IgG antibodies. Although the combination of the tests may provide certain advantage (see preceding text), the value of each separate parameter included to the panel requires a separate judgment.

H. pylori antibody tests are provided by multiple manufacturers; still, all the test systems are not equally good in any territory; therefore, regional validation is required. In clinical practice, ^{13}C-urea breath tests and monoclonal *H. pylori* antigen tests in feces are the tests of choice, while *H. pylori* IgG antibody tests should be reserved only for special situations (Malfertheiner et al., 2012).

13.13 Concluding Remarks

At the moment there are no perfect noninvasive screening tools for gastric cancer available. The most extensive studied of the available tests are pepsinogens; however additional data is necessary prior these can be recommended for the use in organized screening programs.

New and exciting developments are currently under investigation; these include miRNA signatures, cancer autoantibody panels, and volatile components in exhaled breath. However, there is still a long way to go before they could be available to the practice; in addition, the cost-efficacy issues will have to be studied before such tests could be implemented to population-based screening programs for gastric cancer.

Acknowledgments

The authors acknowledge Aija Line for the advice and Ieva Lasina for technical assistance in the manuscript preparation. Special thanks to Dr. Jochen Weigt for the endoscopic images.

References

Agreus, L., E.J. Kuipers et al. 2012. Rationale in diagnosis and screening of atrophic gastritis with stomach-specific plasma biomarkers. *Scand J Gastroenterol* 47(2): 136–147.

Ang, T.L., K.M. Fock et al. 2012. The diagnostic utility of narrow band imaging magnifying endoscopy in clinical practice in a population with intermediate gastric cancer risk. *Eur J Gastroenterol Hepatol* 24(4): 362–367.

Avidan, B., A. Sonnenberg et al. 2002. Hiatal hernia size, Barrett's length, and severity of acid reflux are all risk factors for esophageal adenocarcinoma. *Am J Gastroenterol* 97(8): 1930–1936.

Babu, S.D., V. Jayanthi et al. 2006. Expression profile of mucins (MUC2, MUC5AC and MUC6) in *Helicobacter pylori* infected pre-neoplastic and neoplastic human gastric epithelium. *Mol Cancer* 5: 10.

Backert, S., E. Ziska et al. 2000. Translocation of the *Helicobacter pylori* CagA protein in gastric epithelial cells by a type IV secretion apparatus. *Cell Microbiol* 2(2): 155–164.

Balassiano, K., S. Lima et al. 2011. Aberrant DNA methylation of cancer-associated genes in gastric cancer in the European Prospective Investigation into Cancer and Nutrition (EPIC-EURGAST). *Cancer Lett* 311(1): 85–95.

Baldus, S.E., S.P. Monig et al. 2002. Correlation of MUC5AC immunoreactivity with histopathological subtypes and prognosis of gastric carcinoma. *Ann Surg Oncol* 9(9): 887–893.

Bang, Y.J., E. Van Cutsem et al. 2010. Trastuzumab in combination with chemotherapy versus chemotherapy alone for treatment of HER2-positive advanced gastric or gastro-oesophageal junction cancer (ToGA): A phase 3, open-label, randomised controlled trial. *Lancet* 376(9742): 687–697.

Banno, K., Y. Niwa et al. 2010. Confocal endomicroscopy for phenotypic diagnosis of gastric cancer. *J Gastroenterol Hepatol* 25(4): 712–718.

Barber, M., R.C. Fitzgerald et al. 2006. Familial gastric cancer—Aetiology and pathogenesis. *Best Pract Res Clin Gastroenterol* 20(4): 721–734.

Barresi, V., E. Vitarelli et al. 2006. Relationship between immunoexpression of mucin peptide cores MUC1 and MUC2 and Lauren's histologic subtypes of gastric carcinomas. *Eur J Histochem* 50(4): 301–309.

Basso, D., C.F. Zambon et al. 2008. Clinical relevance of *Helicobacter pylori* cagA and vacA gene polymorphisms. *Gastroenterology* 135(1): 91–99.

Batista, S.A., G.A. Rocha et al. 2011. Higher number of *Helicobacter pylori* CagA EPIYA C phosphorylation sites increases the risk of gastric cancer, but not duodenal ulcer. *BMC Microbiol* 11: 61.

Bertuccio, P., L. Chatenoud et al. 2009. Recent patterns in gastric cancer: A global overview. *Int J Cancer* 125(3): 666–673.

Betterle, C., P.A. Mazzi et al. 1988. Complement-fixing gastric parietal cell autoantibodies. A good marker for the identification of type A chronic atrophic gastritis. *Autoimmunity* 1(4): 267–274.

Blaser, M.J., G.I. Perez-Perez et al. 1995. Infection with *Helicobacter pylori* strains possessing cagA is associated with an increased risk of developing adenocarcinoma of the stomach. *Cancer Res* 55(10): 2111–2115.

Blot, W.J. and J.K. McLaughlin. 1999. The changing epidemiology of esophageal cancer. *Semin Oncol* 26(5 Suppl 15): 2–8.

Borch, K., C.K. Axelsson et al. 1989. The ratio of pepsinogen A to pepsinogen C: A sensitive test for atrophic gastritis. *Scand J Gastroenterol* 24(7): 870–876.

Bornschein, J. and P. Malfertheiner. 2011. Gastric carcinogenesis. *Langenbecks Arch Surg* 396(6): 729–742.

Bornschein, J., M. Selgrad et al. 2010. *H. pylori* infection is a key risk factor for proximal gastric cancer. *Dig Dis Sci* 55(11): 3124–3131.

Bornschein, J., M. Selgrad et al. 2012. Serological assessment of gastric mucosal atrophy in gastric cancer. *BMC Gastroenterol* 12: 10.

Bornschein, J., J. Weight et al. 2009. Molecular aspects in the diagnosis of gastric cancer. *Expert Opin Med Diagn* 3(5): 585–596.

Bosman, F.T., F. Carneiro et al. 2010. *WHO Classification of Tumours of the Digestive System*, 4th edn. Lyon, France: IARC.

Botterweck, A.A., L.J. Schouten et al. 2000. Trends in incidence of adenocarcinoma of the oesophagus and gastric cardia in ten European countries. *Int J Epidemiol* 29(4): 645–654.

Boussioutas, A., H. Li et al. 2003. Distinctive patterns of gene expression in premalignant gastric mucosa and gastric cancer. *Cancer Res* 63(10): 2569–2577.

Bozzetti, C., F.V. Negri et al. 2011. Comparison of HER2 status in primary and paired metastatic sites of gastric carcinoma. *Br J Cancer* 104(9): 1372–1376.

Brandt, S., T. Kwok et al. 2005. NF-kappaB activation and potentiation of proinflammatory responses by the *Helicobacter pylori* CagA protein. *Proc Natl Acad Sci USA* 102(26): 9300–9305.

Brenner, H., V. Arndt et al. 2004. Is *Helicobacter pylori* infection a necessary condition for noncardia gastric cancer? *Am J Epidemiol* 159(3): 252–258.

Brenner, H., D. Rothenbacher et al. 2007. Epidemiologic findings on serologically defined chronic atrophic gastritis strongly depend on the choice of the cutoff-value. *Int J Cancer* 121(12): 2782–2786.

Breurec, S., R. Michel et al. 2012. Clinical relevance of cagA and vacA gene polymorphisms in *Helicobacter pylori* isolates from Senegalese patients. *Clin Microbiol Infect* 18(2): 153–159.

Camargo, M.C., R. Mera et al. 2006. Interleukin-1beta and interleukin-1 receptor antagonist gene polymorphisms and gastric cancer: A meta-analysis. *Cancer Epidemiol Biomarkers Prev* 15(9): 1674–1687.

Cao, Q., Z.H. Ran et al. 2007. Screening of atrophic gastritis and gastric cancer by serum pepsinogen, gastrin-17 and *Helicobacter pylori* immunoglobulin G antibodies. *J Dig Dis* 8(1): 15–22.

Capelle, L.G., A.C. de Vries et al. 2010a. The staging of gastritis with the OLGA system by using intestinal metaplasia as an accurate alternative for atrophic gastritis. *Gastrointest Endosc* 71(7): 1150–1158.

Capelle, L.G., J. Haringsma et al. 2010b. Narrow band imaging for the detection of gastric intestinal metaplasia and dysplasia during surveillance endoscopy. *Dig Dis Sci* 55(12): 3442–3448.

Chang, X., Z. Li et al. 2012. DNA methylation of NDRG2 in gastric cancer and its clinical significance. *Dig Dis Sci* 58: 715–723.

Cheng, A.S., M.S. Li et al. 2012. *Helicobacter pylori* causes epigenetic dysregulation of FOXD3 to promote gastric carcinogenesis. *Gastroenterology* 144: 122–133.

Choi, J.S., M.A. Kim et al. 2009. Mucinous gastric carcinomas: Clinicopathologic and molecular analyses. *Cancer* 115(15): 3581–3590.

Choi, K.S., J.K. Jun et al. 2011. Performance of gastric cancer screening by endoscopy testing through the National Cancer Screening Program of Korea. *Cancer Sci* 102(8): 1559–1564.

Chua, T.C. and N.D. Merrett. 2012. Clinicopathologic factors associated with HER2-positive gastric cancer and its impact on survival outcomes—A systematic review. *Int J Cancer* 130(12): 2845–2856.

Cisco, R.M. and J.A. Norton. 2008. Hereditary diffuse gastric cancer: Surgery, surveillance and unanswered questions. *Future Oncol* 4(4): 553–559.

Corso, G., D. Marrelli et al. 2012. Frequency of CDH1 germline mutations in gastric carcinoma coming from high-and low-risk areas: Metanalysis and systematic review of the literature. *BMC Cancer* 12(1): 8.

Craig, V.J., S.B. Cogliatti et al. 2011. Epigenetic silencing of microRNA-203 dysregulates ABL1 expression and drives *Helicobacter*-associated gastric lymphomagenesis. *Cancer Res* 71(10): 3616–3624.

Crane, S.J., G. Richard Locke, 3rd et al. 2007. The changing incidence of oesophageal and gastric adenocarcinoma by anatomic sub-site. *Aliment Pharmacol Ther* 25(4): 447–453.

Dan, Y.Y., J.B. So et al. 2006. Endoscopic screening for gastric cancer. *Clin Gastroenterol Hepatol* 4(6): 709–716.

Dardaei, L., R. Shahsavani et al. 2011. The detection of disseminated tumor cells in bone marrow and peripheral blood of gastric cancer patients by multimarker (CEA, CK20, TFF1 and MUC2) quantitative real-time PCR. *Clin Biochem* 44(4): 325–330.

Daugule, I., A. Sudraba et al. 2011. Gastric plasma biomarkers and operative link for gastritis assessment gastritis stage. *Eur J Gastroenterol Hepatol* 23(4): 302–307.

Devesa, S.S., W.J. Blot et al. 1998. Changing patterns in the incidence of esophageal and gastric carcinoma in the United States. *Cancer* 83(10): 2049–2053.

Dinis-Ribeiro, M., M. Areia et al. 2012. Management of precancerous conditions and lesions in the stomach (MAPS): Guideline from the European Society of Gastrointestinal Endoscopy (ESGE), European Helicobacter Study Group (EHSG), European Society of Pathology (ESP), and the Sociedade Portuguesa de Endoscopia Digestiva (SPED). *Endoscopy* 44(1): 74–94.

Dinis-Ribeiro, M., G. Yamaki et al. 2004. Meta-analysis on the validity of pepsinogen test for gastric carcinoma, dysplasia or chronic atrophic gastritis screening. *J Med Screen* 11(3): 141–147.

Dixon, M.F., R.M. Genta et al. 1996. Classification and grading of gastritis. The updated Sydney System. International Workshop on the Histopathology of Gastritis, Houston 1994. *Am J Surg Pathol* 20(10): 1161–1181.

Dohi, O., N. Yagi et al. 2012. Recognition of endoscopic diagnosis in differentiated-type early gastric cancer by flexible spectral imaging color enhancement with indigo carmine. *Digestion* 86(2): 161–170.

Douraghi, M., Y. Talebkhan et al. 2009. Multiple gene status in *Helicobacter pylori* strains and risk of gastric cancer development. *Digestion* 80(3): 200–207.

Duraker, N. and A.N. Celik 2001. The prognostic significance of preoperative serum CA 19–9 in patients with resectable gastric carcinoma: Comparison with CEA. *J Surg Oncol* 76(4): 266–271.

Dutta, A.K., K.G. Sajith et al. 2012. Narrow band imaging versus white light gastroscopy in detecting potentially premalignant gastric lesions: A randomized prospective crossover study. *Indian J Gastroenterol* 32: 37–42.

Edge, S.B., D.R. Byrd et al. 2009. *AJCC Cancer Staging Manual*, 7th edn. New York: Springer.

Ekstrom, A.M., M. Held et al. 2001. *Helicobacter pylori* in gastric cancer established by CagA immunoblot as a marker of past infection. *Gastroenterology* 121(4): 784–791.

El Omar, E.M., M. Carrington et al. 2000. Interleukin-1 polymorphisms associated with increased risk of gastric cancer. *Nature* 404: 398–402.

Enroth, H., W. Kraaz et al. 2000. *Helicobacter pylori* strain types and risk of gastric cancer: A case-control study. *Cancer Epidemiol Biomark Prev* 9(9): 981–985.

Eslick, G.D., L.L. Lim et al. 1999. Association of *Helicobacter pylori* infection with gastric carcinoma: A meta-analysis. *Am J Gastroenterol* 94(9): 2373–2379.

Ezoe, Y., M. Muto et al. 2011. Magnifying narrowband imaging is more accurate than conventional white-light imaging in diagnosis of gastric mucosal cancer. *Gastroenterology* 141(6): 2017–2025. e2013.

Fassan, M., L. Mastracci et al. 2012. Early HER2 dysregulation in gastric and oesophageal carcinogenesis. *Histopathology* 61(5): 769–776.

Ferreira, R.M., J.C. Machado et al. 2012a. A novel method for genotyping *Helicobacter pylori* vacA intermediate region directly in gastric biopsy specimens. *J Clin Microbiol* 50: 3983–3989.

Ferreira, R.M., J.C. Machado et al. 2012b. The number of *Helicobacter pylori* CagA EPIYA C tyrosine phosphorylation motifs influences the pattern of gastritis and the development of gastric carcinoma. *Histopathology* 60(6): 992–998.

Fitzgerald, R.C., R. Hardwick et al. 2010. Hereditary diffuse gastric cancer: Updated consensus guidelines for clinical management and directions for future research. *J Med Genet* 47(7): 436–444.

Fock, K.M., P. Katelaris et al. 2009. Second Asia-Pacific Consensus Guidelines for *Helicobacter pylori* infection. *J Gastroenterol Hepatol* 24(10): 1587–1600.

Forman, D. and V.J. Burley. 2006. Gastric cancer: Global pattern of the disease and an overview of environmental risk factors. *Best Pract Res Clin Gastroenterol* 20(4): 633–649.

Forman, D. and P. Pisani. 2008. Gastric cancer in Japan—Honing treatment, seeking causes. *N Engl J Med* 359(5): 448–451.

Fuccio, L., R.M. Zagari et al. 2009. Meta-analysis: Can *Helicobacter pylori* eradication treatment reduce the risk for gastric cancer? *Ann Intern Med* 151(2): 121–128.

Gerhard, M., N. Lehn et al. 1999. Clinical relevance of the *Helicobacter pylori* gene for blood-group antigen-binding adhesin. *Proc Natl Acad Sci USA* 96(22): 12778–12783.

Gigek, C.O., E.S. Chen et al. 2012. Epigenetic mechanisms in gastric cancer. *Epigenomics* 4(3): 279–294.

Gomez-Martin, C., E. Garralda et al. 2012. HER2/neu testing for anti-HER2-based therapies in patients with unresectable and/or metastatic gastric cancer. *J Clin Pathol* 65(8): 751–757.

Graziano, F., B. Humar et al. 2003. The role of the E-cadherin gene (CDH1) in diffuse gastric cancer susceptibility: From the laboratory to clinical practice. *Ann Oncol* 14(12): 1705–1713.

Guilford, P., J. Hopkins et al. 1998. E-cadherin germline mutations in familial gastric cancer. *Nature* 392(6674): 402–405.

Guilford, P., B. Humar et al. 2010. Hereditary diffuse gastric cancer: Translation of CDH1 germline mutations into clinical practice. *Gastric Cancer* 13(1): 1–10.

Guo, Y.T., Y.Q. Li et al. 2008. Diagnosis of gastric intestinal metaplasia with confocal laser endomicroscopy in vivo: A prospective study. *Endoscopy* 40(7): 547–553.

Gupta, N., A. Bansal et al. 2011. Endoscopy for upper GI cancer screening in the general population: A cost-utility analysis. *Gastrointest Endosc* 74(3): 610–624, e612.

Halldorsdottir, A.M., M. Sigurdardottrir et al. 2003. Spasmolytic polypeptide-expressing metaplasia (SPEM) associated with gastric cancer in Iceland. *Dig Dis Sci* 48(3): 431–441.

Hamashima, C., D. Shibuya et al. 2008. The Japanese guidelines for gastric cancer screening. *Jpn J Clin Oncol* 38(4): 259–267.

Han, H.S., S.Y. Lee et al. 2009. Unclassified mucin phenotype of gastric adenocarcinoma exhibits the highest invasiveness. *J Gastroenterol Hepatol* 24(4): 658–666.

Hansen, S., S.E. Vollset et al. 2007. Two distinct aetiologies of cardia cancer; Evidence from premorbid serological markers of gastric atrophy and *Helicobacter pylori* status. *Gut* 56(7): 918–925.

Hassan, C., A. Zullo et al. 2010. Cost-effectiveness of endoscopic surveillance for gastric intestinal metaplasia. *Helicobacter* 15(3): 221–226.

Hatakeyama, M. 2004. Oncogenic mechanisms of the *Helicobacter pylori* CagA protein. *Nat Rev Cancer* 4(9): 688–694.

Hattori, Y., H. Tashiro et al. 1995. Sensitivity and specificity of mass screening for gastric cancer using the measurement of serum pepsinogens. *Jpn J Cancer Res* 86(12): 1210–1215.

Helicobacter and Cancer Collaborative Group. 2001. Gastric cancer and *Helicobacter pylori*: A combined analysis of 12 case control studies nested within prospective cohorts. *Gut* 49(3): 347–353.

Higashi, H., R. Tsutsumi et al. 2002. SHP-2 tyrosine phosphatase as an intracellular target of *Helicobacter pylori* CagA protein. *Science* 295(5555): 683–686.

Higashi, H., K. Yokoyama et al. 2005. EPIYA motif is a membrane-targeting signal of *Helicobacter pylori* virulence factor CagA in mammalian cells. *J Biol Chem* 280(24): 23130–23137.

Hiraiwa, K., H. Takeuchi et al. 2008. Clinical significance of circulating tumor cells in blood from patients with gastrointestinal cancers. *Ann Surg Oncol* 15(11): 3092–3100.

Hishida, A., K. Matsuo et al. 2010. Genetic predisposition to *Helicobacter pylori*-induced gastric precancerous conditions. *World J Gastrointest Oncol* 2(10): 369.

Hoffmann, W. 2012. Stem cells, self-renewal and cancer of the gastric epithelium. *Curr Med Chem* 19: 5975–5983.

Honda, S., T. Fujioka et al. 1998. Development of *Helicobacter pylori*-induced gastric carcinoma in Mongolian gerbils. *Cancer Res* 58(19): 4255–4259.

Huang, F.Y., A.O. Chan et al. 2012. *Helicobacter pylori* induces promoter methylation of E-cadherin via interleukin-1beta activation of nitric oxide production in gastric cancer cells. *Cancer* 118(20): 4969–4980.

Huang, J.Q., S. Sridhar et al. 1998. Meta-analysis of the relationship between *Helicobacter pylori* seropositivity and gastric cancer. *Gastroenterology* 114(6): 1169–1179.

Huang, J.Q., G.F. Zheng et al. 2003. Meta-analysis of the relationship between cagA seropositivity and gastric cancer. *Gastroenterology* 125(6): 1636–1644.

Huntsman, D.G., F. Carneiro et al. 2001. Early gastric cancer in young, asymptomatic carriers of germ-line E-cadherin mutations. *N Engl J Med* 344(25): 1904–1909.

Hur, K., M.K. Kwak et al. 2006. Expression of gastrin and its receptor in human gastric cancer tissues. *J Cancer Res Clin Oncol* 132(2): 85–91.

IARC. 2011. *Monographs on the Evaluation of Carcinogenic Risks to Humans, Volume 100. A Review of Carcinogen—Part B: Biological Agents*. Lyon, France: International Agency for Research on Cancer.

IARC Working Group on the Evaluation of Carcinogenic Risks to Humans. 1994. Schistosomes, liver flukes and *Helicobacter pylori*. *IARC Monogr Eval Carcinog Risks Hum* 61: 1–241.

Ilhan, O., U. Han et al. 2010. Prognostic significance of MUC1, MUC2 and MUC5AC expressions in gastric carcinoma. *Turk J Gastroenterol* 21(4): 345–352.

Ishigami, S., S. Natsugoe et al. 2001. Clinical importance of preoperative carcinoembryonic antigen and carbohydrate antigen 19–9 levels in gastric cancer. *J Clin Gastroenterol* 32(1): 41–44.

Ito, H., H. Inoue et al. 2012. Prognostic impact of detecting viable circulating tumour cells in gastric cancer patients using a telomerase-specific viral agent: A prospective study. *BMC Cancer* 12(1): 346.

Ito, M., K. Haruma et al. 2002. Implication of anti-parietal cell antibody levels in gastrointestinal diseases, including gastric carcinogenesis. *Dig Dis Sci* 47(5): 1080–1085.

Ivanauskas, A., J. Hoffmann et al. 2008. Distinct TPEF/HPP1 gene methylation patterns in gastric cancer indicate a field effect in gastric carcinogenesis. *Dig Liver Dis* 40(12): 920–926.

Jang, S., K.R. Jones et al. 2010. Epidemiological link between gastric disease and polymorphisms in VacA and CagA. *J Clin Microbiol* 48(2): 559–567.

Janjigian, Y.Y., D. Werner et al. 2012. Prognosis of metastatic gastric and gastroesophageal junction cancer by HER2 status: A European and USA International collaborative analysis. *Ann Oncol* 23(10): 2656–2662.

Jemal, A., F. Bray et al. 2011. Global cancer statistics. *CA Cancer J Clin* 61(2): 69–90.

Jeon, S.R., W.Y. Cho et al. 2011. Optical biopsies by confocal endomicroscopy prevent additive endoscopic biopsies before endoscopic submucosal dissection in gastric epithelial neoplasias: A prospective, comparative study. *Gastrointest Endosc* 74(4): 772–780.

Ji, R., X.L. Zuo et al. 2011. Confocal endomicroscopy for in vivo prediction of completeness after endoscopic mucosal resection. *Surg Endosc* 25(6): 1933–1938.

Jia, Y., C. Persson et al. 2010. A comprehensive analysis of common genetic variation in MUC1, MUC5AC, MUC6 genes and risk of stomach cancer. *Cancer Causes Control* 21(2): 313–321.

Jones, K.R., S. Jang et al. 2011. Polymorphisms in the intermediate region of VacA impact *Helicobacter pylori*-induced disease development. *J Clin Microbiol* 49(1): 101–110.

Jorgensen, J.T. and M. Hersom 2012. HER2 as a prognostic marker in gastric cancer—A systematic analysis of data from the literature. *J Cancer* 3: 137–144.

Jung, S.W., K.S. Lim et al. 2011. Flexible spectral imaging color enhancement (FICE) is useful to discriminate among non-neoplastic lesion, adenoma, and cancer of stomach. *Dig Dis Sci* 56(10): 2879–2886.

Kaise, M., M. Kato et al. 2009. Magnifying endoscopy combined with narrow-band imaging for differential diagnosis of superficial depressed gastric lesions. *Endoscopy* 41(4): 310–315.

Kamada, T., J. Hata et al. 2005. Clinical features of gastric cancer discovered after successful eradication of *Helicobacter pylori*: Results from a 9-year prospective follow-up study in Japan. *Aliment Pharmacol Ther* 21(9): 1121–1126.

Kamangar, F., C. Cheng et al. 2006. Interleukin-1B polymorphisms and gastric cancer risk—A meta-analysis. *Cancer Epidemiol Biomark Prev* 15(10): 1920–1928.

Kang, H.M., N. Kim et al. 2008a. Effects of *Helicobacter pylori* infection on gastric mucin expression. *J Clin Gastroenterol* 42(1): 29–35.

Kang, J.M., N. Kim et al. 2008b. The role of serum pepsinogen and gastrin test for the detection of gastric cancer in Korea. *Helicobacter* 13(2): 146–156.

Kataoka, Y., H. Okabe et al. 2012. HER2 expression and its clinicopathological features in resectable gastric cancer. *Gastric Cancer* 16: 84–93.

Kato, M., M. Kaise et al. 2010. Magnifying endoscopy with narrow-band imaging achieves superior accuracy in the differential diagnosis of superficial gastric lesions identified with white-light endoscopy: A prospective study. *Gastrointest Endosc* 72(3): 523–529.

Kikuchi, S., M. Kato et al. 2006. Design and planned analyses of an ongoing randomized trial assessing the preventive effect of *Helicobacter pylori* eradication on occurrence of new gastric carcinomas after endoscopic resection. *Helicobacter* 11(3): 147–151.

Kim, H., J.W. Lim et al. 2001. *Helicobacter pylori*-induced expression of interleukin-8 and cyclooxygenase-2 in AGS gastric epithelial cells: Mediation by nuclear factor-kappaB. *Scand J Gastroenterol* 36(7): 706–716.

Kim, H.H., T.Y. Jeon et al. 2012. Differential expression of ghrelin mRNA according to anatomical portions of human stomach. *Hepatogastroenterology* 59(119): 2217–2221.

Kim, H.S., J.S. Lee et al. 2006. CDX-2 homeobox gene expression in human gastric carcinoma and precursor lesions. *J Gastroenterol Hepatol* 21(2): 438–442.

Kim, N. and H.C. Jung 2010. The role of serum pepsinogen in the detection of gastric cancer. *Gut Liver* 4(3): 307–319.

Kim, S.J., A. Masago et al. 2011. A novel approach using telomerase-specific replication-selective adenovirus for detection of circulating tumor cells in breast cancer patients. *Breast Cancer Res Treat* 128(3): 765–773.

Kitahara, F., K. Kobayashi et al. 1999. Accuracy of screening for gastric cancer using serum pepsinogen concentrations. *Gut* 44(5): 693–697.

Klaamas, K., O. Kurtenkov et al. 2007. Impact of *Helicobacter pylori* infection on the humoral immune response to MUC1 peptide in patients with chronic gastric diseases and gastric cancer. *Immunol Invest* 36(4): 371–386.

Kobara, H., H. Mori et al. 2012. Prediction of invasion depth for submucosal differentiated gastric cancer by magnifying endoscopy with narrow-band imaging. *Oncol Rep* 28(3): 841–847.

Kobayashi, M., M. Takeuchi et al. 2011. Mucin phenotype and narrow-band imaging with magnifying endoscopy for differentiated-type mucosal gastric cancer. *J Gastroenterol* 46(9): 1064–1070.

Kocer, B., A. Soran et al. 2004. Prognostic significance of mucin expression in gastric carcinoma. *Dig Dis Sci* 49(6): 954–964.

Kodera, Y., Y. Yamamura et al. 1996. The prognostic value of preoperative serum levels of CEA and CA19–9 in patients with gastric cancer. *Am J Gastroenterol* 91(1): 49–53.

Kolligs, F.T., G. Bommer et al. 2002. Wnt/beta-catenin/tcf signaling: A critical pathway in gastrointestinal tumorigenesis. *Digestion* 66(3): 131–144.

Konturek, P.C., S.J. Konturek et al. 1999. Role of gastrin in gastric cancerogenesis in *Helicobacter pylori* infected humans. *J Physiol Pharmacol* 50(5): 857–873.

Krebs, M.G., R. Sloane et al. 2011. Evaluation and prognostic significance of circulating tumor cells in patients with non-small-cell lung cancer. *J Clin Oncol* 29(12): 1556–1563.

Kudo, T., S. Kakizaki et al. 2011. Analysis of ABC (D) stratification for screening patients with gastric cancer. *World J Gastroenterol* 17(43): 4793–4798.

Kuipers, E.J. 1999. Review article: Exploring the link between *Helicobacter pylori* and gastric cancer. *Aliment Pharmacol Ther* 13(Suppl 1): 3–11.

Kupcinskas, L., T. Wex et al. 2010. Interleukin-1B and interleukin-1 receptor antagonist gene polymorphisms are not associated with premalignant gastric conditions: A combined haplotype analysis. *Eur J Gastroenterol Hepatol* 22(10): 1189–1195.

Kuzuhara, T., M. Suganuma et al. 2007. *Helicobacter pylori*-secreting protein Tipalpha is a potent inducer of chemokine gene expressions in stomach cancer cells. *J Cancer Res Clin Oncol* 133(5): 287–296.

Kwak, M.S., N. Kim et al. 2010. Predictive power of serum pepsinogen tests for the development of gastric cancer in comparison to the histologic risk index. *Dig Dis Sci* 55(8): 2275–2282.

Laurén, P. 1965. The two histological main types of gastric carcinoma: Diffuse and so-called intestinal-type carcinoma. An attempt at a histo-clinical classification. *Acta Pathol Microbiol Scand* 64: 31–49.

Lee, K.H., J.H. Lee et al. 2001. A prospective correlation of Lauren's histological classification of stomach cancer with clinicopathological findings including DNA flow cytometry. *Pathol Res Pract* 197(4): 223–229.

Lee, O.J., H.J. Kim et al. 2009. The prognostic significance of the mucin phenotype of gastric adenocarcinoma and its relationship with histologic classifications. *Oncol Rep* 21(2): 387–393.

Lee, Y.C., T.H. Chen et al. 2012. The benefit of mass eradication of *Helicobacter pylori* infection: A community-based study of gastric cancer prevention. *Gut* 62: 676–682.

Leja, M., E. Cine et al. 2012. Prevalence of *Helicobacter pylori* infection and atrophic gastritis in Latvia. *Eur J Gastroenterol Hepatol* 24(12): 1410–1417.

Leja, M., L. Kupcinskas et al. 2009. The validity of a biomarker method for indirect detection of gastric mucosal atrophy versus standard histopathology. *Dig Dis Sci* 54(11): 2377–2384.

Leja, M., L. Kupcinskas et al. 2011. Value of gastrin-17 in detecting antral atrophy. *Adv Med Sci* 56(2): 145–150.

Leung, W.K., M.S. Wu et al. 2008. Screening for gastric cancer in Asia: Current evidence and practice. *Lancet Oncol* 9(3): 279–287.

Li, W.B., X.L. Zuo et al. 2011. Diagnostic value of confocal laser endomicroscopy for gastric superficial cancerous lesions. *Gut* 60(3): 299–306.

Li, Z., T. Yu et al. 2010. Confocal laser endomicroscopy for in vivo diagnosis of gastric intraepithelial neoplasia: A feasibility study. *Gastrointest Endosc* 72(6): 1146–1153.

Lim, L.G., K.G. Yeoh et al. 2011. Experienced versus inexperienced confocal endoscopists in the diagnosis of gastric adenocarcinoma and intestinal metaplasia on confocal images. *Gastrointest Endosc* 73(6): 1141–1147.

Link, A., J. Kupcinskas et al. 2012. Macro-role of microRNA in gastric cancer. *Dig Dis* 30(3): 255–267.

Liotta, L.A., J. Kleinerman et al. 1974. Quantitative relationships of intravascular tumor cells, tumor vessels, and pulmonary metastases following tumor implantation. *Cancer Res* 34(5): 997–1004.

Lo, C.C., P.I. Hsu et al. 2005. Implications of anti-parietal cell antibodies and anti-*Helicobacter pylori* antibodies in histological gastritis and patient outcome. *World J Gastroenterol* 11(30): 4715–4720.

Lomba-Viana, R., M. Dinis-Ribeiro et al. 2012. Serum pepsinogen test for early detection of gastric cancer in a European country. *Eur J Gastroenterol Hepatol* 24(1): 37–41.

Lu, J., G. Getz et al. 2005. MicroRNA expression profiles classify human cancers. *Nature* 435(7043): 834–838.

Lu, X.X., J.L. Yu et al. 2012. Stepwise cumulation of RUNX3 methylation mediated by *Helicobacter pylori* infection contributes to gastric carcinoma progression. *Cancer* 118: 5507–5517.

Lynch, H.T., P. Kaurah et al. 2008. Hereditary diffuse gastric cancer: Diagnosis, genetic counseling, and prophylactic total gastrectomy. *Cancer* 112(12): 2655–2663.

Maher, D.M., B.K. Gupta et al. 2011. Mucin 13: Structure, function, and potential roles in cancer pathogenesis. *Mol Cancer Res* 9(5): 531–537.

Maki, S., K. Yao et al. 2012. Magnifying endoscopy with narrow-band imaging is useful in the differential diagnosis between low-grade adenoma and early cancer of superficial elevated gastric lesions. *Gastric Cancer* 16: 140–146.

Malfertheiner, P., F. Megraud et al. 2012. Management of *Helicobacter pylori* infection—The Maastricht IV/ Florence Consensus Report. *Gut* 61(5): 646–664.

Malfertheiner, P., P. Sipponen et al. 2005. *Helicobacter pylori* eradication has the potential to prevent gastric cancer: A state-of-the-art critique. *Am J Gastroenterol* 100(9): 2100–2115.

Manente, L., A. Perna et al. 2008. The *Helicobacter pylori*'s protein VacA has direct effects on the regulation of cell cycle and apoptosis in gastric epithelial cells. *J Cell Physiol* 214(3): 582–587.

Marin, F., C. Bonet et al. 2012. Genetic variation in MUC1, MUC2 and MUC6 genes and evolution of gastric cancer precursor lesions in a long-term follow-up in a high-risk area in Spain. *Carcinogenesis* 33(5): 1072–1080.

di Mario, F. and L.G. Cavallaro 2008. Non-invasive tests in gastric diseases. *Dig Liver Dis* 40(7): 523–530.

Marrelli, D., F. Roviello et al. 1999. Prognostic significance of CEA, CA 19–9 and CA 72–4 preoperative serum levels in gastric carcinoma. *Oncology* 57(1): 55–62.

de Martel, C., J. Ferlay et al. 2012. Global burden of cancers attributable to infections in 2008: A review and synthetic analysis. *Lancet Oncol* 13(6): 607–615.

Maruta, F., A. Sugiyama et al. 2000. Timing of N-methyl-N-nitrosourea administration affects gastric carcinogenesis in Mongolian gerbils infected with *Helicobacter pylori*. *Cancer Lett* 160(1): 99–105.

Mason, J., A.T. Axon et al. 2002. The cost-effectiveness of population *Helicobacter pylori* screening and treatment: A Markov model using economic data from a randomized controlled trial. *Aliment Pharmacol Ther* 16(3): 559–568.

Mejias-Luque, R., S.K. Linden et al. 2010. Inflammation modulates the expression of the intestinal mucins MUC2 and MUC4 in gastric tumors. *Oncogene* 29(12): 1753–1762.

Mesquita, P., A.J. Peixoto et al. 2003. Role of site-specific promoter hypomethylation in aberrant MUC2 mucin expression in mucinous gastric carcinomas. *Cancer Lett* 189(2): 129–136.

Miki, K. 2006. Gastric cancer screening using the serum pepsinogen test method. *Gastric Cancer* 9(4): 245–253.

Miki, K. 2011. Gastric cancer screening by combined assay for serum anti-*Helicobacter pylori* IgG antibody and serum pepsinogen levels–"ABC method". *Proc Jpn Acad Ser B Phys Biol Sci* 87(7): 405–414.

Miki, K. and M. Fujishiro. 2009. Cautious comparison between East and West is necessary in terms of the serum pepsinogen test. *Dig Endosc* 21(2): 134–135.

Miki, K., M. Fujishiro et al. 2009. Long-term results of gastric cancer screening using the serum pepsinogen test method among an asymptomatic middle-aged Japanese population. *Dig Endosc* 21(2): 78–81.

Miyamoto, K. and T. Ushijima. 2005. Diagnostic and therapeutic applications of epigenetics. *Jpn J Clin Oncol* 35(6): 293–301.

Mizuno, S., M. Kobayashi et al. 2009. Validation of the pepsinogen test method for gastric cancer screening using a follow-up study. *Gastric Cancer* 12(3): 158–163.

Mottershead, M., E. Karteris et al. 2007. Immunohistochemical and quantitative mRNA assessment of ghrelin expression in gastric and oesophageal adenocarcinoma. *J Clin Pathol* 60(4): 405–409.

Mueller, D., N. Tegtmeyer et al. 2012. c-Src and c-Abl kinases control hierarchic phosphorylation and function of the CagA effector protein in Western and East Asian *Helicobacter pylori* strains. *J Clin Invest* 122(4): 1553–1566.

Murphy, G., F. Kamangar et al. 2011. The relationship between serum ghrelin and the risk of gastric and esophagogastric junctional adenocarcinomas. *J Natl Cancer Inst* 103(14): 1123–1129.

Naito, M., T. Yamazaki et al. 2006. Influence of EPIYA-repeat polymorphism on the phosphorylation-dependent biological activity of *Helicobacter pylori* CagA. *Gastroenterology* 130(4): 1181–1190.

Nakamura, M., T. Shibata et al. 2010. The usefulness of magnifying endoscopy with narrow-band imaging to distinguish carcinoma in flat elevated lesions in the stomach diagnosed as adenoma by using biopsy samples. *Gastrointest Endosc* 71(6): 1070–1075.

Nakayama, M., J. Hisatsune et al. 2009. *Helicobacter pylori* VacA-induced inhibition of GSK3 through the PI3K/Akt signaling pathway. *J Biol Chem* 284(3): 1612–1619.

Nam, K.T., R.L. O'Neal et al. 2011. Spasmolytic polypeptide-expressing metaplasia (SPEM) in the gastric oxyntic mucosa does not arise from Lgr5-expressing cells. *Gut* 61: 1678–1685.

Nobili, S., L. Bruno et al. 2011. Genomic and genetic alterations influence the progression of gastric cancer. *World J Gastroenterol* 17(3): 290–299.

Nomura, S., T. Baxter et al. 2004. Spasmolytic polypeptide expressing metaplasia to preneoplasia in *H. felis*-infected mice. *Gastroenterology* 127(2): 582–594.

Nozaki, K., M. Ogawa et al. 2008. A molecular signature of gastric metaplasia arising in response to acute parietal cell loss. *Gastroenterology* 134(2): 511–522.

Odenbreit, S., J. Puls et al. 2000. Translocation of *Helicobacter pylori* CagA into gastric epithelial cells by type IV secretion. *Science* 287(5457): 1497–1500.

Okubo, M., T. Tahara et al. 2010. Association between common genetic variants in pre-microRNAs and gastric cancer risk in Japanese population. *Helicobacter* 15(6): 524–531.

Osawa, H., H. Yamamoto et al. 2012a. Diagnosis of depressed-type early gastric cancer using small-caliber endoscopy with flexible spectral imaging color enhancement. *Dig Endosc* 24(4): 231–236.

Osawa, H., H. Yamamoto et al. 2012b. Diagnosis of extent of early gastric cancer using flexible spectral imaging color enhancement. *World J Gastrointest Endosc* 4(8): 356–361.

Oshima, H. and M. Oshima 2010. Mouse models of gastric tumors: Wnt activation and PGE2 induction. *Pathol Int* 60(9): 599–607.

Oz Puyan, F., N. Can et al. 2011. The relationship among PDX1, CDX2, and mucin profiles in gastric carcinomas; correlations with clinicopathologic parameters. *J Cancer Res Clin Oncol* 137(12): 1749–1762.

Pagni, F., S. Zannella et al. 2012. HER2 status of gastric carcinoma and corresponding lymph node metastasis. *Pathol Oncol Res* 19: 103–109.

Park, J.G., H.K. Yang et al. 2000. Report on the first meeting of the International Collaborative Group on Hereditary Gastric Cancer. *J Natl Cancer Inst* 92(21): 1781–1782.

Parkin, D.M. 2006. The global health burden of infection-associated cancers in the year 2002. *Int J Cancer* 118(12): 3030–3044.

Parkin, D.M., F. Bray et al. 2005. Global cancer statistics, 2002. *CA Cancer J Clin* 55: 74–108.

Parsonnet, J., G.D. Friedman et al. 1997. Risk for gastric cancer in people with CagA positive or CagA negative *Helicobacter pylori* infection. *Gut* 40(3): 297–301.

Parsonnet, J., R.A. Harris et al. 1996. Modelling cost-effectiveness of *Helicobacter pylori* screening to prevent gastric cancer: A mandate for clinical trials. *Lancet* 348(9021): 150–154.

Pavicic, W., E. Perkio et al. 2011. Altered methylation at microRNA-associated CpG islands in hereditary and sporadic carcinomas: A methylation-specific multiplex ligation-dependent probe amplification (MS-MLPA)-based approach. *Mol Med* 17(7–8): 726–735.

Peek, R.M., Jr. and M.J. Blaser. 2002. *Helicobacter pylori* and gastrointestinal tract adenocarcinomas. *Nat Rev Cancer* 2(1): 28–37.

Peitz, U. and P. Malfertheiner. 2002. Chromoendoscopy: From a research tool to clinical progress. *Dig Dis* 20(2): 111–119.

Peleteiro, B., N. Lunet et al. 2010. Association between cytokine gene polymorphisms and gastric precancerous lesions: Systematic review and meta-analysis. *Cancer Epidemiol Biomark Prev* 19(3): 762–776.

Pharoah, P.D., P. Guilford et al. 2001. Incidence of gastric cancer and breast cancer in CDH1 (E-cadherin) mutation carriers from hereditary diffuse gastric cancer families. *Gastroenterology* 121(6): 1348–1353.

Pimentel-Nunes, P., M. Dinis-Ribeiro et al. 2012. A multicenter validation of an endoscopic classification with narrow band imaging for gastric precancerous and cancerous lesions. *Endoscopy* 44(3): 236–246.

Pirrelli, M., M.L. Caruso et al. 2012. Are biopsy specimens predictive of HER2 status in gastric cancer patients? *Dig Dis Sci* 58: 397–404.

Preuss, K.D., C. Zwick et al. 2002. Analysis of the B-cell repertoire against antigens expressed by human neoplasms. *Immunol Rev* 188: 43–50.

Price, A.B. and J.J. Misiewicz. 1991. Sydney classification for gastritis. *Lancet* 337(8734): 174.

Prinz, C., N. Hafsi et al. 2003. *Helicobacter pylori* virulence factors and the host immune response: Implications for therapeutic vaccination. *Trends Microbiol* 11(3): 134–138.

Quiroga, A.J., A. Huertas et al. 2010. Variation in the number of EPIYA-C repeats in CagA protein from Colombian *Helicobacter pylori* strains and its ability middle to induce hummingbird phenotype in gastric epithelial cells. *Biomedica* 30(2): 251–258.

Rad, R., M. Gerhard et al. 2002. The *Helicobacter pylori* blood group antigen-binding adhesin facilitates bacterial colonization and augments a nonspecific immune response. *J Immunol* 168(6): 3033–3041.

Rau, T.T., A. Rogler et al. 2012. Methylation-dependent activation of CDX1 through NF-kappaB: A link from inflammation to intestinal metaplasia in the human stomach. *Am J Pathol* 181(2): 487–498.

Retterspitz, M.F., S.P. Monig et al. 2010. Expression of {beta}-catenin, MUC1 and c-met in diffuse-type gastric carcinomas: Correlations with tumour progression and prognosis. *Anticancer Res* 30(11): 4635–4641.

Rugge, M., M. de Boni et al. 2010. Gastritis OLGA-staging and gastric cancer risk: A twelve-year clinico-pathological follow-up study. *Aliment Pharmacol Ther* 31(10): 1104–1111.

Rugge, M. and R.M. Genta 2005. Staging and grading of chronic gastritis. *Hum Pathol* 36(3): 228–233.

Rupnow, M.F., A.H. Chang et al. 2009. Cost-effectiveness of a potential prophylactic *Helicobacter pylori* vaccine in the United States. *J Infect Dis* 200(8): 1311–1317.

Rupnow, M.F., R.D. Shachter et al. 2001. Quantifying the population impact of a prophylactic *Helicobacter pylori* vaccine. *Vaccine* 20(5–6): 879–885.

Saadat, I., H. Higashi et al. 2007. *Helicobacter pylori* CagA targets PAR1/MARK kinase to disrupt epithelial cell polarity. *Nature* 447(7142): 330–333.

Saeki, N., A. Saito et al. 2011. A functional single nucleotide polymorphism in mucin 1, at chromosome 1q22, determines susceptibility to diffuse-type gastric cancer. *Gastroenterology* 140(3): 892–902.

Schmassmann, A., M.G. Oldendorf et al. 2009. Changing incidence of gastric and oesophageal cancer subtypes in central Switzerland between 1982 and 2007. *Eur J Epidemiol* 24(10): 603–609.

Schmidt, N., U. Peitz et al. 2005. Missing gastric cancer in dyspepsia. *Aliment Pharmacol Ther* 21(7): 813–820.

Semb, H. and G. Christofori. 1998. The tumor-suppressor function of E-cadherin. *Am J Hum Genet* 63(6): 1588–1593.

Shigematsu, Y., T. Niwa et al. 2012. Identification of a DNA methylation marker that detects the presence of lymph node metastases of gastric cancers. *Oncol Lett* 4(2): 268–274.

Shimamura, T., H. Ito et al. 2005. Overexpression of MUC13 is associated with intestinal-type gastric cancer. *Cancer Sci* 96(5): 265–273.

Shimizu, N., K. Inada et al. 1999. *Helicobacter pylori* infection enhances glandular stomach carcinogenesis in Mongolian gerbils treated with chemical carcinogens. *Carcinogenesis* 20(4): 669–676.

Shimoyama, T., M. Aoki et al. 2012. ABC screening for gastric cancer is not applicable in a Japanese population with high prevalence of atrophic gastritis. *Gastric Cancer* 15(3): 331–334.

Shiroiwa, T., T. Fukuda et al. 2011. Cost-effectiveness analysis of trastuzumab to treat HER2-positive advanced gastric cancer based on the randomised ToGA trial. *Br J Cancer* 105(9): 1273–1278.

Shiroshita, H., H. Watanabe et al. 2004. Re-evaluation of mucin phenotypes of gastric minute well-differentiated-type adenocarcinomas using a series of HGM, MUC5AC, MUC6, M-GGMC, MUC2 and CD10 stains. *Pathol Int* 54(5): 311–321.

Shitara, K., Y. Yatabe et al. 2012. Prognosis of patients with advanced gastric cancer by HER2 status and trastuzumab treatment. *Gastric Cancer* 16: 261–267.

Sipponen, P., M. Harkonen et al. 2003. Diagnosis of atrophic gastritis from a serum sample. *Minerva Gastroenterol Dietol* 49(1): 11–21.

Sipponen, P., M. Kekki et al. 1991. The Sydney System: Epidemiology and natural history of chronic gastritis. *J Gastroenterol Hepatol* 6(3): 244–251.

Sipponen, P., P. Ranta et al. 2002. Serum levels of amidated gastrin-17 and pepsinogen I in atrophic gastritis: An observational case-control study. *Scand J Gastroenterol* 37(7): 785–791.

Skoog, E.C., A. Sjoling et al. 2012. Human gastric mucins differently regulate *Helicobacter pylori* proliferation, gene expression and interactions with host cells. *PLoS One* 7(5): e36378.

Sonnenberg, A. and J.M. Inadomi. 1998. Review article: Medical decision models of *Helicobacter pylori* therapy to prevent gastric cancer. *Aliment Pharmacol Ther* 12(Suppl 1): 111–121.

Stein, M., F. Bagnoli et al. 2002. c-Src/Lyn kinases activate *Helicobacter pylori* CagA through tyrosine phosphorylation of the EPIYA motifs. *Mol Microbiol* 43(4): 971–980.

Sugiu, K., T. Kamada et al. 2006. Anti-parietal cell antibody and serum pepsinogen assessment in screening for gastric carcinoma. *Dig Liver Dis* 38(5): 303–307.

Sun, M., H. Uozaki et al. 2012. SOX9 expression and its methylation status in gastric cancer. *Virchows Arch* 460(3): 271–279.

Suriano, G., S. Yew et al. 2005. Characterization of a recurrent germ line mutation of the E-cadherin gene: Implications for genetic testing and clinical management. *Clin Cancer Res* 11(15): 5401–5409.

Suzuki, H., E. Yamamoto et al. 2010. Methylation-associated silencing of microRNA-34b/c in gastric cancer and its involvement in an epigenetic field defect. *Carcinogenesis* 31(12): 2066–2073.

Tachibana, M., Y. Takemoto et al. 1998. Serum carcinoembryonic antigen as a prognostic factor in resectable gastric cancer. *J Am Coll Surg* 187(1): 64–68.

Tajima, Y., K. Yamazaki et al. 2006. Gastric and intestinal phenotypic marker expression in early differentiated-type tumors of the stomach: Clinicopathologic significance and genetic background. *Clin Cancer Res* 12(21): 6469–6479.

Take, S., M. Mizuno et al. 2007. Baseline gastric mucosal atrophy is a risk factor associated with the development of gastric cancer after *Helicobacter pylori* eradication therapy in patients with peptic ulcer diseases. *J Gastroenterol* 42(Suppl 17): 21–27.

Takiguchi, S., S. Adachi et al. 2012. Mapping analysis of ghrelin producing cells in the human stomach associated with chronic gastritis and early cancers. *Dig Dis Sci* 57(5): 1238–1246.

Tanaka-Shintani, M. and M. Watanabe. 2005. Distribution of ghrelin-immunoreactive cells in human gastric mucosa: Comparison with that of parietal cells. *J Gastroenterol* 40(4): 345–349.

Tashiro, A., M. Sano et al. 2006. Comparing mass screening techniques for gastric cancer in Japan. *World J Gastroenterol* 12(30): 4873–4874.

Tocchi, A., G. Costa et al. 1998. The role of serum and gastric juice levels of carcinoembryonic antigen, CA19.9 and CA72.4 in patients with gastric cancer. *J Cancer Res Clin Oncol* 124(8): 450–455.

Tsuji, Y., K. Ohata et al. 2012. Magnifying endoscopy with narrow-band imaging helps determine the management of gastric adenomas. *Gastric Cancer* 15(4): 414–418.

Tsukamoto, T., K. Inada et al. 2004. Down-regulation of a gastric transcription factor, Sox2, and ectopic expression of intestinal homeobox genes, Cdx1 and Cdx2: Inverse correlation during progression from gastric/intestinal-mixed to complete intestinal metaplasia. *J Cancer Res Clin Oncol* 130(3): 135–145.

Tsutsumi, R., H. Higashi et al. 2003. Attenuation of *Helicobacter pylori* CagA x SHP-2 signaling by interaction between CagA and C-terminal Src kinase. *J Biol Chem* 278(6): 3664–3670.

Tureci, O., U. Sahin et al. 1997. Serological analysis of human tumor antigens: Molecular definition and implications. *Mol Med Today* 3(8): 342–349.

Ucar, E., E. Semerci et al. 2008. Prognostic value of preoperative CEA, CA 19–9, CA 72–4, and AFP levels in gastric cancer. *Adv Ther* 25(10): 1075–1084.

Uchida, T., L.T. Nguyen et al. 2009. Analysis of virulence factors of *Helicobacter pylori* isolated from a Vietnamese population. *BMC Microbiol* 9: 175.

Ueda, T., S. Volinia et al. 2010. Relation between microRNA expression and progression and prognosis of gastric cancer: A microRNA expression analysis. *Lancet Oncol* 11(2): 136–146.

Uedo, N., M. Fujishiro et al. 2011. Role of narrow band imaging for diagnosis of early-stage esophagogastric cancer: Current consensus of experienced endoscopists in Asia-Pacific region. *Dig Endosc* 23(Suppl 1): 58–71.

Uemura, N., S. Okamoto et al. 2001. *Helicobacter pylori* infection and the development of gastric cancer. *N Engl J Med* 345(11): 784–789.

Vaananen, H., M. Vauhkonen et al. 2003. Non-endoscopic diagnosis of atrophic gastritis with a blood test. Correlation between gastric histology and serum levels of gastrin-17 and pepsinogen I: A multicentre study. *Eur J Gastroenterol Hepatol* 15(8): 885–891.

Volinia, S., G.A. Calin et al. 2006. A microRNA expression signature of human solid tumors defines cancer gene targets. *Proc Natl Acad Sci USA* 103(7): 2257–2261.

Wakatsuki, K., Y. Yamada et al. 2008. Clinicopathological and prognostic significance of mucin phenotype in gastric cancer. *J Surg Oncol* 98(2): 124–129.

Wang, R.Q. and D.C. Fang. 2006. Effects of *Helicobacter pylori* infection on mucin expression in gastric carcinoma and pericancerous tissues. *J Gastroenterol Hepatol* 21(2): 425–431.

Wang, T.C., C.A. Dangler et al. 2000. Synergistic interaction between hypergastrinemia and *Helicobacter* infection in a mouse model of gastric cancer. *Gastroenterology* 118(1): 36–47.

Watabe, H., T. Mitsushima et al. 2005. Predicting the development of gastric cancer from combining *Helicobacter pylori* antibodies and serum pepsinogen status: A prospective endoscopic cohort study. *Gut* 54(6): 764–768.

Watanabe, T., M. Tada et al. 1998. *Helicobacter pylori* infection induces gastric cancer in Mongolian gerbils. *Gastroenterology* 115(3): 642–648.

Watson, S.A., A.M. Grabowska et al. 2006. Gastrin—Active participant or bystander in gastric carcinogenesis? *Nat Rev Cancer* 6(12): 936–946.

Wightman, B., I. Ha et al. 1993. Posttranscriptional regulation of the heterochronic gene lin-14 by lin-4 mediates temporal pattern formation in C. elegans. *Cell* 75(5): 855–862.

Wong, B.C., S.K. Lam et al. 2004. *Helicobacter pylori* eradication to prevent gastric cancer in a high-risk region of China: A randomized controlled trial. *JAMA* 291(2): 187–194.

Wroblewski, L.E., R.M. Peek, Jr. et al. 2010. *Helicobacter pylori* and gastric cancer: Factors that modulate disease risk. *Clin Microbiol Rev* 23(4): 713–739.

Xia, Y., Y. Yamaoka et al. 2009. A comprehensive sequence and disease correlation analyses for the C-terminal region of CagA protein of *Helicobacter pylori*. *PLoS One* 4(11): e7736.

Xie, F., N. Luo et al. 2008. Cost-effectiveness analysis of *Helicobacter pylori* screening in prevention of gastric cancer in Chinese. *Int J Technol Assess Health Care* 24(1): 87–95.

Xu, Z.-Q., Y. Broza et al. 2013. A nanomaterial-based breath test for distinguishing gastric cancer from benign gastric conditions. *Br J Cancer* 108: 941–950.

Xue, L., X. Zhang et al. 2011. Differences of immunophenotypic markers and signaling molecules between adenocarcinomas of gastric cardia and distal stomach. *Hum Pathol* 42(4): 594–601.

Yamaguchi, H., J.R. Goldenring et al. 2002. Identification of spasmolytic polypeptide expressing metaplasia (SPEM) in remnant gastric cancer and surveillance postgastrectomy biopsies. *Dig Dis Sci* 47(3): 573–578.

Yamamoto, K., M. Kato et al. 2011. Clinicopathological analysis of early-stage gastric cancers detected after successful eradication of *Helicobacter pylori*. *Helicobacter* 16(3): 210–216.

Yan, B., E.X. Yau et al. 2010. A study of HER2 gene amplification and protein expression in gastric cancer. *J Clin Pathol* 63(9): 839–842.

Yanaoka, K., M. Oka et al. 2008. Cancer high-risk subjects identified by serum pepsinogen tests: Outcomes after 10-year follow-up in asymptomatic middle-aged males. *Cancer Epidemiol Biomark Prev* 17(4): 838–845.

Yeh, J.M., C. Hur et al. 2010. Cost-effectiveness of treatment and endoscopic surveillance of precancerous lesions to prevent gastric cancer. *Cancer* 116(12): 2941–2953.

Yeh, J.M., K.M. Kuntz et al. 2009. Exploring the cost-effectiveness of *Helicobacter pylori* screening to prevent gastric cancer in China in anticipation of clinical trial results. *Int J Cancer* 124(1): 157–166.

Yokoyama, A., H. Inoue et al. 2010. Novel narrow-band imaging magnifying endoscopic classification for early gastric cancer. *Dig Liver Dis* 42(10): 704–708.

Zayakin, P., G. Ancans et al. 2013. Tumor-associated autoantibody signature for the early detection of gastric cancer. *Int J Cancer* 132(1): 137–147.

Zeng, Y., Q.M. Sun et al. 2010. Correlation between pre-miR-146a C/G polymorphism and gastric cancer risk in Chinese population. *World J Gastroenterol* 16(28): 3578–3583.

Zhang, C., S. Xu et al. 2012. Risk assessment of gastric cancer caused by *Helicobacter pylori* using CagA sequence markers. *PLoS One* 7(5): e36844.

Zhang, J., S.B. Guo et al. 2011. Application of magnifying narrow-band imaging endoscopy for diagnosis of early gastric cancer and precancerous lesion. *BMC Gastroenterol* 11: 135.

Zhang, J.N., Y.Q. Li et al. 2008. Classification of gastric pit patterns by confocal endomicroscopy. *Gastrointest Endosc* 67(6): 843–853.

Zub-Pokrowiecka, A., K. Rembiasz et al. 2010. Ghrelin in diseases of the gastric mucosa associated with *Helicobacter pylori* infection. *Med Sci Monit* 16(10): CR493–CR500.

14

Biomarkers in Esophageal Adenocarcinoma

Simon J.W. Monkhouse, J. Muhlschlegel, and H. Barr

CONTENTS

ABSTRACT Esophageal carcinoma is the ninth most common cancer with a global incidence of 461,000 cases and a lifetime risk of 2%–5%. It is associated with high rates of morbidity and mortality due to late symptomatic presentation and hence diagnosis of the disease. The overall poor survival from this disease means that there is a requirement for early, presymptomatic detection so that treatment can be with curative intent.

Barrett's esophagus (BE), a term used to describe the change in the lower esophageal lining from squamous- to intestinal-type columnar epithelium, is considered to be the main precursor for adenocarcinoma. Although poorly defined, genetic mutations, which over years cause genetic instability, are thought to accumulate within the BE segment and cause transformation from metaplasia through dysplasia to invasive cancer.

Detection and treatment of presymptomatic and pre-invasive disease dramatically improves outcomes. Currently surveillance programs rely on endoscopic biopsies that are costly, invasive, and associated with sampling error. High-grade dysplasia (HGD) is both patchy and macroscopically identical to non dysplastic mucosa. Multiple biopsies have to be taken and may still miss the dysplastic areas, while intrapathologist interpretation of results is highly variable with only 48% concordance demonstrated in studies.

Significant research has been performed to develop biological molecular imaging tools (biomarkers) that could identify those patients at higher risk of neoplastic progression and hence would benefit from further monitoring and/or intervention. The idea is that biomarker detection would replace costly, redundant screening and surveillance programs.

There are many candidate biomarkers including tumor suppressor genes and genes that influence the cell cycle. The targets and the current research will be explored in this chapter.

This is an area of exciting, progressive research. The development of techniques to allow ex vivo cellular analysis in a minimally invasive fashion is rapidly advancing and surely we are not far off developing a rigorous set of easily detectable biomarkers that can identify those at most risk from this devastating condition.

KEY WORDS: *esophageal, adenocarcinoma, Barrett's, epigenetic, biomarkers, dysplasia.*

14.1 Introduction

14.1.1 Importance of Disease, Epidemiology, Disease Progression, and Treatment Strategies

Rates of adenocarcinoma of the esophagogastric junction are increasing annually in the Western world. The peak age of diagnosis is between 50 and 60 years, and males are more susceptible than females with ratios reported in the literature of anywhere between 12:1 and 2:1 in favor of male predominance (Allum et al. 2012).

Symptoms vary but usually involve a degree of dysphagia and weight loss. Often patients are asymptomatic and disease is picked up on a routine scan or endoscopy. The unfortunate feature of most of the patients that present with symptoms is that the disease is frequently at an advanced stage, which means the treatment with curative intent is often futile.

The current hypothesis is that etiology is mainly due to gastroesophageal reflux disease (GERD). Chronic reflux results in the squamous cellular lining of the lower esophagus being exposed to acid. This results in a change of morphology into cells more in keeping with the intestinal tract, which is columnar in nature. Such changes are referred to as metaplasia, and the resulting altered esophageal lining is often referred to as Barrett's esophagus (BE)—see Figure 14.1a continued acid exposure may result in these cells entering the stepwise progression to cancerous cells (Figure 14.1b), a process known as the metaplasia–dysplasia–adenocarcinoma sequence.

This is a similar process to the development of colon cancer—that of acquisition of genetic and epigenetic mutations, which in combination result in genomic instability and ultimately autonomous clonal proliferation of tumor cells.

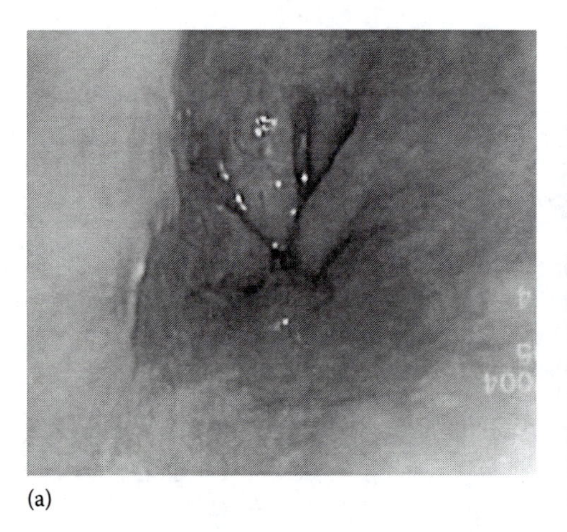

(a)

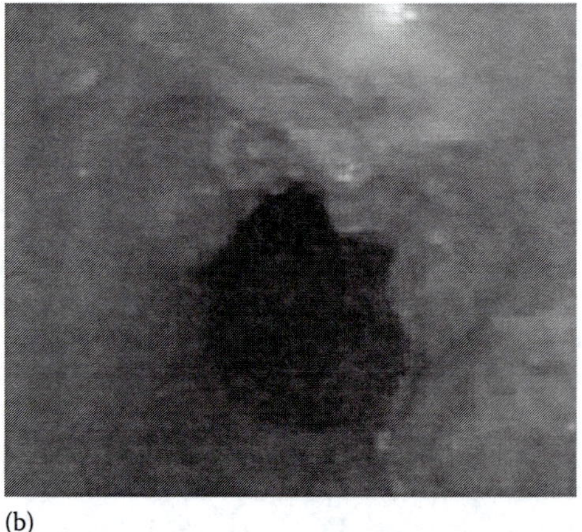

(b)

FIGURE 14.1 (a) BE—Considered to be a potential precursor to esophageal cancer. (Permission granted by free license to reproduce.) (b) Esophageal cancer that can develop in Barrett's segment—treatment options are limited in advanced disease. (Courtesy of Professor Barr.)

Dysplasia is defined as an "unequivocal neoplastic alteration of epithelium which has the potential to progress to invasive malignancy but remains confined within the basement membrane of the epithelium in which it arose" (Barr and Shepherd 2005). It is further categorized into indefinite, low grade, or high grade. Dysplasia develops in 5% of patients with BE (Heading and Attwood 2005). In those with low-grade dysplasia (LGD), 10%–50% may progress to high-grade dysplasia (HGD) and adenocarcinoma over 2–5 years (Heading and Attwood 2005). In the presence of HGD on an endoscopic biopsy, up to 50% will already have a focus of invasive adenocarcinoma in their esophagus—thus, the detection of HGD should prompt a full set of staging investigations and progression to treatment with curative intent. This may be endoscopic mucosal resection, radiofrequency ablation, or indeed formal esophagectomy. The treatment and management of such patients is beyond the scope of this chapter but it highlights that if HGD is detected, treatment needs to be offered.

How can we make detection of dysplasia in BE more accurate? Identifying "biomarkers" within the cells lining the esophagus or indeed in blood may be the answer to more accurate, early diagnosis. They would also be able to identify those at risk allowing for more intensive surveillance strategies.

The ideal biomarker would be sensitive, specific, reproducible, cheap, and acceptable to the patient. The available biomarkers and the future potential biomarkers will now be explored.

14.2 Dysplasia Biomarkers

14.2.1 Dysplasia and Difficulties with Interpretation

Currently, surveillance programs rely on endoscopic biopsies and histological assessment of dysplasia for high-risk screening (Figure 14.2). In patients with BE, these are performed on a periodic basis to assess the risk of progression to adenocarcinoma. The risk of progression to adenocarcinoma rises in a stepwise manner according to the degree of dysplasia (5.98, 16.98, and 65.8 per 1000 patients/year compared to patients with no dysplasia, LGD, and HGD, respectively) (Wani et al. 2009).

Detection and treatment of presymptomatic and preinvasive disease dramatically improves outcomes. Several retrospective studies found that more patients diagnosed with esophageal adenocarcinoma (EAC) on a surveillance program were detected at earlier stages, prior to lymph node involvement, compared with those who were newly diagnosed, and this was associated with improved survival (Fergusen and Durkin 2002; Van Sandick et al. 1998; Wong et al. 2010). Moreover, early tumors without regional or distal metastasis can be treated effectively with endoscopic ablation avoiding the need for surgery. A recent review article however noted that "most of these studies had small sample sizes some had short follow-up intervals and none were randomized control trials" (Reid et al. 2010). Despite all this evidence, there are equally a number of problems that exist fundamentally with this current method of diagnosis.

Primarily, there still appears to be doubt as to the accuracy of degree of dysplasia in determining risk stratification. Varying degrees of correlation between dysplasia and progression to adenocarcinoma have been demonstrated at different research centers, perhaps relating to selection criteria. LGD has a low rate of progression to EAC and a reproducibility that is variable and frequently is not detected in subsequent

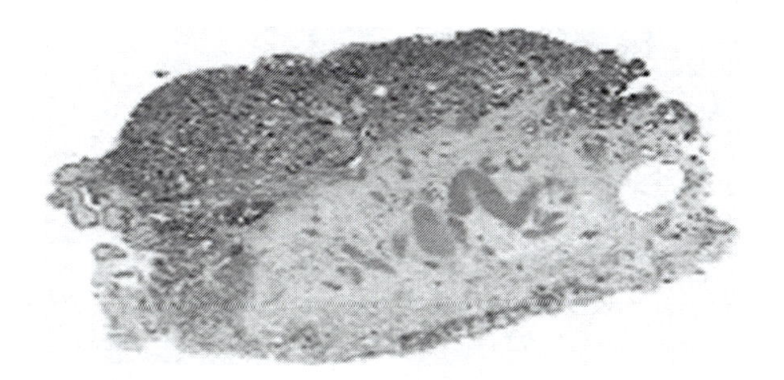

FIGURE 14.2 A histological sample of Barrett's stained showing HGD. (Courtesy of Professor Barr.)

endoscopies (Reid et al. 2000, 2010). The vast majority of patients diagnosed with BE who undergo surveillance programs with endoscopy do not progress to adenocarcinoma, and it has been quoted that 95% die of unrelated causes (Reid et al. 2000). This represents a huge burden on healthcare resources and a small proportion of these people undergoing the potentially unnecessary invasive test will suffer adverse consequences such as perforation and bleeding (Reid et al. 2010).

Using a system of surveillance with endoscopic biopsy, only 1%–2% of early carcinomas and 15% of precancerous lesions in asymptomatic populations are detected. In particular, recent research suggests that there is no evidence that endoscopic investigation for GERD improves detection of BE prior to adenocarcinoma diagnosis. It has been reported that 80% of patients who develop adenocarcinoma have no prior diagnosis of GERD (Cooper et al. 2009), and 48% of those who develop adenocarcinoma report either no or an infrequent history of symptoms associated with GERD (Lagergren et al. 1999). In light of this growing evidence, the American College of Gastroenterology Guidelines withdrew recommendations for endoscopic screening of patients for reflux disease alone (Wang and Sampliner 2008) and recommended a more individualized approach to decisions on who underwent screening.

Dysplasia classification is subjective, and there is significant variability between intrapathologist interpretation of results, with only 48% concordance demonstrated in studies (Reid et al. 2000). It is therefore common practice to seek second opinions on slides with suspected dysplasia, increasing costs and patient anxiety. Indeed it is now recommended in the UK guidelines that dysplasia specimens are dual reported by expert gastrointestinal histopathologists. This is confounded by the fact that HGD is both patchy and macroscopically identical to non-dysplastic mucosa. Large numbers of samples are required to reduce sampling error. Despite the recommendation that systematic four quadrant biopsies should be taken every 1–2 cm in the BE segment, some lesions are still missed.

In addition, a diagnosis of dysplasia does not lead to a low-cost, non invasive intervention to prevent the progression to adenocarcinoma. Esophagectomy is no longer the preferred option for a diagnosis of HGD, due to its high levels of morbidity and mortality. For those patients who present with resectable esophageal cancer, it offers only a limited (25%–35%) chance of cure and is associated with a considerable risk of serious complications (Wu and Poser 2003). Medicare database has quoted the rates of mortality associated with esophagectomy at 8%–23% (Birkmeyer et al. 2002). Ablation therapy for a subset of high-risk patients has been suggested although this has not proved to cause a reduction in mortality in randomized control trials. With the risk of progression from HGD being estimated anywhere from 16% to as high as 59% (Reid et al. 2000, Schnell et al. 2001) and with some of those diagnosed with HGD already harboring invasive adenocarcinoma, it seems that endoscopic or surgical treatment may be unnecessary for some and already too late for others.

Ultimately, recent research suggests that treatment for these surrogate endpoints for EAC (e.g., LGD or HGD) may not be associated with a decreased incidence of adenocarcinoma or a reduction in mortality (Overholt et al. 2007). As such, current research is aiming to develop a primary care risk model, to be used in conjunction with current systems, to better stratify patients into high and low risk for progression to EAC. Consequently, finding a biomarker that is both sensitive and specific will enable the development of programs of prevention and early detection that will hopefully have improved outcomes in terms of adenocarcinoma incidence and mortality.

14.3 Biomarkers under Investigation

Of the many biomarkers that have been suggested, a large body of evidence has been accumulated over the last 20 years implicating chromosomal instability in progression from BE to adenocarcinoma. This was first reported in the 1980s, when a higher proportion of aneuploidy cells in patients with adenocarcinoma was demonstrated using flow cytometry to assess DNA content (Reid et al. 1987). Since then, this evidence has been supported by investigations by a large number of laboratories using various different methods. The number of potential biomarkers has dramatically increased as a result of genomic and proteomic studies that now have been performed using large scale datasets. Loss of heterozygosity (LOH) analysis, FISH, CGH, and single-nucleotide polymorphism (SNP) assays have all been used to accumulate evidence for this process. However, with the ever increasing number of mutations being found, it seems unlikely that one sole event is responsible for the development of adenocarcinoma. The more likely scenario is that many mutations affecting multiple steps in multiple biological pathways are responsible for the pathogenesis. This makes the challenge to find a biomarker capable of detection and risk stratification in this process ever more difficult.

14.3.1 DNA-Ploidy Biomarkers

DNA content abnormalities (aneuploidy and tetraploidy) are perhaps some of the most extensively studied changes in the progression from BE to adenocarcinoma. Aneuploidy is the name given when a cell no longer contains a normal number of chromosomes. In a normal cell there are 46 chromosomes, known as 2N. When this doubles, 4N, it is referred to as tetraploidy.

Numerous studies have correlated aneuploidy and tetraploidy with the progression of BE to EAC.

Reid et al.'s cohort study using DNA flow cytometry in 2000 offers perhaps the most convincing evidence that tetraploidy (classified as a 4N fraction of greater than 6%) and aneuploidy are highly predictive of progression to adenocarcinoma. Their evidence showed that 65% of patients with HGD on biopsy had either aneuploidy, increased level of tetraploidy, or both. In comparison neither aneuploidy nor tetraploidy was present in 92% of patients who were either negative for dysplasia or had only LGD on biopsy. Zero percent of the patients who were both negative for chromosomal abnormalities and only had LGD apparent on biopsy progressed on to adenocarcinoma. Those patients with LGD who demonstrated a chromosomal content abnormality possessed a relative risk of 19 for progression to adenocarcinoma in comparison with those who had normal chromosomal content. They demonstrated that the 5-year cumulative incidence of adenocarcinoma in patients who had normal flow cytometry results at baseline was only 5% in comparison with 62% for those with tetraploidy and 41% with aneuploidy. This represented a relative risk of 7.5 (95% CI 4–14) for those with a 4N fraction of >6% and 5 (95% CT 2.7–9.4) for those with aneuploidy compared to neither.

Further studies on the same population looked at different levels of aneuploidy to determine whether this affected rate of progression (Rabinovitch et al. 2001). Aneuploidy of greater than 2.7N had higher rates of progression, with 75% of patients with tetraploidy and aneuploidy of 2.7N or above developing EAC, compared with 5.2% of those with neither abnormality.

14.3.2 p16

The p16 gene (found on chromosome 9p) and p53 gene (chromosome 17p), are important commonly studied tumor suppressor genes. Abnormalities of these genes, and on the pathways in which they act, are strongly associated with the development of human cancer based upon evidence from numerous studies.

p16 mutations are among the earliest and most common mutations seen in the pathogenesis of adenocarcinoma (Wong et al. 2001). Ninety percent of patients with BE have been shown to possess a p16 lesion. Despite this, no strong evidence has yet demonstrated an association between p16 silencing and grade of dysplasia and is therefore unlikely to be beneficial as a biomarker if used in isolation.

14.3.3 p53

The p53 gene, however, has much stronger evidence and is perhaps among the strongest contenders for use as a biomarker. The p53 gene is a nuclear tumor suppressor protein responsible for the integrity of the genetic sequence. For example, if DNA becomes damaged, it stimulates upregulation of p53 gene, which in turn leads to the arrest of the cell cycle in the G1 phase. This resultant pause in development gives time for the DNA to self-repair. With silencing of the p53 gene, there is loss of the self-repair mechanism and a resultant instability of the cell DNA would arise.

Silencing of the p53 gene can occur for a number of reasons: LOH, mutations, or DNA methylation. Reid et al. (2001) studied the LOH of the 17p chromosome in patients with EAC. In a cohort study of 325 patients, LOH of 17p was associated with a significantly increased risk of developing EAC (RR 16, 95% CI 6.2–39). Of the 269 patients with BE who had 17p LOH, there was a 38% 3-year cumulative incidence of EA in comparison with only 3.3% of those with two normal 17p alleles.

LOH of 17p appears to occur early in the pathogenesis of EA, and it has been postulated that these abnormalities generate DNA instability, eventually resulting in tetraploidy and aneuploidy. This said, not all cases of DNA content abnormalities occur in the context of 17p silencing. It must be deduced therefore, that alternative pathways exist. In addition, these early events, which may simply be arising as an adaptation to reflux as part of the mucosal defense or as a precursor to adenocarcinoma, occur with such high frequency that is unlikely they would be able to act as a sole biomarker given the rarity of progression to adenocarcinoma. As a result, no single biomarker is likely to be adequate to diagnose or stratify adenocarcinoma.

It seems instead that in BE, neoplastic progression occurs by clonal evolution. The latest papers (Reid 2011) suggest that acquired genetic instability generates new variants that undergo stepwise natural selection. These then undergo clonal expansion and eventually new variants arise that in turn undergo further selection. A complex number of changes develop during neoplastic evolution culminating in progression to adenocarcinoma. As such, combinations of chromosomal abnormalities prove to be much more accurate and informative.

14.3.4 Combinations and Loss of Heterozygosity

Galipeau et al. (2007) performed a 10-year prospective biomarker study of BE using adenocarcinoma as an end marker. They evaluated all patients at base line for p53 and p16 abnormalities as well as tetraploidy and aneuploidy. They looked at the risk of progression with all of these markers individually and collectively. They found that individually all abnormalities except for the mutation or methylation of the p16 gene significantly increased the risk of developing adenocarcinoma at 10-years (Table 14.1). However, when these were combined to form a panel, the results were much more significant. The best predictor of adenocarcinoma was a chromosome instability panel made up of a combination of 9p LOH, 17p LOH, and DNA content abnormalities (tetraploidy and aneuploidy). In combination these demonstrated a relative risk of 38.7 (95% CI of 10.8–138.5, $p < 0.001$) of progression to adenocarcinoma. Of those patients who demonstrated all of the previously mentioned abnormalities at baseline, 79.1% developed adenocarcinoma within 5 years. There were no cases of progression to adenocarcinoma within 8 years in any patient who had no biomarker abnormality, reaching only 12% at 10 years (Galipeau et al. 2007; Reid et al. 2000).

14.3.5 SNP Analysis

SNP assays have been shown to closely correlate, and give similar information, to the validated LOH biomarkers previously used (short tandem repeat [STR] polymorphisms) (Kissel et al. 2009; Li et al. 2008).

TABLE 14.1

Biomarkers and Relative Risk of Progression to Adenocarcinoma

a. Category of Biomarker with Associated Risk

Abnormality	Univariate Relative Risk of Developing Adenocarcinoma at 10 Years (95% CI)
17p LOH	10.6
p53 Mutation	7.3
Tetraploidy (4N > 6%)	8.8
Aneuploidy	8.5
9p LOH	2.6

b. Cumulative Incidence of Adenocarcinoma and Relative Risk of Different Baseline Abnormalities

Marker	2 Years	6 Years	10 Years	RR (95% CI) p Value
No abnormalities (n = 85)	0% (0)	0% (0)	12% (3)	Base for RR calculations
One abnormality (n = 104)	0.96% (1)	5.65% (5)	19.88% (8)	RR 1.8, p > 0.38
Two abnormalities (n = 32)	16.83% (5)	28.0% (8)	35.6% (9)	RR 9.0, p < 0.001
Three abnormalities (n = 22)	40.3% (8)	79.1% (14)	(14) Insufficient data	RR 38.7, p < 0.001

The main advantage of SNPs is that they allow chromosomal abnormalities to be detected in whole unprocessed biopsies (Li et al. 2008). In addition, they are present in higher densities than STRs in genomes and can be used in high-throughput methods. STRs have been shown to be problematic with low levels of input DNA or degraded DNA and are limited in use with formalin-fixed samples due to the difficulty with polymerase chain reaction (PCR) amplification required when using STR loci. SNP assays in contrast, can amplify regions surrounding an SNP segment, making them more robust and hence allowing their use with formalin-fixed or degraded DNA.

Measures of chromosomal instability associated with progression can be detected in peripheral blood cells. Mutagen sensitivity to lymphocytes is an indirect measure of an individual's ability to repair DNA damage, and it has been shown that this is associated with an increased risk of developing aneuploidy and hence esophageal cancer (Chao et al. 2006). Shorter telomere lengths, also detectable in peripheral blood cells, are similarly associated with an increased risk of adenocarcinoma ($p = 0.009$) (Risques et al. 2007).

14.3.6 Proliferation Markers

Abnormal cellular proliferation, differentiation, and cell cycle intervals have all been implicated in the pathogenesis of BE. A number of important proto-oncogenes are associated with cell cycle abnormalities. Cell surface expression of cyclin A, an important check mechanism at the G1-S transition of the cell cycle, has been shown to be correlated with degree of dysplasia and a resultant increased risk of progressing to adenocarcinoma (Lao-Sireix et al. 2007). Over expression of cyclin D, a proto-oncogene protein, results in inactivation of p105-R6 due to inappropriate levels of phosphorylation, which has been implicated in transformation of metaplastic epithelium into cancer. Patients whose biopsies were cyclin D positive have been shown to be at significantly higher risk of progressing to adenocarcinoma when compared to those who were negative (Bani-Hani et al. 2000). However, these finding were not replicated in further, larger studies (Murray et al. 2006).

14.3.7 Glyco-Lipids

Glycosylation, the enzymatic addition of a complex carbohydrate to a protein, has been shown to be altered in a number of different cancer groups, including colon, pancreas and stomach. Molecular changes in glycosylation have been implicated in signaling pathways during malignant transformation. This results in increased branching and altered terminal glycan groups that can be measured using mass spectrometry (MS). More recent research suggests that these abundant and diverse structures may also be involved in the pathogenesis of EAC.

These glycomarkers (glycoproteins, proteoglycans, and glycolipids) are more stable than RNA and proteins, making them more suitable for epidemiological studies, whereby human populations can be effectively screened.

In addition, cancerous cells with altered glycosylation shed these proteins or their fragments into circulating fluids and therefore could offer noninvasive sources for detection.

Mechref et al. (2009) used MS to generate glycomic profiles from human blood serum derived from individuals who were known to be either disease-free or have BE, HGD, or EAC. Over 134 different glycans were identified with 26 of these demonstrating statistically significant changes as a result of disease progression. These changes were unique to esophageal cancer with different glycans showing alterations in the previous analysis of samples from patients with breast, prostate, and lung cancers.

Moreover, changes in these glycans could be assessed using endoscopic imaging of mucosal surfaces. Lectins, nonimmune carbohydrate recognition proteins, have well-established binding specificities for particular glycan structures. These proteins are abundant, inexpensive, heat and low pH stable, resistant to proteolysis, and of low toxicity. They may be fluorescently labeled and sprayed on to the mucosal surface of tissue and then detected using fluorescence endoscopy (Figure 14.3). This could be used either to delineate areas of concern to guide biopsy or to demonstrate the extent of disease and therefore determine best treatment (ablation versus surgery). Studies have demonstrated its accuracy but this has only

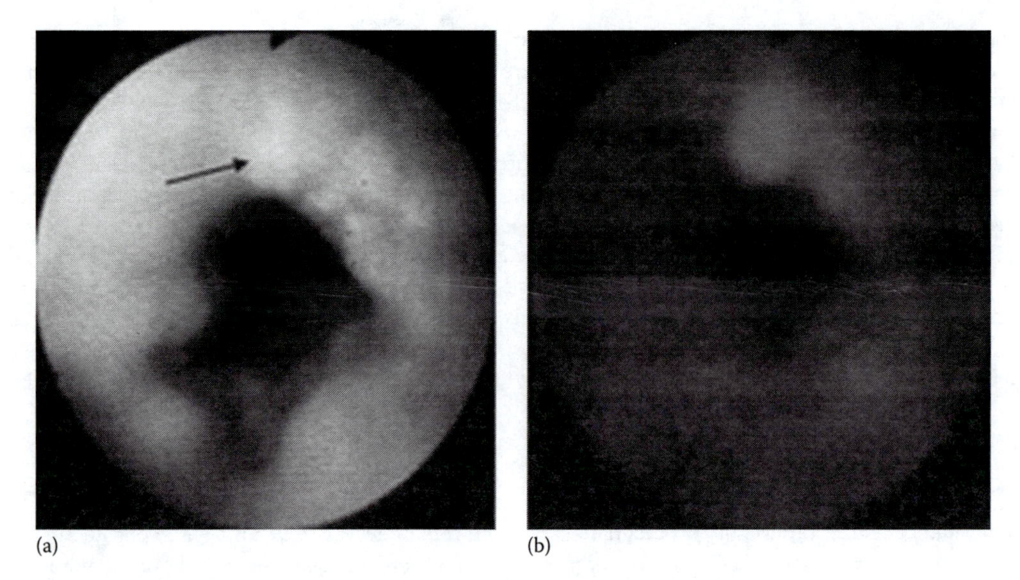

FIGURE 14.3 Fluorescent endoscopy—fluorescence induced with 5-aminolevulinic acid for the endoscopic detection and follow-up of esophageal lesions: (a) endoscopic view and (b) fluorescence view of lesion. (Reprinted from *Gastroint. Endosc.*, 54(5), Mayinger, B., Neidhart, S., Reh, H., Martus, P., and Hahn, E., Fluorescence induced with 5-aminolevulinic acid for the endoscopic detection and follow-up of esophageal lesions, 572–578, November 2001, with permission from Elsevier.)

been conducted ex vivo, using small sample numbers and without real-time sampling (Bird-Lieberman 2012). Significant further research needs to be completed both in vivo and with larger numbers to validate its potential role.

14.3.8 Micro RNAs

Micro ribonucleic acids (miRNAs) are single-stranded, noncoding RNAs of approximately 17–25 ribonucleotides long. They are involved in the regulation of development, differentiation, apoptosis, and proliferation. Since they were first discovered in 1993, in Lin four worms, there have been over 1100 diverse miRNAs identified in humans (Griffiths-Jones et al. 2006).

The international registry miRBase describes their nomenclature, targets, and functions, although the mechanism by which they act is still very much uncertain. Certain miRNAs, when overexpressed, act as tumor promoters through reduced expression of tumor suppressor genes. This is likely related to inhibition of translation and degradation of messenger RNA through imperfect pairing of target mRNAs (Kim and Nam 2006). Suggested targets include BCL2 (B-cell CLL/lymphoma 2), PTEN, and programmed cell death four genes.

Abnormal miRNA expression has been demonstrated in many different cancer subtypes. Changes in miR-196a have been cited in both pancreatic adenocarcinoma and breast carcinoma as well as in BE. Aberrant miRNA expression in esophageal cancer not only enables differentiation between different types of tumor, with an accuracy of 40% (Lu et al. 2005), but also correlates with degree of dysplasia.

miR-194, miR-192, and miR-200c are all raised in EAC but not ESCC (Ogawa et al. 2009), whereas, conversely, there is an increase in aberrant expression of miR-342 in ESCC but not in EAC. miRNA expression, particularly miR-25 and miR-130b, correlates with degree of differentiation (Guo et al. 2008), and expression in BE with HGD significantly differs from corresponding normal tissue or tissue with LGD (Feber et al. 2008; Yang et al. 2009). These studies demonstrated that these miRNAs functioned through downregulation of RAS, mutations of which have already been identified in precancerous tissues and EAC tissues and were predictive of progression from HGD to EAC.

Notably, however, PCR analysis of blood samples has been able to detect and quantify over 100 different miRNAs in healthy patients. Tumor-derived miRNAs appear to be resistant to endogenous ribonuclease activity and consequently studies demonstrated no significant difference in miRNA expression between tumor tissues and its expression in peripheral circulation (Rabinowits et al. 2009; Taylor and Gercel-Taylor 2008). This stability signifies that they can be measured both reproducibly and consistently (Mitchell et al. 2008), indicating that circulating miRNA could act as a surrogate, noninvasive biomarker for high-risk subject screening. Although studies have focused on the functional role of miRNAs in esophageal cancer, there have been no studies to date that have focused on the circulating/serum levels of miRNA in this disease. Significant further research needs to be conducted to confirm their role and potential application in diagnosis and management of esophageal carcinoma.

14.3.9 Epigenetic Biomarkers

Several genetic changes have been described consistently in both adeno- and squamous subtypes. These are predictable and reliable. Epigenetic changes, particularly DNA methylation of the suppressor genes, have been shown not only in both adeno- and squamous varieties but also in the adenocarcinoma precursor, BE (Clement et al. 2006). Some of these abnormal methylations are postulated to be causative for disease progression and it is this fact that makes them potentially useful predictive biomarkers for those at risk.

As previously mentioned, current strategies for identifying those patients at risk rely on the fact that a small proportion of people with BE will progress to fulminant adenocarcinoma. The result of this theory is that huge numbers of people are unnecessarily endoscopically screened. Those that have histological changes of dysplasia are then considered to be on the spectrum towards adenocarcinoma, and appropriate treatment is instituted. This regime is cumbersome and labor intensive so it is hoped that the discovery of these methylation changes may provide a new, more targeted approach.

14.4 Problems with Using Biomarker Panels as Early Biomarkers

These chromosome instability biomarker panels accurately identify patients at high and low risk for progression to adenocarcinoma but rely on a huge number of different technologies to achieve these results, including DNA multiparameter flow cytometry cell sorting for enrichment of cells, STR polymorphisms on chromosomes 9 and 17 for LOH analysis, and DNA flow cytometry analysis of tetraploidy and aneuploidy. These are expensive, time consuming, and difficult to perform outside of research centers, and this has hence hindered their use in the clinical setting. As a result, immunostaining, SNP analysis and image cytometry, have all been trialed to identify alternative methods for detecting these chromosomal abnormalities that can be used in a clinical setting.

14.5 Imaging Biomarkers

14.5.1 Immunostaining and Image Cytometry

The use of immunohistochemical detection of biomarkers has been conducted on a number of potential biomarkers. The presence of a p53 mutation causes protein accumulation that can be detected with immunohistochemistry, and this has been shown to correspond to malignant progression in BE (Murray et al. 2006). This offers the possibility of a biomarker that can be detected in NHS laboratories and can be adapted to the analysis of small routinely fixed and processed biopsies. However, immunostaining for p53 does not correlate with mutation of the p53 gene. Deletions or truncation of p53 are not detected by immunostaining, and increased expression as a result of wild-type p53 due to alterations in other genes produced a positive result. Baseline immunostaining in patients who eventually progressed to malignancy and HGD tested positive for p53 in only one-third of cases (Murray et al. 2006), in contrast with 80% in tumor samples from patients with adenocarcinoma. This may have been due to mutations occurring after biopsy collection or due to sampling limitations or the immunohistochemical assay used. Combining p53 with dysplasia or other markers did not improve its accuracy.

The use of image cytometric DNA analysis has been proposed as an alternative method to assess chromosome content abnormalities. Image cytometry has significant advantages over flow cytometry in that it is cheaper, more easily performed, and readily available in gastroenterology practices. Vogt et al. (2010) conducted a prospective study that demonstrated that histology with image cytometry from brush cytology specimens was a more sensitive marker than dysplasia alone in identifying low- and high-risk groups. No patient with a diploid DNA pattern and negative findings progressed to HGD or adenocarcinoma, whereas patients with aneuploidy DNA pattern had a significantly higher risk (3 of 12) of progressing. These studies indicate that this is a promising method of detection but have only been conducted with a small sample number and with a short follow-up time. Further validation in larger studies is still required.

14.6 Clinically Useful Biomarkers

Among the first genes discovered to be aberrantly methylated in esophageal cancer was CDKN2A, which is a tumor suppressor of the Rb protein in the cell cycle. CDKN2A is inactivated by hypermethylation in some people displaying histological changes of dysplasia. A large study looking at the reliability of this showed that this methylation was present in 15% of those with established BE and not present at all in normal individuals with normal gastric and esophageal tissue (Eads et al. 2001). Another interesting finding was that hypermethylation of this candidate gene was also found alongside established biomarkers such as tetraploidy/aneuploidy and p53 LOH, suggesting that it is one of many changes that occur on the road to cancer. Hypermethylation of CDKN2A seems to occur early in the carcinoma progression pathway, thus making it an ideal potential candidate for screening (Bian et al. 2002).

Another gene that has received much attention is APC gene, another tumor suppressor gene. Hypermethylated APC has been found with incredible consistency in adenocarcinoma (92% of samples tested) and in squamous carcinoma (50% of samples tested) and to a lesser extent in BE (39.5% of samples tested). It was not found in normal individuals. The exciting part of this research is that hypermethylated APC can be detected in the plasma of some patients—representing a unique opportunity to avoid the invasive endoscopy. However, it was not consistent with only 25% of adenocarcinoma sufferers having positive plasma. Those that do have positive plasma seem to exhibit a dose response, that is, the higher the level of hypermethylated APC the poorer the overall survival (Kawakami et al. 2000).

The REPRIMO gene is a tumor suppressor that regulates p53 and inhibition of the cell cycle. It is also methylated and appears to be clonally expanded as the metaplasia–dysplasia–adenocarcinoma pathway progresses. A large-scale study, evaluating 175 endoscopy specimens, showed that hypermethylated REPRIMO was present in 36% of those with BE, 64% of those with high-grade dysplastic changes in BE, and 63% of those with confirmed adenocarcinoma (Hamilton et al. 2006). Other target genes showing positive DNA methylation in similar specimens include somatostatin (SST), tachykinin (TAC-1), NELL1, and AKAP12 (Kaz and Grady 2012).

The ideal biomarker would be one that could risk stratify a patient with BE. Currently all patients are surveyed endoscopically with a consequent huge burden on resources. As mentioned only a small proportion of those with BE progress to full blown cancer, so finding a specific "BE progression" biomarker would have economical and psychological appeal as a large number of patients suffer unnecessary anxiety with current regimes.

One such study looked retrospectively at those individuals with BE who had progressed to HGD or adenocarcinoma and found that hypermethylation of CDKN2A, RUNX3, and HPP1 was positively correlated with this disease progression (Kaz and Grady 2012). Interestingly age, length of BE segment, and hypermethylation of a few other candidate genes such as TIMP-3, and CRBP-1 were not associated with positive progression (Schulmann 2005). Another study looked at the methylation of APC, TIMP-3, and TERT in those who progressed to HGD and beyond compared to those who did not progress. In all three genes, methylation was over three times more likely with progressers than nonprogressers (Clement et al. 2006).

Another useful application of biomarkers would be in quantifying prognosis and survival. Currently, patients are subject to staging investigations that include computed tomography, positron emission tomography, laparoscopy, and endoscopic ultrasound. These are not without risks as there is a small but definite risk of perforation with endoscopic ultrasound and laparoscopy conveys risks that include organ damage and torrential bleeding. Brock and colleagues examined a combination of genes (APC, E-cadherin, MGMT, ER, CDKN2A, DAPK, and TIMP-3) in esophagectomy specimens displaying adenocarcinoma and matched them to normal tissue. They found hypermethylation more abundant in the diseased tissue, but of more importance, they noticed that individuals who had greater than 50% of their target genes aberrantly methylated were more likely to show decreased survival and increased recurrence (Brock et al. 2003; Kaz and Grady 2012). This might have implications for rationing of staging investigations in the future.

Hypermethylation of at least two out of SFRP1, DKK3, and RUNX3 has been shown to be heavily positively correlated with disease recurrence. These methylations are detectable in the plasma of patients, again showing potential for future replacement of invasive surveillance (Liu et al. 2011).

Another useful place for biomarkers on the esophageal cancer treatment pathway would be in detecting response to neoadjuvant chemotherapy. Methylation of the genes that regulate DNA damage may attenuate or restrict the response to chemotherapeutic drugs. A prime candidate is REPRIMO, as one study showed that levels of this methylated gene were significantly lower in chemotherapy responders than nonresponders (Hamilton et al. 2006; Kaz and Grady 2012).

There are hundreds of other hypermethylated genes that could have potential to be used as a detecting biomarker such as SOCS-1, SOCS-3, and NELL-1, but as with all of the others mentioned so far, they have not been subject to validating trials. Their use thus remains experimental.

14.7 Market Players for Molecular Biomarkers

For a suggested biomarker to enter clinical practice, it must be validated—that is to say, it must have gone through a series of rigorous tests to confirm its reproducibility, sensitivity, and specificity. The National Cancer Institute's Early Detection Research Network (EDRN) have outlined a system for validating biomarkers that consists of five phases (expanded to six phases by Jankowski et al. 1999) (Table 14.2), and to date no biomarker candidate in esophageal cancer has progressed beyond phase 3 or at least phase 4. p53 is the biomarker with most potential but will require prospective, multicenter trials before it can be considered as an adjunct, or instead of, dysplasia detection by biopsies. The two stumbling blocks to developing biomarkers for use in clinical practice are the lack of large prospective clinical trials and the lack

TABLE 14.2

Five Phases for Biomarker Validation

Phase	Description	Aim	Example
1	Preclinical and exploratory	Confirm levels are high in adenomatous tissue compared to metaplastic BO	p16
2	Retrospective validation of clinical assay	Optimize a minimally invasive assay, correlate with dysplastic progression, relate to age, sex, etc.	Ki-67
3	Retrospective and longitudinal	Early detection of metaplasia–dysplasia–adenocarcinoma sequence. Define minimum positive level in phase 4	Cyclin D1
4	Prospective screening of large numbers	Determine the biomarkers ability to predict progression of MCS; establish false referral rate	p53
5	Cancer reduction	Verify the impact on cancer mortality by interventions initiated by the detection of the biomarker	Nil
6	Multiple populations	Ascertain whether the biomarker can be applied to all populations with BO	Nil

Source: National Cancer Institutes Early Detection Research Network (EDRN).

of large esophageal tissue stores that include clinical details. This may be addressed by two large-scale prospective trials in BE that are running but still to report. These provide a long-term cohort of patients, in an appropriate research setting, which can be used for analysis. These trials are the Barrett's Oesophagus Surveillance Study (BOSS) and Aspirin and Esomeprazole Chemoprevention Trial (AspECT)—the outcomes of which are eagerly awaited.

14.8 Conclusions and Future Perspectives

At present, detection of patients at risk of adenocarcinoma is reliant on endoscopic biopsies of metaplastic epithelium. This is prone to sampling error, analytical error, and possible overinterpretation of positive results. An alternative strategy is being sought in order to minimize patient discomfort and accurately predict those at risk. There are many promising biomarkers but until the point that they have been formally validated, their use remains experimental. The most useful marker in clinical practice remains detection of dysplasia. Table 14.3 presents a summary of the existing biomarkers.

TABLE 14.3

Summary of Principle Markers and Their Value

Biomarker	Biological Meaning	Validation Phase	Source	Clinical Applicability	Outcome from Studies
Dysplasia	Increased nuclear: cytoplasmic ratio on pathway to adenocarcinoma	4	EB	Yes	Most useful biomarker but difficulty in interpretation
p16	Decelerates cell cycle	1	EB/FC	No	Data in literature lacking but may have value in future
p53	Involved in apoptosis	4	EB/FC	No	More intense staining for p53 in those who progress to adenocarcinoma compared to controls
Cyclin D1	Growth signaling	3	EB/FC	No	Two out of three genotypes confer poor survival
Aneuploidy and LOH	Chromosomal aberrations	3	EB/FC	No	Tetraploidy alone 8× risk of developing adenocarcinoma Aneuploidy alone 8.5× risk LOH at 9p 2.6× risk
Ki-67	Growth signaling	1	EB/FC	No	Low levels associated with poorer survival
APC	Growth inhibitory signaling	2	EB/FC	No	High plasma levels of methylated APC associated with poor survival
microRNA	Regulation of gene expression	—	EB/FC	No	Low miR-3745 levels associated with worse survival
TIMP	Involved in tissue invasion	—	EB/FC	No	Reduction of expression correlates with poor survival

Sources: Jankowski, J.A. et al., *Am. J. Pathol.*, 154, 965, 1999; Ong, C.J. et al., *World J. Gastroenterol.*, 16(45), 5669, 2010.
EB, endoscopic biopsy; FC, flow cytometry.

References

Allum W.H., Blazeby J.M., Griffin S.M. et al. Association of Upper Gastrointestinal Surgeons of Great Britain and Ireland, the British Society of Gastroenterology and the British Association of Surgical Oncology. Guidelines for the management of oesophageal and gastric cancer. *Gut*. November 2011. 60(11):1449–1472.

Bani-Hani K., Martin I.G., Hardie L.J. et al. Prospective study of cyclin D1 overexpression in Barrett's esophagus: Association with increased risk of adenocarcinoma. *J Natl Cancer Inst*. 2000. 92:1316–1321.

Barr H. and Shepherd N. The management of dysplasia. *Guidelines for the diagnosis and management of Barrett's columnar-lined oesophagus a report of the working party of the British Society of Gastroenterology*. August 2005, pp. 32–36. http://www.bsg.org.uk/pdf_word_docs/Barretts_Oes.pdf (last accessed August 2013).

Bian Y.S. et al. P16 inactivation by methylation of CDKN2A promoter occurs early during neoplastic progression in Barrett's oesophagus. *Gastroenterology*. 2002. 122:1113–1121.

Bird-Lieberman E.L., Neves A.A., Lao-Sirleix P., O'Donavan M., Novelli M., Lovat L.B., Eng W.S., Brindle K.M., and Fitzgerald R.C. Molecular imaging using fluorescent lectins permits rapid endoscopic identification of dysplasia in Barrett's esophagus. *Nat Med*. January 2012. 18(2):315–321.

Birkmeyer J.D., Siewers A.E., Finlayson A.E. et al. Hospital volume and surgical mortality in the United States. *N Engl J Med*. 2002. 346:1128–1137.

Brock M.V., Gou M., Akiyama A. et al. Prognostic importance of promoter hypermethylation of multiple genes in oesophageal adenocarcinoma. *Clin Cancer Res*. 2003. 9:2912–2919.

Chao D.L., Maley C.C., Wu X., Farrow D.C., Galipeau P.C., Sanchez C.A., Paulson T.G. et al. Mutagen sensitivity and neoplastic progression in patients with Barrett's esophagus: A prospective analysis. *Cancer Epidemiol Biomarkers Prev*. October 2006. 15(10):1935–1940.

Clement G., Braunschweig N., Pasquier F.T. et al. Methylation of APC, TIMP3 and TERT, a new predictive marker to distinguish Barrett's oesophagus patients at risk of malignant transformation. *J Pathol*. 2006. 208:100–107.

Cooper G.S., Kou T.D., and Chak A. Receipt of previous diagnoses and endoscopy and outcome from esophageal adenocarcinoma: A population-based study with temporal trends. *Am J Gastroenterol*. June 2009. 104(6):1356–1362.

Eads C.A. et al. Epigenetic patterns in the progression of oesophageal adenocarcinoma. *Cancer Res*. 2001. 61:3410–3418.

Feber A., Xi L., Luketich J.D., Pennathur A., Landreneau R.J., Wu M., Swanson S.J., Godfrey T.E., and Litle V.R. Micro RNA expression profiles of esophageal cancer. *J Thorac Cardiovasc Surg*. 2008. 135:255–260.

Ferguson M.K. and Durkin A. Long term survival after esophagectomy for Barrett's esophageal adenocarcinoma in endoscopically surveyed and non surveyed patients. *J Gastrointest Surg*. 2002. 6:29–35.

Galipeau P.C., Li X., Blount P.L., Maley C.C. et al. NSAIDs modulate CDKN2A, TP53, and DNA content risk for progression to esophageal adenocarcinoma. *PLoS Med*. February 2007. 4(2):e67.

Griffiths-Jones S., Grocock R.J., van Dongen S., Bateman A., and Enright A.J. MiRBase: MicroRNA sequences, targets and gene nomenclature. *Nucleic Acid Res*. 2006. 34 Database: D140–D144.

Guo Y., Chen Z., Zhang L., Zhou F., Shi S., Feng X., Li B. et al. Distinctive microRNA profiles relating to patient survival in esophageal squamous cell carcinoma. *Cancer Res*. 2008. 68:26–33.

Hamilton J.P., Sato F. et al. Reprimo methylation is a potential biomarker of Barrett's associated esophageal neoplastic progression. *Clin Cancer Res*. 2006. 12:6637–6642.

Heading R.C. and Attwood S.E.A. Natural history of columnar-lined oesophagus. *Guidelines for the diagnosis and management of Barrett's columnar-lined oesophagus a report of the working party of the British Society of Gastroenterology*. August 2005. 28:18–20. http://www.bsg.org.uk/pdf_word_docs/Barretts_Oes.pdf (last accessed August 2013).

Jankowski J.A., Wright N.A., Meltser S.J. et al. Molecular evolution of the metaplasia–dysplasia-adenocarcinoma sequence in the esophagus. *Am J Pathol*. 1999. 154:965–973.

Kawakami K., Brabender J., Lord R.V. et al. Hypermethylated APC DNA in plasma and prognosis of patients with esophageal adenocarcinoma. *J Natl Cancer Inst*. November 15, 2000. 92(22):1805–1811.

Kaz A.M. and Grady W.M. Epigenetic biomarkers in oesophageal cancer. *Cancer Lett.* 2012. Published online March 2012 Ahead of press. Available at http://www.cancerletters.info/article/S0304-3835%2812%2900158-9/fulltext (last accessed August 2013)

Kim V.N. and Nam J.W. Genomics of microRNA. *Trends Genet.* 2006. 22:165–173.

Kissel H.D., Patricia C., Galipeau Li X., and Reid B. Translation of an STR-based biomarker into a clinically compatible SNP-based platform for loss of heterozygosity. *Cancer Biomarkers.* 2009. 5(3):143–158.

Lagergren J., Bergström R., Lindgren A., and Nyrén O. Symptomatic gastroesophageal reflux as a risk factor for esophageal adenocarcinoma. *N Engl J Med.* March 18, 1999. 340(11):825–831.

Lao-Sirieix P., Rous B., O'Donovan M., Hardwick R.H., Debiram I., and Fitzgerald R.C. Non-endoscopic immunocytological screening test for Barrett's oesophagus. *Gut.* July 2007. 56(7):1033–1034.

Li X., Galipeau P., Sanchez C. et al. Single nucleotide polymorphism-based genome-wide chromosome copy change, loss of heterozygosity, and aneuploidy in BE neoplastic progression. *Cancer Prev Res.* 2008. 1:413–423.

Liu J.B., Qiang J. et al. Plasma DNA methylation of Wnt antagonists predicts recurrence of esophageal squamous cancer. *World J Gastroenterol.* 2011. 17:4917–4921.

Lu J., Getz G., Miska E.A., Alvarez-Saavedra E., Lamb J., Peck D., Sweet-Cordero A. et al. MicroRNA expression profiles classify human cancers. *Nature.* 2005. 435:834–838.

Mayinger B., Neidhart S., Reh H., Martus P., and Hahn E. Fluorescence induced with 5-aminolevulinic acid for the endoscopic detection and follow-up of esophageal lesions. *Gastroint. Endosc.* November 2001. 54(5):572–578.

Mechref Y., Hussein A., Bekesova S., Pungpapong V., Zhang M., Dobrolecki L.E., Hickey R.J., Hammoud Z.T., and Novotny M.V. Quantitative serum glycomics of esophageal adenocarcinoma and other esophageal disease onsets. *J Proteome Res.* June 2009. 8(6):2656–2566.

Mitchell P.S., Parkin R.K., Kroh E.M., Fritz B.R., Wyman S.K., Pogosova-Agadjanyan E.L., Peterson A. et al. Circulating microRNAs as stable blood-based markers for cancer detection. *Proc Natl Acad Sci USA.* 2008. 105:10513–10518.

Murray L., Sedo A., Scott M., McManus D., Sloan J.M., Hardie L.J., Forman D., and Wild C.P. TP53 and progression from Barrett's metaplasia to oesophageal adenocarcinoma in a UK population cohort. *Gut.* October 2006. 55(10):1390–1397. Epub May 8, 2006.

Ogawa R., Ishiguro H., Kuwabara Y., Kimura M., Mitsui A., Katada T., Harata K., Tanaka T., and Fujii Y. Expression profiling of micro-RNAs in human esophageal squamous cell carcinoma using RT-PCR. *Med Mol Morphol.* 2009. 42:102–109.

Overholt B.F., Wang K.K., Burdick J.S., Lightdale C.J., Kimmey M., Nava H.R., Sivak M.V. Jr. et al. International Photodynamic Group for High-Grade Dysplasia in Barrett's Esophagus. Five-year efficacy and safety of photodynamic therapy with Photofrin in Barrett's high-grade dysplasia. *Gastrointest Endosc.* September 2007. 66(3):460–468. Epub July 23, 2007.

Rabinovitch P.S., Longton G., Blount P.L., Levine D.S., and Reid B.J. Predictors of progression in Barrett's esophagus III: Baseline flow cytometric variables. *Am J Gastroenterol.* November 2001. 96(11):3071–3083.

Rabinowits G., Gerçel-Taylor C., Day J.M., Taylor D.D., and Kloecker G.H. Exosomal microRNA: A diagnostic marker for lung cancer. *Clin Lung Cancer.* 2009. 10:42–46.

Reid B.J., Haggit R.C., Rubin C.E., and Rabinovitch P.S. Barrett's esophagus. Correlation between flow cytometry and histology in detection of patients at risk for adenocarcinoma. *Gastroenterology.* 1987. 93(1):1–11.

Reid B.J., Kostadinov R., and Maley C. New strategies in Barrett's esophagus: Integrating clonal evolutionary theory with clinical management. *Clin Cancer Res.* June 1, 2011. 17:3512.

Reid B.J., Levine D.S., Longton G., Blount P.L., and Rabinovitch P.S. Predictors of progression to cancer in Barrett's esophagus: Baseline histology and flow cytometry identify low- and high-risk patient subsets. *Am J Gastroenterol.* 2000. 95:1669–1676.

Reid B.J., Prevo L.J., Galipeau P.C. et al. Predictors of progression in Barrett's esophagus II: Baseline 17p (p53) loss of heterozygosity identifies a patient subset at increased risk for neoplastic progression. *Am J Gastroenterol.* 2001. 96:2839–2848.

Reid B.J., Xiahong L., Galipeau P.C., and Vaughan T. Barrett's oesophagus and oesophageal adenocarcinoma: Time for a new synthesis. *Nat Rev Cancer.* 2010. 10:87–101.

Risques R.A., Vaughan T.L., Li X., Odze R.D., Blount P.L., Ayub K., Gallaher J.L., Reid B.J., and Rabinovitch P.S. Leukocyte telomere length predicts cancer risk in Barrett's esophagus. *Cancer Epidemiol Biomarkers Prev*. December 2007. 16(12):2649–2655.

Schnell T.G., Sontag S.J., Chejfec G., Aranha G., Metz A., O'Connell S., Seidel U.J., and Sonnenberg A. Long term nonsurgical management of Barrett's esophagus with high-grade dysplasia. *Gastroenterology*. 2001. 120:1607–1619.

Schulmann K. Inactivation of p16, RUNX3 and HPP1 occurs early in Barrett's associated neoplastic progression and predicts progression risk. *Oncogene*. 2005. 24:4138–4148.

Taylor D.D. and Gercel-Taylor C. MicroRNA signatures of tumor derived exosomes as diagnostic biomarkers of ovarian cancer. *Gynecol Oncol*. 2008. 110:13–21.

Van Sandick J.W., van Lanschot J.J., Kuiken B.W., Tygat G.N., Offerhaus G.J., and Obertop H. Impact of endoscopic biopsy surveillance of Barrett's oesophagus on pathological stage and clinical outcome of Barrett's carcinoma. *Gut*. 1998. 43:216–222.

Vogt N., Schönegg R., Gschossmann J.M., and Borovicka J. Benefit of baseline cytometry for surveillance of patients with Barrett's esophagus. *Surg Endosc*. May 2010. 24(5):1144–1150. Epub December 8, 2009.

Wang K.K. and Sampliner R.E. Practice Parameters Committee of the American College of Gastroenterology. Updated guidelines 2008 for the diagnosis, surveillance and therapy of Barrett's esophagus. *Am J Gastroenterol*. March 2008. 103(3):788–797.

Wani S., Puli S.R., Shaeen N.J., Westhoff B., Slehria S., Bansal A., Rastogi A., Sayana H., and Sharma P. Esophageal adenocarcinoma in Barrett's esophagus after endoscopic ablative therapy; A meta-analysis and systematic review. *Am J Gastroenterol*. 2009. 104:502–513.

Wong D.J., Paulson T.G., Prevo L.J. et al. p16 (INK4a) lesions are common, early abnormalities that undergo clonal expansion in Barrett's metaplastic epithelium. *Cancer Res*. 2001. 61:8284–8289.

Wong T., Tian J., and Nagar A.B. Barrett's surveillance identifies patients with early esophageal adenocarcinoma. *Am J Med*. 2010. 123:462–467.

Wu P.C. and Posner M.C. The role of surgery in the management of oesophageal cancer. *Lancet Oncol*. August 2003. 4(8):481–488.

Yang H., Gu J., Wang K.K., Zhang W., Xing J., Chen Z., Ajani J.A., and Wu X. MicroRNA expression signatures in Barrett's esophagus and esophageal adenocarcinoma. *Clin Cancer Res*. 2009. 15:5744–5752.

15

Biomarkers for Diagnosis and Metastasis of Hepatocellular Carcinoma

Dengfu Yao, Min Yao, Xiaodi Yan, Li Wang, and Zhizhen Dong

CONTENTS

ABSTRACT Hepatocellular carcinoma (HCC) is one of the most common and rapidly fatal malignancies worldwide. Multiple risk factors are associated with HCC disease etiology, with the highest incidence in patients with chronic hepatitis B virus (HBV) and hepatitis C virus (HCV), although other factors such as genetic makeup, environmental exposure, and lifestyle (alcohol consumption) are involved. As a common malignant solid tumor, HCC is characterized by fast infiltrating growth, early metastasis, high-grade malignancy, and poor therapeutic efficacy. It is a highly vascular tumor dependent on neovascularization and one of the most common and rapidly developing malignancies, especially in Asian countries. HCC treatment options are severely limited by the frequent presence of metastases. HCC is a multifactorial, multistep, and complex process. And multistep malignance of HCC progression with multigene alterations is mostly accompanied with chronic hepatitis and liver cirrhosis. Its prognosis is poor and early diagnosis and monitoring metastasis is of utmost importance. Circulating diagnostic and prognostic biomarkers could be used in proper postoperative treatment of patients at an early stage of HCC development. The chapter summarizes recent studies of the specific biomarkers in diagnosing and monitoring metastasis or postoperative recurrence of HCC. Hepatoma tissues can synthesize various tumor-related proteins, polypeptides, and isoenzymes, such as alpha-fetoprotein (AFP) and hepatoma-specific gamma-glutamyl transferase (HS-GGT), and then secrete them into the blood. The valuable early diagnostic and prognostic biomarkers could predict the development and metastases of HCC. Recent researches have confirmed that circulating hepatoma-specific AFP subfraction, transforming growth factor (TGF)-β1, HS-GGT (85%), and insulin-like growth factor (IGF)-II may be more specific biomarkers than total AFP level for the diagnosis of HCC. The circulating genetic markers such as AFP mRNA, TGF-β1 mRNA, and IGF-II mRNA from peripheral blood mononuclear cells of HCC patients have been most extensively used in monitoring distal metastasis or postoperative recurrence of HCC. Hepatoma tissues synthesize and secrete valuable biomarkers into blood. The analyses of circulating hepatoma-specific biomarkers are useful for the early diagnosis of HCC or monitoring metastasis or postoperative recurrence of HCC.

KEY WORDS: *biomarker, diagnosis, hepatocellular carcinoma, metastasis.*

15.1 Introduction

Hepatocellular carcinoma (HCC) is the third deadliest and fifth most common cancer worldwide. It ranks the second in China among all malignancies, and its mortality is almost equal to its morbidity (Yang and Roberts, 2010; El-Serag, 2012). Carcinogenesis of HCC is a multifactor, multistep, and complex process, which is associated with a background of chronic and persistent infection of hepatitis B virus (HBV) and hepatitis C virus (HCV). Their infections along with alcohol and aflatoxin B1 intake are widely recognized etiological agents in HCC (El-Serag, 2008; Jain, 2010). However, the underlying mechanisms that lead to malignant transformation of infected cells remain unclear. Most of HCC patients died quickly because of the rapid tumor progression, and hepatic resection or transplantation is the only potential curative treatment for HCC patients (Yao and Dong, 2007). Although the mortality of HCC has significantly decreased with the development of surgical techniques, about 60%–100% of the patients suffered from HCC recurrence ultimately even after curative resection, and it has become the most important factor that limits the long-term survival of HCC patients (Aravalli, 2008).

The most urgent needs are to find sensitive biomarkers for early diagnosis and monitoring of postoperative recurrence of HCC and to give adequate treatment for HCC patients. HCC has many characteristics, such as fast infiltrating growth, metastasis in early stage, high-grade malignancy, and poor therapeutic efficacy. HCC prognosis is poor and early detection is of utmost importance (Block et al., 2008). Although serum alpha-fetoprotein (AFP) level is a useful tumor biomarker for the detection and monitoring of HCC, the false-negative rate with AFP level alone may be as high as 40% for patients with early-stage HCC. Even in patients with advanced HCC, the AFP levels may remain normal in 15%–30% of the patients (Volk et al., 2007). New tumor-specific markers (Hayashi et al., 2005; Chen et al., 2011), such as circulating HS-GGT (Yao and Dong, 2007), hepatoma-specific AFP (HS-AFP or AFP-L3, Wu et al., 2006; Kohles et al., 2012), microRNA (miRNA) (Qu et al., 2011), glypican-3 (GPC-3, Wang et al., 2008), and Golgi glycoprotein 73 (Mao et al., 2008; Hu et al., 2010), have been developed to improve the sensitivity, specificity, early detection, and prediction of prognosis. However, the overall results have been unsatisfactory (Zinkin et al., 2008; Imbeaud et al., 2010). This chapter summarizes recent studies of the specific molecular biomarkers in diagnosis and monitoring metastasis or postoperative recurrence of HCC.

15.2 Hepatoma-Specific AFP and AFP mRNA

15.2.1 Serum Total AFP

AFP, a 70 kDa glycoprotein synthesized from fetal yolk sac, liver, and intestines, has a half-life of 5–7 days. Total serum AFP level is a prognostic indicator of the response and survival of germ cell tumors (Nouso et al., 2011). However, when an AFP level is slightly elevated, it may be falsely elevated owing to nonneoplastic liver disease (Yuen and Lai, 2005). Although total AFP is a useful serological marker for the diagnosis of HCC, the false-negative or false-positive rate with AFP level alone may be as high as 40%, especially for its early diagnosis or the finding of small-size HCC (<3 cm). It is sometimes very difficult to make the distinction (Yoshida et al., 2002) between tumors (Figure 15.1A) and falsely elevated AFP levels because of benign liver diseases (Figure 15.1A). Recently, the separation of an HS-AFP subfraction has been reported to be superior to total AFP level in both sensitivity (85% vs. 65%) and specificity (90% vs. 50%) in differentiating between benign and malignant liver disease (El-Serag et al., 2011).

15.2.2 Hepatoma-Specific AFP

Total AFP can be divided into three different glycol forms (Figure 15.1C), AFP-L1, AFP-L2, and AFP-L3 (Figure 15.1D), according to their binding capacity for lens culinaris agglutinin (LCA) or their

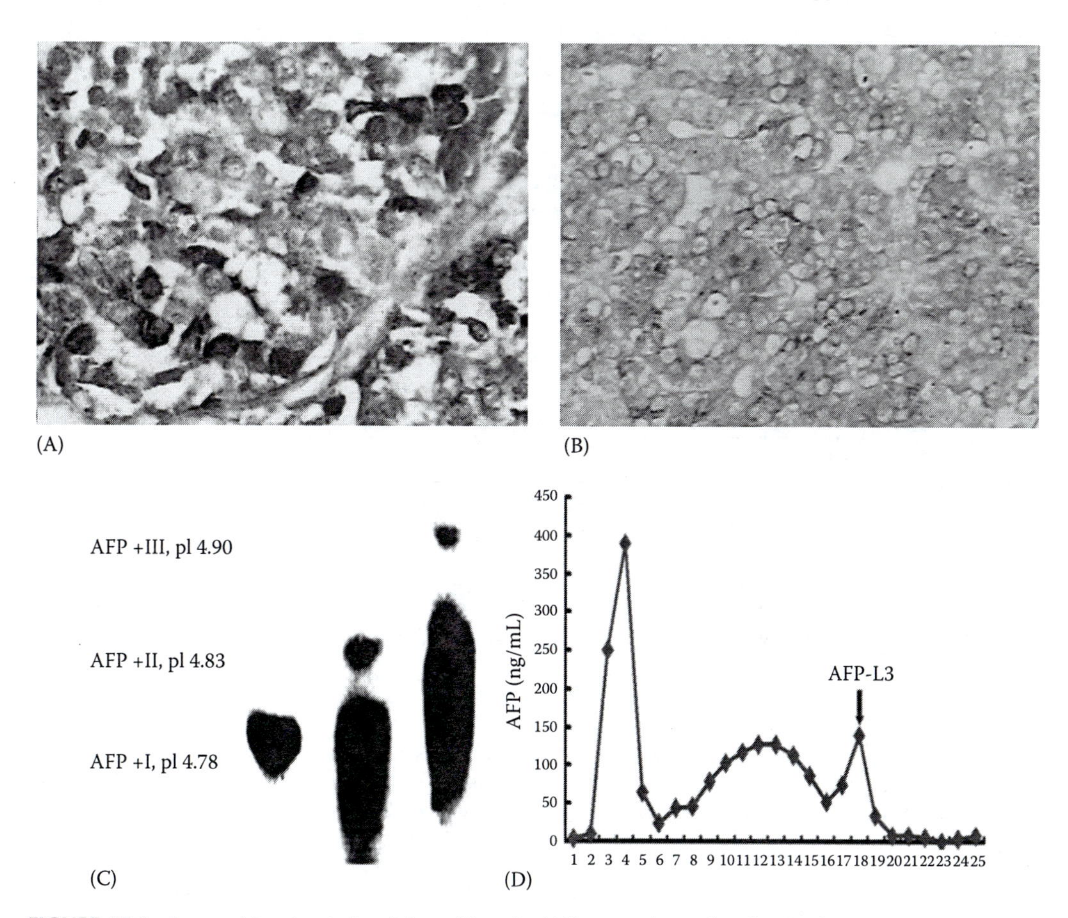

FIGURE 15.1 Immunohistochemical staining of hepatic AFP expression and molecular features in HCC. (A) AFP expression in HCC tissues (SP, original magnification 400×). (B) AFP expression in precancerous tissue (SP, original magnification 400×). (C) Isoelectric point (pI) of AFP protein from different tissues. (D) Separation of HS-AFP-L3 by a minicolumn LCA chromatography.

isoelectric point difference. HS-AFP, as the LCA-bound fraction, is the major glycoform of AFP in the sera of HCC patients. Early diagnosis is very important for HCC. With an HS-AFP of more than 15%, the levels of total serum AFP and HS-AFP fraction in HCC were significantly higher than those in other liver diseases (Li et al., 2001). Although total serum AFP level in liver cirrhosis was significantly higher than in chronic hepatitis and normal control, no significant relationship was found between percentage of HS-AFP and total AFP concentration, HBsAg-positive or HBsAg-negative status, tumor size, or tumor number; however, there was a relation with HCC differentiation, metastasis, and relapse, suggesting that percentage HS-AFP may be a more specific biomarker (85%) than total AFP (65%) for early diagnosis and discovery of recurrence in HCC (Kusaba, 1998; Cheng et al., 2007; Miyaaki et al., 2007).

15.2.3 Circulating AFP mRNA

The genetic markers of HCC or tumor-specific protein can monitor carcinogenesis of hepatocytes and diagnose HCC at an early stage of HCC development. Angiogenesis is necessary for solid tumors larger than 1 × 1 mm, otherwise the tumor remains dormant and does not metastasize (Cheng et al., 2007). As soon as it enters the angiogenesis stage, metastasis potency is exhibited. AFP messenger RNA (mRNA) from peripheral blood mononuclear cells (PBMCs) by reverse transcription-polymerase chain reaction (RT-PCR) has been most extensively studied in recent years (Figure 15.2). Using the appropriate single tumor marker or combination of other markers may improve the effectiveness in screening HCC patients

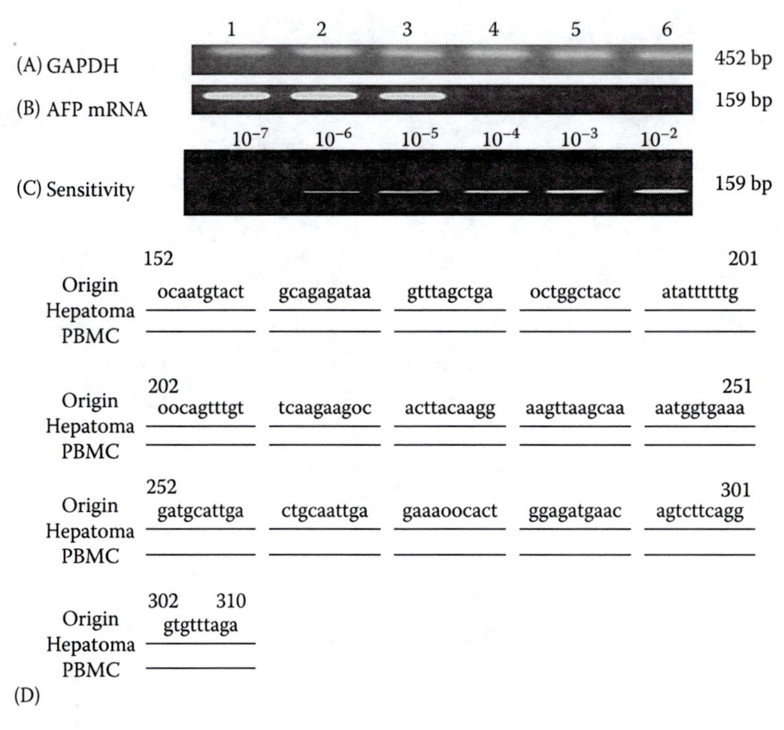

FIGURE 15.2 The amplification of AFP mRNA from liver tissues or PBMCs and the alignment of the amplified sequences. The AFP mRNA was synthesized to AFP complementary DNA and detected by nested PCR (159 bp). (A) The amplified fragments (452 bp) of the glyceraldehyde-3-phosphate dehydrogenase genome from liver or blood was used as a control. (B) The amplification of AFP genomes in liver tissues and circulating blood. Lanes 1 and 2, positive AFP fragments from HCC tissue; lane 3, positive AFP fragments from paracancerous tissue; lane 4, negative result from noncancerous tissue; lane 5, negative result from circulating PBMCs of patients with liver cirrhosis; and lane 6, negative fragments from PBMCs in patients with chronic hepatitis. M, DNA molecular weight marker. (C) The sensitive limitation for AFP mRNA analysis was 2 ng/L in the detection system using total RNA with 10^{-2}–10^{-8}-fold dilution and then amplified by nested PCR. (D) Alignment of nucleotide sequences of the amplified fragments of AFP genome from hepatoma tissues or PMBCs in HCC patients. Origin: the cited sequence (159 bp, nt 152–310) of human AFP genome; hepatoma: the amplification fragment of AFP genome from hepatoma tissue; PBMCs: the amplified fragment of peripheral blood AFP genome from patient with HCC.

(Zhang et al., 2008; Marubashi et al., 2011). If hepatocyte-specific mRNAs are detected in circulating blood, it is possible to infer the presence of circulating, presumably malignant liver cells and predict the likelihood of hematogenous metastasis. By now, many clinical, tumor genetic, and molecular biological markers have been used to diagnose HCC or predict HCC recurrence, but it is a frequently encountered situation that different conclusions were drawn from different researches concerning the value of the same predictor (Yao and Dong, 2007). As the cancer cells in the circulation are an important source for HCC metastasis (because they can be assayed in samples collected noninvasively), the biomarkers that indicate the existence of malignant cells may be a useful predictor for HCC extrahepatic metastasis (Montaser et al., 2007; Debruyne and Delanghe, 2008).

15.3 Hepatoma-Specific GGT Isoenzyme

15.3.1 Serum Total GGT Level

GGT (Enzyme Commission number 2.3.2.2) is a membrane-bound enzyme that catalyzes the degradation of glutathione and other gamma-glutamyl compounds by hydrolysis of the gamma-glutamyl moiety or by its transfer to a suitable acceptor (Wang et al., 2009; Carr et al., 2010). This enzyme exhibits a tissue-specific expression that is modified under various physiologic and pathologic conditions, such as development and carcinogenesis. It is highest in embryo livers and decreases rapidly to the lowest levels after birth, and it is a widely distributed enzyme that has been extensively studied in relation to hepatocarcinogenesis (Yao et al., 2004). GGT is a heterodimeric glycoprotein (Morsi et al., 2006; Ju et al., 2009). Total GGT activities in patients with liver diseases and extrahepatic tumors were abnormally increased. Several studies have demonstrated that these increases are often associated with structural changes in the sugar chains of the enzyme, as evidenced by a variation in the pattern of serum GGT isoforms, suggesting that evaluations of GGT multiple forms might improve the specificity of the GGT measurement and that there might be a correlation between specific patterns and different disease states (West and Hanigan, 2010; Zhang et al., 2011).

15.3.2 Hepatoma-Specific GGT

GGT is reexpressed during the development of HCC and can be divided into several subfractions according to different electrophoresis mobilities. The HS-GGT bands (including I′, II, and II′, HS-GGT) in sera of HCC patients can be separated by a vertical slab electrophoresis assay of polyacrylamide stage gradient gel and have been used in diagnosis of HCC (Yao et al., 1998; Yu et al., 2005). Hepatic GGT with alteration of the gene methylation status is reexpressed during the development of HCC. HS-GGT is a part of total GGT activity that can only be found in sera of HCC patients and has been confirmed a useful specific HCC marker, and its analysis may improve the specificity and sensitivity of HCC diagnosis. The circulating HS-GGT activity was significantly elevated in the HCC patients with an incidence of 86% at the level of over 5.5 IU/L and in patients with other diseases less than 3% (Figure 15.3, Yao et al., 2000).

From liver cancer to distal noncancerous tissues, an increasing tendency of total RNA concentrations was found (Tang et al., 1999; Yao et al., 2004). The frequencies of amplified fragment and hypomethylated M3 site of GGT genes were 100% and 75% in HCC, 85% and 55% in paracancerous tissues, and 75% and 50% in noncancerous tissues, respectively. An inverse correlation was found between methylational degrees of GGT genes and expression levels of GGT. The abnormal alteration of serum HS-GGT level is a sensitive tumor marker for diagnosis or differentiation of HCC, and the overexpression of GGT in HCC may be related to the hypomethylational status of CCGG sites of GGT genes (Yao et al., 2000).

HCC patients are divided into two groups according to the greatest tumor dimension: small-size HCC (less than 5 cm) and large-size HCC (more than 5 cm). Diagnostic values of AFP and HS-GGT levels were 42% (23 of 55) in AFP, 76% (42 of 55) in HS-GGT for small-size HCC, and 83% (84 of 101) in AFP, 92% (93 of 101) in HS-GGT for large-size HCC, respectively. Of the 55 cases with small-size HCC, the frequency of abnormality was significantly higher ($P < 0.01$) in HS-GGT than in AFP. A significant correlation was found between the serum AFP levels and tumor size ($P < 0.01$). The HCC

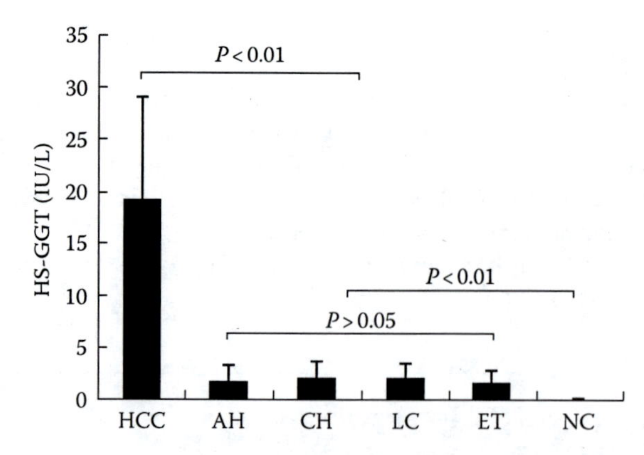

FIGURE 15.3 Diagnostic values of circulating HS-GGT activities in sera of patients with different liver diseases or extrahepatic tumors. HCC, hepatocellular carcinoma; AH, acute hepatitis; CH, chronic hepatitis; LC, liver cirrhosis; ET, extrahepatic tumor; NC, normal controls.

TABLE 15.1

Relation between AFP Levels and HS-GGT Activities

		HS-GGT (≥5.5 IU/L)	
AFP (ng/mL)	n	Positive (%)	Negative (%)
<50	49	39 (79.6)	10 (20.6)
51–499	28	27 (96.4)	1 (3.6)
500–999	18	16 (88.9)	2 (11.1)
>1000	61	53 (86.9)	8 (13.1)
Total	156	135 (86.5)	21 (13.5)

Abbreviations: HS-GGT, hepatoma-specific γ-glutamyl transferase; AFP, α-fetoprotein.

patients were divided into four groups based on their serum AFP concentrations: less than 50, 51–499, 500–999 ng/mL, and more than 1000 ng/mL. The frequency of HS-GGT activity >5.5 IU/mL in HCC patients was 79.6%, 96.4%, 88.9%, and 86.9%, respectively. The positivity rate for the HS-GGT marker was 79.6% (39 of 49) in patients with AFP < 50 ng/mL and 89.7% (96 of 107) in patients with AFP more than 50 ng/mL. No significant relation was found between AFP level and HS-GGT activity. However, the positive result of AFP could be found in HCC patients with low HS-GGT levels. A comparative analysis of HS-GGT and AFP markers for HCC diagnosis is shown in Table 15.1. The sensitivity, specificity, positive predictive value, negative predictive value, and accuracy of HS-GGT quantitative analysis in HCC diagnosis were superior to the same values for the AFP marker (Yao et al., 2000).

15.4 GPC-3 and Its Gene Transcription

15.4.1 GPC-3 in HCC

GPC-3 is a membrane-anchored heparin sulfate proteoglycan normally expressed in fetal liver and placenta, but not in normal adult liver (Filmus and Capurro, 2008; Shafizadeh et al., 2008). It is an oncofetal antigen that is a reliable circulating and biomarker for HCC and hasn't been observed in benign liver lesions by in situ hybridization or immunohistochemistry (Bian et al., 2011). High-grade dysplastic nodules typically express GPC-3 in a weak and focal fashion, although the results have not been consistent across different series (Nassar et al., 2009). GPC-3 expression in hepatocarcinogenesis was previously investigated by rat hepatoma models, with the brown GPC-3-positive expression mainly distributed in

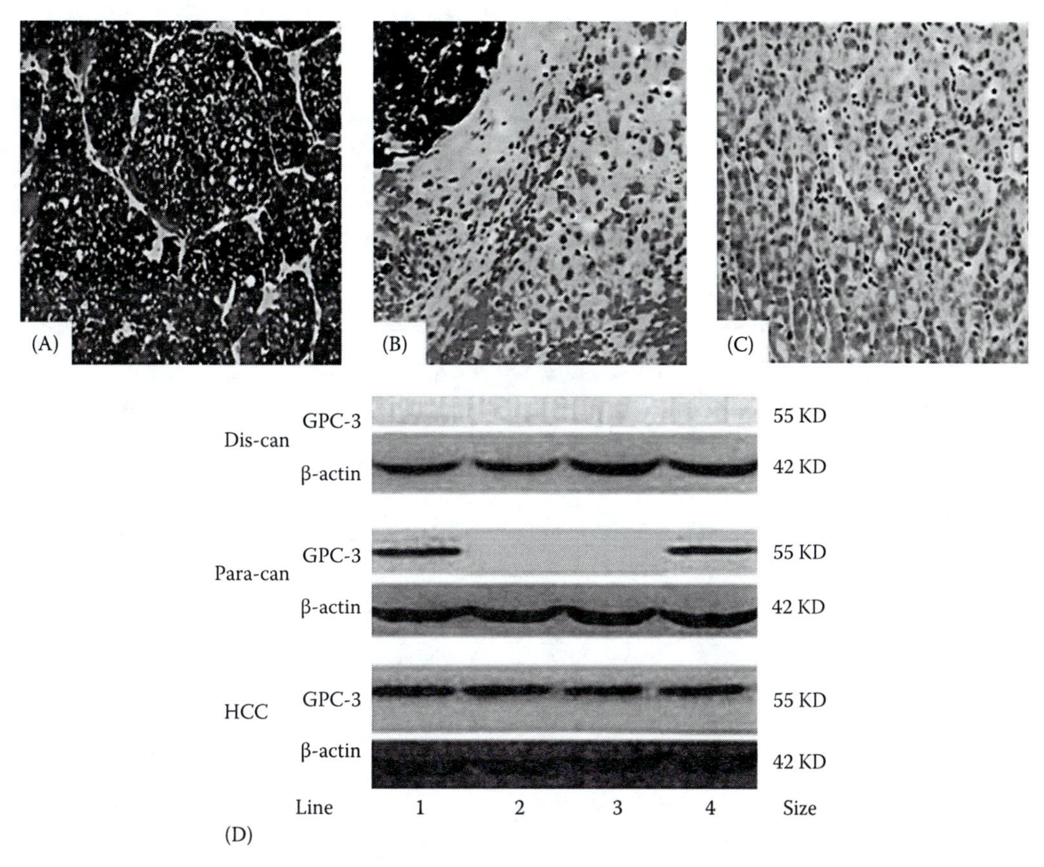

FIGURE 15.4 The immunohistochemical staining and Western blotting analysis of hepatic GPC-3 expression in different parts of human HCC tissues. The cellular distribution of hepatic GPC-3 by immunohistochemical staining with anti-GPC-3 antibody (SP, original magnification 200×). (A) GPC-3 positive in cytoplasm in HCC focus tissues from HCC patients; (B) comparative analysis of GPC-3 expression in cancerous (positive staining) or paracancerous (negative staining) tissues from HCC patients; (C) no GPC-3 expression in distal cancerous tissues from HCC patients; (D) the analysis of hepatic GPC-3 expression in different parts of HCC tissues by Western blotting, GPC-3 expression in cytoplasm of liver analyzed in different parts of HCC. Lanes 1–4, liver tissues from different HCC patients. HCC: the cancerous tissues; para-can: their paracancerous tissues; and dis-can, their distal cancerous tissues. GPC-3, 55 KD; and β-actin, 42 KD as the control protein.

cytosol and membrane. The incidence of GPC-3 expression was 100% in precancerous and cancerous tissues, and its abnormality was associated with hepatocyte malignant transformation, indicating that it is an early biomarker for HCC. The expressions and hepatocyte distribution of GPC-3 in different parts of HCC tissues analyzed by immunohistochemistry with human anti-GPC-3 antibody are shown in Figure 15.4. The positive GPC-3 expression showed brown particles located in cytosol and cell membrane with only a few in cellular nuclei. The GPC-3 staining of HCC tissues (Figure 15.4A) was significantly higher than that in their paracancerous tissues (Figure 15.4B) or distal cancerous tissues (Figure 15.4C). When more positive cells were stained, they were often diffusely localized in HCC tissues. Moreover, the positive GPC-3 was markedly increased by specific expression in HCC tissues and confirmed by Western blotting (Figure 15.4D, Yao et al., 2011).

The incidence of GPC-3 expression in HCC group (80.6%) was significantly higher than that in paracancerous group or distal cancerous groups ($P < 0.001$), and also the paracancerous group was significantly higher than that in the distal cancerous group ($P < 0.001$). The clinicopathological characteristics demonstrated that no significant difference was found between GPC-3 intensity and differentiation degree, age, gender, tumor number, and AFP levels except tumor size (the more than 3 cm group vs. the less than 3 cm group, $P < 0.05$) and HBV infection (Table 15.2).

TABLE 15.2

The Pathological Characteristics of Circulating GPC-3 mRNA in Peripheral Blood Mononuclear Cells from 123 HCC Patients

Group		No. of Cases	GPC-3		χ^2	P
			Positive	Negative		
Sex	Male	103	74	29	0.379	0.538
	Female	20	13	7		
Age	≥60 year	56	39	17	0.059	0.808
	<60 year	67	48	19		
TNM staging	I–II	47	39	8	5.551	0.019
	III–IV	76	48	28		
Tumor size	≥3.0 cm	98	65	33	4.520	0.034
	<3.0 cm	25	22	3		
AFP (ng/mL)	≥400	52	36	16	0.098	0.754
	<400	71	51	20		
HBsAg	Positive	89	79	10	50.571	<0.001
	Negative	34	8	26		
Tumor number	Single	58	40	18	0.165	0.685
	Multiple	65	47	18		
Child-pugh	A	60	40	20	1.005	0.605
	B	45	34	11		
	C	18	13	5		
Periportal cancer embolus	With	44	44	0	28.347	<0.001
	Without	79	43	36		
Extra-hepatic metastasis	With	65	65	0	57.019	<0.001
	Without	58	22	36		

The fragment of GPC-3 mRNA in the PBMCs, the cancerous tissues, and the parts of the paracancerous tissues from HCC patients can be amplified and confirmed by sequencing, but not in the distal cancerous tissues and the PBMCs from patients with benign liver diseases (Shafizadeh et al., 2008; Yan et al., 2011).

15.4.2 GPC-3 mRNA

The incidence of circulating GPC-3 mRNA was 70.7% in HCC and 2.0% in benign liver diseases or non-liver tumors (Shirakawa et al., 2009). The significant higher incidence of GPC-3 mRNA was found in HCC patients with I–II vs. III–IV staging, HBV infection, and small-size tumor, especially in HCC patients with the periportal cancer embolus group or the extrahepatic metastasis group higher than that in the without periportal cancer embolus group or the without extrahepatic metastasis group (Table 15.2) (Qiao et al., 2011). The quantitative GPC-3 levels showed that only GPC-3 was overexpressed in HCC patients (52.8%) and was 1.4% in cases with benign liver diseases or 2.0% in cases with non-liver tumors, with significant differences between the HCC group and each of the study groups. The non-GPC-3 expression in sera of cases with benign liver diseases was detected except of one case with cirrhosis. There were no false-positives among patients with acute hepatitis or chronic hepatitis or among healthy subjects. However, compared with AFP for HCC diagnosis, the higher positive result (14.3%–20.0%) of AFP could be found in patients with benign liver diseases, although the positive rate of serum AFP was higher (70.73%). According to tumor size, the frequency of serum GPC-3 abnormality was significantly higher ($P < 0.01$) in the less than 3 cm group (80.0%) than that in the more than 3 cm group (41.7%).

The combining diagnostic values of circulating GPC-3, GPC-3 mRNA, and AFP levels for HCC are shown in Table 15.3. The positive rate in 123 HCC patients was 52.8% in serum GPC-3, 70.7% in positive-GPC-3 mRNA from circulating PBMC, and 70.7% in serum AFP. Total positive rates of circulating GPC-3 and its gene in combination with AFP level could rise up to 94.3% of HCC diagnosis. The detection of circulating GPC-3 and GPC-3 mRNA quantitative analysis in HCC diagnosis were superior to

TABLE 15.3

Combining Diagnostic Values of Circulating GPC-3, GPC-3 mRNA, and AFP Levels for HCC

GPC-3	GPC-3	GPC-3 mRNA	AFP[a]	Total
Sensitivity (%)	52.8	70.7	70.7	94.3
Specificity (%)	98.8	99.8	86.2	85.8
Diagnostic accuracy (%)	83.5	89.4	81.0	88.6
Positive predictive value (%)	95.6	96.7	71.9	76.8
Negative predictive value (%)	80.7	87.1	85.5	96.8

[a] AFP level was more than 20 ng/mL.

AFP in the sensitivity, specificity, positive predictive value, negative predictive value, and accuracy for HCC diagnosis. The detection of GPC-3 and its gene transcription in hepatoma specificity was superior to serologic AFP alone, with efficacy in differentiating diagnosis and monitoring hematogenous metastasis of HCC. The complementary values of circulating GPC-3 and AFP markers should rise up the diagnostic sensitivity for HCC (Kandil et al., 2007).

15.5 TGF-β_1 and TGF-β_1 mRNA

15.5.1 TGF-β_1 in HCC

TGF-β is a family of related proteins that regulate many cellular processes including growth, differentiation, extracellular matrix formation, and immunosuppression (Morris et al., 2012). Every cell in the body, including epithelial, endothelial, hematopoietic, neuronal, and connective tissue cells, produces TGF-β and has receptors for it. TGF-β_1 is one of the TGF-β isoforms (TGF-β_{1-5}) and arrests the cell cycle in the G1 phase thereof eliciting inhibition of cell proliferation and triggering apoptosis (Blobe et al., 2000; Bissell et al., 2001). In normal liver tissues, TGF-β_1 is produced only by nonparenchymal cells (Kupffer's cell, fat-storing cell, and endothelial cell, El-Serag et al., 2008). Previous studies have shown an upregulated expression of TGF-β_1 in tumor cells, including HCC (Divella et al., 2012). Though a growth inhibitor, the overexpression of hepatic TGF-β_1 was found in HCC tissues and correlated with carcinogenesis, progression, and prognosis of HCC (Figure 15.5) (Lee et al., 2012). TGF-β_1 expression was increased as the HBV-induced disease progressed from chronic hepatitis to cirrhosis, then HCC. In in vitro experiment, immunohistochemistry and in situ hybridization revealed that normal hepatocytes hadn't any TGF-β_1 staining (Yamazaki et al., 2011; Morris et al., 2012). But in regenerative and cirrhotic livers, hepatocytes and HCC cells expressed different degrees of TGF-β_1 and its mRNA.

15.5.2 TGF-β_1 mRNA

As the longevity of cirrhosis and HCC cells was observed compared to normal hepatocytes, it is plausible to propose that TGF-β_1 up-expression in these tumor cells is closely related to the cell survival, thereof possibly escaping the control of cell proliferation by TGF-β (Hoshida, 2011). The incidence of hepatic TGF-β_1 expression was higher in HCC tissues (83%) and lower in their surrounding tissues, and the incidence was 95% in HBV-DNA-positive group and 64% in HBV-DNA-negative one, respectively. The TGF-β_1 expression is associated with degree of HCC differentiation and status of HBV replication, but neither to the size nor to number of the tumor. The levels of circulating TGF-β_1 and TGF-β_1 mRNA were significantly higher in the HCC patients than in any of other patients. The sensitivity and specificity of circulating TGF-β_1 level that was more than 1.2 μg/L were 90% and 94% for HCC diagnosis, respectively, but no significant correlation was found between TGF-β_1 expression and AFP levels or tumor sizes. The combined detection of TGF-β_1 and serum AFP could raise the detection rate of HCC up to 97%. Both of the circulating TGF-β_1 and TGF-β_1 mRNA could be used as sensitive biomarkers for diagnosis and prognosis of HBV-induced HCC (Dong et al., 2007, 2008).

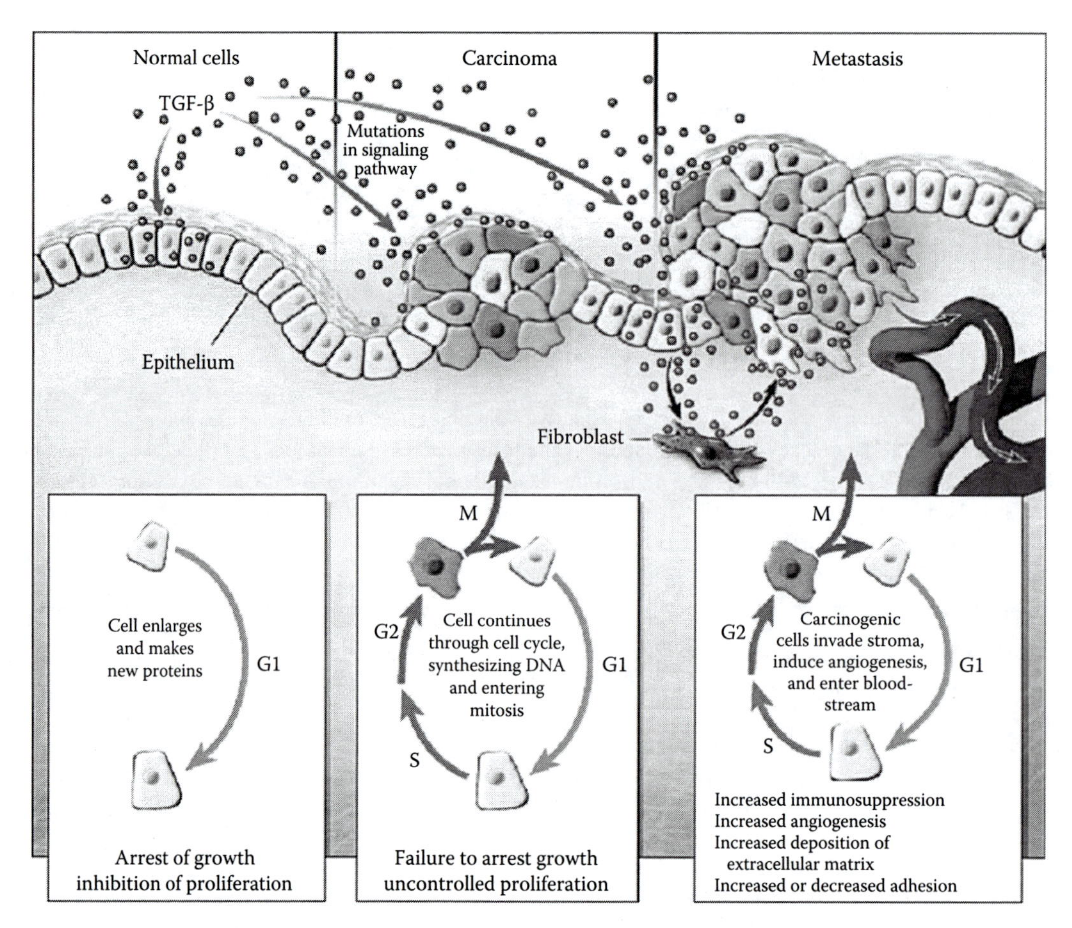

FIGURE 15.5 Role of TGF-β_1 in the occurrence and development of cancer. (From Blobe, G.C. et al., *N. Engl. J. Med.*, 342, 1350, 2000.)

15.6 IGF-II and IGF-II mRNA

15.6.1 IGF-II in HCC

IGF-II is a mitogenic polypeptide closely related to insulin. Its gene has complex regulation of transcription, resulting in multiple mRNA initiated by different promoters (Scharf and Braulke, 2003; Rehem and El-Shikh, 2011). It is speculated to serve as an autocrine growth factor in various cancers because they often coexpress IGF-II and IGF-I receptors, and it is a kind of fetal growth factor and highly expressed during hepatocarcinogenesis (Wang et al., 2003), and reexpression of the IGF-II gene has recently been described in HCC (Scharf et al., 2001; Cantarini et al., 2006; Qiu et al., 2008). HCC is generally considered to be a hypervascular tumor. Although hepatic arterial embolization is widely used as an effective treatment of HCC on the basis of hypervascularization of HCC, IGF-II may play an important role in the development of neovascularization of HCC, because IGF-II substantially increases vascular endothelial growth factor (VEGF) mRNA and protein levels in a time-dependent manner in human hepatoma cells. The induction of VEGF by IGF-II was additively increased by hypoxia, and IGF-II may be a hypoxia-inducible angiogenic factor in HCC and stimulates the growth of HCC cells in vitro. Most of cirrhotic and HCC tissues express IGF-II (Figure 15.6). However, little is known of its circulating IGF-II gene in HCC.

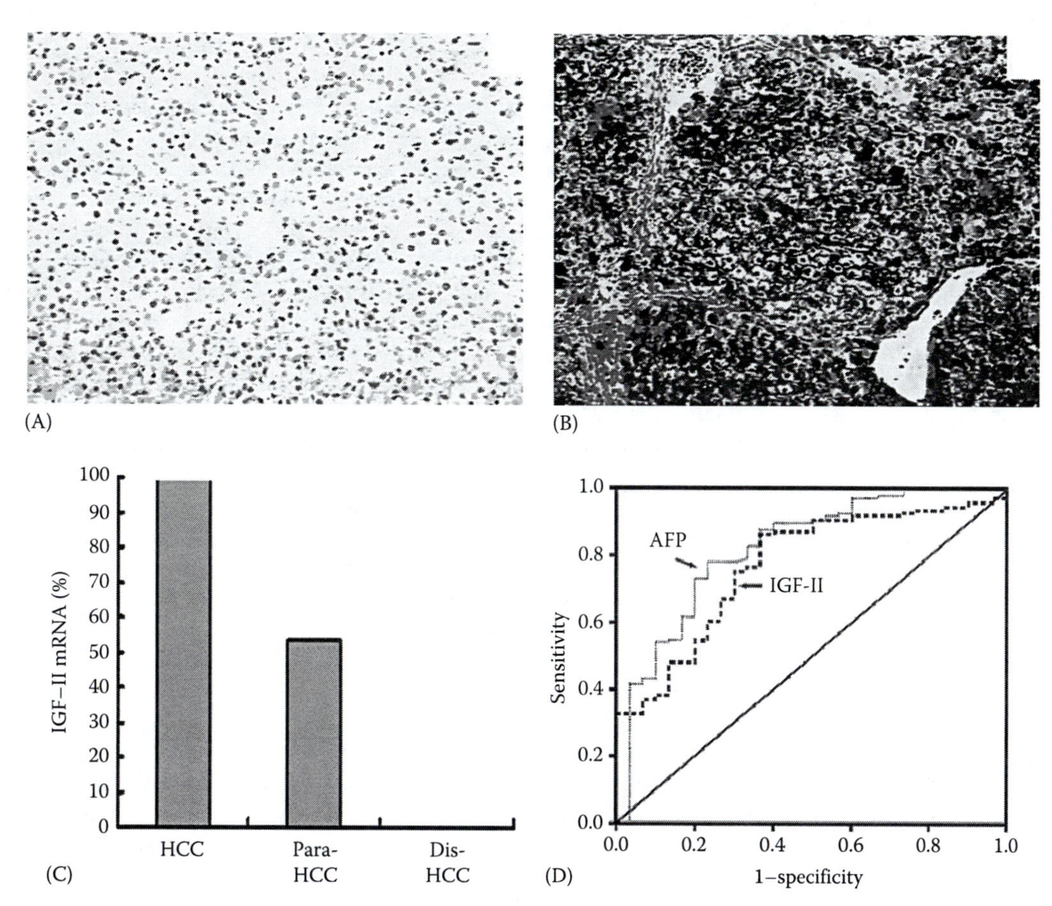

FIGURE 15.6 (See color insert.) IGF-II expression in hepatoma tissues and blood. The expressions of hepatic IGF-II and IGF-II mRNA and diagnostic value of circulating IGF-II level for HCC: (A) without IGF-II expression in the distal cancerous tissues; (B) with the strongest IGF-II expression in HCC tissues (From Dong, Z.Z. et al., *Zhonghua Gan Zang Bing Za Zhi*, 13, 866, 2005a); (C) the percentage of IGF-II mRNA amplification from different liver tissues. HCC, paracancerous tissues, and distal cancerous tissues (From Shafizadeh, N. et al., *Mod. Pathol.*, 21, 1011, 2008; Shirakawa, H. et al., *Cancer Sci.*, 100, 1403, 2009); and (D) receiver operating characteristic (ROC) curves for the serum IGF-II investigated marker for HCC. Sensitivity, true-positive rate; specificity, false-positive rate. The area under the ROC curves was 0.823 for AFP and 0.771 for IGF-II. (From Qian, J. et al., *Am. J. Clin. Pathol.*, 134, 799, 2010.)

15.6.2 IGF-II mRNA

Studies found that the amplified fragments of IGF-II mRNA by RT-PCR were identical to original designed ones with size of 170 base pairs (bp) and confirmed by sequencing analysis. The dilution experiments revealed that the lowest sensitivity of our system was 2 ng/L of total RNA. The positive frequencies of IGF-II mRNA were 100% in HCC, half in paracancerous, and none in noncancerous tissues, respectively (Yao et al., 2003). The circulating free IGF-II levels were significantly higher in HCC than in chronic hepatitis or liver cirrhosis. The positive frequency of circulating IGF-II mRNA was 34% in HCC, and no amplified fragment was found in other liver diseases, extrahepatic tumors, and normal controls. The circulating IGF-II mRNA was correlated with the stage of HCC, and its incidence was 100% in HCC with extrahepatic metastasis and 35% in HCC with negative AFP. No significant difference was found between tumor sizes and circulating IGF-II mRNA fragment. Hence, the abnormal expressions of free IGF-II and IGF-II mRNA are useful tumor markers for HCC diagnosis, differentiation of extrahepatic metastasis, and monitoring postoperative recurrence (Dong et al., 2005b; Qian et al., 2010).

15.7 Genetic Alterations of Telomerase in HCC

Telomerase, an RNA-dependent DNA polymerase, can maintain the telomeric length by acting as a reverse transcriptase. In humans, tumor cells escape programmed cell senescence through reactivation of telomerase (Satyanarayana et al., 2004; Daniel et al., 2012). These immortalized cells can compensate for telomeric shortening at each cell division, leading to progressive neoplastic evolution. Telomerase reexpression was found in 85% of human malignant tumors (Mu and Wei, 2002; Durant, 2012). Maybe HBV infection is merely a carcinogenic factor and is not related to the growth, infiltration, and metastasis of HCC. It is increasingly clear that oncogenesis is driven by the activation of telomerase, a ribonucleoprotein complex that adds telomeric repeats (hexanucleotide 5′-TTAGGG-3′) to the ends of replicating chromosomes. Telomerase is a ribonucleoprotein composed of an essential RNA and a few proteins. It is expressed in embryonic cell and in adult male germ line cells but is undetectable in normal somatic cells except proliferative cells of renewable tissues (Lewis and Wuttke, 2012).

The expression of telomerase is important to cell proliferation, senescence, immortalization, and carcinogenesis. The hepatoma model displayed the dynamic expression of hepatic telomerase during HCC development and up to its highest peak at the stage of HCC formation. The telomerase activities were consistent with liver total RNA levels at the stages of degeneration, precancerosis, and cancerization of hepatocytes. In human HCC tissues, the telomerase levels were also significantly higher than those in their adjacent noncancerous tissues, but liver total RNA levels were lower in the former than in the latter. Although the circulating telomerase of HCC patients was abnormally expressed among patients with chronic liver diseases, the telomerase activity was a nonspecific marker for HCC diagnosis, because the incidence was lower in normal control or in chronic liver disease and 83% in HCC when absorbance value of telomerase activity is more than 0.2, respectively. If the value is over 0.6, the incidence was 63% in the HCC patients and none in any of others except for two patients with liver cirrhosis. However, the analysis of telomerase in combination with AFP could increase the accuracy (93%) of HCC diagnosis. The expression of telomerase was associated with HCC development and its abnormality in liver tissues or in peripheral blood could be a useful marker for diagnosis and prognosis of HCC (Wu et al., 2005; Yao et al., 2006b).

15.8 HSP Expression

15.8.1 HSP in HCC

Heat shock protein (HSP) is a highly conserved protein produced under the perturbation or stressors of many physical and chemical factors. It participates in the complex formation of many proteins, contributes to the folding and extension of proteins as well as the assembly of polycomplex, functions in protein transport between cell organelles, and regulates the target proteins other than changes of their construction (Ciocca and Calderwood, 2005; Lu et al., 2009). Thus, it is defined as a molecular chaperone. HSPs are ubiquitous molecules induced in cells exposed to various stress conditions, including carcinogenesis. Previous studies have shown upregulated expression of gp96 in tumor cells, including those of HCC. As an apoptosis inhibitor, HSP is overexpressed in human HCC tissues and correlated with carcinogenesis, progression, and prognosis of HCC. HSP gp96 (or GRP94) as a putative high-density lipoprotein-binding protein in the liver and a member of the HSP90 family (HSP83, HSP84, HSP87, HSP90 gp96, etc.) binds the repertoires of peptides, thus eliciting peptide-specific T cell immune responses. It predominantly locates inside the endoplasmic reticulum (ER) with some cell surface expression in certain cancerous cells. Enhancement of intracellular HSP is closely related to the formation and development of HCC (Sakamoto et al., 2008) and a vital marker indicating the progression and aggravation of HCC (Wu, 2007; Block et al., 2008).

15.8.2 HSP90

HSP90 is required for the activity of HBV reverse transcriptase. The gp96 expression is increased as the HBV-induced disease progresses from chronic hepatitis to cirrhosis, then HCC. The longevity of cirrhotic and HCC cells compared to normal hepatocytes is plausible to propose that increased gp96 expression in these tumor cells is closely related to the cell survival, thereof possibly by preventing cell apoptosis. The gp96 was strongly expressed in HCC (73.3%) and weakly in noncancerous tissues. The gp96 expression in HCC tissues was correlated with the degree of tumor differentiation and tumor size, but not with tumor number. The data of gp96 immunohistochemical analysis showed that 90% of HCC patients who were HBV-DNA-positive strongly expressed gp96, whereas only 46% of the patients who were HBV-DNA-negative were positive for gp96 (Yao et al., 2006a).

15.8.3 HSP70 and HSP27

HSP70 and HSP27 among HSPs are of special relevance in human cancer inhibiting apoptosis. They were frequently stained in the cytoplasm and nuclei of tumor cells, but not in nonneoplastic hepatocytes. Immunoreactivities of HSP70 and HSP27 were observed in 56.3% and 61.9% of HCCs, respectively. The former was correlated with high Ki-67 labeling indices (LIs), large tumor size, presence of portal vein invasion, and high tumor stage. The latter was significantly related to the subgroup of HBV-associated HCCs, but not to others. Both HSP70 and HSP27 immunoreactivities showed no relation to Apotag LIs or p53 immunoreactivity. Expressions of HSP70 and HSP27 might play an important role in hepatocarcinogenesis, and HSP70 in particular was closely related to the pathological parameters associated with tumor progression (Joo et al., 2005; Luk et al., 2006).

15.9 MicroRNAs in HCC

miRNAs are small noncoding RNAs that function as endogenous silencers of numerous target genes (Gui et al., 2011; Kojima et al., 2011). Hundreds of miRNAs have been identified in the human genome. miRNAs are expressed in a tissue-specific manner and play important roles in cell proliferation, apoptosis, and differentiation of HCC. Aberrant expression of miRNAs may also contribute to the development and progression of human HCC. Recent studies have shown that some miRNAs play roles as tumor suppressors or oncogenes in HCC. *miR-122*, *let-7* family, and *miR-101* are downregulated in HCC, suggesting that it is a potential tumor suppressor of HCC. *miR-221* and *miR-222* are upregulated in HCC and may act as oncogenic miRNAs in hepatocarcinogenesis. miRNA expression profiling may be a powerful clinical tool for diagnosis and regulation of miRNA expression could be a novel therapeutic strategy for HCC (Effendi and Sakamoto, 2010; Augello et al., 2012).

15.10 Perspectives

HCCs exhibit numerous genetic abnormalities as well as epigenetic alterations including modulation of DNA methylation (Couvert et al., 2012; Liao et al., 2012; Yan et al., 2012). Molecular factors are involved in the process of HCC development and metastasis (Gish et al., 2012; Wong and Chan, 2012). Several laboratories have implicated constitutive activation of miRNA as one of the early key events involved in neoplastic progression of the liver (Kohles et al., 2011; Oda et al., 2011; Abdalla and Haj-Ahmad, 2012). Further studies will permit us to analyze the mechanism of human hepatocarcinogenesis and pay attention to these areas (Zhang et al., 2012). However, the combination of pathological features and some biomarkers with high sensitivity and specificity for early diagnosis and metastasis of HCC seems to be more practical up to the present.

Acknowledgments

This work was supported by the Grant BL2012053 and H200925 from the Projects of Jiangsu Medical Science, the Grant PAPD from the Priority Academic Program Development of Jiangsu Higher Education Institution, the Grant HS2011012 from the Program of Nantong Society Undertaking and Technological Innovation, and the Grant ISTCP from International Science and Technology Cooperation Program of China.

References

Abdalla MA, Haj-Ahmad Y. 2012. Promising candidate urinary MicroRNA biomarkers for the early detection of hepatocellular carcinoma among high-risk hepatitis C virus Egyptian patients. *J Cancer* 3: 19–31 [PMID: 22211142].

Aravalli RN, Steer CJ, Cressman EN. 2008. Molecular mechanisms of hepatocellular carcinoma. *Hepatology* 48: 2047–2063 [PMID: 19003900].

Augello C, Vaira V, Caruso L, Destro A et al. 2012. MicroRNA profiling of hepatocarcinogenesis identifies C19MC cluster as a novel prognostic biomarker in hepatocellular carcinoma. *Liver Int.* 32: 772–782 [PMID: 22429613].

Bian YZ, Yao DF, Zhang CG, Li SS, Wu W, Dong ZZ, Qiu LW, Yu DD. 2011. Expression features of glypican-3 and its diagnostic and differential values in hepatocellular carcinoma. *Zhonghua Gan Zang Bing Za Zhi* 19: 260–265 [PMID: 21586223].

Bissell DM, Roulot D, George J. 2001. Transforming growth factor beta and the liver. *Hepatology* 34: 859–967 [PMID: 11679955].

Blobe GC, Schiemann WP, Lodish HF. 2000. Role of transforming growth factor beta in human disease. *N Engl J Med.* 342: 1350–1358 [PMID:10793168].

Block TM, Marrero J, Gish RG, Sherman M, London WT, Srivastava S, Wagner PD. 2008. The degree of readiness of selected biomarkers for the early detection of hepatocellular carcinoma: Notes from a recent workshop. *Cancer Biomark.* 4: 19–33 [PMID: 18334731].

Cantarini MC, de la Monte SM, Pang M, Tong M, D'Errico A, Trevisani F, Wands JR. 2006. Aspartyl-asparagyl beta hydroxylase over-expression in human hepatoma is linked to activation of insulin-like growth factor and notch signaling mechanisms. *Hepatology* 44: 446–457 [PMID: 16871543].

Carr BI, Pancoska P, Branch RA. 2010. Significance of increased serum GGTP levels in HCC patients. *Hepatogastroenterology* 57: 869–874 [PMID: 21033244].

Chen F, Xue J, Zhou L, Wu S, Chen Z. 2011. Identification of serum biomarkers of hepato-carcinoma through liquid chromatography/massspectrometry-based metabonomic method. *Anal Bioanal Chem.* 401: 1899–1904 [PMID: 21833635].

Cheng HT, Chang YH, Chen YY, Lee TH, Tai DI, Lin DY. 2007. AFP-L3 in chronic liver diseases with persistent elevation of alpha-fetoprotein. *J Chin Med Assoc.* 70: 310–317 [PMID: 17698430].

Ciocca DR, Calderwood SK. 2005. Heat shock proteins in cancer: Diagnostic, prognostic, predictive, and treatment implications. *Cell Stress Chaperones* 10: 86–103 [PMID: 16038406].

Couvert P, Carrié A, Tezenas du Montcel S, Vaysse J et al. 2012. Insulin-like growth factor 2 gene methylation in peripheral blood mononuclear cells of patients with hepatitis C related cirrhosis or hepatocellular carcinoma. *Clin Res Hepatol Gastroenterol.* 36: 345–351 [PMID: 22902352].

Daniel M, Peek GW, Tollefsbol TO. 2012. Regulation of the human catalytic subunit of telomerase (hTERT). *Gene* 498: 135–146 [PMID:22381618].

Debruyne EN, Delanghe JR. 2008. Diagnosing and monitoring hepatocellular carcinoma with alpha-fetoprotein: New aspects and applications. *Clin Chim Acta* 395: 19–26 [PMID: 18538135].

Divella R, Daniele A, Gadaleta C, Tufaro A, Venneri MT, Paradiso A, Quaranta M. 2012. Circulating transforming growth factor-β and epidermal growth factor receptor as related to virus infection in liver carcinogenesis. *Anticancer Res.* 32: 141–145 [PMID: 22213299].

Dong ZZ, Yao DF, Wu XH, Shi GS, Qiu LW, Wu W, Su XQ. 2005a. Early diagnostic value of abnormal expression of insulin-like growth factor (IGF)-II and IGF-II-mRNA in hepatocellular carcinoma patients. *Zhonghua Gan Zang Bing Za Zhi* 13: 866–868 [PMID: 16313745].

Dong ZZ, Yao DF, Yao DB, Wu XH, Wu W, Qiu LW, Jiang DR, Zhu JH, Meng XY. 2005b. Expression and alteration of insulin-like growth factor II-messenger RNA in hepatoma tissues and peripheral blood of patients with hepatocellular carcinoma. *World J Gastroenterol.* 11: 4655–4660 [PMID: 16094705].

Dong ZZ, Yao DF, Yao M, Qiu LW, Zong L, Wu W, Wu XH, Yao DB, Meng XY. 2008. Clinical impact of plasma TGF-beta1 and circulating TGF-beta1 mRNA in diagnosis of hepatocellular carcinoma. *Hepatobiliary Pancreat Dis Int.* 7: 288–295 [PMID: 18522884].

Dong ZZ, Yao DF, Zou L, Yao M, Qiu LW, Wu XH, Wu W. 2007. An evaluation of transforming growth factor-beta 1 in diagnosing hepatocellular carcinoma and metastasis. *Zhonghua Gan Zang Bing Za Zhi* 15: 503–508 [PMID: 17669238].

Durant ST. 2012. Telomerase-independent paths to immortality in predictable cancer subtypes. *J Cancer* 3: 67–82 [PMID: 22315652].

Effendi K, Sakamoto M. 2010. Molecular pathology in early hepatocarcinogenesis. *Oncology* 78: 157–160 [PMID: 20389138].

El-Serag HB. 2012. Epidemiology of viral hepatitis and hepatocellular carcinoma. *Gastroenterology* 142: 1264–1273.e1 [PMID: 22537432].

El-Serag HB, Kramer JR, Chen GJ, Duan Z, Richardson PA, Davila JA. 2011. Effectiveness of AFP and ultrasound tests on hepatocellular carcinoma mortality in HCV-infected patients in the USA. *Gut* 60: 992–997 [PMID: 21257990].

El-Serag HB, Marrero JA, Rudolph L, Reddy KR. 2008. Diagnosis and treatment of hepatocellular carcinoma. *Gastroenterology* 134: 1752–1763 [PMID: 18471552].

Filmus J, Capurro M. 2008. The role of glypican-3 in the regulation of body size and cancers. *Cell Cycle* 7: 2787–2790 [PMID: 18787398].

Gish RG, Lencioni R, Di Bisceglie AM, Raoul JL, Mazzaferro V. 2012. Role of the multidisciplinary team in the diagnosis and treatment of hepatocellular carcinoma. *Expert Rev Gastroenterol Hepatol.* 6: 173–185 [PMID: 22375523].

Gui J, Tian Y, Wen X, Zhang W et al. 2011. Serum microRNA characterization identifies miR-885-5p as a potential marker for detecting liver pathologies. *Clin Sci.* 120: 183–193 [PMID: 20815808].

Hayashi E, Kuramitsu Y, Okada F, Fujimoto M, Zhang X, Kobayashi M, Iizuka N, Ueyama Y, Nakamura K. 2005. Protoemics profiling for cancer progression differential display analysis for the expression of intracellular proteins between regressive and progressive cancer cell lines. *Proteomics* 5: 1024–1032 [PMID: 15712240].

Hoshida Y. 2011. Molecular signatures and prognosis of hepatocellular carcinoma. *Minerva Gastroenterol Dietol.* 57: 311–322 [PMID: 21769080].

Hu JS, Wu DW, Liang S, Miao XY. 2010. GP73, a resident Golgi glycoprotein, is sensibility and specificity for hepatocellular carcinoma of diagnosis in a hepatitis B-endemic Asian population. *Med Oncol.* 27: 339–345 [PMID: 19399652].

Imbeaud S, Ladeiro Y, Zucman-Rossi J. 2010. Identification of novel oncogenes and tumor suppressors in hepatocellular carcinoma. *Semin Liver Dis.* 30: 75–86 [PMID: 20175035].

Jain S, Singhal S, Lee P, Xu R. 2010. Molecular genetics of hepatocellular neoplasia. *Am J Transl Res.* 2: 105–118 [PMID: 20182587].

Joo M, Chi JG, Lee H. 2005. Expressions of HSP70 and HSP27 in hepatocellular carcinoma. *J Korean Med Sci.* 20: 829–834 [PMID: 16224158].

Ju MJ, Qiu SJ, Fan J, Zhou J, Gao Q, Cai MY, Li YW, Tang ZY. 2009. Preoperative serum gamma-glutamyl transferase to alanine aminotransferase ratio is a convenient prognostic marker for Child-Pugh A hepatocellular carcinoma after operation. *J Gastroenterol.* 44: 635–642 [PMID: 19387533].

Kandil D, Leiman G, Allegretta M, Trotman W, Pantanowitz L, Goulart R, Evans M. 2007. Glypican-3 immunocytochemistry in liver fine-needle aspirates: A novel stain to assist in the differentiation of benign and malignant liver lesions. *Cancer.* 111: 316–322 [PMID: 17763368].

Kohles N, Nagel D, Jüngst D, Durner J, Stieber P, Holdenrieder S. 2011. Relevance of circulating nucleosomes and oncological biomarkers for predicting response to transarterial chemoem-bolization therapy in liver cancer patients. *BMC Cancer* 11: 202 [PMID: 21615953].

Kohles N, Nagel D, Jüngst D, Durner J, Stieber P, Holdenrieder S. 2012. Prognostic relevance of oncological serum biomarkers in liver cancer patients undergoing transarterial chemo- embolization therapy. *Tumour Biol.* 33: 33–40 [PMID: 21931992].

Kojima K, Takata A, Vadnais C, Otsuka M, Yoshikawa T, Akanuma M, Kondo Y et al. 2011. MicroRNA122 is a key regulator of α-fetoprotein expression and influences the aggressiveness of hepatocellular carcinoma. *Nat Commun.* 2: 338 [PMID: 21654638].

Kusaba T. 1998. Relationship between Lens culinaris agglutinin reactive alpha- fetoprotein and biological features of hepatocellular carcinoma. *Kurume Med J.* 45: 113–120 [PMID: 9658760].

Lee D, Chung YH, Kim JA, Lee YS et al. 2012. Transforming growth factor beta 1 overexpression is closely related to invasiveness of hepatocellular carcinoma. *Oncology* 82: 11–18 [PMID: 22269311].

Lewis KA, Wuttke DS. 2012. Telomerase and telomere-associated proteins: Structural insights into mechanism and evolution. *Structure* 20: 28–39 [PMID: 22244753].

Li D, Mallory T, Satomura S. 2001. AFP-L3: A new generation of tumor marker for hepatocellular carcinoma. *Clin Chim Acta* 313: 15–19 [PMID: 11694234].

Liao SF, Yang HI, Lee MH, Chen CJ, Lee WC. 2012. Fifteen-year population attributable fractions and causal pies of risk factors for newly developed hepatocellular carcinomas in 11,801 men in Taiwan. *PLoS One* 7: e34779 [PMID: 22506050].

Lu WJ, Lee NP, Fatima S, Luk JM. 2009. Heat shock proteins in cancer: Signaling pathways, tumor markers and molecular targets in liver malignancy. *Protein Pept Lett.* 16: 508–516 [PMID: 19442230].

Luk JM, Lam CT, Siu AF, Lam BY, Ng IO, Hu MY, Che CM, Fan ST. 2006. Proteomic profiling of hepatocellular carcinoma in Chinese cohort reveals heat-shock proteins (Hsp27, Hsp70, GRP78) up-regulation and their associated prognostic values. *Proteomics* 6: 1049–1057 [PMID: 16400691].

Mao YL, Yang HY, Xu HF, Sang XT et al. 2008. Significance of Golgi glycoprotein 73, a new tumor marker in diagnosis of hepatocellular carcinoma: A primary study. *Chin Med J.* 88: 945–951 [PMID: 18756964].

Marubashi S, Nagano H, Wada H, Kobayashi S, Eguchi H, Takeda Y, Tanemura M, Umeshita K, Doki Y, Mori M. 2011. Clinical significance of alpha-fetoprotein mRNA in peripheral blood in liver resection for hepatocellular carcinoma. *Ann Surg Oncol.* 18: 2200–2209 [PMID: 21301972].

Miyaaki H, Nakashima O, Kurogi M, Eguchi K, Kojiro M. 2007. Lens culinaris agglutinin-reactive alpha-fetoprotein and protein induced by vitamin K absence II are potential indicators of a poor prognosis: A histopathological study of surgically resected hepatocellular carcinoma. *J Gastroenterol.* 42: 962–968 [PMID: 18085353].

Montaser LM, Abbas OM, Saltah AM, Waked IA. 2007. Circulating AFP mRNA as a possible indicator of hematogenous spread of HCC cells: A possible association with HBV infection. *J Egypt Natl Canc Inst.* 19: 48–60 [PMID: 18839035].

Morris SM, Baek JY, Koszarek A, Kanngurn S, Knoblaugh SE, Grady WM. 2012. Transforming growth factor-beta signaling promotes hepatocarcinogenesis induced by p53 loss. *Hepatology* 55: 121–131 [PMID: 21898503].

Morsi MI, Hussein AE, Mostafa M, El-Abd E, El-Moneim NA. 2006. Evaluation of tumour necrosis factor-alpha, soluble P-selectin, gamma-glutamyl transferase, glutathione S-transferase-pi and alpha-fetoprotein in patients with hepatocellular carcinoma before and during chemotherapy. *Br J Biomed Sci.* 63: 74–78 [PMID: 16871999].

Mu J, Wei LX. 2002. Telomere and telomerase in oncology. *Cell Res.* 12: 1–7 [PMID: 11942406].

Nassar A, Cohen C, Siddiqui MT. 2009. Utility of glypican-3 and survivin in differentiating hepatocellular carcinoma from benign and preneoplastic hepatic lesions and metastatic carcinomas in liver fine-needle aspiration biopsies. *Diagn Cytopathol.* 37: 629–635 [PMID: 19405109].

Nouso K, Kobayashi Y, Nakamura S, Kobayashi S, Takayama H, Toshimori J, Kuwaki K et al. 2011. Prognostic importance of fucosylated alpha-fetoprotein in hepatocellular carcinoma patients with low alpha-fetoprotein. *J Gastroenterol Hepatol.* 26: 1195–1200 [PMID: 21410750].

Oda K, Ido A, Tamai T, Matsushita M, Kumagai K, Mawatari S, Saishoji A et al. 2011. Highly sensitive lens culinaris agglutinin-reactive α-fetoprotein is useful for early detection of hepatocellular carcinoma in patients with chronic liver disease. *Oncol Rep.* 26: 1227–1233 [PMID: 21874252].

Qian J, Yao D, Dong Z, Wu W et al. 2010. Characteristics of hepatic IGF-II expression and monitored levels of circulating IGF-II mRNA in metastasis of hepatocellular carcinoma. *Am J Clin Pathol.* 134: 799–806 [PMID: 20959664].

Qiao SS, Cui ZQ, Gong L, Han H, Chen PC, Guo LM, Yu X et al. 2011. Simultaneous measurements of serum AFP, GPC-3 and HCCR for diagnosing hepatocellular carcinoma. *Hepatogastroenterology* 58: 1718–1724 [PMID: 21940340].

Qiu LW, Yao DF, Zong L, Lu YY, Huang H, Wu W, Wu XH. 2008. Abnormal expression of insulin- like growth factor-II and its dynamic quantitative analysis at different stages of hepatocellular carcinoma development. *Hepatobiliary Pancreat Dis Int.* 7: 406–411 [PMID: 18693177].

Qu KZ, Zhang K, Li H, Afdhal NH, Albitar M. 2011. Circulating microRNAs as biomarkers for hepatocellular carcinoma. *J Clin Gastroenterol.* 45: 355–360 [PMID: 21278583].

Rehem RN, El-Shikh WM. 2011. Serum IGF-1, IGF-2 and IGFBP-3 as parameters in the assessment of liver dysfunction in patients with hepatic cirrhosis and in the diagnosis of hepatocellular carcinoma. *Hepatogastroenterology* 58: 949–954 [PMID: 21830422].

Sakamoto M, Mori T, Masugi Y, Effendi K, Rie I, Du W. 2008. Candidate molecular markers for histological diagnosis of early hepatocellular carcinoma. *Intervirology* 51: 42–45 [PMID: 18544947].

Satyanarayana A, Manns MP, Rudolph KL. 2004. Telomeres and telomerase: A dual role in hepatocarcinogenesis. *Hepatology* 40: 276–283 [PMID: 15368430].

Scharf JG, Braulke T. 2003. The role of the IGF axis in hepatocarcinogenesis. *Horm Metab Res.* 35: 685–693 [PMID: 14710347].

Scharf JG, Dombrowski F, Ramadori G. 2001. The IGF axis and hepatocarcinogenesis. *Mol Pathol.* 54: 138–144 [PMID: 11376124].

Shafizadeh N, Ferrell LD, Kakar S. 2008. Utility and limitations of glypican-3 expression for the diagnosis of hepatocellular carcinoma at both ends of the differentiation spectrum. *Mod Pathol.* 21: 1011–1018 [PMID: 18536657].

Shirakawa H et al. 2009. Glypican-3 expression is correlated with poor prognosis in hepatocellular carcinoma. *Cancer Sci.* 100: 1403–1407 [PMID: 19496787].

Tang QY, Yao DF, Lu JX, Wu XH, Meng XY. 1999. Expression and alterations of different molecular form gamma-glutamyl transferase and total RNA concentration during the carcinogenesis of rat hepatoma. *World J Gastroenterol.* 5: 356–358 [PMID: 11819467].

Volk ML, Hernandez JC, Su GL, Lok AS, Marrero JA. 2007. Risk factors for hepatocellular carcinoma may impair the performance of biomarkers: A comparison of AFP, DCP, and AFP-L3. *Cancer Biomark.* 3: 79–87 [PMID: 17522429].

Wang HL, Anatelli F, Zhai QJ, Adley B, Chuang ST, Yang XJ. 2008. Glypican-3 as a useful diagnostic marker that distinguishes hepatocellular carcinoma from benign hepatocellular mass lesions. *Arch Pathol Lab Med.* 132: 1723–1728 [PMID: 18976006].

Wang NY, Zhang D, Zhao W, Fang GX, Shi YL, Duan MH. 2009. Clinical application of an enzyme-linked immunosorbent assay detecting hepatoma-specific gamma-glutamyl transferase. *Hepatol Res.* 39: 979–987 [PMID: 19624768].

Wang Z, Ruan YB, Guan Y, Liu SH. 2003. Expression of IGF-II in early experimental hepatocellular carcinomas and its significance in early diagnosis. *World J Gastroenterol.* 9: 267–270 [PMID: 12532445].

West MB, Hanigan MH. 2010. γ-Glutamyl transpeptidase is a heavily N-glycosylated heterodimer in HepG2 cells. *Arch Biochem Biophys.* 504: 177–181 [PMID: 20831856].

Wong VW, Chan HL. 2012. Prevention of hepatocellular carcinoma: A concise review of contemporary issues. *Ann Hepatol.* 11: 284–293 [PMID: 22481445].

Wu W, Yao DF, Qiu LW, Wu XH, Yao M, Su XQ, Zou L. 2005. Abnormal expression of hepatomas and circulating telomerase and its clinical values. *Hepatobiliary Pancreat Dis Int.* 4: 544–549 [PMID: 16286259].

Wu W, Yao DF, Yuan YM, Fan JW, Lu XF, Li XH, Qiu LW, Zong L, Wu XH. 2006. Combined serum hepatoma-specific alpha-fetoprotein and circulating alpha- fetoprotein-mRNA in diagnosis of hepatocellular carcinoma. *Hepatobiliary Pancreat Dis Int.* 5: 538–544 [PMID: 17085339].

Wu XH, Yao DF, Su XQ, Tai BJ, Huang H, Qiu LW, Wu W, Shao YX. 2007. Dynamic expression of rat heat shock protein gp96 and its gene during development of hepatocellular carcinoma. *Hepatobiliary Pancreat Dis Int.* 6: 616–621 [PMID: 18086628].

Yamazaki K, Masugi Y, Sakamoto M. 2011. Molecular pathogenesis of hepatocellular carcinoma: Altering transforming growth factor-β signaling in hepatocarcinogenesis. *Dig Dis.* 29: 284–288 [PMID: 21829019].

Yan D, He Q, Chen Y, Wang L, Zhang X. 2011. Detection of α-fetoprotein and glypican-3 mRNAs in the peripheral blood of hepatocellular carcinoma patients by using multiple FQ-RT-PCR. *J Clin Lab Anal.* 25: 113–117 [PMID: 21438004].

Yan J, Lu Q, Dong J, Li X, Ma K, Cai L. 2012. Hepatitis B virus X protein suppresses caveolin-1 expression in hepatocellular carcinoma by regulating DNA methylation. *BMC Cancer* 12: 353 [PMID: 22894556].

Yang JD, Roberts LR. 2010. Hepatocellular carcinoma: A global view. *Nat Rev Gastroenterol Hepatol.* 7: 449–458 [PMID: 20628345].

Yao DF, Dong ZZ. 2007. Hepatoma-related gamma-glutamyl transferase in laboratory or clinical diagnosis of hepatocellular carcinoma. *Hepatobiliary Pancreat Dis Int.* 6: 9–11 [PMID: 17287158].

Yao DF, Dong ZZ, Liu YH, Zhao L, Huang JF, Meng XY. 2003. Amplification of peripheral blood insulin-like growth factor II-mRNA and its clinical significance in the diagnosis of hepatocellular carcinoma. *Zhonghua GanZangBing Za Zhi* 11: 695–696 [PMID: 14636457].

Yao DF, Dong ZZ, Yao DB, Wu XH, Wu W, Qiu LW, Wang HM, Meng XY. 2004. Abnormal expression of hepatoma-derived gamma-glutamyltransferase subtyping and its early alteration for carcinogenesis of hepatocytes. *Hepatobiliary Pancreat Dis Int.* 3: 564–570 [PMID: 15567746].

Yao DF, Huang ZW, Chen SZ, Huang JF, Lu JX, Xiao MB, Meng XY. 1998. Diagnosis of hepatocellular carcinoma by quantitative detection of hepatoma-specific bands of serum gamma- glutamyltransferase. *Am J Clin Pathol.* 110: 743–749 [PMID: 9844586].

Yao DF, Jiang DR, Huang ZW, Lu JX, Tao QY, Yu ZJ, Meng X. 2000. Abnormal expressiom of hepatoma specific γ-glutamyl transferase and alteration of γ-glutamyl transferase gene methylation status in patients with hepatocellular carcinoma. *Cancer* 88: 761–769 [PMID: 10679644].

Yao DF, Wu XH, Su XQ, Yao M, Wu W, Qiu LW, Zou L, Meng XY. 2006a. Abnormal expression of HSP gp96 associated with HBV replication in human hepatocellular carcinoma. *Hepatobiliary Pancreat Dis Int.* 5: 381–386 [PMID: 16911935].

Yao DF, Wu W, Yao M, Qiu LW, Wu XH, Su XQ, Zou L, Yao DB, Meng XY. 2006b. Dynamic alteration of telomerase expression and its diagnostic significance in liver or peripheral blood for hepatocellular carcinoma. *World J Gastroenterol.* 12: 4966–4972 [PMID:16937491].

Yao M, Yao DF, Bian YZ, Zhang CG, Qiu LW, Wu W, Sai WL, Yang JL, Zhang HJ. 2011. Oncofetal antigen glypican-3 as a promising early diagnostic marker for hepatocellular carcinoma. *Hepatobiliary Pancreat Dis Int.* 10: 289–294 [PMID: 21669573].

Yoshida S, Kurokohchi K, Arima K, Masaki T et al. 2002. Clinical significance of lens culinaris agglutinin-reactive fraction of serum alpha-fetoprotein in patients with hepatocellular carcinoma. *Int J Oncol.* 20: 305–309 [PMID: 11788893].

Yu ZJ, Yu JW, Cai W, Yuan HX, Li XY, Yuan Y, Chen JP, Wu XY, Yao DF. 2005. Evaluation of HCPTd1, d14-double passaged intervening chemotherapy protocol for hepatocellular carcinoma. *World J Gastroenterol.* 11: 5221–5225 [PMID: 16127757].

Yuen MF, Lai CL. 2005. Serological markers of liver cancer. *Best Pract Res Clin Gastroenterol.* 19: 91–99 [PMID: 15757806].

Zhang JB, Chen Y, Zhang B, Xie X, Zhang L, Ge N, Ren Z, Ye SL. 2011. Prognostic significance of serum gamma-glutamyl transferase in patients with intermediate hepatocellular carcinoma treated with transcatheter arterial chemoembolization. *Eur J Gastroenterol Hepatol.* 23: 787–793 [PMID: 21730869].

Zhang Y, Li J, Cao L, Xu W, Yin Z. 2012. Circulating tumor cells in hepatocellular carcinoma: Detection techniques, clinical implications, and future perspectives. *Semin Oncol.* 39: 449–460 [PMID: 22846862].

Zhang Y, Li Q, Liu N, Song T, Liu Z, Guo R, Meng L. 2008. Detection of MAGE-1, MAGE-3 and AFP mRNA as multimarker by real-time quantitative PCR assay: A possible predictor of hematogenous micrometastasis of hepatocellular carcinoma. *Hepatogastroenterology* 55: 2200–2206 [PMID: 19260505].

Zinkin NT, Grall F, Bhaskar K, Otu HH, Spentzos D, Kalmowitz B, Wells M et al. 2008. Serum proteomics and biomarkers in hepatocellular carcinoma and chronic liver disease. *Clin Cancer Res.* 14: 470–477 [PMID: 18223221].

16

Noninvasive Early Markers in Gallbladder Cancer

Mumtaz Ahmad Ansari, Ruhi Dixit, and Vijay Kumar Shukla

CONTENTS

16.1 Introduction

Gallbladder cancer (GBC) is the most common biliary tree cancer in the world, but it is only 0.5% of all gastrointestinal cancers with lethal malignancy and marked ethnic and geographical variations. The presenting symptoms are typically vague so patient presents in advanced stage. The overall mean survival rate for patients with advanced GBC is 6 months, with a 5-year survival rate of 5% (Levy et al. 2001). Early GBC (confined to the mucosa), though infrequent, offers the potential for a cure by cholecystectomy. Most (>80%) GBCs are adenocarcinomas that originate from the fundus (60%), body (30%), or neck (10%). The basis likely is genetic susceptibility, perhaps elicited by chronic gallbladder inflammation, often a product of cholelithiasis (Pandey 2003). One reasonable hypothesis focuses on chronic irritation of the mucosa (e.g., from the physical presence of the stones and/or superimposed chronic infection such as from *Salmonella typhi*) leading to dysplasia (perhaps abetted by mutagenic secondary bile acids) and terminating in malignant change.

16.2 Risk Factors

The risk factors for developing GBC therefore include ethnicity, genetic susceptibility, lifestyle factors, and infections. If we see globally, GBC has a low occurrence, <2/100,000, but has a wide variance like in the United States, it only accounts for 0.5% of all gastrointestinal malignancies, accounting for less than 5,000 cases per year (1–2.5/100,000). High annual incidence rates occur in North and South American Indians, generating an inordinate mortality, particularly among women: 15.5/100,000 versus 7.5/100,000 in men from La Paz, Bolivia, and 11.3/100,000 in women versus 4/100,000 in men from New Mexico. Hence, carcinoma of the gallbladder is the leading cause of cancer death in Chilean women, exceeding even breast, lung, and cervical cancers (Serra et al. 1989, Andia et al. 2008). Other high-risk regions are scattered through eastern Europe (14/100,000 in Poland), northern India (as high as 21.5/100,000 for women from Delhi), and south Pakistan (11.3/100,000) (Lazcano-Ponce et al. 2001, Randi et al. 2006). Intermediate incidences (3.7–9.1/100,000) occur elsewhere in South Americans of Indian descent and in Israel (5/100,000) and Japan (7/100,000) (Lazcano-Ponce et al. 2001). The frequency is increasing in Shanghai, China, and now accounts for the most frequent gastrointestinal malignancy and is a substantial cause of mortality (Hsing et al. 2007).

Although the majority of the world has decreasing mortality trends in GBC, Iceland, Costa Rica, and Korea have an increase in mortality for men (Hariharan et al. 2008). There appears to be a modest decline in prevalence over the past two decades (National Cancer Institute: Surveillance, Epidemiology and End Results [SEER] Program). Worldwide, GBC affects females two to three times more frequently than males. To some extent, this distinct gender bias has been attributed to the prevalence of cholelithiasis, which is more pronounced in females (Gabbi et al. 2010). Although the exact etiology of GBC remains indistinct, several factors are known to increase the risk including cholelithiasis, chronic cholecystitis (CC), calcified "porcelain" gallbladder, choledochal cysts, anomalous pancreatobiliary duct junction, and gallbladder polyps (Table 16.1). A number of dietary factors, chronic gallbladder infections, and

TABLE 16.1

Risk Factors for Gallstone Disease

Not Modifiable	Modifiable
Family history	Obesity/metabolic syndrome/diabetes mellitus/dyslipidemia
Genetic predilection	Drugs—ceftriaxone, octreotide, thiazide diuretics, female sex hormones
Ethnic background	Reduced physical activity
Female sex	Rapid weight loss
Age	TPN
	Diet
	Underlying disease: cirrhosis, Crohn's disease

TPN, total parental nutrition.

TABLE 16.2
Risk Factors for GBC

Cancer Risk Factor	Relative Risk	Reference
Gallstones	3.01–23.8	Chow et al. (1999)
		Ishiguro et al. (2008)
		Zatonski et al. (1992)
		Khan et al. (1999)
		Hsing et al. (2007)
Size of gallstones		
2.0–2.9 cm	2.4	Diehl (1983)
>3.0	9.2–10.1	Lowenfels et al. (1989)
Duration of gallstones		
5–19 year	4.9	Zatonski et al. (1997)
>20 year		
BMI	Men/Women	Calle et al. (2002)
30.0–34.9	1.8/2.1	
Infections		
Chronic typhoid and paratyphoid carriers	12.7–16.7	Caygill et al. (1994)
Helicobacter bilis	2.6–6.5	Strom et al. (1995)

environmental exposure to specific chemicals have also been associated with the development of GBC (Srivastava et al. 2011). Increasing risk factors for gallstone diseases like modifiable factors also contribute to development of GBC (Table 16.1). Gender differences exist with geographic variances, generally being unfavorable for women. In those locals with the highest incidence, women have frequency rates greater than men. With age, GBC increases. Size of gallstones and duration of gallstone disease also raise risk to develop cancer. Increased obesity and repeated salmonella infection too increase the risk of GBC (Caygill et al. 1994, Zatonski et al. 1997, Chow et al. 1999, Stinton and Shaffer 2012). Various modifiable and nonmodifiable risk factors have been listed (Table 16.2).

16.3 Genetic Predisposition in GBC

There are undoubtedly genetic and environmental factors that coincide to become expressed as GBC. A family history of GBC is clearly a risk factor (Goldgar et al. 1994, Hemminki and Li 2003). The only responsible gene so far identified seems to be that for apolipoprotein B function (the APOB gene), which influences cholesterol handling yet is not associated with gallstones. In fact, the link between cholesterol, gallstones, and GBC may relate to an interdependent disposal pathway that increases the export of both cholesterol and environmental toxins into bile. As GBC is more common in women, such mutagenic toxins secreted reside longer in the gallbladder due to stasis from impaired contractility associated with the female hormone progesterone. This protracted exposure allows environmental carcinogens to then cause malignant transformation, helping to reconcile the schism of seed versus soil and incorporate the predilection to the development of gallstones (also requiring some gallbladder stasis) and GBC (Venniyoor 2008).

GBC has familial predisposition. The nationwide Swedish Cancer Registry reported high risk for familial GBC and also found maternal transmission favoring over paternal (Hemminki and Li 2003). Another Utah Cancer Registry estimated 26% familial GBC (Jackson et al. 2007). These data suggest a possible role of genetic component in gallbladder carcinogenesis (Lichtenstein et al. 2000). The most frequent molecular alterations in GBC are the mutations in TP53 and K-ras gene, along with loss of cell-cycle regulation, microsatellite instability, and loss of heterozygosity (LOH) (Wistuba and Albores-Saavedra 1999) (Table 16.3). However, most of these mutations account for a small proportion of cases with GBC. Epidemiological studies have identified the role of various low-penetrance variants in GBC susceptibility (Srivastava et al. 2011); however, many more genes with modest effects and their interactions with each

TABLE 16.3

Level of Risk According to Cumulative Risk Factors

Factors	Risk Level
Age: >65 years; exposures: obesity, diabetes, tobacco, estrogen, total carbohydrate intake, 3-methylcholanthrene, nitrosamines, and radon; K-ras, TP53, CDKN2A, and mtDNA D310 mutations; ERBB2, PTGS2, cyclin D1, and cyclin E overexpression; FHIT abnormalities; previous history of GB disease (gallstones, CC, porcelain GB, primary sclerosing cholangitis); increasing number of pregnancies (usu. >5); parity; family history of GBC	Low (<5-fold)
Ethnicity: populations from western parts of the Andes, North American Indians, Mexican Americans, Chile, and Northern India; gender: female; exposures: chronic infection (*S. typhi*, *Salmonella paratyphi*, *H. bilis*, *Helicobacter pylori*)	Moderate (5–10-fold)
Congenital malformation (APBDJ)	High (<10-fold)

APBDJ, anomalous pancreatobiliary duct junction; CC, chronic cholecystitis; GB, gallbladder.

other and with environment are yet to be discovered. Nonetheless, a recent genome-wide association study (GWAS) in the Japanese population (Cha et al. 2012) has identified a single nucleotide polymorphism (SNP) in the deleted in colorectal cancer (DCC) gene to be implicated in GBC.

16.4 Diagnostic Imaging in GBC

Ultrasound, CT scans, MRI, MRCP, MR angiography (Figures 16.1 and 16.2)

Endoscopic retrograde cholangiopancreatography (ERCP)

Percutaneous transhepatic cholangiography

Endoscopic and laparoscopic ultrasound

Diagnostic laparoscopy

Guided biopsies

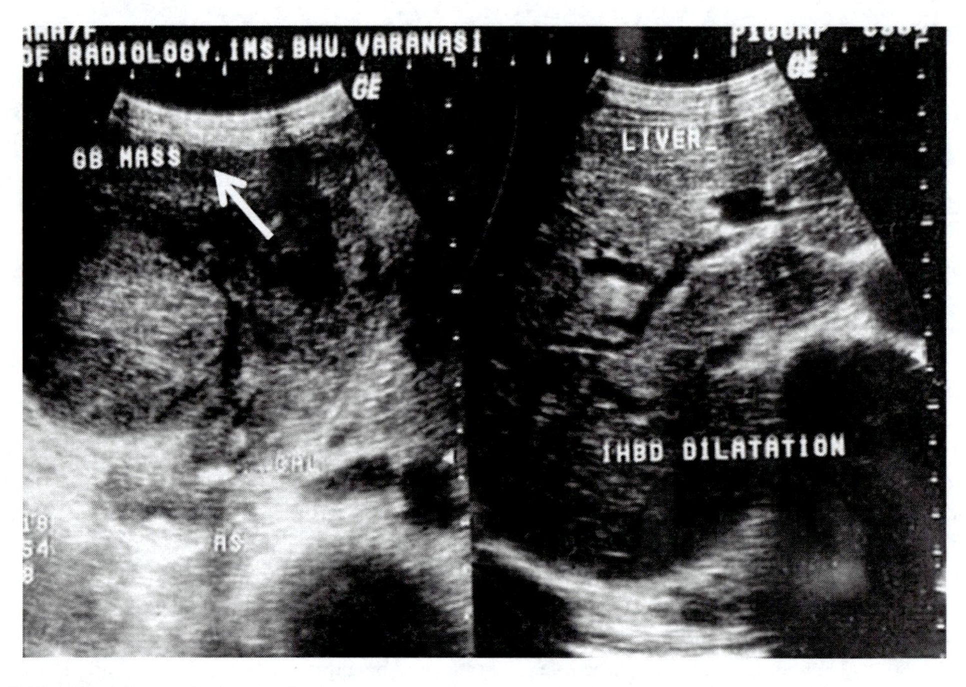

FIGURE 16.1 Ultrasound showing GBC mass.

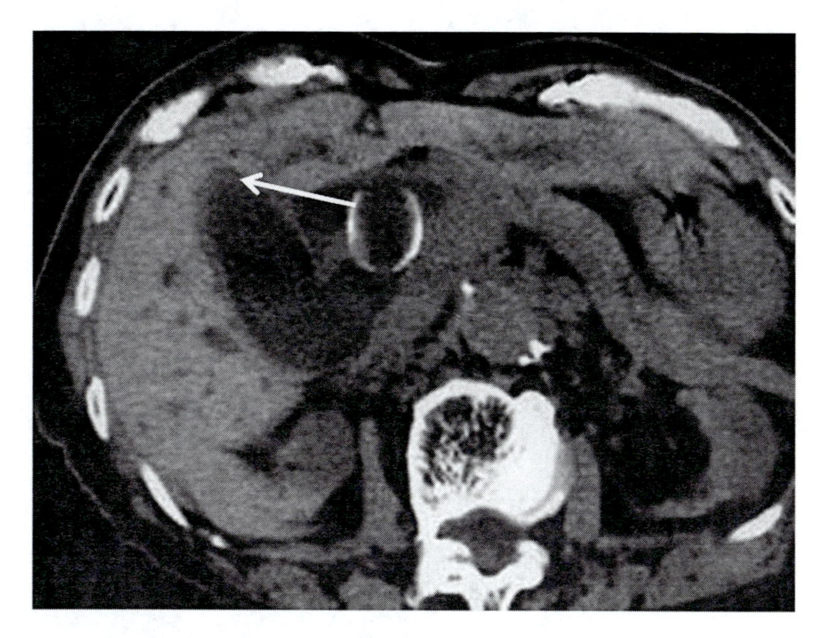

FIGURE 16.2 CT scan showing GBC mass.

16.5 Biomarkers in GBC

Carcinoma of the gallbladder progresses from dysplasia to carcinoma in situ (CIS) advancing to invasive carcinoma in approximately 15 years (Roa et al. 1996). It usually presents as a mass of GBC (Figure 16.3). Despite recent advances and enthusiastic progress toward identifying potential biomarkers for early diagnosis and management, GBC remains a challenging tumor with an overall poor prognosis. So some noninvasive biomarkers are required for early detection of GBC.

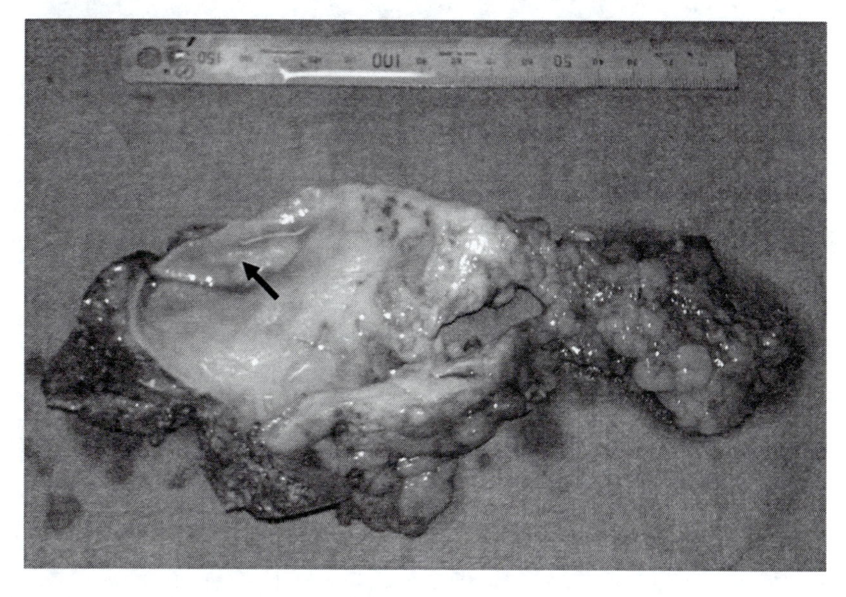

FIGURE 16.3 Photograph of gross specimen of GBC.

There are different types of GBC: adenocarcinoma (well-differentiated, moderately differentiated, and poorly differentiated adenocarcinoma), squamous cell carcinoma, adenosquamous cell carcinoma, CIS, small cell carcinoma, sarcomas, and papillary cancer (Figures 16.4 and 16.5).

Biomarker is a protein whose detection indicates a particular disease state. More specifically, a "biomarker" indicates a change in expression or state of a protein that correlates with the risk or progression of a disease or with the susceptibility of the disease to a given treatment. Biomarkers can

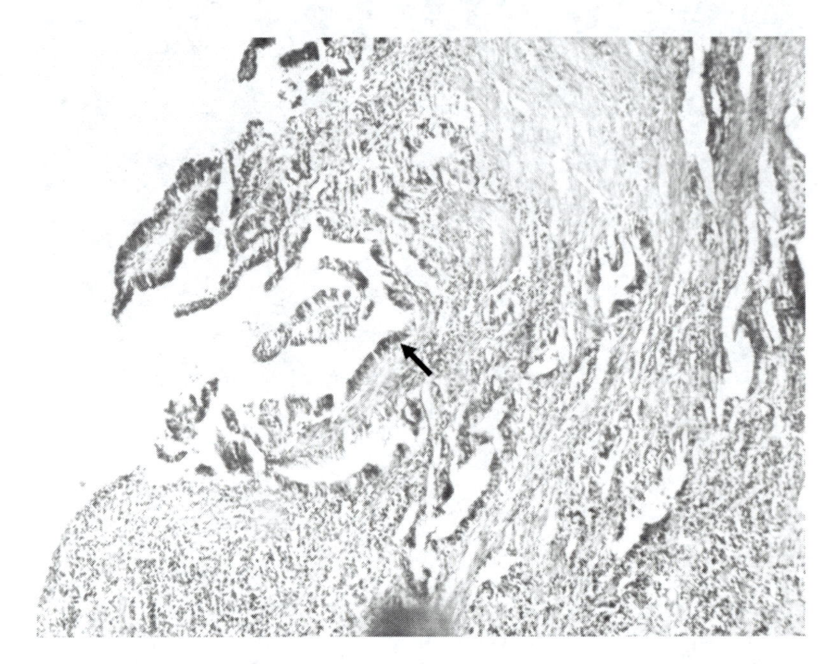

FIGURE 16.4 Well-differentiated adenocarcinoma of the gallbladder infiltrating the muscularis (HXE stain 100×).

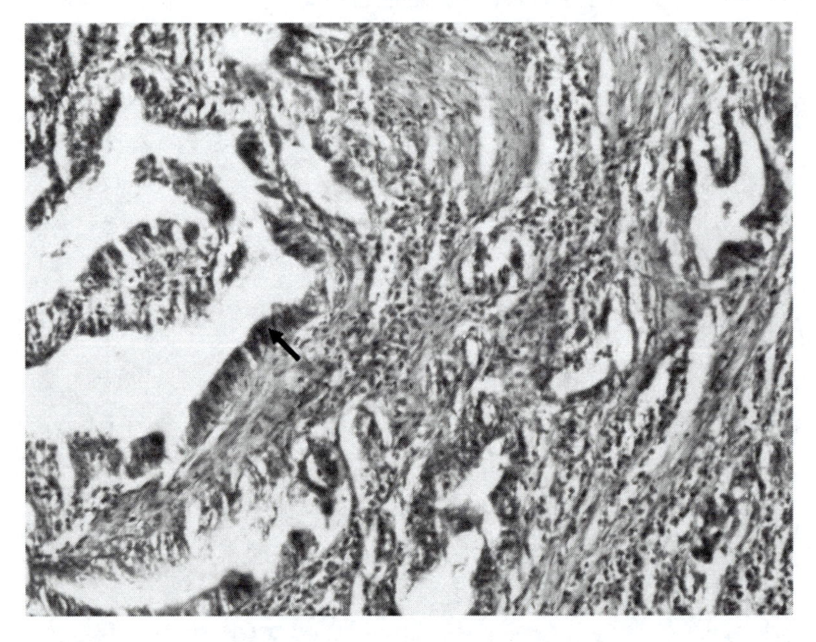

FIGURE 16.5 **(See color insert.)** Well-differentiated adenocarcinoma of the gallbladder infiltrating the muscularis (HXE stain 200×).

be predictive or prognostic. The predictive marker predicts response to treatment like estrogen receptors in breast cancer, while prognostic marker determines prognosis like lymph node status in breast cancer.

A tumor marker is a substance expressed either by a tumor or by the host body in response to a tumor that helps in cancer detection and monitoring. These markers can be normal endogenous products that are produced at a greater rate in cancer cells or the products of newly switched on genes that remained quiescent in the normal cells. A tumor marker produced by the tumor, when present in significant amounts, indicates the presence of a cancer. They may be present as intracellular substances in tissues or may be released into the circulation and appear in serum (Harnden 1985, Bates and Longo 1987, Virji et al. 1988). Along with the serum, other body fluids such as urine, effusions, saliva, cerebrospinal fluid (CSF), and nipple discharge can also be used for evaluation of tumor markers.

Various biomarkers have already been found to be useful in the evaluation of carcinoma of the gallbladder. Important ones are CA242, CA19-9, CA15-3, CA125, CA50, CA72-4, carcinoembryonic antigen (CEA), mucins, proliferating cell nuclear antigen (PCNA), receptor-binding cancer antigen expressed on SiSo cells (RCAS1) (Enjoji et al. 2004, Shukla et al. 2006), and arginase (Shukla et al. 2009) (Table 16.4).

16.5.1 Serological Marker

16.5.1.1 CA19-9

CA19-9 is a first choice biomarker in the gallbladder. It is a 210 kDa tumor-associated glycoprotein antigen present as carbohydrate determinant on glycolipid and glycoprotein. CA19-9 is characterized by monoclonal antibody 1116-NS 19-9 by immunizing BALB/c mice with human colorectal cancer cell line. This antibody reacts with a carbohydrate antigenic determinant (CA19-9) that has been identified as a sialylated lacto-N fucopentaose II, an oligosaccharide sharing structural features with Lewis blood group substances. Appreciable concentration of CA19-9 is also present in mucin-rich saliva, seminal fluid, gastric juice, amniotic fluid, urine, ovarian cyst fluid, pancreatic, gallbladder, and duodenal aspirate (Malati 2007). Shukla et al. studied CA242, CA19-9, CA15-3, and CA125 assay preoperatively in the serum of 39 patients with carcinoma of the gallbladder, 16 patients with cholelithiasis, and 8 healthy controls using the enzyme-linked immunosorbent assay (ELISA) technique. CA19-9 level was 86.06 μm/mL in patients with cholelithiasis as compared to 211.27 μm/mL in patients with GBC, the difference being statistically significant (Shukla et al. 2006). Combining CA19-9 and CA125 gave accuracy of 80.65% in the diagnosis of GBC (Shukla et al. 2006). Sensitivity and specificity of CA19-9 alone and along with CA125, CA15-3, CA242, and CA125 have been listed in Table 16.5.

Akdogan et al. have also shown association of CA19-9 in malignant obstructive jaundice (Akdoğan et al. 2003). Rumalla et al. showed elevated levels of CA19-9 in GBC and found the values of >100 μm/mL in GBC (Rumalla and Petersen 2000).

Noshiro et al., in a retrospective study of 56 patients with GBC, found CA19-9 to be elevated in 30% of the patients. In a univariate analysis, they found it to affect prognosis in these patients (Noshiro et al. 2003). Tasaki et al. reported a case of GBC who had undergone cholecystectomy 5 years ago and reported to them with raised CA19-9 level (136 μm/mL), 5 years after surgery. Investigations later on showed patient had metastasis from GBC. CA19-9 level returned to normal after extrahepatic bile duct resection and lymphadenectomy (Tasaki et al. 2003).

The immunohistochemical expression of CA19-9 in gallbladder lesions was studied by Roa et al. (1992). CA19-9 staining was found to be positive in over 90% of cancer. CA19-9 has been found to have a progressively increasing expression in the various degrees of dysplasia (Pingitore et al. 1992). Stefanovic et al. found CA19-9 to be of most clinical significance as it was increased in CIS and stage I GBC (Stefanovic et al. 1993).

16.5.1.2 RCAS1

RCAS1 is a type II membrane protein that is expressed by a variety of human cancer cells. Expression of RCAS1 inhibits growth and induces apoptosis in immune cell such as T, B, and natural killer (NK) cells (Nakashima et al. 1999). Immunohistochemical studies have shown that RCAS1 is expressed

TABLE 16.4

Carcinoma of the Gallbladder and Different Noninvasive Biomarkers

	Biomarkers
Serological biomarkers of carcinoma of the gallbladder	CA242
	CA19-9
	CA15-3
	CA125
	CA50
	CA72-4
	Mucins
	PCNA
	RCAS1
	Arginase
	Carcinoembryonic antigen (CEA)
Molecular biomarkers of carcinoma of the gallbladder	p53
	p16INK4/CDKN2
	K-ras mutations
	LOH
	Mutation in FHIT gene
	Polypeptide (CD antigen)
	HER2/neu
	Heat shock protein
	Chromosomal aberrations
	COX enzymes
	APC gene
	HLA
	Growth factor
	Angiogenesis/VEGF
Others	Pteridines
	cFNA
	Mitochondria DNA copy number
	Plasma membrane proteins
	Autoantibody signatures
	Circulating tumor cells
	Laminin-5γ2 (TME biomarker)
	miRNAs
	E-cadherin expression
	Vimentin
	Somatostatin
	Gastrin
	Human chorionic gonadotropin, serotonin, and pancreatic polypeptide

with a high frequency in uterine, ovarian, and lung cancers and that expression of this antigen correlates with a poor prognosis (Sasaki 1989, Pingitore et al. 1992, Roa et al. 1992, Stefanovic et al. 1993). Enjoji et al. have reported RCAS1 expression in a high percentage of biliary carcinomas (88.7%) (Enjoji et al. 2002).

Oshikiri et al. studied RCAS1 expression by immunohistochemistry in 60 patients with EBDC (extra hepatic bile duct cancer). High expression of RCAS1 was detected in 76.7% cases. High RCAS1 expression was an independent negative predictor for survival (Oshikiri et al. 2001). Sensitivity and specificity are 74.4% and 91%, respectively (Table 16.5).

TABLE 16.5
Sensitivity and Specificity in Selected Tumor Markers in GBC

Tumor Marker	Sensitivity (%)	Specificity (%)	Source	Reference
CA19-9				
Alone	77.5	68.7	Serum	Shukla et al. (2006)
Combination with CA125	75	90.9	Serum	Shukla et al. (2006)
Combination with CA15-3	70	91.7	Serum	Shukla et al. (2006)
Combination with CA242	73.1	86.7	Serum	Shukla et al. (2006)
Combination with CA125 and CA15-3	84.6	88.8	Serum	Shukla et al. (2006)
RCAS1	74.4	91.0	Tissue	Enjoji et al. (2002)
			Tissue	Enjoji et al. (2004)
CA125				
Alone	64	90	Tissue	Chaube et al. (2006)
Combination with CA15-3	65.2	84.6	Serum	Shukla et al. (2006)
Combination with CA242	87.5	85.7	Serum	Shukla et al. (2006)
CA242				
Alone	64	83	Tissue	Rana et al. (2012)
Combination with CA15-3	73.7	84.6	Serum	Shukla et al. (2006)
CEA	61	44	Tissue	Rana et al. (2012)
Mac-2BP	69	67	Serum	Koopmann et al. (2004)

Note: CA, carbohydrate antigen; CEA, carcinoembryonic antigen; RCAS1, receptor-binding cancer antigen expressed on SiSo cells; Mac-2BP, macrophage galactose-specific lectin-2 binding protein.

16.5.1.3 CA125

CA125 is a tumor-associated glycoprotein of more than 200 kDa. It was detected by using murine monoclonal antibody OC125 generated by immunization against histologically well-defined ovarian adenocarcinoma cell line (Bast et al. 1981, Magnani et al. 1982, Davis et al. 1986, O'Brien et al. 1991).

CA125 level was significantly higher in patients with GBC (253.6 μm/mL) as compared to patients with cholelithiasis (65.5 μm/mL) ($p < 0.05$). Combining CA125 with CA19-9 gave a diagnostic accuracy of 80.65% (Shukla et al. 2006). Chaube et al. measured CA125 level in 64 patients with GBC, 47 patients with gallstone disease, and 23 healthy volunteers. It found a cutoff value of 11 μm/mL that yielded sensitivity and specificity of 64% and 90%, respectively, and in combination with CA15-3 and CA242, as listed in Table 16.5 (Chaube et al. 2006). Though CA125 is a relatively nonspecific marker of malignancy as it is raised in different type of neoplasm, it holds promise in combination with other tumor markers (Table 16.5).

16.5.1.4 CA15-3

CA15-3 is a heterogeneous 300 kDa glycoprotein antigen. It is elevated in serum in patients with carcinoma of the breast. This marker has not been extensively evaluated in GBC; however, Atkinson BF reported significantly elevated levels of CA15-3 in patients with carcinoma of the gallbladder (Atkinson et al. 1982). These results need to be validated in larger studies to establish its usefulness in early detection of carcinoma of the gallbladder (Table 16.5).

16.5.1.5 CA242

CA242 antigen is defined by a monoclonal antibody, which was obtained by immunizing mice with a human colorectal carcinoma cell line (COLO 205) (Lindholm et al. 1983). The chemical structure of the antigenic determinant is not exactly described, but it seems to be a sialylated carbohydrate structure, possibly a type I chain (Johansson et al. 1991a). CA242 is related, but not identical, to the epitope of CA19-9 and CA50 (Johansson et al. 1991b). CA242 is found on the same macromolecular mucin complex as CA19-9. Shukla et al. found significantly high serum level of CA242 (42.19 µm/mL) in carcinoma of the gallbladder as compared to 12.10 µm/mL in cholelithiasis (Shukla et al. 2006). A high positive correlation between CA242 values and serum bilirubin or alkaline phosphatase levels has also been earlier reported (Pasanen et al. 1995). Therefore, when interpreting the serum CA242 values, more research is needed to evaluate its usefulness in GBC. Sensitivity and specificity of CA242 alone and in combination with CA15-3 are listed in Table 16.5.

16.5.1.6 CA50

CA50 can be used to differentiate between benign and malignant diseases of the gallbladder. Sera from patients with diseases in the pancreas, gallbladder, and bile duct were analyzed for the tumor marker CA-50, and it was found to be valuable in differentiating malignant from benign disease in the gallbladder. Though the usefulness of this marker is well established in pancreatic cancer, not much work has been done in GBC (Johnson et al. 1991).

16.5.1.7 CA72-4

Analysis of CA72-4 gives an opportunity for improvement in the detection of cancers of the pancreatobiliary system. Bile from resected gallbladders of patients suffering from carcinomas of the pancreatobiliary system was analyzed for CA72-4 and CA125. CA72-4 antigen in gallbladder bile was found to be superior to any serum and pancreatic juice examination with respect to sensitivity and specificity (Brockmann et al. 2000). CA72-4 was found to be of most important clinical significance and was increased in CIS and carcinoma of the first stage (Stefanovic et al. 1993).

16.5.1.8 Arginase

Arginase is a manganese-containing enzyme. The reaction catalyzed by this enzyme is arginine + $H_2O \rightarrow$ ornithine + urea. It is the final enzyme of the urea cycle. Stage III gallbladder carcinoma showed maximum tissue arginase activity (142.00 ± 21.68 unit/g of tissue) followed by stage II (15 ± 19.88) and stage I (108.46 ± 6.73). The increase in tissue arginase activity was statistically significant ($p < 0.05$) from stage I to stage II and from stage I to stage III (Shukla et al. 2009).

16.5.1.9 Carcinoembryonic Antigen

The cellular demonstration of CEA and its role in the diagnosis of premalignant and malignant lesions of the intestinal tract has been well established (Bordes et al. 1973, Isaacson 1976, O'Brien et al. 1981). The progression from normal tissue to invasive adenocarcinoma results in increased levels of serum CEA (Strom et al. 1989).

Okami et al. (2000) evaluated the role of RT-polymerase chain reaction (PCR)-based CEA mRNA evaluation to detect micrometastasis in lymph nodes from biliary tract cancers (BTCs).

Kanthan et al. (2000) evaluated CEA expression by immunohistochemistry and found a positive CEA staining in 89% of carcinoma and 84% of the in situ lesions. The moderate to strong staining was associated with a mean survival of 10.6 months in 76% of the cases (Kanthan et al. 2000). Dowaki et al. (2000) examined CEA expression in human gallbladder adenocarcinomas and its clinicopathological significance. Lymph node metastasis was frequently found in the cytoplasmic CEA- and stromal CEA-positive GBCs (44.1% and 62.5%, respectively) (Dowaki et al. 2000). The sensitivity and specificity alone and in combination with Mac-2BP are listed in Table 16.5.

16.5.1.10 Mucins

Mucins are a group of high molecular weight glycoproteins consisting of a mucin core protein and O-linked carbohydrates. To date, nine apomucins (MUCl–8 and MUC5B) have been identified. Recent studies have demonstrated that MUC1 is expressed in tumors of various human organs and may function as an antiadhesion molecule that inhibits cell-to-cell adhesion, inducing tumor metastasis (Kashiwagi et al. 2001). Kashiwagi et al. examined MUC1 and MUC2 expression in human gallbladder adenocarcinoma. MUC1 immunoreactivity was detected in the cancer cells and in the cancer stroma and was significantly related to lymphatic invasion, lymph node metastasis ($p < 0.001$), and a poor outcome. On the other hand, MUC2 was rarely expressed and had no prognostic significance with its immunoreactivity detected only in the cancer goblet cells (Kashiwagi et al. 2001).

16.5.1.11 Proliferating Cell Nuclear Antigen

PCNA positivity rate is an indicator of cell proliferation activity and, hence, indirect measure of cell kinetics. Isozaki et al. studied PCNA expression in GBC patients with pancreaticobiliary maljunction (PBM) and found a 14.2% positivity rate in cancerous lesion with maljunction compared to 3.9% among cancer patients with normal pancreaticobiliary junction. They further observed an 11.6% positivity rate among noncancer patients with maljunction and 1.5% positivity among normal subjects (Isozaki et al. 1997). These findings suggest higher cell kinetics in cancerous gallbladder compared to normal gallbladder and a higher turnover among patients with anomalous pancreaticobiliary junction with or without carcinoma. They presented a strong case for maljunction to be a possible etiological factor as no attempt was made to correlate these findings with survival; hence, the effect of cell kinetics on outcome of patients with GBC in their study is unknown.

Lee et al. studied PCNA and MIB-1 indices in patients with CC and GBC. Both were significantly higher ($p < 0.001$) in both moderately and poorly differentiated carcinoma of the gallbladder. Similarly, cases of ampullary and GBC in situ had significantly lower PCNA and MIB-1 indices than the invasive carcinoma cases ($p < 0.001$) (Lee 1996). Qing et al. found PCNA index to be significantly higher in malignant lesions than in benign ones (Qing et al. 1995).

E-cadherin expression has been demonstrated in 17/49 cases of GBC (Wistuba et al. 1995a). This expression was not found to correlate with age, sex, tumor dimension, grading, and lymph node status (Sasatomi et al. 1993).

Vimentin, somatostatin, gastrin, human chorionic gonadotropin, serotonin, and pancreatic polypeptide have also been studied; however, their exact role in gallbladder carcinogenesis is not clear.

16.5.2 Molecular Basis

16.5.2.1 p53

Molecular studies in several neoplasms have demonstrated their association with the activation of dominant proto-oncogenes and inactivation of recessive tumor suppressor genes. Tumor suppressor genes are frequently inactivated by a mutation at one allele and deletion at another allele (Knudson 1989). It plays a major role in maintaining the integrity of genome. Mutations in p53 are among the most frequent genetic changes in many different cancers including GBC (Greenblatt et al. 1994, Harris 1996). Most of these mutations are missense and prolong the half-life of protein by several hours, which can be detected by immunohistochemistry.

p53 overexpression has been immunohistochemically detected in early phases of gallbladder carcinogenesis (Kamb et al. 1994, Wistuba et al. 1995a). Itoi et al. reported that p53 overexpression correlates well with p53 mutations in GBC (Itoi et al. 1997). The close relationship between 17p LOH and p53 overexpression, ranging from 53% to 74%, has been reported in various types of malignancies (Cunningham et al. 1992, Wagata et al. 1993, Wistuba et al. 1995a, Hidaka et al. 1999). Wistuba et al. (1995a) found that LOH at the p53 gene (91%) was more frequent than protein overexpression (59%) in invasive carcinomas. Therefore, LOH is more sensitive than immunohistochemical detection of protein overexpression.

While immunohistochemical detection was limited to dysplasia, CIS, and invasive tumors, LOH was detected at earlier stages, including normal-appearing epithelium and metaplasia.

Ajika et al. found p53 expression in 39.6% of GBC cases but none in adenoma or dysplasia. p53 overexpression correlated well with DNA aneuploidy and absence of stones and not with clinical stage or lymph node metastasis (Ajiki et al. 1996). Billo et al. (2000) found p53 overexpression in 64% of the GBC. Misra et al. (2000) studied overexpression of p53 in 20 cases of GBC from North India and observed p53 overexpression in 70% cases of GBC. Moreno et al. (2005) studied LOH and TP53 mutations in 30 cases of GBC. LOH was found in 95% of tumors and high frequency of TP53 abnormalities were found in 75% of tumors (Moreno et al. 2005). They also observed a significant correlation of p53 expression with the presence of gallstones, T-stage, grade of the tumor, and liver invasion (Billo et al. 2000, Misra et al. 2000, Moreno et al. 2005).

16.5.2.2 p16INK4/CDKN2

Allelic loss on the short arm of chromosome 9 (9p) has been identified in many cancers. A tumor suppressor gene has been identified near the interferon gene cluster in chromosome region 9p21–22. The gene *CDKN2* also known as MTS1 or p16INK4 inhibits a previously known inhibitor (p16) of cyclin-dependent kinase 4 (Kamb et al. 1994, Okamoto et al. 1994). Wistuba et al. (1995b) in their study of 22 invasive GBCs found deletions in region 9p21–22 in 100% of CIS and 50% invasive carcinoma. This shows that this is involved in the pathogenesis of early GBC. Yoshida et al. found mutation in CDKN2 in 8 out of 10 GBCs in their study (Yoshida et al. 1995). Hidaka et al., however, found LOH at 9p to be more frequent in the intramucosal portion of invasive GBC than in in situ lesions (Hidaka et al. 1999). Yoshida et al. (1995) examined 25 BTCs for somatic mutations in p16INK4/CDKN2, p15INK4B/MTS2, and allelic loss of 9p21 y microsatellite analysis. Four BTC cell lines were also analyzed for homozygous deletions and point mutations.

16.5.2.3 K-ras Mutations

The ras gene family is a group of three closely related proto-oncogenes that are involved in the pathogenesis of many cancers. The three members of this family are H-ras, K-ras, and N-ras (Barbacid 1987). They code for homologous proteins of 21 kDa that are involved in the signal transduction pathway. The ras gene family is activated for point mutation at codons 12, 13, and 61 (Bos 1988).

The immunohistochemical expression of the ras oncogene in human gallbladder adenocarcinoma (n = 13), dysplasia (n = 3), and CC (n = 11) was examined by Lee. They concluded that ras p21 expression might be important in the development of GBC but not in its progression. In a previous study, the authors failed to detect any K-ras gene mutation in periampullary cancers (21 ampulla of Vater cancers, 2 common bile duct cancers, and 2 duodenal cancers), 2 GBC, and 6 cholangiocarcinomas (Lee et al. 1995).

Epithelial dysplasia of the gallbladder is an important precancerous lesion in gallbladder carcinogenesis. Mutations were detected in 59% (30 of 51) of GBC, in 73% (8 of 11) of gallbladder dysplasia in gallstone cases, and in none of the cases with normal gallbladder epithelium.

K-ras and p53 mutations in stage I GBC of patients with PBM were compared with those in patients without PBM by Hanada et al. The incidence of K-ras mutation in GBC of patients with PBM (50%) was significantly higher than in patients without PBM (6%) ($p < 0.05$). Their results suggested that K-ras mutation might be important in the early stage of carcinogenesis of the gallbladder mucosa with PBM, as observed earlier in patients without PBM (Hanada et al. 1996).

16.5.2.4 Loss of Heterozygosity

Allelic losses of the short arm of chromosome 8 are common in colorectal and other malignancies (Harnden 1985). There is evidence that there are two distinct regions of 8p LOH (8p21 and 8p22) involved in colon carcinoma, suggesting the existence of two independent tumor suppressor genes (Harnden 1985). Wistuba et al. detected a high incidence of LOH at the 8p22 locus in GBC (44%), suggesting that a putative suppressor oncogene located in this region may play an important role in its pathogenesis (Wistuba et al. 1995b). Mutations of the DCC (18q21) gene are associated with the development of sporadic colon cancer (Fearon et al. 1990). In a study by Wistuba et al., LOH of the DCC gene was a relatively frequent (31%) and early event, detected even in normal and metaplastic epithelia (Wistuba et al. 1995b). This suggested that it is an early event in the pathogenesis of GBC.

They concluded that in GBC at least 21 chromosomal regions with frequent allele losses are involved (Wistuba et al. 2001).

Yoshida et al. examined LOH in the p53, APC, DCC, RB, and NM23-H1 gene regions. LOH was found at p53 in 9 of 15 informative cases (60%), at DCC in 10 of 22 (45%), at APC in 5 of 15 (33%), at RB in 1 of 8 (13%), and at NM23-H1 in 1 of 15 (7%) (Yoshida et al. 2000). Matsuo et al. got high incidences of LOH at 1p36 (19/36: 53%), 9p21 (12/32: 38%), 13q14 (20/36: 56%), 16q24 (31/54: 61%), and 17p13 (15/36: 42%). However, only LOH at 16q24 had a high incidence (5/6: 83%) at an early stage of GBC (Matsuo et al. 2002).

16.5.2.5 FHIT Gene Mutation

Fragile histidine triad (FHIT) is present at chromosome 3p14.2 spanning the FRA3B common fragile site (Tanaka et al. 1998). Highly frequent abnormal transcripts are found in a variety of human cancers including those of the digestive tract, lung, breast, and head and neck (Tanaka et al. 1998, Zöchbauer-Muller et al. 2001, Wistuba et al. 2002). The majority of these abnormalities include aberrant mRNA transcripts with the absence of one or more exons. Genomic analysis demonstrated frequent allelic loss and homozygous deletions (Tanaka et al. 1998, Zöchbauer-Muller et al. 2001). In addition, tumor-specific promoter methylation and epigenetic inactivation of the FHIT gene have also established the important role of FHIT in tumorigenesis (Tanaka et al. 1998, Zöchbauer-Muller et al. 2001).

Wistuba et al. 2002 reported that reduced or loss of FHIT immunostaining and allelic loss were detected in 79% and 76% of GBC, respectively. Moreover, they also demonstrated that FHIT expression correlates with allelic loss. Masaharu Koda et al., however, found absence of staining of FHIT in 9 out of 20 cases (45%) of GBC examined (Koda et al. 2003). Riquelme et al. detected very high frequency of GBC methylation (66%) of FHIT in GBC (Riquelme et al. 2007).

16.5.2.6 CD Antigen

Yamaguchi et al. studied CD44v8-10 expression in 37 GBC patients. It was seen in 18 of 37 GBC tissues. A significant correlation was observed between CD44v8-10 immunoreactivity and perineural invasion, venous invasion, and lymph node metastasis. Patients with CD44 polypeptide antigen positivity showed poor prognosis, whereas those negative had favorable prognosis. Multivariate analysis showed the immunoreactivity in GBC, suggesting this expression may be a biological marker of prognostic significance in GBC (Yamaguchi et al. 2000).

HCAM or CD44 is a multifunctional cell adhesion molecule, related to cell–cell and cell–extracellular matrix interactions and involved in tumor invasion. To study the importance of CD44 expression in subserous GBC, 105 samples of subserous GBC and 33 nontumoral gallbladder were studied by Roa et al. Eighty subjects with carcinoma were followed for a period up to 105 months. CD44 was expressed in all controls and 91% of the expression was normal. In 57% of cancer samples, CD44 expression was abnormal. In 50%, its expression was less, and in 24%, it was not expressed at all. The 5 years survival was 40%. No significant differences in survival were observed in those tumors with a lower or absent CD44 expression (Roa et al. 2001).

Studies have suggested a correlation between increased or decreased expression of CD44 variant molecules and tumor metastasis. To study this further, Yanagisawa et al. studied 83 GBC, 17 gallbladder adenoma, and 66 normal mucosa samples. Normal gallbladder mucosa showed strong, membranous staining for CD44. It was stained as strongly as it was in normal mucosa, but immunoreactivity for CD44v3 and CD44v6 also was significant. Immunoreactivity for CD44v3 and CD44v6 in moderately and poorly differentiated areas was significantly higher than that in well-differentiated areas

($p < 0.0001$ and $p = 0.0378$, respectively). Contrary to earlier study, the results of this study suggested that the prognosis of patients with GBC was not associated with altered expression of CD44s, CD44v3, or CD44v6 (Yanagisawa et al. 2001).

16.5.2.7 HER2/neu

The c-erb B-2/HER2/neu proto-oncogene encodes for the tyrosine kinase receptor p185neu and has been observed frequently in cisplatin-resistant human tumors, such as colorectal and non-small cell lung cancers. It is known to induce resistance to cisplatin (CDDP) in vitro (Boudny et al. 1999), suggesting that the overexpression of beta fibroblast growth factor (β-FGF), platelet-derived growth factor (PDGF), and HER2/neu and the presence of the K-ras mutation are important for the carcinogenesis of bile duct cancers, and detection of the aforementioned abnormalities in bile is helpful for early diagnosis (Su et al. 2001).

16.5.2.8 Heat Shock Protein

Expression of pS2 (an estrogen-induced gene isolated from breast carcinoma MCF7 cells) and of the human spasmolytic polypeptide (hSP) gene was analyzed in 21 human biliary tract and GBC and 16 nonneoplastic gallbladders by Seitz et al. (1991). Eighteen carcinomas and 14 nonneoplastic gallbladders showed pS2 activity. In addition, in samples with pS2 expression, hSP RNA was demonstrated. Northern blots showed weak (basal) level of activity for pS2 and hSP. The genes' increased expression in correlation to inflammatory and neoplastic processes, by now observed in several carcinomas and idiopathic inflammatory bowel disease, hints to their essential role in such diseases (Seitz et al. 1991).

16.5.2.9 Chromosomal Aberrations

Chromosome banding analysis of 11 short-term cultured GBCs revealed acquired clonal aberrations in 7 tumors (5 primary and 2 metastases). Three of these had 1 clone, whereas the remaining 4 were cytogenetically heterogeneous, displaying 2–7 aberrant clones. Of a total of 21 abnormal clones, 18 had highly complex karyotypes and 3 exhibited simple numerical deviations. Chromosome 7 was rearranged most frequently, followed by chromosomes 1, 3, 11, 6, 5, and 8. The bands preferentially involved were 1p36, 1q32, 3p21, 6p21, 7p13, 7q11, 7q32, 19p13, 19q13, and 22q13. Nine recurrent abnormalities could, for the first time, be identified in GBC: del (3) (p13), i (5) (p10), del (6) (q13), del (9) (p13), del (16) (q22), del (17) (p11), i (17) (q10), del (19) (p13), and i (21) (q10). The most common partial or whole-arm gains involved 3q, 5p, 7p, 7q, 8q, 11q, 13q, and 17q, and the most frequent partial or whole-arm losses affected 3p, 4q, 5q, 9p, 10p, 10q, 11p, 14p, 14q, 15p, 17p, 19p, 21p, 21q, and Xp. These chromosomal aberrations and imbalances provide some starting points for molecular analyses of genomic regions that may harbor genes of pathogenetic importance in gallbladder carcinogenesis (Gorunova et al. 1999).

16.5.2.10 Cyclooxygenase Enzymes

Acute cholecystitis is associated with increased gallbladder prostanoid formation, and the inflammatory changes and prostanoid increases can be inhibited by nonsteroidal antiinflammatory drugs (NSAIDs). Recent information indicates that prostanoids are produced by two cyclooxygenase (COX) enzymes, COX-1 and COX-2. Kanoh et al. examined 88 cases with CC, 28 of which showed a thick and sclerotic wall caused by recurrent inflammation, for example, contracted cholecystitis, for the malignant potential of these lesions. Severe dysplasia or CIS in a very small portion of the specimen was identified with hematoxylin–eosin staining in four cases (14.3%) of contracted cholecystitis. These specimens revealed a positive expression of p53, Ki-67, iNOS, and COX-2, suggesting contracted cholecystitis to be an early changed leading to carcinogenesis (Kanoh et al. 2001).

Kawamoto et al. (2002) studied the expression levels of COX-2 in the subserosal layer of 33 cases of pT(2) GBC in which curative resections had been performed and correlated the expression levels of COX-2 with mode of recurrence and postsurgical survival. Intense staining was observed in large percentages of hyperplastic lesions (65%), pT(2) carcinoma specimens (76%), and pT(3) and pT(4) carcinoma specimens (64%) compared to the percentages of normal epithelia and other pathological lesions (0%–25%). Intense staining was also observed in the adjacent stroma in pT(2) carcinoma specimens (33%) and in those in pT(3) and pT(4) carcinoma specimens (43%) but only in small percentages of the stroma adjacent to normal epithelia and pathological lesions (0%–8%) (Kawamoto et al. 2002).

16.5.2.11 APC Gene

APC gene mutations were examined by RNase protection analysis in both tumors and benign lesions of the gallbladder. APC mutation was not found in 16 de novo carcinomas or the one pyloric gland-type adenoma examined (Itoi et al. 1996).

In a study on 30 GBCs, LOH in the APC, DCC, RB, and NM23-H1 gene regions was studied. LOH was found at p53 in 9 of 15 informative cases (60%), at DCC in 10 of 22 (45%), at APC in 5 of 15 (33%), at RB in 1 of 8 (13%), and at NM23-H1 in 1 of 15 (7%). MSI was observed in 5 of 30 cases (17%) in at least 1 chromosomal locus of these 9 microsatellite markers (Su et al. 2001).

16.5.2.12 HLA Antigens

Monoclonal antibody HI-531 of immunoglobulin G2b subclass was produced against a human GBC cell line and was investigated for reactivity by Yamamoto et al., with a panel comprising 10 types of different origins in fluorescence-activated cell sorter analysis.

Tamiolakis et al. (2003) evaluated 31 cases of dysplasia of the gallbladder, 12 cases of CIS, and 39 cases of invasive carcinoma for the detection of HLA-DR monoclonal antigen. This shows decreased expression of HLA-DR and increased expression of CD4 as the lesion progressed to malignancy (Tamiolakis et al. 2003).

16.5.2.13 Growth Factor

The expression of several growth factors and K-ras gene mutation in bile has helped to better understand the pathogenesis and improve early diagnosis of bile duct cancers. The highest mean value of TGF-β in bile was in patients with biliary tract; the mean levels of bFGF and PDGF were highest in cholangiocarcinoma. The results suggest that the overexpression of bFGF, PDGF, and HER2/neu, and the presence of K-ras mutation are important for carcinogenesis of bile duct cancers, and detection of the aforementioned abnormalities in bile is helpful for early diagnosis (Su et al. 2001).

16.5.2.14 Angiogenesis/Vascular Endothelial Growth Factor

Angiogenesis must occur for malignant tumors to proliferate and vascular endothelial growth factor (VEGF) is now believed to be central to this process. Comparison of clinicopathologic parameters between the groups with and without VEGF expression showed significant differences in tumor size, lymphatic invasion, and disease stage. Survival rate was worse in the patients whose tumors demonstrated VEGF expression. It is suggested that VEGF is correlated with tumor progression and may be used as a prognostic indicator (Okita et al. 1998). GBC expressed VEGF far more often than adenoma or cholecystitis ($p = 0.001$); VEGF-positive rates were lower in Nevin staging S1, S2, and S3 than in S4 and S5 of GBC ($p = 0.044$) (Quan et al. 2001).

16.5.3 More Recent GBC Biomarkers

A solid-state 13C nuclear magnetic resonance (NMR) analysis of human gallbladder stones in patients with malignant and benign gallbladder disease was recently published by Jayalakshmi et al. (2009). Differences were identified in the 13C chemical shift between stones from cholecystitis patients and from GBC patients. The study also performed qualitative and quantitative 1H NMR analysis of lipid extracts of gallbladder tissue in CC, xanthogranulomatous cholecystitis (XGC), and

GBC patients (Jayalakshmi et al. 2011). They identified alterations in various gallbladder tissue lipid components in CC, XGC, and GBC patients.

The chemical profile of bile exhibits metabolic processes associated with hepatobiliary organs including the gallbladder (Kristiansen et al. 2004). Thus, various studies have investigated the components of bile for potential biomarkers in hepatobiliary diseases including GBC (Uchida et al. 2003, Park et al. 2006, Somashekar et al. 2007, Gowda et al. 2010).

A malignancy-related protein, Mac-2-binding protein (Mac-2BP), expressed in several tumors was analyzed in a study by Koopmann et al. (2004). The authors concluded Mac-2BP levels in conjunction with biliary CA19-9 levels as a novel diagnostic marker for GBC. Wen et al. (2010) applied a metabolomic approach to develop an effective diagnostic tool in BTC utilizing the metabolite richness of bile. Their NMR-based metabolomic approach was able to discriminate between cancer and benign biliary duct diseases furnishing a greater sensitivity and specificity than bile cytology.

Tan et al. (2010) analyzed total proteins from GBC tissue and benign gallbladder tissue using 2D gel electrophoresis (2-DGE) for potential biomarker identification. They identified 17 differentially expressed proteins and characterized them by comparative proteomic analysis.

Tan et al. (2011) further studied to identify new serum biomarkers using 2-DGE and matrix assisted laser desorption ionization-time of flight mass spectroscopy (MALDI-TOF MS) for the early detection of GBC. They successfully identified a total of 24 differentially expressed proteins, including 12 upregulated proteins and 12 downregulated proteins, between GBC patients and healthy cancer-free controls. This was the first study in Chinese population using proteomic-based analysis for serum biomarker identification in GBC. Some of the upregulated proteins in GBC, such as splicing factor 3B subunit 5, cystatin B, S100A10 protein, histone H2B type 2-E, profilin-1, eukaryotic translation initiation factor 1A, isoform 1 of eukaryotic translation initiation factor 5A-1, FERM domain-containing 3, glyceraldehyde-3-phosphate dehydrogenase, serum amyloid P-component precursor, and harmonin isoform b3, were firstly identified in GBC, among which, two upregulated proteins S100A10 and haptoglobin were further validated in GBC samples. Using Western blotting, they demonstrated elevated protein levels. In this study, all of the patients with GBC had a small, surgically resectable tumor, suggesting that the differentially expressed proteins can be potentially used as biomarkers for the early diagnosis of GBC.

Mou et al. (2012) also used MALDI-TOF MS to profile and compare the serum proteins from GBC patients and healthy controls. An optimal proteomic pattern composed of three statistically different protein peaks was identified that distinguished GBC group from the control group. Wang et al. (2009) used comparative proteomic analysis in GBC-SD cell lines to identify metastasis-associated proteins between high and low metastatic potential cell lines.

The role of stem cells in mediating metastasis, invasion, and resistance to therapy has been studied in few reports. Shi et al. (2010) identified CD44+CD133+ subpopulation exhibiting cancer stem cell (CSC)-like characteristics in primary GBC and in GBC-SD cell line representing a novel diagnostic and therapeutic target (Shi et al. 2011). Another study by Li et al. (2012) used flow cytometry to sort side population cells from human GBC cell line, which displayed CSC characteristics including higher proliferative, stronger clonal-generating, more migratory, and more invasive capacities.

Ueki et al. (2004) evaluated alterations in p16 gene as a prognostic marker in 68 GBC patients. The authors observed high percentage of p16 gene nonsilent mutations, p16 methylation, and loss of chromosome 9p21–22 in GBC cases. There were also significant differences between the mean survival of GBC patients without p16 alterations and patients with p16 alterations ($p < 0.02$). Quan et al. (2001) and Ma et al. (2005) also observed mutations in p53, p16, and Rb genes correlating with the progression of GBC.

A recent article by Heaphy et al. (2011) has demonstrated alternative lengthening of telomeres (ALT) phenotype in GBC, which warrants further studies to evaluate the plausible prognostic significance of ALT-positive gallbladder tumors.

Langner et al. (2004) performed a systematic analysis of KIT immunoreactivity in both primary and metastatic GBCs using tissue microarray (TMA). The authors concluded KIT immunoreactivity to be infrequent in GBCs as against those reported by Aswad et al. (2002) who advocated it as a potential therapeutic target for biliary carcinomas.

Tumor-related mRNAs in the serum/plasma of cancer patients have emerged as a potential diagnostic tool with greater sensitivity in various malignancies (Miura et al. 2008). Kawahara et al. (2007)

measured hTERT mRNA levels in bile samples from 19 patients with BTC including 6 patients with GBC. The combination of cytological examination and hTERT mRNA analysis significantly improved the diagnostic accuracy (positive rate of 78.9%) in GBC.

Epigenetic changes such as promoter hypermethylation of cell cycle, DNA mismatch repair, apoptosis, and protein degradation pathway genes have also been reported to play a crucial role in the development of GBC (Wistuba and Gazdar 2004). Various studies have been carried out for screening aberrant methylation of CpG islands to identify gallbladder-specific epigenetic markers. García et al. (2009), House et al. (2003), and Takahashi et al. (2004) investigated the potential role of promoter methylation in GBC. The authors examined promoter methylation profile of tumor suppressor genes and observed an increase of multigenic methylation during tumoral progression hyper methylation of promoter regions to be an early, progressive, and cumulative event in gallbladder carcinogenesis.

Kee et al. (2007) suggested downregulation of ras association domain family 1A expression by DNA hypermethylation in GBC. Epigenetic inactivation by abnormal promoter methylation was also found to be a frequent event in chromosome 3p candidate tumor suppressor genes (SEMA3B [3p21.3] and FHIT [3p14.2]) in GBC pathogenesis (Riquelme et al. 2007). Lee et al. (2006) proposed promoter hypomethylation of the protein gene product 9.5 (PGP9.5) gene, a neurospecific peptide, as a reliable marker for GBC.

Several studies have shown neovascularization to be directly associated with growth, invasion, metastasis, staging, and prognosis of tumors (Tanaka et al. 2003). Similar studies in GBC have also shown angiogenesis to be strongly correlated with the Nevin staging and tumor differentiation (Tian et al. 2006) and also as an important parameter to predict the degree of malignancy, prognosis, and drug resistance (Giatromanolaki et al. 2002).

16.6 Gene Expression and Potential Biomarker

In GBC, multiple gene expression profiles have been done to examine differential gene expression patterns between normal and tumor cells to identify potential biomarkers for GBC progression. Predictions of clinical behavior in GBC patients can also be identified from expression signatures of cancer behavior using microarray expression data from other cancer types. Alvarez et al. (2008) generated serial analysis of gene expression (SAGE) libraries from GBC and nonneoplastic gallbladder mucosa and identified overexpression of connective tissue growth factor (CTGF), which was significantly associated with better overall survival. Swierczynski et al. (2004) used TMA to study the expression pattern of selected markers in pathogenesis and neoplastic progression of GBC and found novel tumor markers.

16.7 Gene Expression Biomarkers and Drug Responsiveness in the Clinical Setting

Surgery is the first-line treatment for patients with GBC followed by radiation and chemotherapy. Because of limited knowledge about the predictors of response, it is difficult to treat individual patients. Mutations in various oncogenes are frequently found to be associated with GBC that can predict prognosis and drug response. Identifying potential predictive gene or protein biomarkers for the mechanisms of resistance to anticancer agents could be gradually applied for individualized drug selection in patients receiving GBC chemotherapy (Robert et al. 2004). Several diseases such as breast cancer (Nagasaki and Miki 2008) and colon cancer (Schetter et al. 2008) have been benefitted using this approach in the treatment response. Studies in GBC have analyzed the role of proteins involved in drug responsiveness including ribonucleotide reductase subunit M1 (Ohtaka et al. 2008); hMLH1 (Kohya et al. 2002, Sato et al. 2007); Nrf2 and Kelch-like ECH-associating protein 1 (Keapl) (Shibata et al. 2008); multidrug resistance mRNA and P-glycoprotein (Cao et al. 1998); and dihydropyrimidine dehydrogenase (DPD) (Sato et al. 2006). Relationships between various genetic mutations and the efficacy of molecular targeted agents have also been studied in GBC (Furuse 2010). However, due to limited information on the genetic architecture of GBC, there are only few potential therapeutically beneficial molecular targeted agents (Zhu and Hezel 2011). Further understanding of the gallbladder tumor

TABLE 16.6
Selected Global Gene Expression Studies in GBC

No. of Samples	Microarray Platform	Findings	References
12	Oligonucleotide	Identified 2270 upregulated genes and 2412 downregulated genes	Kim et al. (2008)
11	Oligonucleotide	Identified 282 genes upregulated and 513 genes downregulated in primary resected cancers and biliary cancer cell lines vs. normal epithelial scrapings	Hansel et al. (2003)
11	cDNA	118 genes identified with a predictive value	Murakawa et al. (2004)
12	Oligonucleotide	Four cell-cycle-related genes and one metabolism-related gene were found to be upregulated.	Washiro et al. (2008)
9	Oligonucleotide	Identified 1281 genes with altered expression	Miller et al. (2009)

genetic profile and its role in drug sensitivity will facilitate in the evaluation of tailored first-line treatment with targeted agents based on the molecular signature (Table 16.6).

16.8 Current Research Trend in Biomarkers of GBC

Alternative splice variants and GBC bioinformatics analysis suggest that up to 65% of human genes are alternatively spliced (Mironov et al. 1999). Alternative splice variants have been detected in many cancers as well as in a large number of cancer-related genes (Brinkmann et al. 2004). These splice variants could either modify the cancer susceptibility or act as surrogate markers. An in-depth analysis of proteins coded by mRNA transcript variants of well-known as well as in less well-annotated genes may advance the discovery of novel diagnostic and prognostic biomarkers, including potentially new drug targets in GBC. MicroRNAs (miRNAs) and GBC miRNAs are small (18–25 nt), noncoding, single-stranded RNA molecules that regulate gene expression posttranscriptionally (Bartel 2004). Nearly 30% of the global gene expression is probably regulated by miRNAs. Aberrant expression of multiple miRNAs has been reported to be associated with many human cancers, and >50% of miRNA genes are found to be present with a satisfactory response to chemotherapy located in cancer-related chromosomal regions (Pang et al. 2010). Although there are currently no large-scale miRNA expression profiling studies in GBC, Braconi et al. (2010) recently analyzed aberrant miRNA expression patterns in Mz-ChA-1 cells (derived from metastatic GBC) overexpressing interleukin 6. The authors noticed decreased expression of miR-148a and miR-152 in Mz-ChA-1 cells relative to H69 nonmalignant human cholangiocytes in vitro as well as in tumor xenografts in vivo. Thus, miRNAs represent a novel class of biomarkers in clinical diagnostic applications, and whether they can be used as surrogate markers for GBC or response to therapy is an area of active research.

16.8.1 Tumor Microenvironment Biomarkers in GBC

Stephen Paget, in 1889, put forward the "Seed and Soil" theory, which is the basis of the present tumor microenvironment (TME) model of cancer metastasis (Paget 1889). TME provides survival signals and proangiogenic factors, which are essential for tumor growth and metastasis (Ribatti and Vacca 2008). Characterization of biomarkers that govern the molecular mechanisms involved in TME might elucidate the interplay between tumor cells and their microenvironment and lead to advances in early detection or prevention of metastasis.

The presence of inflammatory elements such as a multitude of signaling molecules has been linked to promote tumor growth and metastasis in GBC (Kiguchi and DiGiovanni 2008). Okada et al.

(2009) demonstrated stromal staining of laminin-5γ2, a component of extracellular matrix and cancer invasiveness marker, demonstrating an interaction between cancer cells and stromal tissue. Further studies of TME in GBC will enhance our understanding of the molecular mechanisms underlying GBC development potentially leading to the identification of biomarkers and drug targets.

16.8.2 Other Potential Biomarkers

In addition to the aforementioned potential opportunities, recent studies have identified a class of low molecular weight metabolites, known as pteridines, to be significantly elevated in various cancers accentuating as a promising tool in cancer diagnosis (Koslinski et al. 2011). The metabolic phenotyping can also provide important information, which is distinct from the genetic or proteomic profile of an individual. In addition to the open-ended genome-wide expression microarray analyses, specific gene families can also be used to identify and interrogate prognostic markers in GBC (Jeong et al. 2010). The transgenic mouse model (BK5.ErbB-2A mice) for GBC also represents a promising tool for the development of new treatment and/or prevention strategies (Kiguchi et al. 2001).

The tumor role of cell-free nucleic acids (cfNAs), mitochondrial DNA copy number, plasma membrane proteins, autoantibody signatures, and circulating tumor cells (CTCs) as cancer biomarkers for diagnostic applications has also attracted the scientific community (Punnoose et al. 2010, Desmetz et al. 2011, Man 2011, Schwarzenbach et al. 2011, Sun et al. 2011). Network mining algorithms and mathematical models are also being developed and studied to identify highly connected gene coexpression networks to prognosticate clinical outcome in cancer patients (Karrila et al. 2011).

At present, the main prognostic factors for GBC are resection status and TNM stage (North et al. 1998). Because the underlying molecular processes often go on for decades until the initial clinical symptoms surface, the prognosis of GBC is generally poor and it is difficult to cure by surgery alone. Identification of new prognostic biomarkers would help identify patients who might benefit from additional treatment. The present article reviewed published studies in GBC on potential gene expression biomarkers. To infer, none of the markers identified in GBC are specific or effective as a routine screening test in a clinical setting. Further efforts are required to better understand the prognostic value of gene expression biomarkers in gallbladder malignancy.

16.8.3 Remarks

GBC is the most common cause of mortality among BCTs. Patients with GBC often present in an advanced stage and are treated palliatively. In spite of years of research with multiple studies on prognostic value of markers, to date there are no 100% sensitive and specific biomarkers for GBC. Recent advances in the field of protein microarray expression analyses have identified novel markers that, when correlated with clinical data, can be used as genetic signatures for the precise diagnosis and prediction of clinical outcomes in GBC (Matarraz et al. 2011). Although the results have provided us with vital information about the molecular biology of GBC, they have not yet been translated into clinical use. The strategy group of "Program for the Assessment of Clinical Cancer Tests" and a working group of "The National Cancer Institute–European Organisation for Research and Treatment of Cancer" have developed guidelines for the reporting of tumor marker studies to provide relevant information about the study design, hypotheses, patient and specimen characteristics, assay methods, and statistical methods (McShane et al. 2006).

Thus, the accumulating knowledge about the gene expression patterns in malignant versus premalignant gallbladder epithelium might eventually provide us with objective analytical tools and more precise markers with better sensitivity and specificity and expedite the discovery of novel therapeutic opportunities for the management of GBC. Nomograms and multivariable tests such as artificial neural networks combining variables such as tumor grade/stage and biomarkers will provide physicians with standardized patient care. Finally, an international coordination and amalgamation in basic and clinical research is required for further progress in the field of GBC diagnosis and treatment.

References

Ajiki T, Onoyama H, Yamamoto M, Asaka K, Fujimori T, Maeda S, and Saitoh Y. p53 protein expression and prognosis in gallbladder carcinoma and premalignant lesions. *Hepatogastroenterology*. 1996;43(9):521–526.

Akdoğan M, Parlak E, Kayhan B, Balk M, Saydam G, and Sahin B. Are serum and biliary carcinoembryonic antigen and carbohydrate antigen 19–9 determinations reliable for differentiation between benign and malignant biliary disease? *Turk J Gastroenterol*. 2003;14(3):181–184.

Alvarez H, Corvalan A, Roa JC et al. Serial analysis of gene expression identifies connective tissue growth factor expression as a prognostic biomarker in gallbladder cancer. *Clin Cancer Res*. 2008;14(9):2361–2368.

Andia ME, Hsing AW, Andreotti G, and Ferreccio C. Geographic variation of gallbladder cancer mortality and risk factors in Chile: A population-based ecologic study. *Int J Cancer*. September 15, 2008;123(6):1411–1416.

Aswad B, Constantinou M, Iannitti D et al. KIT is a potential therapeutic target for biliary carcinomas. *Proc Am Soc Clin Oncol*. 21:103b, 2002 (abstr 2227).

Atkinson BF, Ernst CS, Herlyn M, Steplewski Z, Sears HF, and Koprowski H. Gastrointestinal cancer-associated antigen in immunoperoxidase assay. *Cancer Res*. 1982;42:4820–4823.

Barbacid M. Ras genes. *Ann Rev Biochem*. 1987;56:779–827.

Bartel DP. MicroRNAs: Genomics, biogenesis, mechanism, and function. *Cell*. 2004;116:281–297.

Bast RC, Jr. Freeney M, Lazarus H et al. Reactivity of a monoclonal antibody with human ovarian carcinoma. *J Clin Invest*. 1981;68:1331–1337.

Bates SE and Longo DL. Use of serum tumor markers in cancer diagnosis and management. *Semin Oncol*. 1987;14:102–138.

Billo P, Marchegiani C, Capella C, and Sessa F. Expression of p53 in gallbladder carcinoma and in dysplastic and metaplastic lesions of the surrounding mucosa. *Pathologica*. 2000;92(4):249–256.

Bordes M, Michiels R, and Martin F. Detection by immunofluorescence of carcinoembryonic antigen in colonic carcinoma, other malignant and benign tumor and non-cancerous tissues. *Digestion*. 1973;9:106–115.

Bos JL. The ras gene family and human carcinogenesis. *Mutat Res*. 1988;195(3):255–271.

Boudny V, Murakami Y, Nakano S, and Niho Y. Expression of activated c-erbB-2 oncogene induces sensitivity to cisplatin in human gallbladder adenocarcinoma cells. *Anticancer Res*. 1999;19(6B):5203–5206.

Braconi C, Huang N, and Patel T. MicroRNA-dependent regulation of DNA methyltransferase-1 and tumor suppressor gene expression by interleukin-6 in human malignant cholangiocytes. *Hepatology*. 2010;51:881–890.

Brinkmann D, Ryan A, Ayhan A, McCluggage WG, Feakins R, Santibanez-Koref MF, Mein CA, Gayther SA, and Jacobs IJ. A molecular genetic and statistical approach for the diagnosis of dual-site cancers. *J Natl Cancer Inst*. October 6, 2004;96(19):1441–1446.

Brockmann J, Emparan C, Hernandez CA et al. Gallbladder bile tumor marker quantification for detection of pancreatico-biliary malignancies. *Anticancer Res*. 2000;20:4941–4947.

Calle EE, Rodriguez C, Jacobs EJ et al. The American Cancer Society Cancer Prevention Study II Nutrition Cohort: Rationale, study design, and baseline characteristics. *Cancer*. 2002;94:2490–2501.

Cao L, Duchrow M, Windhövel U, Kujath P, Bruch HP, and Broll R. Expression of MDR1 mRNA and encoding P-glycoprotein in archival formalin-fixed paraffin-embedded gall bladder cancer tissues. *Eur J Cancer*. 1998;34:1612–1617.

Caygill CP, Hill MJ, Braddick M, and Sharp JC. Cancer mortality in chronic typhoid and paratyphoid carriers. *Lancet*. 1994;343:83–84.

Cha PC, Zembutsu H, Takahashi A, Kubo M, Kamatani N, and Nakamura Y. A genome-wide association study identifies SNP in DCC is associated with gallbladder cancer in the Japanese population. *J Hum Genet*. April 2012;57(4):235–237.

Chaube A, Tewari M, Singh U et al. CA 125. A potential tumor marker for gallbladder cancer. *J Surg Oncol*. 2006;93(8):665–669.

Chow WH, Johansen C, Gridley G, Mellemkjaer L, Olsen JH, and Fraumeni JF Jr. Gallstones, cholecystectomy and risk of cancers of the liver, biliary tract and pancreas. *Br J Cancer*. 1999;79(3–4):640–644.

Cunningham J, Lust JA, Schaid DJ, Bren GD, Carpenter HA, Rizza E, Kovach JS, and Thibodeau SN. Expression of p53 and 17p allelic loss in colorectal carcinoma. *Cancer Res*. 1992;52(7):1974–1980.

Davis HM, Zurawski VR, Bast RC et al. Characterization of the CA 125 antigen associated with human epithelial ovarian carcinomas. *Cancer Res*. 1986;46:6143–6148.

Desmetz C, Mange A, Maudelonde T, and Solassol J. Autoantibody signatures: Progress and perspectives for early cancer detection. *J Cell Mol Med*. 2011;15:2013–2024.

Diehl AK. Gallstone size and the risk of gallbladder cancer. *JAMA*. 1983;250:2323–2326.

Dowaki S, Kijima H, Kashiwagi H et al. immunohistochemical localization is correlated with growth and metastasis of human gallbladder carcinoma. *Int J Oncol*. 2000;16(1):49–53.

Enjoji M, Nakashima M, Nishi H et al. The tumor-associated antigen, RCAS1, can be expressed in immune-mediated diseases as well as in carcinomas of biliary tract. *J Hepatol*. 2002;36(6):786–792.

Enjoji M, Yamaguchi K, Nakamuta M, Nakashima M, Kotoh K, Tanaka M, Nawata H, and Watanabe T. Movement of a novel serum tumour marker, RCAS1, in patients with biliary diseases. *Dig Liver Dis*. 2004;36(9):622–627.

Fearon ER, Cho KR, Nigro JM et al. Identification of a chromosome 18q gene that is altered in colorectal cancers. *Science*. 1990;247(4938):49–56.

Furuse J. Targeted therapy for biliary-tract cancer. *Lancet Oncol*. 2010;11:5–6.

Gabbi C, Kim HJ, Barros R, Korach-Andrè M, Warner M, and Gustafsson JA. Estrogen-dependent gallbladder carcinogenesis in LXRbeta-/- female mice. *Proc Natl Acad Sci USA*. 2010;107:14763–14768.

García P, Manterola C, Araya JC, Villaseca M, Guzmán P, Sanhueza A, Thomas M, Alvarez H, and Roa JC. Promoter methylation profile in preneoplastic and neoplastic gallbladder lesions. *Mol Carcinog*. 2009;48:79–89.

Giatromanolaki A, Sivridis E, Koukourakis MI, Polychronidis A, and Simopoulos C. Prognostic role of angiogenesis in operable carcinoma of the gallbladder. *Am J Clin Oncol*. 2002;25:38–41.

Goldgar DE, Easton DF, Cannon-Albright LA, and Skolnick MH. Systematic population-based assessment of cancer risk in first-degree relatives of cancer probands. *J Natl Cancer Inst*. 1994;86:1600–1608.

Gorunova L, Parada LA, Limon J, Jin Y, Hallén M, Hägerstrand I, Iliszko M, Wajda Z, and Johansson B. Nonrandom chromosomal aberrations and cytogenetic heterogeneity in gallbladder carcinomas. *Genes Chromosomes Cancer*. 1999;26(4):312–321.

Gowda GA. Human bile as a rich source of biomarkers for hepatopancreatobiliary cancers. *Biomark Med*. 2010;4(2):299–314.

Greenblatt MS, Bennett WP, Hollstein M, and Harris CC. Mutations in the p53 tumor suppressor gene: Clues to cancer etiology and molecular pathogenesis. *Cancer Res*. 1994;54(18):4855–4878.

Hanada K, Itoh M, Fujii K, Tsuchida A, Ooishi H, and Kajiyama G. K-ras and p53 mutations in stage I gallbladder carcinoma with an anomalous junction of the pancreaticobiliary duct. *Cancer*. 1996;77(3):452–458.

Hansel DE, Rahman A, Hidalgo M et al. Identification of novel cellular targets in biliary tract cancers using global gene expression technology. *Am J Pathol*. 2003;163:217–229.

Hariharan D, Saied A, and Kocher HM. Analysis of mortality rates for gallbladder cancer across the world. *HPB (Oxford)*. 2008;10:327–331.

Harnden DG. Human tumor markers. Biological basis and clinical relevance. *J Roy Soc Med*. 1985;78:1071–1072.

Harris CC. p53 Tumor suppressor gene from the basic research laboratory to the clinic—An abridged historical perspective. *Carcinogenesis*. 1996;17:1187–1198.

Heaphy CM, Subhawong AP, Hong SM et al. Prevalence of the alternative lengthening of telomeres telomere maintenance mechanism in human cancer subtypes. *Am J Pathol*. October 2011;179(4):1608–1615.

Hemminki K and Li X. Familial liver and gall bladder cancer: A nationwide epidemiological study from Sweden. *Gut*. 2003;52:592–596.

Hidaka E, Yanagisawa A, Sakai Y, Seki M, Kitagawa T, Setoguchi T, and Kato Y. Losses of heterozygosity on chromosomes 17p and 9p/18q may play important roles in early and advanced phases of gallbladder carcinogenesis. *J Cancer Res Clin Oncol*. 1999;125(8–9):439–443.

House MG, Wistuba II, Argani P, Guo M, Schulick RD, Hruban RH, Herman JG, and Maitra A. Progression of gene hypermethylation in gallstone disease leading to gallbladder cancer. *Ann Surg Oncol*. 2003;10:882–889.

Hsing AW, Bai Y, Andreotti G et al. Family history of gallstones and the risk of biliary tract cancer and gallstones: A population-based study in Shanghai, China. *Int J Cancer*. 2007;121:832–838.

Isaacson P. The demonstration of carcinoembryonic antigen (CEA) in ulcerative colitis. *Gut*. 1976;17: 561–567.

Ishiguro S, Inoue M, Kurahashi N, Iwasaki M, Sasazuki S, and Tsugane S. Risk factors of biliary tract cancer in a large-scale population-based cohort study in Japan (JPHC study); with special focus on cholelithiasis, body mass index, and their effect modification. *Cancer Causes Control*. 2008;19:33–41.

Isozaki H, Okajima K, Hara H, Sako S, and Mabuchi H. Proliferating cell nuclear antigen expression in the gallbladder with pancreaticobiliary maljunction. *J Surg Oncol*. 1997;65(1):46–49.

Itoi T, Watanabe H, Ajioka Y, Oohashi Y, Takel K, Nishikura K, Nakamura Y, Horil A, and Saito T. APC, K-ras codon 12 mutations and p53 gene expression in carcinoma and adenoma of the gall-bladder suggest two genetic pathways in gall-bladder carcinogenesis. *Pathol Int*. 1996;46(5):333–340.

Itoi T, Watanabe H, Yoshida M, Ajioka Y, Nishikura K, and Saito T. Correlation of p53 protein expression with gene mutation in gall-bladder carcinomas. *Pathol Int*. 1997;47(8):525–530.

Jackson HH, Glasgow RE, Mulvihill SJ, and Cannon-Albright LA. Familial risk in gallbladder cancer. *J Am Coll Surg*. 2007;205:S38.

Jayalakshmi K, Sonkar K, Behari A, Kapoor VK, and Sinha N. Solid state (13)C NMR analysis of human gallstones from cancer and benign gall bladder diseases. *Solid State Nucl Magn Reson*. 2009;36(1):60–65.

Jayalakshmi K, Sonkar K, Behari A, Kapoor VK, and Sinha N. Lipid profiling of cancerous and benign gallbladder tissues by 1H NMR spectroscopy. *NMR Biomed*. 2011;24(4):335–342.

Jeong Y, Xie Y, Xiao G, Behrens C, Girard L, Wistuba II, Minna JD, and Mangelsdorf DJ. Nuclear receptor expression defines a set of prognostic biomarkers for lung cancer. *PLoS Med*. 2010;7:e1000378.

Johansson C, Nilsson O, and Bäckström D. Novel epitopes on the CA50-carrying antigen: Chemical and immunochemical studies. *Tumour Biol*. 1991a;12:159–170.

Johansson C, Nilsson O, and Lindholm L. Comparison of serological expression of different epitopes on the CA50 carrying antigen CanAg. *Int J Cancer*. 1991b;48:757–763.

Kamb A, Gruis NA, Weaver-Feldhaus J, Liu Q, Harshman K, Tavtigian SV, Stockert E, Day RS 3rd, Johnson BE, and Skolnick MH. A cell cycle regulator potentially involved in genesis of many tumor types. *Science*. April 15, 1994;264(5157):436–440.

Kanoh K, Shimura T, Tsutsumi S, Suzuki H, Kashiwabara K, Nakajima T, and Kuwano H. Significance of contracted cholecystitis lesions as high risk for gallbladder carcinogenesis. *Cancer Lett*. 2001;169(1):7–14.

Kanthan R, Radhi JM, and Kanthan SC. Gallbladder carcinomas: An immunoprognostic evaluation of P53, Bcl-2, CEA and alpha-fetoprotein. *Can J Gastroenterol*. 2000;14(3):181–184.

Karrila S, Lee JH, and Tucker-Kellogg G. A comparison of methods for data-driven cancer outlier discovery, and an application scheme to semisupervised predictive biomarker discovery. *Cancer Inform*. 2011;10:109–120.

Kashiwagi H, Kijima H, Dowaki S et al. MUC1 and MUC2 expression in human gallbladder carcinoma: A clinicopathological study and relationship with prognosis. *Oncol Rep*. 2001;8(3):485–489.

Kawahara R, Odo M, Kinoshita H, Shirouzu K, and Aoyagi S. Analysis of hTERT mRNA expression in biliary tract and pancreatic cancer. *J Hepatobiliary Pancreat Surg*. 2007;14:189–193.

Kawamoto T, Shoda J, Asano T, Ueda T, Furukawa M, Koike N, Tanaka N, Todoroki T, and Miwa M. Expression of cyclooxygenase-2 in the subserosal layer correlates with postsurgical prognosis of pathological tumor stage 2 carcinoma of the gallbladder. *Int J Cancer*. 2002;98(3):427–434.

Kee SK, Lee JY, Kim MJ et al. Hypermethylation of the Ras association domain family 1A (RASSF1A) gene in gallbladder cancer. *Mol Cells*. 2007;24:364–371.

Khan ZR, Neugut AI, Ahsan H, and Chabot JA. Risk factors for biliary tract cancers. *Am J Gastroenterol*. 1999;94:149–152.

Kiguchi K, Carbajal S, Chan K, Beltrán L, Ruffino L, Shen J, Matsumoto T, Yoshimi N, and DiGiovanni J. Constitutive expression of ErbB-2 in gallbladder epithelium results in development of adenocarcinoma. *Cancer Res*. 2001;61:6971–6976.

Kiguchi K and DiGiovanni J. Role of growth factor signaling pathways. In *Biliary Tract and Gallbladder Cancer: Diagnosis & Therapy*. Thomas CR and Fuller CD (eds.), New York: Demos Medical, 2008, pp. 19–36.

Kim JH, Kim HN, Lee KT, Lee JK, Choi SH, Paik SW, Rhee JC, and Lowe AW. Gene expression profiles in gallbladder cancer: The close genetic similarity seen for early and advanced gallbladder cancers may explain the poor prognosis. *Tumour Biol*. 2008;29:41–49.

Knudson AG Jr. The ninth Gordon Hamilton-Fairley memorial lecture. Hereditary cancers: Clues to mechanisms of carcinogenesis. *Br J Cancer*. 1989;59(5):661–666.

Koda M, Yashima K, Kawaguchi K, Andachi H, Hosoda A, Shiota G, Ito H, and Murawaki Y. Expression of Fhit, Mlh1, and P53 protein in human gallbladder carcinoma. *Cancer Lett.* 2003;199(2):131–138.

Kohya N, Miyazaki K, Matsukura S, Yakushiji H, Kitajima Y, Kitahara K, Fukuhara M, Nakabeppu Y, and Sekiguchi M. Deficient expression of O(6)-methylguanine-DNA methyltransferase combined with mismatch-repair proteins hMLH1 and hMSH2 is related to poor prognosis in human biliary tract carcinoma. *Ann Surg Oncol.* 2002;9:371–379.

Koopmann J, Thuluvath PJ, Zahurak ML et al. Mac-2-binding protein is a diagnostic marker for biliary tract carcinoma. *Cancer.* October 1. 2004;101(7):1609–1615.

Koslinski P, Bujak R, Daghir E, and Markuszewski MJ. Metabolic profiling of pteridines for determination of potential biomarkers in cancer diseases. *Electrophoresis.* 2011;32:2044–2054.

Kristiansen TZ, Bunkenborg J, Gronborg M, Molina H, Thuluvath PJ, Argani P, Goggins MG, Maitra A, and Pandey A. A proteomic analysis of human bile. *Mol Cell Proteomics.* 2004;3(7):715–728.

Langner C, Lemmerer M, and Kornprat P. Analysis of KIT (CD117) expression in gallbladder carcinomas by tissue microarray. *Eur J Surg Oncol.* 2004;30:847–850.

Lazcano-Ponce EC, Miquel JF, Muñoz N et al. Epidemiology and molecular pathology of gallbladder cancer. *CA Cancer J Clin.* 2001;51:349–364.

Lee CS. Differences in cell proliferation and prognostic significance of proliferating cell nuclear antigen and Ki-67 antigen immunoreactivity in in situ and invasive carcinomas of the extrahepatic biliary tract. *Cancer.* 1996;78(9):1881–1887.

Lee JC, Lin PW, Lin YJ, Lai J, Yang HB, and Lai MD. Analysis of K-ras gene mutations in periampullary cancers, gallbladder cancers and cholangiocarcinomas from paraffin-embedded tissue sections. *J Formos Med Assoc.* 1995;94(12):719–723.

Lee YM, Lee JY, Kim MJ, Bae HI, Park JY, Kim SG, and Kim DS. Hypomethylation of the protein gene product 9.5 promoter region in gallbladder cancer and its relationship with clinicopathological features. *Cancer Sci.* 2006;97(11):1205–1210.

Levy AD, Murakata LA, and Rohrmann CA Jr. Gallbladder carcinoma: Radiologic-pathologic correlation. *Radiographics.* 2001;21:295–314.

Li XX, Wang J, Wang HL, Wang W, Yin XB, Li QW, Chen YY, and Yi J. Characterization of cancer stem-like cells derived from a side population of a human gallbladder carcinoma cell line, SGC-996. *Biochem Biophys Res Commun.* 2012;419:728–734.

Lichtenstein P, Holm NV, Verkasalo PK et al. Environmental and heritable factors in the causation of cancer—analyses of cohorts of twins from Sweden, Denmark, and Finland. *N Engl J Med.* 2000;343(2):78–85.

Lindholm L, Holmgren J, Svennerholm L et al. Monoclonal antibodies against gastrointestinal tumour-associated antigens isolated as monosialogangliosides. *Int Arch Allergy Appl Immun.* 1983;71:178–181.

Lowenfels AB, Walker AM, Althaus DP, Townsend G, and Domellöf L. Gallstone growth, size, and risk of gallbladder cancer: An interracial study. *Int J Epidemiol.* 1989;18:50–54.

Ma HB, Hu HT, Di ZL, Wang ZR, Shi JS, Wang XJ, and Li Y. Association of cyclin D1, p16 and retinoblastoma protein expressions with prognosis and metastasis of gallbladder carcinoma. *World J Gastroenterol.* 2005;11:744–747.

Magnani J, Nilsson B, Brockhous M et al. The antigen of a tumor specific monoclonal antibody is a ganglioside containing sialylated lacto-N-fucopentaose II. *Fed Proc.* 1982;41:898.

Malati T. Tumor markers: An overview. *Indian J Clin Biochem.* 2007;22(2):17–31.

Man Y. Generation, function and diagnostic value of mitochondrial DNA copy number alterations in human cancers. *Life Sci.* 2011;89:65–71.

Matarraz S, González-González M, Jara M, Orfao A, and Fuentes M. New technologies in cancer. Protein microarrays for biomarker discovery. *Clin Transl Oncol.* 2011;13:156–161.

Matsuo K, Kuroki T, Kitaoka F, Tajima Y, and Kanematsu T. Loss of heterozygosity of chromosome 16q in gallbladder carcinoma. *J Surg Res.* 2002;102(2):133–136.

McShane LM, Altman DG, Sauerbrei W, Taube SE, Gion M, and Clark GM, Statistics Subcommittee of NCI-EORTC Working Group on Cancer Diagnostics. Reporting recommendations for tumor marker prognostic studies (REMARK). *Breast Cancer Res Treat.* 2006;100:229–235.

Miller G, Socci ND, Dhall D et al. Genome wide analysis and clinical correlation of chromosomal and transcriptional mutations in cancers of the biliary tract. *J Exp Clin Cancer Res.* 2009;28:62.

Mironov AA, Fickett JW, and Gelfand MS. Frequent alternative splicing of human genes. *Genome Res.* 1999;9:1288–1293.

Misra S, Chaturvedi A, Goel MM, Mehrotra R, Sharma ID, Srivastava AN, and Misra NC. Overexpression of p53 protein in gallbladder carcinoma in North India. *Eur J Surg Oncol.* 2000;26(2):164–167.

Miura N, Hasegawa J, and Shiota G. Serum messenger RNA as a biomarker and its clinical usefulness in malignancies. *Clin Med Oncol.* 2008;2:511–527.

Moreno M, Pimentel F, Gazdar AF, Wistuba II, and Miquel JF. TP53 abnormalities are frequent and early events in the sequential pathogenesis of gallbladder carcinoma. *Ann Hepatol.* 2005;4(3): 192–199.

Mou Y, Xing R, and Liu C. Diagnosis of gallbladder cancer using matrix-assisted laser desorption/ionization time-of-flight profiling. *Am J Med Sci.* 2012;343(2):119–123.

Murakawa K, Tada M, Takada M et al. Prediction of lymph node metastasis and perineural invasion of biliary tract cancer by selected features from cDNA array data. *J Surg Res.* 2004;122:184–194.

Nagasaki K and Miki Y. Molecular prediction of the therapeutic response to neoadjuvant chemotherapy in breast cancer. *Breast Cancer.* 2008;15:117–120.

Nakashima M, Sonoda K, and Watanabe T. Inhibition of cell growth and induction of apoptotic cell death by the human tumor-associated antigen RCAS1. *Nat Med.* 1999;5:938–942.

North JH Jr, Pack MS, Hong C, and Rivera DE. Prognostic factors for adenocarcinoma of the gallbladder: An analysis of 162 cases. *Am Surg.* 1998;64:437–440.

Noshiro H, Chijiiwa K, Yamaguchi K et al. Factors affecting surgical outcome for gallbladder carcinoma. *Hepatogastroenterology.* 2003;50(52):939–944.

O'Brien MJ, Zamcheck N, Burke B et al. Immunocytochemical localization of carcinoembryonic antigen in benign and malignant colorectal tissues: Assessment of diagnostic value. *Am J Clin Pathol.* 1981;75:283–290.

O'Brien TJ, Raymond LM, and Bannon GA. New monoclonal antibodies identify the glycoprotein carrying the CA 125 epitope. *Am J Obstet Gynecol.* 1991;165:1857–1864.

Ohtaka K, Kohya N, Sato K, Kitajima Y, Ide T, Mitsuno M, and Miyazaki K. Ribonucleotide reductase subunit M1 is a possible chemoresistance marker to gemcitabine in biliary tract carcinoma. *Oncol Rep.* 2008;20:279–286.

Okada K, Kijima H, Imaizumi T et al. Stromal laminin-5gamma2 chain expression is associated with the wall-invasion pattern of gallbladder adenocarcinoma. *Biomed Res.* 2009;30:53–62.

Okami J, Dohno K, Sakon M et al. Genetic detection for micrometastasis in lymph node of biliary tract carcinoma. *Clin Cancer Res.* 2000;6(6):2326–2332.

Okamoto A, Demetrick DJ, Spillare EA et al. Mutations and altered expression of p16INK4 in human cancer. *Proc Natl Acad Sci USA.* 1994;91(23):11045–11049.

Okita S, Kondoh S, Shiraishi K, Kaino S, Hatano S, and Okita K. Expression of vascular endothelial growth factor correlates with tumor progression in gallbladder cancer. *Int J Oncol.* 1998;12(5):1013–1038.

Oshikiri T, Hida Y, Miyamoto M et al. RCAS1 expression as a prognostic factor after curative surgery for extrahepatic bile duct cancer. *Br J Cancer.* 2001;85:1922–1927.

Paget S. The distribution of secondary growths in cancer of the breast. *Lancet.* 1889;133:571–573.

Pandey M. Risk factors for gallbladder cancer: A reappraisal. *Eur Pancreat Surg.* 2003;6:237–244.

Pang Y, Young CY, and Yuan H. MicroRNAs and prostate cancer. *Acta Biochim Biophys Sin (Shanghai).* 2010;42:363–369.

Park JY, Park BK, Ko JS, Bang S, Song SY, and Chung JB. Bile acid analysis in biliary tract cancer. *Yonsei Med J.* 2006;47(6):817–825.

Pasanen PA, Eskelinen M, Partanen K, Pikkarainen P, Penttilä I, and Alhava E. Multivariate analysis of six serum tumor markers (CEA, CA 50, CA 242, TPA, TPS, TATI) and conventional laboratory tests in the diagnosis of hepatopancreatobiliary malignancy. *Anticancer Res.* 1995;15(6B):2731–2737.

Pingitore R, Bonucci M, Bigini D et al. Chronic calculous cholecystitis: Elementary and dysplastic lesions, echographic correlations and immunohistochemical approach. *Pathologica.* 1992;84:171–185.

Punnoose EA, Atwal SK, Spoerke JM et al. Molecular biomarker analyses using circulating tumor cells. *PLoS One.* 2010;5:e12517.

Qing D, Xia L, and Zhang X. The expressions of proliferating cell nuclear antigen (PCNA) in primary gallbladder carcinoma and its significance. *Zhonghua Wai Ke Za Zhi.* 1995;33(2):102–104.

Quan ZW, Wu K, Wang J, Shi W, Zhang Z, and Merrell RC. Association of p53, p16, and vascular endothelial growth factor protein expressions with the prognosis and metastasis of gallbladder cancer. *J Am Coll Surg*. 2001;193(4):380–383.

Rana S, Dutta U, Kochhar R et al. Evaluation of CA 242 as a tumor marker in gallbladder cancer. *Gastrointest Cancer*. 2012;43(2):267–271.

Randi G, Randi G, Franceschi S, and La Vecchia C. Gallbladder cancer worldwide: Geographical distribution and risk factors. *Int J Cancer*. 2006;118:1591–1602.

Ribatti D and Vacca A. The role of microenvironment in tumor angiogenesis. *Genes Nutr*. 2008;3:29–34.

Riquelme E, Tang M, Baez S, Diaz A, Pruyas M, Wistuba II, and Corvalan A. Frequent epigenetic inactivation of chromosome 3p candidate tumor suppressor genes in gallbladder carcinoma. *Cancer Lett*. 2007;250(1):100–106.

Roa I, Arya JC, Shirasch T et al. Gallbladder cancer: Immunohistochemical expression of CA 19–9, epithelial membrane antigen, dupin-2 and CEA. *Rev Med Chil*. 1992;120:1218–1226.

Roa I, Araya JC, Villaseca M, De Aretxabala X, Riedemann P, Endoh K, Roa J. Preneoplastic lesions and gallbladder cancer: An estimate of the period required for progression. *Gastroenterology*. 1996;111:232–236.

Roa I, Villaseca M, Araya J, Roa J, de Aretxabala X, Ibacache G, and García M. CD44 (HCAM) expression in subserous gallbladder carcinoma. *Rev Med Chil*. 2001;129(7):727–734.

Robert J, Vekris A, Pourquier P, and Bonnet J. Predicting drug response based on gene expression. *Crit Rev Oncol Hematol*. 2004;51:205–227.

Rumalla A and Petersen BT. Diagnosis and therapy of biliary tract malignancy. *Semin Gastrointest Dis*. 2000;11(3):168–173.

Sasaki R. Immunohistochemical study of cancer-associated carbohydrate antigens in carcinoma of the biliary tract. *Nippon Geka Gakkai Zasshi*. 1989;90:1976–1988.

Sasatomi E, Tokunaga O, and Miyazaki K. Spontaneous apoptosis in gallbladder carcinoma. Relationship with clinicopathologic factors, expression of E-cadherin, bcl2 protooncogene, and p53 oncosuppressor gene. *Cancer*. 1993;78:2101–2110.

Sato K, Kitajima Y, Kohya N, Koga Y, Ohtaka K, and Miyazaki K. CPT-11 (SN-38) chemotherapy may be selectively applicable to biliary tract cancer with low hMLH1 expression. *Anticancer Res*. 2007;27:865–872.

Sato K, Kitajima Y, Miyoshi A, Koga Y, and Miyazaki K. Deficient expression of the DPD gene is caused by epigenetic modification in biliary tract cancer cells, and induces high sensitivity to 5-FU treatment. *Int J Oncol*. 2006;29:429–435.

Schetter AJ, Leung SY, and Sohn JJ et al. MicroRNA expression profiles associated with prognosis and therapeutic outcome in colon adenocarcinoma. *JAMA*. 2008;299:425–436.

Schwarzenbach H, Hoon DS, and Pantel K. Cell-free nucleic acids as biomarkers in cancer patients. *Nat Rev Cancer*. 2011;11:426–437.

Seitz G, Thelsinger B, Tomasetto G, Rio MC, Chambon P, Blin N, and Welter G. Breast cancer-associated protein pS2 expression in tumors of the biliary tract. *Am J Gastroenterol*. October 1991;86(10):1491–1494.

Serra I, Calvo A, Csendes A, and Sharp A. Gastric and gallbladder carcinoma in Chile: Epidemiological changes and control programs. *Rev Med Chil*. 1989;117:834–836.

Shi CJ, Gao J, Wang M, Wang X et al. CD133(+) gallbladder carcinoma cells exhibit self-renewal ability and tumorigenicity. *World J Gastroenterol*. 2011;17:2965–2971.

Shi CJ, Tian R, Wang M, Wang X, Jiang J, Zhang Z, Li X, He Z, Gong W, and Qin R. CD44+ CD133+ population exhibits cancer stem cell-like characteristics in human gallbladder carcinoma. *Cancer Biol Ther*. 2010;10:1182–1190.

Shibata T, Kokubu A, Gotoh M, Ojima H, Ohta T, Yamamoto M, and Hirohashi S. Genetic alteration of Keap1 confers constitutive Nrf2 activation and resistance to chemotherapy in gallbladder cancer. *Gastroenterology*. 2008;135:1358–1368, 1368.e1.

Shukla VK, Gurubachan, Sharma D, Dixit VK, and Usha. Diagnostic value of serum CA242, CA 19–9, CA 15–3 and CA 125 in patients with carcinoma of the gallbladder. *Trop Gastroenterol*. October–December 2006;27(4):160–165.

Shukla VK, Tandon A, Ratha BK, Sharma D, Singh TB, and Basu S. Arginase activity in carcinoma of the gallbladder. A pilot study. *Eur J Cancer Prev*. 2009;18(3):199–202.

Somashekar BS, Ijare OB, and Gowda GA. Analysis of bile and gallbladder tissue by NMR: A route for diagnosis of gallbladder cancer. *Proc Intl Soc Mag Reson Med*. 2007;15:127.

Srivastava K, Srivastava A, Sharma KL, and Mittal B. Candidate gene studies in gallbladder cancer: A systematic review and meta-analysis. *Mutat Res*. 2011;728:67–79.

Stefanovic D, Novakovic R, Perisic-Savic M et al. The evaluation of tumor markers levels in determination of surgical procedure in patients with gallbladder carcinoma. *Med Pregl*. 1993;46(Suppl 1):58–59.

Stinton LM and Shaffer EA. Epidemiology of gallbladder disease: Cholelithiasis and cancer. *Gut Liver*. 2012;6(2):172–187.

Strom BL, Soloway RD, Rios-Dalenz JL et al. Risk factors for gallbladder cancer. An international collaborative case-control study. *Cancer*. 1995;76:1747–1756.

Strom BL, Uiopoulos D, Atkinson B et al. Pathophysiology of tumor progression in human gallbladder: Flow cytometry CEA and CA 19–9 levels in bile and serum in different stages of gallbladder diseases. *J Natl Cancer Inst*. 1989;81:1575–1580.

Su WC, Shiesh SC, Liu HS, Chen CY, Chow NH, and Lin XZ. Expression of oncogene products HER2/Neu and Ras and fibrosis-related growth factors bFGF, TGF-beta, and PDGF in bile from biliary malignancies and inflammatory disorders. *Dig Dis Sci*. 2001;46(7):1387–1392.

Sun YF, Yang XR, Zhou J, Qiu SJ, Fan J, and Xu Y. Circulating tumor cells: Advances in detection methods, biological issues, and clinical relevance. *J Cancer Res Clin Oncol*. 2011;137:1151–1173.

Swierczynski SL, Maitra A, Abraham SC et al. Analysis of novel tumor markers in pancreatic and biliary carcinomas using tissue microarrays. *Hum Pathol*. 2004;35:357–366.

Takahashi T, Shivapurkar N, Riquelme E et al. Aberrant promoter hypermethylation of multiple genes in gallbladder carcinoma and chronic cholecystitis. *Clin Cancer Res*. 2004;10:6126–6133.

Tamiolakis D, Simopoulos C, Kotini A, Venizelos J, Jivannakis T, Skaphida P, and Papadopoulos N. Prognostic significance of HLA-DR antigen in dysplasia, carcinoma in situ and invasive carcinoma of the gallbladder. *East Afr Med J*. 2003;80(11):554–558.

Tan Y, Ma SY, Wang FQ, Meng HP, Mei C, Liu A, and Wu HR. Proteomic-based analysis for identification of potential serum biomarkers in gallbladder cancer. *Oncol Rep*. 2011;26:853–859.

Tan Y, Meng HP, Wang FQ, Cheng ZN, Wu Q, and Wu HR. Comparative proteomic analysis of human gallbladder carcinoma. *Zhonghua Zhong Liu Za Zhi*. 2010;32:29–32.

Tanaka H, Shimada Y, Harada H, Shinoda M, Hatooka S, Imamura M, and Ishizaki K. Methylation of the 5′ CpG island of the FHIT gene is closely associated with transcriptional inactivation in esophageal squamous cell carcinomas. *Cancer Res*. 1998;58(15):3429–3434.

Tanaka S, Takahashi R, Kitadai Y, Sumii M, Yoshihara M, Haruma K, and Chayama K. Expression of vascular endothelial growth factor and angiogenesis in gastrointestinal stromal tumor of the stomach. *Oncology*. 2003;64:266–274.

Tasaki K, Yamamoto H, Watanabe K et al. Successful treatment of lymph node metastases recurring from gallbladder cancer. *J Hepatobiliary Pancreat Surg*. 2003;10(1):113–117.

Tian Y, Ding RY, Zhi YH, Guo RX, and Wu SD. Analysis of p53 and vascular endothelial growth factor expression in human gallbladder carcinoma for the determination of tumor vascularity. *World J Gastroenterol*. 2006;12:415–419.

Uchida N, Tsutsui K, Ezaki T et al. Combination of assay of human telomerase reverse transcriptase mRNA and cytology using bile obtained by endoscopic transpapillary catheterization into the gallbladder for diagnosis of gallbladder carcinoma. *Am J Gastroenterol*. 2003;98:2415–2419.

Ueki T, Hsing AW, Gao YT, Wang BS, Shen MC, Cheng J, Deng J, Fraumeni JF Jr, and Rashid A. Alterations of p16 and prognosis in biliary tract cancers from a population-based study in China. *Clin Cancer Res*. 2004;10:1717–1725.

Venniyoor A. Cholesterol gallstones and cancer of gallbladder (CAGB): Molecular links. *Med Hypotheses*. 2008;70(3):646–653.

Virji MA, Mercer DW, and Herberman RB. Tumor Markers and their measurements. *Pathol Res Pract*. 1988;183:95–99.

Wagata T, Shibagaki I, Imamura M, Shimada Y, Toguchida J, Yandell DW, Ikenaga M, Tobe T, and Ishizaki K. Loss of 17p, mutation of the p53 gene, and overexpression of p53 protein in esophageal squamous cell carcinomas. *Cancer Res*. 1993;53(4):846–850.

Wang X, Huang K, and Xu L. Interaction among Rb/p16, Rb/E2F1 and HDAC1 proteins in gallbladder carcinoma. *J Huazhong Univ Sci Technolog Med Sci*. 2009;29(6):729–731.

Washiro M, Ohtsuka M, Kimura F, Shimizu H, Yoshidome H, Sugimoto T, Seki N, and Miyazaki M. Upregulation of topoisomerase IIalpha expression in advanced gallbladder carcinoma: A potential chemotherapeutic target. *J Cancer Res Clin Oncol*. 2008;134:793–801.

Wen H, Yoo SS, Kang J et al. A new NMR-based metabolomics approach for the diagnosis of biliary tract cancer. *J Hepatol*. 2010;52:228–233.

Wistuba I, Gazdar AF, Sugio K et al. Abnormalities of p53 and K-ras gene in the pathogenesis of endemic gallbladder carcinoma (GBC) in Chile [abstract]. *Lab Invest*. 1995a;72:70A.

Wistuba II and Albores-Saavedra J. Genetic abnormalities involved in the pathogenesis of gallbladder carcinoma. *J Hepatobiliary Pancreat Surg*. 1999;6:237–244.

Wistuba II, Ashfaq R, Maitra A, Alvarez H, Riquelme E, and Gazdar AF. Fragile histidine triad gene abnormalities in the pathogenesis of gallbladder carcinoma. *Am J Pathol*. 2002;160(6):2073–2079.

Wistuba II and Gazdar AF. Gallbladder cancer: Lessons from a rare tumour. *Nat Rev Cancer*. 2004;4(9):695–706.

Wistuba II, Sugio K, Hung J, Kishimoto Y, Virmani AK, Roa I, Albores-Saavedra J, and Gazdar AF. Allele-specific mutations involved in the pathogenesis of endemic gallbladder carcinoma in Chile. *Cancer Res*. 1995b;55(12):2511–2515.

Wistuba II, Tang M, Maitra A, Alvarez H, Troncoso P, Pimentel F, and Gazdar AF. Genome-wide allelotyping analysis reveals multiple sites of allelic loss in gallbladder carcinoma. *Cancer Res*. 2001;61(9):3795–3800.

Yamaguchi A, Zhang M, Goi T, Fujita T, Niimoto S, Katayama K, and Hirose K. Expression of variant CD44 containing variant exon v8–10 in gallbladder cancer. *Oncol Rep*. 2000;7(3):541–544.

Yanagisawa N, Mikami T, Mitomi H, Saegusa M, Koike M, and Okayasu I. CD44 variant overexpression in gallbladder carcinoma associated with tumor dedifferentiation. *Cancer*. 2001;91(2):408–416.

Yoshida S, Todoroki T, Ichikawa Y, Hanai S, Suzuki H, Hori M, Fukao K, Miwa M, and Uchida K. Mutations of p16Ink4/CDKN2 and p15Ink4B/MTS2 genes in biliary tract cancers. *Cancer Res*. 1995;55(13):2756–2760.

Yoshida T, Sugai T, Habano W, Nakamura S, Uesugi N, Funato O, and Saito K. Microsatellite instability in gallbladder carcinoma: Two independent genetic pathways of gallbladder carcinogenesis. *J Gastroenterol*. 2000;35(10):768–774.

Zatonski WA, La Vecchia C, Przewozniak K, Maisonneuve P, Lowenfels AB, and Boyle P. Risk factors for gallbladder cancer: A Polish case-control study. *Int J Cancer*. 1992;51:707–711.

Zatonski WA, Lowenfels AB, Boyle P et al. Epidemiologic aspects of gallbladder cancer: A case-control study of the SEARCH Program of the International Agency for Research on Cancer. *J Natl Cancer Inst*. 1997;89:1132–1138.

Zhu AX and Hezel AF. Development of molecularly targeted therapies in biliary tract cancers: Reassessing the challenges and opportunities. *Hepatology*. 2011;53:695–704.

Zöchbauer-Müller S, Fong KM, Maitra A, Lam S et al. 5′ CpG island methylation of the FHIT gene is correlated with loss of gene expression in lung and breast cancer. *Cancer Res*. 2001;61(9):3581–3585.

17

Noninvasive Early Markers in Pancreatic Cancer

Aleksandra Nikolic

CONTENTS

ABSTRACT The development of early detection biomarkers is of special importance for pancreatic cancer, a devastating disease with poor prognosis and one of the most aggressive human malignancies. Despite considerable development in sophisticated imaging techniques and cytological examination, pancreatic cancer is most often diagnosed late in the course of the disease, after local spread and distant metastases have already occurred. Since pancreatic cancer is very difficult to treat, the key to the management of this disease are understanding of the molecular basis of transformation into malignant tumor of the pancreas and identification of molecular markers that can be used for early detection of the disease in the clinical practice. Although many molecular markers have been examined in pancreatic cancer, none are considered to be sufficiently specific and sensitive for preoperative diagnosis. Altered serum levels of CA 19-9 and mutated *K-RAS* gene are often used in clinical practice as markers of pancreatic malignancy. However, their sensitivity and specificity are relatively low and the use of other markers in combination with these two is necessary to improve diagnostic accuracy.

Of several tumor suppressor genes inactivated in pancreatic tumors, *SMAD4* genetic alterations appear to be the landmark of pancreatic tumorigenesis and they may prove to have high diagnostic value for this type of malignancy. Latest studies are directed toward the discovery of altered levels of proteins other than CA 19-9 and other molecules in serum samples of pancreatic cancer patients as early markers of malignant process. Diagnostics based on such markers would be noninvasive, and these markers would also be useful for disease monitoring and assessment of the response to therapy. However, altered serum levels of proteins and other molecules are not reliable diagnostic markers, since they may vary due to factors other than malignancy, inflammation above all. Genetic and epigenetic markers are much more reliable, but their analysis currently requires tumor tissue samples, which can only be obtained during invasive procedures, such as surgical procedure or biopsy. Considering the previously mentioned limitations, the most promising approach in early diagnosis of pancreatic cancer appears to be the analysis of circulating DNA in serum samples of pancreatic cancer patients. Fragments of DNA released in the blood flow of patients with malignancy by necrotic pancreatic cancer cells represent the largest portion of cell-free DNA. Since cell-free DNA reflects the genetic status of the tumor, it can be analyzed for the presence of mutations in specific genes and for methylation of various gene promoters, which would produce the most accurate and specific diagnostic information. Methodological improvements in molecular diagnosis of pancreatic cancer remain to change the way this disease is discovered and treated.

17.1 Outline

This chapter will give the overview of molecular profile of pancreatic cancer, current and potential biomarkers for this disease, and existing and developing methods for their analysis. Markers currently used in clinical practice, CA 19-9 and *K-RAS* mutations, will be presented and their limitations will be discussed. Latest studies on pancreatic cancer biomarkers development will be summarized and proteins and other molecules of potential importance will be pointed out. This topic will be concluded by presenting the most promising approach in early diagnosis of pancreatic cancer, analysis of serum DNA, which can produce the most accurate and specific diagnostic information and can also be used for prognosis, disease monitoring, and assessment of the response to therapy.

17.2 Pancreatic Cancer

Pancreatic ductal adenocarcinoma, usually referred to as pancreatic cancer, is the most common malignant pancreatic neoplasm, accounting for 90% of all pancreatic tumors (Mergo et al., 1997). It is a highly malignant disease and the fourth cause of cancer-related deaths in the world (Siegel et al., 2012). The disease is characterized by poor prognosis, due to rapid progression, highly invasive tumor phenotype, and resistance to chemotherapy. Despite continuous research efforts and significant advances in treatment of the disease during the past few decades, clinical outcome of pancreatic cancer has only marginally improved with minor overall changes in survival rate. With a median survival of less than 6 months after initial diagnosis and an average 5-year survival rate below 5%, the mortality–incidence ratio for pancreatic cancer patients is about 0.99 (Hayat et al., 2007).

An understanding of the molecular basis of transformation into malignant tumor of the pancreas may provide a basis for the development of more effective strategies for the prevention, diagnosis, and treatment of this cancer. The disease develops through several phases of pancreatic intraepithelial neoplasia (PanIN) lesions from benign to fully malignant. There are three PanIN stages through which the disease progresses, marked by worsening histologic dysplasia and the accumulation of genetic defects. Although biological mechanisms still remain largely unclear, research is showing different genetic alternations during different phases, which is of importance for disease prognosis and monitoring (Iacobuzio-Donahue, 2012) (Figure 17.1).

Major contributory factor to the poor outcome of pancreatic cancer is the lack of appropriate sensitive and specific biomarkers for early diagnosis. Furthermore, efficient biomarkers for population

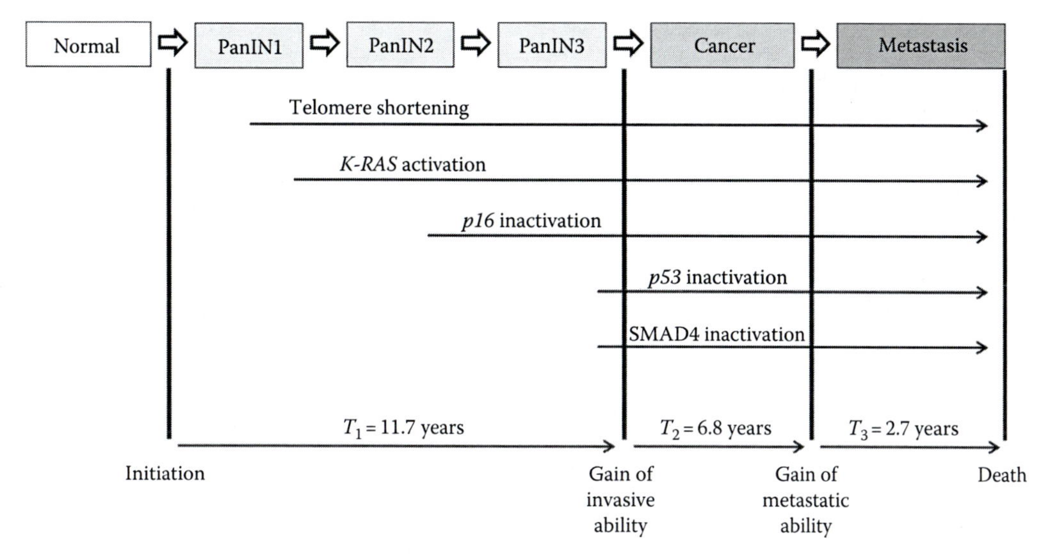

FIGURE 17.1 Chronology of key molecular events in the development of pancreatic cancer.

screening, targeting, directing, and assessing therapeutic intervention, as well as for detection of residual or recurrent disease, are absent. Up to now, despite the development of novel techniques and potential markers reported, only a limited number may be of potential use in the clinical setting. Of many candidate markers for pancreatic cancer currently under investigation, CA 19-9 remains the only one routinely used in clinical practice, in spite of its imperfections. Additional markers are needed not only to facilitate the early diagnosis of pancreatic cancer but also to help diagnose pancreatic cancer precursor lesions. Our knowledge of pancreatic neoplasia and evidence from clinical studies conducted in high-risk individuals support the idea that the best way to reduce the mortality of pancreatic cancer is to use molecular markers and pancreatic imaging to identify patients with precancerous lesions of the pancreas.

Research on pancreatic cancer biomarkers is intensive and the use of novel technologies may provide completely novel tools and possibilities of potential improvement, achieving early diagnosis, targeted therapy, and discovery of recurrence in patients with pancreatic cancer. Considering the characteristics of pancreatic cancer, with often vague symptoms but associated tumor aggressiveness, resistance to standard therapy, and a poor prognosis, the identification of adequate biomarkers is of extreme importance for improving clinical management and therapeutic outcome in pancreatic cancer patients.

17.2.1 Pancreatic Cancer Diagnosis

Despite considerable development in sophisticated imaging techniques and cytological examination, pancreatic cancer is most often diagnosed after local spread and distant metastases have already occurred. Most symptoms, including profound weight loss, abdominal pain, new-onset type 2 diabetes mellitus, jaundice, and nausea, are usually vague and occur late during the course of disease. Only in a minority of cases, the diagnosis is made at a very early stage, when curative surgery might significantly ameliorate the 5-year survival rate. Also, chronic pancreatitis can be difficult to distinguish from pancreatic cancer with the use of clinical, imaging, and biochemical parameters routinely used for diagnostic purposes. Available diagnostic tools for pancreatic cancer include several advanced techniques (Table 17.1) (Bhat et al., 2012). However, these techniques are costly and require access to highly specialized facilities and therefore are not readily available for detecting the disease at an early stage. In general, the diagnosis is most often established using computerized tomography (CT) with histological or cytological confirmation upon biopsy (Figure 17.2) (Cascinu et al., 2010).

TABLE 17.1
Available Diagnostic Tools for Pancreatic Cancer

Diagnostic Tool	Application and Advantages	Limitations
Transabdominal ultrasound (US)	Visualization of bile duct and liver	Poor visualization of pancreas
CT	Diagnosis and staging	Nephrotoxicity of iodine contrast agent; potential side effects from exposure to radiation
Magnetic resonance imaging (MRI)	Superior imaging of pancreas and bile duct; iodine-free contrast agent; no radiation	Expensive; less availability
Positron emission tomography (PET)	Metastatic disease assessment; monitoring recurrence and response to adjuvant therapy	Expensive; less availability
EUS	Imaging of pancreatic masses and lymph nodes	Expensive; less availability
Endoscopic ultrasound–fine-needle aspiration (EUS-FNA)	Specific detection; safe and less invasive; imaging of lesions from 3 to 4 mm upward; puncturing of lymph nodes >5 mm	Access only to posterior mediastinum
Magnetic resonance cholangiopancreatography (MRCP)	Imaging of fluid in the pancreatic ducts in a noninvasive manner	Lower resolution; no biopsy; expensive
ERCP	Imaging strictures	Complications like bleeding and infection
Cholangiopancreatoscopy	Site-directed biopsies of strictures	Fragile equipment

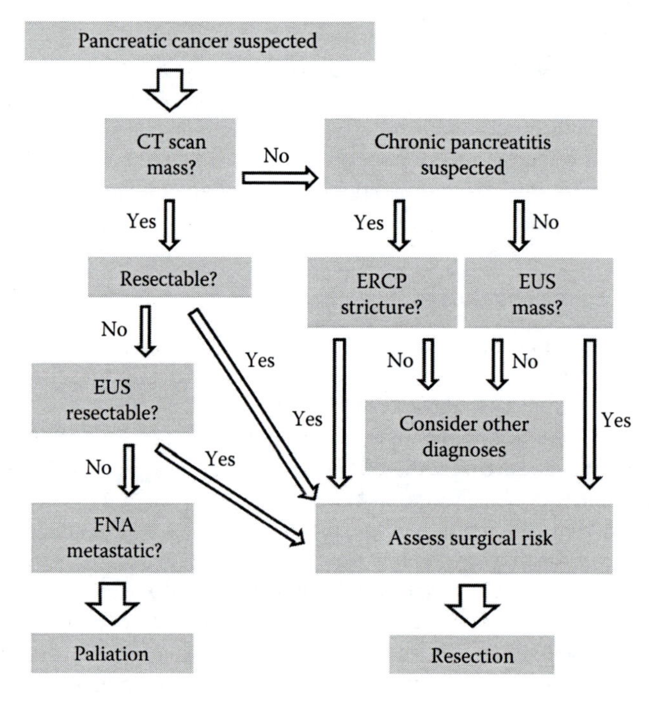

FIGURE 17.2 Diagnostic and treatment strategy for pancreatic cancer.

17.2.2 Pancreatic Cancer Treatment

The treatment of pancreatic cancer is undertaken with two different aims. In patients with early stage of disease, the aim is removal of the tumor by radical surgery. In all other cases, the aim of the treatment is the palliation of the several distressing symptoms related to the pancreatic cancer. The only potentially curative approach is surgical resection, which is often unsuccessful because the invasive and metastatic nature of the pancreatic tumor masses makes their complete removal difficult. Resectable pancreatic cancer is associated with an improved outcome, especially if the diagnosis is obtained in an early phase, but less than 20% of patients are candidates for a potentially curative resection, which makes pancreatic cancer extremely difficult to treat (Wray et al., 2005). Treatment options other than surgical resection include chemotherapy protocols that routinely use gemcitabine and 5-fluorouracil and often include radiotherapy (Saif, 2011). Numerous clinical trials have compared multiple drugs in combination with gemcitabine, but all the drug combinations have failed despite costly clinical trials involving thousands of patients. Most physicians, particularly oncologists, treating patients with pancreatic cancer are largely focused on treating their patients in the palliative setting.

17.3 Sources of Samples for Pancreatic Cancer Marker Analysis

Sample source is of special importance in the search for biomarkers to detect and diagnose early pancreatic cancer. Pancreatic biopsy samples are reliable sources for diagnosis, but there is great need and ongoing research for samples that could be obtained less invasively. Except in the pancreatic tissue, potential molecular markers are sought in pancreatic juice as well as other body fluids including blood and urine (Table 17.2) (Bhat et al., 2012). To minimize invasive procedures, ideal markers should optimally be detected in the blood. An important consideration is that pancreatic tumor cells and secreted molecules are found in markedly higher concentrations in the pancreas and pancreatic juice compared to the blood. For example, CA 19-9 levels in the pancreatic juice are 30–1000 times higher than in serum (Zhou et al., 2007). Thus, it is logical to first obtain pancreas tissue to identify differential markers of pancreatic cancer and then look for their presence further from the pancreas. Endoscopic ultrasound-guided fine-needle aspiration (EUS-FNA) can be used to readily and safely obtain pancreatic tissue to enable this process and has an important role in biomarker discovery (Laurell et al., 2006).

Pancreatic cancer tissue is the most direct source of biomarkers, as it is likely to have the highest concentrations of pancreatic cancer-specific markers. However, invasive biopsy material for screening is usually not readily available, and percutaneous biopsies might even result in seeding of cancer cells. For these reasons, invasive biopsy material is not used for cancer screening and final diagnosis is based on pathological evaluation of the pancreatic cancer tissue obtained on surgery. Ongoing biomarker research obtained from pancreatic cancer tissue is not often done for diagnostic purposes but rather for the development of potential future targeted therapies.

Pancreatic juice, a fluid from the pancreatic duct, has recently been identified as an alternative source for biomarker discovery (Chen et al., 2006; Gao et al., 2010). Pancreatic juice is rich in DNA/RNA/

TABLE 17.2

Sources of Specimens for Pancreatic Cancer Biomarker Research

Sample Source	Detection Method
Tissue	Immunohistochemistry, PCR-based techniques, microarray
Pancreatic juice	Quantitative proteomics
Serum	Quantitative proteomics, ELISA
Plasma	Functional genomics
Saliva	Human genome array
Stool	PCR

protein markers directly shed into the ductal lumen from pancreatic ductal cancer cells and should therefore constitute a perfect source for specific biomarkers for pancreatic cancer detection. To date approximately 170 proteins have been identified in human pancreatic juice, one-third of which are enzymes (Sun et al., 2011). However, pancreatic juice is not readily accessible, and in addition, the procedure used in order to obtain pancreatic juice, endoscopic retrograde cholangiopancreatography (ERCP), may induce side effects. Pure pancreatic juice collection requires ERCP, but pancreatic juice can also be collected in the duodenum and assayed for the presence of markers during routine upper gastrointestinal endoscopy after secretin stimulation without the need for ERCP. Pancreatic juice markers and the assays designed for their detection are currently still undergoing evaluation and have not yet been demonstrated to be useful in clinical practice.

Blood is the most frequently used source for biomarkers, being minimally invasive, easily accessible, generally inexpensive, and reproducible to obtain and analyze. Molecules (DNA, RNA, protein), disseminated tumor cells (DTCs), and circulating tumor cells (CTCs) from plasma/serum are frequently used for biomarker detection (Ehmann et al., 2007; Hanash et al., 2008). However, some highly abundant proteins, such as albumin or globulin, can affect the detection of less abundant, but for the diagnosis, valuable proteins.

Saliva has also been exploited as a source of pancreatic cancer biomarkers and genes have been detected with potential for classification of resectable disease (Zhang et al., 2010).

Stool samples were suggested by a recent study as a sample source for the analysis of genetic markers such as *K-RAS* and *p53* mutations that might enable the detection of early pancreatic cancer (Haug et al., 2008).

Urine is a potential source of biomarkers for pancreatic cancer, as it is easily and noninvasively available. However, a limitation of urine is the dilution of the proteins of potential interest. Secondly, the urine is derived from the kidneys, only being in contact with the pancreas through blood, and most of the proteomic information exists in circulating blood.

17.4 Markers Used for Pancreatic Cancer

Over the last three decades, several markers have been proposed for pancreatic cancer, but no specific markers have been found that could be helpful in diagnostics and there are no population-wide screening tests for this disease. The most widely used and best validated marker for pancreatic cancer is CA 19-9, but inadequate sensitivity and specificity limit its use in the early diagnosis of pancreatic cancer. Mutations in the *K-RAS* gene are routinely detected in tumor tissue samples obtained on either resective surgery or FNA but are rarely used for early diagnosis of pancreatic cancer. In most cases, by the time tumor is resected and genetically analyzed, the malignancy is already in an advanced stage. Analysis of *K-RAS* mutations in samples obtained noninvasively, such as serum and plasma, would have been of substantial help in pancreatic cancer screening, but such methods have not yet been developed and validated for clinical use. Of the commercially available genetic tests for pancreatic cancer susceptibility, analyses of mutations in the genes *BRCA2*, *PALB2*, and *PALLD* are offered (GeneTests, 2012). Although several potential markers for pancreatic cancer are currently undergoing evaluation, none are sufficiently validated for routine clinical use. Therefore, in spite of its inadequacies, CA 19-9 remains the pancreatic cancer marker against which new markers for this malignancy should be judged.

17.4.1 Carbohydrate Antigen 19-9

Carbohydrate antigen 19-9 (CA 19-9) is the most widely used and the most thoroughly evaluated biochemical marker for pancreatic cancer. It is a high molecular weight (MW) glycolipid defined from the culture medium of a colorectal cancer cell line (Koprowski et al., 1981). In clinical practice, CA 19-9 is routinely measured in serum by radioimmunoassay method (Farini et al., 1985). However, serum levels of CA 19-9 are not sensitive or specific enough to use as a screening test for cancer and are not diagnostic of a specific type of cancer.

The utility of serum CA 19-9 in the diagnosis of pancreatic cancer has been extensively investigated in numerous retrospective and prospective studies that have enrolled multiple control groups (chronic pancreatitis, obstructive jaundice, abdominal pain, healthy subjects). Sensitivity of CA 19-9 marker varies from 69% to 94%, specificity from 44% to 96%, while diagnostic accuracy varies from 49% to 81% (Farini et al., 1985; Del Favero et al., 1986a,b; Molina et al., 1990, 2012; DelMaschio et al., 1991; Banfi et al., 1996; Safi et al., 1998). The principal limitation of CA 19-9 use in pancreatic cancer diagnostics is its low specificity due to the fact that it can be temporarily elevated in many nonmalignant conditions that affect the liver or pancreas (Del Favero et al., 1986a; Haglund et al., 1986b). Taking the recommended cutoff value of 37 U/mL, the test may be falsely normal (false negative) in many cases or abnormally elevated in people who have no cancer at all (false positive). Among patients with resectable pancreatic cancer, CA 19-9 levels are not elevated in up to 35% of the patients (Goggins, 2005). Also, the expression of the CA 19-9, defined by the monoclonal antibody and immunoperoxidase staining in formalin-fixed, paraffin-embedded tissue sections, demonstrated a correlation between the degree of differentiation of the ductal adenocarcinomas and the expression of CA 19-9, whereas the correlation between tissue expression and serum levels of CA 19-9 was poor (Haglund et al., 1986a).

Serum levels of CA 19-9 may be used as a tumor marker to help differentiate between cancer of the pancreas and other conditions, such as pancreatitis, to monitor response to pancreatic cancer treatment and/or cancer progression and to watch for pancreatic cancer recurrence. Guidelines on pancreatic cancer diagnostics discourage the use of CA 19-9 as a screening test, because its specificity and sensitivity for this purpose are not adequate for accurate diagnosis (Table 17.3) (Locker et al., 2006; Goggins et al., 2007). According to the guidelines from the American Society of Clinical Oncology, CA 19-9 can be measured every 1–3 months for patients with locally advanced or metastatic disease receiving active therapy. As a biomarker, CA 19-9 is primarily used clinically to follow the response to therapy, both before and after surgical resection and chemoradiotherapy (Sperti et al., 1993; Safi et al., 1996; Ishii et al., 1997; Halm et al., 2000; Rocha Lima et al., 2002; Saad et al., 2002, 2010; Kang et al., 2007; Berger et al., 2008; Hess et al., 2008; Nakai et al., 2008; Koom et al., 2009; Vormittag et al., 2009; Wasan et al., 2009; Bernhard et al., 2010; Katz et al., 2010; Kondo et al., 2010; Hata et al., 2012). Measurement of CA 19-9 serum levels is useful as a prognostic index after resection for pancreatic carcinoma and as a surveillance test in monitoring the efficacy of treatment. If CA 19-9 is initially elevated in pancreatic cancer, then it may be ordered several times during cancer treatment to monitor response and on a regular basis following treatment to help detect recurrence or confirm effect of the therapy. Kinetics of CA 19-9 in serum serves as an early and reliable indicator of response and helps to predict survival

TABLE 17.3

Recommendations by Different Expert Groups for Use of CA 19-9 as a Tumor Marker for Pancreatic Cancer

Application	European Group on Tumor Markers (1999)	American Gastroenterological Association (1999)	National Academy of Clinical Biochemistry (2005)
Screening	No specific recommendations	No specific screening method for high-risk subjects recommended, clinical benefit unproven	Not for screening of the general population, often normal in high-risk subjects
Diagnosis	Diagnostic aid with limited value, especially in early stages and the presence of cholestasis	No specific recommendations	Should be used in conjunction with an imaging test, can guide further testing in the appropriate clinical context
Prognosis	Routine use for prognosis of unproven value	No specific recommendations	Has independent prognostic value with regard to respectability and survival
Monitoring	Routine use for monitoring of unproven value	Not an accepted test for antitumor efficacy	Serial measurements during palliative chemotherapy can be used in conjunction with imaging tests to determine response, recommended for follow-up after surgery

in patients with advanced pancreatic cancer receiving treatment (Stemmler et al., 2003; Boeck et al., 2007, 2010). The recommendations of the American Society of Clinical Oncology include that CA 19-9 determinations by themselves cannot provide definitive evidence of disease recurrence without seeking confirmation with imaging studies for clinical findings and/or biopsy (Locker et al., 2006). In people with pancreatic masses, CA 19-9 can be useful in distinguishing between cancer and other diseases of the gland. Also, preoperative CA 19-9 levels may be a useful marker for determining preoperatively which patients have unresectable disease despite the demonstration of resectable disease on CT (Kilic et al., 2006). The use of CA 19-9 can satisfactorily discriminate between pancreatic cancer and chronic pancreatitis; in contrast, the discrimination is poor for other gastrointestinal diseases, mainly of a malignant nature (Farini et al., 1985).

For a long time, during which many other markers have been evaluated, none was regarded as consistently superior to CA 19-9, although most clinicians would gladly eliminate CA 19-9 for a more reliable biomarker. The variability in CA 19-9 serum levels is not only detected in the patient population but can be variable throughout the course of treatment of an individual. This lack of reproducible quantitative measurement may give a false sense of hope to patients with dramatic drop in CA 19-9 levels, who are often faced with the finding of a high CA 19-9 value on follow-up visits. Although useful as an additional diagnostic tool for the detection and monitoring of pancreatic cancer, CA 19-9 is of no value for the early detection of the disease (Frebourg et al., 1988). By the time a person has symptoms and significantly elevated levels of CA 19-9, pancreatic cancer is usually at an advanced stage. A common current approach is to use CA 19-9 in combination with other markers. Available data are insufficient to recommend the routine use of serum CA 19-9 alone for monitoring response to treatment and it appears that the time has come to abandon the routine use of CA 19-9 determination in the suspicion of pancreatic cancer.

17.4.2 *K-RAS* Gene Mutations

The *K-RAS* protein plays a key role in signal transduction, and point mutations resulting in the constitutive activation of the *K-RAS* oncogene make it independent of growth factor stimulation (Malumbres and Barbacid, 2003). The result of *K-RAS* constitutive activation is an uncontrolled mediation of a variety of cellular functions including unchecked proliferation and survival, as well as angiogenesis.

Mutations in the *K-RAS* gene occur at high frequency in pancreatic neoplasias and represent a critical event in the development of pancreatic cancer. In the classic PanIN model of tumor progression, *K-RAS* mutation is one of the earliest genetic events to occur, which predisposes cells toward further mutations, resulting in tumor development and maintenance of advanced tumor (Figure 17.1). Mutated *K-RAS* gene is the first known and the most prevalent genetic alteration in pancreatic cancer, occurring sporadically in normal pancreatic tissue, and is detected in 30% of early neoplasms, with the frequency rising to nearly 100% in advanced tumors (Almoguera et al., 1988; Berrozpe et al., 1994; Parker et al., 2011; Pellegata et al., 1994; Watanabe et al., 1996a,b; Uehara et al., 1996; Evans et al., 1997; Wenger et al., 1999; Li et al., 2002). The point mutation of *K-RAS* in pancreatic cancer typically occurs in codon 12. Alteration of GGT to GAT, GTT, or rarely to CGT results in the substitution of glycine with aspartate, valine, or arginine, respectively (Evans et al., 1997).

The sensitivity and specificity of *K-RAS* mutations are not sufficiently high for independent diagnostic use (Rifa et al., 2011). Relatively high sensitivity and specificity of 70% and 100% have been reported for *K-RAS* mutations in pancreatic cancer (Salek et al., 2007). However, they have also been detected in patients with chronic pancreatitis with relatively high frequency, of up to 30% (Uehara et al., 1996; Watanabe et al., 1996b). Since *K-RAS* gene mutations occur in chronic pancreatitis and are associated with evolution toward pancreatic cancer, they can precede clinical evidence of pancreatic cancer, but the clinical implications of this finding need further study. The absence of pancreatic calcifications and the presence of exocrine insufficiency were identified as additional predictive factors for the development of pancreatic cancer in patients with chronic pancreatitis carrying *K-RAS* codon 12 mutation (Arvanitakis et al., 2004). Also, smoking and diabetes diagnosed 5 or more years before were associated with pancreatic cancer patients positive for *K-RAS* codon 12 mutations, but not with those who tested negative (Fryzek et al., 2006).

Clinical samples obtained by noninvasive methods, such as pancreatic juice and plasma, represent easily obtainable source of tumor-specific DNA and can serve as valuable material for *K-RAS* mutation analysis. Patients showing a *K-RAS* alteration in pancreatic juice represent a subset of high-risk individuals and may be followed up closely (Boadas et al., 2001). Identification of *K-RAS* mutations in samples of pancreatic juice can provide a tool for screening and early detection of pancreatic cancer and may be useful in differentiating between pancreatic cancer and noncancerous pancreatic diseases (Berthelemy et al., 1995; Lu et al., 2002). *K-RAS* mutations in plasma DNA are a predictive biomarker for a poor prognosis of unresectable pancreatic cancer patients (Chen et al., 2010). Between 29% and 100% of patients with a tumor *K-RAS* mutation presented the same mutation in peripheral blood, while only 2% presented blood *K-RAS* mutation in the absence of the same tumor mutation, possibly due to sampling errors (Rogosnitzky and Danks, 2010). A big leap forward in the clinical use of *K-RAS* is that circulating *K-RAS* in the peripheral blood of patients with locally advanced pancreatic cancer has been taken as a potential biomarker for the response to combined radiotherapy and chemotherapy in a phase 1 clinical trial (Olsen et al., 2009). Rapid changes in the levels of *K-RAS* in plasma proved to be useful in determining the efficacy of a novel agent and this property of *K-RAS* can be used to measure the efficacy of novel therapeutic agents in the future. The main disadvantage of cell-free DNA analysis is the small amount of available tumor DNA, especially if the tumor is in the early stage of development and mutant cell line DNA is diluted in the DNA from wild-type cells. This problem may be overcome by application of advance methods based on detection of fluorescently labeled DNA, which are under development.

17.4.3 Testing for Pancreatic Cancer Predisposition

While there is no population screening for pancreatic cancer, surveillance programs are widely used to evaluate individuals with genetic syndromes strongly associated with pancreatic malignancy and those with extensive family history.

The most common germ line mutations associated with pancreatic cancer occur in *BRCA2* gene. Mutations in the *BRCA2* gene are among the initial mutations in PanIN progression of pancreatic cancer (Hruban et al., 2000). This gene plays a role in regulating the pathways involved in cell proliferation and differentiation (Rajan et al., 1996). It acts as a transcriptional factor, is essential for cell division by cytokinesis, and participates in homologous repair of DNA double-strand breaks (Milner et al., 1997; Xia et al., 2001; Daniels et al., 2004).

Familial aggregation of pancreatic cancer with other cancers, such as breast cancers or melanomas, has been linked to the presence of *BRCA2* mutations in them (Shi et al., 2009; Stracci et al., 2009). It is estimated that 10% of inherited cases and 5% of apparently sporadic pancreatic cancer cases are due to mutations in *BRCA2* (Couch et al., 2007; Stracci et al., 2009). The risk of pancreatic cancer is increased in individuals with *BRCA2* mutations, and germ line *BRCA2* mutations represent the most common inherited genetic alteration yet identified in familial pancreatic cancer (Murphy et al., 2002; Kim et al., 2009). Therefore, families with familial pancreatic cancer, or early onset of pancreatic cancer, should be considered for *BRCA2* testing for risk stratification of these individuals. A genetic survey of *BRCA2* gene based on a simple blood test may aid physicians and families at risk in their decision making.

The results of *BRCA2* testing may be used not only for preventive surgical options such as prophylactic resection but also for treatment options such as targeted chemotherapy. Some pancreatic cancers with mutated *BRCA2* tend to change from being chemosensitive to chemoresistant to DNA intercalating agents (Edwards et al., 2008). In such exceptional cases, mutated *BRCA2* undergoes either a deletion of mutation or a secondary mutation, each of which would restore the wild-type *BRCA2* reading frame (Sakai et al., 2008). Carcinomas that harbor *BRCA2* mutations are susceptible to the effects of an emerging class of targeted agents, namely, poly (ADP-ribose) polymerase (PARP) inhibitors (Fogelman et al., 2011).

Apart from *BRCA2* gene, sequence analysis of the entire coding region is available commercially for *PALB2* and *PALLD* (Greenhalf et al., 2009; GeneTests, 2012). While PALB3 is a partner and localizer of *BRCA2*, PALLD is a component of actin-containing microfilaments that control cell shape, adhesion, and contraction (Landi, 2009; Tischkowitz and Xia, 2010).

17.5 Markers under Development for Pancreatic Cancer

17.5.1 Genetic Markers

Pancreatic cancer originates in the ductal epithelium and evolves from premalignant lesions to fully invasive cancer through a series of mutations that affect various genes. Typical molecular profile of malignant pancreatic tumor comprises of genetic defects that lead to four characteristic molecular events in the majority of cases: activation of the *K-RAS* oncogene and inactivation of the tumor suppressor genes *p16*, *p53*, and *SMAD4* (Moore et al., 2001; Sun et al., 2001; Hong et al., 2011) (Table 17.4). The progression from minimally dysplastic epithelium (PanIN1) to more severe dysplasia (PanIN2 and PanIN3) and,

TABLE 17.4

List of Genes Commonly Altered in Pancreatic Cancer

Gene Symbol	Genetic Alteration Type	Genetic Alteration Mechanism	Location	Known or Predicted Function	Alteration in Primary Pancreatic Cancer (%)
p16	Inactivation	Homozygous deletion Intragenic mutation	9p21	Cyclin-dependent kinase inhibitor	95
KRAS2	Activation	Point mutation	12p12.1	Signal transduction, proliferation, cell survival, motility	>90
P53	Inactivation	Intragenic mutation + LOH	17p13.1	Cell cycle arrest, apoptosis, senescence, DNA repair, metabolism change	50–70
SMAD4	Inactivation	Homozygous deletion Intragenic mutation + LOH	18q21.1	Signal transmission	55
AKT2	Activation	Amplification	19q13.1–19q13.2	AKT pathway, hormone metabolism	10–20
MLH1	Inactivation	Heterozygous mutation	3p21.3	DNA mismatch repair	3–15
BRCA2	Inactivation	Homozygous deletion	13q12.3	DNA repair, proliferation, differentiation	7
STK11	Inactivation	Homozygous deletion Intragenic mutation + LOH	19p13.3	Apoptosis regulation	5
BRAF	Activation	Point mutation	7q34	Signal transduction, cell growth	5
TGFBR2	Inactivation	Homozygous deletion Homozygous mutation	3p22	Signal transduction	4
MAP24K	Inactivation	Homozygous deletion Homozygous mutation	17p11.2	MAPK pathway	2

LOH, loss of heterozygosity.

finally, to invasive carcinoma is paralleled by the successive accumulation of mutations in these genes (Figure 17.1). Since the presence of mutations in the four listed genes represents typical genetic profile of pancreatic cancer, these mutations have been widely investigated as potentially useful diagnostic markers for pancreatic cancer, but their prognostic value is variably reported (Smith et al., 2011). For the time being, *K-RAS* mutations are analyzed from various tissue types by polymerase chain reaction (PCR)-based methods, while aberrations in the expression of tumor suppressors p16, p53, and SMAD4 are commonly investigated by immunohistochemistry in resected pancreatic cancer. However, the absence of the protein that can be detected by the immunohistochemical analysis is not always in correlation with genetic defects, making genetic analysis of these markers necessary in order to establish their exact status in pancreatic tumor tissue. Currently, genetic analysis of these markers is performed only in the samples of tumor tissue obtained by biopsy or FNA, making them undesirable as biomarkers for routine diagnosis and screening in clinical practice. Further development of methods for sensitive noninvasive analysis of these genetic markers in cell-free DNA from plasma/serum and pancreatic juice could potentially be exploited in clinical practice for diagnosis and screening of pancreatic cancer.

17.5.1.1 p16 Gene Mutations

Tumor suppressor p16 (p16INK4A) is encoded by the *CDKN2A* locus on chromosome 9q21 (Serrano et al., 2000). It regulates cell cycle progression by inhibiting cyclin D/CDK4/6 complexes leading to p53 activation. In pancreatic cancer development, germ line and sporadic mutations have been identified that inactivate p16INK4A. Germ line mutations in *p16INK4A* are associated with a high incidence of melanoma, as well as a 13-fold increased risk of pancreatic cancer (Goldstein et al., 1995; Whelan et al., 1995). This suggests that a surveillance program for individuals with a family history of melanoma would be useful in detecting their predisposition to the development of pancreatic cancer.

In sporadic pancreatic cancer, loss of *p16INK4A* function by mutation, deletion, or promoter hypermethylation occurs in up to 95% of cases (Hustinx et al., 2005). The loss of *p16INK4A* occurs at one of the earlier stages of PanIN and is generally seen in moderately advanced lesions that show features of dysplasia (Hruban et al., 2000). Alterations of *p16INK4A* were also observed in chronic pancreatitis tissues not associated with pancreatic cancer. Therefore, *p16INK4A* alterations, especially promoter methylation, might indicate high-risk precursors in chronic pancreatitis that might progress to cancer (Gerdes et al., 2001). Methylation in the *p16INK4A* gene may also be a useful indicator of the potential malignancy of pancreatic epithelial cells (Fukushima et al., 2002).

Alterations of *p16INK4A* were shown to have a bearing on the aggressiveness of pancreatic cancer, either alone or in combination with other polymorphisms in other genes such as *K-RAS*, *cyclin D1*, *SMAD4*, and *p53* (Ohtsubo et al., 2003). Its role in prognosis is conflicting. One study has linked *p16INK4A* alterations to significantly shorter survival, whereas another study did not find any significant correlation between the two (Ohtsubo et al., 2003; Jeong et al., 2005).

Methylation status of *p16INK4A* has been proposed to be a diagnostic marker in the endoscopic differentiation of benign and malignant pancreatic disease (Klump et al., 2003). Simultaneous measurement of *K-RAS* and *p16INK4A* mutations may provide an additional tool in the differential diagnosis of chronic pancreatitis and pancreatic adenocarcinoma (Talar-Wojnarowska et al., 2004). EUS-guided fine-needle aspiration cytology (FNAC) combined with screening of *K-RAS* mutations and allelic losses of tumor suppressors p16 and SMAD4 has been suggested as a screening approach, particularly in cases where FNAC has been inconclusive (Salek et al., 2007). Detection of mutations in *p16* and/or *p53*, in clinical samples of pancreatic tissue, using limiting dilution PCR, is suggested to help distinguish patients with pancreatic cancer from those without evidence of pancreatic neoplasia (Bian et al., 2006). Polymorphic genotypes of p16 were significantly associated with shorter time to tumor progression (Chen et al., 2009a). Also, it was observed that carriers of a *p16*-Leiden mutation develop aggressive tumors (Vasen et al., 2011).

17.5.1.2 p53 Gene Mutations

Stress-inducible transcription factor p53 exerts its protective effect through the induction of either cell cycle arrest or programmed cell death in damaged, stressed cells (Seoane et al., 2002; Vousden, 2002).

In normal, unstressed conditions, p53 levels are kept very low by its negative regulator mdm2, while in tumors with mutated *p53* gene, high levels of inactive p53 accumulate (Selivanova and Wiman, 2007). Loss of p53 function in tumors results in cell survival and progression through the cell cycle, even after serious cellular insult that may have caused genomic damage.

Inactivation of *p53* by somatic mutation occurs in 50%–75% of pancreatic cancers (Scarpa et al., 1993). Depending on their impact on structure and function, *p53* mutations fall into two general classes: DNA contact mutations, which change the residues directly involved in contact with DNA but have modest impact on *p53* conformation, and structural mutations that dramatically alter the conformation of *p53*. Mutations in the *p53* gene generally occur relatively late in the neoplastic to invasive pancreatic cancer, and the detection of *p53* gene mutations has been widely investigated as a potentially specific diagnostic marker in various cancers, including pancreatic cancer. Although a few authors have shown a significant correlation of p53 expression with patient survival, for the most part it is conflicting, probably because *p53* mutational status was not resolved in these studies (Nio et al., 1999; Jinfeng et al., 2007; Hermanova et al., 2009; Salek et al., 2009). The *p53* mutations alone are unlikely to offer useful prognostic information in patients with pancreatic cancer but may be useful in stratifying patients for more effective adjuvant chemotherapy. Although *K-RAS* mutations occur earlier in the PanIN progression of pancreatic cancer, lesions bearing *K-RAS* mutations do not progress into full-blown carcinoma unless *p53* is mutated. The crosstalk between *K-RAS* and p53 is mediated by p120 catenin along with N-cadherin or by Snail (Deramaudt et al., 2006; Lee et al., 2009a,b). It has been proposed that this *K-RAS*–Snail–p53 pathway can be used in diagnosis.

Although a few nucleotide hot spots of *p53* gene mutation are known to exist, mutations occur throughout the gene (Hainaut and Hollstein, 2000). Most studies of *p53* mutations as a cancer marker have used assays such as chip technologies, single-strand conformational polymorphism, and temperature gradient capillary electrophoresis that have the potential to identify the complete spectrum of *p53* gene mutations. The sensitivity and limit of detection of these technologies are not as good as of those that detect single-nucleotide mutations. Assays such as single-strand conformational polymorphism and temperature gradient capillary electrophoresis can detect mutations that are present in at least 1% and more often 5%–10% of the total DNA (Kaino et al., 1999; Yamaguchi et al., 1999). Using this technique, investigators have reported the presence of *p53* gene mutations within exons 5–8 in pancreatic juice samples and in brush cytology specimens of 40%–50% of patients with pancreatic cancers, and this figure is close to the number of mutations that one would expect to find in the primary pancreatic cancers from these patients (Sturm et al., 1998). One study using temperature gradient gel electrophoresis demonstrated that pancreatic juice from patients with chronic pancreatitis rarely harbors *p53* gene mutations (Lohr et al., 2001). Gene chip technology has also been used for *p53* gene mutation detection and it has the advantage that it can identify in a single assay a large percentage of possible *p53* gene mutations in a given DNA sample as long as the mutation is present in the sample at sufficient concentration relative to normal DNA (>1% of DNA) (Wikman et al., 2000). Although these gene chips are very effective in identifying missense mutations, they may miss the small deletions and insertions that represent 10%–20% of all *p53* gene mutations. The concentration of mutant DNA in the pancreatic juice of patients with pancreatic cancer can be less than 1% of total DNA, so the utility of using *p53* gene chip assays for pancreatic cancer diagnosis remains to be determined (Shi et al., 2004).

17.5.1.3 SMAD4 Gene Mutations

Protein SMAD4 is a member of the SMAD family of signal transduction proteins, important mediators of transforming growth factor (TGF)-beta signaling (Heldin et al., 1997). Protein SMAD4 is a common TGF-beta mediator, which forms a heteromeric complex with phosphorylated SMADs and translocates to the nucleus, where along with other cofactors regulates transcription, mainly of the genes encoding for cell cycle regulatory proteins such as p53, p15, p21, and p27 (Liu et al., 1997; Robson et al., 1999). It is inactivated in 55% of pancreatic cancers either by deletion of both alleles (35%) or by intragenic mutation in one allele coupled with the loss of the other allele (20%) (Hahn et al., 1996; Schutte et al., 1996).

Loss of SMAD4 protein expression occurs at a later stage of PanIN (Hruban et al., 2000). It is highly correlated with the presence of widespread metastasis but not with locally destructive tumors

(Iacobuzio-Donahue et al., 2009). Protein SMAD4 is thought to be dispensable for normal pancreas but critical for the progression of tumors with mutated *K-RAS* gene (Bardeesy et al., 2006). Inactivation of the *SMAD4* gene is associated with poorer prognosis in patients with surgically resected tumor (Hua et al., 2003; Blackford et al., 2009). Determination of *SMAD4* status at initial diagnosis may be of value in determining the stage and metastatic status of disease and will help in stratifying patients into treatment regimens accordingly (Iacobuzio-Donahue et al., 2009; Ali et al., 2007).

The phenomenon of haploinsufficiency, or dosage dependence, is increasingly being taken into consideration when evaluating relevance of the *SMAD4* gene both as a possible cause of malignant transformation and as a potential biomarker. Currently, *SMAD4* gene is not considered to be a classic tumor suppressor gene, considering that it was found that, in addition to loss of both copies of the gene, decrease in *SMAD4* gene expression levels may also have serious consequences for the cell (Ando et al., 2005; Alberici et al., 2008). These data shed new light on mutations in *SMAD4* gene regulatory elements as well, since they can significantly affect *SMAD4* expression. Preliminary results indicate that SMAD4 gene promoter haplotype-462T(14)/-4T(10) may represent an early genetic marker of potential relevance for pancreatic cancer (Nikolic et al., 2011).

Mutations occurring in the *SMAD4* gene have not been considered as pancreatic cancer biomarkers due to the fact that loss of *SMAD4* protein occurs late in the pancreatic carcinogenesis. However, the haploinsufficiency phenomenon indicates that some aberrations in *SMAD4* gene function may occur early and be potentially useful as biomarkers. They may be of special value in pancreatic cancer diagnostics and monitoring, since *SMAD4* gene aberrations are generally rare in other diseases (Van Heek et al., 2002). Translational research aimed at investigating potential application of *SMAD4* gene mutations as early molecular markers for pancreatic cancer may yet prove useful.

17.5.1.4 Single-Nucleotide Polymorphisms

Genome-wide association studies have been employed to identify certain single-nucleotide polymorphisms (SNPs) associated with pancreatic cancer (Petersen et al., 2010; Li et al., 2012; Pierce et al., 2012; Willis et al., 2012). Focusing association studies on certain regions and conducting larger genome-wide association studies can reveal susceptibility loci for this disease and identify potential markers for early diagnosis and monitoring of therapy. Genome-wide association studies may provide the foundation for testing the biology and clinical effects of novel genes and their heritable variants through mechanistic and confirmatory studies in pancreatic cancer (You et al., 2011; Innocenti et al., 2012).

An association was identified between a locus on 9q34 and pancreatic cancer, marked by the SNP rs505922 that maps to the first intron of the ABO blood group gene, suggesting that people with blood group O may have a lower risk of pancreatic cancer than those with groups A or B (Amundadottir et al., 2009). It was found that SNP rs8028529 was weakly associated with a better overall survival, while NR5A2 rs12029406_T allele was associated with a shorter survival (Rizzato et al., 2011). Association studies in a large pancreatic case–control study indicate that SNPs in mitotic regulation pathway genes previously found to be associated with breast cancer may also be associated with pancreatic cancer susceptibility and survival (Couch et al., 2009, 2010). It was observed that polymorphic variations of drug metabolic genes and DNA damage response genes may be associated with toxicity of gemcitabine-based chemoradiotherapy and clinical outcome in patients with resectable pancreatic cancer (Okazaki et al., 2008, 2010; Tanaka et al., 2011).

17.5.1.5 Mitochondrial Mutations

Analysis of the complete 16.5 kb mitochondrial genome (mtDNA) structure and function in 15 pancreatic cancer cell lines and xenografts has revealed somatic mutations and novel variants in nearly all samples, as well as a great (six- to eightfold) increase in intracellular mass of mtDNA in pancreatic cancer cells in relation to corresponding normal cells (Jones et al., 2001). No association was observed between mtDNA mutations and overall survival in pancreatic cancer (Halfdanarson et al., 2008). Since automated sequencing of 16.5 kb of mtDNA poses a difficult task, a high-throughput array-based platforms for mtDNA mutational analyses of human cancers have been developed (Maitra et al., 2004; Kassauei et al., 2006).

The nearly ubiquitous prevalence of somatic mtDNA mutations in pancreatic cancers, as well as their high copy number, suggests that they should be considered as promising biomarkers for early detection of the disease.

17.5.2 Methylated DNA

Since aberrant hypermethylation of tumor suppressor genes is common during carcinogenesis, DNA methylation abnormalities may be particularly suitable for use in early detection strategies (Jones and Baylin, 2002). Several dozen genes have been identified as aberrantly methylated in pancreatic cancer, and some of these markers are aberrantly methylated in 90% of cases (Sato et al., 2003). Initial studies in patients with pancreatic disease have demonstrated that aberrant DNA methylation patterns can be detected in pancreatic juice samples from patients with pancreatic cancer and are only rarely found in pancreatic juice samples from patients without pancreatic cancer (Fukushima et al., 2003; Sato et al., 2003, 2005). Aberrant DNA methylation has been detected in PanIN precursor lesions, suggesting epigenetic changes occur early in pancreatic carcinogenesis (Sato et al., 2008).

Methylation-specific PCR (MSP) and bisulfite-sequencing PCR (BSP) have been used to analyze DNA from different samples of patients with pancreatic cancer (Iacobuzio-Donahue et al., 2003; Gao et al., 2010). MSP is the method of choice if a small number of genes are tested in a larger set of patient samples. After DNA isolation by standard procedure, the DNA is then modified using sodium bisulfite to convert all unmethylated cytosines to uracils and can then be used in qualitative and quantitative PCR assays (Herman et al., 1996; Biewusch et al., 2012). High sensitivity of these methods enables their application in analysis of noninvasive samples, such as pancreatic juice (Fukushima et al., 2003). This method has been used successfully to identify methylated DNA in most biologic fluids, including blood and fine-needle aspirates from cancer patients (Esteller et al., 2001). In addition, use of real-time quantitative MSP (QMSP) for the detection and quantification of aberrantly methylated DNA in pancreatic juice is a promising approach for the diagnosis of pancreatic cancer (Matsubayashi et al., 2006; Park et al., 2007).

Aberrant DNA methylation offers several advantages as a potential biomarker. Identification of promoter hypermethylation is readily accomplished in a cost-effective manner with PCR-based technologies that have the sensitivity to detect 1 cancer cell among 1,000–10,000 normal cells, which is favorable for the detection of cancer cells or cancer cell DNA in body fluids (Sidransky, 2002). A relatively small number of hypermethylated genes characterize a particular tumor type, allowing one to potentially screen a limited panel of less than 10–20 genes as markers to identify a suitable tumor-specific marker for each patient, which is advantageous for high-throughput technologies (Esteller et al., 2001). Although these data are promising, several biologic features of DNA methylation require consideration when DNA methylation markers are considered for use in clinical practice as cancer markers. These include tissue-specific differences in normal methylation patterns, increases in DNA methylation with patient age, and the potential for methylated DNA markers to detect early neoplasia with little propensity for cancer (Issa et al., 1994; Nguyen et al., 2001; Pao et al., 2001; Matsubayashi et al., 2003, 2005). Because MSP requires a bisulfate modification step that causes DNA degradation, MSP is not as sensitive as simple PCR and has a lower limit of detection of 10–20 copies (Fukushima et al., 2003). Even at this level of detection, MSP may detect low-level methylation that arises either from normal aging or in lesions of low malignant potential. Low-grade PanINs develop with increasing frequency in the pancreas with increasing age, and some of these PanINs harbor methylation changes that are not found in normal pancreatic epithelium. For this reason, genes that only undergo methylation in high-grade PanINs and invasive cancers are likely to have more diagnostic accuracy for detecting pancreatic cancer as opposed to those that are methylated in early PanIN (Sato et al., 2004, 2008).

Methylated DNA is one of the most promising markers for pancreatic cancer and one of the present research challenges is to identify candidate methylated genes (Corn, 2008; Tan et al., 2009). Differential methylation profiling of plasma DNA can detect ductal adenocarcinoma of the pancreas with significant accuracy and is currently under investigation as a detection tool for pancreatic cancer (Melnikov et al., 2009). Knowledge about the CpG island methylation status of pancreatic cancer-specific genes could support the development of earlier diagnostic assays and finding new treatment strategies. Several recent patents have been published, for either methods for detection of the methylation status of CpG sites or therapeutic approaches based on applying modulators of DNA cytosine-5 methyltransferase such as decitabine or C-5 methylcytosine (Wehrum et al., 2008). These patents provide new methods in fighting pancreatic cancer by focusing on methylated CpG islands in pancreatic cancer-related genes.

17.5.3 MicroRNAs

Recent studies have revealed that expression patterns of microRNAs rather than messenger RNAs (mRNAs) appear to be more informative as tumorigenic events for human cancers (Lu et al., 2005; Rachagani et al., 2010). MicroRNAs are short, functional, noncoding RNAs that negatively regulate gene expression, and their aberrant expression has recently been implicated in the initiation and progression of malignant diseases, including pancreatic cancer. A number of studies have demonstrated different roles of various types of microRNAs in the progression and survival of pancreatic cancer. A recent report claims that aberrant microRNA production is an early event in the development of PanIN (Du Rieu et al., 2010). The deregulated microRNAs expression profiles have been proposed to represent helpful markers for differential diagnosis of pancreatic cancer from chronic inflammatory disease of the pancreas and other tumors. Plasma microRNA profiling can be developed as a sensitive and specific blood-based biomarker assay for pancreatic cancer.

Previous studies have identified microRNA signatures specific for normal pancreas, chronic pancreatitis, and cancer tissues using microarray technology. A set of aberrantly expressed microRNAs was found in the plasma of pancreatic cancer patients (Wang et al., 2009; Wang and Sen, 2011). The presence of microRNA-216 and microRNA-217 and absence of microRNA-133a are characteristic of pancreatic tissue, and a total of 26 microRNAs are aberrantly expressed in pancreatic cancer (Lu et al., 2005). Among these, only downregulation of microRNA-217 and elevated expression of microRNA-196a can discriminate normal pancreas and chronic pancreatitis from pancreatic cancer. Additionally, eight differentially expressed microRNAs were reported to differentiate pancreatic cancer from chronic pancreatitis (Szafranska et al., 2007; Zhang et al., 2009). Upregulation of these eight microRNAs occurs in the most of pancreatic cancer tissues and cell types. The incidence of upregulation of these eight genes between normal controls and tumor cells or tissues was ranging from 70% to 100%. The magnitude of increase of these microRNAs in pancreatic cancer samples was ranging from 3- to over 2000-fold of normal controls. Pancreatic cancer tissues or cell lines have a unique microRNA profiling pattern at the individual basis as compared with relatively normal pancreatic tissues or cells.

A number of studies have suggested prognostic significance of microRNA expression profiles in pancreatic carcinomas. A subgroup of six microRNAs was reported to distinguish long-term survivors with node-positive disease from those succumbing within 2 years and elevated expression of microRNA-196a-2 was predictive of median survival differing by about a year among pancreatic cancer patients (Bloomston et al., 2007). Furthermore, the upregulation of microRNA-155, microRNA-203, microRNA-210, and microRNA-222 was also found to be significantly associated with poorer survival of patients with pancreatic carcinomas (Greither et al., 2010). MicroRNA-21, which is significantly overexpressed in pancreatic cancer, has been most extensively studied. Its strong expression predicts reduced survival in patients with node-negative disease and may be an important biologic marker for outcome (Dillhoff et al., 2008). It contributes to cell proliferation, invasion, and chemoresistance of the disease (Moriyama et al., 2009).

17.5.4 Protein Biomarkers for Pancreatic Cancer

Of the currently available tools to evaluate pancreatic cancer, CA 19-9 is the only protein marker in routine clinical use, despite of its lack of sensitivity and specificity. Many other candidate serum markers for pancreatic cancer have been evaluated using specific assays, but none are superior to CA 19-9. Recently, accompanying the development of proteomic technology and devices, more and more potential biomarkers for pancreatic cancer have appeared and are being reported (Sun et al., 2011). The development of proteomic techniques has increased the interest for clinical applications of biomarkers in pancreatic cancer. However, the identification of suitable biomarkers with good sensitivity and specificity for clinical use in pancreatic cancer has been sparse.

TABLE 17.5

Overview of Commonly Studied Protein Markers in Pancreatic Cancer

Marker	Designation	Sensitivity (%)	Specificity (%)
Carbohydrate antigen 19-9	CA 19-9	69–94	44–96
Carbohydrate antigen 50	CA 50	78–84	70–85
Carbohydrate antigen 242	CA 242	57–82	76–93
Carbohydrate antigen 195	CA 195	76–82	73–85
Carbohydrate antigen 125	CA 125	45–57	76–78
Carcinoembryonic antigen	CEA	25–54	75–91
Pancreatic oncofetal antigen	POA	68–81	88–96
Tissue polypeptide antigen	TPA	48–96	67–85
Tissue polypeptide-specific antigen	TPS	50–98	22–70
Pancreatic cancer-associated antigen Du-PAN 2	Du-PAN 2	48–72	85–94
Pancreatic cancer-associated antigen SPan-1	SPan-1	81–92	76–85
Antimucin antibody CAM 17.1	CAM17.1	67–78	76–100

A panel of proteomic biomarkers with the appropriate combination of high sensitivity and specificity will likely be better than a single biomarker. Many researchers have focused on proteomic profiling for pancreatic cancer detection using a combined biomarker approach and results so far have gained interest. Compared with other types of cancers, pancreatic cancer is probably one of the solid tumors with the highest levels of genetic alterations resulting in aberrant expression of a large number of proteins.

In spite of extensive research in this field, there is no protein tumor marker, apart from CA 19-9, that has experienced broad clinical application until today. The most commonly studied molecules are tumor-associated antigens, but some candidate tumor markers were also found among enzymes and oncofetal antigens. The sensitivity and specificity of serum markers depend on the determination of cutoff values derived from different studies. An overview of established and experimental protein markers in the diagnosis of pancreatic cancer is given in Table 17.5 (Ruckert et al., 2010).

17.5.5 Circulating Tumor Cells

CTCs are tumor cells detached from primary tumor sites that circulate through normal vessels and capillaries and neovessels formed by tumor-induced angiogenesis leading to distant metastasis (Fidler, 2003; Allard et al., 2004). They are detected in the blood of patients with metastatic malignancies but are a rare finding in people without cancer (Allard et al., 2004; Nagrath et al., 2007; Stott et al., 2010). Recent progress in molecular oncology enables us to detect the CTCs in blood with high sensitivity and specificity. They are typically present at low concentrations in cancer patients and numerous assays for their detection have been developed.

The current common approach for detection of CTCs in patients with pancreatic cancer is based on immunological assays using antibodies directed against cell-surface antigen (Nagrath et al., 2007; Kurihara et al., 2008; Stott et al., 2010). Pancreatic cancer cells express tumor-associated antigens such as Wilms' tumor gene 1 (WT1) (75%), mucin 1 (MUC1) (85%), human telomerase reverse transcriptase (hTERT) (88%), mutated *K-RAS* (73%), survivin (77%), carcinoembryonic antigen (CEA) (90%), HER-2/neu (61%), or p53 (67%) (Cen et al., 2012). The weakness of antibody-based immunological assays is the potential loss of any subpopulation of CTCs that do not express the specific antigens used in the capture protocol, making this method incapable of sampling the entire population of CTCs. The other often used methods for detection of CTCs are PCR-based molecular assays for tumor-derived DNA or RNA originating from CTCs (Soeth et al., 2005; Hoffmann et al., 2007; Sergeant et al., 2011). The pitfall of PCR-based approaches is that the origin of the nucleic acids is not clear and the results may not represent actual CTCs. This limitation could be overcome by performing an initial purification of nucleated cells from the circulation followed by extraction of nucleic acids from the cells prior to performing PCR.

Technologies based on physical or biological properties of cancer cells, such as differences in morphological and electrical conductivity, are antibody independent but have not been yet extensively studied in patients with pancreatic cancer (Hsieh et al., 2006; Gascoyne et al., 2009).

Preliminary results suggest the prognostic and predictive values of CTCs in pancreatic cancer (De Albuquerque et al., 2011; Ren et al., 2011; Xu et al., 2011; Cen et al., 2012; Khoja et al., 2012). The qualitative and quantitative monitoring of CTCs could serve as a noninvasive tool to monitor changes in tumor biology throughout the disease and thereby improve the understanding of the processes of dissemination and therapeutic resistance. Detection of CTCs is also suggested to provide useful information for the tumor staging and anticancer treatments in clinical practices in the near future. CTCs are a potential marker for pancreatic cancer not only because of their specificity but also because CTCs allow repeated study of tumor genetics, proteomics, and molecular biology of the cancer cells as well as pharmacodynamics throughout a patient's clinical course. If CTCs are shown to correlate with the risk of distant metastasis, isolation of CTCs would also allow more accurate study of drug targets in the disseminated cancer cells and thus allow a more rational selection of adjuvant therapy for localized pancreatic cancer. Also, CTCs have the potential to provide a surrogate for real-time biopsy thus allowing assessment of the tumor biological activity. As such, enumeration and characterization of CTCs in pancreatic cancer could have important role in the diagnosis, predicting risk for postsurgical recurrence, examining pharmacodynamic biomarkers, detecting treatment resistant profiles, assisting in response measurements to therapies, and identifying prognostic and predictive molecular features. Also, CTCs could potentially help in the diagnosis of metastatic pancreatic cancer, especially in cases where the primary tumor was small possibly not even apparent on scans or in cases where neither the metastatic nor the primary lesion is accessible for biopsy. They can be used to identify the specific molecules driving metastasis and chemoresistance and thus allow targeted interventions in neoadjuvant and adjuvant therapy. Study of CTCs allows the oncology team to potentially identify the metastatic potential of the patient as CTCs likely vary in risk from innocent bystanders to those seed metastasis thus allowing identifying and targeting high-risk patients as well as targeting CTCs by using the most sensitive chemotherapy agents. The tumor response to preoperative treatment might be predictable prior to surgery by noting a drop in CTC count, and this allows improved choice of the best timing of surgery. After surgery, CTCs can be examined in terms of pharmacodynamic biomarkers to choose or change to the most sensitive chemotherapy agents and assist in decision on the duration of adjuvant therapy. As a bridge between metastatic tumors and the primary tumors, CTCs can help discover discrepancies in their phenotypes or genotypes. Genotyping and phenotyping of CTCs can be repeated at therapeutic decision-making points during a patient's course of therapy in the management of pancreatic cancer to ensure that resistance has not developed and to guide changes in chemotherapy agents when resistant clone is found. The detailed molecular analysis on the gene profiling and microRNA profiling of CTCs may lead to new insights and novel therapeutic strategies for pancreatic cancer.

17.6 Technologies for Pancreatic Cancer Marker Discovery and Validation

Important technological innovations made in the past several decades have provided significant leads in search for potential pancreatic cancer biomarkers (Table 17.6) (Bhat et al., 2012). There are two major approaches to molecular marker discovery. In the high-throughput "shotgun" strategies, thousands of contenders are screened simultaneously. In the traditional hypothesis-driven approach, interactions between molecules known to be important for pancreatic cancer development are studied. The underlying principle of both strategies is to comparatively analyze malignant and normal tissue of the pancreas. While high-throughput techniques have generated several important candidates, much work remains. Problems with high-throughput methods include reproducibility and in particular identification of markers that can be measured by readily available clinical laboratory methods.

17.6.1 Genomics Techniques

Microarray enables the study of thousands of genes simultaneously and has allowed the identification of hundreds of genes that are differentially expressed in pancreatic cancer (Harada et al., 2009; Lopez-Casas and Lopez-Fernandez, 2010). The study of pancreatic cancer that makes use of the whole-genome technologies

TABLE 17.6
Available Diagnostic Tools for Pancreatic Cancer

Technology	Applications and Advantages	Limitations
Microarray	Chip-based concurrent analysis of thousands of genes	Frequent identification of false positives
RT-PCR/PCR/MSP	Multiple target analysis in a single, multiplexed reaction	Sensitive, can generate false-positive results
2DE	Separation of proteins by isoelectric point (IP) and MW	Permits detection of very basic or acidic proteins only
DIGE	Co-separation of multiple samples and visualization on one 2D gel	Changes in labeling can markedly alter position of migration of specific proteins
Multidimensional protein identification technology (MudPIT)	Nongel approach for the identification of proteins from complex mixtures	Inability to directly measure the relative abundance of proteins
Isotope-coded affinity tag (ICAT)	Measurement of relative abundance of proteins labeled at cysteine residues	Suitable only for proteins with labeling-accessible cysteines
Isobaric tags for relative and absolute quantification (iTRAQ)	Identification and quantification of proteins by labeling both whole and subcellular proteomes	Unlikely to reveal basic information on proteins of interest
MALDI	Identification of proteins isolated through gel electrophoresis	Quantitation difficult
SELDI	Analysis of protein mixtures by MS ionization method	Low reproducibility and low resolution

has revealed several molecular mechanisms that affect pancreatic cancer development. Additionally, microRNAs have emerged as a potential source of variation between cancer and normal samples, and several of them have been identified as being deregulated in pancreatic tumors. However, validation of these genes as biomarkers for early diagnosis, prognosis, or treatment efficacy is still incomplete. The use of microarray for pancreatic cancer research is mainly for the evaluation of prognostic markers and in guiding treatment for recurrent and resistant malignancy (Zhao et al., 2007; Lopez-Casas and Lopez-Fernandez, 2010). While still in its infancy as a technique and with a number of barriers to be overcome, microarray is allowing scientists to thoroughly examine the molecular pathways of pancreatic cancer pathogenesis. However, the adoption of microarray as a clinically applicable technique has been slow coming.

The DNA arrays involve the use of microchips to which are appended the "negative" sequences to thousands of portions of genes (Iacobuzio-Donahue et al., 2003). Tissue from those with and without pancreatic cancer is processed to yield RNA that is used to generate cDNA sequences that are differentially marked using fluorescence tags. The cDNA is then exposed to the microchips that anneal to the corresponding negative sequences. Differences in the fluorescence pattern between the pancreatic cancer and control can be used to rapidly identify differential gene expression.

High-throughput analysis can also be performed to look at messenger RNA and microRNA (Lee et al., 2007). Arrays containing probes for hundred of known microRNAs are being used to study their role in pancreatic cancer with encouraging results (Szafranska et al., 2007). Major challenges include correctly identifying the genes with which specific microRNA interacts. mRNA has also been evaluated using microarray technology (Zhang et al., 2010). Subsequently, expression of potentially important genes and protein levels, as well as epigenetic markers, from patients with pancreatic cancer, control, and those with benign pancreatic disease, particularly chronic pancreatitis, must be compared among groups of patients.

Quantitative real-time reverse transcription (RT)-PCR, as the most sensitive technique for mRNA detection and quantification, complements arrays for the confirmation of individual transcripts in larger sample cohorts (Streit et al., 2009). Microarray and quantitative RT-PCR or PCR are frequently used to analyze the variations of RNA/microRNA or DNA in the tumor tissues and other types of specimens from patients and healthy individuals (Laurell et al., 2006; Liang et al., 2009; Lopez-Casas and Lopez-Fernandez, 2010). Gene expression profiling and tissue microarray have been used to identify novel cell-surface targets (Morse et al., 2010).

17.6.2 Proteomics Techniques

Since the serum proteome contains many potential biomarkers for disease detection, several proteomic approaches are being used to identify novel protein markers of pancreatic cancer. New equipment and techniques have been developed to systematically search for protein markers in specimens, including differential in-gel electrophoresis (DIGE), tandem mass spectrometry (MS/MS), reverse-phase protein array (RPPA), time-of-flight mass spectroscopy (TOF-MS), matrix-assisted laser desorption/ionization (MALDI), surface-enhanced laser desorption/ionization (SELDI), and quantitative proteomics (Yu et al., 2005; Grote et al., 2008; Ma et al., 2008; Wong et al., 2009; Tambor et al., 2010; Xue et al., 2010).

Comparative proteomic analysis using 2D gel electrophoresis (2DE) and MALDI-TOF-MS and/or SELDI-TOF-MS is an effective method for identifying differentially expressed proteins that may be the potential diagnostic serum biomarkers and therapeutic targets for pancreatic cancer. Pilot studies utilizing MALDI-TOF-MS and SELDI-TOF-MS have identified candidate biomarkers in pancreatic cancer by comparing serum samples of pancreatic cancer patients and healthy individuals (Rosty et al., 2002; Koopmann et al., 2004a–c; Chen et al., 2009b; Cui et al., 2009; Fiedler et al., 2009; Walsh et al., 2009). Also, these techniques can be applied for analysis of biomarkers in pancreatic juice (Park et al., 2011). Additionally, this approach can be exploited for investigating molecular mechanisms of therapeutic resistance in pancreatic cancer cells and potential follow-up of therapeutic response in patients undergoing treatment (Chen et al., 2009b). In a case–control study, serum samples from patients with resectable pancreatic cancer were compared using SELDI to those of a variety of disease and healthy controls (Koopmann et al., 2004c). They found that two discriminating peptide peaks could differentiate patients with pancreatic cancer from healthy controls with a sensitivity of 78% and specificity of 97%, outperforming CA 19-9 ($p < 0.05$). The diagnostic accuracy of these two peptides was improved by using them in combination with CA 19-9. These markers were also better than CA 19-9 in distinguishing patients with pancreatic cancer from those with pancreatitis. The combination of the SELDI panel and CA 19-9 was superior to CA 19-9 alone in distinguishing individuals with pancreatic cancer from the healthy subject group, patients with chronic pancreatitis, and patients with type 2 diabetes mellitus (Navaglia et al., 2009; Gao et al., 2012). The results obtained by this method can further be improved by depleting serum of high-abundance proteins in order to minimize the interference and by the use of magnetic beads to pretreat the serum in order to achieve higher sensitivity (Qian et al., 2012; Xue et al., 2012). In general, SELDI system requires less sample as well as less extensive sample preparation and less sample cleanup than MALDI system and also increases reproducibility (Borgaonkar et al., 2010). Although these results suggest that high-throughput proteomic profiling has the capacity to provide new biomarkers for the early detection and diagnosis through assaying small serum peptide markers of pancreatic cancer, large multicenter studies are needed to confirm these findings and to precisely identify peptide markers so that more specific assays can be designed for their detection.

Another critical high-throughput technique is quantitative proteomics, based on the fact that protein levels may be more clinically relevant as gene expression does not necessarily correlate with the quantity and nature of the proteins they encode (Petricoin et al., 2002; Chen et al., 2005a; Paradis et al., 2005). While there are several methods, most rely on an initial fractionation step whether by 2D electrophoresis or more sophisticated methods such as protein chip technology (Scarlett et al., 2006). In most cases the samples are then analyzed by MS in which the components are separated based on MWs and the quantities of different mass size can be compared between malignant and control samples, while the proteins are subsequently identified by sequencing (Gygi et al., 1999; Link et al., 1999; Chen et al., 2005b, 2006).

17.7 Future Perspectives for Pancreatic Cancer Marker Discovery

Future exploratory work in pancreatic cancer markers should satisfy the need for the integration of emerging technologies and systems biology to help create roadmaps for early diagnosis and prediction of therapy (Harsha et al., 2009; Brody et al., 2011). Large amounts of money and resources are being invested into direct sequencing and genome-wide expression analyses of pancreatic cancer genomes and transcriptomes. The promise of this work is that commonly found genetic alterations in pancreatic cancer will, in part, aid in the discovery of novel biomarkers for disease monitoring and novel targets that are susceptible to drugs. In the near future, sequencing of the entire genome could become routine practice on a visit to the clinic by a patient with pancreatic cancer. As technologies advance and sequencing becomes less expensive, major medical centers will most likely be able to integrate and use direct sequencing of patient samples. Currently, the common goal of molecular biologists and pathologists should be to prove the validity of gene mutations, SNPs, and altered gene expression patterns as guides for the clinical management of patients with pancreatic cancer. Presently, high-throughput, genome-wide analyses of cancer genomes are taking place in multiple institutions. These studies should incorporate innovative molecular techniques with novel techniques in pathology to search for and validate robust biomarkers for this disease. Combining these results with computational programming should enhance the pace of biomarker discovery and expose uncharted regions and patterns of the genome that are important for the clinical management of pancreatic cancer. An interdisciplinary and systems biology approach of combining biochemical techniques with sequencing of laser capture microdissected materials, along with cutting-edge, automated image analysis allowing for the objective quantitative analysis of protein expression in subcellular compartments in tumor samples, could identify biomarkers that conventional screening methods would be unable to detect. However, the paucity of funds available for pancreatic cancer research leaves only a small amount for the validation and large-scale studies that are necessary for the success of this line of work. Integration of previous studies with high-throughput technologies and more sophisticated biobanking should create a landscape in which realistic and reproducible biomarkers can be generated by the pancreatic cancer research community.

17.8 Concluding Remarks

Pancreatic cancer has the darkest prognosis of all gastrointestinal cancers, with the mortality approaching the incidence. There is a great necessity to develop sensitive and specific biomarkers for this disease that would lead to earlier disease detection and more efficient therapies. Currently, the only biomarker in routine clinical use is CA 19-9, which most clinicians would gladly eliminate from the practice due to its unsatisfactory sensitivity and specificity. However, of many other biomarkers of different types that have been evaluated in the past decades, none was regarded as consistently superior to CA 19-9. The greatest resources supporting pancreatic cancer research are dedicated to the identification of two types of biomarkers: early detection markers that provide a timely opportunity for curative therapy and predictive markers that may help in selection and optimization of adjuvant therapies. The best scenario would be to identify biomarkers that are both prognostic and predictive in value, which at the same time facilitate tumorigenesis and represent a target that responds to drugs. Although several reliable genetic markers emerged, their analysis is still based on tumor tissue analysis and due to the invasiveness of the techniques used for their detection they cannot be considered adequate for routine use in clinical practice. Recent development in pancreatic cancer research indicates that, after search for various types of markers in various types of samples, attention of researchers has turned back to blood, as an easily and noninvasively obtainable source of various types of molecules that could serve as biomarkers for clinical practice. The most promising biomarkers seem to be small molecules, DNA, and malignant cells released in the blood stream by the tumor. There is a constant discovery of novel methods for pancreatic cancer biomarkers search and validation. Since a variety of candidate markers has already been identified, advancement of existing methods in order to adjust their use for routine clinical practice is as necessary as methodology improvement. Based on previous experience during several decades long search for pancreatic cancer biomarkers, it is highly unlikely that a single marker with high sensitivity and specificity will be found. The future quest for pancreatic cancer early markers appears to lie in the development of assays based on noninvasive analysis of blood samples for the presence of different markers whose combined analysis could provide sufficient information for diagnostic purposes and that could be successfully adjusted for routine use in clinical practice.

References

Alberici, P., Gaspar, C., Franken, P. et al. 2008. Smad4 haploinsufficiency: A matter of dosage. *Pathogenetics* 1(1):2.

Ali, S., Cohen, C., Little, J.V. et al. 2007. The utility of SMAD4 as a diagnostic immunohistochemical marker for pancreatic adenocarcinoma, and its expression in other solid tumors. *Diagn Cytopathol* 35(10):644–648.

Allard, W.J., Matera, J., Miller, M.C. et al. 2004. Tumor cells circulate in the peripheral blood of all major carcinomas but not in healthy subjects or patients with nonmalignant diseases. *Clin Cancer Res* 10(20):6897–6904.

Almoguera, C., Shibata, D., Forrester, K. et al. 1988. Most human carcinomas of the exocrine pancreas contain mutant c-K-ras genes. *Cell* 53(4):549–554.

Amundadottir, L., Kraft, P., Stolzenberg-Solomon, R.Z. et al. 2009. Genome-wide association study identifies variants in the ABO locus associated with susceptibility to pancreatic cancer. *Nat Genet* 41(9):986–990.

Ando, T., Sugai, T., Habano, W., Jiao, Y.F., and K. Suzuki. 2005. Analysis of SMAD4/DPC4 gene alterations in multiploid colorectal carcinomas. *J Gastroenterol* 40(7):708–715.

Arvanitakis, M., Van Laethem, J.L., Parma, J., De Maertelaer, V., Delhaye, M., and J. Deviare. 2004. Predictive factors for pancreatic cancer in patients with chronic pancreatitis in association with K-ras gene mutation. *Endoscopy* 36(6):535–542.

Banfi, G., Bravi, S., Ardemagni, A., and A. Zerbi. 1996. CA 19.9, CA 242 and CEA in the diagnosis and follow-up of pancreatic cancer. *Int J Biol Markers* 11(2):77–81.

Bardeesy, N., Cheng, K.H., Berger, J.H. et al. 2006. Smad4 is dispensable for normal pancreas development yet critical in progression and tumor biology of pancreas cancer. *Genes Dev* 20(22):3130–3146.

Berger, A.C., Garcia, M. Jr., Hoffman, J.P. et al. 2008. Postresection CA 19-9 predicts overall survival in patients with pancreatic cancer treated with adjuvant chemoradiation: A prospective validation by RTOG 9704. *J Clin Oncol* 26(36):5918–5922.

Bernhard, J., Dietrich, D., Glimelius, B. et al. 2010. Estimating prognosis and palliation based on tumour marker CA 19-9 and quality of life indicators in patients with advanced pancreatic cancer receiving chemotherapy. *Br J Cancer* 103(9):1318–1324.

Berrozpe, G., Schaeffer, J., Peinado, M.A., Real, F.X., and M. Perucho. 1994. Comparative analysis of mutations in the p53 and K-ras genes in pancreatic cancer. *Int J Cancer* 58(2):185–191.

Berthelemy, P., Bouisson, M., Escourrou, J., Vaysse, N., Rumeau, J.L., and L. Pradayrol. 1995 Identification of K-ras mutations in pancreatic juice in the early diagnosis of pancreatic cancer. *Ann Intern Med* 123(3):188–191.

Bhat, K., Wang, F., Ma, Q. et al. 2012. Advances in biomarker research for pancreatic cancer. *Curr Pharm Des* 18(17):2439–2451.

Bian, Y., Matsubayashi, H., Li, C.P. et al. 2006. Detecting low-abundance p16 and p53 mutations in pancreatic juice using a novel assay: Heteroduplex analysis of limiting dilution PCRs. *Cancer Biol Ther* 5(10):1392–1399.

Biewusch, K., Heyne, M., Grutzmann, R., and C. Pilarsky. 2012. DNA methylation in pancreatic cancer: Protocols for the isolation of DNA and bisulfite modification. *Methods Mol Biol* 863:273–280.

Blackford, A., Serrano, O.K., Wolfgang, C.L. et al. 2009. SMAD4 gene mutations are associated with poor prognosis in pancreatic cancer. *Clin Cancer Res* 15(14):4674–4679.

Bloomston, M., Frankel, W.L., Petrocca, F. et al. 2007. MicroRNA expression patterns to differentiate pancreatic adenocarcinoma from normal pancreas and chronic pancreatitis. *JAMA* 297:1901–1908.

Boadas, J., Mora, J., Urgell, E. et al. 2001. Clinical usefulness of K-ras gene mutation detection and cytology in pancreatic juice in the diagnosis and screening of pancreatic cancer. *Eur J Gastroenterol Hepatol* 13(10):1153–1159.

Boeck, S., Haas, M., Laubender, R.P. et al. 2010. Application of a time-varying covariate model to the analysis of CA 19-9 as serum biomarker in patients with advanced pancreatic cancer. *Clin Cancer Res* 16(3):986–994.

Boeck, S., Schulz, C., Stieber, P., Holdenrieder, S., Weckbach, S., and V. Heinemann. 2007. Assessing prognosis in metastatic pancreatic cancer by the serum tumor marker CA 19-9: Pretreatment levels or kinetics during chemotherapy? *Onkologie* 30(1–2):39–42.

Borgaonkar, S.P., Hocker, H., Shin, H., and M.K. Markey. 2010. Comparison of normalization methods for the identification of biomarkers using MALDI-TOF and SELDI-TOF mass spectra. *OMICS* 14(1):115–126.

Brody, J.R., Witkiewicz, A.K., and C.J. Yeo. 2011. The past, present, and future of biomarkers: A need for molecular beacons for the clinical management of pancreatic cancer. *Adv Surg* 45:301–321.

Cascinu, S., Falconi, M., Valentini, V., and S. Jelic; ESMO Guidelines Working Group. 2010. Pancreatic cancer: ESMO Clinical Practice Guidelines for diagnosis, treatment and follow-up. *Ann Oncol* 21 (Suppl 5):v55–v58.

Cen, P., Ni, X., Yang, J., Graham, D.Y., and M. Li. 2012. Circulating tumor cells in the diagnosis and management of pancreatic cancer. *Biochim Biophys Acta* 1826(12):350–356.

Chen, H., Tu, H., Meng, Z.Q., Chen, Z., Wang, P., and L.M. Liu. 2010. K-ras mutational status predicts poor prognosis in unresectable pancreatic cancer. *Eur J Surg Oncol* 36(7):657–662.

Chen, J., Li, D., Killary, A.M. et al. 2009a. Polymorphisms of p16, p27, p73, and MDM2 modulate response and survival of pancreatic cancer patients treated with preoperative chemoradiation. *Ann Surg Oncol* 16(2):431–439.

Chen, J.H., Ni, R.Z., Xiao, M.B., Guo, J.G., and J.W. Zhou. 2009b. Comparative proteomic analysis of differentially expressed proteins in human pancreatic cancer tissue. *Hepatobiliary Pancreat Dis Int* 8(2):193–200.

Chen, R., Pan, S., Brentnall, T.A., and R. Aebersold. 2005a. Proteomic profiling of pancreatic cancer for biomarker discovery. *Mol Cell Proteomics* 4:523–533.

Chen, R., Pan, S., Yi, E.C. et al. 2006. Quantitative proteomic profiling of pancreatic cancer juice. *Proteomics* 6:3871–3879.

Chen, R., Yi, E.C., Donohoe, S. et al. 2005b. Pancreatic cancer proteome: The proteins that underlie invasion, metastasis, and immunologic escape. *Gastroenterology* 129:1187–1197.

Corn, P.G. 2008. Genome-wide profiling of methylated promoters in pancreatic adenocarcinoma: Defining the pancreatic cancer [corrected] epigenome. *Cancer Biol Ther* 7(7):1157–1159.

Couch, F.J., Johnson, M.R., Rabe, K.G. et al. 2007. The prevalence of BRCA2 mutations in familial pancreatic cancer. *Cancer Epidemiol Biomarkers Prev* 16(2):342–346.

Couch, F.J., Wang, X., Bamlet, W.R., de Andrade, M., Petersen, G.M., and R.R. McWilliams. 2010. Association of mitotic regulation pathway polymorphisms with pancreatic cancer risk and outcome. *Cancer Epidemiol Biomarkers Prev* 19(1):251–257.

Couch, F.J., Wang, X., McWilliams, R.R., Bamlet, W.R., de Andrade, M., and G.M. Petersen. 2009. Association of breast cancer susceptibility variants with risk of pancreatic cancer. *Cancer Epidemiol Biomarkers Prev* 18(11):3044–3048.

Cui, Y., Wu, J., Zong, M. et al. 2009. Proteomic profiling in pancreatic cancer with and without lymph node metastasis. *Int J Cancer* 124(7):1614–1621.

Daniels, M.J., Wang, Y., Lee, M., and A.R. Venkitaraman. 2004. Abnormal cytokinesis in cells deficient in the breast cancer susceptibility protein BRCA2. *Science* 306(5697):876–879.

De Albuquerque, A., Kubisch, I., Ernst, D., Breier, G., Kaul, S., and N. Fersis. 2011. Prognostic significance of multimarker circulating tumor cells analysis in patients with advanced pancreatic cancer. *J Clin Oncol* 29(Suppl.):e14657.

Del Favero, G., Fabris, C., Panucci, A. et al. 1986a. Carbohydrate antigen 19-9 (CA 19-9) and carcinoembryonic antigen (CEA) in pancreatic cancer. Role of age and liver dysfunction. *Bull Cancer* 73(3):251–255.

Del Favero, G., Fabris, C., Plebani, M. et al. 1986b. CA 19-9 and carcinoembryonic antigen in pancreatic cancer diagnosis. *Cancer* 57(8):1576–1579.

DelMaschio, A., Vanzulli, A., Sironi, S. et al. 1991. Pancreatic cancer versus chronic pancreatitis: Diagnosis with CA 19-9 assessment, US, CT, and CT-guided fine-needle biopsy. *Radiology* 178(1):95–99.

Deramaudt, T.B., Takaoka, M., Upadhyay, R. et al. 2006. N-cadherin and keratinocyte growth factor receptor mediate the functional interplay between Ki-RASG12V and p53V143A in promoting pancreatic cell migration, invasion, and tissue architecture disruption. *Mol Cell Biol* 26(11):4185–4200.

Dillhoff, M., Liu, J., Frankel, W. et al. 2008. MicroRNA-21 is overexpressed in pancreatic cancer and a potential predictor of survival. *J Gastrointest Surg* 12(12):2171–2176.

Du Rieu, M.C., Torrisani, J., Selves, J. et al. 2010. MicroRNA-21 is induced early in pancreatic ductal adenocarcinoma precursor lesions. *Clin Chem* 56(4):603–612.

Edwards, S.L., Brough, R., Lord, C.J. et al. 2008. Resistance to therapy caused by intragenic deletion in BRCA2. *Nature* 451(7182):1111–1115.

Ehmann, M., Felix, K., Hartmann, D. et al. 2007. Identification of potential markers for the detection of pancreatic cancer through comparative serum protein expression profiling. *Pancreas* 34:205–214.

Esteller, M., Corn, P.G., Baylin, S.B., and J.G. Herman. 2001. A gene hypermethylation profile of human cancer. *Cancer Res* 61(8):3225–3229.

Evans, T., Faircloth, M., Deery, A., Thomas, V., Turner, A., and A. Dalgleish. 1997. Analysis of K-ras gene mutations in human pancreatic cancer cell lines and in bile samples from patients with pancreatic and biliary cancers. *Oncol Rep* 4(6):1373–1381.

Farini, R., Fabris, C., Bonvicini, P. et al. 1985. CA 19-9 in the differential diagnosis between pancreatic cancer and chronic pancreatitis. *Eur J Cancer Clin Oncol* 21(4):429–432.

Fidler, I.J. 2003. The pathogenesis of cancer metastasis: The 'seed and soil' hypothesis revisited. *Nat Rev Cancer* 3(6):453–458.

Fiedler, G.M., Leichtle, A.B., Kase, J. et al. 2009. Serum peptidome profiling revealed platelet factor 4 as a potential discriminating peptide associated with pancreatic cancer. *Clin Cancer Res* 15(11):3812–3819.

Fogelman, D.R., Wolff, R.A., Kopetz, S. et al. 2011. Evidence for the efficacy of Iniparib, a PARP-1 inhibitor, in BRCA2-associated pancreatic cancer. *Anticancer Res* 31(4):1417–1420.

Frebourg, T., Bercoff, E., Manchon, N. et al. 1988. The evaluation of CA 19-9 antigen level in the early detection of pancreatic cancer. A prospective study of 866 patients. *Cancer* 62(11):2287–2290.

Fryzek, J.P., Garabrant, D.H., Schenk, M., Kinnard, M., Greenson, J.K., and F.H. Sarkar. 2006. The association between selected risk factors for pancreatic cancer and the expression of p53 and K-ras codon 12 mutations. *Int J Gastrointest Cancer* 37(4):139–145.

Fukushima, N., Sato, N., Ueki, T. et al. 2002. Aberrant methylation of preproenkephalin and p16 genes in pancreatic intraepithelial neoplasia and pancreatic ductal adenocarcinoma. *Am J Pathol* 160(5):1573–1581.

Fukushima, N., Walter, K.M., Uek, T. et al. 2003. Diagnosing pancreatic cancer using methylation specific PCR analysis of pancreatic juice. *Cancer Biol Ther* 2(1):78–83.

Gao, H., Zheng, Z., Yue, Z., Liu, F., Zhou, L., and X. Zhao. 2012. Evaluation of serum diagnosis of pancreatic cancer by using surface-enhanced laser desorption/ionization time-of-flight mass spectrometry. *Int J Mol Med* 30(5):1061–1068.

Gao, J., Zhu, F., Lv, S. et al. 2010. Identification of pancreatic juice proteins as biomarkers of pancreatic cancer. *Oncol Rep* 23:1683–1692.

Gascoyne, P.R., Noshari, J., Anderson, T.J., and F.F. Becker. 2009. Isolation of rare cells from cell mixtures by dielectrophoresis. *Electrophoresis* 30:1388–1398.

GeneTests. 2012. http://www.ncbi.nlm.nih.gov/sites/GeneTests/?db = GeneTests (accessed November 7, 2012).

Gerdes, B., Ramaswamy, A., Kersting, M. et al. 2001. p16(INK4a) alterations in chronic pancreatitis-indicator for high-risk lesions for pancreatic cancer. *Surgery* 129(4):490–497.

Goggins, M. 2005. Molecular markers of early pancreatic cancer. *J Clin Oncol* 23:4524–4531.

Goggins, M., Koopmann, J., Yang, D., Canto, M.I., and R. Hruban. 2007. National Academy of Clinical Biochemistry (NACB) guidelines for the use of tumor markers in pancreatic ductal adenocarcinoma. American Association for Clinical Chemistry. http://www.aacc.org/sitecollectiondocuments/nacb/lmpg/tumor/chp3i_pancreatic.pdf (accessed November 7, 2012).

Goldstein, A.M., Fraser, M.C., Struewing, J.P. et al. 1995. Increased risk of pancreatic cancer in melanoma-prone kindreds with p16INK4 mutations. *N Engl J Med* 333(15):970–974.

Greenhalf, W., Grocock, C., Harcus, M., and J. Neoptolemos. 2009. Screening of high-risk families for pancreatic cancer. *Pancreatology* 9(3):215–222.

Greither, T., Grochola, L.F., Udelnow, A., Lautenschlager, C., Wurl, P., and H. Taubert. 2010. Elevated expression of microRNAs 155, 203, 210 and 222 in pancreatic tumors is associated with poorer survival. *Int J Cancer* 126:73–80.

Grote, T., Siwak, D.R., Fritsche, H.A. et al. 2008. Validation of reverse phase protein array for practical screening of potential biomarkers in serum and plasma: Accurate detection of CA19-9 levels in pancreatic cancer. *Proteomics* 8(15):3051–3060.

Gygi, S.P., Rist, B., Gerber, S.A., Turecek, F., Gelb, M.H., and R. Aebersold. 1999. Quantitative analysis of complex protein mixtures using isotope-coded affinity tags. *Nat Biotechnol* 17:994–999.

Haglund, C., Lindgren, J., Roberts, P.J., and S. Nordling. 1986a. Gastrointestinal cancer-associated antigen CA 19-9 in histological specimens of pancreatic tumours and pancreatitis. *Br J Cancer* 53(2):189–195.

Haglund, C., Roberts, P.J., Kuusela, P., Scheinin, T.M., Makela, O., and H. Jalanko. 1986b. Evaluation of CA 19-9 as a serum tumour marker in pancreatic cancer. *Br J Cancer* 53(2):197–202.

Hahn, S.A., Schutte, M., Hoque, A.T. et al. 1996. DPC4, a candidate tumor suppressor gene at human chromosome 18q21.1. *Science* 271(5247):350–353.

Hainaut, P. and M. Hollstein. 2000. p53 and human cancer: The first ten thousand mutations. *Adv Cancer Res* 77:81–137.

Halfdanarson, T.R., Wang, L., Bamlet, W.R. et al. 2008. Mitochondrial genetic polymorphisms do not predict survival in patients with pancreatic cancer. *Cancer Epidemiol Biomarkers Prev* 17(9):2512–2513.

Halm, U., Schumann, T., Schiefke, I., Witzigmann, H., Mossner, J., and V. Keim. 2000. Decrease of CA 19-9 during chemotherapy with gemcitabine predicts survival time in patients with advanced pancreatic cancer. *Br J Cancer* 82(5):1013–1016.

Hanash, S.M., Pitteri, S.J., and V.M. Faca. 2008. Mining the plasma proteome for cancer biomarkers. *Nature* 452:571–579.

Harada, T., Chelala, C., Crnogorac-Jurcevic, T., and N.R. Lemoine. 2009. Genome-wide analysis of pancreatic cancer using microarray-based techniques. *Pancreatology* 9(1–2):13–24.

Harsha, H.C., Kandasamy, K., Ranganathan, P. et al. 2009. A compendium of potential biomarkers of pancreatic cancer. *PLoS Med* 6(4):e1000046.

Hata, S., Sakamoto, Y., Yamamoto, Y. et al. 2012. Prognostic impact of postoperative serum CA 19-9 levels in patients with resectable pancreatic cancer. *Ann Surg Oncol* 19(2):636–641.

Haug, U., Wente, M.N., Seiler, C.M., Jesnowski, R., and H. Brenner. 2008. Stool testing for the early detection of pancreatic cancer: Rationale and current evidence. *Expert Rev Mol Diagn* 8:753–759.

Hayat, M.J., Howlader, N., Reichman, M.E., and B.K. Edwards. 2007. Cancer statistics, trends, and multiple primary cancer analyses from the Surveillance, Epidemiology, and End Results (SEER) Program. *Oncologist* 12(1):20–37.

Heldin, C.H., Miyazono, K., and P. ten Dijke P. 1997. TGF-beta signalling from cell membrane to nucleus through SMAD proteins. *Nature* 390(6659):465–471.

Herman, J.G., Graff, J.R., Myohanen, S., Nelkin, B.D., and S.B. Baylin. 1996. Methylation-specific PCR: A novel PCR assay for methylation status of CpG islands. *Proc Natl Acad Sci USA* 93(18):9821–9826.

Hermanova, M., Karasek, P., Nenutil, R. et al. 2009. Clinicopathological correlations of cyclooxygenase-2, MDM2, and p53 expressions in surgically resectable pancreatic invasive ductal adenocarcinoma. *Pancreas* 38(5):565–571.

Hess, V., Glimelius, B., Grawe, P. et al. 2008. CA 19-9 tumour-marker response to chemotherapy in patients with advanced pancreatic cancer enrolled in a randomised controlled trial. *Lancet Oncol* 9(2):132–138.

Hoffmann, K., Kerner, C., Wilfert, W. et al. 2007. Detection of disseminated pancreatic cells by amplification of cytokeratin-19 with quantitative RT-PCR in blood, bone marrow and peritoneal lavage of pancreatic carcinoma patients. *World J Gastroenterol* 13:257–263.

Hong, S.M., Park, J.Y., Hruban, R.H., and M. Goggins. 2011. Molecular signatures of pancreatic cancer. *Arch Pathol Lab Med* 135(6):716–727.

Hruban, R.H., Goggins, M., Parsons, J., and S.E. Kern. 2000. Progression model for pancreatic cancer. *Clin Cancer Res* 6(8):2969–2972.

Hsieh, H.B., Marrinucci, D., Bethel, K. et al. 2006. High speed detection of circulating tumor cells. *Biosens Bioelectron* 21:1893–1899.

Hua, Z., Zhang, Y.C., Hu, X.M. et al. 2003. Loss of DPC4 expression and its correlation with clinicopathological parameters in pancreatic carcinoma. *World J Gastroenterol* 9(12):2764–2767.

Hustinx, S.R., Leoni, L.M., Yeo, C.J. et al. 2005. Concordant loss of MTAP and p16/CDKN2A expression in pancreatic intraepithelial neoplasia: Evidence of homozygous deletion in a noninvasive precursor lesion. *Mod Pathol* 18(7):959–963.

Iacobuzio-Donahue, C.A. 2012. Genetic evolution of pancreatic cancer: Lessons learnt from the pancreatic cancer genome sequencing project. *Gut* 61(7):1085–1094.

Iacobuzio-Donahue, C.A., Fu, B., Yachida, S. et al. 2009. DPC4 gene status of the primary carcinoma correlates with patterns of failure in patients with pancreatic cancer. *J Clin Oncol* 27(11):1806–1813.

Iacobuzio-Donahue, C.A., Maitra, A., Olsen, M. et al. 2003. Exploration of global gene expression patterns in pancreatic adenocarcinoma using cDNA microarrays. *Am J Pathol* 162:1151–1162.

Innocenti, F., Owzar, K., Cox, N.L. et al. 2012. A genome-wide association study of overall survival in pancreatic cancer patients treated with gemcitabine in CALGB 80303. *Clin Cancer Res* 18(2):577–584.

Ishii, H., Okada, S., Sato, T. et al. 1997. CA 19-9 in evaluating the response to chemotherapy in advanced pancreatic cancer. *Hepatogastroenterology* 44(13):279–283.

Issa, J.P., Ottaviano, Y.L., Celano, P., Hamilton, S.R., Davidson, N.E., and S.B. Baylin. 1994. Methylation of the oestrogen receptor CpG island links ageing and neoplasia in human colon. *Nat Genet* 7(4):536–540.

Jeong, J., Park, Y.N., Park, J.S. et al. 2005. Clinical significance of p16 protein expression loss and aberrant p53 protein expression in pancreatic cancer. *Yonsei Med J* 46(4):519–525.

Jinfeng, M., Kimura, W., Sakurai, F. et al. 2007. Prognostic role of angiogenesis and its correlations with thymidine phosphorylase and p53 expression in ductal adenocarcinoma of the pancreas. *Hepatogastroenterology* 54(78):1635–1640.

Jones, J.B., Song, J.J., Hempen, P.M., Parmigiani, G., Hruban, R.H., and S.E. Kern. 2001. Detection of mitochondrial DNA mutations in pancreatic cancer offers a "mass"-ive advantage over detection of nuclear DNA mutations. *Cancer Res* 61(4):1299–1304.

Jones, P.A. and S.B. Baylin. 2002. The fundamental role of epigenetic events in cancer. *Nat Rev Genet* 3(6):415–428.

Kaino, M., Kondoh, S., Okita, S. et al. 1999. Detection of K-ras and p53 gene mutations in pancreatic juice for the diagnosis of intraductal papillary mucinous tumors. *Pancreas* 18(3):294–299.

Kang, C.M., Kim, J.Y., Choi, G.H. et al. 2007. The use of adjusted preoperative CA 19-9 to predict the recurrence of resectable pancreatic cancer. *J Surg Res* 140(1):31–35.

Kassauei, K., Habbe, N., Mullendore, M.E., Karikari, C.A., Maitra, A., and G. Feldmann. 2006. Mitochondrial DNA mutations in pancreatic cancer. *Int J Gastrointest Cancer* 37(2–3):57–64.

Katz, M.H., Varadhachary, G.R., Fleming, J.B. et al. 2010. Serum CA 19-9 as a marker of resectability and survival in patients with potentially resectable pancreatic cancer treated with neoadjuvant chemoradiation. *Ann Surg Oncol* 17(7):1794–1801.

Khoja, L., Backen, A., Sloane, R. et al. 2012. A pilot study to explore circulating tumour cells in pancreatic cancer as a novel biomarker. *Br J Cancer* 106(3):508–516.

Kilic, M., Gocmen, E., Tez, M., Ertan, T., Keskek, M., and M. Koc. 2006. Value of preoperative serum CA 19-9 levels in predicting resectability for pancreatic cancer. *Can J Surg* 49(4):241–244.

Kim, D.H., Crawford, B., Ziegler, J., and M.S. Beattie. 2009. Prevalence and characteristics of pancreatic cancer in families with BRCA1 and BRCA2 mutations. *Fam Cancer* 8(2):153–158.

Klump, B., Hsieh, C.J., Nehls, O. et al. 2003. Methylation status of p14ARF and p16INK4a as detected in pancreatic secretions. *Br J Cancer* 88(2):217–222.

Kondo, N., Murakami, Y., Uemura, K. et al. 2010. Prognostic impact of perioperative serum CA 19-9 levels in patients with resectable pancreatic cancer. *Ann Surg Oncol* 17(9):2321–2329.

Koom, W.S., Seong, J., Kim, Y.B., Pyun, H.O., and S.Y. Song. 2009. CA 19-9 as a predictor for response and survival in advanced pancreatic cancer patients treated with chemoradiotherapy. *Int J Radiat Oncol Biol Phys* 73(4):1148–1154.

Koopmann, J., Buckhaults, P., Brown, D.A. et al. 2004a. Serum macrophage inhibitory cytokine 1 as a marker of pancreatic and other periampullary cancers. *Clin Cancer Res* 10(7):2386–2392.

Koopmann, J., Fedarko, N.S., Jain, A. et al. 2004b. Evaluation of osteopontin as biomarker for pancreatic adenocarcinoma. *Cancer Epidemiol Biomarkers Prev* 13(3):487–491.

Koopmann, J., Zhang, Z., White, N. et al. 2004c. Serum diagnosis of pancreatic adenocarcinoma using surface-enhanced laser desorption and ionization mass spectrometry. *Clin Cancer Res* 10(3):860–868.

Koprowski, H., Herlyn, M., Steplewski, Z., and H.F. Sears. 1981. Specific antigen in serum of patients with colon carcinoma. *Science* 212(4490):53–55.

Kurihara, T., Itoi, T., Sofuni, A. et al. 2008. Detection of circulating tumor cells in patients with pancreatic cancer: A preliminary result. *J Hepatobiliary Pancreat Surg* 15:189–195.

Landi, S. 2009. Genetic predisposition and environmental risk factors to pancreatic cancer: A review of the literature. *Mutat Res* 681(2–3):299–307.

Laurell, H., Bouisson, M., Berthelemy, P. et al. 2006. Identification of biomarkers of human pancreatic adenocarcinomas by expression profiling and validation with gene expression analysis in endoscopic ultrasound-guided fine needle aspiration samples. *World J Gastroenterol* 12:3344–3351.

Lee, E.J., Gusev, Y., Jiang, J. et al. 2007. Expression profiling identifies microRNA signature in pancreatic cancer. *Int J Cancer* 120:1046–1054.

Lee, S.H., Lee, S.J., Chung, J.Y. et al. 2009a. p53, secreted by *K-Ras*-Snail pathway, is endocytosed by *K-Ras*-mutated cells; implication of target-specific drug delivery and early diagnostic marker. *Oncogene* 28(19):2005–2014.

Lee, S.H., Lee, S.J., Jung, Y.S. et al. 2009b. Blocking of p53-Snail binding, promoted by oncogenic *K-Ras*, recovers p53 expression and function. *Neoplasia* 11(1):22–31.

Li, D., Duell, E.J., Yu, K. et al. 2012. Pathway analysis of genome-wide association study data highlights pancreatic development genes as susceptibility factors for pancreatic cancer. *Carcinogenesis* 33(7):1384–1390.

Li, D., Firozi, P.F., Zhang, W., Shen, J. et al. 2002. DNA adducts, genetic polymorphisms, and K-ras mutation in human pancreatic cancer. *Mutat Res* 513(1–2):37–48.

Liang, J.J., Kimchi, E.T., Staveley-O'Carroll, K.F., and D. Tan. 2009. Diagnostic and prognostic biomarkers in pancreatic carcinoma. *Int J Clin Exp Pathol* 2:1–10.

Link, A.J., Eng, J., Schieltz, D.M. et al. 1999. Direct analysis of protein complexes using mass spectrometry. *Nat Biotechnol* 17:676–682.

Liu, F., Pouponnot, C., and J. Massague. 1997. Dual role of the Smad4/DPC4 tumor suppressor in TGFbeta-inducible transcriptional complexes. *Genes Dev* 11(23):3157–3167.

Locker, G.Y., Hamilton, S., Harris, J. et al. for the American Society of Clinical Oncology Tumor Markers Expert Panel. 2006. American Society of Clinical Oncology 2006 update of recommendations for the use of tumor markers in gastrointestinal cancer. *J Clin Oncol* 24(33):5313–5327.

Lohr, M., Muller, P., Mora, J. et al. 2001. p53 and K-ras mutations in pancreatic juice samples from patients with chronic pancreatitis. *Gastrointest Endosc* 53(7):734–743.

Lopez-Casas, P.P. and L.A. Lopez-Fernandez. 2010. Gene-expression profiling in pancreatic cancer. *Expert Rev Mol Diagn* 10:591–601.

Lu, J., Getz, G., Miska, E.A. et al. 2005. MicroRNA expression profiles classify human cancers. *Nature* 435:834–838.

Lu, X., Xu, T., Qian, J. et al. 2002. Detecting K-ras and p53 gene mutation from stool and pancreatic juice for diagnosis of early pancreatic cancer. *Chin Med J (Engl)* 115(11):1632–1636.

Ma, N., Ge, C.L., Luan, F. et al. 2008. Serum protein fingerprint of patients with pancreatic cancer by SELDI technology. *Chinese J Cancer Res* 20:171–176.

Maitra, A., Cohen, Y., Gillespie, S.E. et al. 2004. The human MitoChip: A high-throughput sequencing microarray for mitochondrial mutation detection. *Genome Res* 14(5):812–819.

Malumbres, M. and M. Barbacid. 2003. RAS oncogenes: The first 30 years. *Nat Rev Cancer* 3(6):459–465.

Matsubayashi, H., Canto, M., Sato, N. et al. 2006. DNA methylation alterations in the pancreatic juice of patients with suspected pancreatic disease. *Cancer Res* 66(2):1208–1217.

Matsubayashi, H., Sato, N., Brune, K. et al. 2005. Age- and disease-related methylation of multiple genes in nonneoplastic duodenum and in duodenal juice. *Clin Cancer Res* 11(2 Pt 1):573–583.

Matsubayashi, H., Sato, N., Fukushima, N. et al. 2003. Methylation of cyclin D2 is observed frequently in pancreatic cancer but is also an age-related phenomenon in gastrointestinal tissues. *Clin Cancer Res* 9(4):1446–1452.

Melnikov, A.A., Scholtens, D., Talamonti, M.S., Bentrem, D.J., and V.V. Levenson. 2009. Methylation profile of circulating plasma DNA in patients with pancreatic cancer. *J Surg Oncol* 99(2):119–122.

Mergo, P.J., Helmberger, T.K., Buetow, P.C., Helmberger, R.C., and P.R. Ros. 1997. Pancreatic neoplasms: MR imaging and pathologic correlation. *Radiographics* 17(2):281–301.

Milner, J., Ponder, B., Hughes-Davies, L., Seltmann, M., and T. Kouzarides. 1997. Transcriptional activation functions in BRCA2. *Nature* 386(6627):772–773.

Molina, L.M., Diez, M., Cava, M.T. et al. 1990. Tumor markers in pancreatic cancer: A comparative clinical study between CEA, CA 19-9 and CA 50. *Int J Biol Markers* 5(3):127–132.

Molina, V., Visa, L., Conill, C. et al. 2012. CA 19-9 in pancreatic cancer: Retrospective evaluation of patients with suspicion of pancreatic cancer. *Tumour Biol* 33(3):799–807.

Moore, P.S., Sipos, B., Orlandini, S. et al. 2001. Genetic profile of 22 pancreatic carcinoma cell lines. Analysis of *K-ras*, p53, p16 and DPC4/Smad4. *Virchows Arch* 439(6):798–802.

Moriyama, T., Ohuchida, K., Mizumoto, K. et al. 2009. MicroRNA-21 modulates biological functions of pancreatic cancer cells including their proliferation, invasion, and chemoresistance. *Mol Cancer Ther* 8(5):1067–1074.

Morse, D.L., Balagurunathan, Y., Hostetter, G. et al. 2010. Identification of novel pancreatic adenocarcinoma cell-surface targets by gene expression profiling and tissue microarray. *Biochem Pharmacol* 80:748–754.

Murphy, K.M., Brune, K.A., Griffin, C. et al. 2002. Evaluation of candidate genes MAP2K4, MADH4, ACVR1B, and BRCA2 in familial pancreatic cancer: Deleterious BRCA2 mutations in 17%. *Cancer Res* 62(13):3789–3793.

Nagrath, S., Sequist, L.V., Maheswaran, S. et al. 2007. Isolation of rare circulating tumour cells in cancer patients by microchip technology. *Nature* 450(7173):1235–1239.

Nakai, Y., Kawabe, T., Isayama, H. et al. 2008. CA 19-9 response as an early indicator of the effectiveness of gemcitabine in patients with advanced pancreatic cancer. *Oncology* 75(1–2):120–126.

Navaglia, F., Fogar, P., Basso, D. et al. 2009. Pancreatic cancer biomarkers discovery by surface-enhanced laser desorption and ionization time-of-flight mass spectrometry. *Clin Chem Lab Med* 47(6):713–723.

Nguyen, C., Liang, G., Nguyen, T.T. et al. 2001. Susceptibility of nonpromoter CpG islands to de novo methylation in normal and neoplastic cells. *J Natl Cancer Inst* 93(19):1465–1472.

Nikolic, A., Kojic, S., Knezevic, S., Krivokapic, Z., Ristanovic, M., and D. Radojkovic. 2011. Structural and functional analysis of SMAD4 gene promoter in malignant pancreatic and colorectal tissues: Detection of two novel polymorphic nucleotide repeats. *Cancer Epidemiol.* 35(3):265–271.

Nio, Y., Dong, M., Uegaki, K. et al. 1999. Comparative significance of p53 and WAF/1-p21 expression on the efficacy of adjuvant chemotherapy for resectable invasive ductal carcinoma of the pancreas. *Pancreas* 18(2):117–126.

Ohtsubo, K., Watanabe, H., Yamaguchi, Y. et al. 2003. Abnormalities of tumor suppressor gene p16 in pancreatic carcinoma: Immunohistochemical and genetic findings compared with clinicopathological parameters. *J Gastroenterol* 38(7):663–671.

Okazaki, T., Javle, M., Tanaka, M., Abbruzzese, J.L., and D. Li. 2010. Single nucleotide polymorphisms of gemcitabine metabolic genes and pancreatic cancer survival and drug toxicity. *Clin Cancer Res* 16(1):320–329.

Okazaki, T., Jiao, L., Chang, P., Evans, D.B., Abbruzzese, J.L., and D. Li. 2008. Single-nucleotide polymorphisms of DNA damage response genes are associated with overall survival in patients with pancreatic cancer. *Clin Cancer Res* 14(7):2042–2048.

Olsen, C.C., Schefter, T.E., Chen, H. et al. 2009. Results of a phase I trial of 12 patients with locally advanced pancreatic carcinoma combining gefitinib, paclitaxel, and 3-dimensional conformal radiation: Report of toxicity and evaluation of circulating K-ras as a potential biomarker of response to therapy. *Am J Clin Oncol* 32(2):115–121.

Pao, M.M., Tsutsumi, M., Liang, G., Uzvolgyi, E., Gonzales, F.A., and P.A. Jones. 2001. The endothelin receptor B (EDNRB) promoter displays heterogeneous, site specific methylation patterns in normal and tumor cells. *Hum Mol Genet* 10(9):903–910.

Paradis, V., Degos, F., Dargere, D. et al. 2005. Identification of a new marker of hepatocellular carcinoma by serum protein profiling of patients with chronic liver diseases. *Hepatology* 41:40–47.

Park, J.K., Ryu, J.K., Lee, K.H. et al. 2007. Quantitative analysis of NPTX2 hypermethylation is a promising molecular diagnostic marker for pancreatic cancer. *Pancreas* 35(3):e9–e15.

Park, J.Y., Kim, S.A., Chung, J.W. et al. 2011. Proteomic analysis of pancreatic juice for the identification of biomarkers of pancreatic cancer. *J Cancer Res Clin Oncol* 137(8):1229–1238.

Parker, L.A., Porta, M., Lumbreras, B. et al. 2011. Clinical validity of detecting K-RAS mutations for the diagnosis of exocrine pancreatic cancer: A prospective study in a clinically-relevant spectrum of patients. *Eur J Epidemiol* 26(3):229–236.

Pellegata, N.S., Sessa, F., Renault, B. et al. 1994. K-ras and p53 gene mutations in pancreatic cancer: Ductal and nonductal tumors progress through different genetic lesions. *Cancer Res* 54(6):1556–1560.

Petersen, G.M., Amundadottir, L., Fuchs, C.S. et al. 2010. A genome-wide association study identifies pancreatic cancer susceptibility loci on chromosomes 13q22.1, 1q32.1 and 5p15.33. *Nat Genet* 42(3):224–228.

Petricoin, E.F., Ardekani, A.M., Hitt, B.A. et al. 2002. Use of proteomic patterns in serum to identify ovarian cancer. *Lancet* 359:572–577.

Pierce, B.L., Tong, L., Kraft, P., and H. Ahsan. 2012. Unidentified genetic variants influence pancreatic cancer risk: An analysis of polygenic susceptibility in the PanScan study. *Genet Epidemiol* 36(5):517–524.

Qian, J.Y., Mou, S.H., and C.B. Liu. 2012. SELDI-TOF MS combined with magnetic beads for detecting serum protein biomarkers and establishment of a boosting decision tree model for diagnosis of pancreatic cancer. *Asian Pac J Cancer Prev* 13(5):1911–1915.

Rachagani, S., Kumar, S., and S.K. Batra. 2010. MicroRNA in pancreatic cancer: Pathological, diagnostic and therapeutic implications. *Cancer Lett* 292(1):8–16.

Rajan, J.V., Wang, M., Marquis, S.T., and L.A. Chodosh. 1996. Brca2 is coordinately regulated with Brca1 during proliferation and differentiation in mammary epithelial cells. *Proc Natl Acad Sci USA* 93(23):13078–13083.

Ren, C., Han, C., Zhang, J. et al. 2011. Detection of apoptotic circulating tumor cells in advanced pancreatic cancer following 5-fluorouracil chemotherapy. *Cancer Biol Ther* 12(8):700–706.

Rifa, J., Fernandez, E., Alguacil, J., Malats, N., and F.X. Real. 2011. Clinical validity of detecting K-ras mutations for the diagnosis of exocrine pancreatic cancer: A prospective study in a clinically-relevant spectrum of patients. *Eur J Epidemiol* 26(3):229–236.

Rizzato, C., Campa, D., Giese, N. et al. 2011. Pancreatic cancer susceptibility loci and their role in survival. *PLoS One* 6(11):e27921.

Robson, C.N., Gnanapragasam, V., Byrne, R.L. et al. 1999. Transforming growth factor-beta1 up-regulates p15, p21 and p27 and blocks cell cycling in G1 in human prostate epithelium. *J Endocrinol* 160(2):257–266.

Rocha Lima, C.M., Savarese, D., Bruckner, H. et al. 2002. Irinotecan plus gemcitabine induces both radiographic and CA 19-9 tumor marker responses in patients with previously untreated advanced pancreatic cancer. *J Clin Oncol* 20(5):1182–1191.

Rogosnitzky, M. and R. Danks. 2010. Validation of blood testing for K-ras mutations in colorectal and pancreatic cancer. *Anticancer Res* 30(7):2943–2947.

Rosty, C., Christa, L., Kuzdzal, S. et al. 2002. Identification of hepatocarcinoma-intestine-pancreas/pancreatitis-associated protein I as a biomarker for pancreatic ductal adenocarcinoma by protein biochip technology. *Cancer Res* 62(6):1868–1875.

Ruckert, F., Pilarsky, C., and R. Grutzmann. 2010. Serum tumor markers in pancreatic cancer—Recent discoveries. *Cancers* 2(2):1107–1124.

Saad, E.D., Machado, M.C., Wajsbrot, D. et al. 2002. Pretreatment CA 19-9 level as a prognostic factor in patients with advanced pancreatic cancer treated with gemcitabine. *Int J Gastrointest Cancer* 32(1):35–41.

Saad, E.D., Reis, P.T., Borghesi, G. et al. 2010. Further evidence of the prognostic role of pretreatment levels of CA 19-9 in advanced pancreatic cancer. *Rev Assoc Med Bras* 56(1):22–26.

Safi, F., Schlosser, W., Falkenreck, S., and H.G. Beger. 1996. CA 19-9 serum course and prognosis of pancreatic cancer. *Int J Pancreatol* 20(3):155–161.

Safi, F., Schlosser, W., Falkenreck, S., and H.G. Beger. 1998. Prognostic value of CA 19-9 serum course in pancreatic cancer. *Hepatogastroenterology* 45(19):253–259.

Saif, M.F. 2011. Pancreatic neoplasm in 2011: An update. *JOP* 12(4):316–321.

Sakai, W., Swisher, E.M., Karlan, B.Y. et al. 2008. Secondary mutations as a mechanism of cisplatin resistance in BRCA2-mutated cancers. *Nature* 451(7182):1116–1120.

Salek, C., Benesova, L., Zavoral, M. et al. 2007. Evaluation of clinical relevance of examining *K-ras*, p16 and p53 mutations along with allelic losses at 9p and 18q in EUS-guided fine needle aspiration samples of patients with chronic pancreatitis and pancreatic cancer. *World J Gastroenterol* 13(27):3714–3720.

Salek, C., Minarikova, P., Benesova, L. et al. 2009. Mutation status of *K-ras*, p53 and allelic losses at 9p and 18q are not prognostic markers in patients with pancreatic cancer. *Anticancer Res* 29(5):1803–1810.

Sato, N., Fukushima, N., Hruban, R.H., and M. Goggins. 2008. CpG island methylation profile of pancreatic intraepithelial neoplasia. *Mod Pathol* 21(3):238–244.

Sato, N., Fukushima, N., Maitra, A. et al. 2003. Discovery of novel targets for aberrant methylation in pancreatic carcinoma using high-throughput microarrays. *Cancer Res* 63(13):3735–3742.

Sato, N., Parker, A.R., Fukushima, N. et al. 2004. Epigenetic inactivation of TFPI-2 as a common mechanism associated with growth and invasion of pancreatic ductal adenocarcinoma. *Oncogene* 24(5):850–858.

Sato, N., Parker, A.R., Fukushima, N. et al. 2005. Epigenetic inactivation of TFPI-2 as a common mechanism associated with growth and invasion of pancreatic ductal adenocarcinoma. *Oncogene* 24(5):850–858.

Scarlett, C.J., Smith, R.C., Saxby, A. et al. 2006. Proteomic classification of pancreatic adenocarcinoma tissue using protein chip technology. *Gastroenterology* 130:1670–1678.

Scarpa, A., Capelli, P., Mukai, K. et al. 1993. Pancreatic adenocarcinomas frequently show p53 gene mutations. *Am J Pathol* 142(5):1534–1543.

Schutte, M., Hruban, R.H., Hedrick, L. et al. 1996. DPC4 gene in various tumor types. *Cancer Res* 56(11):2527–2530.

Selivanova, G. and K.G. Wiman. 2007. Reactivation of mutant p53: Molecular mechanisms and therapeutic potential. *Oncogene* 26(15):2243–2254.

Seoane, J., Le, H.V., and J. Massague 2002. Myc suppression of the p21(Cip1) Cdk inhibitor influences the outcome of the p53 response to DNA damage. *Nature* 419(6908):729–734.

Sergeant, G., Roskams, T., van Pelt, J., Houtmeyers, F., Aerts, R., and B. Topal. 2011. Perioperative cancer cell dissemination detected with a real-time RT-PCR assay for EpCAM is not associated with worse prognosis in pancreatic ductal adenocarcinoma. *BMC Cancer* 11:47.

Serrano, J., Goebel, S.U., Peghini, P.L. et al. 2000. Alterations in the p16INK4a/CDKN2A tumor suppressor gene in gastrinomas. *J Clin Endocrinol Metab* 85(11):4146–4156.

Shi, C., Eshelman, S.H., Jones, D. et al. 2004. LigAmp for sensitive detection of single-nucleotide differences. *Nat Methods* 1:141–147.

Shi, C., Hruban, R.H., and A.P. Klein. 2009. Familial pancreatic cancer. *Arch Pathol Lab Med* 133(3):365–374.

Sidransky, D. 2002. Emerging molecular markers of cancer. *Nat Rev Cancer* 2:210–219.

Siegel, R., Naishadham, D., and A. Jemal. 2012. Cancer statistics, 2012. *CA Cancer J Clin* 62(1):10–29.

Smith, R.A., Tang, J., Tudur-Smith, C., Neoptolemos, J.P., and P. Ghaneh. 2011. Meta-analysis of immunohistochemical prognostic markers in resected pancreatic cancer. *Br J Cancer* 104(9):1440–1451.

Soeth, E., Grigoleit, U., Moellmann, B. et al. 2005. Detection of tumor cell dissemination in pancreatic ductal carcinoma patients by CK 20 RT-PCR indicates poor survival. *J Cancer Res Clin Oncol* 131:669–676.

Sperti, C., Pasquali, C., Catalini, S. et al. 1993. CA 19-9 as a prognostic index after resection for pancreatic cancer. *J Surg Oncol* 52(3):137–141.

Stemmler, J., Stieber, P., Szymala, A.M. et al. 2003. Are serial CA 19-9 kinetics helpful in predicting survival in patients with advanced or metastatic pancreatic cancer treated with gemcitabine and cisplatin? *Onkologie* 26(5):462–467.

Stott, S.L., Hsu, C.H., Tsukrov, D.I. et al. 2010. Isolation of circulating tumor cells using a microvortex-generating herringbone-chip. *Proc Natl Acad Sci USA* 107(43):18392–18397.

Stracci, F., D'Alo, D., Cassetti, T., Scheibel, M., and F. La Rosa. 2009. Incidence of multiple primary malignancies in women diagnosed with breast cancer. *Eur J Gynaecol Oncol* 30(6):661–663.

Streit, S., Michalski, C.W., Erkan, M., Friess, H., and J. Kleeff. 2009. Confirmation of DNA microarray-derived differentially expressed genes in pancreatic cancer using quantitative RT-PCR. *Pancreatology* 9(5):577–582.

Sturm, P.D., Hruban, R.H., Ramsoekh, T.B. et al. 1998. The potential diagnostic use of K-ras codon 12 and p53 alterations in brush cytology from the pancreatic head region. *J Pathol* 186(3):247–253.

Sun, C., Rosendahl, A.H., Ansari, D., and R. Andersson. 2011. Proteome-based biomarkers in pancreatic cancer. *World J Gastroenterol* 17(44):4845–4852.

Sun, C., Yamato, T., Furukawa, T., Ohnishi, Y., Kijima, H., and A. Horii. 2001. Characterization of the mutations of the *K-ras*, p53, p16, and SMAD4 genes in 15 human pancreatic cancer cell lines. *Oncol Rep* 8(1):89–92.

Szafranska, A.E., Davison, T.S., John, J. et al. 2007. MicroRNA expression alterations are linked to tumorigenesis and non-neoplastic processes in pancreatic ductal adenocarcinoma. *Oncogene* 26:4442–4452.

Talar-Wojnarowska, R., Gasiorowska, A., Smolarz, B. et al. 2004. Usefulness of p16 and K-ras mutation in pancreatic adenocarcinoma and chronic pancreatitis differential diagnosis. *J Physiol Pharmacol* 55(Suppl 2):129–138.

Tambor, V., Fucikova, A., Lenco, J. et al. 2010. Application of proteomics in biomarker discovery: A primer for the clinician. *Physiol Res* 59:471–497.

Tan, A.C., Jimeno, A., Lin, S.H. et al. 2009. Characterizing DNA methylation patterns in pancreatic cancer genome. *Mol Oncol* 3(5–6):425–438.

Tanaka, M., Okazaki, T., Suzuki, H., Abbruzzese, J.L., and D. Li. 2011. Association of multi-drug resistance gene polymorphisms with pancreatic cancer outcome. *Cancer* 117(4):744–751.

Tischkowitz, M. and B. Xia. 2010. PALB2/FANCN: Recombining cancer and Fanconi anemia. *Cancer Res* 70(19):7353–7359.

Uehara, H., Nakaizumi, A., Baba, M. et al. 1996. Diagnosis of pancreatic cancer by K-ras point mutation and cytology of pancreatic juice. *Am J Gastroenterol* 91(8):1616–1621.

Van Heek, T., Rader, A.E., Offerhaus, G.J. et al. 2002. *K-ras*, p53, and DPC4 (MAD4) alterations in fine-needle aspirates of the pancreas: A molecular panel correlates with and supplements cytologic diagnosis. *Am J Clin Pathol* 117(5):755–765.

Vasen, H.F., Wasser, M., van Mil, A. et al. 2011. Magnetic resonance imaging surveillance detects early-stage pancreatic cancer in carriers of a p16-Leiden mutation. *Gastroenterology* 140(3):850–856.

Vormittag, L., Gleiss, A., Scheithauer, W., Lang, F., Laengle, F., and G.V. Kornek. 2009. Limited value of CA 19-9 in predicting early treatment failure in patients with advanced pancreatic cancer. *Oncology* 77(2):140–146.

Vousden, K.H. 2002. Switching from life to death: The Miz-ing link between Myc and p53. *Cancer Cell* 2(5):351–352.

Walsh, N., O'Donovan, N., Kennedy, S. et al. 2009. Identification of pancreatic cancer invasion-related proteins by proteomic analysis. *Proteome Sci* 7:3.

Wang, J., Chen, J., Chang, P. et al. 2009. MicroRNAs in plasma of pancreatic ductal adenocarcinoma patients as novel blood-based biomarkers of disease. *Cancer Prev Res (Phila)* 2:807–813.

Wang, J. and S. Sen. 2011. MicroRNA functional network in pancreatic cancer: From biology to biomarkers of disease. *J Biosci* 36(3):481–491.

Wasan, H.S., Springett, G.M., Chodkiewicz, C. et al. 2009. CA 19-9 as a biomarker in advanced pancreatic cancer patients randomised to gemcitabine plus axitinib or gemcitabine alone. *Br J Cancer* 101(7):1162–1167.

Watanabe, H., Miyagi, C., Yamaguchi, Y. et al. 1996a. Detection of K-ras point mutations at codon 12 in pancreatic juice for the diagnosis of pancreatic cancer by hybridization protection assay: A simple method for the determination of the types of point mutation. *Jpn J Cancer Res* 87(5):466–474.

Watanabe, H., Sawabu, N., Songur, Y. et al. 1996b. Detection of K-ras point mutations at codon 12 in pure pancreatic juice for the diagnosis of pancreatic cancer by PCR-RFLP analysis. *Pancreas* 12(1):18–24.

Wehrum, D., Grutzmann, R., Hennig, M., Saeger, H.D., and C. Pilarsky. 2008. Recent patents concerning diagnostic and therapeutic applications of aberrantly methylated sequences in pancreatic cancer. *Recent Pat DNA Gene Seq* 2(2):97–106.

Wenger, F.A., Zieren, J., Peter, F.J., Jacobi, C.A., and J.M. Maller. 1999. K-ras mutations in tissue and stool samples from patients with pancreatic cancer and chronic pancreatitis. *Langenbecks Arch Surg* 384(2):181–186.

Whelan, A.J., Bartsch, D., and P.J. Goodfellow. 1995. Brief report: A familial syndrome of pancreatic cancer and melanoma with a mutation in the CDKN2 tumor-suppressor gene. *N Engl J Med* 333(15):975–977.

Wikman, F.P., Lu, M.L., Thykjaer, T. et al. 2000. Evaluation of the performance of a p53 sequencing microarray chip using 140 previously sequenced bladder tumor samples. *Clin Chem* 46(10):1555–1561.

Willis, J.A., Olson, S.H., Orlow, I. et al. 2012. A replication study and genome-wide scan of single-nucleotide polymorphisms associated with pancreatic cancer risk and overall survival. *Clin Cancer Res* 18(14):3942–3951.

Wong, S.C.C., Chan, C.M.L., Ma, B.B.Y. et al. 2009. Advanced proteomic technologies for cancer biomarker discovery. *Expert Rev Proteomics* 6:123–134.

Wray, C.J., Ahmad, S.A., Matthews, J.B., and A.M. Lowy. 2005. Surgery for pancreatic cancer: Recent controversies and current practice. *Gastroenterology* 128(6):1626–1641.

Xia, F., Taghian, D.G., DeFrank, J.S. et al. 2001. Deficiency of human BRCA2 leads to impaired homologous recombination but maintains normal nonhomologous end joining. *Proc Natl Acad Sci USA* 98(15):8644–8649.

Xu, X., Strimpakos, A.S., and M.W. Saif. 2011. Biomarkers and pharmacogenetics in pancreatic cancer. Highlights from the "2011 ASCO Annual Meeting". *JOP* 12(4):325–329.

Xue, A., Gandy, R.C., Chung, L., Baxter, R.C., and R.C. Smith. 2012. Discovery of diagnostic biomarkers for pancreatic cancer in immunodepleted serum by SELDI-TOF MS. *Pancreatology* 12(2):124–129.

Xue, A., Scarlett, C.J., Chung, L. et al. 2010. Discovery of serum biomarkers for pancreatic adenocarcinoma using proteomic analysis. *Br J Cancer* 103:391–400.

Yamaguchi, Y., Watanabe, H., Yrdiran, S. et al. 1999. Detection of mutations of p53 tumor suppressor gene in pancreatic juice and its application to diagnosis of patients with pancreatic cancer: Comparison with K-ras mutation. *Clin Cancer Res* 5(5):1147–1153.

You, L., Chang, D., Du, H.Z., and Y.P. Zhao. 2011. Genome-wide screen identifies PVT1 as a regulator of Gemcitabine sensitivity in human pancreatic cancer cells. *Biochem Biophys Res Commun* 407(1):1–6.

Yu, K.H., Rustgi, A.K., and I.A. Blair. 2005. Characterization of proteins in human pancreatic cancer serum using differential gel electrophoresis and tandem mass spectrometry. *J Proteome Res* 4:1742–1751.

Zhang, L., Farrell, J.J., Zhou, H. et al. 2010. Salivary transcriptomic biomarkers for detection of resectable pancreatic cancer. *Gastroenterology* 138:949–957.

Zhang, Y., Li, M., Wang, H., Fisher, W.E., Lin, P.H., Yao, Q., and C. Chen. 2009. Profiling of 95 microRNAs in pancreatic cancer cell lines and surgical specimens by real-time PCR analysis. *World J Surg* 33(4):698–709.

Zhao, Y.P., Chen, G., Feng, B., Zhang, T.P., Ma, E.L-., and Y.D. Wu. 2007. Microarray analysis of gene expression profile of multidrug resistance in pancreatic cancer. *Chin Med J (Engl)* 120:1743–1752.

Zhou, L., Lu, Z., Yang, A. et al. 2007. Comparative proteomic analysis of human pancreatic juice: Methodological study. *Proteomics* 7:1345–1355.

Part IV

Lung Cancer and Mesothelioma

18

Noninvasive Early Markers in Lung Cancer

Mukesh Verma, Debmalya Barh, and Neha Jain

CONTENTS

ABSTRACT Lung cancer early markers are needed to develop strategies for prevention and treatment. A number of genetic, epigenetic, proteomic, metabolomic, and imaging biomarkers have been identified for lung cancer. Among proteomic biomarkers, GSTP1, HSPB1, and CKB showed promise because their levels increased with the progression of the disease, and these markers could be measured quantitatively with minimum amount of samples. Among epigenomic biomarkers, *PAX5alpha*, *GATA5*, and *SULF2* methylation exhibited promise in lung cancer early diagnosis when sputum samples were analyzed. A systematic evaluation of biomarkers, their strengths and weaknesses, and potential use in early detection of lung cancer is discussed in this chapter. The importance of analytical and clinical validation of biomarkers and the challenges and opportunities in this field is also discussed. The emphasis is on minimally invasive biomarkers, which could be detected easily in biological fluids and can be used for screening and early diagnostics of lung cancer, before clinical manifestation.

KEY WORDS: *biomarker, cancer, chromatin, diagnosis, early detection, epigenetics, genomic instability, histone, methylation, microRNA, prognosis, proteomics, surveillance, validation.*

18.1 Introduction

Lung cancer is one of the leading cancers in the United States with a high rate of mortality (D'Urso et al., 2013). Approximately 1 million new cases of lung cancer are diagnosed each year worldwide, resulting in more than 900,000 deaths, and approximately 220,000 new cases and 160,000 deaths occur annually in the United States (Hoque et al., 2010). Adenocarcinoma (ADC) is the most common type of lung cancer with maximum deaths in the United States and around the world (Yu et al., 2010). The need of identification and characterization of early cancer diagnostic biomarker is high because cancer is a heterogeneous disease, and patient's individual molecular profiling due to tumor microenvironment determines the disease development and response to treatment (Verma et al., 2006; Verma, 2012). Tumor microenvironment is affected by several factors including epigenetic factors of the cell. A number of noninvasive biomarkers of early detection of lung cancers have been identified. We have evaluated the current status of their implication in clinical practice and also proposed various panels for assay development.

18.2 Genomic Biomarkers

Genomic markers include single nucleotide polymorphisms (SNPs), addition and deletion mutations, recombinations, and change in copy number (Jacobson et al., 1995; Wiest et al., 1997; Oyama et al., 2005; Chorostowska-Wynimko and Szpechcinski, 2007; Li et al., 2007; Gill et al., 2008; Adams and Harvey, 2010; Ponomareva et al., 2011). Generally, lung cancer is diagnosed as a tumor micrometastasis when gene alterations such as *p53*, *KRAS*, and *p16* mutations and telomerase activity are observed in samples of sputum, peripheral blood, and bronchoalveolar lavage fluid (Osaki et al., 2001; Mitsudomi and Oyama, 2002). When a gain in copy number was evaluated in chromosome 1q32, 3q26, 5p15, and 8q24 in fine-needle aspiration samples, distinction could be made between normal and lung cancer patients (Gill et al., 2008). SNP loci occur once per approximately 1000 nucleotides in an individual, and there are approximately 3–10 million SNP loci scattered throughout the human genome (Ingelman-Sundberg, 2001; Oyama et al., 2003). Polymorphisms in *GSTP1* were observed when blood DNA was analyzed in a case–control study in a Polish population with age and sex matched 404 cases and 410 noncancer patient samples (Reszka et al., 2007). Deletion in *HYAL2* and *FHIT* was observed in sputum samples of 36 cancer patients compared to 28 healthy nonsmokers detected by in situ hybridization (Li et al., 2007). A six-gene signature mini-chip (*ENO1*, *SKP2*, *FHIT p16*, *14-3-3zeta*, and *HYAL2*) is reported to detect non-small cell lung carcinoma (NSCLC) at stage I with 93.9% specificity and 86.7% sensitivity in sputum samples (Jiang et al., 2010). Sidransky's group reported deletion of *SH3GL2* gene in NSCLC when patients' samples were analyzed by genome-wide analysis on Affymetrix 250K NSp1 array platform (Dasgupta et al., 2013). *SH3GL2* is located on chromosome 9p22 and is involved in cellular growth and invasion by modulating epidermal growth factor receptor (EGRF) function. Gene expression biomarkers in RNA-stabilized whole blood from NSCLC were reported by Zander's group (Zander et al., 2011). Initial results from one set of patients were validated successfully in another set of patients. Other groups have also

TABLE 18.1

Genomic Biomarkers of Lung Cancer

Biomarkers	Sample	Comments	References
SH3GL2	Tissue	SH3GL2 is involved in cellular growth and invasion by modulating EGRF function.	Dasgupta et al. (2013)
p53, *KRAS*, and *p16* mutations and telomerase activity	Sputum, peripheral blood, and bronchoalveolar lavage fluid	Multiple markers were followed.	Osaki et al. (2001), Mitsudomi and Oyama (2002)
Gain in copy number in chromosome 1q32, 3q26, 5p15, and 8q24	Fine-needle aspirations	Biomarker multiplexing was successful for lung cancer detection.	Gill et al. (2008)
Polymorphisms in *GSTP1*	Blood	Low-penetrance genes involved in cancer were identified.	Reszka et al. (2007)
Deletion in *HYAL2* and *FHIT*	Sputum	Diagnosis was based on in situ hybridization.	Li et al. (2007)
RNA-expression array	RNA-stabilized whole blood	Multiple markers.	Zander et al. (2011)

Note: The list of biomarkers is very long and only few biomarkers that are fairly characterized are shown in the table.

tried to analyze gene expression profiling as a biomarker for lung cancer diagnosis. A 29-gene signature is shown to detect NSCLC with 91% sensitivity and 80% specificity in peripheral blood mononuclear cell samples (Showe et al., 2009). Three small nucleolar RNA (snoRNA) genes (*SNORD33*, *SNORD66*, and *SNORD76*) are highly upregulated in NSCLC patient's plasma and can distinguish NSCLC cases from COPD and healthy individual with 81.1% sensitivity and 95.8% specificity (Liao et al., 2010). Cytological atypia in sputum can be considered as an independent risk factor in lung cancer (Fan et al., 2009), and sputum cytology-based detection of lung is reported to have 100% sensitivity for squamous cell lung cancer and 71% for other lung cancer subtypes (Lam et al., 2009). Selected genomic biomarkers of lung cancer diagnosis are presented in Table 18.1.

18.3 Epigenomic Biomarkers

18.3.1 Methylation Markers

Epigenetics is an integral part of cancer initiation, development, and recurrence (Verma, 2003; Verma et al., 2003, 2004; Jones, 2005; Kumar and Verma, 2009; Khare and Verma, 2012; Mishra and Verma, 2012). It involves alterations in promoter, histones, microRNA (miRNA) expression, and chromatin structure (sometimes called "epimutations") (Baylin and Jones, 2011; Han et al., 2012; Peltomaki, 2012). Cancer-specific methylation alterations are hallmark of different cancers (Fang et al., 2011). Alteration in methylation may cause genomic instability, genomic alterations, and change in gene expression (Jones and Baylin, 2007; Fang et al., 2011; Melichar and Kroupis, 2012). A systematic approach to determine epigenetic changes in tumor development may lead to identify biomarkers needed for cancer diagnosis. Baylin's group suggested that an integration of genome and hypermethylome might provide insight into major pathways of cancer development, which in turn might help us identify new biomarkers of cancer diagnosis and prognosis (Yi et al., 2011). Methylation and miRNA alterations are the main biomarkers, which can be assayed easily in samples noninvasively (Xing et al., 2010; Yu et al., 2010). Because of their small size and stable secondary structure, miRNAs are stable in sputum.

Hypermethylation of *RUNX-3* was useful not only in lung cancer diagnosis but also in characterizing clinical stage, lymph node metastasis, and degree of differentiation (Yu et al., 2012). In a case–control study comprised of 125 cases and 125 controls, bronchial aspirate samples were analyzed by methylation analysis (Dietrich et al., 2012). Results indicated hypermethylation of *SHOX2* with 78% sensitivity and 96% specificity. In another study, blood plasma samples from 371 cases and controls were analyzed to follow *SHOX2* methylation, and results showed a difference in the methylation patterns of cases and controls with a sensitivity of 60% and specificity of 90% (Kneip et al., 2011) (Table 18.2). In a cohort of 247 lung cancer patients, bronchial lavage was analyzed for methylation status of *adenomatous polyposis coli (APC), cyclin-dependent kinase inhibitor-2A (p16(INK4a)), retinoic acid receptor beta*, and *RAS-associated domain family protein 1* (*RASSF1*) (Schmiemann et al., 2005). A combination of *APC*, *p16(INK4a)*, and *RASSF1A* hypermethylation could distinguish normal from benign and primary lung cancer. Hypermethylation of *p16* gene in sputum can be detected 5–35 months before any cytological changes can be found in the sputum sample of lung cancer (Shames et al., 2006). Therefore, methylation status of *p16* alone can be useful in early detection and risk assessment. Belinsky's group evaluated methylation levels of 31 genes in sputum as biomarkers of lung cancer detection in a case–control study from the Colorado cohort (Leng et al., 2012). Results from this study identified 17 genes with odd ratios of 1.5–3.6. These genes were used for validation in a different set of population in the New Mexico study. Outcomes from both studies were similar, and the largest increase in case discrimination was observed for genes *PAX5alpha*, *GATA5*, and *SULF2* with odd ratios ranging from 3.2 to 4.2. This was the largest study to date where results of one population were validated in another population. In one study to follow derepression of lung cancer, brother of the regulator of imprinted sites (BORIS) binding to chromatin resulted in its opening and hypomethylation of the gene *MAGEA3* (Bhan et al., 2011). When a group of genes (*APC*, *CDH1*, *MGMT*, *DCC*, *RASSF1A*, and *AIM1*) was evaluated for their ability to detect lung cancer in serum of normal and lung cancer patients by quantitative methylation analysis, sensitivity from 35.5% to 75% and specificity from 73% to 100% were observed in a series of experiments (Begum et al., 2011).

TABLE 18.2
Epigenetic Biomarkers in Lung Cancer

Biomarkers	Sample	Comments	References
Panel of miRNAs (miR-21, miR-486, miR-375, miR-200b)	Sputum	Noninvasively collected samples from lung cancer patients	Xing et al. (2010), Yu et al. (2010)
miR-21, miR-451, miR-451, miR-485-5p	Formalin-fixed tissues	Differential expression of miRNAs in lung cancer	Solomides et al. (2012)
APC, cyclin-dependent kinase inhibitor-2A (p16(INK4a)), retinoic acid receptor beta, and *RASSF1*	Bronchial lavage	A panel of gene hypermethylation as a diagnostic tool for lung cancer	Schmiemann et al. (2005)
PAX5alpha, GATA5, and *SULF2*	Sputum	Validation of results from one population was performed in a different population	Leng et al. (2012)
RUNX-3	Blood	Useful not only in lung cancer diagnosis but to characterize clinical stage, lymph node metastasis, and degree of differentiation	Yu et al. (2012)
SHOX2	Bronchial aspirate	Lung cancer diagnosis with 78% sensitivity and 96% specificity	Dietrich et al. (2012), Schmidt et al. (2010)

In one interesting study, early lung cancer detection markers were used to evaluate cancerous and noncancerous abnormal computer tomography (CT) findings (Ostrow et al., 2010). A panel of four genes, *DCC*, *Kif1a*, *NISCH*, and *Rarb*, were chosen for the study using plasma samples; results indicated a specificity of 71%–100% based on inclusion or exclusion of the smoking history.

18.3.2 miRNA Markers

Several panels of miRNAs were reported in sputum, serum, or blood samples of lung cancer patients. miR-21, miR-486, miR-375, and miR-200b showed excellent prediction values for early lung cancer detection with 80.6% sensitivity and 91.7% specificity (Yu et al., 2010). According to Xing et al. (2010), expression level of three miRs (miR-205, miR-210, and miR-708) can detect stage I squamous cell lung carcinoma with 73% sensitivity and 96% specificity in real-time polymerase chain reaction (RT-PCR)-based assay. Similarly, expression profile of four plasma miRs (miR-21, miR-126, miR-210, and miR-486-5p) reported to detect NSCLC with 86.22% sensitivity and 96.55% specificity. Ten-serum miRNA profiling by Chen et al. (2012) is highly accurate in diagnosis and risk prediction of NSCLC.

Microarray analysis of miRNAs from formalin-fixed normal lung squamous cell carcinoma (SQCC) and ADC tissues indicated increased expression of miR-21 in both tumor types, whereas levels of miR-451 and miR-485-5p were reduced compared to other miRNAs (Solomides et al., 2012). Furthermore, SQCC showed clear distinction from normal and ADC based on higher expression of miR-205 and lower expression of miR-26b. Circulating miRNA levels were associated with survival in NSCLC (Hu et al., 2010). In this study, serum miRNA signatures were identified in a genome-wide serum miRNA profiling of patients with stages I to IIIa lung ADC and squamous carcinoma (treated with both surgery and adjuvant chemotherapies). Four specific miRNA signatures were identified that could be used to follow survival of lung cancer. A total of 303 patients were included in this analysis: 60 patients were selected for Solexa sequencing during the discovery stage, 30 patients who had survived more than 30 months during the last follow-up were classified as the longer survival group, 30 patients who had survived less than 25 months were classified as the shorter survival group, and the remaining 243 participants were classified in the training or testing group. Another group of investigators reported similar results with the additional information that histology was associated with miRNA expression (Landi et al., 2010). miRNA profile is also useful in prognosis of lung cancer. Low hsa-let-7a-2 and high hsa-mir-155 expression correlate with poor survival even in stage I lung ADCs (Yanaihara et al., 2006).

18.4 Proteomic Biomarkers

Recently, patient samples from laser-capture microdissected purified normal bronchial epithelium (NBE), squamous metaplasia (SM), atypical hyperplasia (AH), carcinoma in situ (CIS), and invasive lung cancer squamous cells (LSCC) were analyzed using iTRAQ-tagging combined with 2D liquid chromatography tandem mass spectrometry (MS) to identify differentially expressed proteomic biomarkers (Zeng et al., 2012). Out of 102 differentially expressed proteins, *GSTP1*, *HSPB1*, and *CKB* exhibited quantitative association with progression of the diseases (Table 18.3). Validation of these biomarkers was done by Western blot analysis and immunohistochemistry. In an independent set of samples of formalin-fixed tissues, these markers could be detected in lung cancer patients. Receiver operating characteristics (ROC) curves indicated a sensitivity of 96% and a specificity of 92%. Discrimination of NBE with preneoplastic lesions could be achieved in these experiments indicating that these markers could be used for early detection of cancer. Serine protease inhibitors, such as alpha-1 antitrypsin, were shown to detect lung cancer (Zelvyte et al., 2004). Biomarkers such as ectopic atrial natriuretic peptide (ANP) were used for the management of lung cancer and hyponatremia

TABLE 18.3

Proteomic Biomarkers

Biomarkers	Expressed in	Comments	References
Antithrombin protein III	Plasma	Higher levels were observed when higher platelet aggregation and vascular endothelial growth factor expression were observed in lung cancer patients	Roselli et al. (2003, 2004), Seitz et al. (1993)
AVP	Plasma	Levels increased with disease progression	Chute et al. (2006)
ANP	Plasma	To follow up management of patients with lung cancer and hyponatremia	Chute et al. (2006)
CD40 ligand	Plasma	Cytokine levels increased with higher stages of lung cancer	Roselli et al. (2004)
CHGA	Plasma	Prognostic biomarker of lung cancer	Drivsholm et al. (1999)
Colony-stimulating factor (CSF)	Plasma	Diagnostic and prognostic marker in lung cancer patients with neutrophilia	Adachi et al. (1994)
Gelatinase B	Plasma	Diagnosis marker	Farias et al. (2000)
Ghrelin	Plasma	Levels of ghrelin increased in lung cancer patients with anorexia undergoing chemotherapy	Shimizu et al. (2003)
GM-CSF	Plasma	Increased levels of GM-CSF were observed in neutrophilia patients	Adachi et al. (1994)
GSTP1, HSPB1, and CKB	Plasma	Quantitative increment of markers with progression of disease	Zeng et al. (2012)
Insulin-like growth factor B	Plasma	Biomarker for lung cancer risk	Yu et al. (1999)
Panel of markers in microarray analysis	Endobronchial ELF	Main genes in the panel were tenascin-C ligand 14, S100 calcium binding protein A9, and keratin 17	Kahn et al. (2012)
Serine proteases (alpha-1 antitrypsin)	Plasma	For cancer detection and progression	Zelvyte et al. (2004)
Autoantibody-based test	Blood	Six autoantibodies were used for detecting NSCLC in a population-based study	Wu et al. (2010)
Annexin II and MUC5AC	Blood	Early lung cancer diagnosis biomarkers	Kim et al. (2009)
MTAP, fumarate hydratase, endoplasmic reticulum protein 29	Blood	Circulating autoantibodies to detect NSCLC	

Note: The list of biomarkers is very long and only few biomarkers that are fairly characterized are shown in the table.

with no evidence of ectopic arginine vasopressin (AVP) (Chute et al., 2006). This information helped in understanding kidney metabolism associated with sodium excretion and free water clearance during the disease. In one study of factors affecting lung cancer progression, antiprothrombin complex III correlated with the progression of the disease (Roselli et al., 2003). Chromogranin A (CHGA) is a protein present in neuroendocrine vesicles and its levels in plasma increased in lung cancer. CHGA was used for disease prognosis (Drivsholm et al., 1999). Microarray analysis indicated higher levels of a group of proteins containing tenascin-C ligand 14, S100 calcium binding protein A9, and keratin 17 in endobronchial epithelial lining fluid (ELF) collected by bronchoscopic microsampling (Kahn et al., 2012). The idea of circulating tumor-specific autoantibodies stems from the popular notion that although a cancer cannot be detected by histopathological and other tests due to its early stage of development, autoantibodies produced in response to cancer-specific antigens may be detectable due to signal amplification from the humoral immune response. Serum based multi-analyte immunoassay with a panel of six proteins TNF-α, IL-1ra, MMP-2, CYFRA21.1, sE-selectin, and MCP-1 is reported to detect NSCLC with 95% specificity and 99% sensitivity by the same research group. A multiplexed tumor-associated autoantibody-based blood test was developed to detect NSCLC (Wu et al., 2010). A sensitivity of 92% and specificity of 85% were observed in a six-phage peptide autoantibody-based assays for early NSCLC diagnosis (Wu et al., 2010). Serum autoantibodies to SOX2, Hu-D, TP53, NY-ESO-1, CAGE, and GBU 4-5 have been described to detect small cell lung cancer with 99% specificity in ELISA assay (Chapman et al., 2011).

18.5 Imaging Biomarkers

Diagnosis of lung cancer is routinely conducted by different imaging technologies. Over the past decade, diagnostic imaging of lung and other cancers has improved tremendously (Mulshine et al., 2010). For example, a knowledge-based coherent anti-Stokes Raman scattering (CARS) microscopy for label-free imaging system was developed, which can distinguish nonneoplastic lung cancer cells and their subtypes with cancerous cells (Gao et al., 2011). After developing the learning system, this method was applied in clinical samples and a specificity of 91% and sensitivity of 92% was reported. Distinction of small cell carcinoma and non-small cell carcinoma was achieved with 100% sensitivity and specificity. This advancement in technology system may provide the first step needed for in vivo point-of-care diagnosis of precancerous and cancerous lung cancer lesions. Quantitative imaging and management and dissemination of data have been the topic of interest among clinicians, academicians, and societies such as Radiological Society of North America, The Optical Society, and Quantitative Imaging Biomarker Alliance in recent years. Quantitative imaging involves some key features including the following: How was the image acquired, how was that process quality controlled, what was the frequency of equipment calibration, who did the calibration, what were the controls, and how many repeats were performed? Imaging technologies such as positron emission tomography (PET) with fluorine-18-deoxyglucose (PET-FDGE) are used to evaluate metastasis of lung cancer (Ohno et al., 2007).

18.6 Mesothelioma Biomarkers

Mesothelioma is a highly aggressive tumor with poor prognosis. Pleural mesothelioma patients suffer from chest wall pain and shortness of breath due to pleural effusion, which induces fluid between lung and the chest wall. Prolonged exposure of asbestos contributes to the development of mesothelioma, a type of lung cancer that is detected very late because early detection markers are not available. It develops from transformed cells originating from mesothelium (in this case pleural mesothelium), which is a protective lining that covers many internal organs including lungs. Pleura is the outer lining of the lungs and internal chest wall. Mesothelioma and lung cancer are different in case of risk factors because smoking does not contribute to mesothelioma but lung cancer.

The incidence rate of mesothelioma is increasing rapidly. Recently, a panel of proteomic biomarkers, called SOMAmer panel, was developed, which can detect cancer with a sensitivity of 97% and specificity of 92% (Ostroff et al., 2012). Initially, serum samples from 117 mesothelioma cases and 142 asbestos-exposed control individuals were analyzed, and 64 candidate biomarkers were identified. Later on blinded validation studies were performed with different sets of samples, and a candidate panel of biomarkers consisting of both inflammatory and proliferative proteins was developed, which showed a sensitivity of 90% and specificity of 89%. A correlation of pathological stage and sensitivity indicated 77% of stage I, 93% of stage II, 96% stage III, and 96% of stage IV cases. This panel of marker can be used for diagnosis and surveillance purposes. In another study, a panel of biomarkers CEA, CD15, calretinin, and CK5/6 could distinguish between lung ADC and pleural mesothelioma (Mohammad et al., 2012). Current diagnosis of mesothelioma is by chest x-ray, CT scan, and tissue biopsies and all these procedures are considered invasive. In terms of treatment, gemcitabine is used, and one recent report indicated that polymorphism in the gene deoxycytidine kinase, ribonucleotide reductase M1 (RRM1), showed association with the efficiency of treatment (Erculj et al., 2012). Intelectin-1 is another biomarker that helped in histological-based diagnosis of mesothelioma, but its specificity is not very good (Washimi et al., 2012). Blanquart's group identified another set of biomarker panel (CCL2, galectin-3, and SMRP) for mesothelioma diagnosis (Blanquart et al., 2012). Among miRNAs, miR-625-3p seems promising for mesothelioma diagnosis in plasma samples (Kirschner et al., 2012; Tomasetti et al., 2012). Individual patient data meta-analysis of serum mesothelin indicated no added value in currently available early diagnostic biomarkers of pleural mesothelioma (Hollevoet et al., 2012).

18.7 Invasive and Noninvasive Biomarkers: Advantages and Disadvantages

Tissues are the best source of material to assay early detection cancer biomarkers because they represent true expression of biomarkers during cancer development. However, tissue collection is a noninvasive procedure and it is difficult to get healthy tissue for comparison. Therefore, such biomarkers are preferred, which can be assayed in samples collected noninvasively. Biofluids (urine, blood, sputum) and exfoliated cells are good examples of noninvasive source of biomarkers for lung cancer early diagnosis. Imaging is a good biomarker for lung cancer, but radiations may be damaging if repeated exposure is conducted. Furthermore, chest x-ray and sputum cytology for screening techniques have been ineffective in increasing patient survival (Ellis and Gleeson, 2001, 2002; Ellis et al., 2001; Marcus, 2001). In fact, spiral CT in screening lung cancer among smokers was not very beneficial in increasing mortality (Lu et al., 2004; Singhal et al., 2005). When the response of treatment is followed in a patient, samples are collected several times. In that situation, noninvasive biomarkers are the best (Begum et al., 2011). The complexity and heterogeneity of cancer progression suggest that a combination of single and small panel of biomarkers may be able to characterize cancer stages (Srivastava et al., 2001; Negm et al., 2002; Srinivas et al., 2002; Verma and Srivastava, 2003; Verma, 2004, 2012; Wagner et al., 2004; Banerjee and Verma, 2006; Verma and Manne, 2006; Verma et al., 2006; Kelloff and Sigman, 2012). A combination of low-dose spiral CT with serum biomarkers should give high sensitivity and specificity. They may also distinguish indolent and aggressive form of cancers. If study design is conducted properly, plasma samples and extracellular nucleic acids (circulating DNAs and RNAs including miRNAs) are an excellent source of material for the early diagnosis and also for prediction of antitumor treatment efficiency, posttreatment monitoring, and prognosis.

18.8 Suggested Markers for Assay Development

Based on the published literatures and our experience here, we propose sample- and assay-specific panels of markers for early diagnosis and prognosis of lung cancer. The markers have been selected based on their highest specificity and sensitivity. Table 18.4 represents these markers.

TABLE 18.4

Suggested Noninvasive Markers for Assay Development

Assay	Sample Source	Marker Panel	Sensitivity (%)	Specificity (%)	Reference
Methylation	Tissue	*LOX, BNC1, CCNA1, NRCAM,* and *SOX15*			Belinsky et al. (2007)
	Tissue, sputum, and serum	*p16, MGMT, RASSF1A, DAPK, PAX5α, PAX5β, H-Cadherin,* and *GATA5*	>60	>80	Inferred
	Sputum	*GATA5, MGMT,* and *p16*	>60	>70	Inferred
	Sputum	*SFRP1, TCF21, RARβ, FHIT,* and *GSTP1*	>60	>70	Inferred
	Serum/plasma	*BLU, CDH13, FHIT, p16, RARβ,* and *RASSF1A*	73	>72	Inferred
	Serum/plasma	*p16, MGMT, DAPK, PAX5β,* and *GATA5*	>65	>79	Inferred
	Serum/plasma	*APC, AIM1, CDH1, DCC, MGMT,* and *RASSF1A*	>60	90–100	Begum et al. (2011)
	Plasma	*KIF1A, DCC, RARβ,* and *NISCH*	73	71	Ostrow et al. (2010)
	Serum	*MGMT, p16, DAPK, CHAD, GATA5, PAX5a, ZMYND10, FHIT,* and *CDH13*	>60	73–98	Inferred
	Bronchoalveolar lavage	*SEMA3B, SOCS1,* and *PTGS2*	>60	>70	Inferred
RNA signatures	Plasma	*SNORD33, SNORD66,* and *SNORD76* for non-small cell lung carcinoma	81.1	95.8	Liao et al. (2010)
mRNA/gene expression	Sputum	*ENO1, FHIT, HYAL2, SKP2, p16,* and 14-3-3zeta for stage I NSCLC	86.7	93.9	Jiang et al. (2010)
	Peripheral blood mononuclear cells	Twenty-nine gene signature *RSF1, DYRK2, YY1, C19orf12, THEM2, TRIO, MYADM, BAIAP2, ROGDI, DNAJB14, BRE, TMEM41A, C9orf64, FAM110A, PCNXL2, REST, C19orf62, C13orf27, ASCC3, SLC1A5, PTPLAD1, MRE11A, GTPBP10, BX118737, SERPINI2, CREB1, CCDC53, USP48,* and *ZSCAN2* for non-small cell lung carcinoma	91	80	Showe et al. (2009)

18.9 Patents of Lung Cancer Biomarkers

A list of patents of lung biomarkers and assays is shown in Table 18.5. One of the patents (US 5455159) claimed that lung cancer could be detected 2 years before clinical diagnosis of the disease. Another patent described about the prediction of lung cancer based on the levels of selected biomarkers (US 2010/0179067 A1). Treatment follow-up was the focus of one patent (US 7785821). Methylation biomarkers also were patented (US 0027796 A1, US 0117551 A1). miRNAs were also potential biomarkers of cancer detection (US 0117565 A1). In another patent (US 6939675), mutational analysis was helpful in identification of a variety of cancers.

TABLE 18.5
Patents in Lung Cancer Biomarkers

Patent No.	Inventors and Assignee	Title of Patents	Filling Date	Expiry Date	Remarks
US 5455159	Melvyn et al.	Method for early detection of lung cancer	Nov. 16, 1993	Oct. 3, 2012	Sputum or bronchial fluid sample; detection of antigen markers; early diagnosis
US 6312390	Michael Phillips (NJ)	Breath test for detection of lung cancer	Oct. 1, 1999	Oct. 16, 2017	Alveolar breath sample; measuring the presence of volatile organic markers heptane, 2,2,4,6,6-pentamethyl; heptane, 2-methyl; cyclopentane, methyl; octane, 3-methyl; nonane, 3-methyl; and heptane, 2,4-dimethyl; detection of probable presence of lung cancer
US 7214485	Belinsky et al. Lovelace Respiratory Research Institute, Albuquerque, NM (United States)	Nested methylation-specific PCR cancer detection method	Aug. 24, 2001	Aug. 24, 2021	Tissue plasma, ejaculate, cerebrospinal fluid, serum, mammary duct fluid, urine, fecal stool, and sputum samples; nested PCR-based promoter methylation assay for p16, MGMT, RASSF1A, CDH13, RARB, and FHIT genes; screening for the detection
US 2010/ 0179067	Patz et al.	Serum biomarkers for the early detection of lung cancer	May 19, 2008		Serum sample; panel of salpha-1-antitrypsin, carcinoembryonic antigen, SQCC antigen, retinol binding protein, transferrin, and haptoglobin; probability of lung cancer
US 7785821	Wolfgang et al. Roche Diagnostics Operations Inc., Indianapolis, IN (United States)	Measurement of nicotinamide N-methyl transferase in diagnosis of lung cancer	Jan. 30, 2009	Jul. 30, 2027	Whole blood, serum, plasma, bronchial lavage, and sputum samples; measuring the level of NNMT in addition with CYFRA 21-1, CEA, NSF, and SCC; early detection
US 2011/ 0053156 A1	Vander-Borght et al.	Small cell lung carcinoma biomarker panel	Feb. 19, 2009		Blood, serum, plasma, urine, saliva, semen, breast exudates, cerebrospinal fluid, tears, sputum, mucous, lymph, pleural effusions, tumor tissue, and bronchoalveolar lavage samples
	Mubio Products BV, Maastricht (NL)				Expression of NCAM 180, CK4, CK5, CK6, CK7, CK8, CK10, CK13, CK14, CK15, CK16, CK17, CK18, CK19, CK20, NSP, SYPH, CHGA, RTN1, and HSP47 proteins; detection, diagnosis, subtyping, and staging

(continued)

TABLE 18.5 (continued)
Patents in Lung Cancer Biomarkers

Patent No.	Inventors and Assignee	Title of Patents	Filling Date	Expiry Date	Remarks
US 2011/ 0117551 A1	Van Criekinge et al. OncoMethylome Sciences SA (BE) and Johns Hopkins University (United States)	Detection and prognosis of lung cancer	Feb. 19, 2009		Biopsy, sputum, pleural fluid, bronchoalveolar lavage samples; hypermethylation of ACSL6, ALS2CL, APC2, ART-S1, BEX1, BMP7, BNIP3, CBR3, CD248, CD44, CHD5, DLK1, DPYSL4, DSC2, EDNRB, EPB41L3, EPHB6, ERBB3, FBLN2, FBN2, FOXL2, GNAS, GSTP1, HS3ST2, HPN, IGFBP7, IRF7, JAM3, LOX, LY6D, LY6K, MACF1, MCAM, NCBP1, NEFH, NID2, PCDHB15, PCDHGA12, PFKP, PGRMC1, PHACTR3, PHKA2, POMC, PRKCA, PSEN1, RASSF1A, RASSF2, RBP1, RRAD, SFRP1, SGK, SOD3, SOX17, SULF2, TIMP3, TJP2, TRPV2, UCHL1, WDR69, ZFP42, ZNF442, and ZNF655; early detection and prediction
US 2011/ 0097756 A1	Marie-Luise et al.	APEX as a marker for lung cancer	Sep. 10, 2009		Body fluid samples; in vitro assessment of concentration of APEX along with CYFRA 21-1, CEA, NSE, proGRP, and SCC; diagnosis
US 2011/ 0117565 A1	Zhang et al. Micromedmark Biotech Co., Ltd., Beijing (China)	Serum or plasma miRNA as biomarkers for non-small cell lung carcinoma	Dec. 14, 2009		Serum or plasma sample; expression of a panel of 26 miRNA; detection, diagnosis, and prognosis of non-small cell lung carcinoma
US 2011/ 0053158 A1	Mambo et al. Asuragen, Inc., Austin TX (United States)	miRNA biomarkers of lung disease	Aug. 27, 2010		Serum sample; alone or in combination with miRs expression; early detection, diagnosis, and prognosis

18.10 Treatment Strategies

Since the major factor in the high mortality of lung cancer is the presence of metastatic tumors in approximately two-thirds of patients and no curative therapies exist for metastasis, individualized therapy is needed to intervene lung cancer, which requires precise molecular information. In one study, a panel of biomarkers in ELF collected by bronchoscopic microsampling (BMS) was useful in preoperative diagnosis of malignant pulmonary nodules (Kahn et al., 2012). In another study, integration of genetic and epigenetic biomarkers was achieved where mutations and methylation profiling of *EGFR*, *RASSF1A*, and *BRAF* were evaluated in order to find out whether targeted therapy would be benefited from this information in NSCLC (Hoque et al., 2010). The mutation status of *KRAS* and *p53* was already known in samples (primary NSCLC, ADC, and SQCC) in this study. Results indicated genetic and epigenetic alterations in the erbB pathway in 80% ADC and 50% primary ADC. The epidermal growth factor receptor (ERBB) pathway was selected for these studies because it involved tyrosine kinases, which contributed to resistance to radiation and chemotherapy in different tumor types including lung tumors (Chakravarti et al., 2002). Therapeutic investigations are ongoing in future studies by these investigators. Imaging technologies are used in lung cancer diagnosis as well as follow-up of treatment.

18.11 Concluding Remarks and Perspective

Lung cancer is the world's most lethal cancer and has attracted pharmaceutical industry, clinicians, and academicians. Lung cancer early detection by noninvasive methods aims at achieving efficient intervention and subsequent reduction in death rate due to this disease. Plasma and serum are the best sources of biomarkers as they are collected noninvasively. However, for microarray analysis, ELF was collected by BMS and the procedure was found equally effective. Sputum was used to determine miRNA profiling for early detection of lung cancer successfully. Results discussed earlier indicate that there are potential biomarkers that can be collected from a variety of biospecimens noninvasively, and assays have been developed, which have reasonable sensitivity and specificity to detect lung cancer. The main areas that need progress/attention are the cost and high throughput. Another area where adequate progress has not been made is the application of lung cancer biomarkers in clinic. Proper analytical and clinical validation of early markers has not been achieved. Clinical validation of identified biomarkers is especially the key challenge in the field. The National Cancer Institute has developed guidelines for the analytical and clinical validation of biomarkers, but none of the biomarkers has been validated to date (Srivastava et al., 2001; Srinivas et al., 2002; Verma and Srivastava, 2003; Verma et al., 2006; Srivastava, 2007; Verma, 2012). Integration of genomic and proteomic markers with epigenetic markers may help us subtyping different cancers and cancer stages (Yi et al., 2011; Kelloff and Sigman, 2012). Many times results of methylation profiling from blood and tissues are different. Koestler et al. conducted a systematic epigenome-wide methylation analysis and demonstrated that shifts in leukocyte subpopulations might account for a considerable proportion of variability in these patterns (Koestler et al., 2012). Multiplexing of biomarkers may reduce false-positive results in screening studies where intention is to identify populations that are at high risk of developing lung cancer. Quantitative imaging data storage and maintenance have their own challenges as I discussed previously.

After identifying lung cancer biomarkers, the assay and the biomarker have to be approved by the Food and Drug Administration (FDA) so that these biomarkers can be assayed in clinical samples. FDA has provided guidelines in this direction. If biomarkers, assays, or devices are planned for clinical use in patient samples, they should be reviewed by the FDA's Center for Devices and Radiological Health (CDRH) for their ability to analytically measure the biomarker. Biomarkers and devices for quantification are expected to yield equivalent results. Biomarkers should have passed analytical and clinical validation tests specified by the FDA. Analytical validity in this context is defined as the ability of an assay to accurately and reliably measure the analyte in the laboratory as well as in the clinical sample. Clinical validation requires the detection or prediction of the associated disease (cancer) in specimens from targeted patient. Biomarker qualification by FDA enables collaboration among stakeholders, reduces cost for individual stakeholders, and provides biomarkers that are useful for general public and private parties.

Epigenomic biomarkers have enormous potential of clinical implication in cancer diagnosis and prognosis. Because of the availability of genome-wide methylation, histone, and miRNA analysis technologies, and our rapidly accumulating knowledge regarding epigenome, the translation of findings discussed in this chapter may be possible in the near future. Epigenetic biomarkers may also help in identifying patients who will benefit from the therapy and will not develop resistance to drugs. Recently developed drugs for cancer treatment are based on specific pathways and may be useful for those individuals where those pathways are altered. This approach can be designed for personalized medicine and precision medicine. Epigenetic biomarkers may help in such approaches. All potential lung cancer biomarkers have by no means been exhausted, and it is expected that additional high penetrance markers will be identified.

Based on the information provided previously, I am sure that we have made progress in early lung cancer diagnosis using different biomarkers. After we met the challenges of clinical validation of these biomarkers, precise intervention and therapeutic approaches can be developed.

Acknowledgment

We are thankful to Joanne Brodsky of the Scientific Consulted Group (SCG), Inc., for reading the manuscript and providing their suggestions.

References

Adachi N, Yamaguchi K, Morikawa T, Suzuki M, Matsuda I, Abe MK. Constitutive production of multiple colony-stimulating factors in patients with lung cancer associated with neutrophilia. *British Journal of Cancer* 1994;69:125–129.

Adams VR, Harvey RD. Histological and genetic markers for non-small-cell lung cancer: Customizing treatment based on individual tumor biology. *American Journal of Health-System Pharmacy* 2010;67:S3–S9, quiz S15–S16.

Anglim PP, Alonzo TA, Laird-Offringa IA. DNA methylation-based biomarkers for early detection of non-small cell lung cancer: An update. *Molecular Cancer* 2008 Oct 23;7:81. doi: 10.1186/1476-4598-7-81.

Banerjee HN, Verma M. Use of nanotechnology for the development of novel cancer biomarkers. *Expert Review of Molecular Diagnostics* 2006;6:679–683.

Baylin SB, Jones PA. A decade of exploring the cancer epigenome—Biological and translational implications. *Nature Reviews Cancer* 2011;11:726–734.

Begum S, Brait M, Dasgupta S, Ostrow KL, Zahurak M, Carvalho AL et al. An epigenetic marker panel for detection of lung cancer using cell-free serum DNA. *Clinical Cancer Research* 2011;17:4494–4503. doi: 10.1158/1078-0432.CCR-10-3436. Epub 2011 May 24.

Belinsky SA, Grimes MJ, Casas E, Stidley CA, Franklin WA, Bocklage TJ, Johnson DH, Schiller JH. Predicting gene promoter methylation in non-small-cell lung cancer by evaluating sputum and serum. *British Journal of Cancer* 2007 Apr 23;96(8):1278–1283. Epub 2007 Apr 3.

Belinsky SA, Klinge DM, Dekker JD, Smith MW et al. Gene promoter methylation in plasma and sputum increases with lung cancer risk. *Clinical Cancer Research* 2005 Sep 15;11(18):6505–6511.

Bhan S, Negi SS, Shao C, Glazer CA, Chuang A, Gaykalova DA et al. BORIS binding to the promoters of cancer testis antigens, MAGEA2, MAGEA3, and MAGEA4, is associated with their transcriptional activation in lung cancer. *Clinical Cancer Research* 2011;17:4267–4276.

Blanquart C, Gueugnon F, Nguyen JM, Roulois D, Cellerin L, Sagan C et al. CCL2, galectin-3, and SMRP combination improves the diagnosis of mesothelioma in pleural effusions. *Journal of Thoracic Oncology* 2012;7:883–889.

Chakravarti A, Chakladar A, Delaney MA, Latham DE, Loeffler JS. The epidermal growth factor receptor pathway mediates resistance to sequential administration of radiation and chemotherapy in primary human glioblastoma cells in a RAS-dependent manner. *Cancer Research* 2002;62:4307–4315.

Chapman CJ, Thorpe AJ, Murray A, Parsy-Kowalska CB et al. Immunobiomarkers in small cell lung cancer: Potential early cancer signals. *Clinical Cancer Research* 2011 Mar 15;17(6):1474–1480.

Chen X, Hu Z, Wang W, Ba Y, Ma L, Zhang C et al. Identification of ten serum microRNAs from a genome-wide serum microRNA expression profile as novel noninvasive biomarkers for nonsmall cell lung cancer diagnosis. *International Journal of Cancer* 2012 Apr 1;130(7):1620–1628.

Chorostowska-Wynimko J, Szpechcinski A. The impact of genetic markers on the diagnosis of lung cancer: A current perspective. *Journal of Thoracic Oncology* 2007;2:1044–1051.

Chute JP, Taylor E, Williams J, Kaye F, Venzon D, Johnson BE. A metabolic study of patients with lung cancer and hyponatremia of malignancy. *Clinical Cancer Research* 2006;12:888–896.

Dasgupta S, Jang JS, Shao C, Mukhopadhyay ND, Sokhi UK, Das SK et al. SH3GL2 is frequently deleted in non-small cell lung cancer and downregulates tumor growth by modulating EGFR signaling. *Journal of Molecular Medicine (Berlin, Germany)* 2013 Mar;91(3):381–393. doi: 10.1007/s00109-012-0955-3. Epub 2012 Sep 12.

Dietrich D, Kneip C, Raji O, Liloglou T, Seegebarth A, Schlegel T et al. Performance evaluation of the DNA methylation biomarker SHOX2 for the aid in diagnosis of lung cancer based on the analysis of bronchial aspirates. *International Journal of Oncology* 2012;40:825–832.

Drivsholm L, Paloheimo LI, Osterlind K. Chromogranin A, a significant prognostic factor in small cell lung cancer. *British Journal of Cancer* 1999;81:667–671.

D'Urso V, Doneddu V, Marchesi I, Collodoro A, Pirina P, Giordano A et al. Sputum analysis: Non-invasive early lung cancer detection. *Journal of Cellular Physiology* 2013 May;228(5):945–951. doi: 10.1002/jcp.24263.

Ellis JR, Gleeson FV. Lung cancer screening. *The British Journal of Radiology* 2001;74:478–485.

Ellis JR, Gleeson FV. New concepts in lung cancer screening. *Current Opinion in Pulmonary Medicine* 2002;8:270–274.

Ellis SM, Husband JE, Armstrong P, Hansell DM. Computed tomography screening for lung cancer: Back to basics. *Clinical Radiology* 2001;56:691–699.

Erculj N, Kovac V, Hmeljak J, Franko A, Dodic-Fikfak M, Dolzan V. The influence of gemcitabine pathway polymorphisms on treatment outcome in patients with malignant mesothelioma. *Pharmacogenetics and Genomics* 2012;22:58–68.

Esteller M, Sanchez-Cespedes M, Rosell R, Sidransky D, Baylin SB, Herman JG. Detection of aberrant promoter hypermethylation of tumor suppressor genes in serum DNA from non-small cell lung cancer patients. *Cancer Research* 1999 Jan 1;59(1):67–70.

Fan YG, Hu P, Jiang Y, Chang RS, Yao SX, Wang W et al. Association between sputum atypia and lung cancer risk in an occupational cohort in Yunnan, China. *Chest* 2009;135:778–785.

Fang F, Turcan S, Rimner A, Kaufman A, Giri D, Morris LG et al. Breast cancer methylomes establish an epigenomic foundation for metastasis. *Science Translational Medicine* 2011;3:75ra25.

Farias E, Ranuncolo S, Cresta C, Specterman S, Armanasco E, Varela M et al. Plasma metalloproteinase activity is enhanced in the euglobulin fraction of breast and lung cancer patients. *International Journal of Cancer* 2000;89:389–394.

Gao L, Li F, Thrall MJ, Yang Y, Xing J, Hammoudi AA et al. On-the-spot lung cancer differential diagnosis by label-free, molecular vibrational imaging and knowledge-based classification. *Journal of Biomedical Optics* 2011;16:096004.

Gill RK, Vazquez MF, Kramer A, Hames M, Zhang L, Heselmeyer-Haddad K et al. The use of genetic markers to identify lung cancer in fine needle aspiration samples. *Clinical Cancer Research* 2008;14:7481–7487.

Han H, Wolff EM, Liang G. Epigenetic alterations in bladder cancer and their potential clinical implications. *Advances in Urology* 2012;2012:546917.

Hollevoet K, Reitsma JB, Creaney J, Grigoriu BD, Robinson BW, Scherpereel A et al. Serum mesothelin for diagnosing malignant pleural mesothelioma: An individual patient data meta-analysis. *Journal of Clinical Oncology* 2012;30:1541–1549.

Hoque MO, Brait M, Rosenbaum E, Poeta ML, Pal P, Begum S et al. Genetic and epigenetic analysis of erbB signaling pathway genes in lung cancer. *Journal of Thoracic Oncology* 2010;5:1887–1893.

Hsu HS, Chen TP, Hung CH, Wen CK, Lin RK, Lee HC, Wang YC. Characterization of a multiple epigenetic marker panel for lung cancer detection and risk assessment in plasma. *Cancer* 2007 Nov 1;110(9):2019–2026.

Hu Z, Chen X, Zhao Y, Tian T, Jin G, Shu Y et al. Serum microRNA signatures identified in a genome-wide serum microRNA expression profiling predict survival of non-small-cell lung cancer. *Journal of Clinical Oncology* 2010;28:1721–1726.

Ingelman-Sundberg M. Genetic susceptibility to adverse effects of drugs and environmental toxicants. The role of the CYP family of enzymes. *Mutation Research* 2001;482:11–19.

Jacobson DR, Fishman CL, Mills NE. Molecular genetic tumor markers in the early diagnosis and screening of non-small-cell lung cancer. *Annals of Oncology* 1995;6(Suppl 3):S3–S8.

Jiang F, Todd NW, Li R, Zhang H, Fang H, Stass SA. A panel of sputum-based genomic marker for early detection of lung cancer. *Cancer Prevention Research (Philadelphia, PA)* 2010; 3(12):1571–1578.

Jones PA. Overview of cancer epigenetics. *Seminars in Hematology* 2005;42:S3–S8.

Jones PA, Baylin SB. The epigenomics of cancer. *Cell* 2007;128:683–692.

Kahn N, Meister M, Eberhardt R, Muley T, Schnabel PA, Bender C et al. Early detection of lung cancer by molecular markers in endobronchial epithelial-lining fluid. *Journal of Thoracic Oncology* 2012;7:1001–1008.

Kelloff GJ, Sigman CC. Cancer biomarkers: Selecting the right drug for the right patient. *Nature Reviews Drug Discovery* 2012;11:201–214.

Khare S, Verma M. Epigenetics of colon cancer. *Methods in Molecular Biology (Clifton, NJ)* 2012;863:177–185.

Kim DM, Noh HB, Park DS, Ryu SH, Koo JS, Shim YB. Immunosensors for detection of Annexin II and MUC5AC for early diagnosis of lung cancer. *Biosensors & Bioelectronics* 2009;25:456–462.

Kirschner MB, Cheng YY, Badrian B, Kao SC, Creaney J, Edelman JJ et al. Increased circulating miR-625-3p: A potential biomarker for patients with malignant pleural mesothelioma. *Journal of Thoracic Oncology* 2012;7:1184–1191.

Kneip C, Schmidt B, Seegebarth A, Weickmann S, Fleischhacker M, Liebenberg V et al. SHOX2 DNA methylation is a biomarker for the diagnosis of lung cancer in plasma. *Journal of Thoracic Oncology* 2011;6:1632–1638.

Koestler DC, Marsit CJ, Christensen BC, Accomando W, Langevin SM, Houseman EA et al. Peripheral blood immune cell methylation profiles are associated with nonhematopoietic cancers. *Cancer Epidemiology, Biomarkers & Prevention* 2012;21:1293–1302.

Kumar D, Verma M. Methods in cancer epigenetics and epidemiology. *Methods in Molecular Biology (Clifton, NJ)* 2009;471:273–288.

Lam B, Lam SY, Wong MP, Ooi CG, Fong DY, Lam DC et al. Sputum cytology examination followed by autofluorescence bronchoscopy: A practical way of identifying early stage lung cancer in central airway. *Lung Cancer* 2009;64:289–294.

Landi MT, Zhao Y, Rotunno M, Koshiol J, Liu H, Bergen AW et al. MicroRNA expression differentiates histology and predicts survival of lung cancer. *Clinical Cancer Research* 2010;16:430–441.

Leng S, Do K, Yingling CM, Picchi MA, Wolf HJ, Kennedy TC et al. Defining a gene promoter methylation signature in sputum for lung cancer risk assessment. *Clinical Cancer Research* 2012;18:3387–3395.

Li R, Todd NW, Qiu Q, Fan T, Zhao RY, Rodgers WH et al. Genetic deletions in sputum as diagnostic markers for early detection of stage I non-small cell lung cancer. *Clinical Cancer Research* 2007;13:482–487.

Liao J, Yu L, Mei Y, Guarnera M, Shen J, Li R, Liu Z, Jiang F. Small nucleolar RNA signatures as biomarkers for non-small-cell lung cancer. *Molecular Cancer* 2010 Jul 27;9:198.

Liu Y, An Q, Li L, Zhang D, Huang J, Feng X, Cheng S, Gao Y. Hypermethylation of p16INK4a in Chinese lung cancer patients: Biological and clinical implications. *Carcinogenesis* 2003 Dec;24(12):1897–1901. Epub 2003 Sep 11.

Lu C, Soria JC, Tang X, Xu XC, Wang L, Mao L et al. Prognostic factors in resected stage I non-small-cell lung cancer: A multivariate analysis of six molecular markers. *Journal of Clinical Oncology* 2004;22:4575–4583.

Marcus PM. Lung cancer screening: An update. *Journal of Clinical Oncology* 2001;19:83S–86S.

Melichar B, Kroupis C. Cancer epigenomics: Moving slowly, but at a steady pace from laboratory bench to clinical practice. *Clinical Chemistry and Laboratory Medicine* 2012;50:1699–1701.

Mishra A, Verma M. Epigenetics of solid cancer stem cells. *Methods in Molecular Biology (Clifton, NJ)* 2012;863:15–31.

Mitsudomi T, Oyama T. [Molecular diagnosis in lung cancer]. *Nihon Rinsho Japanese Journal of Clinical Medicine* 2002;60(Suppl. 5):233–237.

Mohammad T, Garratt J, Torlakovic E, Gilks B, Churg A. Utility of a CEA, CD15, calretinin, and CK5/6 panel for distinguishing between mesotheliomas and pulmonary adenocarcinomas in clinical practice. *The American Journal of Surgical Pathology* 2012;36:1503–1508.

Mulshine JL, Baer TM, Avila RS. Introduction: Imaging in diagnosis and treatment of lung cancer. *Optics Express* 2010;18:15242–15243.

Negm RS, Verma M, Srivastava S. The promise of biomarkers in cancer screening and detection. *Trends in Molecular Medicine* 2002;8:288–293.

Ohno Y, Koyama H, Nogami M, Takenaka D, Yoshikawa T, Yoshimura M et al. Whole-body MR imaging vs. FDG-PET: Comparison of accuracy of M-stage diagnosis for lung cancer patients. *Journal of Magnetic Resonance Imaging* 2007;26:498–509.

Osaki T, Oyama T, Inoue M, Gu CD, Kodate M, Aikawa M et al. Molecular biological markers and micrometastasis in resected non-small-cell lung cancer. Prognostic implications. *The Japanese Journal of Thoracic and Cardiovascular Surgery* 2001;49:545–551.

Ostroff RM, Mehan MR, Stewart A, Ayers D, Brody EN, Williams SA et al. Early detection of malignant pleural mesothelioma in asbestos-exposed individuals with a noninvasive proteomics-based surveillance tool. *PLoS One* 2012;7:e46091.

Ostrow KL, Hoque MO, Loyo M, Brait M, Greenberg A, Siegfried JM et al. Molecular analysis of plasma DNA for the early detection of lung cancer by quantitative methylation-specific PCR. *Clinical Cancer Research* 2010;16:3463–3472.

Oyama T, Matsumoto A, Isse T, Kim YD, Ozaki S, Osaki T et al. Evidence-based prevention (EBP): Approach to lung cancer prevention based on cytochrome 1A1 and cytochrome 2E1 polymorphism. *Anticancer Research* 2003;23:1731–1737.

Oyama T, Osaki T, Baba T, Nagata Y, Mizukami M, So T et al. Molecular genetic tumor markers in non-small cell lung cancer. *Anticancer Research* 2005;25:1193–1196.

Peltomaki P. Mutations and epimutations in the origin of cancer. *Experimental Cell Research* 2012;318:299–310.

Ponomareva AA, Rykova E, Cherdyntseva NV, Choinzonov EL, Laktionov PP, Vlasov VV. [Molecular-genetic markers in lung cancer diagnostics]. *Molekuliarnaia biologiia* 2011;45:203–217.

Reszka E, Wasowicz W, Gromadzinska J. Antioxidant defense markers modulated by glutathione S-transferase genetic polymorphism: Results of lung cancer case-control study. *Genes & Nutrition* 2007;2:287–294.

Roselli M, Mineo TC, Basili S, Mariotti S, Martini F, Bellotti A et al. Vascular endothelial growth factor (VEGF-A) plasma levels in non-small cell lung cancer: Relationship with coagulation and platelet activation markers. *Thrombosis and Haemostasis* 2003;89:177–184.

Roselli M, Mineo TC, Basili S, Martini F, Mariotti S, Aloe S et al. Soluble CD40 ligand plasma levels in lung cancer. *Clinical Cancer Research* 2004;10:610–614.

Schmidt B, Liebenberg V, Dietrich D, Schlegel T, Kneip C, Seegebarth A et al. SHOX2 DNA methylation is a biomarker for the diagnosis of lung cancer based on bronchial aspirates. *BMC Cancer* 2010;10:600.

Schmiemann V, Bocking A, Kazimirek M, Onofre AS, Gabbert HE, Kappes R et al. Methylation assay for the diagnosis of lung cancer on bronchial aspirates: A cohort study. *Clinical Cancer Research* 2005;11:7728–7734.

Seitz R, Rappe N, Kraus M, Immel A, Wolf M, Maasberg M et al. Activation of coagulation and fibrinolysis in patients with lung cancer: Relation to tumour stage and prognosis. *Blood Coagulation & Fibrinolysis* 1993;4:249–254.

Shames DS, Girard L, Gao B, Sato M, Lewis CM, Shivapurkar N et al. A genome-wide screen for promoter methylation in lung cancer identifies novel methylation markers for multiple malignancies. *PLoS Medicine* 2006 Dec;3(12):e486.

Shimizu Y, Nagaya N, Isobe T, Imazu M, Okumura H, Hosoda H et al. Increased plasma ghrelin level in lung cancer cachexia. *Clinical Cancer Research* 2003;9:774–778.

Showe MK, Vachani A, Kossenkov AV, Yousef M, Nichols C, Nikonova EV et al. Gene expression profiles in peripheral blood mononuclear cells can distinguish patients with non-small cell lung cancer from patients with nonmalignant lung disease. *Cancer Research* 2009;69:9202–9210.

Singhal S, Vachani A, Antin-Ozerkis D, Kaiser LR, Albelda SM. Prognostic implications of cell cycle, apoptosis, and angiogenesis biomarkers in non-small cell lung cancer: A review. *Clinical Cancer Research* 2005;11:3974–3986.

Solomides CC, Evans BJ, Navenot JM, Vadigepalli R, Peiper SC, Wang ZX. MicroRNA profiling in lung cancer reveals new molecular markers for diagnosis. *Acta Cytologica* 2012;56:645–654.

Srinivas PR, Verma M, Zhao Y, Srivastava S. Proteomics for cancer biomarker discovery. *Clinical Chemistry* 2002;48:1160–1169.

Srivastava S. Cancer biomarker discovery and development in gastrointestinal cancers: Early detection research network—A collaborative approach. *Gastrointestinal Cancer Research* 2007;1:S60–S63.

Srivastava S, Verma M, Henson DE. Biomarkers for early detection of colon cancer. *Clinical Cancer Research* 2001;7:1118–1126.

Tomasetti M, Staffolani S, Nocchi L, Neuzil J, Strafella E, Manzella N et al. Clinical significance of circulating miR-126 quantification in malignant mesothelioma patients. *Clinical Biochemistry* 2012;45:575–581.

Ulivi P, Zoli W, Calistri D, Fabbri F, Tesei A, Rosetti M, Mengozzi M, Amadori D. p16INK4A and CDH13 hypermethylation in tumor and serum of non-small cell lung cancer patients. *Journal of Cellular Physiology* 2006 Mar;206(3):611–615.

Usadel H, Brabender J, Danenberg KD, Jerónimo C, Harden S, Engles J, Danenberg PV, Yang S, Sidransky D. Quantitative adenomatous polyposis coli promoter methylation analysis in tumor tissue, serum, and plasma DNA of patients with lung cancer. *Cancer Research* 2002 Jan 15;62(2):371–375.

Verma M. Viral genes and methylation. *Annals of the New York Academy of Sciences* 2003;983:170–180.

Verma M. Biomarkers for risk assessment in molecular epidemiology of cancer. *Technology in Cancer Research & Treatment* 2004;3:505–514.

Verma M. Epigenetic biomarkers in cancer epidemiology. *Methods in Molecular Biology (Clifton, NJ)* 2012;863:467–480.

Verma M, Dunn BK, Ross S, Jain P, Wang W, Hayes R et al. Early detection and risk assessment: Proceedings and recommendations from the Workshop on Epigenetics in Cancer Prevention. *Annals of the New York Academy of Sciences* 2003;983:298–319.

Verma M, Manne U. Genetic and epigenetic biomarkers in cancer diagnosis and identifying high risk populations. *Critical Reviews in Oncology/Hematology* 2006;60:9–18.

Verma M, Maruvada P, Srivastava S. Epigenetics and cancer. *Critical Reviews in Clinical Laboratory Sciences* 2004;41:585–607.

Verma M, Seminara D, Arena FJ, John C, Iwamoto K, Hartmuller V. Genetic and epigenetic biomarkers in cancer: Improving diagnosis, risk assessment, and disease stratification. *Molecular Diagnosis & Therapy* 2006;10:1–15.

Verma M, Srivastava S. New cancer biomarkers deriving from NCI early detection research. *Recent Results in Cancer Research* 2003;163:72–84; discussion 264–266.

Wagner PD, Verma M, Srivastava S. Challenges for biomarkers in cancer detection. *Annals of the New York Academy of Sciences* 2004;1022:9–16.

Washimi K, Yokose T, Yamashita M, Kageyama T, Suzuki K, Yoshihara M et al. Specific expression of human intelectin-1 in malignant pleural mesothelioma and gastrointestinal goblet cells. *PLoS One* 2012;7:e39889.

Wiest JS, Franklin WA, Drabkin H, Gemmill R, Sidransky D, Anderson MW. Genetic markers for early detection of lung cancer and outcome measures for response to chemoprevention. *Journal of Cellular Biochemistry Supplement* 1997;28–29:64–73.

Wu L, Chang W, Zhao J, Yu Y, Tan X, Su T et al. Development of autoantibody signatures as novel diagnostic biomarkers of non-small cell lung cancer. *Clinical Cancer Research* 2010;16:3760–3768.

Xing L, Todd NW, Yu L, Fang H, Jiang F. Early detection of squamous cell lung cancer in sputum by a panel of microRNA markers. *Modern Pathology* 2010;23:1157–1164.

Yanaihara N, Caplen N, Bowman E, Seike M, Kumamoto K, Yi M et al. Unique microRNA molecular profiles in lung cancer diagnosis and prognosis. *Cancer Cell* 2006 Mar;9(3):189–198.

Yi JM, Dhir M, Van Neste L, Downing SR, Jeschke J, Glockner SC et al. Genomic and epigenomic integration identifies a prognostic signature in colon cancer. *Clinical Cancer Research* 2011;17:1535–1545.

Yu GP, Ji Y, Chen GQ, Huang B, Shen K, Wu S et al. Application of RUNX3 gene promoter methylation in the diagnosis of non-small cell lung cancer. *Oncology Letters* 2012;3:159–162.

Yu H, Spitz MR, Mistry J, Gu J, Hong WK, Wu X. Plasma levels of insulin-like growth factor-I and lung cancer risk: A case-control analysis. *Journal of the National Cancer Institute* 1999;91:151–156.

Yu L, Todd NW, Xing L, Xie Y, Zhang H, Liu Z et al. Early detection of lung adenocarcinoma in sputum by a panel of microRNA markers. *International Journal of Cancer* 2010;127:2870–2878.

Zander T, Hofmann A, Staratschek-Jox A, Classen S, Debey-Pascher S, Maisel D et al. Blood-based gene expression signatures in non-small cell lung cancer. *Clinical Cancer Research* 2011;17:3360–3367.

Zelvyte I, Wallmark A, Piitulainen E, Westin U, Janciauskiene S. Increased plasma levels of serine proteinase inhibitors in lung cancer patients. *Anticancer Research* 2004;24:241–247.

Zeng GQ, Zhang PF, Deng X, Yu FL, Li C, Xu Y et al. Identification of candidate biomarkers for early detection of human lung squamous cell cancer by quantitative proteomics. *Molecular & Cellular Proteomics* 2012;11:M111 013946.

19

Exhaled Volatile Organic Compounds as Noninvasive Early Molecular Markers in Lung Cancer: Bridging the Gap from Bench to Bedside

Meggie Hakim, Ulrike Tisch, Michael Unger, and Hossam Haick

CONTENTS

ABSTRACT Lung cancer (LC) remains one of the deadliest cancers worldwide, with a 5-year survival rate as low as 13%. Reliable and cost-effective LC markers are urgently needed for early LC diagnosis through population-based screening. Certain volatile organic compounds (VOCs) (alkanes, alkenes, alcohols, aldehydes, ketones, and their collective patterns) in exhaled breath are interesting candidates as LC markers for malignancy, staging, histology, genotype, and distinction from other malignant and benign disease. VOC LC markers can be derived either as LC-specific compounds by analytical chemistry or as collective breath prints by statistical treatment of the output of sensor arrays. Direct breath printing using sensor arrays is better suited for clinical applications than chemical analysis of the breath VOCs.

However, breath VOCs that could serve as LC markers have not yet left the realm of research and entered clinical practice, despite intensive research for over three decades. This is mainly due to lack of standardization of the experimental techniques. In this chapter, we will outline the vast potential of exhaled VOCs as a novel class of molecular LC markers and describe the challenges on the way from bench to bedside. A didactic approach is provided to the state-of-the-art experimental techniques for breath collection, sample storage, analysis of the breath VOCs, and direct sensor-based breath printing. Selected pilot studies are presented as representative examples that have demonstrated the feasibility of exhaled VOCs as future noninvasive markers for diagnosing LC, identifying LC phenotypes, and monitoring treatment response.

19.1 Introduction

19.1.1 Lung Cancer

Lung cancer (LC) is the leading cause of cancer mortality in both women and men, with approximately 1.4 million fatalities worldwide per year (Jemal et al., 2011). Most LCs are carcinomas originating from epithelial cells. Lung carcinomas are classified, according to their histology, either as small cell lung carcinoma (SCLC) (ca. 15% of all LCs), adenocarcinoma (ADCA), squamous cell carcinoma (SqCC), or large cell carcinoma. Prognosis and management of the latter three histological types (together ca. 80% of all LCs) are often similar, so that they are usually grouped together as non-small cell lung carcinoma (NSCLC). SCLC and squamous cell carcinoma are most strongly linked with smoking, and ADCA is the most common type of LC in patients who have never smoked (Culter, 2008, Jemal et al., 2010).

The evaluation of a patient's prognosis and treatment options requires confirmation of lung malignancy; determination of its stage according to the tumor size, node, and metastasis (TNM) classification; and identification of the tumor's histology (Detterbeck et al., 2009). The 5-year survival rate of LC is only 13%, even though about 80% of early LCs are curable, either through lung resection alone or through lung resection followed by adjuvant chemotherapy (Amann et al., 2011). The high LC mortality is associated with three factors: (1) late diagnosis, since LC usually is not symptomatic at its early, treatable stage; (2) inadequate staging and histological evaluation of the tumor; and (3) advanced age and general state of bad health among patients, with comorbidities, which prevent radical lung resection.

Hence, population-based screening programs of at-risk populations are necessary to identify presymptomatic patients with treatable LC at the earliest possible stage. However, there are currently no cost-effective methods with sufficient sensitivity and specificity available to achieve this goal. Volatile organic compound (VOC)-based breath prints that are detectable by sensor arrays could provide a satisfactory method for early diagnosis and screening of LC in the future and, hence, may soon enter clinical practice as LC markers.

19.1.2 Conventional Imaging LC Markers for Diagnosis and Screening

The most widely available methods for LC diagnosis and staging in clinical practice, besides tumor marker (TM) blood tests of limited sensitivity and specificity (see Section 19.1.3), are imaging tests such as chest x-ray (Todd and McGrath, 2011), computed tomography (CT) (Brandman and Ko, 2011), magnetic resonance imaging (MRI) (Hochhegger et al., 2011), and positron emission tomography (PET) (Truong et al., 2011). Detection and diagnosis of LC rely heavily on CT and/or PET, which have excellent detection limits for small lung nodules (2 and 8–10 mm for state-of-the-art CT and PET scanners, respectively). However, these techniques involve exposure to x-ray radiation and/or radioactive substances. In addition, they have limited specificity for detecting malignancies (the positive predictive value of a CT scan is <10%) (McWilliams and Lam, 2005, Szulejko et al., 2010). The overwhelming majority of the lung nodules detected through imaging are benign granulomas or scars that confound the analysis of small tumors. Confirmation of malignancy and differential diagnosis require additional invasive and potentially risky procedures for tissue sampling from the tumor and histopathological evaluation of the sample. The tissue specimen can be obtained by biopsy that is guided by fiber-optic bronchoscopy (Rossi et al., 2004) or by CT scan-guided needle biopsy (Wu et al., 2011). Biopsy samples are examined under the microscope to determine the cell morphology, as well as specific immunohistochemical markers and other parameters that could be relevant for the choice of treatment (Hamilton, 2012).

One of the major impediments in developing a feasible imaging-based screening program for LC lies in the definition of the at-risk populations. Smoking is the most important single risk factor of LC. However, about 15% of LC cases occur in nonsmokers. Additional environmental risk factors include, for example, exposure to radon or asbestos. Risk assessment models are based on factoring these and some other components for calculating the probability of developing LC. However, these calculations do not necessarily reflect clinical reality (Cassidy et al., 2007, Spitz et al., 2007, D'Amelio et al., 2010, Etzel and Bach, 2011, Tammemagi et al., 2011). The number of potential at-risk subjects is staggering, raising the issue of cost-effectiveness. Recently, a large study in the United States has documented for the first time that low-dose CT screening of a very specific at-risk population (subjects aged between 55 and 74 years with a history of smoking of at least an equivalent of one pack of cigarettes per day for 30 years) reduced mortality from LC within this group by 20% (Aberle et al., 2011). About 25% of the screened individuals had positive CT findings, out of which about 3% were diagnosed with LC after biopsies. In a wider screening population that also includes nonsmokers, the percentage of LC cases would be even smaller. CT has insufficient imaging criteria for distinguishing benign from malignant pulmonary nodules (Bach et al., 2012). Hence, CT screening could expose large populations to unnecessary, invasive, potentially risky, and costly diagnostic follow-up tests. The Fleischner Society has published detailed recommendations for the follow-up and management of small, indeterminate lung nodules above 4 mm, in order to minimize unnecessary recalls. However, following the current guidelines bears the risk of missing treatable early-state cancers (MacMahon, 2010).

A further problematic aspect of the imaging techniques lies in their inability to determine the biological activity of malignant lung tumors, which is another important parameter for treatment decisions (Greenberg et al., 2012). Indeed, LC aggressiveness and treatment response may vary dramatically from patient to patient, even if their disease is at the same stage, because of the histological and molecular heterogeneity of the LC cells (Pleasance et al., 2010).

19.1.3 Emerging Molecular LC Markers for Personalized Medicine: Impact on Treatment Decisions

There is currently a trend toward personalized medicine in LC care, with individualized treatment plans for patients (based on the molecular specification of the LC cells) to optimize clinical response and minimize toxicity (Modak, 2010). The trend toward personalized medicine drives the search for molecular markers of LC that could complement conventional diagnostic methods and improve their diagnostic yield. Clinically accessible sources for LC markers can be exhaled air, saliva, sputum or bronchoalveolar lavage, blood, urine, stools, and tumor tissue. For example, histopathological examination of biopsy samples that are taken from suspected LC patients is already helping to tailor the therapeutic approach according to the LC cell histology, but discrepancies among pathologists can be in excess of 15% (Hamilton, 2012). A broad spectrum of molecules, produced or induced by the tumor, may reflect its growth and activity. These molecules are therefore utilized as TMs. Table 19.1 lists the TMs used to aid LC diagnosis, prognosis, and treatment choice. Several different algorithms of TM use have been suggested, but the usefulness of TMs in LC is debated and virtually no guidelines for clinical use exist. False-positive results are frequently present due to drug interaction or interference with normal bodily functions or through unrelated benign and malignant diseases. Most of the TMs are catabolized in the liver and excreted via the renal route. Therefore, pathological changes in the liver and kidneys impede the use of TMs.

More sophisticated methods such as gene expression profiling and protein profiling are currently gaining acceptance for a more accurate prediction of an individual patient's treatment response (Beer et al., 2002, Olaussen et al., 2006, Potti et al., 2006b, Taguchi et al., 2007, Yanagisawa et al., 2007, Guo et al., 2008). Recently developed microarray techniques can be used to profile gene expressions in LC cells that have been associated with tumor heterogeneity and treatment outcome (Beer et al., 2002, Potti et al., 2006a,b, Chen et al., 2007a). Protein profiling may provide important additional information to the treating physician, as most targeted therapeutic agents are designed to inhibit the activity of proteins

TABLE 19.1

TMs That Are Currently Used in Clinical Practice to Aid LC Diagnosis

Marker	Normal Value	False-Positives	Other Cancers
CA15-3	<35 U/mL	Infectious lung disease, renal failure, megaloblastic anemias, drug treatment	Breast, ovarian, lymphoma
CA 125	<35 U/mL	Female menstrual cycle, infectious lung disease, COPD, liver disease, fluid retention	Ovarian and endometrial carcinomas
Calcitonin	<15 pg/mL (males) <7 pg/mL (females)	Renal failure, sepsis	Thyroid, Zollinger–Ellison syndrome
NSE	<25 ng/mL	Liver disease, renal failure, hemolysis, cerebral hemorrhage, cerebral ischemia	Neuroblastomas, Wilms' tumor
ProGRP	<50 pg/mL	Chronic disorders, liver disease, renal failure	Neuroblastomas, Wilms' tumor
SCCA	<25 ng/mL	5%–10% of pulmonary or hepatic diseases, renal failure, psoriasis, eczema, pemphigus	None (specific marker for NSCLC)
CA72-4	<6 U/mL	COPD, treatment with NSAIDs, corticosteroids, or omeprazole	Gastrointestinal, ovarian

Abbreviations: CA, cancer antigen; LC, lung cancer; NSE, neuron-specific enolase; ProGRP, pro-gastrin-releasing peptide; SCCA, squamous cell carcinoma antigen; TM, tumor marker.

(Olaussen et al., 2006, Yildiz et al., 2007, Weiss et al., 2008, Yu et al., 2008). Already today, physicians often rely on genetic mutation testing of cancer cells that lead to changes in their protein levels. Clinicians look at posttranslational protein modifications when determining the individual prognosis of NSCLC patients, and they increasingly design their patients' treatment plans according to these tests (Pleasance et al., 2010). For example, advanced NSCLC patients with mutated epidermal growth factor receptor (EGFR*mut*) could benefit from first-line EGFR TKI treatment, which compares favorably to chemotherapy in terms of efficacy, toxicity, and quality of life (Jackman et al., 2006, Cappuzzo et al., 2007). On the other hand, patients with fusion of the echinoderm microtubule-associated protein-like 4 gene to the anaplastic lymphoma kinase gene (EML4-ALK), which has been associated with 5%–13% of LCs (Mano, 2008, Shaw et al., 2009, Wong et al., 2009), might benefit from crizotinib (Shaw et al., 2009, Shaw and Solomon, 2011), but not from EGFR TKI. However, profiling of gene expression and proteins requires sophisticated, expensive techniques, which are available only in specialized laboratories and usually require tissue samples (Kumar et al., 2006, Yang and Schwartz, 2011).

It should also be noted that despite recent progress in the identification of molecular LC markers, gene mutations, and genomic signatures, these approaches still face formidable obstacles, including tumor heterogeneity, high complex interplay between the environment and host, and complexity, multiplicity, and redundancy of tumor cell signaling networks involving genetic, epigenetic, and microenvironmental effects. As of today, no reliable markers of any sort are available for the early detection of LC, and no single marker or combination of markers in screening lead to a reduction of the LC mortality as a whole.

19.1.4 Volatile Organic Compounds as Potential Future Noninvasive Molecular LC Markers

Volatile organic compounds (VOCs) are emerging as potential future molecular markers of LC (Gordon et al., 1985, O'Neill et al., 1988, Mendis et al., 1994, Phillips et al., 1994, 1999, 2003, 2008, Smith et al., 2003, Deng et al., 2004, Miekisch et al., 2004, Poli et al., 2005, 2010, Buszewski et al., 2007, Cao and Duan, 2007, Wehinger et al., 2007, Filipiak et al., 2008, 2010, Patel et al., 2008, Peng et al., 2008, 2009a,b, 2010, Bajtarevic et al., 2009, Barash et al., 2009, 2012, Horvath et al., 2009, Sponring et al., 2009, 2010, Sulé-Suso et al., 2009, Amann et al., 2010a, 2011, Brunner et al., 2010, Kischkel et al., 2010, Tisch and Haick, 2010, Hakim et al., 2011). VOCs have a relatively high vapor pressure (>0.1 mm Hg) and, hence, tend to be excreted with the exhaled breath after alveolar exchange from the blood. This means that VOCs could be derived noninvasively from exhaled breath. Molecularly different phenotypes and genotypes of LC are expected to generate distinguishable VOC profiles. Impressive empirical data have confirmed the potential of VOCs to serve as a basis for a noninvasive, simple, inexpensive, and easy-to-use diagnostic tool. Hence, monitoring of VOCs in the breath may soon become an interesting supplement (or even alternative) to conventional medical diagnostics and follow-up of therapeutic effects, thanks to the rapid advances in the techniques for breath collection and gas analysis during the past two decades. This novel approach could revolutionize personalized LC care and management and has potential for becoming an integral part of population-based LC screening in the future, even though the technique is not yet mature enough for imminent clinical use (Tisch et al., 2012).

19.2 Volatile Organic Compounds in Exhaled Breath

Exhaled breath is potentially the most easily clinically accessible source for LC markers that would allow noninvasive sampling and even continuously online sampling in the future (King et al., 2010b, 2012a). In addition, the matrix of exhaled breath is less complex than that of saliva, sputum or bronchoalveolar lavage, blood, urine, stools, and tumor tissue and, hence, would be easier to analyze. Human exhaled breath is a diverse mixture of inorganic and organic molecules in the gas phase (Miekisch et al., 2004). Its main constituents are nitrogen, oxygen, carbon dioxide, water, and inert gases. Exhaled breath is almost fully humidified with high and extremely variable values of relative humidity (RH ~40%–80%). The humidity in breath samples decreases with age and may vary considerably as a result of benign and malignant pulmonary diseases, as well as diet and lifestyle. In addition to the inorganic gases, thousands of VOCs may be detected at very low concentrations in the breath of different persons, in parts-per-billion with respect to volume (ppb_v) or even parts per trillion (ppt_v). The VOCs in the exhaled breath stem from blood-borne VOCs that are either generated by the various cellular biochemical processes of the body or absorbed from the environment through ingestion, inhalation, or skin contact (Amann et al., 2007, Buszewski et al., 2007). The analysis of these VOCs can serve as a window into the metabolic activity and toxicological state of the body. Pathological processes such as LC affect a small fraction of the blood-borne VOCs by producing new compounds or changing their normal concentration ratios. Hence, molecular markers of LC could be derived from the disease-specific changes of an organism's VOC patterns.

The VOC profiles of LC patients can be detected via the exhaled breath (Gordon et al., 1985), since the changes of the blood chemistry are reflected in measurable changes of the chemical composition of the alveolar exhaled breath through exchange via the lung (Preti et al., 1988, Sponring et al., 2009). It was found that some gases exchange in the airways, rather than the alveoli, depending on the blood/air partition coefficient, $\lambda_{b:a}$. Gases with low solubility in blood, mainly nonpolar VOCs ($\lambda_{b:a} < 10$), exchange almost solely in the alveoli, while highly blood-soluble gases, mainly polar VOCs ($\lambda_{b:a} > 100$), tend to exchange in the airways (Anderson et al., 2003). Furthermore, VOCs with $10 < \lambda_{b:a} < 100$ interact significantly both with the airways and with the alveoli (Anderson et al., 2003). Hence, the airways may play a larger role in pulmonary gas exchange than has generally been assumed (King et al., 2011, 2012a), and the implications of pulmonary tests and breath tests might have to be reevaluated (Anderson et al., 2003). The VOC profile is also influenced by the retention of VOCs in the lungs, viz., the fraction of the molecules that remains in the respiratory tract at any time, after inhalation and exhalation, because of the blood/air partition coefficient (Kalliomäki et al., 1978). Thus, the final partition and exhalation of the VOCs depends on their physical and chemical properties and on their interaction with the different alveolar clearance processes (Kalliomäki et al., 1978, Jakubowski and Czerczak, 2009).

It is important to note that several other parameters, besides diseases, may also affect the VOC concentrations in a person's breath. These include both permanent/long-term body states and short-term dynamic changes. The resulting changes of the VOC profiles are sometimes substantial and could therefore confound the disease-induced VOC profiles. Confounding factors such as age, gender, lifestyle, nutrition, medication, medical history, smoking habits, and alcohol consumption can alter the concentration of certain breath VOCs (Mendis et al., 1994, Lechner et al., 2006, Kushch et al., 2008, Kischkel et al., 2010). For example, exhaled isoprene levels change with a person's age and gender or can be altered through therapeutic intervention (Amann et al., 2011). One of the most critical confounding factors in LC patients is smoking. Several studies have identified long-term VOC markers of smoking, including acetonitrile and toluene (Bajtarevic et al., 2009, Hakim et al., 2012).

19.3 Potential Future LC Markers Derived from Exhaled Breath VOCs

19.3.1 Future Clinical Potential

The disease-specific changes of a small fraction (ca. 1%) of the exhaled VOCs could be used to derive molecular markers of LC in the future (Pennazza et al., 2013). LC-specific breath VOCs or compositional changes in VOCs that are present in everyone's breath may either be products of the metabolic activity of the tumor itself, or by-products of bacteria and necrotic reactions caused by local inflammation in the microenvironment of the tumor, or else they could be partially re-emitted environmental toxins that were previously adsorbed to the body (Tisch et al., 2012). In addition, systemic breath VOCs may be produced or consumed because of cancer-related changes elsewhere in the body, affecting the blood chemistry, and eventually being expired via the respiratory system (Tisch et al., 2012).

Breath VOCs of both exogenous and endogenous origin could be utilized for LC diagnostics and management. The following molecular LC markers could in principle be derived:

1. Risk markers of developing LC in healthy subjects
2. Markers indicating the presence of measurable disease in the early or more advanced stage, including staging information
3. Markers for different phenotypes (including histology and presence of oncogenes) with prediction of prognosis and/or response to therapy
4. Markers for monitoring of the responses to therapy such as surgery, radiation therapy, immunotherapy, or chemotherapy

Breath-based LC markers would have many advantages: their noninvasive acquisition would be safe and convenient for the patient; sampling and analysis would be fast and could be performed in nonspecialist settings, for example, in local GP clinics; and the method could be potentially cost-effective (if sensor arrays were used) and, hence, could be accessible also in the developing world and for use in future population-based LC screening programs.

19.3.2 Analysis of Separate LC-Specific VOCs versus Direct Breath Printing by Sensor Arrays

There are two fundamentally different approaches for deriving LC markers from the exhaled breath VOCs. The first approach consists in the identification and quantification of the LC-specific VOCs, using techniques of analytical chemistry. Table 19.2 provides an overview over the strengths and weaknesses of three different analytical methods that have been used for exhaled VOC analysis, viz., gas chromatography linked with mass spectrometry (GC-MS), proton transfer reaction mass spectrometry (PTR-MS), and ion mobility spectrometry coupled with mass spectrometry (IMS-MS). In this case the LC markers would be identical with the (concentrations of the) actual breath VOCs that characterize LC patients. However, the compositional changes of the separate VOCs are not distinct enough for reliable LC classification. Furthermore, available techniques either require additional experimental procedures (e.g., sample preconcentration and system calibration in the case of GC-MS) or are sensitive only to specific classes of breath VOCs. The analytical techniques are described in detail in Section 19.5. Collective breath VOC patterns can in principle be derived through additional statistical analysis of the concentration profiles of preselected VOCs, but the entire process is tedious and time consuming. To summarize, analytical chemical analysis of the exhaled breath may yield highly accurate concentration profiles of separate LC-specific VOCs that provide interesting input for studying biochemical pathways of LC. However, the experimental procedures involved would not be practical for real-world LC diagnosis or screening.

The second approach consists in the direct detection of collective breath VOC patterns (without actually identifying the constituent compounds), using arrays of broadly cross-reactive sensors (Persaud and Dodd, 1982, Röck et al., 2008). These patterns have been termed *breath prints*. Sensor arrays mimic the mammalian sense of smell and are therefore often called *electronic noses*. Each sensor in the array responds to all or part of the VOCs in the breath sample. Breath prints are then derived from the collective numerical output

TABLE 19.2

A Comparison of the Methods of Analytical Chemistry and of Sensor Arrays That Have Been Used for Studying Breath VOC of LC

	Methods of Analytical Chemistry			
Characteristic	**GC-MS**	**PTR-MS**	**IMS-MS**	**Sensor Arrays**
Compounds	Volatile and semivolatile compounds	VOCs with proton affinity higher than water	Specific compounds	Tunable through choice of sensors
Accuracy of compound identification	Very high	Does not distinguish between compounds of the same mass	High	No compound identification
Detection limit	~ single ppm_v, can be improved to ~ single ppb_v through sample preconcentration	~10 ppt_v	~0.1 ppb_v	Strongly varies for different types of sensors: from single ppb_v to more than 1 ppm_v; tunable for specific VOC mixtures
Compound quantification	Requires calibration	Real times	Yes	N/A
Speed	Off-line	Real time	High	High
Required user skill level	High	Medium	Medium	None
Sample preparation	Preconcentration of breath VOCs necessary	None	None	None
Possibility of direct breath sampling	No	Yes	Yes	Yes
Breath print/VOC pattern determination	Separate statistical treatment of VOC concentration profiles; requires quantification	N/A	Separate statistical treatment of VOC concentration profiles	Directly through built-in statistical treatment of the collective sensing signals
Size of equipment	Typically very large	Compact, transportable units are available	Compact, transportable units are available	Small, portable
Maintenance	High	Medium	Medium	Low
Consumable costs per sample	\$40–\$150	\$1–\$9	\$1–\$9	\$1–\$5

Abbreviations: GC-MS, gas chromatography linked with mass spectrometry; IMS-MS, ion mobility spectrometry coupled with mass spectrometry; LC, lung cancer; PTR-MS, proton transfer reaction mass spectrometry; VOC, volatile organic compound.

of the sensors that interact with the breath VOCs, using methods of statistical data analysis. The breath print LC markers are dimensionless parameters. This approach avoids expensive equipment and, therefore, has realistic potential for future fast, cost-effective, and high-throughput LC diagnostics. Preconcentration is generally not necessary, because additive signals are monitored that stem from a wide range of breath VOCs, at total concentrations of at least 1 ppm_v or above. In principle, this approach can be adapted for direct sampling of patients' breath, but until now indirect sampling of pre-collected breath samples has been more feasible, since the sensor arrays are usually operated in a research laboratory. Sensor arrays are therefore ideally suited for direct LC marker breath printing (Mazzone, 2008, Peng et al., 2009a,b, Tisch and Haick, 2010, Hakim et al., 2011). Types of sensors that have been used for breath printing will be described in Section 19.6. However, breath printing is essentially a black box approach to chemical sensing, which bears the risk of over-fitting small data sets during the statistical analysis (Tisch and Haick, 2010). Therefore, careful validation of the study results, preferably with a blinded validation sample set, should be an integral part both of limited proof-of-concept studies and of large-scale clinical trials.

19.3.3 Challenges on the Way to Clinical Practice

Breath VOCs that might indicate LC have attracted much research interest during the past decades, and impressive preliminary results have been achieved both in the chemical analysis of exhaled breath and in the sensor-based breath printing. However, no viable and generally accepted LC markers have yet been established, and LC breath markers are still entirely confined to research. This is due to the complexity of the process of breath collection and analysis, insufficient attention to confounding factors in proof-of-concept studies, and the wide variety of techniques that have been developed and used by different researchers in the course of their studies. The lack of standardization pertains to each step of the multi-step process toward the establishment of reliable LC markers from exhaled VOCs. Scheme 19.1 provides an overview over the breath LC marker development—from bench to bedside. Inconsistent findings of different study groups in limited pilot trials could be attributed to one or more of the following problematic aspects of current breath marker research:

1. Inconsistencies in the preselection of the rather small control groups used in the proof-of-concept clinical studies. For example, control groups might consist of healthy nonsmokers, healthy smokers, age-matched groups, chronic obstructive pulmonary disease (COPD) groups, hospital personnel, and relatives and spouses of the patients. Clinical studies investigating exhaled VOCs of LC, especially proof-of-concept studies of limited size, should be carefully designed to avoid biased results, by using well-matched study populations.
2. Inconsistent breath sampling and VOC preconcentration procedures used in various studies (see Section 19.4). Breath collection should be standardized and either one universally accepted

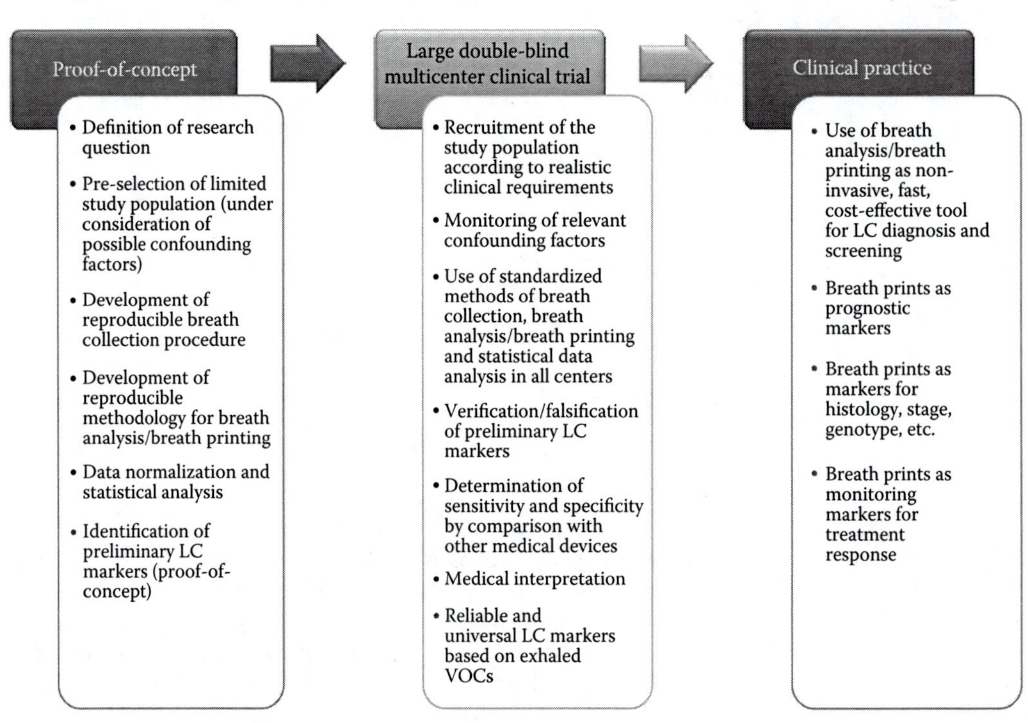

SCHEME 19.1 Steps toward the development of reliable VOC-based breath LC markers for clinical practice—from bench to bedside. LC, lung cancer; VOC, volatile organic compound.

method should be adapted by all researchers in the field or a small number of well-defined techniques should be established for use. In addition, a breath collection protocol should be followed, which minimizes the effect of nutrition, smoking habits, and medication.

3. Use of different analytical methods including different equipments (e.g., GC-MS [Phillips et al., 2003, Kischkel et al., 2010] PTR-MS [Wehinger et al., 2007, Brunner et al., 2010]). Note that the identification of the VOCs by GC-MS or PTR-MS is not 100% certain, even if the identification by spectral library match and retention time for GC-MS is quite reliable (Filipiak et al., 2008, 2010, Sponring et al., 2009).
4. Use of different sensor arrays for breath print detection (e.g., nanomaterial-based chemiresistive layers [Peng et al., 2009a, 2010, Hakim et al., 2011], colometric sensors [Mazzone et al., 2011], polymer sensors [Dragonieri et al., 2009], quartz microbalance [QMB] sensors [Di Natale et al., 2003]). Different sensing transducers and chemisensitive materials interact differently with the same breath VOCs. Special attention must be paid to confounding factors when using sensor arrays. The response of the sensor array to the relevant confounding factors should be studied in order to exclude biased results.
5. Inconsistencies in the normalization procedures of the raw data. While part of the studies normalized the data according to the concentration of a specific VOC in the exhaled breath (Wehinger et al., 2007, Bajtarevic et al., 2009), other studies have normalized the data according to the difference between the concentrations in the exhaled and the inhaled air (Phillips et al., 1999, 2003, 2008). Non-normalized data were reported as well. Normalization for sensor arrays is even more challenging, because long-term and short-term sensor drift has to be considered (Konvalina and Haick, 2012).
6. Inconsistent data analysis. For instance, the analysis of the GC-MS raw data includes identification, separation, and area integration of the peaks in the chromatograms for each sample, as well as quantitative comparisons of the chromatogram peak areas or compound concentrations between different study groups, using statistical algorithms. Patterns distinguishing the study groups may be obtained from in the collective GC-MS results through a variety of supervised or non-supervised statistical pattern recognition algorithms. For example, forward stepwise multi-linear regression, a supervised method, was used by Phillips et al. (Poli et al., 2005, Peng et al., 2009a) in order to establish LC patterns based on (unidentified) chromatogram peaks (Phillips et al., 2007). VOC patterns of LC and histologically different types of LC were studied using non-supervised methods such as principal component analysis. Also the data analysis of the collective sensor array output involves multivariant statistical analysis of the raw data.

The following sections are designed to provide the reader with a detailed understanding of the key components of the experimental process in state-of-the-art breath LC marker research that may affect the results of experimental studies: different methods of breath sample collection with their strength and limitations are discussed in Section 19.4; methods of analytical breath VOC analysis, together with selected studies, are presented in Section 19.5; and sensor arrays that were developed for and/or have been applied to LC marker breath printing will be described in Section 19.6.

19.4 Breath Collection, Sample Storage, and Possible Sources of Contamination

Exhaled breath samples are rather delicate. Special attention should be paid during sample collection and storage (1) to preserve the highly volatile disease markers and (2) to avoid contamination with confounding or environmental VOCs from external sources. The study of biomarkers in exhaled breath still suffers from a lack of standardization of the breath collection and analysis. Amann and co-workers have recently proposed a standardization of the breath collection process that might be generally accepted in the future (Amann et al., 2010b).

Several different procedures of direct and indirect breath collection are currently being used. Sampling procedures include, but are not limited to, mixed expiratory breath collection, end-tidal breath collected with CO_2-controlled sampling (Wehinger et al., 2007), sampling with Tedlar or Mylar bags (Kischkel et al., 2010), and portable breath collection apparatus (BCA), which was developed and used by Phillips et al. (Musa-Veloso et al., 2002, Wehinger et al., 2007).

During direct breath sampling, air exhaled by the subject is introduced into the measuring system without any intermediate steps (Phillips et al., 2003). This approach would be most convenient for a future clinical device. Breath print analyzers based on sensor arrays could in principle be adapted to direct sampling. In contrast, direct sampling cannot be used in combination with the most important method of chemical analysis (GC-MS). During indirect sampling, the exhaled air is stored on an adequate medium and analyzed later. Indirect sampling is still by far more widely used method in research settings, both for chemical analysis of breath and sensor array studies.

Several VOC collection media for indirect breath sampling are being used: bags of Tedlar, Mylar, or other (almost) chemically inert, low-emission plastic materials; empty glass vials; and stainless steel containers or glass cartridges containing adsorbent substances (so-called adsorbent traps). Tedlar bags and adsorbent traps are currently most widely used (Pennazza et al., 2013). Adsorbent traps are commercially available as thin glass or stainless steel tubes containing a single resin or resin mixture. Resins that can adsorb VOCs include, for example, carboxene, Tenax® TA, and Tenax® GR, which is a composite material of Tenax® TA and 30% graphite. The selection should be made according to material parameters such as breakthrough volume and retention time (Pennazza et al., 2013). Breath VOCs can be trapped at room temperature, if the retention volume for the compounds of interest is sufficiently high to prevent VOCs from being released during collection. Since the retention volume decreases strongly with temperature, the trapped VOCs can be fully and immediately thermally desorbed from the adsorbent trap at elevated temperatures around 200°C–300°C, allowing sample analysis several days or even weeks after sample collection.

Adsorbent traps offer numerous advantages over sample bags, for example, higher sample storage stability, easier transport, and preconcentration of the breath VOCs. The latter enhances the ability of the analytical equipment to detect VOCs at very low concentrations (typically of the order of magnitude of single ppb_v). However, while bags can be easily filled by the test persons during exhalation, adsorbent traps offer such a high resistance to air transit that a pump device is required for pushing exhaled air into the cartridge (Pennazza et al., 2013). This methodology is rather complex and may affect the overall reliability of the collection procedure. Hence, adsorbent traps are often used in combination with collection bags: the breath sample is initially collected into a bag, while the test person exhales. The content of the bag is then transferred immediately after the breath collection into the adsorbent trap, using a syringe or an electrical pump. This method combines the advantages of bags and adsorbent tubes and does not require the use of sophisticated equipment. Other methods of preconcentrating VOCs from breath samples in collection bags are available as well, for example, solid-phase microextraction (SPME) that uses a fused-silica optical fiber coated with a thin film polymeric stationary phase or a mixture of polymers and is based on the preferential partitioning of the VOCs by adsorption from the gas phase or from the solution to the stationary phase. However, the intermediate steps of sample transfer and preconcentration may increase the risk of information loss and/or external contamination.

It is especially challenging to avoid exogenous VOCs that are exhaled by the test person during the collection process, after being adsorbed to the body via previous inhalation, ingestion, or skin contact. Exogenous VOCs or their metabolic products are either exhaled immediately (e.g., highly volatile room air contaminates in a hospital environment) or within a short period of time of 1–2 h (e.g., some ingredients of coffee, food, or cigarette smoke) or they are stored in the body's fatty tissue and are released over an extended period of weeks or even years, depending on each VOC's vapor pressure and alveolar gradient (viz., the difference between the amounts of each VOC in breath and in the room air).

Figure 19.1 shows a schematic representation of a BCA for alveolar air that was designed to minimize sample contamination during the collection process. When using this device, the inhaled air is cleared of such ambient contaminants that are exhaled immediately by means of a so-called lung washout. During this procedure the test person inhales repeatedly to total lung capacity for 3 min through a mouthpiece with a filter cartridge on the inspiratory port mouthpiece (can be obtained, e.g., from Eco Medics, Duerten, Switzerland). It was shown that the lung washout greatly reduces the concentration of exogenous VOCs (Peng et al., 2009a, 2010). Following the lung washout, subjects inhaled to full lung capacity and exhaled slowly through the mouthpiece into a separate exhalation port against 10–15 cm H_2O pressure. This

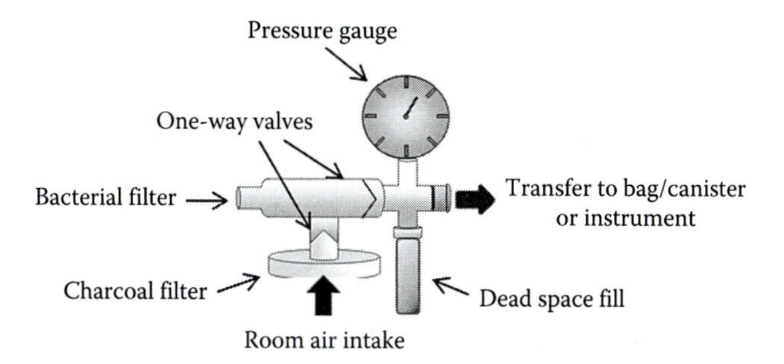

FIGURE 19.1 Example of a BCA. The system allows performing a lung washout from highly volatile room air contaminants prior to the collection of the breath sample, whereby the test person inhales several times through a charcoal filter. Thereafter the test person exhales through a bacterial filter. The system automatically separates alveolar air and air from the respiratory dead space. A pressure gauge ensures closure of the vellum. The sampled alveolar air can be collected in an inert bag, canister or transferred directly into the instrument. The system was used in several studies. (Hakim, M. et al., *Br. J. Cancer,* 104, 1649, 2011; Hakim, M. et al., *Chem. Rev.,* 112, 5949, 2012; Peng, G. et al., *Nano. Lett.,* 8, 3631, 2008; Peng, G. et al., *Nat. Nanotechnol,* 4, 669, 2009a; Peng, G. et al., *Nano. Lett.,* 9, 1362, 2009b; Peng, G. et al., *Br. J. Cancer,* 103, 542, 2010.)

ensures the closure of the vellum in order to exclude contamination through nasal entrainment. Exhaled breath consists of respiratory dead space air that is exhaled first (i.e., the volume of air that is inhaled, but does not take part in gas exchange region of the lung), followed by the alveolar air from the lungs. The collection apparatus in Figure 19.1 automatically fills the dead space into a designated dead space bag that can later be removed. Although the dead space air is usually not analyzed for VOCs, it should be taken into consideration that certain gases exchange in the airways, rather than the alveoli, depending on the blood/air partition coefficient, $\lambda_{b:a}$. For example, highly blood-soluble, polar VOCs tend to exchange in the airways (Anderson et al., 2003). The alveolar breath from the end of the exhalation can be sampled indirectly into an inert bag or canister or directly into the analyzing equipment.

Exogenous contaminants with intermediate release times from nutrition, smoking, medication, or body care products can be minimized by following a breath collection protocol. For example, the test persons can be instructed to fast for 1–2 h prior to the breath collection and to refrain from smoking, drinking coffee, taking medication, using perfume, etc. However, some contaminants with longer release times, mainly those originating in cigarette smoke or from continuous uptake of a certain VOC through long-term occupational exposure, cannot be avoided altogether (Hakim et al., 2012). Indeed, some of these VOCs are known carcinogens and may be utilized, for example, as exogenous markers of developing LC.

19.5 Chemical Analysis: Identification of Specific LC Marker VOCs

Over the past three decades, hundreds of studies have addressed the identification and quantification of a wide variety of separate breath and headspace VOCs. This section will briefly present the different analytical techniques that have been used for the chemical analysis of breath samples. Examples of important studies will be provided, and the state-of-the-art understanding of the biochemical pathways will be presented.

19.5.1 Analytical Techniques

19.5.1.1 Gas Chromatography Linked with Mass Spectrometry (GC-MS)

GC-MS is the gold standard for determining the composition of breath samples and has been used in most studies on LC marker VOCs (Preti et al., 1988, Phillips et al., 1999, 2003, 2007, Bajtarevic et al., 2009, Amann et al., 2010a, Kischkel et al., 2010). The gas chromatograph separates the VOCs according to their volatility: the sample is carried in a helium stream through a long, heated capillary column, whereby more volatile compounds travel faster than less volatile ones. The separating ability of the GC depends on the column's dimensions (length, diameter, film thickness). The retention time in the column is a measure for the volatility. The mass spectrometer determines molecular mass and chemical structure of the breath VOCs, after they have been broken up into characteristic fragments and ionized. In the mass analyzer, the ions are filtered by an electrical field according to their mass charge ration (m/e). The range of masses can be adjusted to the compounds of interest, or, on the other hand, known contaminants can be excluded. The compounds are identified according to the masses of their fragments and their retention times in the GC column. Combining GC and MS reduces the possibility of error considerably, as it is extremely unlikely that two different molecules have the same mass and the same retention time. Tentative compound identification can either be achieved through spectral library match, using tabulated values from the literature. However, verification of compound identity can only be achieved experimentally, through calibration of the actual GC-MS instrument for each compound of interest, using highly pure laboratory standards.

Although GC-MS yields highly accurate results and presents a wealth of information for basic research, the method has several prominent disadvantages for use as a clinical point-of-care tool (see Table 19.2). First and foremost, it still requires sophisticated, expensive equipment that would only be available in large, well-equipped laboratories. The first GC-MS instruments were slow and bulky, but speed and sensitivity have been greatly improved during the past decades, and miniaturized equipment for limited, well-defined applications will most probably become available during the next decade (Amann et al., 2010a). The second setback of GC-MS lies in the high expertise that is required to interpret the GC-MS raw data. Third, the analysis of breath VOCs at ppb_v/ppt_v concentrations requires pre-concentration prior to GC-MS—for example, onto SPME fibers or to other suitable absorption media (Amann et al., 2010a) or by cryo-focusing (Phillips et al., 1999), as described in Section 19.4. The pre-concentration methods complicate the overall experimental procedure. Furthermore, they selectively enhance the signals of certain VOCs, while potentially missing others. All in all, the method would be too time-consuming and expensive for clinical application in high-throughput LC diagnosis and screening and does not allow direct breath sampling.

Empirical data from hundreds of GC-MS studies on LC marker VOCs in exhaled breath have been accumulated for over three decades, and over 100 different VOCs have been identified in the breath of LC patients (Phillips et al., 1999, Risby and Solga, 2006, Amann et al., 2007, 2010a, 2011, Buszewski et al., 2007, Mazzone, 2008, Poli et al., 2008, Bajtarevic et al., 2009, Peng et al., 2009a, 2010, Szulejko et al., 2010, Darwiche et al., 2011, Hakim et al., 2011, 2012). Figure 19.2 shows the results of one such study (Amann et al., 2010a). The distribution of 28 breath VOCs in 65 LC patients and 31 healthy controls is illustrated using a hotplot representation. The test population included smokers, ex-smokers, and nonsmokers (Bajtarevic et al., 2009, Ligor et al., 2009). 2-Butanone, 2,3-butanedione, 3-butyn-2-ol, and tetramethyl-urea appeared in the exhaled breath of patients with LC, but did not appear in the exhaled breath of healthy volunteers with the same smoking habits (Bajtarevic et al., 2009, Ligor et al., 2009, Amann et al., 2010a).

A recent rigorous meta-analysis of all the available data from GC-MS studies on breath samples, cancer cells, blood samples, and, in few cases, urine samples and saliva has yielded 16 VOCs that have been positively associated with LC in at least 2 separate studies (see Table 19.3) (Hakim et al., 2012). These include alkanes, alkenes, alcohols, aldehydes, and ketones.

The biochemical pathways leading to the release of these VOCs in exhaled breath are still subject to controversy. The optimal approach to determine the biochemical pathways for the production of the LC VOCs would be to compare VOC profiles from different sources (organs or clinical samples) in the same LC patient and/or the same animal model. However, many technical challenges have been hindering the implementation of such an approach. Despite the inconsistency in experimental methods, interesting conclusions could be drawn from the meta-study about possible biochemical pathways, and the following hypothesis was offered (see Scheme 19.2) (Hakim et al., 2012): both endogenous and exogenous compounds could be interesting candidates for LC biomarkers. Hydrocarbons, aldehydes, and some ketones are produced in the body as a result of oxidative stress, which occurs when increased quantities of reactive oxygen species (ROS), originating mainly from exogenous sources, are produced in the mitochondria. Exogenous sources of VOCs include cigarette smoking, alcohol consumption, air pollution, and radiation. The reactive nature of these exogenous molecules can cause peroxidative damage to biological organelles, stimulating cancer, and, hence, are of great interest. The body reacts to this by activating the detoxification process, in which the liver enzyme cytochrome p450 catalyzes the addition of an oxygen

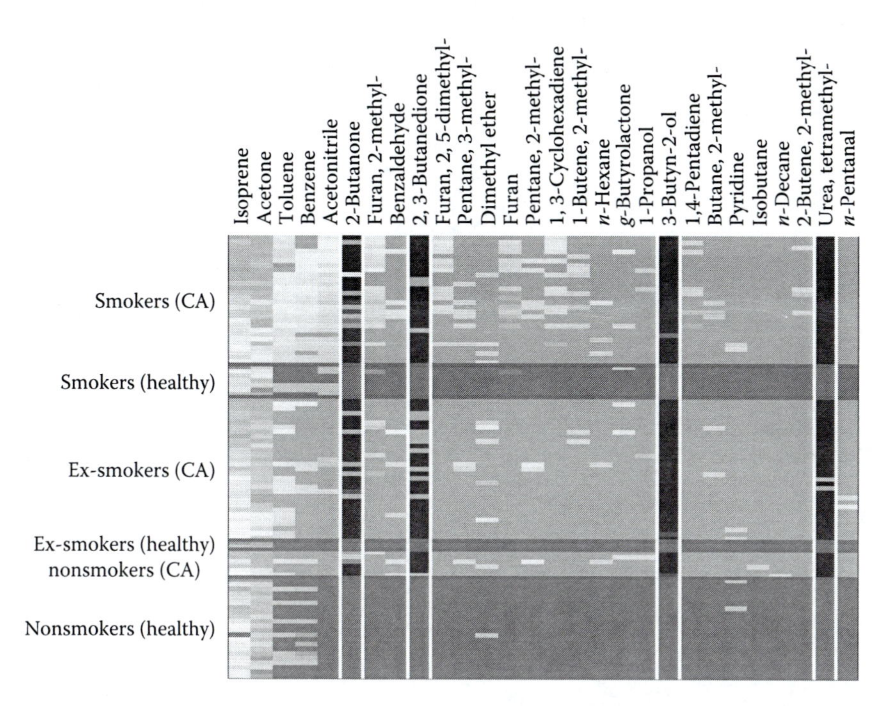

FIGURE 19.2 Hotplot of VOCs in exhaled breath. Hotplot showing the distribution of 28 VOCs in exhaled breath of 65 LC patients and 31 healthy volunteers (patients and volunteers were a mixture of smokers, ex-smokers, and nonsmokers). Several VOCs appear in cancer patients, but do not appear in the exhaled breath of healthy volunteers. These VOCs (2-butanone, 2,3-butanedione, 3-butyn-2-ol, and tetramethyl-urea) are emphasized in the plot. VOC, volatile organic compound. (With kind permission from Springer and memo: *Memo,* Analysis of exhaled breath for screening of lung cancer patients, 3, 2010a, 106–112, Amann, A., Ligor, M., Ligor, T., Bajtarevic, A., Ager, C., Pienz, M., Denz, H. et al.)

atom to the foreign compound, thus turning it to a more soluble substance in water—an alcohol and as by-products aldehydes are formed. Other liver enzymes may also alter the concentration of the VOCs such as alcohol dehydrogenase (ADH), which turns alcohols to aldehydes, and aldehyde dehydrogenase (ALDH), which oxidizes aldehydes into carboxylic acids. Some aldehydes are emitted via the breath as a result of signal transduction during the cancerous pathological process.

Based on empirical results of the analytical studies, LC patient classification was attempted by statistical analysis of the observed VOC concentration profiles, and collective VOC patterns of LC were indeed derived in a few cases (Phillips et al., 1999, 2003, 2008, Risby and Sehnert, 1999, Poli et al., 2005, 2008, 2010, Risby and Solga, 2006, Amann et al., 2007, 2010a, 2011, Buszewski et al., 2007, Bajtarevic et al., 2009, Modak, 2010). Several of these studies have used reasonably large study groups of over 400 LCs and healthy participants and have validated the VOC pattern LC markers using blind validation sets (see Table 19.4).

Differences in LC histology and response to treatment by surgery also lead to statistically significant differences in the concentration of certain VOCs in exhaled breath, as some empirical data indicates (see Table 19.3). Furthermore, statistically significant differences between the VOC of some alkanes, alkenes, and aromatic compounds were observed when directly comparing between the breath of LC patients and the breath of patients with another smoking-related cancer (viz., head-and-neck cancer), as well as patients with benign lung disease (viz., COPD) (see Table 19.3).

One GC-MS study has shown encouraging results for identifying specifically NSCLC patients by collective breath VOC patterns (see Table 19.4), but such breath VOC patterns of LC histology have not yet been studied systematically, and VOC concentration profiles of LC genotypes have not yet been studied at all. However, the potential of VOC concentration profiles for the identification of LC phenotypes and genotypes was demonstrated in several in vitro studies using cell lines with different histology and/or gene expressions (see Table 19.3) (Chen et al., 2007b, Filipiak et al., 2008, 2010,

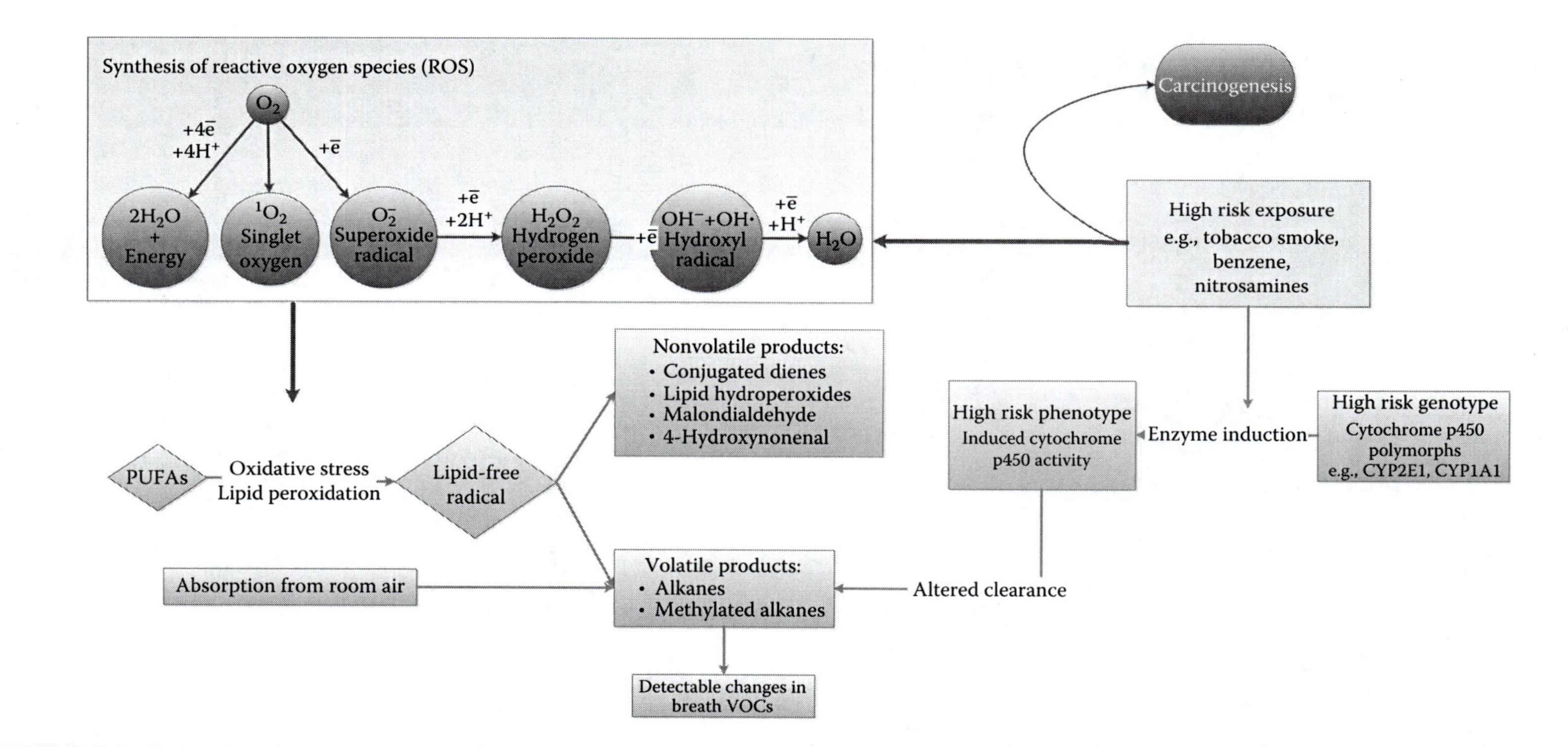

SCHEME 19.2 Hypothetical biochemical origin of the exhaled LC marker VOCs: LC may result from the interaction of hereditary and environmental factors. Several cytochrome p450 mixed oxidases are activated by exposure to environmental toxins such as tobacco smoke. The induced phenotype may increase the LC risk due to increased conversion of precursors to carcinogens. An altered pattern of cytochrome p450 mixed oxidase activity could potentially modulate catabolism of endogenous VOC products of oxidative stress and generate an altered pattern of breath VOCs. (Reprinted with permission from Hakim, M. et al., 5949–5966. Copyright 2012 American Chemical Society.) LC, lung cancer; VOC, volatile organic compound.

TABLE 19.3

Breath VOCs as Potential LC Markers

Type of Marker	Tentative Compounds	Chemical Class	Sample Source
Lung malignancy	Heptane (Phillips et al., 2003, Poli et al., 2005); decane (Phillips et al., 1999, Poli et al., 2005); 2-methylpentane (Poli et al., 2005, Sponring et al., 2009); isoprene (Poli et al., 2005, Bajtarevic et al., 2009); 1-propanol (Bajtarevic et al., 2009, Sponring et al., 2009, Kischkel et al., 2010); 2-ethyl-1-hexanol (Sponring et al., 2009, Barash et al., 2012, Sanchez et al., 2012); formaldehyde (Wehinger et al., 2007, Fuchs et al., 2010); propanal (Kischkel et al., 2010, Poli et al., 2010); butanal (Kischkel et al., 2010, Poli et al., 2010); pentanal (Fuchs et al., 2010, Poli et al., 2010); hexanal (Deng et al., 2004, Fuchs et al., 2010, Kischkel et al., 2010, Lili et al., 2010, Poli et al., 2010); heptanal (Brunner et al., 2010, Deng et al., 2004, Yazdanpanah et al., 1997, Poli et al., 2010); octanal (Fuchs et al., 2010, Lili et al., 2010, Poli et al., 2010); nonanal (Fuchs et al., 2010, Poli et al., 2010, Barash et al., 2012); acetone (Bajtarevic et al., 2009, Sulé-Suso et al., 2009, Fuchs et al., 2010, Kischkel et al., (2010), Poli et al., (2010), Barash et al., 2012); 2-butanone (Filipiak et al., 2008, Bajtarevic et al., 2009, Sponring et al., 2009)	Alkanes; alkenes; alcohols; aldehydes; ketones	Breath; cell lines; blood
Distinction from other malignancy (HNC)	Ammonium acetate (Hakim et al., 2011); 3-methyl-hexane (Hakim et al., 2011); 2,4-dimethyl-heptane (Hakim et al., 2011); 4-methyl-octane (Hakim et al., 2011); p-xylene (Hakim et al., 2011); 2,6,6-trimethyl-octane (Hakim et al., 2011); 3-methyl-nonane (Hakim et al., 2011)	Alkanes; aromatic compounds	Breath
Distinction from nonmalignant lung conditions (COPD)	Isoprene (Poli et al., 2005) 2-Methyl-pentane (Poli et al., 2005) Ethylbenzene (Poli et al., 2005) Styrene (Poli et al., 2005)	Alkanes; alkenes; aromatic compounds	Breath
LC histology: SqCC vs. ADCA	1-Butanol (Song et al., 2010) 3-Hydroxy 2-butanone (Song et al., 2010)	Alcohols; ketones	Breath
LC histology: SCLC vs. NSCLC	Hexanal (Fuchs et al., 2010)	Aldehyde	
Genotype: EGFR*mut*	Triethylamine; styrene; decanal	Amines; aromatic compounds; aldehydes	Cell lines
Genotype: KRAS*mut*	Triethylamine; benzaldehyde	Amines; aldehydes	
Genotype: EML4-ALK	Toluene; decanal	Aromatic compounds; aldehydes	

(*continued*)

TABLE 19.3 (continued)

Breath VOCs as Potential LC Markers

Type of Marker	Tentative Compounds	Chemical Class	Sample Source
Treatment response (surgery): Long term (3 years after surgery)	Isoprene (Poli et al., 2005) Decane (Poli et al., 2005) 2-Methyl-1-pentene (Broza et al., 2012)	Alkanes; alkenes	Breath
Treatment response (surgery): Short term (1 month after surgery)	2-Hexanone (Broza et al., 2012) 3-Heptanone (Broza et al., 2012) Styrene (Broza et al., 2012) 2,2,4-Trimethyl-hexane (Broza et al., 2012)	Alkanes; alkenes; ketones; aromatic compounds	

All listed compounds showed statistically significant differences of the average concentration between the studied LC states and control states in at least one study. The presented choice of 16 lung malignancy marker VOCs is the result of a recent comparative meta-study of all previous experimental studies in the field. (From Hakim, M. et al., *Chem. Rev.*, 112, 5949, 2012.) These VOCs were reported by at least two research groups (as following the same compositional trends). All VOCs were detected in exhaled human breath, except for the genotype markers, which were identified in the headspace of human LC cell lines having specific oncogenes.

ADCA, adenocarcinoma; COPD, chronic obstructive pulmonary disease; EGFR*mut*, mutated epidermal growth factor receptor; EML4-ALK, echinoderm microtubule-associated protein-like 4 (EML4) gene fused to the anaplastic lymphoma kinase (ALK) gene; HNC, head-and-neck cancer; KRAS*mut*, mutated V-Ki-ras2 Kirsten rat sarcoma viral oncogene homolog; LC, lung cancer; NSCLC, non-small cell lung cancer; SCLC, small cell lung cancer; SqCC, squamous cell carcinoma; VOC, volatile organic compound.

Barash et al., 2009, Sponring et al., 2009, 2010). Analysis of headspace samples from cell lines (the mixture of VOCs trapped above the cell lines in a sealed vessel/tool) showed significant concentration differences of a number of VOCs between SCLC and NSCLC (Barash et al., 2012) and has identified characteristic compositional fluctuation in the concentrations of certain amines, aromatic compounds, and aldehydes for different genotypes that are relevant for the treatment approach, including EGFR*mut*, mutated V-Ki-ras2 Kirsten rat sarcoma viral oncogene homolog (KRAS*mut*), and EML4-ALK, as Table 19.3 shows (Peled et al., 2013). Distinct VOC profiles have also been observed for cell lines that differed in the mutational status of two important signaling molecules, RAS and RAF (Filipiak et al., 2008, 2010, Sponring et al., 2009, 2010). However, statistical analysis of these genotype-specific VOC concentration profiles in order to obtain collective patterns has so far been impeded the rather small sample size of cell line studies.

19.5.1.2 Alternative Analytical Methods

MS techniques that do not separate or preconcentrate the compounds before the MS analysis may overcome part of the setbacks of GC-MS, such as PTR-MS and ion mobility spectrometry (IMS) (Wehinger et al., 2007, Bajtarevic et al., 2009, King et al., 2009, 2010a, 2012a,b, Amann et al., 2011). PTR-MS allows real-time measurement and quantification of VOCs with concentrations as low as few tens of ppt_v (see Table 19.2) (Wehinger et al., 2007). The main constituents of a PTR-MS apparatus are the ion source, a reaction region, and a mass analyzer. A chemical ionization system based on proton-transfer reactions, with H_3O^+ as the primary reactant ion, is considered the most suitable system when air samples containing a wide variety VOCs at trace levels are to be analyzed (Lindinger and Jordan, 1998).

PTR-MS employs smaller and more robust equipment than GC-MS and is easier to operate. The short measurement times allow true direct breath sampling in real time (see Section 19.4). Hence, real-time monitoring of the concentration levels of specific VOCs is possible and has been performed during physical exercise or sleep (King et al., 2009, 2010a, 2011, 2012b). Real-time monitoring could be of interest for

TABLE 19.4

Examples for Experimental Studies of LC Specific VOC Patterns, Using Different Analytical Techniques

Determination of VOC Pattern			Study Population				Future Potential as Marker for		
Analytical Method	**VOC as Input for Algorithm**	**Statistical Algorithm**	**Target**	**Control**	**Sensitivity (%)**	**Specificity (%)**	**Lung Malignancy**	**Histology**	**Principal Investigator**
GC-MS	16 VOCs	Fuzzy logic	193 LC	211 H	84.6	80.0	x		Phillips (Phillips et al., 2007)
	9 VOCs	Forward stepwise discriminant analysis	178 LC	102 H	85.1	80.5	x		Phillips (Phillips et al., 2003)
	30 VOCs	Weighted digital analysis	193 LC	211 H	84.5	81.0	x		Phillips (Phillips et al., 2008)
	15 VOCs	N/A	65 LC	31 H	71.0	100	x		Amann (Bajtarevic et al., 2009)
	7 VOCs (aldehydes)	Multivariate analysis	40 NSCLC	38 H	90.0	92.1	x	x	Poli (Poli et al., 2010)
PTR-MS	2 VOCs (tentatively formaldehyde and isopropanol)	Fisher's quadric discriminant method	17 LC	170 H	54.0	99.0	x		Amnn (Wehinger et al., 2007)
IMS-MS	23 peak regions	Discriminant analysis	32 LC	54 H	100	100	x		Westhoff (Westhoff et al., 2009)

The VOC patterns were calculated from the concentration profiles of specific VOCs. The possible future potential as specific LC markers is indicated that could be highly relevant for prognosis, choice of treatment, and treatment follow-up.

short-term treatment response in LC therapy, for example, to monitor life-threatening toxicity of chemotherapy treatments. One major setback of this method lies in the difficulty to unambiguously identify the breath VOCs, because compounds that have similar molecular mass cannot be distinguished. Also, the range of detectable masses is considerably smaller than for GC-MS, because only molecules with a proton affinity higher than water can be detected by PTR-MS. For example, most alkanes cannot be detected, which constitute an important class of LC marker VOCs (see Table 19.2) (Wehinger et al., 2007). Chemical analysis by PTR-MS of exhaled VOCs in LC patients yielded LC-related compositional changes of several VOCs, for example, increased levels of two VOCs, tentatively identified as isopropanol and formaldehyde, as well as decreased levels of (tentatively identified) isoprene (Wehinger et al., 2007, Bajtarevic et al., 2009, Fedrigo et al., 2010). Attempts of LC patient classification based on the statistical treatment of the concentration profiles of the two increased VOCs have not been successful (see Table 19.4).

IMS can separate ionized breath VOCs in the exhaled breath sample based on their mobility in a carrier buffer gas. When coupled with mass spectrometry (IMS-MS), the method represents a highly sensitive analytical technique for detection, identification, and monitoring of chemicals (see Table 19.2) (Karpas, 2009, Westhoff et al., 2009). In contrast to other analytical methods, IMS enables the detection and separation of all breath VOCs and their visualization in a three dimensional IMS chromatogram. However, IMS does not yield chemical identification of the VOCs, but rather detects a disease-specific combination of VOC peaks, using pattern recognition algorithms. ION-MS was used in a pioneering study of respiratory air that was collected via bronchoscopy directly from the tumor-bearing lung and from the opposite, unaffected lung of patients with histologically confirmed NSCLC (Bajtarevic et al., 2009). Characteristic VOC profiles from the tumor-bearing lung were observed, which could classify correctly all the 86 (LC and healthy) participants of a pilot study (see Table 19.4). Hence, IMS-MS concentration profiles of selected breath VOCs could be interesting candidates for markers for the short-term monitoring of the treatment success.

However, despite some encouraging results in patient classification, it is overall questionable whether analytical methods based on MS could provide sufficiently inexpensive, high-throughput, portable point-of-care devices that would be useful for clinical practice.

19.6 Sensor Arrays for LC Marker Breath Printing

Direct breath printing using sensor arrays is better suited for clinical applications than breath analysis. Implementations of sensor arrays for breath printing can be quite diverse. The sensors should meet the following requirements: Since the sensor arrays would be exposed directly to the breath samples in an anticipated future clinical application, the constituent sensors should be sensitive to very low concentrations of the VOCs in exhaled breath in the presence of water vapor, because breath samples are fully humidified. Secondly, each sensor should respond rapidly to small changes in the concentrations of the LC-specific breath VOCs, so that the sensor array output is specific to a given disease state. Ideally the sensors should relax rapidly to their baseline states when removed from the breath sample. Alternatively, disposable sensor arrays could be used, if the device fabrication is reproducible and simple enough that large quantities of identical units could be manufactured at acceptable costs.

The most important studies of LC breath prints have used sensors with electronic, colorimetric, or electroacoustic transduction mechanisms (see Table 19.5). The following sections will provide a brief description of the working principle of the different sensors, their advantages, and limitations for use in breath testing, supported by pertinent examples of actual LC marker breath print research.

19.6.1 Chemiresistors

Chemiresistors are simple electronic devices that consist of a chemiresistive material between two metal electrodes (see Table 19.5). The electrical resistance of a chemiresistor varies when its active material interacts with the breath VOCs. The change of the resistance upon exposure to the breath sample can easily be probed, either by applying a constant DC bias, V, and monitoring the current change, ΔI, or, alternatively, by supplying a constant current, I, and measuring the change in voltage drop, ΔV, across the chemiresistor.

TABLE 19.5

Examples for Experimental Studies of LC Breath Prints, Using Sensor Arrays

Sensor Array			Study Population					
Sensor Type	**Sensing Material**	**Statistical Algorithm**	**Target**	**Control**	**Sensitivity (%)**	**Specificity (%)**	**Future Potential as Marker for**	**Principal Investigator**
Chemiresistor	GNP and RN-SWCNT layers	DFA	53 LC	19 H	86.0	96.0	Lung malignancy	Haick (Peled et al., 2012)
		DFA	30 ADCA	13 SqCC	92.0	78.0	Histology	Haick (Peled et al., 2012)
	GNP layers	DFA	23 stages I–II	30 stages III–V	86.0	88.0	Staging	Haick (Peled et al., 2012)
		PCA and SVM	25 LC	40 H	100	92.3	Lung malignancy	Haick (Hakim et al., 2011)
		PCA and SVM	20 LC	16 HNC	100	100	Lung malignancy; distinction from other malignancy	Haick (Hakim et al., 2011)
		PCA	30 LC	18 PC, 22 BC, 26 CC	N/A	N/A	Lung malignancy; distinction from other malignancy	Haick (Peng et al., 2010)
		PCA	40 LC	56 H	N/A	N/A	Lung malignancy	Haick (Peng et al., 2010)
	GNP and PtNP layers	DFA	12 LC	5 H	100	80.0	Lung malignancy	Haick (Broza et al., 2012)
		DFA	12 LC presurgery	11 LC postsurgery	83.0	75.0	Treatment response	Haick (Broza et al., 2012)
	GNP layers	DFA	10 EGFR*mut*	14 KRAS*mut*, 8 EML4-ALK, 5 wt to all	70.0	100	Genotype	Haick (Peled et al., 2013)
			14 KRAS*mut*	10 EGFR*mut*, 8 EML4-ALK, 5 wt to all	93.0	78.0	Genotype	

(*continued*)

TABLE 19.5 (continued)

Examples for Experimental Studies of LC Breath Prints, Using Sensor Arrays

Sensor Array			Study Population					
Sensor Type	Sensing Material	Statistical Algorithm	Target	Control	Sensitivity (%)	Specificity (%)	Future Potential as Marker for	Principal Investigator
			8 EML4-ALK	10 EGFR*mut*, 14 KRAS*mut*, 5 wt to all	63.0	100	Genotype	
	Polymers	PCA and SVM	14 LC	62 H	71.4	91.9	Lung malignancy	Erzurum (Machado et al., 2005)
		PCA and CDA	10 LC	10 COPD and other benign lung diseases	CVV = 85%		Lung malignancy; distinction from other lung deficiency	Erzurum (Dragonieri et al., 2009)
Colorimetric	Dyes	Four logistic prediction models	83 NSCLC	137 H	70.0	86.0	Lung malignancy; histology	Mazzone (Mazzone et al., 2011)
			50 ADCA	137 H	80.0	86.0	Lung malignancy; histology	
			23 SqCC	137 H	91.0	73.0	Lung malignancy; histology	
			9 SCLC	137 H	89.0	85.0	Lung malignancy; histology	
	Dyes	The random forest algorithm	49 NSCLC	18 COPD[(l)] 21 H, 55 benign lung disorders	73.3	72.4	Lung malignancy; distinction from other lung deficiency; histology	Mazzone (Mazzone et al., 2007)

Electroacoustic: QMB (Quartz; Electrodes (Au))	Metal-loporphyrins	BP-ANN	35 LC	18 H	100	94.4	Lung malignancy	Di Natale (Di Natale et al., 2003)
		PLS-DA	9 postsurgery	18 H	44.4	94.4	Lung malignancy; treatment response	
		DFA	28 LC	36 H	85.7	100	Lung malignancy	Pennazza (D'Amico et al., 2010)
			28 LC	28 benign lung disorders	92.8	78.6	Lung malignancy; distinction from other lung deficiency	
Electroacoustic: SAW	PIB layer	BP-ANN	5 LC	5 H	80.0	80.0	Lung malignancy	Wang (Chen et al., 2005)

The possible future potential as specific LC markers is indicated that could be highly relevant for prognosis, choice of treatment, and treatment follow-up. One in vitro study of LC cell lines was included as an example for possible LC genotype markers, since no studies of breath samples are available yet.

ADCA, adenocarcinoma; ANN, back propagation artificial neural network; BC, breast cancer; BP-ANN, back propagation artificial neural network; CC, colon cancer; COPD, chronic obstructive pulmonary disease; CVV, cross-validation value; EGFR*mut*, mutated epidermal growth factor receptor; EML4-ALK, echinoderm microtubule-associated protein-like 4 (EML4) gene fused to the anaplastic lymphoma kinase (ALK) gene; GNP, gold nanoparticles; H, healthy controls; HNC, head-and-neck cancer; KRAS*mut*, mutated V-Ki-ras2 Kirsten rat sarcoma viral oncogene homolog; LC, lung cancer; NSCLC, non-small cell lung cancer; PC, prostate cancer; PCA, principal component analysis; PIB, polyisobutylene; PLS-DA, partial least squares discriminant; PtNP, platinum nanoparticles; QMB, quartz microbalance; RN-SWCNT, random network of single-walled carbon nanotubes; SAW, surface acoustic wave; SCLC, small cell lung cancer; SqCC, squamous cell carcinoma; SVM, supported vector machine; wt, wild type.

Chemiresistors are very attractive for breath printing applications, because of their simplicity, ease of fabrication and use, small size and weight, fast response, and reliability. Furthermore, automatic packaging of sensor arrays at wafer level, on-chip integration, and mass production of portable systems with integrated readout electronics are easily possible at low cost (Schoening, 2005).

19.6.1.1 Polymer Composite Sensors

Polymer composite sensors incorporate a chemisensitive polymer network with a 3D continuous porous structure filled with conducting carbon black (Machado et al., 2005, Dragonieri et al., 2009). Upon exposure, the VOCs land on the sensing surface, and the reaction between the VOC molecules and the functional group(s) at the polymers causes a volume expansion in the polymer network. As a consequence, the connection between carbon black blocks filling in the polymer network structure becomes loose, and the conductivity decreases. The chemical diversity of the functional group(s) at the macromolecules can in principle be tailored for each sensor type, with the aim that each sensor will respond to a particular VOC or class of VOCs in a different way (Machado et al., 2005). These sensors have been applied to LC marker breath printing and have shown reasonable differentiating ability between LC patients and healthy controls, as well as between LC patients and a control group containing COPD patients and patients with other benign lung diseases in several proof-of-concept studies with small study populations (Machado et al., 2005, Dragonieri et al., 2009). The details of the studies are listed in Table 19.5. However, it should be noted that polymer composite sensors show a high response to water vapor and that the sensing responses to separate breath VOCs have not been established in an atmosphere of high humidity. The high and variable humidity levels in the breath of patients suffering from different lung diseases may introduce a bias into the results, because the humidity response of the constituent sensors could obscure their responses to the much smaller levels of breath VOCs. It must be considered that breath printing is essentially a black box approach to chemical sensing, which bears the risk of overfitting small data sets during the statistical analysis (Tisch and Haick, 2010). These limitations of polymer composite sensors should be carefully considered when using them for diagnostic breath printing.

19.6.1.2 Nanomaterial-Based Chemiresistors

Incorporating nanomaterials into chemiresistors may help to overcome many limitations of bulk sensing layers. Nanomaterials offer several important advantages for sensing applications. Most importantly, their small characteristic dimensions (1–100 nm) increase the active surface-to-volume ratio and generate novel interfaces, yielding excellent sensitivity as well as rapid response and recovery times. In addition, nanomaterials offer high flexibility in their chemical and physical properties, which can be tailored to achieve unusual target-binding properties, including a reduced sensitivity to water molecules. This is especially attractive for the sensing of breath VOCs. This section focuses on sensors comprising layers of gold or platinum nanoparticles (GNPs and PtNPs, respectively) and on layers of random networks of single-walled carbon nanotubes (RN-SWCNTs) capped by organic films (see inset in Table 19.5). In these films the inorganic nanomaterials provide the electrical conductivity, and the organic film component provides sites for the sorption of VOCs. Gold and platinum are preferred choices of NP metal cores because of their chemical inertness.

GNP and PtNP films exhibit two countering effects during the adsorption of VOCs: a 3D swelling of the film, which increases the inter-particle tunneling distance for charge carriers and, hence, the film resistance, and an increase in the permittivity of the organic matrix around the metal cores, which decreases the potential barriers between the metal cores and consequently, the film resistance. These two mechanisms enable metal NP layers to sense the breath VOCs for LC marker breath printing (Peng et al., 2009a, 2010, Peled et al., 2012). The sensitivity of the sensor array can be tuned depending on the choice of the organic ligand through the variety of available ones (e.g., alkylthiols, alkylamines, para-thiophenols, carboxylates, organodithiols). Different combinations of GNP, PtNP, and RN-SWCNT sensors have been used to derive breath prints for lung malignancy, distinction from other cancers, benign lung deficiency, staging, histology, and treatment response, with impressive values for sensitivities and specificities (see Table 19.5). Figure 19.3 shows some examples for breath print LC markers for prognosis and prediction of treatment response. The sensor arrays could distinguish patterns of malignancy among

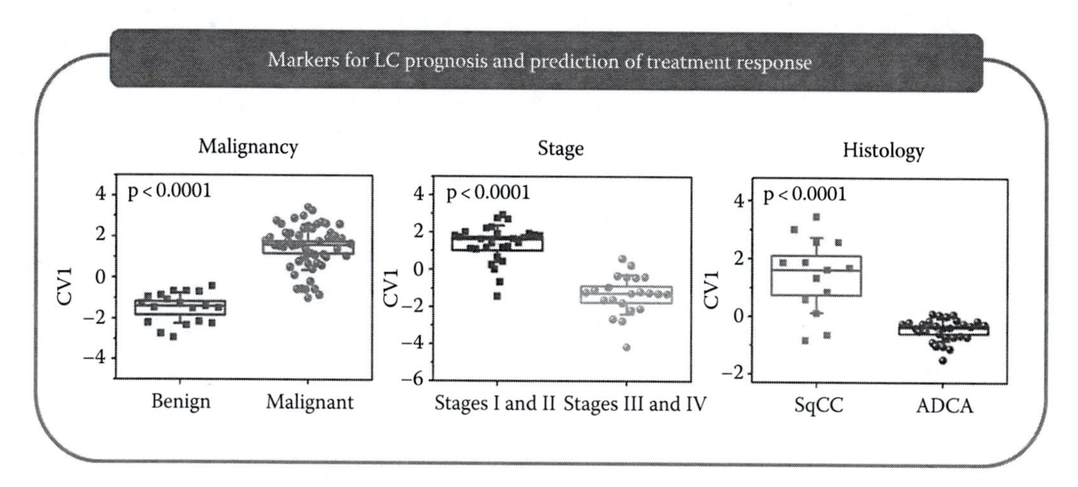

FIGURE 19.3 Examples for breath print LC markers for prognosis and prediction of treatment response (derived from exhaled VOC patterns, using sensor arrays comprising GNP chemiresistors): Breath prints for lung malignancy, LC stage, and NSCLC histology. The graphs show the first canonical score values that were calculated using a DFA for statistical data analysis. Each point represents one patient. The boxes correspond to their 95% confidence limits, corresponding to 1.96* SE, and the error bars correspond to the SDs. Further details of the experiment are given in Table 19.5. (Reproduced from Peled, N. et al., *J. Thorac. Oncol.*, 7, 1528, 2012. With kind permission from Walters Kluwer Health.) ADCA, adenocarcinoma; DFA, discriminant factor analysis; CV1, first canonical variable; GNP, gold nanoparticle; LC, lung cancer; NSCLC, non-small cell lung carcinoma; SD, standard deviation; SE, standard error; SqCC, squamous cell carcinoma; VOC, volatile organic compound.

patients with different lung diseases, identify the stage of the disease, and distinguish between two types of NSCLC that require different therapeutic approach, viz., SqCC and ADCA. In addition, the potential of GNP sensors for LC genotyping was demonstrated by analyzing the headspace of LC cell lines (see Figure 19.4).

All GNP, PtNP, and RN-SWCNT sensors in these studies have been tested under laboratory conditions prior to their application in clinical studies to ensure that they have sufficient detection limits, sensitivities, resolutions, and dynamic ranges for the very low concentrations of the VOCs in the breath of patients with LC. The sensors all had low, well-defined responses of water vapor. It is particularly relevant that the same breath samples were analyzed both with GC-MS and with sensor arrays. The breath VOCs identified by GC-MS were used to optimize the sensor arrays and validated the sensor-arrays' results by considerably reducing the risk of false-positive sample identification.

Finally, arrays that incorporate GNPs, PtNPs, and RN-SWCNTs can be designed in such a way that they are insensitive to important confounding factors, which could be relevant to future diagnostic breath printing. Figure 19.5 illustrates the stability of the breath prints against some important confounding factors, including age, gender, family cancer history, place of birth, ethnicity, smoking habits, work pollution, and consumption of food additives, among a population of 52 healthy subjects.

Nanomaterial-based chemiresistors seem to have realistic potential of becoming the preferred choice in future LC breath printing, based on their excellent performance in laboratory settings that were demonstrated by the presented pilot studies.

19.6.2 Colorimetric Sensors

Colorimetric sensors are composed of a diverse range of chemically responsive dyes, whose colors depend on their chemical environment. Since the measurable responses of the sensors are the color changes in each of the dyes, a colorimetric sensor array can easily be read out with the naked eye. Alternatively, auxiliary equipment such as a spectrometer can be used. Another advantage of colorimetric sensor arrays is their ease of fabrication: they can simply be printed on a variety of substrates using a disposable cartridge printer.

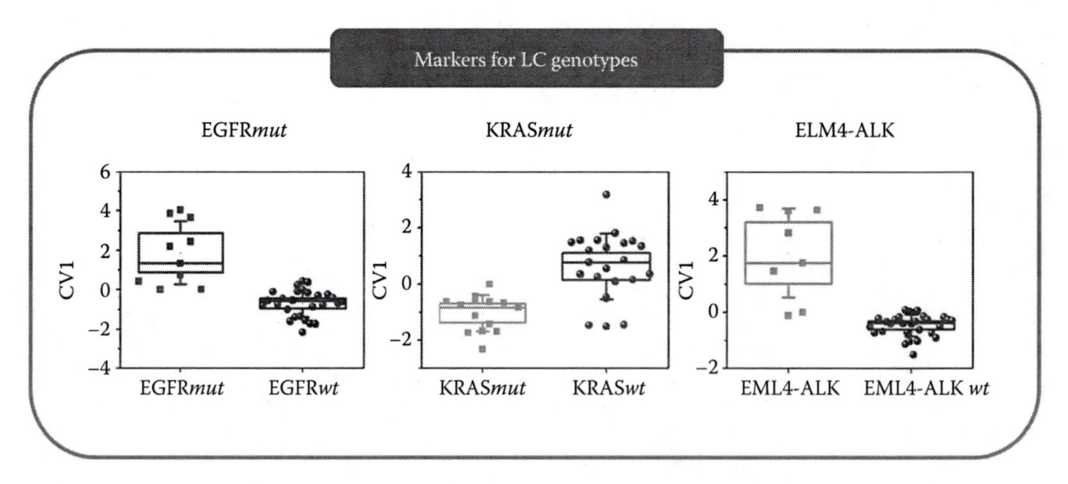

FIGURE 19.4 Examples for in-vitro LC markers for LC genotypes (derived from VOC patterns in the headspace of cell lines, using sensor arrays comprising GNP chemiresistors): in-vitro VOC headspace prints for the oncogenes EGFR*mut*, KRAS*mut*, and EML4-ALK. The graphs show the first canonical score values that were calculated using a DFA algorithm for statistical data analysis. The samples were obtained from multiple replicas of three cell lines with EGFR*mut*, four cell lines with KRAS*mut*, one cell line with EML4-ALK fusion, and eight cell lines with other oncogene. (From Peled, N. et al., *Nanomedicine*, 9, 758, 2013.) The graphs shows the CV1 values that were calculated using DFA. The boxes correspond to their 95% confidence limits, corresponding to 1.96* SE, and the error bars correspond to the SDs. Each point in the graph represents one headspace sample. Further details of the experiment are given in Table 19.4. DFA, discriminant factor analysis; CV1, first canonical variable; EGFR*mut*, mutated epidermal growth factor receptor; EML4-ALK, fusion of the echinoderm microtubule-associated protein-like 4 gene to the anaplastic lymphoma kinase gene; GNP, gold nanoparticle; LC, lung cancer; KRAS*mut*, mutated V-Ki-ras2 Kirsten rat sarcoma viral oncogene homolog; SD, standard deviation; SE, standard error; VOC, volatile organic compound; wt, wild type.

Colorimetric sensor arrays have been applied successfully to LC breath printing, using different classes of chemically responsive dyes (Mazzone et al., 2011). These were dyes containing metal ions (e.g., metalloporphyrins) that respond to Lewis basicity, pH indicators that respond to Bronsted acidity/basicity, and dyes with large permanent dipoles that respond to the polarity of the breath VOCs. The sensitivity of the system was in the low ppm_v range for many relevant VOCs. However, it was not established for humid gas mixtures. An array of 24 colorimetric sensors was used in a clinical trial on 229 subjects (92 LC with different histologies, 137 healthy controls; see Table 19.5). The potential for measuring LC marker breath prints for malignancy, histology, and exclusion of benign lung conditions was successfully demonstrated with acceptable sensitivity and specificity (see Table 19.5).

The colorimetric sensor arrays persuade especially by their ease of fabrication and use. These properties would be extremely useful for a future high-throughput LC screening test. However, the issue of co-sensitivity to water vapor should be addressed if the technology will be used for direct breath sampling.

19.6.3 Electroacoustic Sensors

Electroacoustic sensors measure the electrical response to applied mechanical stress: mechanical stress generates a voltage in piezoelectric materials and vice versa. An oscillating potential near the material's resonant frequency induces a variety of wave modes (Grate et al., 1993). Covering piezoelectric substrates with organic films provides the moderate chemical selectivity that is required for sensor array elements. The electroacoustic sensors use either bulk acoustic waves (BAKs) or surface acoustic waves (SAWs).

19.6.3.1 Quartz Microbalance Sensors

Quartz crystal microbalance (QCM) sensors constitute the simplest implementations of BAK sensors (see inset of Table 19.5). In a QCM, the acoustic wave propagates through the bulk of the crystal in a direction perpendicular to the surface. QCMs with chemoactive coatings of their membranes have been

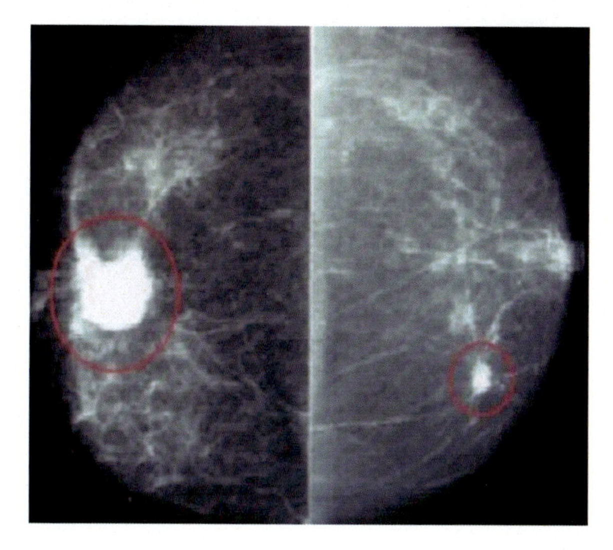

FIGURE 2.1 A mammogram showing cancer in both breasts. (Reprinted from Weinstein Imaging Associates, Pittsburgh, PA.)

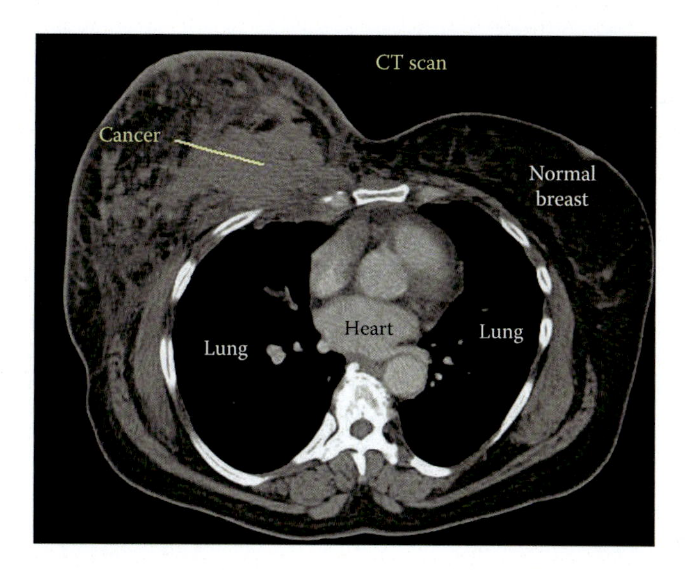

FIGURE 2.2 CT scan of advanced inflammatory breast cancer (cancer of the right breast invading into chest wall). (Reprinted with permission from Dr. Robert Miller.)

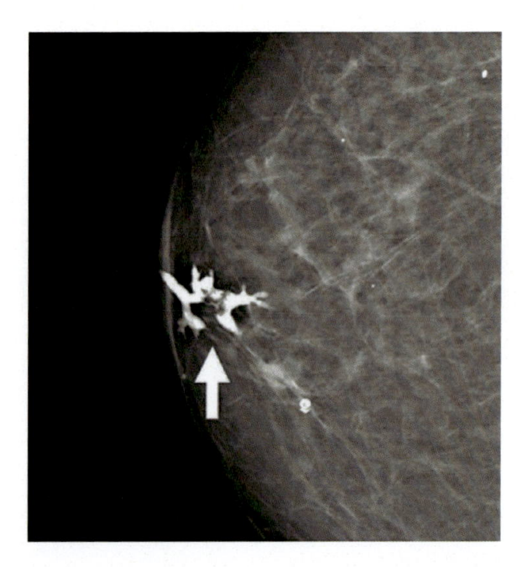

FIGURE 2.3 Conventional craniocaudal galactogram (in a 76-year-old woman with pathologic nipple discharge) shows a retromammillary, solitary intraductal papilloma (arrow). (Reprinted from Schwab, S. et al., *Radiobiology,* 249(1), 54, 2008. With permission.)

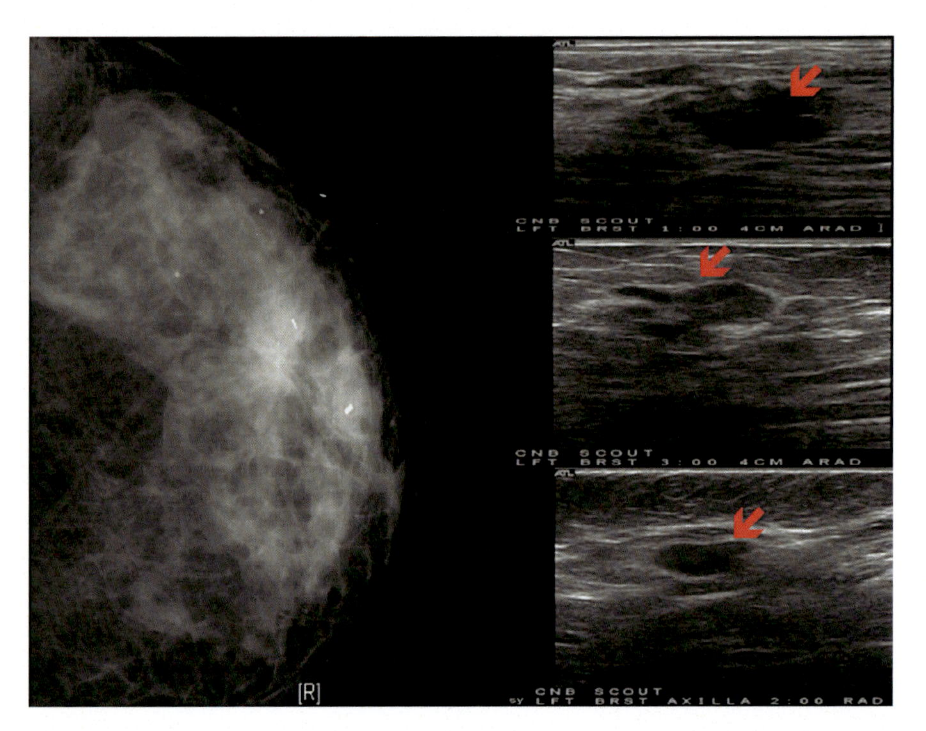

FIGURE 2.4 Sonogram of left breast at 1 o'clock demonstrates a hypoechoic lesion with angular margins highly suspicious for malignancy. Sonogram of left breast at 3 o'clock shows a hypoechoic lesion with what appears to be a duct leading into it. Sonogram of the left axilla shows a lymph node with very prominent cortex highly suggestive of tumor involvement.

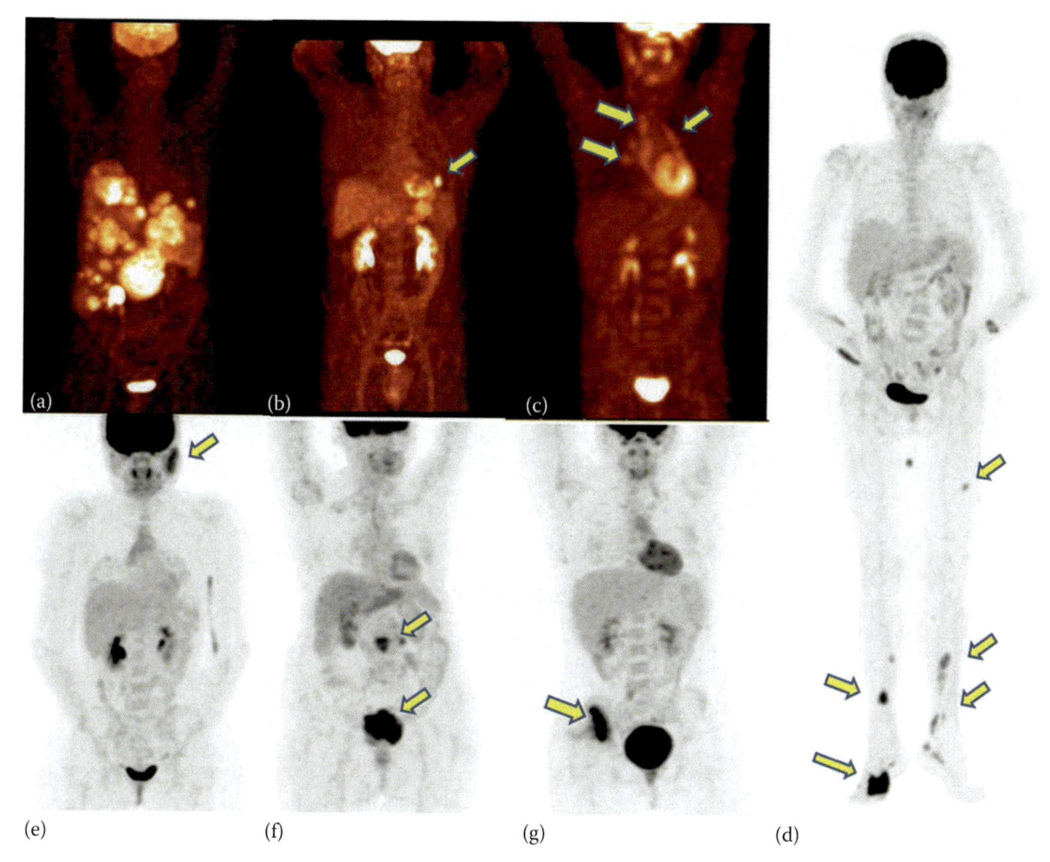

FIGURE 3.1 ^{18}F-FDG PET scans showing (a) multiple liver metastases in a patient with colon cancer, (b) a solitary malignant pulmonary nodule, (c) multiple hypermetabolic mediastinal lymph node in a patient with lymphoma, (d) several cutaneous localizations in a patient with melanoma, (e) lymph nodal metastases in a patient with head and neck tumor, (f) an advanced endometrial cancer with lymph nodal metastases, and (g) a bone localization in a patient with osteosarcoma.

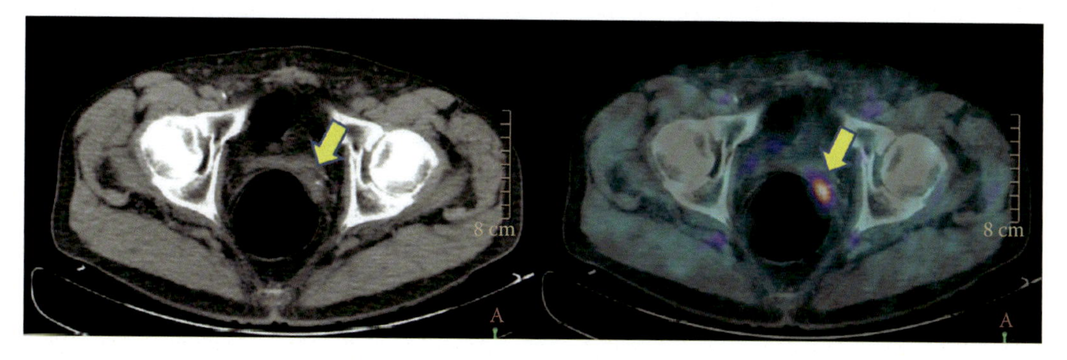

FIGURE 3.2 ^{18}F-choline PET/CT showing a recurrence of prostate cancer (arrow).

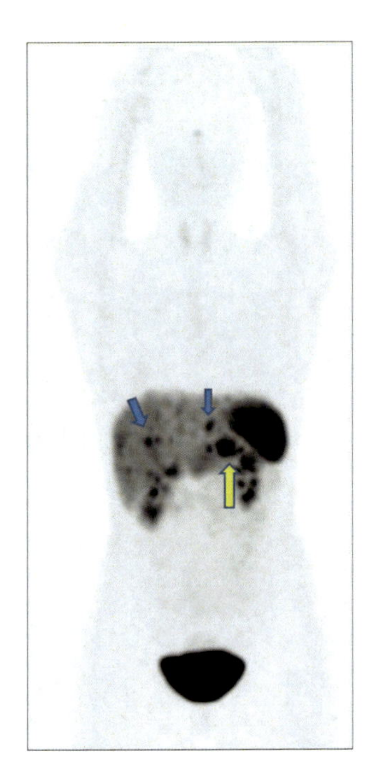

FIGURE 3.3 Somatostatin receptor PET showing a NET of the pancreas (yellow arrow) with multiple liver metastases (blue arrows).

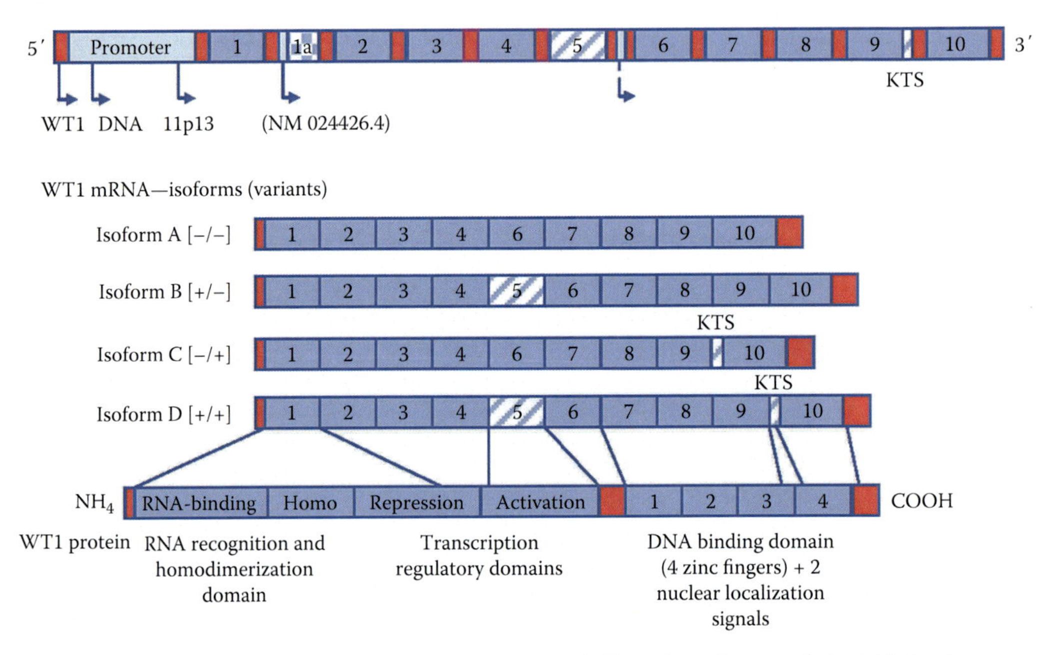

FIGURE 4.1 Alternative splice sites are crosshatched. Blue arrows indicate alternative transcription initiation sites.

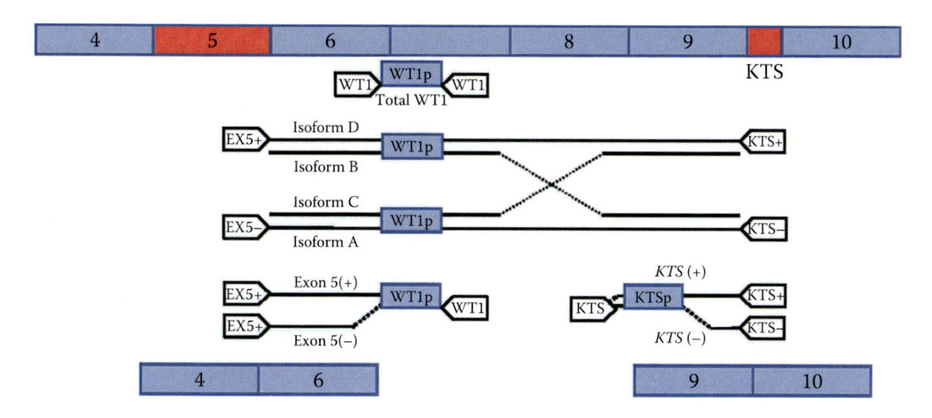

FIGURE 4.2 qPCR detection systems for total WT1 and its four isoforms (primers are indicated by gray arrows and probes by black rectangles).

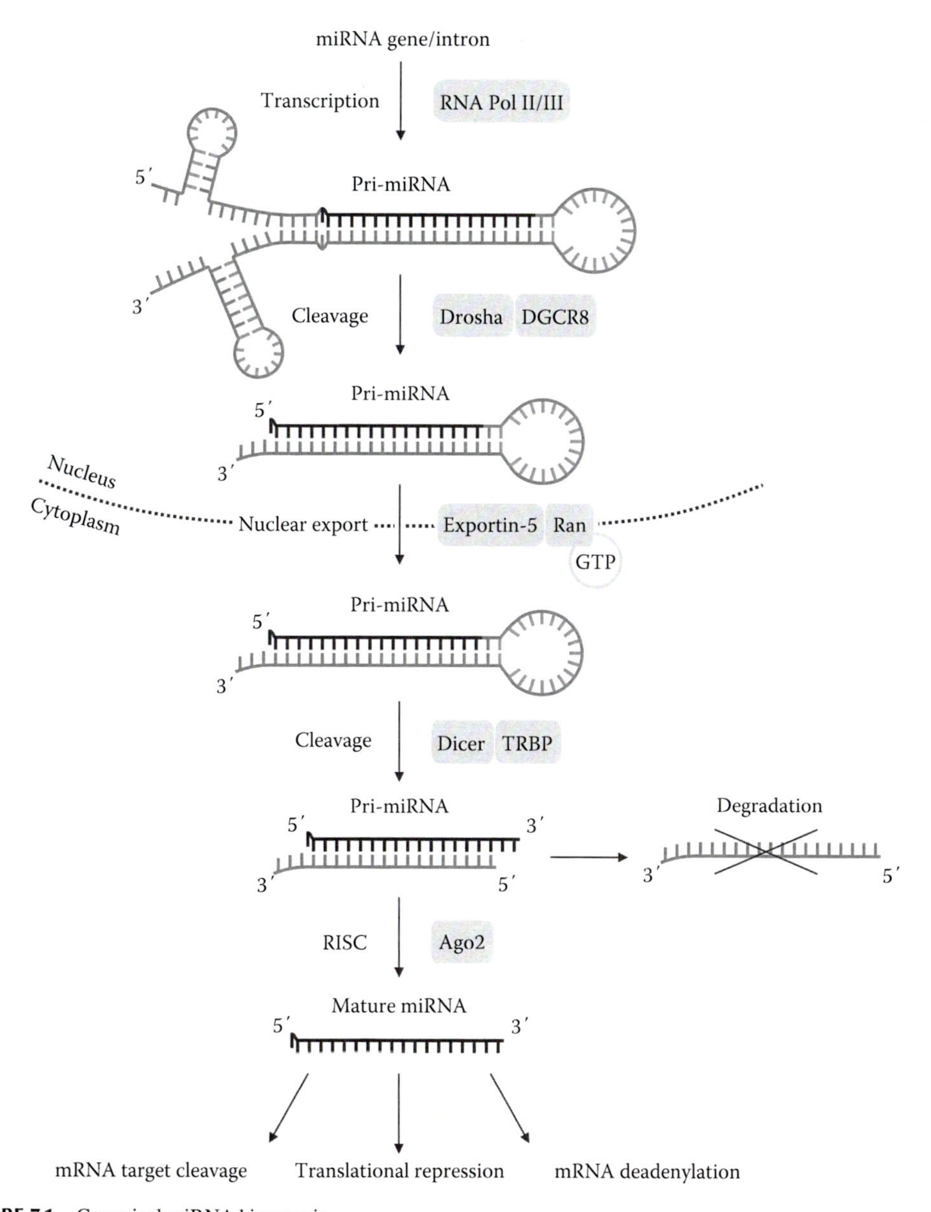

FIGURE 7.1 Canonical miRNA biogenesis.

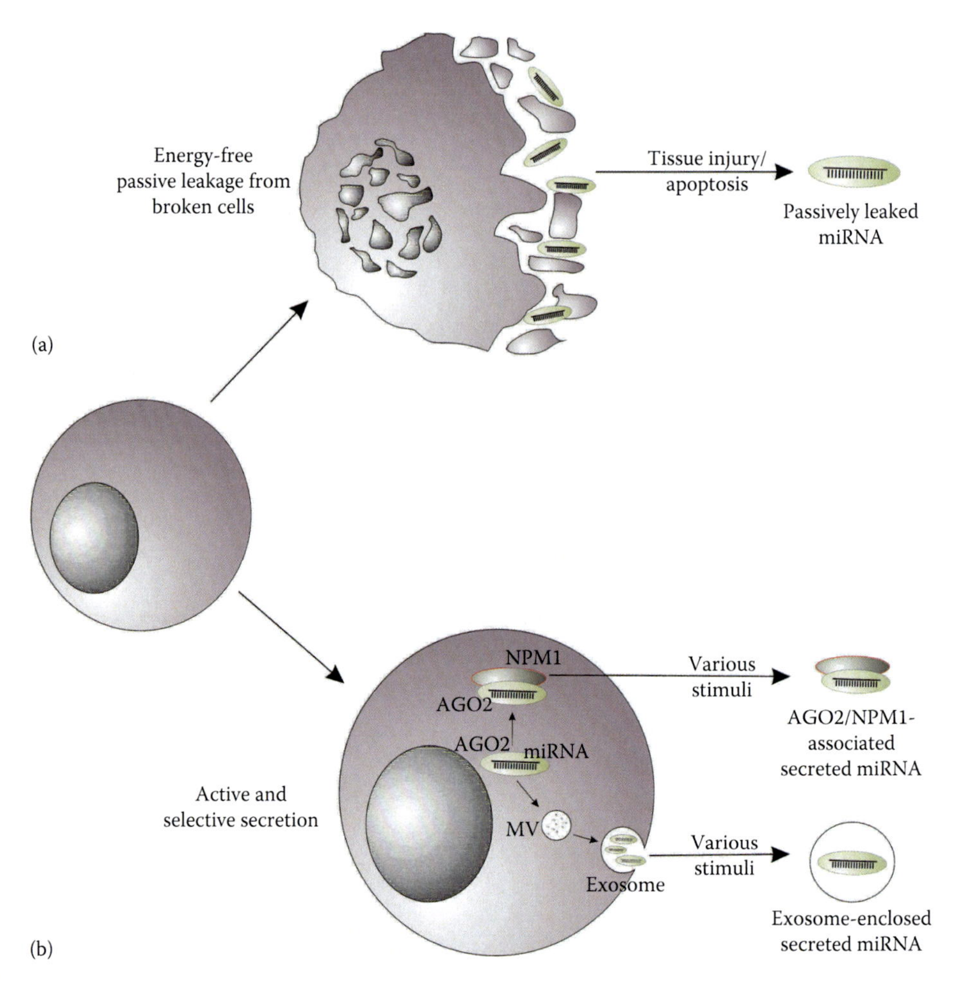

FIGURE 7.2 Sources of circulating miRNAs: miRNAs may enter the circulation by (a) energy-free passive leakage from broken cells under conditions of tissue injury or apoptosis or by (b) active and selective secretion by cells as a response to various stimuli. This second pathway is ATP- and temperature-dependent and is similar to the release of certain hormones and cytokines. miRNAs could be released as MV-free nonmembrane-bound miRNAs associated with various multiprotein complexes or via cell-derived MVs (microparticles and exosomes).

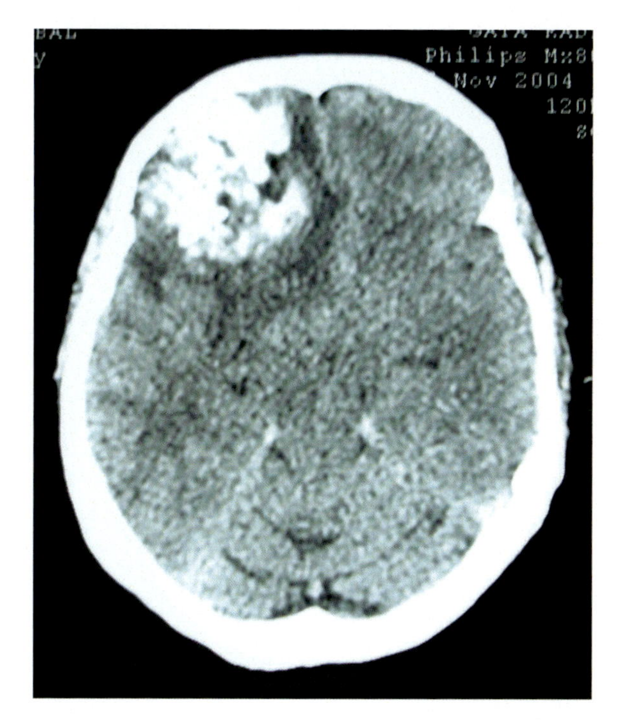

FIGURE 10.3 The axial CT scan of a patient with left frontal calcified mass lesion. The diagnosis was oligodendroglioma.

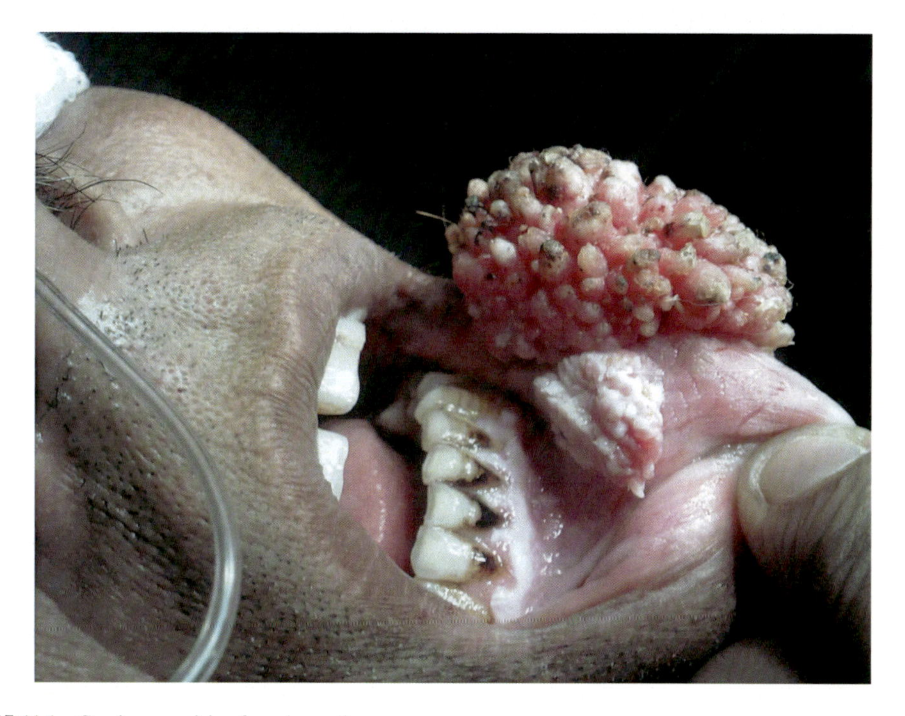

FIGURE 11.1 Carcinoma arising from lower lip.

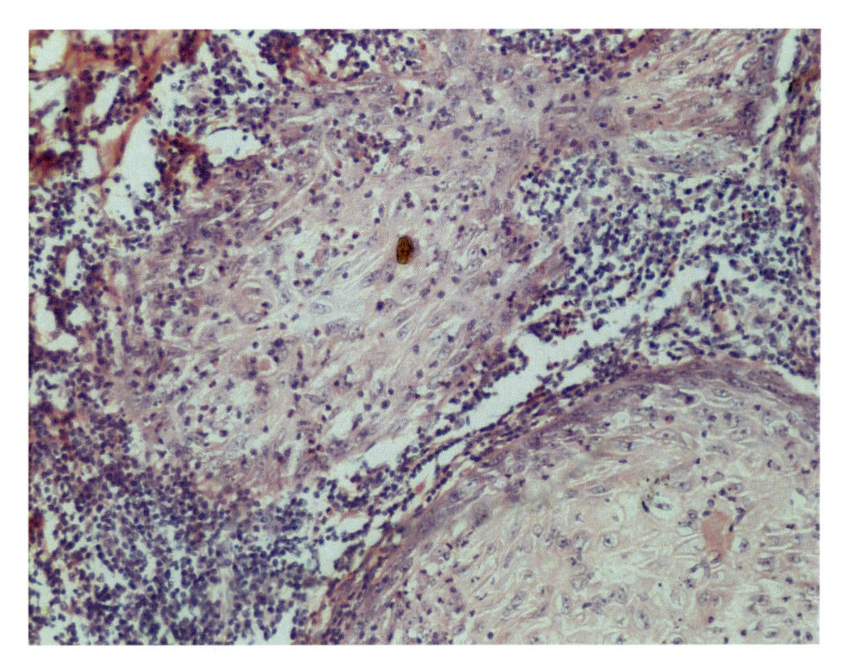

FIGURE 11.3 Section under 20× magnification showing intact basal epithelial cells with variable shape and size with high nucleocytoplasmic ratio and hyperchromatic nuclei. There are dense mononuclear inflammatory infiltrates.

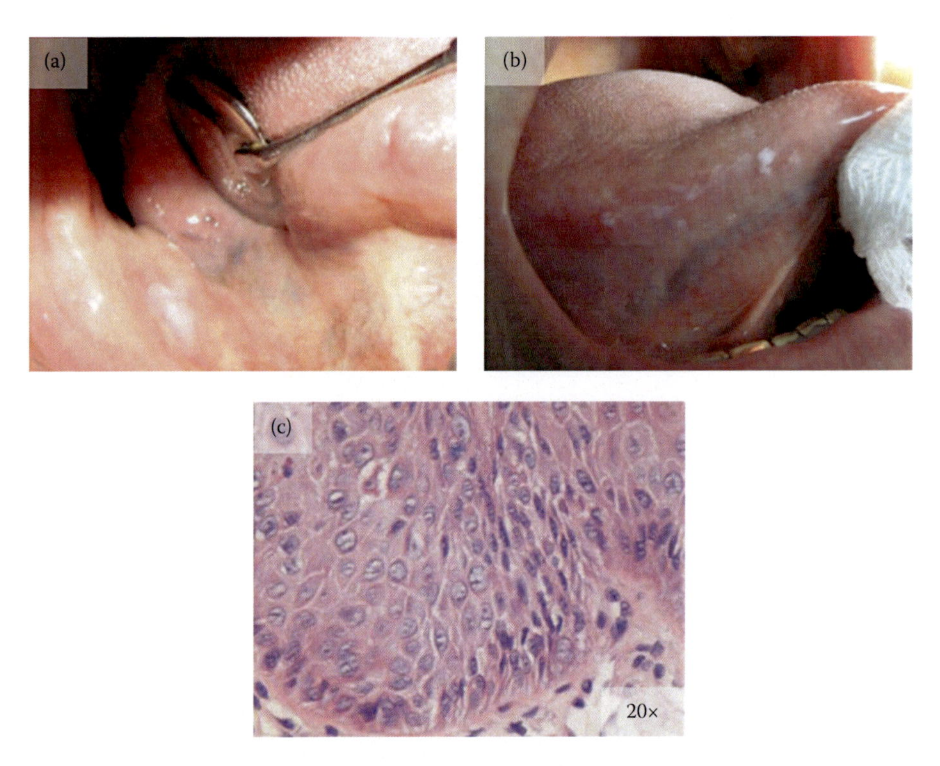

FIGURE 12.1 Early diagnosis for OSCC relies on the detection of potentially malignant disorders and early-stage carcinomas. Discrete homogeneous oral leukoplakias are observed on the (a) floor of the mouth and (b) border of the tongue, which are high-risk areas for malignant transformation. (c) Dysplasia—as noted on routine hematoxylin and eosin histopathological analysis—is still the best available predictor of malignant transformation.

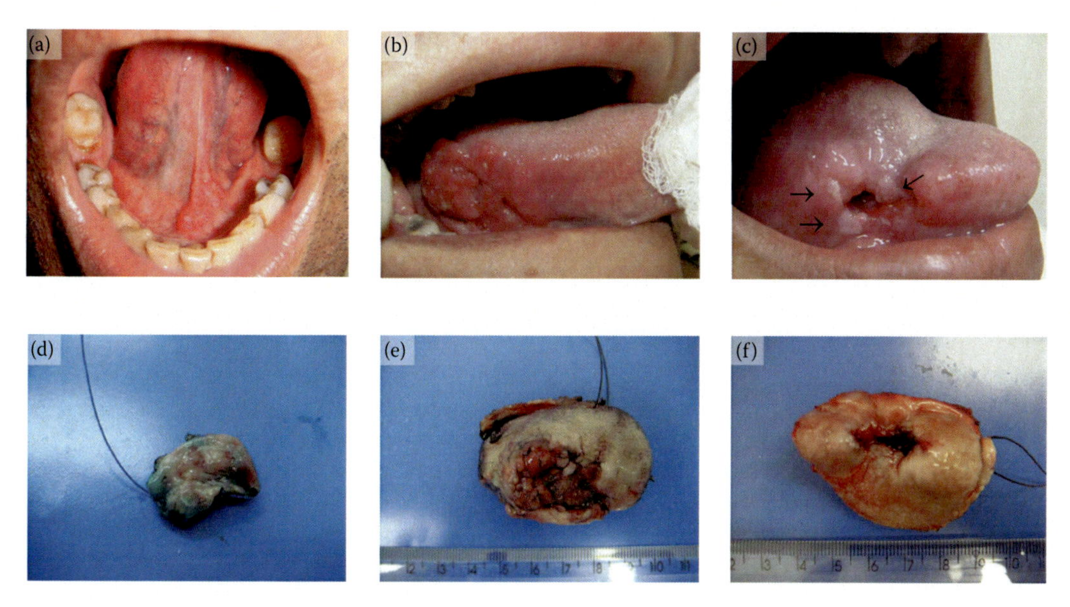

FIGURE 12.2 Clinical aspect of stages I and II SCC and surgical specimens obtained after treatment: (a) Stage I SCC of the mouth floor. (b) Stage II SCC of the tongue. (c) Stage II SCC of the tongue with an adjacent area of leukoplakia (arrows). All patients were submitted to primary surgery followed by neck dissection, because tongue and floor of mouth SCC are predisposed to develop early cervical metastases. (d–f) Surgical specimens show about 1 cm free margins. Depending on histopathological analysis of the specimen and lymph node status, patients were referred to adjuvant radiation.

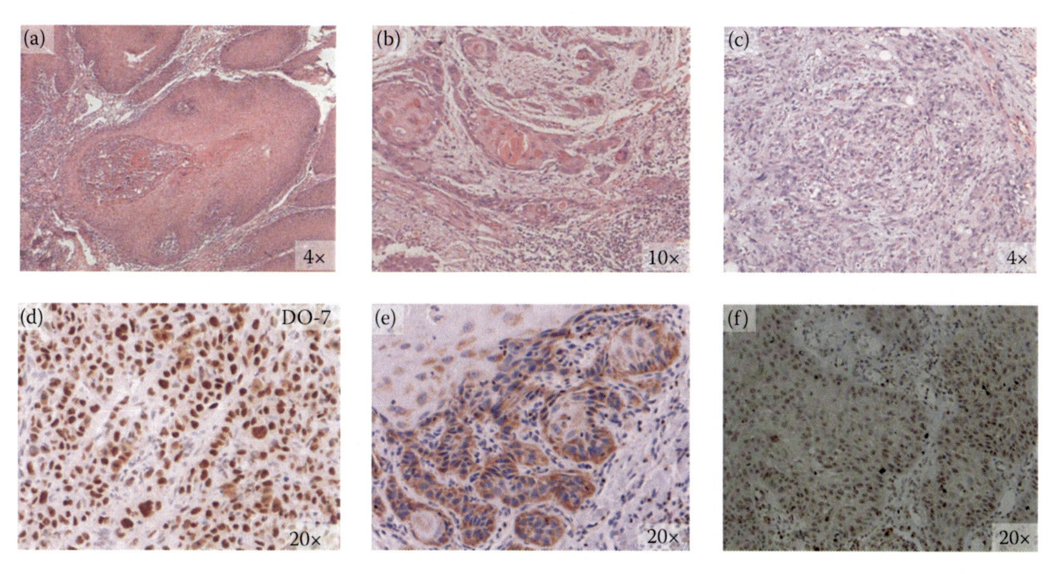

FIGURE 12.3 OSCC histopathological grading and immunohistochemical staining. Usually OSCC is graded as (a) well, (b) moderately, and (c) poorly differentiated, according to keratinocyte resemblance with normal epithelium and as suggested by WHO guidelines. Immunohistochemistry is widely used in researches in an attempt to establish markers of malignant transformation, as well as prognostic markers. Clone DO-7 for p53 protein was extensively studied in leukoplakias and (d) OSCC. Bcl-2 protein, along with other family members, (e) shows prognostic value, and (f) p16 is used in association with HPV-16 to try to determine HPV activity in the tissue.

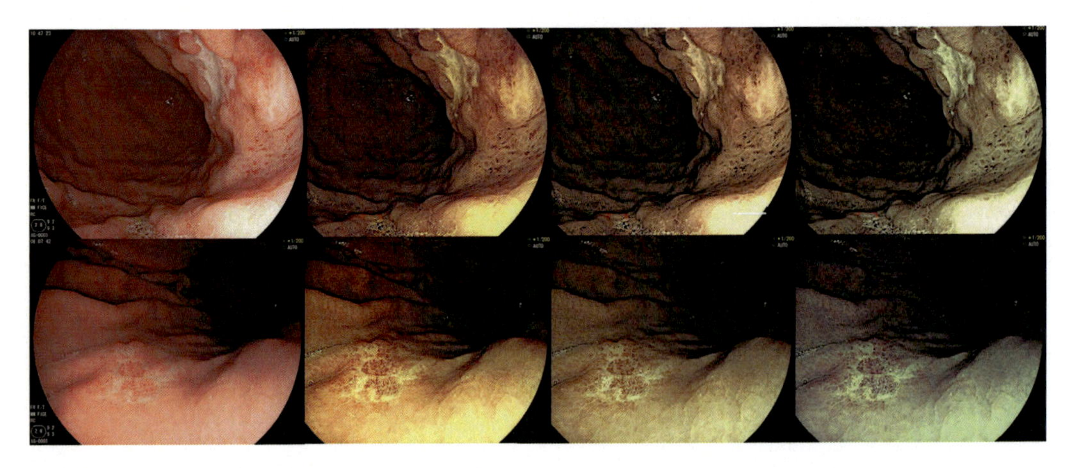

FIGURE 13.1 FICE imaging: Endoscopic image of a gastric cancer (top line) as well as a focal area with intestinal metaplasia in high-resolution white light endoscopy (left panels) and in different filter channels of an FICE device.

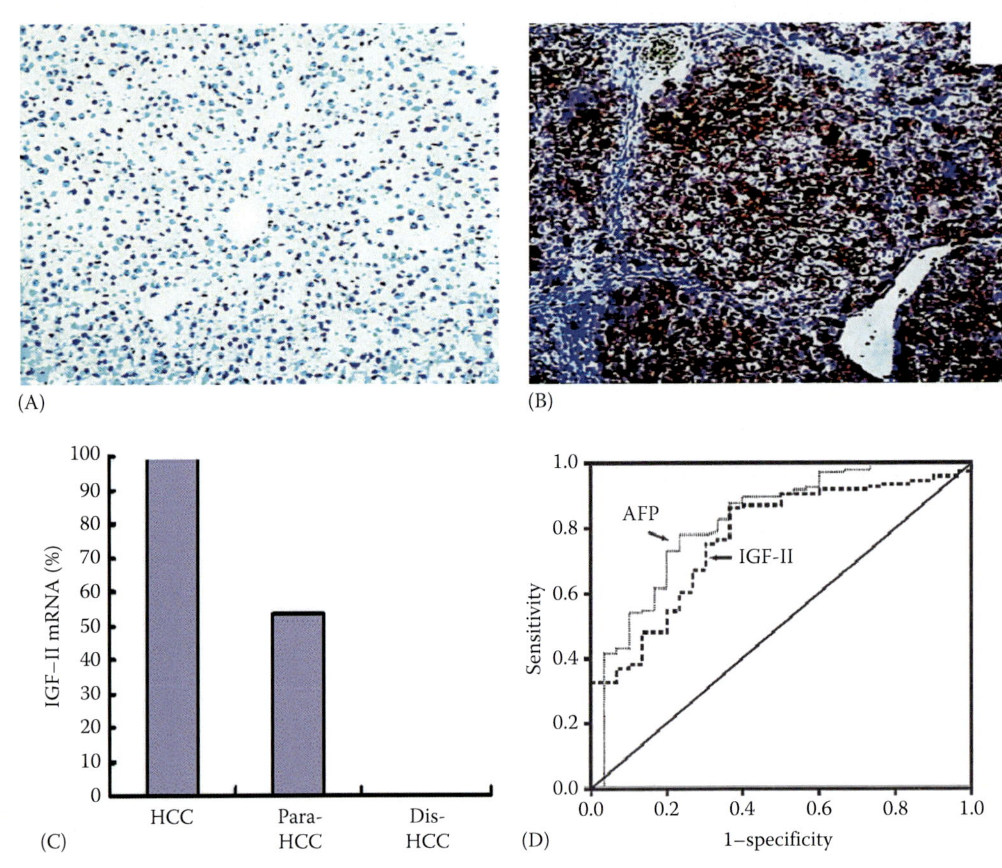

FIGURE 15.6 IGF-II expression in hepatoma tissues and blood. The expressions of hepatic IGF-II and IGF-II mRNA and diagnostic value of circulating IGF-II level for HCC: (A) without IGF-II expression in the distal cancerous tissues; (B) with the strongest IGF-II expression in HCC tissues (From Dong, Z.Z. et al., *Zhonghua Gan Zang Bing Za Zhi*, 13, 866, 2005a); (C) the percentage of IGF-II mRNA amplification from different liver tissues. HCC, paracancerous tissues, and distal cancerous tissues (From Shafizadeh, N. et al., *Mod. Pathol.*, 21, 1011, 2008; Shirakawa, H. et al., *Cancer Sci.*, 100, 1403, 2009) and (D) receiver operating characteristic (ROC) curves for the serum IGF-II investigated marker for HCC. Sensitivity, true-positive rate; specificity, false-positive rate. The area under the ROC curves was 0.823 for AFP and 0.771 for IGF-II. (From Qian, J. et al., *Am. J. Clin. Pathol.*, 134, 799, 2010.)

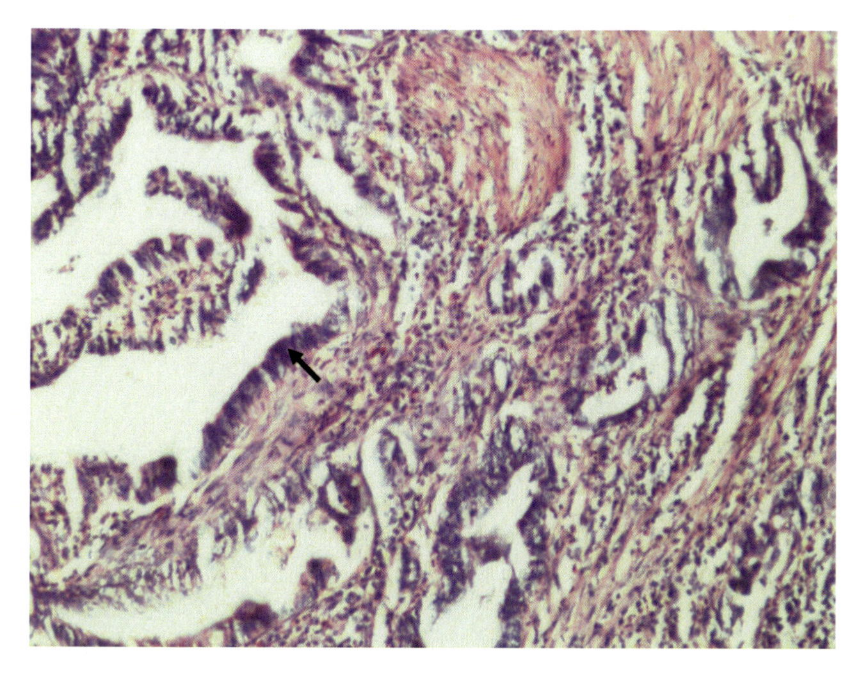

FIGURE 16.5 Well-differentiated adenocarcinoma of the gallbladder infiltrating the muscularis (HXE stain 200×).

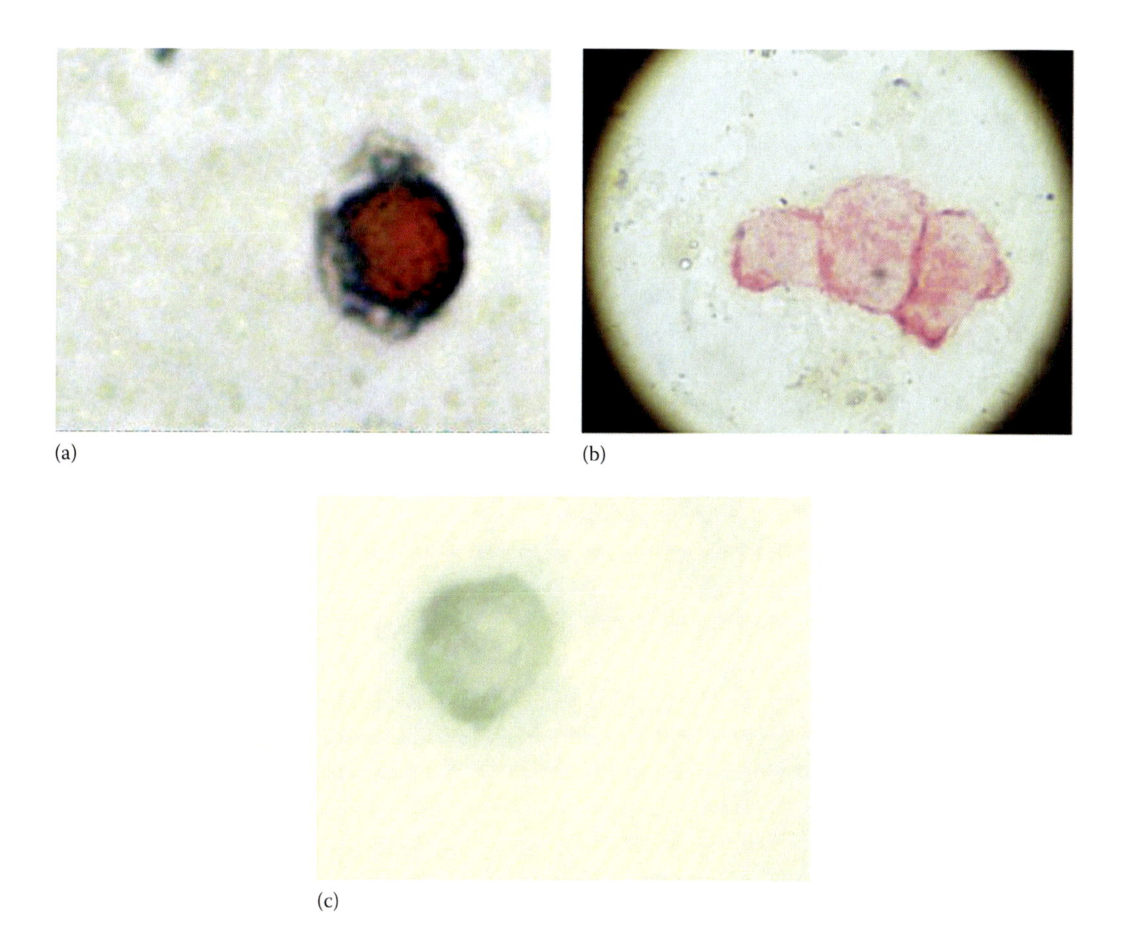

FIGURE 22.7 (a) Malignant CPC PSA (+) red and P504S (+) black. (b) Benign CPC PSA (+) red and P504S (−). (c) Leukocyte PSA (−) P504S (−).

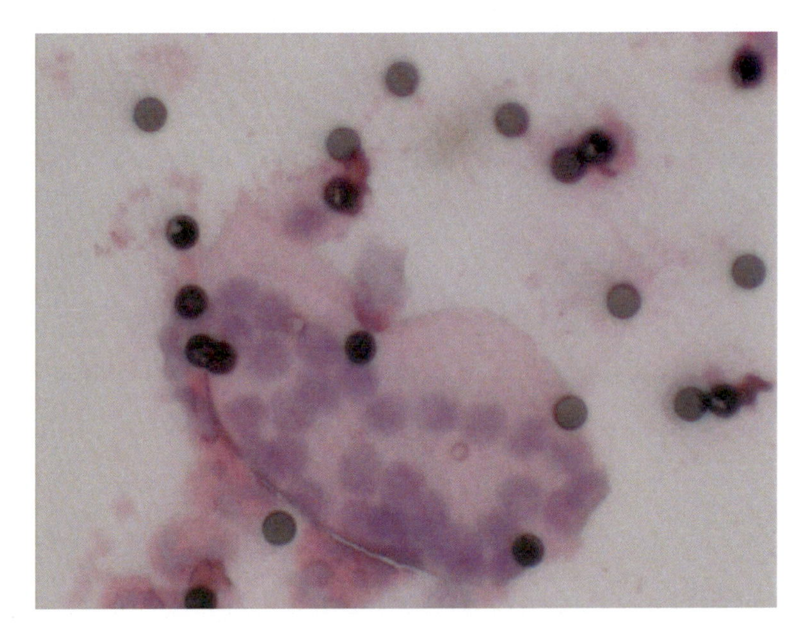

FIGURE 24.4 Capture of CTCs from an ovarian cancer patient using the ScreenCell device.

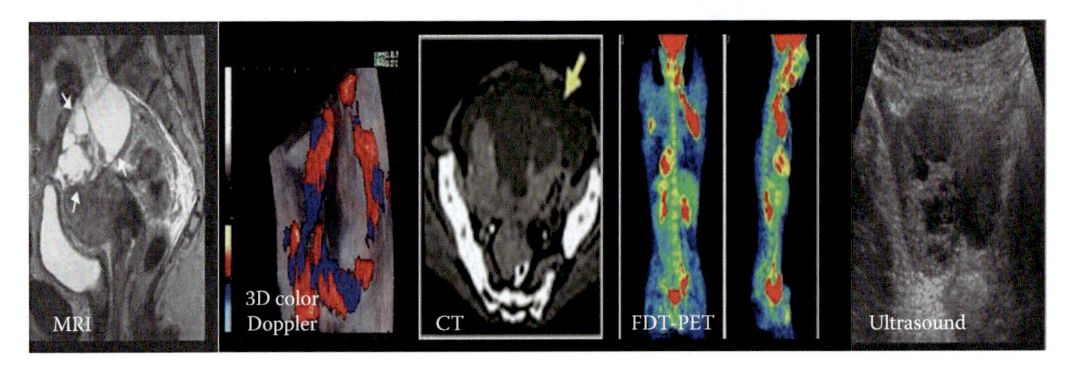

FIGURE 24.5 Different imaging methodologies used in ovarian cancer diagnosis and monitoring: MRI, 3D color Doppler, CT, FDG-PET, and ultrasound. The arrows in CT and MRI point to presumed tumor. The color Doppler shows blood flow: red for arterial and blue for venous. In the FDG-PET image, the red is activity, presumed tumor. The ultrasound shows what appears to be a normal right ovary and queries pelvic fluid/mass on the left.

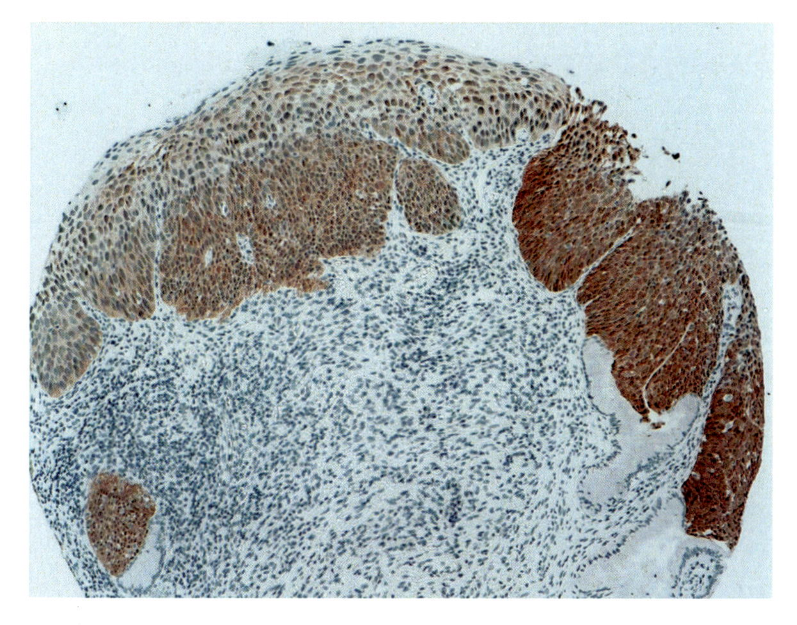

FIGURE 25.4 Tissue microarray core showing cellular localization of p16 in HSIL. Note predominant cytoplasmic staining in the lower third of the epithelium and main nuclear stain in the upper layers (H&E counterstain, ×10).

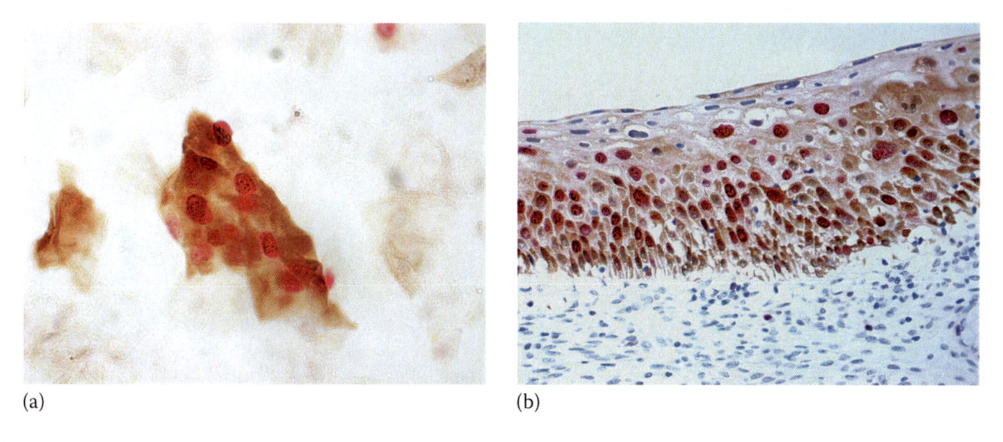

FIGURE 25.6 p16/Ki-67 dual staining: (a) Cytological specimen showing a positive dysplastic cell (middle) with both Ki-67 nuclear red and p16 cytoplasmic brown stainings surrounded by negative squamous cells (H&E counterstain, ×40). (b) Histological specimen with dual positive staining in the lower two-thirds of the epithelium (H&E counterstain, ×20).

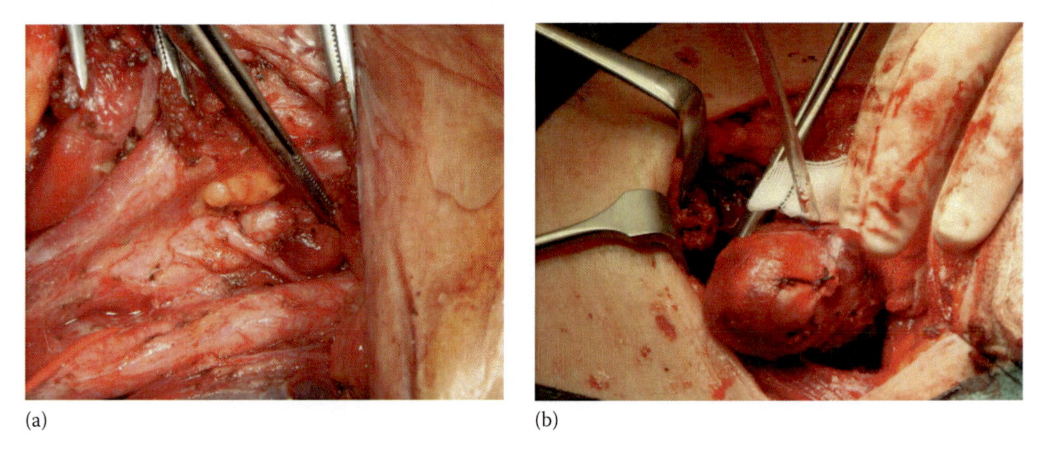
(a) (b)

FIGURE 26.1 Surgery images of PTC: (a) metastatic lymph nodes adjacent to right recurrent nerve in a case of PTC and (b) a case of PTC invading internal left jugular vein.

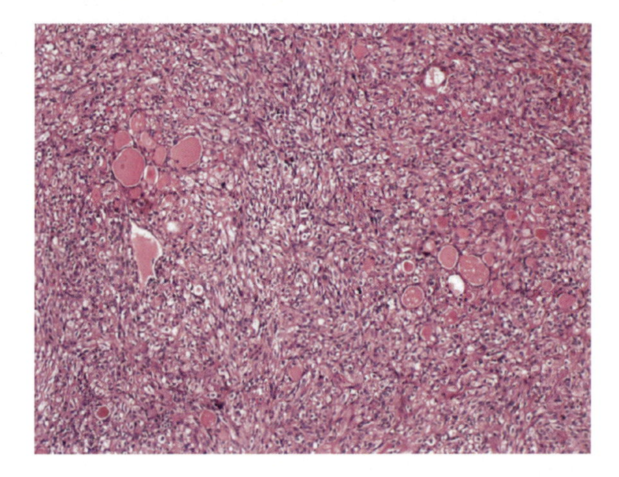

FIGURE 27.1 Hematoxylin–eosin stain of a patient with MTC. Cancer cells destructing the normal thyroid follicular patterns are seen.

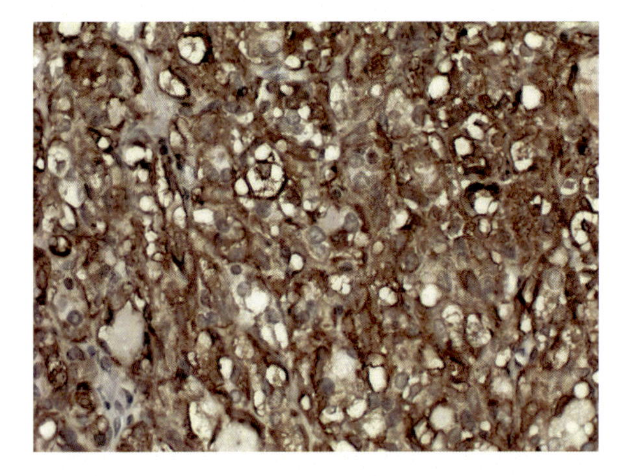

FIGURE 27.2 Immunohistochemistry with Ct. Tumor cells stained positive. Diagnosis confirmed as MTC.

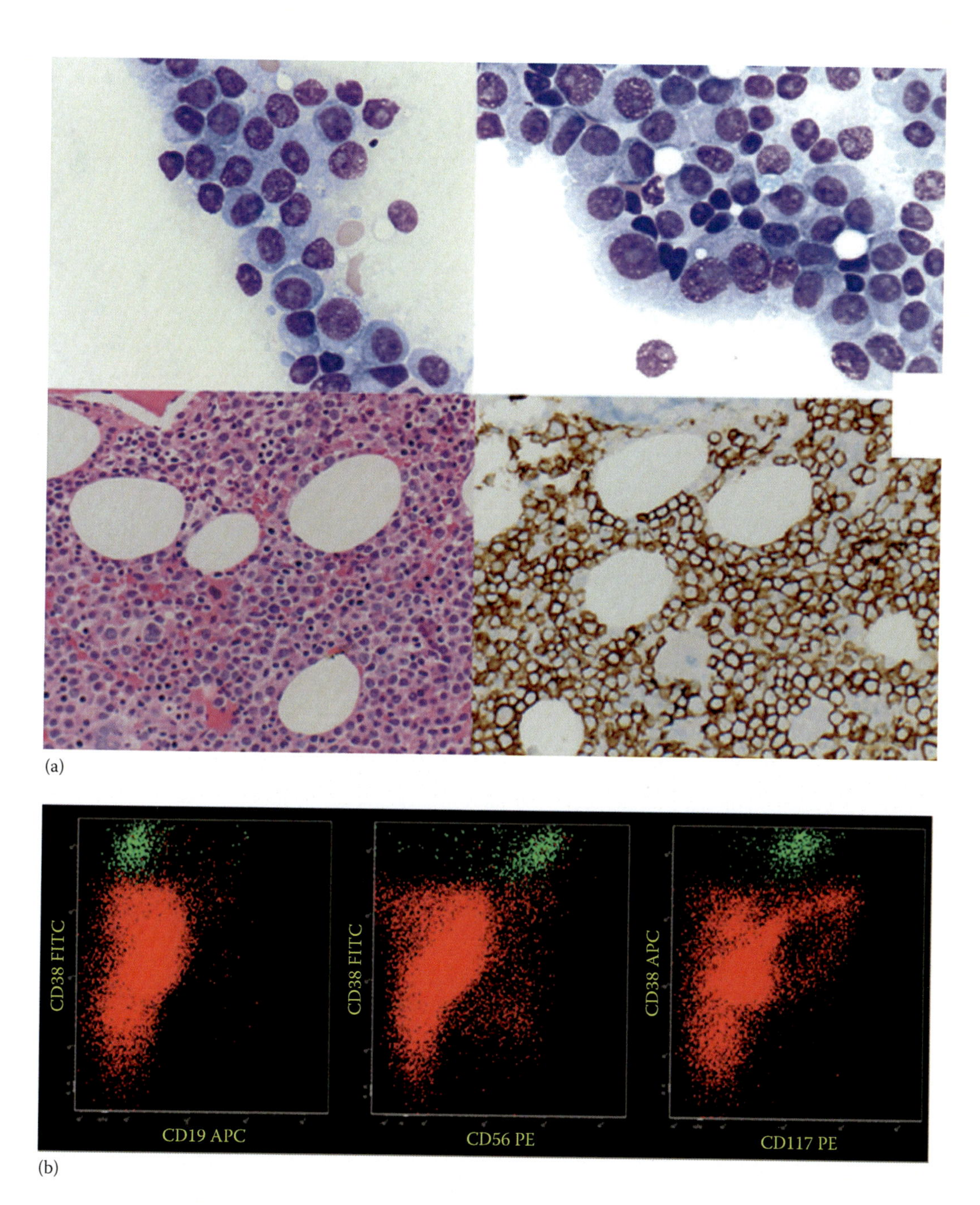

FIGURE 31.2 The essentials for the diagnosis of MM: (a) The top panels show cell morphology of BM aspirate with sheets of atypical PCs displaying big nucleoli. The lower left panel is hypercellular BM with extensive involvement with myeloma as seen in BM biopsy. The right lower panel is IHC staining for CD138 of the same BMB. (b) This panel shows the results of flow cytometry analysis documenting the abnormal phenotype of $CD38^{+}$ myeloma cells, which include $CD56^{+}$/$CD19^{-}$/$CD117^{+}$ (photographs in a and b were generously provided by Dr. Samer Al-Quran, Department of Pathology, University of Florida).

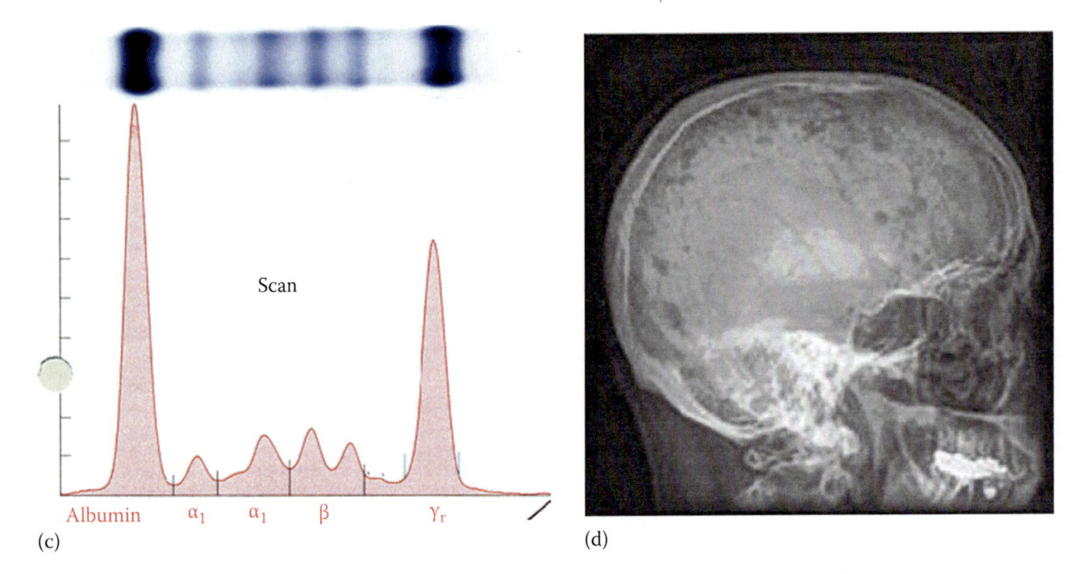

FIGURE 31.2 (continued) The essentials for the diagnosis of MM: (c) This panel shows the results of SPEP. (This example was provided generously by Dr. Neil Harris, Department of Pathology and Laboratory Medicine, University of Florida.) (d) Skull plain x-ray as part of skeletal survey performed, and it shows multiple lytic lesions typical of MM.

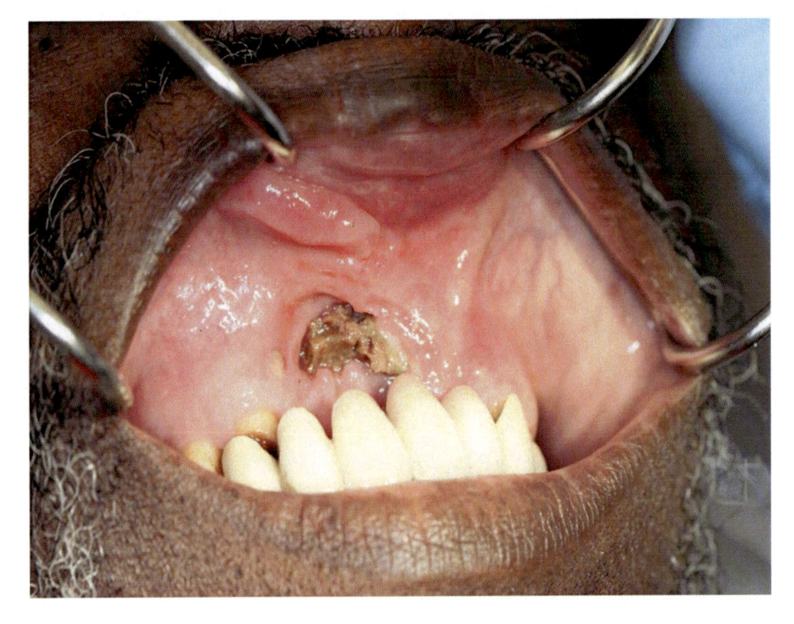

FIGURE 31.3 This photograph is of an MM patient who developed bisphosphonate-induced osteonecrosis of the upper jaw while receiving monthly intravenous zoledronic acid as part of his MM treatment.

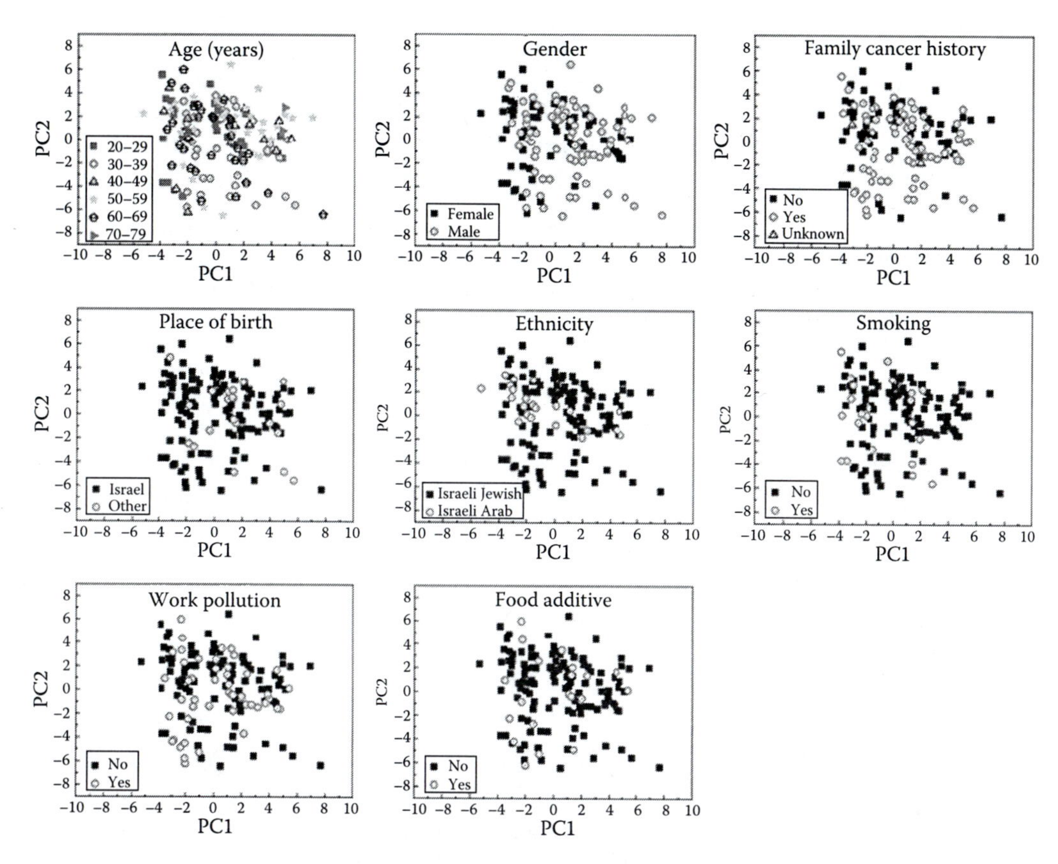

FIGURE 19.5 Stability of the breath prints obtained by sensor arrays against confounding factors. PCA plots of a sensor array comprising GNP chemiresistors, exposed to VOCs in the breath of 52 healthy subjects. Two breath samples were analyzed per test person; each point in the plot represents one breath sample. The plots were analyzed according to important confounding factors that could be relevant to future diagnostic breath testing: age, gender, family cancer history, place of birth, ethnicity, smoking habits, work pollution, and consumption of food additives. (Reprinted with permission from Macmillan Publishers Ltd. *British Journal of Cancer*, Peng et al., Copyright 2010. Nature). GNP, gold nanoparticle; PCA, principle component analysis; VOC, volatile organic compound; PC1, first principle component; PC2, second principal component.

widely used in gas and vapor sensing: adsorption and desorption of the breath VOCs from the coated membrane causes changes in its mass, which, in turn, gives rise to shifts in the resonator's frequency. However, the resonant frequency is also affected by variation in temperature and humidity, which could be important confounding factors during direct breath sampling. These two parameters should be controlled when using QCM sensor arrays for breath testing, in order to minimize their effect during the exposure to the samples. Commercial QCM sensor systems are available out on the market. Most of them are indeed designated for moisture and inorganic gas detection; for example, the Model 3050 Moisture Analyzer from Ametek is used for moisture trace detection.

Table 19.5 shows that LC markers for malignancy have been successfully demonstrated in a small-scale pilot study, using QCM sensor arrays with metal loporphyrin coatings. It was also attempted to derive a breath print marker for monitoring treatment response (lung resection), but the sensitivity of the method was very low.

19.6.3.2 Surface Acoustic Wave Sensors

In a SAW device, wave motion occurs only at the surface, penetrating to a depth of approximately one acoustic wavelength into the crystal. The direction of propagation is parallel to the surface, which can be covered with different chemiselective films. Adsorption and desorption of the breath VOCs from the coated membrane causes changes in its mass and results in a change in the mass (acoustic field of the SAW) and in the electrical conductivity (electric field of the SAW, associated with the acoustic field) of the chemical interface, influencing the SAW amplitude and phase velocity (Venema et al., 1986). SAW sensors have a higher sensitivity to most analytes than QMB sensors and the devices offer better possibilities for surface modifications. Preliminary results showed promise for deriving a breath print marker for LC malignancy, using a pair of chemically modified (polyisobutylene) SAW sensors, but the study population was too small to draw far-reaching conclusions.

19.7 Concluding Remarks and Outlook toward Future Clinical Use

Exhaled breath VOCs hold great potential for providing a new class of molecular LC markers in the near future. Either LC-specific concentration profiles of specific breath VOCs or breath prints from collective VOC patterns could be used to establish novel markers for early LC, for different pheno- and genotypes, for LC risk assessment in healthy individuals, and for monitoring treatment response. LC-specific VOC profiles may represent products of metabolic tumor activity or by-products of local inflammation in and around the tumor. Those VOC profiles could also contain partially re-emitted environmental toxins and/or could be of systemic origin. Both breath prints and individual VOCs have been studied intensively as markers of LC and of different LC phenotypes in numerous proof-of-concept studies. However, this research effort has not yet resulted in the establishment of reliable LC markers for clinical use. Insufficient attention to confounding factors in the preselected study population of small studies, and inconsistencies in the experimental techniques used for breath collection, sample storage, breath gas analysis and sensor-based breath printing, as well as disparities in the statistical analysis of the experimental data have impeded any clinical impact of the LC breath VOC marker research. Issues of standardization have to be prioritized in order to progress the field.

Breath printing by sensor arrays would be better suited than breath gas analysis for real-world clinical applications, because it is fast and potentially cost-effective and allows direct breath sampling with online results. Arrays of nanomaterial-based chemiresistors and colorimetric sensor arrays would be best suited for diagnostic breath printing. This noninvasive approach has realistic potential for becoming an integral part of population-based LC screening, posttreatment follow-up, and personalized LC management in the near future, even though the technique is not yet mature enough for imminent clinical use.

References

Aberle, D.R., Adams, A.M., Berg, C.D., Black, W.C., Clapp, J.D., Fagerstrom, R.M., Gareen, I.F. et al. 2011. Reduced lung-cancer mortality with low-dose computed tomographic screening. *N Engl J Med,* 365, 395–409.

Amann, A., Corradi, M., Mazzone, P., and Mutti, A. 2011. Lung cancer biomarkers in exhaled breath. *Expert Rev Mol Diagn,* 11, 207–217.

Amann, A., Ligor, M., Ligor, T., Bajtarevic, A., Ager, C., Pienz, M., Denz, H. et al. 2010a. Analysis of exhaled breath for screening of lung cancer patients. *Memo,* 3, 106–112.

Amann, A., Miekisch, W., Pleil, J., Risby, T., and Schubert, J. 2010b. Chapter 7: Methodological issues of sample collection and analysis of exhaled breath. *Eur Respir Monogr,* 49, 96–114.

Amann, A., Spaněl, P., and Smith, D. 2007. Breath analysis: The approach towards clinical applications. *Mini Rev Med Chem,* 7, 115–129.

Anderson, J.C., Babb, A.L., and Hlastala, M.P. 2003. Modeling soluble gas exchange in the airways and alveoli. *Ann Biomed Eng,* 31, 1402–1422.

Bach, P.B., Mirkin, J.N., Oliver, T.K., Azzoli, C.G., Berry, D.A., Brawley, O.W., Byers, T. et al. 2012. Benefits and harms of CT screening for lung cancer. *J Am Med Assoc,* 307, 2418–2429.

Bajtarevic, A., Ager, C., Pienz, M., Klieber, M., Schwarz, K., Ligor, M., Ligor, T. et al. 2009. Noninvasive detection of lung cancer by analysis of exhaled breath. *BMC Cancer,* 9, 348.

Barash, O., Peled, N., Hirsch, F.R., and Haick, H. 2009. Sniffing the unique "odor print" of non-small-cell lung cancer with gold nanoparticles. *Small,* 5, 2618–2624.

Barash, O., Peled, N., Tisch, U., Bunn, P.A., Hirsch, F.R., and Haick, H. 2012. Classification of the lung cancer histology by gold nanoparticle sensors. *Nanomed: Nanotechnol Biol Med,* 8, 580–589.

Beer, D., Kardia, S.L., Huang, C.C., Giordano, T.J., Levin, A.M., Misek, D.E., Lin, L. et al. 2002. Gene-expression profiles predict survival of patients with lung adenocarcinoma. *Nat Med,* 8, 816–824.

Brandman, S. and Ko, J.P. 2011. Pulmonary nodule detection, characterization, and management with multidetector computed tomography. *J Thorac Imaging,* 26, 90–105.

Broza, Y.Y., Kremer, R., Tisch, U., Gevorkyan, A., Shiban, A., Best, L.A., and Haick, H. 2012. A nanomaterial-based breath test for short-term follow-up after lung tumor resection. *Nanomed: Nanotechnol Biol Med,* 9, 15–21.

Brunner, C., Szymczak, W., Höllriegl, V., Mörtl, S., Oelmez, H., Bergner, A., Huber, R.M., Hoeschen, C., and Oeh, U. 2010. Discrimination of cancerous and non-cancerous cell lines by headspace-analysis with PTR-MS. *Anal Bioanal Chem,* 397, 2315–2324.

Buszewski, B., Kesy, M., Ligor, T., and Amann, A. 2007. Human exhaled air analytics: Biomarkers of diseases. *Biomed Chromatogr,* 21, 553–566.

Cao, W. and Duan, Y. 2007. Current status of methods and techniques for breath analysis. *Crit Rev Anal Chem,* 37, 3–13.

Cappuzzo, F., Ligorio, C., Toschi, L., Rossi, E., Trisolini, R., Paioli, D., Magrini, E. et al. 2007. EGFR and HER2 gene copy number and response to first-line chemotherapy in patients with advanced non-small cell lung cancer (NSCLC). *J Thorac Oncol,* 2, 423–429.

Cassidy, A., Duffy, S.W., Myles, J.P., Liloglou, T., and Field, J.K. 2007. Lung cancer risk prediction: A tool for early detection. *Int J Cancer,* 120, 1–6.

Chen, H.Y., Yu, S.L., Chen, C.H., Chang, G.C., Chen, C.Y., Yuan, A., Cheng, C.L. et al. 2007a. A five-gene signature and clinical outcome in non-small-cell lung cancer. *N Engl J Med,* 356, 11–20.

Chen, X., Cao, M., Hu, W., Wang, P., Ying, K., and Pan, H. 2005. A study of an electronic nose for detection of lung cancer based on a virtual SAW gas sensors array and imaging recognition method. *Meas Sci Technol,* 16, 1535–1546.

Chen, X., Xu, F., Wang, Y., Pan, Y., Lu, D., Wang, P., Ying, K., Chen, E., and Zhang, W. 2007b. A study of the volatile organic compounds exhaled by lung cancer cells in vitro for breath diagnosis. *Cancer,* 110, 835–844.

Culter, D.M. 2008. Are we finally winning the war on cancer? *J Eco Perspec,* 22, 3–26.

D'Amelio, A.M., Cassidy, A., Asomaning, K., Raji, O.Y., Duffy, S.W., Field, J.K., Spitz, M.R., Christiani, D., and Etzel, C.J. 2010. Comparison of discriminatory power and accuracy of three lung cancer risk models. *Br J Cancer,* 103, 423–429.

D'Amico, A., Penazza, G., Santonico, M., Martinelli, E., Roscioni, C., Galluccio, G., Paolesse, R., and Di Natale, C. 2010. An investigation on electronic nose diagnosis of lung cancer. *Lung Cancer,* 68, 170–176.

Darwiche, K., Baumbach, J.I., Sommerwerck, U., Teschler, H., and Freitag, L. 2011. Bronchoscopically obtained volatile biomarkers in lung cancer. *Lung,* 189, 445–452.

Deng, C., Zhang, X., and Li, N. 2004. Investigation of volatile biomarkers in lung cancer blood using solid-phase microextraction and capillary gas chromatography-mass spectrometry. *J Chromatogr B,* 808, 269–277.

Detterbeck, F.C., Boffa, D.J., and Tanoue, L.T. 2009. The new lung cancer staging system. *Chest,* 136, 260–271.

Di Natale, C., Macagnano, A., Martinelli, E., Paolesse, R., D'Arcangelo, G., Roscioni, C., Finazzi-Agro, A., and D'Amico, A. 2003. Lung cancer identification by the analysis of breath by means of an array of non-selective gas sensors. *Biosens Bioelectron,* 18, 1209–1218.

Dragonieri, S., Annema, J.T., Schot, R., van der Schee, M.P.C., Spanevello, A., Carratú, P., Resta, O., Rabe, K.F., and Sterk, P.J. 2009. An electronic nose in the discrimination of patients with non-small cell lung cancer and COPD. *Lung Cancer,* 64, 166–170.

Etzel, C.J. and Bach, P.B. 2011. Estimating individual risk for lung cancer. *Semin Respir Crit Care Med,* 32, 3–9.

Fedrigo, M., Hoeschen, C., and Oeh, U. 2010. Multidimensional statistical analysis of PTR-MS breath samples: A test study on irradiation detection. *Int J Mass Spectrom,* 295, 13–20.

Filipiak, W., Sponring, A., Filipiak, A., Ager, C., Schubert, J., Miekisch, W., Amann, A., and Troppmair, J. 2010. TD-GC-MS analysis of volatile metabolites of human lung cancer and normal cells in vitro. *Cancer Epidemiol Biomarkers Prev,* 19, 182–195.

Filipiak, W., Sponring, A., Mikoviny, T., Ager, C., Schubert, J., Miekisch, W., Amann, A., and Troppmair, J. 2008. Release of volatile organic compounds (VOCs) from the lung cancer cell line CALU-1 in vitro. *Cancer Cell Int,* 8, 17.

Fuchs, P., Loeseken, C., Schubert, J.K., and Miekisch, W. 2010. Breath gas aldehydes as biomarkers of lung cancer. *Int J Cancer,* 126, 2663–2670.

Gordon, S.M., Szidon, J.P., Krotoszynski, B.K., Gibbons, R.D., and O'Neill, H.J. 1985. Volatile organic compounds in exhaled air from patients with lung cancer. *Clin Chem,* 31, 1278–1282.

Grate, J.W., Martin, S.J., and White, R.M. 1993. Acoustic wave microsensors, Part 1. *Anal Chem,* 65, 940A–948A.

Greenberg, A.K., Lu, F., Goldberg, J.D., Eylers, E. et al. 2012. CT scan screening for lung cancer: Risk factors for nodules and malignancy in a high-risk urban cohort. *PLoS One,* 7, e39403.

Guo, A., Villén, J., Kornhauser, J., Lee, K.A., Stokes, M.P., Rikova, K., Possemato, A. et al. 2008. Signaling networks assembled by oncogenic EGFR and c-Met. *Proc Natl Acad Sci USA,* 105, 692–697.

Hakim, M., Billan, S., Tisch, U., Peng, G., Dvrokind, I., Marom, O., Abdah-Bortnyak, R., Kuten, A., and Haick, H. 2011. Diagnosis of head-and-neck cancer from exhaled breath. *Br J Cancer,* 104, 1649–1655.

Hakim, M., Broza, Y.Y., Barash, O., Peled, N., Phillips, M., Amann, A., and Haick, H. 2012. Volatile organic compounds of lung cancer and possible biochemical pathways. *Chem Rev,* 112, 5949–5966.

Hamilton, S.R. 2012. Molecular pathology. *Mol Oncol,* 6, 177–181.

Hochhegger, B., Marchiori, E., Sedlaczek, O., Irion, K., Heussel, C.P., Ley, S., Ley-Zaporozhan, J., Soares, S.A.J., and Kauczor, H.U. 2011. MRI in lung cancer: A pictorial essay. *Br J Radiol,* 84, 661–668.

Horvath, L., Lazar, Z., Gyulai, N., Kollai, M., and Losonczy, G. 2009. Exhaled biomarkers in lung cancer. *Eur Respir J,* 34, 261–275.

Jackman, D.M., Yeap, B.Y., Sequist, L.V., Lindeman, N., Holmes, A.J., Joshi, V.A., Bell, D.W. et al. 2006. Exon 19 deletion mutations of epidermal growth factor receptor are associated with prolonged survival in non-small cell lung cancer patients treated with gefitinib or erlotinib. *Clin Cancer Res,* 12, 3908–3914.

Jakubowski, M. and Czerczak, S. 2009. Calculating the retention of volatile organic compounds in the lung on the basis of their physicochemical properties. *Environ Toxicol Pharmacol,* 28, 311–315.

Jemal, A., Bray, F., Center, M.M., Ferlay, J., Ward, E., and Forman, D. 2011. Global cancer statistics. *CA Cancer J Clin,* 61, 69–90.

Jemal, A., Siegel, R., Xu, J., and Ward, E. 2010. Cancer statistics, 2010. *CA Cancer J Clin,* 60, 277–300.

Kalliomäki, P.-L., Korhonen, O., Vaaranen, V., Kalliomäki, K., and Koponen, M. 1978. Lung retention and clearance of shipyard arc welders. *Int Arch Occur Environ Health,* 42, 83–90.

Karpas, Z. 2009. Ion mobility spectrometry: A tool in the war against terror. *Bull Israel Chem Soc,* 24, 26–30.

King, J., Koc, H., Unterkofler, K., Mochalski, P., Kupferthaler, A., Teschl, G., Teschl, S., Hinterhuber, H., and Amann, A. 2010a. Physiological modeling of isoprene dynamics in exhaled breath. *J Theor Biol,* 267, 626–637.

King, J., Kupferthaler, A., Frauscher, B., Hackner, H., Unterkofler, K., Teschl, G., Hinterhuber, H., Amann, A., and Högl, B. 2012a. Measurement of endogenous acetone and isoprene in exhaled breath during sleep. *Physiol Meas,* 33, 413–428.

King, J., Kupferthaler, A., Unterkofler, K., Koç, H., Teschl, S., Teschl, G., Miekisch, W. et al. 2009. Isoprene and acetone concentration profiles during exercise on an ergometer. *J Breath Res,* 3, 027006.

King, J., Mochalski, P., Kupferthaler, A., Unterkofler, K., Filipiak, W., Teschl, S., Teschl, G., Hinterhuber, H., and Amann, A. 2010b. Dynamic profiles of volatile organic compounds in exhaled breath as determined by a coupled PTR-MS/GC-MS study. *Physiol Meas,* 31, 1169–1184.

King, J., Unterkofler, K., Teschl, G., Teschl, S., Koc, H., Hinterhuber, H., and Amann, A. 2011. A mathematical model for breath gas analysis of volatile organic compounds with special emphasis on acetone. *J Math Biol,* 63, 959–999.

King, J., Unterkofler, K., Teschl, G., Teschl, S., Mochalski, P., Koç, H., Hinterhuber, H., and Amann, A. 2012b. A modeling-based evaluation of isothermal rebreathing for breath gas analyses of highly soluble volatile organic compounds. *J Breath Res,* 6, 016005.

Kischkel, S., Miekisch, W., Sawacki, A., Straker, E.M., Trefz, P., Amann, A., and Schubert, J.K. 2010. Breath biomarkers for lung cancer detection and assessment of smoking related effects—Confounding variables, influence of normalization and statistical algorithms. *Clin Chim Acta,* 411, 1637–1644.

Konvalina, G. and Haick, H. 2012. Effect of humidity on nanoparticle-based chemiresistors: A comparison between synthetic and real-world samples. *ACS Appl Mater Interfaces,* 4, 317–325.

Kumar, S., Mohan, A., and Guleria, R. 2006. Biomarkers in cancer screening, research and detection: Present and future: A review. *Biomarkers,* 11, 385–405.

Kushch, I., Arendacká, B., Štolc, S., Mochalski, P., Filipiak, W., Schwarz, K., Schwentner, L. et al. 2008. Breath isoprene–aspects of normal physiology related to age, gender and cholesterol profile as determined in a proton transfer reaction mass spectrometry study. *Clin Chem Lab Med,* 46, 1011–1018.

Lechner, M., Moser, B., Niederseer, D., Karlseder, A., Holzknecht, B., Fuchs, M., Colvin, S., Tilg, H., and Rieder, J. 2006. Gender and age specific differences in exhaled isoprene levels. *Respir Physiol Neurobiol,* 154, 478–483.

Ligor, M., Ligor, T., Bajtarevic, A., Ager, C., Pienz, M., Klieber, M., Denz, H. et al. 2009. Determination of volatile organic compounds appearing in exhaled breath of lung cancer patients by solid phase microextraction and gas chromatography mass spectrometry. *Clin Chem Lab Med,* 47, 550–560.

Lili, L., Xu, H., Song, D., Cui, Y., Hu, S., and Zhang, G. 2010. Analysis of volatile aldehyde biomarkers in human blood by derivatization and dispersive liquid–liquid microextraction based on solidification of floating organic droplet method by high performance liquid chromatography. *J Chromatogr A,* 1217, 2365–2370.

Lindinger, W. and Jordan, A. 1998. Proton-transfer-reaction mass spectrometry (PTR–MS): On-line monitoring of volatile organic compounds at pptv levels. *Chem Soc Rev,* 27, 347–375.

Machado, R.F., Laskowski, D., Deffenderfer, O., Burch, T., Zheng, S., Mazzone, P.J., Mekhail, T. et al. 2005. Detection of lung cancer by sensor array analyses of exhaled breath. *Am J Respir Crit Care Med,* 171, 1286–1291.

Macmahon, H. 2010. Compliance with fleischner society guidelines for management of lung nodules: Lessons and opportunities. *Radiology,* 255, 14–15.

Mano, H. 2008. Non-solid oncogenes in solid tumors: EML4-ALK fusion genes in lung cancer. *Cancer Sci,* 99, 2349–2355.

Mazzone, P. 2008. Progress in the development of a diagnostic test for lung cancer through the analysis of breath volatiles. *J Breath Res,* 2, 037014.

Mazzone, P.J., Hammel, J., Dweik, R., Na, J., Czich, C., Laskowski, D., and Mekhail, T. 2007. Diagnosis of lung cancer by the analysis of exhaled breath with a colorimetric sensor array. *Thorax,* 62, 565–568.

Mazzone, P.J., Wang, X.F., Xu, Y., Mekhail, T., Beukemann, M.C., Na, J., Kemling, J.W., Suslick, K.S., and Sasidhar, M. 2011. Exhaled breath analysis with a colorimetric sensor array for the identification and characterization of lung cancer. *J Thorac Oncol,* 7, 137–142.

McWilliams, A. and Lam, S. 2005. Lung cancer screening. *Curr Opin Pulm Med,* 11, 272–277.

Mendis, S., Sobotka, P.A., and Euler, D.E. 1994. Pentane and isoprene in expired air from humans: Gas-chromatographic analysis of single breath. *Clin Chem,* 40, 1485–1488.

Miekisch, W., Schubert, J.K., and Noeldge-Schomburg, G.F.E. 2004. Diagnostic potential of breath analysis–Focus on volatile organic compounds. *Clin Chim Acta,* 347, 25–39.

Modak, A.S. 2010. Breath biomarkers for personalized medicine. *Pers Med,* 7, 643–653.

Musa-Veloso, K., Likhodii, S.S., and Cunnane, S.C. 2002. Breath acetone is a reliable indicator of ketosis in adults consuming ketogenic meals. *Am J Clin Nut,* 76, 65–70.

Olaussen, K.A., Dunant, A., Fouret, P., Brambilla, E., André, F., Haddad, V., Taranchon, E. et al. 2006. DNA repair by ERCC1 in non-small-cell lung cancer and cisplatin-based adjuvant chemotherapy. *N Engl J Med,* 355, 983–991.

O'Neill, H.J., Gordon, S.M., O'Neill, M.H., Gibbons, R.D., and Szidon, J.P. 1988. A computerized classification technique for screening for the presence of breath biomarkers in lung cancer. *Clin Chem,* 34, 1613–1618.

Patel, M., Lu, L., Zander, D. S., Sreerama, L., Coco, D., and Moreb, J.S. 2008. ALDH1A1 and ALDH3A1 expression in lung cancers: Correlation with histologic type and potential precursors. *Lung Cancer,* 59, 340–349.

Peled, N., Barash, O., Tisch, U., Ionescu, R., Broza, Y.Y., Ilouze, M., Mattei, J. et al. 2013. Volatile fingerprints of cancer specific genetic mutations. *Nanomedicine,* 9, 758–766.

Peled, N., Hakim, M., Bunn, Jr., P.A., Miller, Y.E., Kennedy, T.C., Mattei, J., Mitchell, J.D., Hirsch, F.R., and Haick, H. 2012. Non-invasive breath analysis of pulmonary nodules. *J Thorac Oncol,* 7, 1528–1533.

Peng, G., Hakim, M., Broza, Y.Y., Billan, S., Abdah-Bortnyak, R., Kuten, A., Tisch, U., and Haick, H. 2010. Detection of lung, breast, colorectal, and prostate cancers from exhaled breath using a single array of nanosensors. *Br J Cancer,* 103, 542–551.

Peng, G., Tisch, U., Adams, O., Hakim, M., Shehada, N., Broza, Y.Y., Billan, S. et al. 2009a. Diagnosing lung cancer in exhaled breath using gold nanoparticles. *Nature Nanotech,* 4, 669–673.

Peng, G., Tisch, U., and Haick, H. 2009b. Detection of nonpolar molecules by means of carrier scattering in random networks of carbon nanotubes: Toward diagnosis of diseases via breath samples. *Nano Lett,* 9, 1362–1368.

Peng, G., Trock, E., and Haick, H. 2008. Detecting simulated patterns of lung cancer biomarkers by random network of single-walled carbon nanotubes coated with non-polymeric organic materials. *Nano Lett,* 8, 3631–3635.

Pennazza, G., Santonicoa, M., and Agròb, A.F. 2013. Narrowing the gap between breathprinting and disease diagnosis, a sensor perspective. *Sensor Actuat B-Chem,* 179, 270–275.

Persaud, K. and Dodd, G. 1982. Analysis of discrimination mechanisms in the mammalian olfactory system using a model nose. *Nature,* 299, 352–355.

Phillips, M., Altorki, N., Austin, J.H.M., Cameron, R.B. et al. 2007. Prediction of lung cancer using volatile biomarkers in breath. *Cancer Biomarkers,* 3, 95–109.

Phillips, M., Altorki, N., Austin, J.H.M., Cameron, R.B., Cataneo, R.N., Kloss, R., Maxfield, R.A. et al. 2008. Detection of lung cancer using weighted digital analysis of breath biomarkers. *Clin Chim Acta,* 393, 76–84.

Phillips, M., Cataneo, R.N., Cummin, A.R., Gagliardi, A.J., Gleeson, K., Greenberg, J., Maxfield, R.A., and Rom, W.N. 2003. Detection of lung cancer with volatile markers in the breath. *Chest,* 123, 2115–2123.

Phillips, M., Gleeson, K., Hughes, J.M., Greenberg, J., Cataneo, R.N., Baker, L., and Mcvay, W.P. 1999. Volatile organic compounds in breath as markers of lung cancer: A cross-sectional study. *Lancet,* 353, 1930–1933.

Phillips, M., Greenberg, J., and Awad, J. 1994. Metabolic and environmental origins of volatile organic compounds in breath. *J Clin Pathol,* 47, 1052.

Pleasance, E.D., Cheetham, R.K., Stephens, P.J., Mcbride, D.J., Humphray, S.J., Greenman, C.D., Varela, I. et al. 2010. A comprehensive catalogue of somatic mutations from a human cancer genome. *Nature,* 463, 191–196.

Poli, D., Carbognani, P., Corradi, M., Goldoni, M., Acampa, O., Balbi, B., Bianchi, L., Rusca, M., and Mutti, A. 2005. Exhaled volatile organic compounds in patients with non-small cell lung cancer: Cross sectional and nested short-term follow-up study. *Respir Res,* 6, 71.

Poli, D., Goldoni, M., Caglieri, A., Ceresa, G., Acampa, O., Carbognani, P., Rusca, M., and Corradi, M. 2008. Breath analysis in non small cell lung cancer patients after surgical tumour resection. *Acta Biomed,* 79, 64–72.

Poli, D., Goldoni, M., Corradi, M., Acampa, O., Carbognani, P., Internullo, E., Casalini, A., and Mutti, A. 2010. Determination of aldehydes in exhaled breath of patients with lung cancer by means of on-fiber-derivatisation SPME-GC/MS. *J Chromatogr B Analyt Technol Biomed Life Sci,* 878, 2643–2651.

Potti, A., Dressman, H.K., Bild, A., Riedel, R.F., Chan, G., Sayer, R., Cragun, J. et al. 2006a. Genomic signatures to guide the use of chemotherapeutics. *Nat Med,* 12, 1294–1300.

Potti, A., Mukherjee, S., Petersen, R., Dressman, H.K., Bild, A., Koontz, J., Kratzke, R. et al. 2006b. A genomic strategy to refine prognosis in early-stage non-small-cell lung cancer. *N Engl J Med,* 355, 570–580.

Preti, G., Labows, J.N., Kostelc, J.G., Aldinger, S., and Daniele, R. 1988. Analysis of lung air from patients with bronchogenic carcinoma and controls using gas chromatography-mass spectrometry. *J Chromatogr,* 432, 1–11.

Risby, T.H. and Sehnert, S.S. 1999. Clinical application of breath biomarkers of oxidative stress status. *Free Radic Biol Med,* 27, 1182–1192.

Risby, T.H. and Solga, S.F. 2006. Current status of clinical breath analysis. *Appl Phys B,* 85, 421–426.

Röck, F., Barsan, N., and Weimar, U. 2008. Electronic nose: Current status and future trends. *Chem Rev,* 108, 705–725.

Rossi, E.D., Mulè, A., Maggiore, C., Miraglia, A., Lauriola, L., Vecchio, F.M., and Fadda, G. 2004. Bronchofiberscopy. *Rays,* 29, 357–361.

Sanchez, M.D.N., Garcia, E.H., Pavon, J.L.P., and Cordero, B.M. 2012. Fast analytical methodology based on mass spectrometry for the determination of volatile biomarkers in saliva. *Anal Chem,* 84, 379–385.

Schoening, M.J. 2005. "Playing around" with field-effect sensors on the basis of EIS structures, LAPS and ISFETs. *Sensors* 5, 126–138.

Shaw, A.T., and Solomon, B. 2011. Targeting anaplastic lymphoma kinase in lung cancer. *Clin Cancer Res,* 17, 2081–2086.

Shaw, A.T., Yeap, B.Y., Mino-Kenudson, M., Digumarthy, S.R., Costa, D.B., Heist, R.S., Solomon, B. et al. 2009. Clinical features and outcome of patients with non-small-cell lung cancer who harbor EML4-ALK. *J Clin Oncol,* 27, 4247–4253.

Smith, D., Wang, T., Sulé-Suso, J., Spanel, P., and El Haj, A. 2003. Quantification of acetaldehyde released by lung cancer cells in vitro using selected ion flow tube mass spectrometry. *Rapid Commun Mass Spectrom,* 17, 845–850.

Song, G., Qin, T., Liu, H., Xu, G.B., Pan, Y.Y., Xiong, F.X., Gu, K.S., Sun, G.P., and Chen, Z.D. 2010. Quantitative breath analysis of volatile organic compounds of lung cancer patients. *Lung Cancer,* 67, 227–231.

Spitz, M.R., Hong, W.K., Amos, C.I., Wu, X., Schabath, M.B., Dong, Q., Shete, S., and Etzel, C.J. 2007. A risk model for prediction of lung cancer. *J Natl Cancer Inst,* 99, 715–726.

Sponring, A., Filipiak, W., Ager, C., Schubert, J., Miekisch, W., Amann, A., and Troppmair, J. 2010. Analysis of volatile organic compounds (VOCs) in the headspace of NCI-H1666 lung cancer cells. *Cancer Biomarkers,* 7, 153–161.

Sponring, A., Filipiak, W., Mikoviny, T., Ager, C., Schubert, J., Miekisch, W., Amann, A., and Troppmair, J. 2009. Release of volatile organic compounds from the lung cancer cell line NCI-H2087 in vitro. *Anticancer Res,* 29, 419–426.

Sulé-Suso, J., Pysanenko, A., Španěl, L.P., and Smith, D. 2009. Quantification of acetaldehyde and carbon dioxide in the headspace of malignant and non-malignant lung cells in vitro by SIFT-MS. *Analyst,* 134, 2419–2425.

Szulejko, J.E., Mcculloch, M., Jackson, J., Mckee, D.L., Walker, J.C., and Solouki, T. 2010. Evidence for cancer biomarkers in exhaled breath—A review. *IEEE Sens J,* 10, 185–210.

Taguchi, F., Solomon, B., Gregorc, V., Roder, H., Gray, R., Kasahara, K., Nishio, M. et al. 2007. Mass spectrometry to classify non-small-cell lung cancer patients for clinical outcome after treatment with epidermal growth factor receptor tyrosine kinase inhibitors: A multicohort cross-institutional study. *J Natl Cancer Inst,* 99, 838–846.

Tammemagi, C.M., Pinsky, P.F., Caporaso, N.E., Kvale, P.A., Hocking, W.G., Church, T.R., Riley, T.L. et al. 2011. Lung cancer risk prediction: Prostate, lung, colorectal and ovarian cancer screening trial models and validation. *J Natl Cancer Inst* 103, 1058–1068.

Tisch, U., Billan, S., Ilouze, M., Phillips, M., Peled, N., and Haick, H. 2012. Volatile organic compounds in exhaled breath as biomarkers for the early detection and screening of lung cancer. *CML-Lung Cancer,* 5, 107–117.

Tisch, U. and Haick, H. 2010. Arrays of chemisensitive monolayer-capped metallic nanoparticles for diagnostic breath testing. *Rev Chem Eng,* 26, 171–179.

Todd, J. and Mcgrath, E.E. 2011. Chest x-ray mass in a patient with lung cancer. *QJM,* 104, 903–904.

Truong, M.T., Viswanathan, C., and Erasmus, J.J. 2011. Positron emission tomography/computed tomography in lung cancer staging, prognosis, and assessment of therapeutic response. *J Thorac Imaging,* 26, 132–146.

Venema, A., Nieuwkoop, E., Vellekoop, M.J., Nieuwenhuizen, M.S., and Barendsz, A.W. 1986. Design aspects of SAW gas sensors. *Sens Actuat,* 10, 47–64.

Wehinger, A., Schmid, A., Mechtcheriakov, S., Ledochowski, M., Grabmer, C., Gastl, G.A., and Amann, A. 2007. Lung cancer detection by proton transfer reaction mass-spectrometric analysis of human breath gas. *Int J Mass Spectrom,* 265, 49–59.

Weiss, G.J., Bemis, L.T., Nakajima, E., Sugita, M., Birks, D.K., Robinson, W.A., Varella-Garcia, M. et al. 2008. EGFR regulation by microRNA in lung cancer: Correlation with clinical response and survival to gefitinib and EGFR expression in cell lines. *Ann Oncol,* 19, 1053–1059.

Westhoff, M., Litterst, P., Freitag, L., Urfer, W., Bader, S., and Baumbach, J.I. 2009. Ion mobility spectrometry for the detection of volatile organic compounds in exhaled breath of patients with lung cancer: Results of a pilot study. *Thorax,* 64, 744–748.

Wong, D.W., Leung, E.L., So, K.K., Tam, I.Y., Sihoe, A.D., Cheng, L.C., Ho, K.K. et al. 2009. The EML4-ALK fusion gene is involved in various histologic types of lung cancers from nonsmokers with wild-type EGFR and KRAS. *Cancer,* 115, 1723–1733.

Wu, C.C., Maher, M.M., and Shepard, J.A. 2011. CT-guided percutaneous needle biopsy of the chest: Preprocedural evaluation and technique. *Am J Roentgenol,* 196, W511–W514.

Yanagisawa, K., Tomida, S., Shimada, Y., Yatabe, Y., Mitsudomi, T., and Takahashi, T. 2007. A 25-signal proteomic signature and outcome for patients with resected non-small-cell lung cancer. *J Natl Cancer Inst,* 99, 858–867.

Yang, I.V. and Schwartz, D.A. 2011. Epigenetic control of gene expression in the lung. *Am J Respir Crit Care Med,* 183, 1295–1301.

Yazdanpanah, M., Luo, X., Lau, R., Greenberg, M., Fischer, L.J., and Lehotay, D.C. 1997. Cytotoxic aldehydes as possible markers for childhood cancer. *Free Radic Biol Med,* 23, 870–878.

Yildiz, P.B., Shyr, Y., Rahman, J.S., Wardwell, N.R., Zimmerman, L.J., Shakhtour, B., Gray, W.H. et al. 2007. Diagnostic accuracy of MALDI mass spectrometric analysis of unfractionated serum in lung cancer. *J Thorac Oncol,* 2, 893–901.

Yu, S.L., Chen, H.Y., Chang, G.C., Chen, C.Y., Chen, H.W., Singh, S., Cheng, C.L. et al. 2008. MicroRNA signature predicts survival and relapse in lung cancer. *Cancer Cell,* 13, 48–57.

Part V

Urological Cancers

20

Noninvasive Early Molecular Biomarkers in Kidney Cancer

Brian W. Cross, Jonathan Huang, and Viraj A. Master

CONTENTS

ABSTRACT Among the adult population, renal cell carcinoma (RCC) continues to be the most prevalent form of kidney cancer with over 200,000 cases diagnosed worldwide each year. Unfortunately, RCC is a relatively asymptomatic disease, and many tumors are found incidentally upon workup for other unrelated diseases. By the time symptoms develop, many renal tumors are advanced past the stage of curability. Approximately 30% of patients will present with metastatic disease. With numerous recent advances in targeted therapies for RCC, extensive research has focused on the prognostic utility of serum and urinary biomarkers, as well as tissue-staining biomarkers from pathologic specimens. Historically, prognostic information has been obtained from clinicopathologic features, but as the molecular basis of RCC has been elucidated, many studies have focused on the discovery of reliable serum and urinary biomarkers that could have a substantial impact on diagnosis, prognosis, as well as prediction of therapeutic benefit of various treatment options. Initially, most biomarker research focused on the products of the von Hippel–Lindau (VHL) pathway, such as VHL mutations, vascular endothelial growth factor, hypoxia-inducible factor, and carbonic anhydrase IX. More recently, other serum biomarkers of the systemic inflammatory response have been investigated, including C-reactive protein and the erythrocyte sedimentation rate. Previous investigations that used tissue-based expression assays have shown increased expression of certain proteins in surgically excised tissue. On the basis of urinary excretion of these proteins, urinary biomarkers have also been studied, including NMP-22, extracellular matrix proteins, aquaporin-1, adipophilin, and cathepsin D. This chapter examines these potential noninvasive serum and urinary biomarkers and their utility in diagnosis and prognostic models for kidney cancer.

KEY WORDS: *kidney, cancer, biomarkers.*

20.1 Introduction

Over 50,000 Americans are diagnosed with renal cell carcinoma (RCC) each year, approximately 30% of whom will ultimately develop metastatic progression of their disease despite apparent curative nephrectomy for localized cancer at the time of clinical presentation (Jemal et al. 2005; Leibovich et al. 2003). Metastatic RCC, untreated, has a dismal 5-year survival rate of <10% and a median overall survival of less than 1 year (Klatte et al. 2008; Ljungberg 2007; Ramsey et al. 2008; Zisman et al. 2002). As such, there has been a long-standing interest in accurately identifying those patients most likely to suffer from postoperative disease progression, and much research in recent years has focused on the development of prognostic models to aid in surveillance strategies and patient counseling. In highly selected cases, aggressive treatment following early detection of recurrence can improve the 5-year survival to 25%–60% (Kavolius et al. 1998). Thus, investigators have sought biomarkers of relapse-free survival (RFS) to identify high-risk patients for increased surveillance or adjuvant therapy, patient counseling, and enrollment in trials.

Currently, the most commonly used tool to predict outcome in RCC is the TNM staging system. However, there is considerable overlap in survival between stages (Ramsey et al. 2008), and this has fostered the search for other prognostic biomarkers to more clearly stratify those patients in whom a poor outcome can be expected.

Recently, efforts at identifying biomarkers of disease progression in RCC have focused on the readily available and cost-effective clinical indices of preoperative laboratory values (Magera et al. 2008). It is becoming increasingly clear that neoplastic progression depends on an orchestrated interface between tumor biology and the host inflammatory response (Lamb et al. 2008). The systemic inflammatory response, as represented by aberrations in circulating levels of acute-phase reactants, has previously been shown to be a predictor of poor overall survival in a variety of advanced malignancies (Bromwich et al. 2004; McMillan et al. 2001; O'Gorman et al. 2000). The beneficial role of biomarkers in RCC is challenged by the relatively low prevalence of disease, as evidenced by the fact that even if a biomarker for RCC had 100% specificity and 99.4% specificity, the positive predictive value in men over 65 would only be 10% (Tunuguntla and Jorda 2008).

20.2 Renal Cell Carcinoma

20.2.1 Clear Cell RCC

Clear cell RCC is the most common histologic subtype of RCC. This form accounts for 70%–80% of RCC (Rini et al. 2009). Grossly, these tumors have a yellow appearance. On microscopic examination, clear cell RCC originates from the proximal convoluted tubule of the nephron of the kidney. The tumor was aptly named for the abundant clear cells present after the solvents used in tissue processing have washed away the glycogen and lipids. Granular cells possessing eosinophilic cytoplasm can also be present. This tumor is highly vascular, with networks of capillaries surrounding sheets and nests of clear cells.

Clear cell RCC has been associated with abnormalities, including deletions and translocations, mostly commonly on chromosome 3. von Hippel–Lindau (VHL) and familial non-VHL clear cell RCC, diseases also associated with abnormalities on chromosome 3, are inherited diseases that increase the patient's chance of acquiring clear cell RCC. In VHL disease, a mutation in the VHL tumor suppressor gene leads to the formation of various solid vascular tumors, including RCC (Linehan et al. 1995).

The mutation also activates the transcription of genes, such as vascular endothelial growth factor, platelet-derived growth factor-β (PDGF-β), and erythropoietin (Pavlovich and Schmidt 2004). This may be the reason why highly vascular tumors, such as hemangioblastomas, are frequently found in patients with VHL disease. A familial pattern of inheritance, unrelated to abnormalities on chromosome 3, of clear cell RCC has also been reported in cohort of 60 families (Woodward et al. 2000). The individuals in these families developed clear cell RCC at an earlier age and the tumors were more likely to be bilateral and multicentric. Research is still being conducted to find a genetic link to familial non-VHL clear cell RCC.

Commercial genetic testing for hereditary leiomyomatosis and renal cell cancer is available at various laboratory sites. A list of genetic laboratories offering such testing can be found in Table 20.1. The most recent US patent information from 2012 for molecular diagnostic testing for renal cancer can be found in Table 20.2.

20.2.2 Papillary RCC

Papillary RCC is the second most common form of RCC, comprising about 10%–15% of RCC (Storkel et al. 1997). As with familial clear cell RCC, bilateral and multicentric tumors are frequently found in the papillary subtype of RCC (Cheng et al. 1991; Chow et al. 2001). Microscopically, papillary RCC originates from the proximal convoluted tubules. The tumor can be observed growing from a connective tissue stalk, hence its name. Papillary RCC is subdivided into two classes: type 1 and type 2. Histologically, type 1 papillary RCC contains basophilic cells, whereas type 2 papillary RCC contains eosinophilic cells. Type 1 papillary RCC is more common, thought to be less aggressive, and associated with a better prognosis (Rini et al. 2009).

This type of RCC is often associated with mutations in chromosome 7, 17, as well as the Y chromosome (Kovacs et al. 1989). Hereditary papillary RCC (HPRCC) is a familial disease associated with a mutation in the c-*MET* proto-oncogene, found on chromosome 7. The mutation leads to the activation of a tyrosine kinase receptor, which subsequently produces tumor cell proliferation (Vira et al. 2007). One study demonstrated a total of 41 individuals in 10 families who were thought to have HPRCC (Zbar et al. 1994). This inheritable disease is associated with the type 1 form of papillary RCC. Hereditary leiomyomatosis and RCC (HLRCC) is a syndrome that is associated with leiomyomas and papillary RCC. While cutaneous and uterine leiomyomas are commonly found in families with HLRCC, papillary RCC is only found in approximately one-third of these families (Wei et al. 2006). The renal tumors associated with this syndrome are typically type 2 papillary RCC. These tumors tend to be aggressive and metastasize early. In a cohort of 13 patients, from families with HLRCC, 9 of the individuals died of metastatic disease within 5 years of onset (Toro et al. 2003). As such, early surgical management is recommended.

20.2.3 Chromophobe RCC

Chromophobe RCC accounts for approximately 3%–5% of RCCs (Cheville et al. 2003). Grossly, these tumors appear light brown in color and are well circumscribed. Microscopically, chromophobe RCC originates from the intercalated cells in the collecting ducts of the nephron. These tumor cells typically have a pale cytoplasm. The defining characteristic of these cells is the presence of intracytoplasmic microvesicles, ranging between 250 and 400 nm in diameter, that stain positively for Hale colloidal iron (Prasad et al. 2006; Wu et al. 2002).

While most cases of chromophobe RCC are sporadic, these tumors can be associated with Birt–Hogg–Dubé (BHD) syndrome. This syndrome is associated with a mutation of the BHD gene, located on chromosome 17, which normally produces folliculin, a possible tumor suppressor gene (Toro et al. 2008). Manifestations include fibrofolliculomas and lung cysts, which are associated spontaneous pneumothoraces (Toro et al. 1999). Renal tumors, such as chromophobe RCC and oncocytomas, can also be present. Chromophobe RCC, including the tumors associated with BHD syndrome, tends to be less aggressive and associated with a better outcome than other RCC subtypes. A 5-year disease-free survival of 83.9% was found in one study (Patard et al. 2005).

TABLE 20.1

Genetic Laboratories Offering Testing for HLRCC

Laboratory	Sequence Analysis of the Entire Coding Region	Mutation Scanning of Entire Coding Region	Enzyme Assay	Deletion/ Duplication Analysis	Prenatal Diagnosis	Gene Product
Baylor College of Medicine, Houston, TX	X				X	Locus 1q43, mitochondrial fumarate hydratase
Center for Nephrology and Metabolic Disorders, Weisswasser, Sachsen, Germany	X				X	Locus 1q43, mitochondrial fumarate hydratase
Centogene AG, Rostock, Germany	X			X		Locus 1q43, mitochondrial fumarate hydratase
Children's Hospital of Philadelphia, Philadelphia, PA		X		X		Locus 1q43, mitochondrial fumarate hydratase
Dr. Eberhard & Partner Dortmund, Nordrhein-Westfalen, Germany	X					Locus 1q43, mitochondrial fumarate hydratase
Emory University, School of Medicine, Atlanta, GA	X			X	X	Locus 1q43, mitochondrial fumarate hydratase
GeneDx, Gaithersburg, MD	X			X	X	Locus 1q43, mitochondrial fumarate hydratase
Innovagenomics S.L Salamanca, Castilla y Leon, Spain		X				Locus 1q43, mitochondrial fumarate hydratase
Institut de Cancérologie Gustave Roussy, Villejuif, France	X		X	X		Locus 1q43, mitochondrial fumarate hydratase
Klinikum Stuttgart Stuttgart, Baden-Wurttemberg, Germany	X					Locus 1q43, mitochondrial fumarate hydratase
MGZ München, Munich, Germany	X			X		Locus 1q43, mitochondrial fumarate hydratase
Praxis fuer Humangenetik Wien, Vienna, Wien, Austria	X				X	Locus 1q43, mitochondrial fumarate hydratase

TABLE 20.1 (continued)

Genetic Laboratories Offering Testing for HLRCC

Laboratory	Sequence Analysis of the Entire Coding Region	Mutation Scanning of Entire Coding Region	Enzyme Assay	Deletion/ Duplication Analysis	Prenatal Diagnosis	Gene Product
Radboud University Nijmegen Medical Centre, Nijmegen, the Netherlands	X			X		Locus 1q43, mitochondrial fumarate hydratase
Sheffield Children's NHS Foundation Trust, Sheffield, United Kingdom	X			X		Locus 1q43, mitochondrial fumarate hydratase
University Hospitals—University Hospitals Laboratory Service Foundation	X					Locus 1q43, mitochondrial fumarate hydratase
University of Oklahoma Health Sciences Center, Oklahoma City, OK	X					Locus 1q43, mitochondrial fumarate hydratase

TABLE 20.2

2012 US Patent Information for Molecular Diagnostic Testing for RCC

Title	Applicants	Publication Date	Application Number
Biomarkers for predicting and assessing responsiveness of thyroid and kidney cancer subjects to lenvatinib compounds	Funahashi, Yasuhiro; Kadowaki, Tadashi; Matsui, Junji; Simon, Jason; Xu, Lucy; Eisai R&D Management Co., LTD, Tokyo, Japan	December 6, 2012	US2012/040183
Systems and methods for diagnosing kidney cancer	Kruger, Warren; Mustafa, Aladdin; Fox Chase Cancer Center, Philadelphia, PA	July 19, 2012	US2012/021228
Methods for diagnosis and treatment of epithelial-derived cancers, such as colorectal cancers and kidney cancers	Terrett, J.A., Oxford GlycoSciences (UK) Ltd., Abingdon, Oxfordshire	June 13, 2012	02779771.1
Molecular markers in kidney cancer	Smit, Fanciscus Petrus; Schalken, Jack; Nijmegen (NL)	June 7, 2012	13379823
Anaplastic lymphoma kinase in kidney cancer	Haack, Herbert; Crosby, Katherine; Rimkunas, Victoria; Silver, Matthew; Cell Signaling Technology; Danvers, MA	April 26, 2012	13204342

20.2.4 Other Subtypes of RCC

While clear cell, papillary, and chromophobe RCCs comprise the three most common forms of RCC, rarer forms have been reported, including collecting duct RCC, medullary RCC, and RCC with sarcomatoid differentiation.

Collecting duct RCC, also known as Bellini duct carcinoma, comprises approximately 1%–2% of RCCs (Mejean et al. 2003; Peyromaure et al. 2003). Grossly, these tumors have a gray-white-tan appearance and are usually located near the junction of the medulla and renal pelvis (Kennedy et al. 1990). Microscopically, tubular and papillary structures can be seen, as in papillary RCC. However, unlike papillary RCC, collecting duct RCC arises from the collecting ducts and has distinct features, such as desmoplasia, atypia in the collecting ducts, and intratubular spread (Kennedy et al. 1990). Collecting duct RCC is an aggressive subtype of RCC, usually diagnosed at later stages of the disease. One study showed an overall survival in 10 patients at 2 years of 20% (Mejean et al. 2003).

Medullary RCC is typically associated with African-Americans who possess the sickle cell trait or disease (Davis et al. 1995). Grossly, this tumor appears gray white and is poorly circumscribed. Microscopically, medullary RCC commonly has a cribriform appearance. In a study of 40 cases, other common features included desmoplasia, chronic inflammatory infiltrate, and infiltrative borders (Swartz et al. 2002). The tumor develops near the renal papilla. It is hypothesized that the hypoxic nature of this location induces various transcription factors that contribute to tumor angiogenesis and growth (Davis et al. 1995). This disease is usually diagnosed at a late stage and patients have a mean survival of approximately 4 months (Swartz et al. 2002).

Approximately 1%–5% RCC will have sarcomatoid differentiation (Cheville et al. 2004; Kuroda et al. 2003). This is a modifying characteristic of the primary RCC, which can be any of the previous subtypes. Microscopically, tumors of cells from the primary RCC can usually be found, along with the spindle cells of the sarcomatoid differentiation. It is hypothesized that the sarcomatoid differentiation may represent poorly differentiated primary tumors (Delahunt 1999). RCCs with this feature are aggressive and metastasize early. One study reported that the median overall survival in a cohort of 108 patients with RCC with sarcomatoid differentiation was 9 months (Mian et al. 2002).

20.3 Serum Biomarkers

20.3.1 C-Reactive Protein

Recent studies have identified systemic inflammatory biomarkers of poor outcomes, in particular C-reactive protein (CRP) (Ljungberg 2007). Produced in response to cytokines such as IL-6, CRP is an acute-phase reactant that has been associated with poor outcomes in nearly all malignancies. In RCC, increased plasma IL-6 levels induce increased hepatic and intratumoral production of CRP. Although RCC cells express IL-6, it remains unclear whether these cells or surrounding host tissue are responsible for the cytokines that promote CRP production. Nonetheless, increased IL-6 and CRP levels have both been associated with increased tumor stage, grade, tumor burden, and metastatic progression.

Although the biomarker CRP does reflect inflammation and therefore the risk of poor outcomes, the vast majority of investigations of RCC outcomes have focused on preoperative CRP as a biomarker. Clearly, there is an increased risk of poor outcomes among patients with preoperative elevations in CRP. However, the significance of postoperative CRP after potentially curative nephrectomy for localized RCC remains unknown. Anecdotally, an increased risk of metastases in patients with elevations in postoperative CRP regardless of preoperative CRP has been noted by Johnson and colleagues. A prospective study to assess the predictive ability of pre- and postoperative CRP levels in patients undergoing potentially curative nephrectomy for localized RCC was performed with the hypothesis that both CRP values would be independent predictors of a 1-year RFS and overall survival. This study cohort consisted of 110 consecutive patients who underwent potentially curative nephrectomy for clear cell RCC. Of all patients, 16.4% developed metastases, and 6.4% died within 1 year of surgery. The mean (SD) preoperative and postoperative CRP values for patients who developed metastases were 87.04 (73.95) and 69.06 (73.55) mg/L, respectively, whereas these values for patients who did not develop metastases were 9.24 (30.77) and 5.27 (7.80), respectively. Mean (SD) preoperative and postoperative CRP values for patients who died were 102.61 (77.32) and 89.31 (69.51) mg/L, respectively, whereas these values for patients who survived were 19.52 (46.10) and 10.88 (30.32), respectively (Johnson et al. 2010). As demonstrated in Figure 20.1, the odds ratio of metastases compared with a postoperative CRP of 1 mg/L increases with increasing postoperative CRP levels. Similarly, as demonstrated in Figure 20.2, the odds ratio of mortality compared with a postoperative CRP of 1 mg/L increases with increasing postoperative CRP levels.

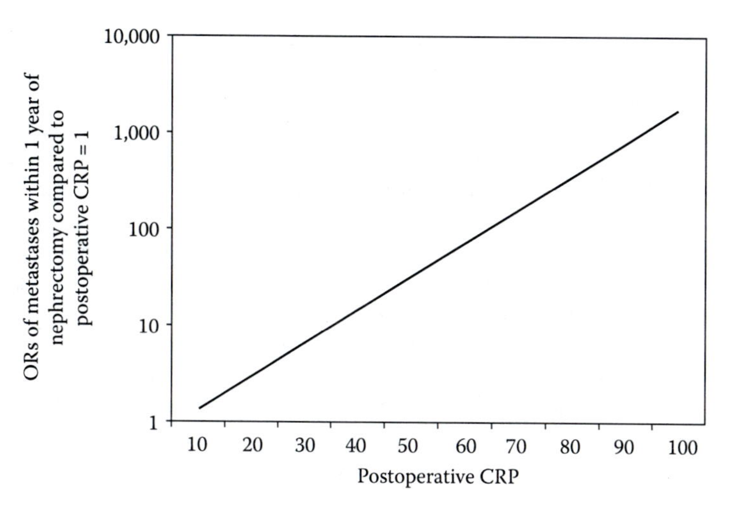

FIGURE 20.1 Odds ratios of developing metastases within 1 year of potentially curative nephrectomy for varying postoperative CRP levels compared with postoperative CRP = 1.

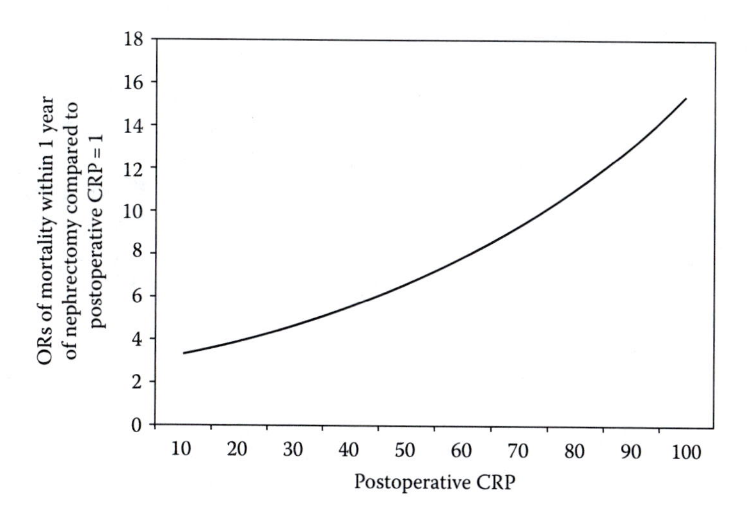

FIGURE 20.2 Odds ratios of mortality within 1 year of potentially curative nephrectomy for varying postoperative CRP levels compared with postoperative CRP = 1.

These findings suggest that patients with elevations in postoperative CRP levels remain at increased risk for developing metastases after potentially curative nephrectomy. This increase in risk is almost logarithmic, as demonstrated in Figure 20.1. For example, compared with patients with a preoperative CRP of 1 mg/L, patients with a preoperative CRP of 10 and 100 mg/L are 1.3 times (95% CI: 0.83–2.30) and 1792 times (95% CI: 14.74–396,725.51) more likely to develop metastases within the first year after surgery, respectively.

As reviewed previously, several studies have investigated the prognostic relationship between both preoperative and postoperative CRP values and mortality. However, the majority of these studies categorized CRP dichotomously, typically elevated versus normal categories (≥10 vs. <10 mg/L, respectively) (Komai et al. 2007; Lamb et al. 2008; Ramsey et al. 2007, 2008). Clinically, however, dichotomous variables may be less useful than trichotomous variables (such as low, intermediate, and high risk). Dividing patients into three (or more) groups may potentially better allocate resources to patients based on risk.

In 2007, Karakiewicz and colleagues separated patients based on preoperative CRP into low- (≤4.0 mg/L), intermediate- (4.1–23.0), and high-risk (>23.0 mg/L) groups (Karakiewicz et al. 2007). In multivariate analysis, they found CRP to be an independent predictor of RCC-specific mortality

($p = 0.003$). Moreover, the model with CRP performed 2.4% and 4.6% better than the UCLA Integrated Staging System (UISS) at, respectively, 2 and 5 years.

In 2010, Johnson and colleagues performed a similar study to assess how to maximize preoperative CRP's prognostic potential as a trinary variable. They evaluated 173 consecutive patients who underwent potentially curative radical nephrectomy for clear cell RCC. Frequency and descriptive analyses were conducted to characterize the patient population. Receiver operating characteristics (ROC) curves were constructed to assess the potential of preoperative CRP to predict overall survival. ROC curves are interpreted as the probability that the modeled phenotype can correctly discriminate subjects developing end points from those without end points, where 0.5 is chance discrimination and 1.0 is perfect discrimination. ROC curves were used to determine the area under the curve (AUC) and relative sensitivity and specificity of the preoperative CRP cutoffs relative to overall survival. Based on these cutoffs, patients were categorized into low-, intermediate-, and high-risk groups. The Kaplan–Meier survival curves were constructed to assess the impact of different cutoffs on overall survival. In this analysis, survival was defined as overall survival.

Low-risk (≤4.0 mg/L), intermediate-risk (4.1–10.0 mg/L), and high-risk (>10.0 mg/L) groups were constructed. The Kaplan–Meier analysis was conducted to assess the probability of overall survival by preoperative CRP risk category (Figure 20.3). Median (95% CI) survival for low-, intermediate-, and high-risk patients was 43.4 (42.2–44.6) months, 41.8 (38.6–45.1) months, and 31.4 (39.8–43.4) months, respectively. The curve for high-risk patients differed significantly from low-risk ($p < 0.001$) and intermediate-risk ($p = 0.009$) population curves. The low- and intermediate-risk curves approached statistical significance ($p = 0.06$).

Overall survival of the low-risk (CRP: 0.0–4.0 mg/L) and intermediate-risk (CRP: 4.1–10.0 mg/L) groups was significantly higher than the survival of the high-risk (CRP: >10.0 mg/L) group ($p < 0.001$ and $p = 0.009$, respectively). Additionally, the difference in survival among low- and intermediate-risk groups trended toward statistical significance ($p = 0.06$). It should be noted that the maximum follow-up was 46 months. Therefore, the median survival of the low-risk group (43.4 months) was likely higher. The sensitivity and specificity of serum CRP values >5 mg/L for renal capsular invasion, lymph node metastases, and distant metastases can be seen in Table 20.3 (Masuda et al. 1997).

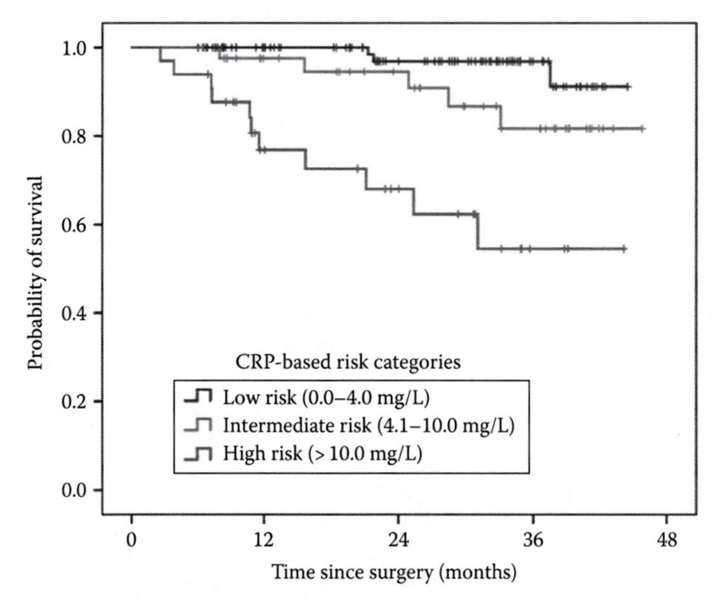

FIGURE 20.3 The Kaplan–Meier survival analysis of probability of survival versus time since surgery (days) by preoperative CRP risk category among patients diagnosed with localized clear cell RCC undergoing potentially curative nephrectomy. Patients categorized into low risk (≤4.0 mg/L), intermediate risk (4.1–10.0 mg/L), and high risk (>10.0 mg/L) based on preoperative CRP levels. Log-rank: low risk versus high risk ($p < 0.001$), low risk versus intermediate risk ($p = 0.06$), intermediate risk versus high risk ($p = 0.009$).

TABLE 20.3

Sensitivity and Specificity of Urinary and Serum Biomarkers for RCC

Biomarker	Sensitivity (%)	Specificity (%)
Serum		
CRP (> 5.0 mg/L)		
Renal capsular invasion	54	84
Lymph node metastases	57	77
Distant metastases	74	81
ESR (>30 mm/h)		
Renal capsular invasion	54	84
Lymph node metastases	57	80
Distant metastases	63	83
CAIX	49	98
Urinary		
NMP-22 (>4.2 U/mL)	95	65
NMP-22 (>4.9 U/mL)	87	80
NMP-22 (>5.8 U/mL)	78	90
NMP-22 (>8.0 U/mL)	60	90
NMP-22 (>9.6 U/mL)	47	90
NMP-22 (>11.3 U/mL)	34	90
ECM proteins	95	96
AQP-1	100	100
ADP	100	100
Cathepsin D	Unreported	Unreported

These survival differences, along with the 1:2:4 ratio in number of deaths and 2:1:1 ratio in population size, underscore the potential need for a risk-based approach to postoperative management of patients with localized RCC that other groups have also reported. Only 3% of the low-risk group died from all causes. During the nearly 4-year study, the high-risk group suffered a nearly 10-fold greater risk of overall mortality. Yet, both groups received the same postoperative management, meaning no adjuvant therapy is given for localized renal cancer. Both groups received restaging CT scans every 3–6 months, at least for the first 2 years.

Postoperative imaging is not without consequence. For example, each restaging abdominal CT scan (not study) exposes the patient's stomach and liver each to approximately 15 milli-Sieverts (mSv) (Brenner and Hall 2007)—the annual limit for radiation workers is 20 mSv (Brenner et al. 2003). Epidemiological data suggest that as few as 10 mSv is the lowest dose for an acute exposure to increase the risk of cancer in humans (Brenner et al. 2003). Consequently, in a patient over 30 years of age, each abdominal CT scan increases the patient's estimated lifetime attributable risk of all cancers by about 0.02%. According to the National Academies' Biological Effects of Ionizing Radiation 7th Report, this risk of cancer proceeds in linear fashion with no lower threshold (Einstein et al. 2007; Health Risks from Exposure to Low Levels of Ionizing Radiation: BEIR VII Phase 2. 2006). However, this linearity assumption may be faulty and in fact underrepresent the true cumulative risk of radiation exposure (Brenner et al. 2003). Regardless, some if not all of this exposure appears to be unnecessary in approximately half of patients with localized RCC.

The potential benefits of lifestyle modifications on CRP have been borne out in several studies. Researchers have examined the efficacy of a variety of exercise programs. In one study conducted over 6 months, participants exercised three times weekly for an average of 70 min per session. Authors noted significant decreases in CRP, BMI, body fat mass, and waist-to-hip ratio (Meyer et al. 2006). Importantly, this study did not involve any dietary intervention. Several trials that have combined diet and exercise have demonstrated robust results. This impact has been shown even in studies of relatively short duration.

For example, Roberts et al. conducted a 2-week trial involving diet and exercise. Subjects were placed on a high-fiber diet and participated in daily exercise for 2–2.5 h. This study design is admittedly unusual because of its high volume of exercise; however, it quickly produced tangible benefits. Participants experienced significant reductions body weight and BMI. More impressively, authors pointed to a greater than 40% reduction in CRP (Roberts et al. 2007). While this study's design might not seem feasible for many, its findings have been mirrored by other trials with less stringent programs. Rosenbaum et al. implemented their program in eighth-grade students. This protocol involved a once-weekly lifestyle class and three weekly sessions of dance/kickboxing. After this 3- to 4-month trial, the intervention group had significantly lowered its CRP, percent body fat, and BMI (Rosenbaum et al. 2007). Kelishadi et al. showed positive benefits, including reduced CRP, BMI, weight, and waist-to-hip ratio, from 6 weeks of diet and exercise. Specifically, participants exercised for three times weekly for an hour (Kelishadi et al. 2008). The work of Rosenbaum and Kelishadi shows that significant, beneficial CRP reduction is possible with realistic lifestyle modifications.

20.3.2 von Hippel–Lindau

A significant breakthrough in the understanding of the molecular mechanisms of RCC came with the discovery of the VHL pathway. Renal cancer, like other malignancies, can occur in sporadic and inherited forms. Inherited renal cancer is estimated to occur in approximately 4%–5% of cases (Linehan et al. 1995), including those associated with VHL disease.

The VHL disease, which has an estimated incidence of 1 in 36,000 live births, is an inherited cancer syndrome characterized by inactivation of the VHL tumor suppressor gene located on chromosome 3. These patients often develop a combination of multifocal tumors, including central nervous system and retinal hemangioblastomas, RCC as well as renal cysts, pheochromocytoma, pancreatic cysts and tumors, endolymphatic sac tumors, and papillary cystadenoma in the epididymis and broad ligament (Wu et al. 2012). RCC is reported to occur in approximately 40% of individuals and is often bilateral and multifocal and most often occurs as clear cell histology. These tumors tend to occur earlier than sporadic RCC, with a mean age of presentation of approximately 39 years and often metastasize (Linehan et al. 1995). Nephron-sparing surgical approaches are often undertaken in these patients to preserve renal function for as long as possible.

The VHL gene product regulates the hypoxia-inducible factor (HIF) transcription factor and plays a critical role in the cellular adaptation to hypoxia. In the presence of oxygen, the VHL protein binds to HIF-α and the resultant polyubiquitination marks HIF-α for proteasomal degradation. In the absence of a functional VHL protein, such as with a mutated VHL gene, HIF-α is allowed to bind to HIF-β. This heterodimer translocates to the nucleus and binds specific DNA sequences that activate transcription of genes encoding potent angiogenic factors, such as VEGF-A, PDGF-β, and transforming growth factor-α (TGF-α) (Vickers and Heng 2010).

Exploration of the prognostic utility of the VHL gene mutation in renal cancer has yielded conflicting results. Early studies suggested VHL gene mutations to portend a poorer prognosis. Brauch and colleagues performed DNA analysis of 227 RCC tumor specimens and found 45% of the clear cell tumors harbored VHL mutations and hypermethylations, while more than 90% had 3p loss of heterozygosity. VHL gene mutations/hypermethylation was shown to be prognostic for advanced tumor stage (pT3) ($p = 0.009$) in patients with clear cell RCC (Brauch et al. 2000).

Other more recent studies have suggested a positive prognostic role for the VHL gene mutation in clear cell RCC. Patard and colleagues examined a series of 100 radical nephrectomy specimens and found VHL mutations in 58% of the specimens. Absence of VHL mutation was associated with more advanced tumors, higher T-stages, and presence of metastases. VHL mutation predicted a longer progression-free survival (76% vs. 51%, $p = 0.037$) (Patard et al. 2008). Additional studies have shown improved cancer-specific survival in patients with stage I–III clear cell RCC, but no association with stage IV disease (Yao et al. 2002). Other studies have further complicated the picture, with larger studies showing no prognostic utility of VHL mutation (Baldewijns et al. 2009; Gimenez-Bachs et al. 2006; Kondo et al. 2002; Smits et al. 2008).

Certainly, the discovery and elucidation of the VHL pathway was a major breakthrough in the understanding of the molecular mechanisms of RCC development, but larger prospective studies are needed to clarify the role of the VHL gene mutation on prognosis in patients with RCC.

20.3.3 Modified Glasgow Prognostic Score

While CRP remains a potent predictor of outcomes, several studies have noted the added benefit of considering hypoalbuminemia with CRP, as measured by the modified Glasgow Prognostic Score (mGPS) as first described by McMillan and colleagues (Al Murri et al. 2006; Crumley et al. 2006; Forrest et al. 2003, 2004; Glen et al. 2006; Roxburgh and McMillan 2010). The mGPS scores patients based on CRP (CRP > 10 mg/L = 1 point) and albumin (albumin <3.5 g/dL = 1 point) and categorizes them as low risk (0 points), intermediate risk (1 point), and high risk (2 points). Patients with a CRP concentration elevations (>10 mg/L) and a decreased serum albumin concentration (<3.5 mg/L) score 2. Those patients with an elevated CRP concentration (>10 mg/L) score 1, and finally patients with a CRP concentration of <10 mg/L and any albumin level score 0 (Table 20.4).

Ramsey and colleagues noted the mGPS' potential for predicting outcomes in patients with metastatic RCC (Ramsey et al. 2007). In a study of 119 patients, intermediate- and high-risk mGPS scores were associated with significantly poorer cancer-specific survival.

Recent data from Johnson et al. followed 129 patients for 1 year following potentially curative radical nephrectomy with negative surgical margins for clear cell RCC. Of the 129 patients in the study, 23.3% developed metastases. Of the low-, intermediate-, and high-risk patients, 10.1%, 38.9%, and 89.9% recurred during the study (Figure 20.4). After accounting for various patient and tumor characteristics in multivariate analysis including stage and grade, only mGPS was significantly associated with RFS. Compared to low-risk patients, intermediate- and high-risk patients experienced a fourfold

TABLE 20.4
The mGPS

Laboratory Values	mGPS
CRP ≤ 10 mg/L + any albumin level	0
CRP > 10 mg/L	1
CRP > 10 mg/L + albumin < 3.5 g/dL	2
Low risk	0
Intermediate risk	1
High risk	2

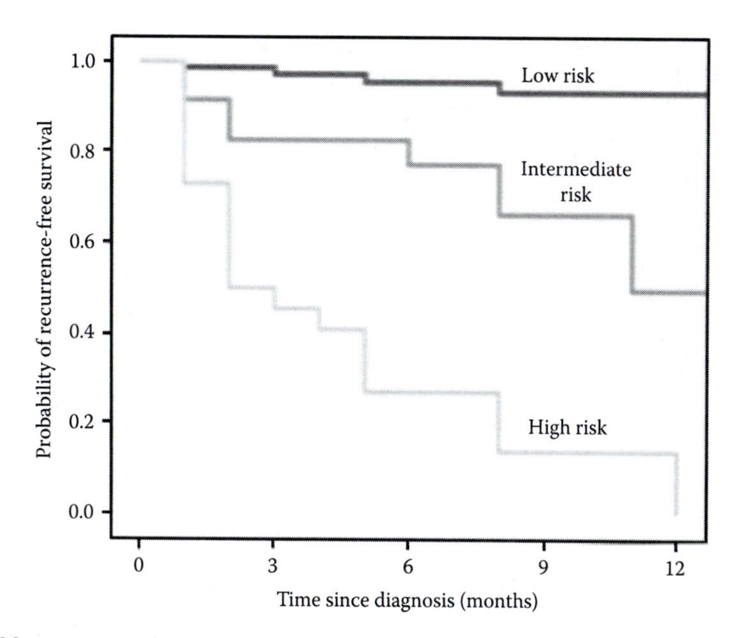

FIGURE 20.4 Mean recurrence-free survival based on mGPS risk categories.

(HR: 4.035, 95% CI: 1.312–12.415, $p = 0.015$) and sevenfold (HR: 7.012, 95% CI: 2.126–23.123 $p < 0.001$) risk of metastasis, respectively (unpublished).

20.3.4 Erythrocyte Sedimentation Rate

The determination of the erythrocyte sedimentation rate (ESR) is a simple and inexpensive laboratory test introduced by Westergren in 1921. It measures the distance erythrocytes have fallen after 1 h in a vertical column of anticoagulated blood under the influence of gravity (Brigden 1999). Though its clinical usefulness as a diagnostic tool has diminished as more intricate methods of analysis have emerged, it remains paramount in the specific diagnosis of a few conditions, including temporal arteritis, polymyalgia rheumatica, and rheumatoid arthritis. Moreover, an extreme elevation is mostly associated with infection or malignancy (Brigden 1999). Numerous studies over three decades have substantiated the prognostic utility of ESR in patients with RCC (Hannisdal et al. 1989; Hoffmann et al. 1999; Hop and van der Werf-Messing 1980; Kawai et al. 2009; Lehmann et al. 2004; Ljungberg et al. 1997, 2000; Magera et al. 2008; Roosen et al. 1994; Sene et al. 1992; Sengupta et al. 2006), with recent data from the Mayo Clinic showing elevated ESR levels predicting the presence of aggressive disease and poorer outcomes (Sengupta et al. 2006).

Despite these numerous observations, the ESR level is not routinely incorporated into current prognostic models for RCC, likely due to the nonspecific nature of its elevation (Frank et al. 2002; Kattan et al. 2001; Zisman et al. 2001), and the relationship between ESR and survival in localized RCC following potentially curative nephrectomy has not been fully elucidated.

Data from Cross et al. reviewed 167 patients undergoing nephrectomy for localized RCC. These patients had ESR levels measured preoperatively and were stratified into either low (0.0–20.0 mm/h), intermediate (20.1–50.0 mm/h), or high risk (>50.0 mm/h) based on their ESR level. The Kaplan–Meier analysis was conducted to assess the univariate impact of these ESR-based groups on overall survival. Overall, 55.2% were low risk, while 27.0% and 17.8% were intermediate and high risk, respectively. Median (95% CI) survival was 44.1 (42.6–45.5) months, 35.5 (32.3–38.8) months, and 32.1 (25.5–38.6) months, for the low-, intermediate-, and high-risk groups, respectively. After controlling for other patient and tumor characteristics, intermediate- and high-risk groups experienced a 4.5-fold (HR: 4.509, 95% CI: 0.735–27.649) and 18.5-fold (HR: 18.531, 95% CI: 2.117–162.228) increased risk of overall mortality, respectively (Figure 20.5) (Cross et al. 2012). The sensitivity and specificity of serum ESR values >30 mm/h for renal capsular invasion, lymph node metastases, and distant metastases can be seen in Table 20.3 (Masuda et al. 1997).

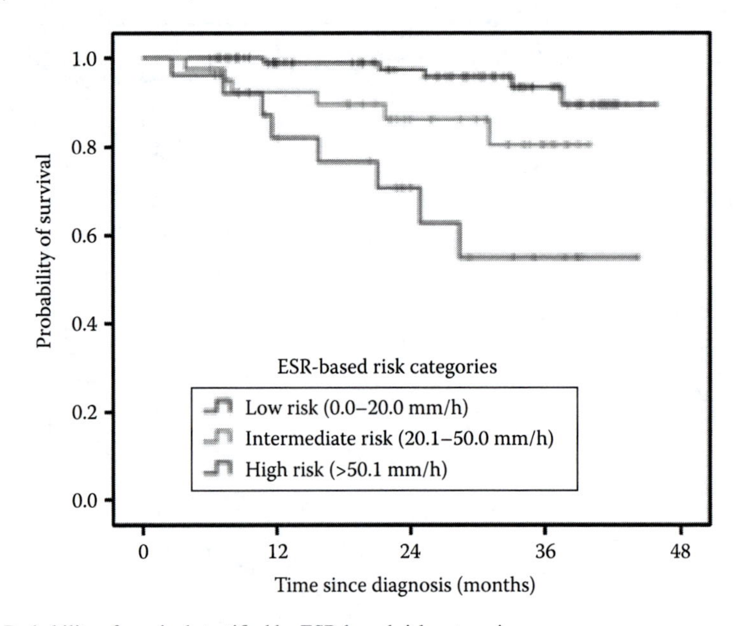

FIGURE 20.5 Probability of survival stratified by ESR-based risk categories.

20.3.5 Peritumoral CRP

Although the prognostic utility of circulating levels of serum acute-phase reactants has been well elucidated in multiple malignancies, the role of tumor and peritumoral expression of inflammatory biomarkers has not been as well studied. Smoldering inflammation is a key component of the tumor microenvironment, and inflammation has been suggested to represent the seventh hallmark of cancer. Tumor-associated macrophages have served as a paradigm for cancer-promoting inflammation and are a major component of leukocytic infiltration of tumors (Mantovani and Sica 2010), though they have the potential to express both pro- and antitumoral effects depending on various intracellular signaling pathways. As such, inflammatory reactions can exert a dual influence on tumor growth, and diversity is a characteristic of cancer-related inflammation. In other words, certain forms of inflammation have long been known to promote metastasis, such as macrophages and their interleukin products. Alternatively, other forms of inflammation offer a protective response. It has been shown that dying tumor cells can be cross-presented by dendritic cells and trigger a protective immune response via toll-like receptor pathways (Apetoh et al. 2007). Accordingly, the effect of CRP secretion on human myeloid dendritic cells (MDCs) in head and neck squamous cell carcinoma has been investigated. CRP has been shown to decrease migration of human MDC in head and neck cancer, mitigating this protective effect of MDC (Frenzel et al. 2007). This functional modulation of immune cells represents a critical escape mechanism for human carcinoma cells. The development of effective therapies to shift the balance from cancer-promoting inflammation to protective immunity requires a better understanding of the tissue microenvironment within as well as around the tumor itself.

In patients with colorectal cancer, there is good evidence that, on simple staining of the tumor specimens, a pronounced lymphocytic infiltrate within the tumor is associated with improved survival (Ropponen et al. 1997) and growth of the primary tumor and metastatic spread are associated with decreased intratumoral immune T-cell densities. The immune status of the tumor outperforms both stage and grade in predicting disease-free survival, disease-specific survival, and overall survival (Mlecnik et al. 2011).

Similarly, cellular accumulation of CRP has been noted in adenocarcinoma of the rectum and squamous cell carcinoma of the esophagus, and increased expression of CRP in tumor cells has been found to be independently linked to patient prognosis (Nozoe et al. 2003). Prior studies by our group and others have shown increased expression of CRP by RCC cells as well as unaffected surrounding tissue (Jabs et al. 2005), and we have shown that increased CRP staining in renal cancer cells is independently associated with prognosis. But, no studies to date have linked expression of *both* CRP and other inflammatory biomarkers by tumor cells and leukocyte infiltration in surrounding tissue to patient prognosis and outcome in RCC.

Recent data show that immunohistochemical staining of intratumoral CRP can be stratified into different categories consisting of grade 0 (negative staining), grade 1+ (weak staining), grade 2+ (moderate staining), and grade 3+ (strong staining) (Figure 20.6). In a recent cohort of patients, these staining patterns have shown prognostic utility, with patients in the high-risk group (grade 3+) showing a 27-fold increased risk of overall mortality compared to the low-risk group (grades 0 and 1+) on multivariate analysis (Johnson et al. 2011).

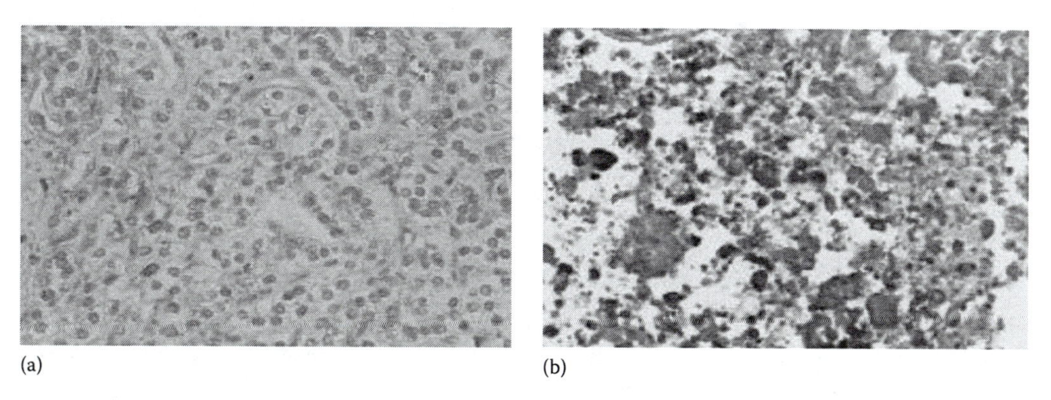

FIGURE 20.6 Intratumoral CRP staining of grade 1+ (a) and 3+ (b).

20.3.6 Carbonic Anhydrase IX

The development of solid tumors in humans can be thought to develop in two distinct stages. Initially, malignant cells transform into small tumors that ultimately cease to grow due to an inadequate supply of oxygen. Thereafter, this tissue hypoxia triggers a drastic change in gene expression and subsequent clonal selection for those cells most adapted to this change in the local oxygen supply. This ultimately results in angiogenesis, a hallmark of the local peritumoral environment. These changes further lead to a new compromised tumor microenvironment with a resultant acidic extracellular pH. The HIF-1 gene can be thought of as a master regulator in this acidic, hypoxic tumor microenvironment and controls the expression of a host of target genes involved in tumor growth. Among them are the surface transmembrane carbonic anhydrases (Ivanov et al. 2001). Induction of carbonic anhydrase IX (CAIX) is thought to maintain an acidic tissue environment and allow tumor cells to grow and ultimately metastasize.

Prior pathologic studies utilizing molecular techniques such as Northern blot RNA analysis and immunostaining of various tumor types (including RCC) have shown that the *trans*membrane carbonic anhydrases, IX and XII, are overexpressed in many different tumor types. Additionally, their expression was markedly increased under hypoxic conditions (Ivanov et al. 2001).

Increased CAIX expression is correlated with a worse prognosis in several malignancies, such as lung, breast, and cervical/ovarian (Chia et al. 2001; Giatromanolaki et al. 2001; Loncaster et al. 2001). Conversely, expression of CAIX in clear cell RCC has shown promise as a predictor of improved prognosis (Atkins et al. 2005; Bui et al. 2003). Sandlund and colleagues examined RCC specimens from 228 patients and found that CAIX expression was significantly higher in 183 conventional than in 31 papillary and 14 chromophobe RCC specimens ($p < 0.001$). Additionally, CAIX expression seemed to correlate with prognosis and median overall survival. Patients with tumors with 0%–10% CAIX expression had a median overall survival of 13.5 months, compared to 41 months for patients with tumors with 91%–100% CAIX expression ($p = 0.001$) (Sandlund et al. 2007).

Though the soluble form of CAIX is found in serum, the immunohistochemical and molecular techniques utilized to evaluate the tissue expression of CAIX are of course limited to surgical or biopsy specimens. Limited data exist regarding the prognostic or diagnostic utility of *serum* CAIX. Li and colleagues examined 91 patients with clear cell RCC as well as 32 healthy individuals as controls. They found that the mean preoperative serum carbonic anhydrase level was significantly higher in patients with metastatic (216.68 ± 67.02 pg/mL) or localized (91.65 ± 13.29 pg/mL) conventional RCC than in healthy individuals (14.59 ± 6.22 pg/mL, $p < 0.001$ and $p = 0.001$, respectively). Additionally, the mean serum CAIX level was significantly higher in those patients with metastatic disease than in those with localized disease ($p = 0.004$). Furthermore, in patients with localized RCC, those with recurrence during the follow-up period had a significantly higher preoperative serum CAIX level than those without recurrence ($p = 0.001$) (Li et al. 2008). The sensitivity and specificity of serum CAIX for RCC can be seen in Table 20.3 (McKiernan et al. 1999).

20.4 Urinary Biomarkers

20.4.1 Nuclear Matrix Protein-22

Nuclear matrix proteins (NMPs) comprise a set of structures in the cellular nucleus that provides 3D organization of the DNA and facilitates DNA replication, RNA synthesis, and gene expression (Pienta et al. 1989). NMP-22, or the nuclear mitotic apparatus protein, is an integral part of mitosis, functioning at the spindle poles to distribute chromatin to daughter cells (Lydersen and Pettijohn 1980). As cancerous cells undergo apoptosis and lyse, NMPs are released into the surrounding tissues. Significant elevations in the urinary concentrations of NMP-22 have been shown in transitional cell carcinoma (TCC) of the bladder, when compared to controls (Hosseini et al. 2012; Jeong et al. 2012). As such, NMP-22 is thought to be useful in diagnosing TCC. However, factors like infection, inflammation, instrumentation of the bladder, and renal calculi, associated with increased cellular turnover, have also been shown to increase the urinary concentration of NMP-22 (Sharma et al. 1999; Todenhofer et al. 2012).

Urinary NMP-22's diagnostic utility in TCC of bladder has prompted studies into its sensitivity and utility in detecting RCC. One study compared the urinary concentration of NMP-22 in patients who were diagnosed with RCC postoperatively and a control group, which included patients with a normal kidney or an oncocytoma, a benign renal mass. Chi-square analysis showed that 12/30 of RCC patients and 2/35 of control patients had a positive urinary NMP-22 specimen, at a cutoff of 10 U/mL (Huang et al. 2000). Their null hypothesis, stating that the number of positive results would not differ, was rejected significantly. Another study compared the pre- and postnephrectomy urine specimens from 25 RCC patients with a urine specimen from 20 control patients, for urinary concentration of NMP-22. The pre-nephrectomy urinary concentration was 10.65 ± 5.49 U/mL and the post-nephrectomy urinary concentration was 5.98 ± 3.86 U/mL, which was statistically significant. The NMP-22 concentration for the control group was 4.64 ± 3.10, which was not statistically different from the post-nephrectomy concentration of the RCC group (Ozer et al. 2002). These results were also shown in a study of 38 RCC patient and 30 control patients, who had kidney stones and simple renal cysts. The former group had significantly higher urinary NMP-22 positivity, measured by a urinary concentration of NMP-22 greater than 10 U/mL (Kaya et al. 2005). The results of these three studies show that there is a significant increase in the urinary concentration of NMP-22 between RCC and healthy patients.

These studies also investigated whether there was any correlation between a patient's urinary concentration of NMP-22 and the Fuhrman grade and the stage of the tumor. While the results of Huang et al.'s study suggested a positive correlation between urinary NMP-22 and Fuhrman grade and tumor stage, the sample size was too small to provide more conclusive evidence. Ozer et al. and Kaya et al. both found no significant difference in the urinary concentration of NMP-22 between Fuhrman grades and between tumor stages.

Limitations of these studies include a small sample size and NMP-22 not being specific to RCC. Each of these studies had less than 50 patients in the RCC arm. A larger sample size would have provided increased power to this study and may have even allowed for stratification by different RCC subtypes. The presence of various NMPs, including NMP-22, in different tissues and tumors may influence the results of these studies. More research needs to be performed before NMP-22 can be utilized regularly as a diagnostic test for RCC.

20.4.2 Extracellular Matrix Proteins

The extracellular matrix (ECM) is a network that provides structural support and maintains an environment suitable for cellular growth. In normal renal tubules, the components of the ECM are secreted by the epithelial cells away from the lumen and toward the interstitium (Sherief et al. 2003; Weimbs et al. 1997). Malignant transformation into RCC causes these epithelial cells to lose this polarity, resulting in the secretion of ECM proteins multidirectionally, including into the urine.

This distinction between normal and malignant cells led one group of investigators to hypothesize that the urinary concentration of ECM proteins would be greater in RCC patients than in healthy individuals. As diseases of the kidney, including diabetic nephropathy and renal damage secondary to toxins, can also lead to an increase in ECM proteins in the urine, the controls did not have any renal disease or take medications that could affect renal function (Price et al. 1995; Watanabe et al. 2000). They specifically tested for the presence of laminin, collagen IV, and fibronectin, which are normally secreted away from the lumen of the renal tubules. Their results showed that, instead of an increase in ECM proteins, there was a significant decrease of these proteins in the RCC patients' urine specimens (Sherief et al. 2003). A subsequent hypothesis, which would support the initial hypothesis, was then proposed: urine specimens from RCC patients contain a greater concentration of matrix metalloproteinase (MMP), which degrade ECM proteins, than healthy individuals. An equivalent amount of fibronectin was incubated in the urine specimens of the same RCC patients and healthy individuals. A Western blot assay demonstrated a decrease of full-length fibronectin in the RCC patients' urine specimens. Furthermore, collagen IV labeled with fluorescein was incubated in RCC patients' and healthy individuals' urine specimens. The thought was that if proteinases were present, they would degrade the fluorescein into peptides that would have fluorescent activity. Their results showed an average of 3.4-fold increase in fluorescent activity when the urine specimens were measured with a fluorescence reader. They concluded that the urine of RCC patients have increased MMP activity, leading to a decrease in ECM proteins.

An interesting point to note is that while all of the healthy individuals' urine demonstrated, at minimum, mild detection of either laminin, collagen IV, or fibronectin, all the RCC patients with the lowest clinical stage (T1N0M0) did not have any detectable ECM proteins in their urine. The investigators suggest that this difference may prove to be of value for detecting early stage RCC. The reported sensitivity and specificity of urinary-based ECM proteins for RCC is 95% and 96%, respectively (Tunuguntla and Jorda 2008).

20.4.3 Aquaporin-1

Aquaporins (AQPs) are membrane channel proteins whose function is to help transport water molecules and small solutes across cellular membranes (Magni et al. 2008). They belong to the larger family of major intrinsic proteins (MIPs), which are membrane channels found in various organisms. AQP1 was the first of 13 AQPs to be identified. This protein is found in many epithelial tissues and endothelium. Changes in AQP1 expression have been noted in various disease processes and cancers (Tamai et al. 2006; Zador et al. 2007). In the normal kidney, AQP1 is found in the extraglomerular capillaries, the glomerular endothelial cells, the proximal renal tubule epithelium, and the descending limb of the loop of Henle (Mazal et al. 2005). When investigators examined primary renal tumors, they found that there was increased expression of AQP1 in the clear cell and papillary subtypes of RCC, albeit at values lower than in normal kidneys, when compared to chromophobe RCC, collecting duct carcinomas, and oncocytomas (Huang et al. 2009; Mazal et al. 2005). Their study also suggested an inverse correlation between the level of AQP1 expression and tumor grade for the clear cell and papillary subtypes of RCC.

Based on the preceding data of increased AQP1 tissue expression in certain subtypes of RCC, one group of investigators tested the hypothesis that there would be a concomitant increase in urinary excretion of AQP1. Urine samples from patients with renal masses and a presumptive renal cancer diagnosis, patients undergoing a non-nephrectomy operation, and healthy controls were compared. When the pre- and post-nephrectomy urine samples of the patients with renal masses, which were postoperatively determined to have clear cell and papillary subtypes of RCC, were compared, there was a 95% and 97% decrease in the urinary concentrations of AQP1 in the clear cell and papillary subtypes of RCC, respectively (Morrissey et al. 2010). It should be noted that the post-nephrectomy urinary concentrations of AQP1 were slightly higher than the healthy controls' level, possibly due to microscopic residual tumor still present in the normal kidney tissue. The pre- and post-nephrectomy urinary samples in patients with renal masses determined to be chromophobe RCC, oncocytomas, and nonmalignant renal masses contained significantly lower concentrations of AQP1 than the clear cell and papillary subtypes and were comparable to the healthy controls. The pre- and postoperative urine samples from patients undergoing a non-nephrectomy operation were stable and comparable to the healthy controls. Their conclusion from this study was that urinary AQP1 may be considered a specific and sensitive noninvasive biomarker for RCCs that arise from the proximal tubule, such as clear cell RCC and papillary RCC.

Additionally, there appears to be a correlation between the urinary concentration of AQP1 and the tumor size in patients with clear cell RCC and papillary cell RCC (Morrissey et al. 2010). With prior studies showing an inverse correlation between the tissue expression of AQP1 and tumor grade (Huang et al. 2009), the urinary concentration of AQP1 may provide further insight to the grading and staging of RCC. However, more investigation with a larger sample size is needed before this can be concluded with more certainty.

While urinary AQP1 may have the potential to be a biomarker for clear cell RCC and papillary RCC, there have been questions directed toward this biomarker's utility. These questions stem from the fact that AQP1 is not a kidney-specific protein and that AQP1 is not only present in diseased renal tissue. Their thought is that increased urinary concentration of AQP1 may have a source other than the kidney or that it may be hard to distinguish whether the presence of AQP1 in the urine is truly related to renal disease processes or simply a result of stress placed on normal renal tissue (Grebe and Erickson 2010).

20.4.4 Adipophilin

Adipophilin, or adipose differentiation-related protein (ADFP), is a protein that is found on the surface of adipocytes and other cells, such as lactating mammary epithelial cells, adrenal cortex cells, and Sertoli and Leydig cells (Yao et al. 2007). It functions in facilitating the uptake of fatty acids and formation and storage of lipid droplets in these cells (Gao and Serrero 1999). The ADFP protein has also been shown to be a potential plasma biomarker for colorectal cancer and to be expressed in sebaceous tumors and cutaneous metastatic RCCs and was found to be elevated in the diabetic kidneys of rat models (Matsubara et al. 2011; Mishra et al. 2004; Ostler et al. 2010). Furthermore, clear cell RCC was named for the lipid droplets, formed with the help of ADFP, which are present in the tumor (Grebe and Erickson 2010). Immunohistochemical staining has shown increased expression of ADFP in primary tumors of the proximal tubules of the kidney, such as clear cell and papillary subtypes of RCC (Yao et al. 2005). It should be noted that clear cell RCC had significantly more positive staining than papillary RCC, but both had increased staining when compared to chromophobe RCC, oncocytomas, and normal kidneys.

Due to ADFP's tissue expression in these subtypes of RCC, the same group that investigated the presence of ADP1 in the urine of RCC patients also tested the same specimens for the ADFP protein. The result of their study indicated that there was a decrease from pre- to postnephrectomy of 88% and 92% of ADFP concentration in the urine samples from clear cell RCC and papillary RCC patients, respectively (Morrissey et al. 2010). The postnephrectomy urine concentrations of ADFP were slightly higher than the healthy controls. This could possibly be due to microscopic residual tumor still present in the kidneys. Both sets of urine samples from the clear cell RCC and papillary RCC patients also contained an increased ADFP concentration, when compared to the corresponding urine samples in the chromophobe RCC, oncocytoma, nonmalignant renal mass, and surgical control patients and the urine samples from the healthy control patients. Based on these results, their conclusion was that ADFP is a specific and sensitive noninvasive biomarker for diagnosing the clear cell and papillary subtypes of RCC.

When assessing, by Spearman analysis, whether there was a correlation between urinary concentration of ADFP and tumor size in patients with clear cell RCC and papillary RCC, investigators found the correlation coefficient to be 0.31 for ADFP, which was not significant at $p = 0.08$ (Morrissey et al. 2010). A larger sample size is needed to determine whether the urinary ADFP concentration is related to tumor size, along with other factors like tumor grade and stage. One confounding factor is that obesity is a known risk factor for clear cell RCC (McGuire and Fitzpatrick 2011). With an increase of ADFP in obese patients and those with obesity-related disease, a greater variety of patients will help decide if an increase in ADFP is simply linked to obesity or a result of the cancer (Matsubara et al. 2011; Yao et al. 2005).

20.4.5 Cathepsin D

Cathepsin D is a protease located in lysosomes. It normally plays a role in the degradation of proteins and other cellular processes, such as apoptosis (Diment et al. 1989; Yin et al. 2005). In cancer cells, cathepsin D has been shown to be involved in a number of key roles, such as cellular proliferation, tumor angiogenesis, and inhibition of apoptosis (Berchem et al. 2002). Furthermore, elevated tissue expression of cathepsin D has been reported in RCC and differences in blood cell gene expression of this protease have been reported in bladder cancer patients, when compared to healthy control (Merseburger et al. 2005; Osman et al. 2006). Cathepsin D may also be of value in determining the prognosis of RCC patients. One study revealed that patients with high tissue-expression of cathepsin D had improved long-term survival and a decreased chance of distant metastases (Merseburger et al. 2005).

With increased tissue expression of cathepsin D in RCC, one group investigated whether urinary levels of cathepsin D are useful in diagnosing this form of cancer. They obtained pre-nephrectomy urine specimens from patients with untreated clear cell RCC and urine specimens from patient with benign urological conditions and healthy controls. The concentration of cathepsin D in these groups, normalized to urinary creatinine, was compared. Though the clear cell RCC patients had a wider range of urinary cathepsin D, there was minimal significant difference between the three groups; the urine specimens of the benign and healthy controls revealed comparable levels of cathepsin D. ROC analysis showed no diagnostic utility when the clear cell RCC patients were compared to the other patients (Vasudev et al. 2009). There have been no studies investigating the utility of urinary cathepsin D in the diagnosis of papillary RCC.

The cathepsin D concentration in these urine specimens was also analyzed to see if any correlations with prognosis could be made. There appeared to be an association between overall survival, measured out to 8 years, and urinary cathepsin D concentration, based on univariate analysis (hazard ratio 1.33, 95% CI [1.09–1.63], $p = 0.005$) (Vasudev et al. 2009). This differs from the results for overall survival in RCC, based on tissue-expression of cathepsin D, where high levels of cathepsin D correlated with a decreased overall survival. It is thought that intracellular levels of cathepsin D do not influence the amount that becomes extracellular (Merseburger et al. 2005). The urinary cathepsin D concentration was also elevated in patients with nodal disease, metastatic disease, and clear cell RCC with sarcomatoid changes, when compared to clear cell RCC patient without these features. However, a larger patient population will be needed to provide stronger evidence of prognostic correlations and more power to this study. The sensitivity and specificity of urinary cathepsin D for RCC are unreported.

20.5 Conclusions

A large number of molecules are currently being studied as potential biomarkers for kidney cancer diagnosis, prognosis, and recurrence, with selected by-products of the VHL pathway and biomarkers of the systemic inflammatory response receiving the most attention. RCC biomarkers have the potential to serve a complementary role in conjunction with established clinical variables for improving early detection, prognostication, risk stratification, as well as patient counseling. They may also contribute to the selection of patients for targeted therapy regimens. Attempts to include biomarkers in select prognostic nomograms have shown promise thus far, but certainly more prospective trials are needed to prove their validity in the clinical setting. Molecular expression has also shown promise in more fully elucidating the underlying pathogenesis of kidney cancer and identifying additional prognostic biomarkers. While there are no standard biomarkers currently in use in the clinical management of patients with kidney cancer, previous studies have been encouraging and future studies promise to expand the understanding of the molecular basis of kidney cancer and provide additional data to use in tailoring treatment strategies for individual patients.

REFERENCES

Al Murri, A.M., J.M. Bartlett, P.A. Canney, J.C. Doughty, C. Wilson, and D.C. McMillan. 2006. Evaluation of an inflammation-based prognostic score (GPS) in patients with metastatic breast cancer. *Br J Cancer* 94 (2):227–230.

Apetoh, L., F. Ghiringhelli, A. Tesniere, M. Obeid, C. Ortiz, A. Criollo, G. Mignot et al. 2007. Toll-like receptor 4-dependent contribution of the immune system to anticancer chemotherapy and radiotherapy. *Nat Med* 13 (9):1050–1059.

Atkins, M., M. Regan, D. McDermott, J. Mier et al. 2005. Carbonic anhydrase IX expression predicts outcome of interleukin 2 therapy for renal cancer. *Clin Cancer Res* 11 (10):3714–3721.

Baldewijns, M.M., I.J. van Vlodrop, K.M. Smits, P.B. Vermeulen et al. 2009. Different angiogenic potential in low and high grade sporadic clear cell renal cell carcinoma is not related to alterations in the von Hippel–Lindau gene. *Cell Oncol* 31 (5):371–382.

Berchem, G., M. Glondu, M. Gleizes, J.P. Brouillet, F. Vignon, M. Garcia, and E. Liaudet-Coopman. 2002. Cathepsin-D affects multiple tumor progression steps in vivo: Proliferation, angiogenesis and apoptosis. *Oncogene* 21 (38):5951–5955.

Brauch, H., G. Weirich, J. Brieger, D. Glavac, H. Rodl, M. Eichinger, M. Feurer et al. 2000. VHL alterations in human clear cell renal cell carcinoma: Association with advanced tumor stage and a novel hot spot mutation. *Cancer Res* 60 (7):1942–1948.

Brenner, D.J. and E.J. Hall. 2007. Computed tomography—An increasing source of radiation exposure. *N Engl J Med* 357 (22):2277–2284.

Brenner, D.J., R. Doll, D.T. Goodhead, E.J. Hall, C.E. Land, J.B. Little, J.H. Lubin et al. 2003. Cancer risks attributable to low doses of ionizing radiation: Assessing what we really know. *Proc Natl Acad Sci U S A* 100 (24):13761–13766.

Brigden, M.L. 1999. Clinical utility of the erythrocyte sedimentation rate. *Am Fam Physician* 60 (5):1443–1450.

Bromwich, E., D.C. McMillan, G.W. Lamb, P.A. Vasey, and M. Aitchison. 2004. The systemic inflammatory response, performance status and survival in patients undergoing alpha-interferon treatment for advanced renal cancer. *Br J Cancer* 91 (7):1236–1238.

Bui, M.H., D. Seligson, K.R. Han, A.J. Pantuck, F.J. Dorey, Y. Huang, S. Horvath et al. 2003. Carbonic anhydrase IX is an independent predictor of survival in advanced renal clear cell carcinoma: Implications for prognosis and therapy. *Clin Cancer Res* 9 (2):802–811.

Cheng, W.S., G.M. Farrow, and H. Zincke. 1991. The incidence of multicentricity in renal cell carcinoma. *J Urol* 146 (5):1221–1223.

Cheville, J.C., C.M. Lohse, H. Zincke, A.L. Weaver, and M.L. Blute. 2003. Comparisons of outcome and prognostic features among histologic subtypes of renal cell carcinoma. *Am J Surg Pathol* 27 (5):612–624.

Cheville, J.C., C.M. Lohse, H. Zincke, A.L. Weaver, B.C. Leibovich, I. Frank, and M.L. Blute. 2004. Sarcomatoid renal cell carcinoma: An examination of underlying histologic subtype and an analysis of associations with patient outcome. *Am J Surg Pathol* 28 (4):435–441.

Chia, S.K., C.C. Wykoff, P.H. Watson, C. Han, R.D. Leek, J. Pastorek, K.C. Gatter, P. Ratcliffe, and A.L. Harris. 2001. Prognostic significance of a novel hypoxia-regulated marker, carbonic anhydrase IX, in invasive breast carcinoma. *J Clin Oncol* 19 (16):3660–3668.

Chow, G.K., J. Myles, and A.C. Novick. 2001. The Cleveland clinic experience with papillary (chromophil) renal cell carcinoma: Clinical outcome with histopathological correlation. *Can J Urol* 8 (2):1223–1228.

Cross, B.W., T.V. Johnson, A.B. Derosa, K. Ogan, J.G. Pattaras, P.T. Nieh, O. Kucuk, W.B. Harris, and V.A. Master. 2012. Preoperative erythrocyte sedimentation rate independently predicts overall survival in localized renal cell carcinoma following radical nephrectomy. *Int J Surg Oncol* 2012:524981.

Crumley, A.B., D.C. McMillan, M. McKernan, A.C. McDonald, and R.C. Stuart. 2006. Evaluation of an inflammation-based prognostic score in patients with inoperable gastro-oesophageal cancer. *Br J Cancer* 94 (5):637–641.

Davis, C.J. Jr., F.K. Mostofi, and I.A. Sesterhenn. 1995. Renal medullary carcinoma. The seventh sickle cell nephropathy. *Am J Surg Pathol* 19 (1):1–11.

Delahunt, B. 1999. Sarcomatoid renal carcinoma: The final common dedifferentiation pathway of renal epithelial malignancies. *Pathology* 31 (3):185–190.

Diment, S., K.J. Martin, and P.D. Stahl. 1989. Cleavage of parathyroid hormone in macrophage endosomes illustrates a novel pathway for intracellular processing of proteins. *J Biol Chem* 264 (23):13403–13406.

Einstein, A.J., M.J. Henzlova, and S. Rajagopalan. 2007. Estimating risk of cancer associated with radiation exposure from 64-slice computed tomography coronary angiography. *JAMA* 298 (3):317–323.

Forrest, L.M., D.C. McMillan, C.S. McArdle, W.J. Angerson, and D.J. Dunlop. 2003. Evaluation of cumulative prognostic scores based on the systemic inflammatory response in patients with inoperable non-small-cell lung cancer. *Br J Cancer* 89 (6):1028–1030.

Forrest, L.M., D.C. McMillan, C.S. McArdle, W.J. Angerson, and D.J. Dunlop. 2004. Comparison of an inflammation-based prognostic score (GPS) with performance status (ECOG) in patients receiving platinum-based chemotherapy for inoperable non-small-cell lung cancer. *Br J Cancer* 90 (9):1704–1706.

Frank, I., M.L. Blute, J.C. Cheville, C.M. Lohse, A.L. Weaver, and H. Zincke. 2002. An outcome prediction model for patients with clear cell renal cell carcinoma treated with radical nephrectomy based on tumor stage, size, grade and necrosis: The SSIGN score. *J Urol* 168 (6):2395–2400.

Frenzel, H., R. Pries, C.P. Brocks, W.J. Jabs, N. Wittkopf, and B. Wollenberg. 2007. Decreased migration of myeloid dendritic cells through increased levels of C-reactive protein. *Anticancer Res* 27 (6B):4111–4115.

Gao, J. and G. Serrero. 1999. Adipose differentiation related protein (ADRP) expressed in transfected COS-7 cells selectively stimulates long chain fatty acid uptake. *J Biol Chem* 274 (24):16825–16830.

Giatromanolaki, A., M.I. Koukourakis, E. Sivridis, J. Pastorek, C.C. Wykoff, K.C. Gatter, and A.L. Harris. 2001. Expression of hypoxia-inducible carbonic anhydrase-9 relates to angiogenic pathways and independently to poor outcome in non-small cell lung cancer. *Cancer Res* 61 (21):7992–7998.

Gimenez-Bachs, J.M., A.S. Salinas-Sanchez, F. Sanchez-Sanchez, J.G. Lorenzo-Romero, M.J. Donate-Moreno, H. Pastor-Navarro, D.C. Garcia-Olmo, J. Escribano-Martinez, and J.A. Virseda-Rodriguez. 2006. Determination of vhl gene mutations in sporadic renal cell carcinoma. *Eur Urol* 49 (6):1051–1057.

Glen, P., N.B. Jamieson, D.C. McMillan, R. Carter, C.W. Imrie, and C.J. McKay. 2006. Evaluation of an inflammation-based prognostic score in patients with inoperable pancreatic cancer. *Pancreatology* 6 (5):450–453.

Grebe, S.K. and L.A. Erickson. 2010. Screening for kidney cancer: Is there a role for aquaporin-1 and adipophilin? *Mayo Clin Proc* 85 (5):410–412.

Hannisdal, E., L. Bostad, K.A. Grottum, and F. Langmark. 1989. Erythrocyte sedimentation rate as a prognostic factor in renal cell carcinoma. *Eur J Surg Oncol* 15 (4):333–336.

Health Risks From Exposure to Low Levels of Ionizing Radiation: BEIR VII Phase 2. 2006. Washington, D.C.: Committee to Assess Health Risks from Exposure to Low Levels of Ionizing Radiation; Nuclear and Radiation Studies Board, Division on Earth and Life Studies, National Research Council of the National Academies.

Hoffmann, R., A. Franzke, J. Buer, S. Sel et al. 1999. Prognostic impact of in vivo soluble cell adhesion molecules in metastatic renal cell carcinoma. *Br J Cancer* 79 (11–12):1742–1745.

Hop, W.C. and B.H. van der Werf-Messing. 1980. Prognostic indexes for renal cell carcinoma. *Eur J Cancer* 16 (6):833–840.

Hosseini, J., A.R. Golshan, M.M. Mazloomfard, A.R. Mehrsai, M.A. Zargar, M. Ayati, S. Shakeri, M. Jasemi, and M. Kabiri. 2012. Detection of recurrent bladder cancer: NMP22 test or urine cytology? *Urol J* 9 (1):367–372.

Huang, S., E. Rhee, H. Patel, E. Park, and J. Kaswick. 2000. Urinary NMP22 and renal cell carcinoma. *Urology* 55 (2):227–230.

Huang, Y., T. Murakami, F. Sano, K. Kondo, N. Nakaigawa, T. Kishida, Y. Kubota, Y. Nagashima, and M. Yao. 2009. Expression of aquaporin 1 in primary renal tumors: A prognostic indicator for clear-cell renal cell carcinoma. *Eur Urol* 56 (4):690–698.

Ivanov, S., S.Y. Liao, A. Ivanova, A. Danilkovitch-Miagkova, N. Tarasova, G. Weirich, M.J. Merrill et al. 2001. Expression of hypoxia-inducible cell-surface transmembrane carbonic anhydrases in human cancer. *Am J Pathol* 158 (3):905–919.

Jabs, W.J., M. Busse, S. Kruger, D. Jocham, J. Steinhoff, and C. Doehn. 2005. Expression of C-reactive protein by renal cell carcinomas and unaffected surrounding renal tissue. *Kidney Int* 68 (5):2103–2110.

Jemal, A., T. Murray, E. Ward, A. Samuels, R.C. Tiwari, A. Ghafoor, E.J. Feuer, and M.J. Thun. 2005. Cancer statistics, 2005. *CA Cancer J Clin* 55 (1):10–30.

Jeong, S., Y. Park, Y. Cho, Y.R. Kim, and H.S. Kim. 2012. Diagnostic values of urine CYFRA21-1, NMP22, UBC, and FDP for the detection of bladder cancer. *Clin Chim Acta* 414C:93–100.

Johnson, T.V., A. Abbasi, A. Owen-Smith, A.N. Young, O. Kucuk, W.B. Harris, A.O. Osunkoya et al. 2010. Postoperative better than preoperative C-reactive protein at predicting outcome after potentially curative nephrectomy for renal cell carcinoma. *Urology* 76 (3):766 e1–e5.

Johnson, T.V., S. Ali, A. Abbasi, O. Kucuk, W.B. Harris, K. Ogan, J. Pattaras et al. 2011. Intratumor C-reactive protein as a biomarker of prognosis in localized renal cell carcinoma. *J Urol* 186 (4):1213–1217.

Karakiewicz, P.I., G.C. Hutterer, Q.D. Trinh, C. Jeldres, P. Perrotte, A. Gallina, J. Tostain, and J.J. Patard. 2007. C-reactive protein is an informative predictor of renal cell carcinoma-specific mortality: A European study of 313 patients. *Cancer* 110 (6):1241–1247.

Kattan, M.W., V. Reuter, R.J. Motzer, J. Katz, and P. Russo. 2001. A postoperative prognostic nomogram for renal cell carcinoma. *J Urol* 166 (1):63–67.

Kavolius, J.P., D.P. Mastorakos, C. Pavlovich, P. Russo, M.E. Burt, and M.S. Brady. 1998. Resection of metastatic renal cell carcinoma. *J Clin Oncol* 16 (6):2261–2266.

Kawai, Y., H. Matsuyama, Y. Korenaga, T. Misumi et al. 2009. Preoperative erythrocyte sedimentation rate is an independent prognostic factor in Japanese patients with localized clear cell renal cell carcinoma. *Urol Int* 83 (3):306–310.

Kaya, K., S. Ayan, G. Gokce, H. Kilicarslan, E. Yildiz, and E.Y. Gultekin. 2005. Urinary nuclear matrix protein 22 for diagnosis of renal cell carcinoma. *Scand J Urol Nephrol* 39 (1):25–29.

Kelishadi, R., M. Hashemi, N. Mohammadifard, S. Asgary, and N. Khavarian. 2008. Association of changes in oxidative and proinflammatory states with changes in vascular function after a lifestyle modification trial among obese children. *Clin Chem* 54 (1):147–153.

Kennedy, S.M., M.J. Merino, W.M. Linehan, J.R. Roberts, C.N. Robertson, and R.D. Neumann. 1990. Collecting duct carcinoma of the kidney. *Hum Pathol* 21 (4):449–456.

Klatte, T., J.S. Lam, B. Shuch, A.S. Belldegrun, and A.J. Pantuck. 2008. Surveillance for renal cell carcinoma: Why and how? When and how often? *Urol Oncol* 26 (5):550–554.

Komai, Y., K. Saito, K. Sakai, and S. Morimoto. 2007. Increased preoperative serum C-reactive protein level predicts a poor prognosis in patients with localized renal cell carcinoma. *BJU Int* 99 (1):77–80.

Kondo, K., M. Yao, M. Yoshida, T. Kishida, T. Shuin, T. Miura, M. Moriyama et al. 2002. Comprehensive mutational analysis of the VHL gene in sporadic renal cell carcinoma: Relationship to clinicopathological parameters. *Genes Chromosomes Cancer* 34 (1):58–68.

Kovacs, G., P. Brusa, and W. De Riese. 1989. Tissue-specific expression of a constitutional 3;6 translocation: Development of multiple bilateral renal-cell carcinomas. *Int J Cancer* 43 (3):422–427.

Kuroda, N., M. Toi, M. Hiroi, and H. Enzan. 2003. Review of sarcomatoid renal cell carcinoma with focus on clinical and pathobiological aspects. *Histol Histopathol* 18 (2):551–555.

Lamb, G.W., P.A. McArdle, S. Ramsey, A.M. McNichol, J. Edwards, M. Aitchison, and D.C. McMillan. 2008. The relationship between the local and systemic inflammatory responses and survival in patients undergoing resection for localized renal cancer. *BJU Int* 102 (6):756–761.

Lehmann, J., M. Retz, N. Nurnberg, U. Schnockel et al. 2004. The superior prognostic value of humoral factors compared with molecular proliferation markers in renal cell carcinoma. *Cancer* 101 (7):1552–1562.

Leibovich, B.C., M.L. Blute, J.C. Cheville, C.M. Lohse, I. Frank, E.D. Kwon, A.L. Weaver, A.S. Parker, and H. Zincke. 2003. Prediction of progression after radical nephrectomy for patients with clear cell renal cell carcinoma: A stratification tool for prospective clinical trials. *Cancer* 97 (7):1663–1671.

Li, G., G. Feng, A. Gentil-Perret, C. Genin, and J. Tostain. 2008. Serum carbonic anhydrase 9 level is associated with postoperative recurrence of conventional renal cell cancer. *J Urol* 180 (2):510–513; discussion 513–514.

Linehan, W.M., M.I. Lerman, and B. Zbar. 1995. Identification of the von Hippel–Lindau (VHL) gene. Its role in renal cancer. *JAMA* 273 (7):564–570.

Ljungberg, B. 2007. Prognostic markers in renal cell carcinoma. *Curr Opin Urol* 17 (5):303–308.

Ljungberg, B., K. Grankvist, and T. Rasmuson. 1997. Serum interleukin-6 in relation to acute-phase reactants and survival in patients with renal cell carcinoma. *Eur J Cancer* 33 (11):1794–1798.

Ljungberg, B., G. Landberg, and F.I. Alamdari. 2000. Factors of importance for prediction of survival in patients with metastatic renal cell carcinoma, treated with or without nephrectomy. *Scand J Urol Nephrol* 34 (4):246–251.

Loncaster, J.A., A.L. Harris, S.E. Davidson, J.P. Logue et al. 2001. Carbonic anhydrase (CA IX) expression, a potential new intrinsic marker of hypoxia: Correlations with tumor oxygen measurements and prognosis in locally advanced carcinoma of the cervix. *Cancer Res* 61 (17):6394–6399.

Lydersen, B.K. and D.E. Pettijohn. 1980. Human-specific nuclear protein that associates with the polar region of the mitotic apparatus: Distribution in a human/hamster hybrid cell. *Cell* 22 (2 Pt 2):489–499.

Magera, J.S. Jr., B.C. Leibovich, C.M. Lohse, S. Sengupta, J.C. Cheville, E.D. Kwon, and M.L. Blute. 2008. Association of abnormal preoperative laboratory values with survival after radical nephrectomy for clinically confined clear cell renal cell carcinoma. *Urology* 71 (2):278–282.

Magni, F., C. Chinello, F. Raimondo, P. Mocarelli, M.G. Kienle, and M. Pitto. 2008. AQP1 expression analysis in human diseases: Implications for proteomic characterization. *Expert Rev Proteomics* 5 (1):29–43.

Mantovani, A. and A. Sica. 2010. Macrophages, innate immunity and cancer: Balance, tolerance, and diversity. *Curr Opin Immunol* 22 (2):231–237.

Masuda, H., Y. Kurita, K. Suzuki, K. Fujita, and Y. Aso. 1997. Predictive value of serum immunosuppressive acidic protein for staging renal cell carcinoma: Comparison with other tumour markers. *Br J Urol* 80 (1):25–29.

Matsubara, J., K. Honda, M. Ono, S. Sekine, Y. Tanaka, M. Kobayashi, G. Jung et al. 2011. Identification of adipophilin as a potential plasma biomarker for colorectal cancer using label-free quantitative mass spectrometry and protein microarray. *Cancer Epidemiol Biomarkers Prev* 20 (10):2195–2203.

Mazal, P.R., M. Stichenwirth, A. Koller, S. Blach, A. Haitel, and M. Susani. 2005. Expression of aquaporins and PAX-2 compared to CD10 and cytokeratin 7 in renal neoplasms: A tissue microarray study. *Mod Pathol* 18 (4):535–540.

McGuire, B.B. and J.M. Fitzpatrick. 2011. BMI and the risk of renal cell carcinoma. *Curr Opin Urol* 21 (5):356–361.

McKiernan, J.M., R. Buttyan, N.H. Bander, A. de la Taille, M.D. Stifelman, E.R. Emanuel, E. Bagiella et al. 1999. The detection of renal carcinoma cells in the peripheral blood with an enhanced reverse transcriptase-polymerase chain reaction assay for MN/CA9. *Cancer* 86 (3):492–497.

McMillan, D.C., M.M. Elahi, N. Sattar, W.J. Angerson, J. Johnstone, and C.S. McArdle. 2001. Measurement of the systemic inflammatory response predicts cancer-specific and non-cancer survival in patients with cancer. *Nutr Cancer* 41 (1–2):64–69.

Mejean, A., M. Roupret, F. Larousserie, V. Hopirtean, N. Thiounn, and B. Dufour. 2003. Is there a place for radical nephrectomy in the presence of metastatic collecting duct (Bellini) carcinoma? *J Urol* 169 (4):1287–1290.

Merseburger, A.S., J. Hennenlotter, P. Simon, P.A. Ohneseit et al. 2005. Cathepsin D expression in renal cell cancer-clinical implications. *Eur Urol* 48 (3):519–526.

Meyer, A.A., G. Kundt, U. Lenschow, P. Schuff-Werner, and W. Kienast. 2006. Improvement of early vascular changes and cardiovascular risk factors in obese children after a six-month exercise program. *J Am Coll Cardiol* 48 (9):1865–1870.

Mian, B.M., N. Bhadkamkar, J.W. Slaton, P.W. Pisters, D. Daliani, D.A. Swanson, and L.L. Pisters. 2002. Prognostic factors and survival of patients with sarcomatoid renal cell carcinoma. *J Urol* 167 (1):65–70.

Mishra, R., S.N. Emancipator, C. Miller, T. Kern, and M.S. Simonson. 2004. Adipose differentiation-related protein and regulators of lipid homeostasis identified by gene expression profiling in the murine db/db diabetic kidney. *Am J Physiol Renal Physiol* 286 (5):F913–F921.

Mlecnik, B., M. Tosolini, A. Kirilovsky, A. Berger, G. Bindea, T. Meatchi, P. Bruneval et al. 2011. Histopathologic-based prognostic factors of colorectal cancers are associated with the state of the local immune reaction. *J Clin Oncol* 29 (6):610–618.

Morrissey, J.J., A.N. London, J. Luo, and E.D. Kharasch. 2010. Urinary biomarkers for the early diagnosis of kidney cancer. *Mayo Clin Proc* 85 (5):413–421.

Nozoe, T., D. Korenaga, M. Futatsugi, H. Saeki, Y. Maehara, and K. Sugimachi. 2003. Immunohistochemical expression of C-reactive protein in squamous cell carcinoma of the esophagus—Significance as a tumor marker. *Cancer Lett* 192 (1):89–95.

O'Gorman, P., D.C. McMillan, and C.S. McArdle. 2000. Prognostic factors in advanced gastrointestinal cancer patients with weight loss. *Nutr Cancer* 37 (1):36–40.

Osman, I., D.F. Bajorin, T.T. Sun, H. Zhong et al. 2006. Novel blood biomarkers of human urinary bladder cancer. *Clin Cancer Res* 12 (11 Pt 1):3374–3380.

Ostler, D.A., V.G. Prieto, J.A. Reed, M.T. Deavers, A.J. Lazar, and D. Ivan. 2010. Adipophilin expression in sebaceous tumors and other cutaneous lesions with clear cell histology: An immunohistochemical study of 117 cases. *Mod Pathol* 23 (4):567–573.

Ozer, G., M. Altinel, B. Kocak, A. Yazicioglu, and F. Gonenc. 2002. Value of urinary NMP-22 in patients with renal cell carcinoma. *Urology* 60 (4):593–597.

Patard, J.J., P. Fergelot, P.I. Karakiewicz, T. Klatte, Q.D. Trinh, N. Rioux-Leclercq, J.W. Said, A.S. Belldegrun, and A.J. Pantuck. 2008. Low CAIX expression and absence of VHL gene mutation are associated with tumor aggressiveness and poor survival of clear cell renal cell carcinoma. *Int J Cancer* 123 (2):395–400.

Patard, J.J., E. Leray, N. Rioux-Leclercq, L. Cindolo, V. Ficarra, A. Zisman, A. De La Taille et al. 2005. Prognostic value of histologic subtypes in renal cell carcinoma: A multicenter experience. *J Clin Oncol* 23 (12):2763–2771.

Pavlovich, C.P. and L.S. Schmidt. 2004. Searching for the hereditary causes of renal-cell carcinoma. *Nat Rev Cancer* 4 (5):381–393.

Peyromaure, M., N. Thiounn, F. Scotte, A. Vieillefond, B. Debre, and S. Oudard. 2003. Collecting duct carcinoma of the kidney: A clinicopathological study of 9 cases. *J Urol* 170 (4 Pt 1):1138–1140.

Pienta, K.J., A.W. Partin, and D.S. Coffey. 1989. Cancer as a disease of DNA organization and dynamic cell structure. *Cancer Res* 49 (10):2525–2532.

Prasad, S.R., P.A. Humphrey, J.R. Catena, V.R. Narra, J.R. Srigley, A.D. Cortez, N.C. Dalrymple, and K.N. Chintapalli. 2006. Common and uncommon histologic subtypes of renal cell carcinoma: Imaging spectrum with pathologic correlation. *Radiographics* 26 (6):1795–1806; discussion 1806–1810.

Price, R.G., S.A. Taylor, E. Crutcher, E. Bergamaschi, I. Franchini, and A.D. Mackie. 1995. The assay of laminin fragments in serum and urine as an indicator of renal damage induced by toxins. *Toxicol Lett* 77 (1–3):313–318.

Ramsey, S., G.W. Lamb, M. Aitchison, J. Graham, and D.C. McMillan. 2007. Evaluation of an inflammation-based prognostic score in patients with metastatic renal cancer. *Cancer* 109 (2):205–212.

Ramsey, S., G.W. Lamb, M. Aitchison, and D.C. McMillan. 2008. Prospective study of the relationship between the systemic inflammatory response, prognostic scoring systems and relapse-free and cancer-specific survival in patients undergoing potentially curative resection for renal cancer. *BJU Int* 101 (8):959–963.

Rini, B.I., S.C. Campbell, and B. Escudier. 2009. Renal cell carcinoma. *Lancet* 373 (9669):1119–1132.

Roberts, C.K., A.K. Chen, and R.J. Barnard. 2007. Effect of a short-term diet and exercise intervention in youth on atherosclerotic risk factors. *Atherosclerosis* 191 (1):98–106.

Roosen, J.U., U. Engel, R.H. Jensen, E. Kvist, and G. Schou. 1994. Renal cell carcinoma: Prognostic factors. *Br J Urol* 74 (2):160–164.

Ropponen, K.M., M.J. Eskelinen, P.K. Lipponen, E. Alhava, and V.M. Kosma. 1997. Prognostic value of tumour-infiltrating lymphocytes (TILs) in colorectal cancer. *J Pathol* 182 (3):318–324.

Rosenbaum, M., C. Nonas, R. Weil, M. Horlick, I. Fennoy, I. Vargas, and P. Kringas. 2007. School-based intervention acutely improves insulin sensitivity and decreases inflammatory markers and body fatness in junior high school students. *J Clin Endocrinol Metab* 92 (2):504–508.

Roxburgh, C.S. and D.C. McMillan. 2010. Role of systemic inflammatory response in predicting survival in patients with primary operable cancer. *Future Oncol* 6 (1):149–163.

Sandlund, J., E. Oosterwijk, K. Grankvist, J. Oosterwijk-Wakka, B. Ljungberg, and T. Rasmuson. 2007. Prognostic impact of carbonic anhydrase IX expression in human renal cell carcinoma. *BJU Int* 100 (3):556–560.

Sene, A.P., L. Hunt, R.F. McMahon, and R.N. Carroll. 1992. Renal carcinoma in patients undergoing nephrectomy: Analysis of survival and prognostic factors. *Br J Urol* 70 (2):125–134.

Sengupta, S., C.M. Lohse, J.C. Cheville, B.C. Leibovich et al. 2006. The preoperative erythrocyte sedimentation rate is an independent prognostic factor in renal cell carcinoma. *Cancer* 106 (2):304–312.

Sharma, S., C.D. Zippe, L. Pandrangi, D. Nelson, and A. Agarwal. 1999. Exclusion criteria enhance the specificity and positive predictive value of NMP22 and BTA stat. *J Urol* 162 (1):53–57.

Sherief, M.H., S.H. Low, M. Miura, N. Kudo, A.C. Novick, and T. Weimbs. 2003. Matrix metalloproteinase activity in urine of patients with renal cell carcinoma leads to degradation of extracellular matrix proteins: Possible use as a screening assay. *J Urol* 169 (4):1530–1534.

Smits, K.M., L.J. Schouten, B.A. van Dijk, C.A. Hulsbergen-van de Kaa, K.A. Wouters, E. Oosterwijk, M. van Engeland, and P.A. van den Brandt. 2008. Genetic and epigenetic alterations in the von Hippel–Lindau gene: The influence on renal cancer prognosis. *Clin Cancer Res* 14 (3):782–787.

Storkel, S., J.N. Eble, K. Adlakha, M. Amin, M.L. Blute, D.G. Bostwick, M. Darson, B. Delahunt, and K. Iczkowski. 1997. Classification of renal cell carcinoma: Workgroup No. 1. Union Internationale Contre le Cancer (UICC) and the American Joint Committee on Cancer (AJCC). *Cancer* 80 (5):987–989.

Swartz, M.A., J. Karth, D.T. Schneider, R. Rodriguez, J.B. Beckwith, and E.J. Perlman. 2002. Renal medullary carcinoma: Clinical, pathologic, immunohistochemical, and genetic analysis with pathogenetic implications. *Urology* 60 (6):1083–1089.

Tamai, K., K. Fukushima, Y. Ueno, Y. Moritoki, Y. Yamagiwa, N. Kanno, D.M. Jefferson, and T. Shimosegawa. 2006. Differential expressions of aquaporin proteins in human cholestatic liver diseases. *Hepatol Res* 34 (2):99–103.

Todenhofer, T., J. Hennenlotter, U. Kuhs, V. Tews, G. Gakis, S. Aufderklamm, A. Stenzl, and C. Schwentner. 2012. Influence of urinary tract instrumentation and inflammation on the performance of urine markers for the detection of bladder cancer. *Urology* 79 (3):620–624.

Toro, J.R., G. Glenn, P. Duray, T. Darling, G. Weirich, B. Zbar, M. Linehan, and M.L. Turner. 1999. Birt–Hogg–Dube syndrome: A novel marker of kidney neoplasia. *Arch Dermatol* 135 (10):1195–1202.

Toro, J.R., M.L. Nickerson, M.H. Wei, M.B. Warren, G.M. Glenn, M.L. Turner, L. Stewart et al. 2003. Mutations in the fumarate hydratase gene cause hereditary leiomyomatosis and renal cell cancer in families in North America. *Am J Hum Genet* 73 (1):95–106.

Toro, J.R., M.H. Wei, G.M. Glenn, M. Weinreich, O. Toure, C. Vocke, M. Turner et al. 2008. BHD mutations, clinical and molecular genetic investigations of Birt–Hogg–Dube syndrome: A new series of 50 families and a review of published reports. *J Med Genet* 45 (6):321–331.

Tunuguntla, H.S. and M. Jorda. 2008. Diagnostic and prognostic molecular markers in renal cell carcinoma. *J Urol* 179 (6):2096–2102.

Vasudev, N.S., S. Sim, D.A. Cairns, R.E. Ferguson et al. 2009. Pre-operative urinary cathepsin D is associated with survival in patients with renal cell carcinoma. *Br J Cancer* 101 (7):1175–1182.

Vickers, M.M. and D.Y. Heng. 2010. Prognostic and predictive biomarkers in renal cell carcinoma. *Target Oncol* 5 (2):85–94.

Vira, M.A., K.R. Novakovic, P.A. Pinto, and W.M. Linehan. 2007. Genetic basis of kidney cancer: A model for developing molecular-targeted therapies. *BJU Int* 99 (5 Pt B):1223–1229.

Watanabe, H., H. Sanada, S. Shigetomi, T. Katoh, and T. Watanabe. 2000. Urinary excretion of type IV collagen as a specific indicator of the progression of diabetic nephropathy. *Nephron* 86 (1):27–35.

Wei, M.H., O. Toure, G.M. Glenn, M. Pithukpakorn, L. Neckers, C. Stolle, P. Choyke et al. 2006. Novel mutations in FH and expansion of the spectrum of phenotypes expressed in families with hereditary leiomyomatosis and renal cell cancer. *J Med Genet* 43 (1):18–27.

Weimbs, T., S.H. Low, S.J. Chapin, and K.E. Mostov. 1997. Apical targeting in polarized epithelial cells: There's more afloat than rafts. *Trends Cell Biol* 7 (10):393–399.

Woodward, E.R., S.C. Clifford, D. Astuti, N.A. Affara, and E.R. Maher. 2000. Familial clear cell renal cell carcinoma (FCRC): Clinical features and mutation analysis of the VHL, MET, and CUL2 candidate genes. *J Med Genet* 37 (5):348–353.

Wu, P., N. Zhang, X. Wang, X. Ning, T. Li, D. Bu, and K. Gong. 2012. Family history of von Hippel–Lindau disease was uncommon in Chinese patients: Suggesting the higher frequency of de novo mutations in VHL gene in these patients. *J Hum Genet* 57 (4):238–243.

Wu, S.L., I.J. Fishman, and R.L. Shannon. 2002. Chromophobe renal cell carcinoma with extensive calcification and ossification. *Ann Diagn Pathol* 6 (4):244–247.

Yao, M., Y. Huang, K. Shioi, K. Hattori, T. Murakami, N. Nakaigawa, T. Kishida, Y. Nagashima, and Y. Kubota. 2007. Expression of adipose differentiation-related protein: A predictor of cancer-specific survival in clear cell renal carcinoma. *Clin Cancer Res* 13 (1):152–160.

Yao, M., H. Tabuchi, Y. Nagashima, M. Baba, N. Nakaigawa, H. Ishiguro, K. Hamada et al. 2005. Gene expression analysis of renal carcinoma: Adipose differentiation-related protein as a potential diagnostic and prognostic biomarker for clear-cell renal carcinoma. *J Pathol* 205 (3):377–387.

Yao, M., M. Yoshida, T. Kishida, N. Nakaigawa, M. Baba, K. Kobayashi, T. Miura et al. 2002. VHL tumor suppressor gene alterations associated with good prognosis in sporadic clear-cell renal carcinoma. *J Natl Cancer Inst* 94 (20):1569–1575.

Yin, L., R. Stearns, and B. Gonzalez-Flecha. 2005. Lysosomal and mitochondrial pathways in H_2O_2-induced apoptosis of alveolar type II cells. *J Cell Biochem* 94 (3):433–445.

Zador, Z., O. Bloch, X. Yao, and G.T. Manley. 2007. Aquaporins: Role in cerebral edema and brain water balance. *Prog Brain Res* 161:185–194.

Zbar, B., K. Tory, M. Merino, L. Schmidt, G. Glenn, P. Choyke, M.M. Walther, M. Lerman, and W. M. Linehan. 1994. Hereditary papillary renal cell carcinoma. *J Urol* 151 (3):561–566.

Zisman, A., A.J. Pantuck, F. Dorey, J.W. Said, O. Shvarts, D. Quintana, B.J. Gitlitz, J.B. deKernion, R.A. Figlin, and A.S. Belldegrun. 2001. Improved prognostication of renal cell carcinoma using an integrated staging system. *J Clin Oncol* 19 (6):1649–1657.

Zisman, A., A.J. Pantuck, J. Wieder, D.H. Chao, F. Dorey, J.W. Said, J.B. deKernion, R.A. Figlin, and A.S. Belldegrun. 2002. Risk group assessment and clinical outcome algorithm to predict the natural history of patients with surgically resected renal cell carcinoma. *J Clin Oncol* 20 (23):4559–4566.

21

Novel Oncomarkers Used for Earlier Detection of Bladder Carcinoma

Miroslava Bilecová-Rabajdová, Peter Urban, Mária Mareková, and Vincent Nagy

CONTENTS

ABSTRACT Bladder cancer is the fourth most common cancer in men and the eighth most common in women. Oncomarkers play a crucial role in early detection of bladder cancer, as well as in treatment response monitoring and prognosis. Searching for a new marker by molecular analysis is in progress because any diagnostic sensitivity and specificity enhancement is a great benefit for clinical practice.

This chapter consists of reviews of the latest markers of early stages of bladder cancer. Carcinoembryonic antigen (*CEA*) and tissue polypeptide-specific antigen (*TPS*) are tumor markers used in clinical diagnostics. The aim of oncomarkers' diagnostic is usually detection of early stages of the disease. These markers are mostly used for systematically observing of patients (2–3 months interval). The newer markers with unconfirmed sensitivity and specificity are fragments of cytokeratin 19 (*CYFRA 21-1*), cytokeratin 20 (*CK20*), nuclear matrix protein 22 (*NMP22*), bladder tumor antigen (*BTA*), bladder cancer-specific NMP (*BLCA-4*), fibroblasts growth factor (*FGFr*), tumor necrosis factor alpha (*TNF*-α), vascular endothelial growth factor (*VEGF*) and their receptors. In the last couple of years, some very promising markers for early stages bladder cancer from biological liquids were discovered. Molecular and proteomic assessments of these markers are frequently implemented to clinical urological diagnostics. The confirmation of high specificity and relative sensitivity of new markers are described.

KEY WORDS: *bladder cancer, early detection, diagnostics, molecular biomarkers.*

21.1 Introduction

21.1.1 Bladder Cancer

Survival in patients with bladder cancer is strongly associated with stage at diagnosis. Although most cancers are superficial at time of diagnosis, currently 10%–20% of all cases of bladder cancer have invaded the muscular wall of the bladder when first diagnosed, with a much worse prognosis (Leliveld et al., 2011). Five-year survival for patients with superficial disease is over 90% but falls to less than 50% with invasive disease (Ploeg et al., 2009). Survival rate according to the stages of bladder cancer is shown in Table 21.1. Routine screening for bladder cancer with microscopic urinalysis, urine dipstick, or urine cytology is not recommended in asymptomatic persons. Dipstick and microscopic urinalysis are simple and sensitive tests for detecting hematuria from early tumors, but they are not sufficiently specific to be practical for screening for bladder cancer in the general population. Even among older high-risk populations, the predictive value of a positive screening test is low (5%–8%). This chapter summarizes all recent and relevant information including classical screening methods and their effectiveness in comparing to commonly used biomarkers for invasive and noninvasive form of bladder malignancies. This chapter also promotes experimental and potential biomarkers suitable for detection of earlier stages of bladder cancer, which could help to reduce morbidity and mortality from this type of cancer in relation to the benefits, costs, and risks of screening tests and early treatment.

21.1.2 Epidemiology

Bladder cancer is the most common malignancy involving the urinary system and the ninth most common malignancy worldwide (Ploeg et al., 2009). Urothelial (transitional cell) carcinoma is the predominant histological type in the United States and Western Europe, where it accounts for approximately 90% of

TABLE 21.1

Table Describes a 5-Year Survival Rate after Detection of Earlier and Advanced Stages of Bladder Cancer

Stage	Relative 5-Year Survival Rate
0	98%
I	88%
II	63%
III	46%
IV	15%

bladder cancers. During the year 2012 about 73,510 new cases of bladder cancer (about 55,600 in men and 17,910 in women) had been diagnosed in the United States. Approximately 70% of newly diagnosed bladder tumors are non-muscle invasive at diagnosis. Ninety percent of bladder cancers are transitional cell carcinoma. The other 10% are squamous cell carcinoma, adenocarcinoma, sarcoma, small cell carcinoma, and secondary deposits from cancers elsewhere in the body. Mortality is about 14,880 deaths from bladder cancer (about 10,510 in men and 4,370 in women) (Siegel et al., 2012). The rates of new cancers and of cancer deaths have been fairly stable over the past 20 years. More than 500,000 people in the United States are bladder cancer survivors. Bladder cancer occurs mainly in older people. About 9 out of 10 people with this cancer are over the age of 55. The average age at the time of diagnosis is 73. In about half of all cases, patients are first diagnosed with bladder cancer while it is still confined to the inner layer of the bladder (noninvasive or in situ cancer). About 35% have bladder cancer that has invaded into deeper layers but is still contained in the bladder. In most of the remaining cases, the cancer has spread to nearby tissues outside the bladder. Rarely (in about 4% of cases), it has spread to distant sites (Jemal et al., 2011).

21.1.3 Bladder Cancer Staging

The classification of the American Urological Association (AUA) considers all T1, high-grade Ta, and carcinoma in situ (CIS) as high risk of recurrence and progression. Long-term follow-up of series of T1G3 patients treated with Bacillus Calmette-Guérin (BCG) reports that despite the treatment, there is a 45% rate of recurrence and a 17% rate of progression (American Urological Association, 2010). Bladder cancer is staged on the degree of tumor invasion into the bladder wall (Lamm and Torti, 1996). CIS (Tis), and Stages Ta and T1 are grouped as superficial bladder cancers because they are restricted to the inner epithelial lining of the bladder and do not involve the bladder cancers because they are restricted to the inner epithelial lining of the bladder and do not involve the muscle wall. Of the "nonmuscle-invasive" tumors, Stage Ta tumors are confined to the mucosa, while Stage T1 tumors superficially invade the lamina propria. T1 tumors are regarded as being more aggressive than Ta tumors (4). Invasive tumors (Stages T2, T3, and T4) extend into the muscle (Stage T2) and into the perivesical fat layer beyond the muscle (Stage T3), with metastatic tumors (Stage T4) involving local nodes or distant organs. The most common cell type of bladder cancer is transitional cell carcinoma, although adenocarcinomas, squamous cell carcinomas, and sarcomas also occur. The cellular morphology of superficial bladder tumors is graded on the degree of cellular differentiation. The grading consists of well-differentiated (Grade 1), moderately differentiated (Grade 2), and poorly differentiated (Grade 3) tumors. Grading of cell morphology is important for establishing prognosis, as Grade 3 tumors are the most aggressive and the most likely to become invasive (Fritsche et al., 2006). Staging is shown in Table 21.2.

21.1.4 Treatment

The yield of onetime screening for bladder cancer (for occurrence of microscopic hematuria) in the general outpatient population appears to be much lower. In a retrospective review of over 20,000 men over 35 and women over 55 receiving a personal health appraisal, dipstick screening detected only 3 cases of cancer (1 bladder, 2 prostate) (Rigaud et al., 2002). Prevalence of positive dipstick results ranged from 3% to 9% over a 7-year period. In a second study of almost 2700 outpatients, 13% of screened men and women had hematuria, but only 2% of those with microscopic hematuria had serious urology disease (Gaya et al., 2012).

Urine cytology is more specific but less sensitive than microscopic hematuria as a screen for early bladder cancer. Because cytology is technically difficult and significantly more expensive than dipstick urinalysis, its use as an initial screening test has been limited to high-risk occupational screening programs. Specificity and sensitivity for cytology has been estimated to be as high as 90.9% and 98.0%, respectively (Kim et al., 2011). Among men with dipstick hematuria in one screening study, urine cytology detected 10 of 17 patients with bladder cancer with a specificity of 96%; 6 of the 7 cases missed were well-differentiated, superficial lesions with a good prognosis (Schips et al., 2002). Transurethral resection (TURB) is recommended as the gold standard for diagnosis and treatment for non-muscle-invasive bladder cancer (Nieder et al., 2005). Although there have been described novel approaches to perform a good-quality transurethral en bloc resection (Nagele et al., 2011), especially

TABLE 21.2

Histological Grading of Nonmuscle-Invasive Bladder Urothelial Carcinomas

T (primary tumor)	
TX	Primary tumor cannot be assessed
T0	No evidence of primary tumor
Ta	Noninvasive papillary carcinoma
Tis	CIS ("flat tumor")
T1	Tumor invades subepithelial connective tissue
T2a	Tumor invades superficial muscle (inner half)
T2b	Tumor invades deep muscle (outer half)
T3	Tumor invades perivesical tissue
T3a	Microscopically
T3b	Macroscopically (extravesical mass)
T4a	Tumor invades prostate, uterus, or vagina
T4b	Tumor invades pelvic wall or abdominal wall
N (lymph nodes)	
NX	Regional lymph nodes cannot be assessed
N0	No regional lymph node metastasis
N1	Metastasis in a single lymph node 2 cm or less in greatest dimension
N2	Metastasis in a single lymph node more than 2 cm, but not more than 5 cm in greatest dimension, or multiple lymph nodes, not more than 5 cm in greatest dimension
N3	Metastasis in a lymph node more than 5 cm in greatest dimension
M (distant metastasis)	
MX	Distant metastasis cannot be assessed
M0	No distant metastasis
M1	Distant metastasis

Note: Classification of noninvasive urothelial tumors was proposed by the World Health Organization (WHO) and the International Society of Urological Pathology (ISUP) (1998 WHO/ISUP classification).

for small tumors (1 cm) (Wolters et al., 2011), TURB has been associated with a high rate of residual tumor (from 30% to 70%) (Jahnson et al., 2005), and this is also true of understaging of T2 disease (from 5% to 27%) (Rigaud et al., 2002). For this reason, European guidelines for high-risk bladder cancer (HRBC) recommend a second TURB, 2–6 weeks after initial resection when there is a high grade or T1 tumor (Babjuk et al., 2011), in case of an initial incomplete resection, multiple or large tumors, or when there is no muscle tissue in the specimen (Babjuk et al., 2011). Due to the low incidence of concomitant CIS in HRBC (3.5%–14%) (Meijer et al., 2011), European guidelines recommend biopsies of the normal-looking mucosa only in case of positive cytology and when an exophytic tumor has a nonpapillary appearance. Flow chart of the Bladder Cancer Treatment Guide is shown in Figure 21.1. Biopsy of the prostatic urethra has to be included in cases of bladder neck tumor when CIS is present or suspected and in cases of positive cytology with normal cystoscopy (Babjuk et al., 2011). During the recent years, numerous urinary tests have been developed for early diagnosis of bladder cancer (Vrooman et al., 2008; Lotan et al., 2010). Almost all molecular markers have been tested in clinical trials, and for a variety of reasons, many are unsuitable for clinical practice (Shirodkar and Lokeshwar, 2009). Sensitivity and specificity of detection techniques and molecular markers are shown in Table 21.3. NMP22, UroVysion, and ImmunoCyt (Hajdinjak, 2008; Mowatt et al., 2010) are the most promising tests. While the value of UroVysion seems to be limited in HRBC (66%–70% sensitivity) (Babjuk et al., 2011), it can replace cytology for high-grade tumors when experience with

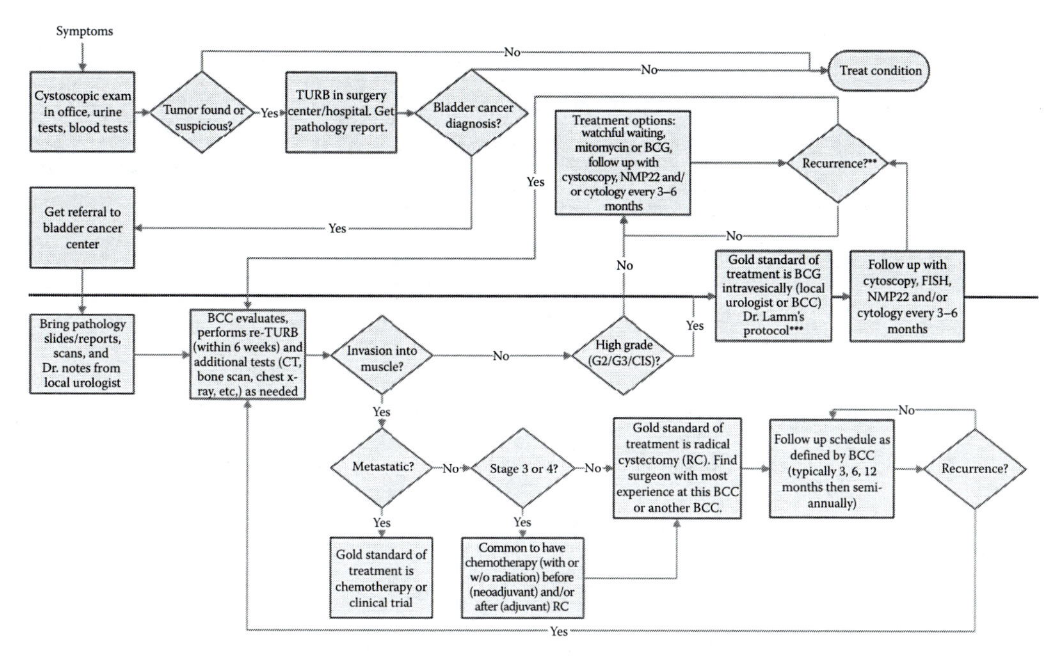

FIGURE 21.1 Flow diagram describes the usual procedure after microhematuria occurs. ** means that in the case of high grade recurrence is advised to use radical cystectomy, *** means that you can follow advice of your private doctor or Dr. Lamms protocol. (According to Schenkman, E. and Lamm, DL., *Sci. World J.* 1(Suppl), 387, 2004.)

TABLE 21.3

Table Describes Sensitivities and Specificities for Current Detection Methods and Markers

Marker	No. of Patients	Median Sensitivity	No. of Patients	Median Specificity
BTAstst	1377	58	2084	73
BTAtrak	360	71	195	66
NMP22	838	71	1203	73
ImmunoCyt	276	67	683	75
Cytometry	364	60	98	82
Hb-dipstick	117	40	113	87
LewisX	95	75	215	85
FISH	165	79	147	70
Telomerase	146	39	—	Na
MSI	108	82	153	89
CYFRA21-1	156	85	323	82
Cytokeratin20	117	85	61	76
BTA	436	48	216	92
Cytology	2213	35	3322	94

Source: According to van Rhijn, B.W. et al., *J. Clin. Oncol.*, 21, 1912, 2003.

urinary cytology is lacking or when the results of cytology are inconclusive (Schmitz-Drager et al., 2007). These markers also provide closer look for determination of grading (shown in Table 21.4). As a treatment of HRBC type is recommend at least 1 year of BCG instillations plus maintenance (Babjuk et al., 2011), but the AUA proposes just three weekly instillations (i.e., each week for 3 weeks) at 3 and 6 months after induction and every 6 months thereafter for 3 years (Lamm et al., 2000). A published meta-analysis has shown a 32% reduction in the risk of recurrence with BCG maintenance compared to mitomycin C (Malstrom et al., 2009). In another study, BCG maintenance was associated with a 37% reduction in the risk of progression compared with control groups (Cliff et al., 2000).

TABLE 21.4

Comparison of Sensitivity and Specificity to Grading of Bladder Tumors

No. of Patients/Median Sensitivity			
Marker	**G1**	**G2**	**G3**
BTAstst	288/45	206/60	208/75
BTAtrak	60/55	61/59	101/74
NMP22	56/41	77/53	81/80
ImmunoCyt	23/78	10/90	18/100
Cytometry	18/11	54/41	38/66
Hb-dipstick	13/15	36/39	22/73
FISH	25/56	9/78	20/95
MSI	27/67	21/86	30/93
Cytokeratin20	14/71	35/80	35/100
BTA	31/16	43/47	50/52
Cytology	239/17	274/34	201/58

Source: According to van Rhijn, B.W. et al., *J. Clin. Oncol.*, 21, 1912, 2003.

This immunotherapy is also used to treat and prevent the recurrence of superficial tumors (Alexandroff et al., 1999). BCG immunotherapy is effective in up to 2/3 of the cases at this stage. Instillations of chemotherapy, such as valrubicin (Valstar) into the bladder can also be used to treat BCG-refractory CIS disease when cystectomy is not an option.

21.2 Markers Based on Source

The urine markers used in patient surveillance have on occasion been criticized for their low sensitivity in detecting disease, but in most studies they have significantly improved the detection of bladder cancer when used in conjunction with cytology and cystoscopy. Voided urine cytology has its own limitations in detecting CIS (Tis) and low-grade bladder tumors (Malik and Murphy, 1999). It appears that urine markers can assist in the early detection of recurrence in patients with CIS and low-grade superficial tumors (van der Poel and Debruyne, 2001). All recently used of experimental markers could be detected from urine, exfoliated cells, or from blood and tissue itself. The list of all markers and their nature and detection methods are shown in Table 21.5.

21.2.1 Urine Markers

Because urine comes into contact with bladder tumors, many tests of voided urine have been designed to detect molecules that may be associated with tumor growth or invasion. At present, the standard noninvasive bladder tumor test is voided urine cytology. A number of markers that take advantage of exfoliated cells in the urine for detection of cell surface antigens, nuclear morphology, or gene expression have been studied in bladder cancer. The most common urine test is bladder tumor antigen (BTA) TRAK test. It is a quantitative test that requires trained personnel and a reference laboratory. These assays detect human complement factor H-related protein (as well as complement factor H), which is present in the urine of patients with bladder cancer (Kinders et al., 1998). It is believed that complement factor H production by tumor cells may prevent tumor cell lysis by immune cells. Both tests have sensitivity comparable to that of cytology for high-grade tumors and better for low-grade tumors. Another possible marker, the nuclear matrix protein 22 (*NMP22*), is a protein that localizes with the spindle poles during mitosis and thus regulates chromatid and daughter cell separation (Shelfo and Soloway, 1997). There is a substantially higher level of *NMP22* in the urine of patients with bladder cancer. However, because this protein is released from dead and dying urothelial cells, many benign conditions of the urinary tract, such as stones, infection,

TABLE 21.5

The List of All Markers, Their Nature, and Detection Methods

Marker	Type of Marker	Material for Detection	Detection Methods
BTA	Antigen, glycoprotein	Urine	Immunoassay
UroVysion	DNA/chromosomes	Urine, exfoliated cells	FISH
NMP22	Protein	Urine	ELISA
ImmunoCyt	Antigen, glycoprotein	Urine, exfoliated cells	Immunoassay
sFas	Protein	Urine	ELISA, RT-PCR
Telomerase	Enzyme/protein	Urine, exfoliated cells	TRAP
MSI	DNA repeats	Urine, blood exfoliated cells	PCR
Cytokeratin20	Protein	Urine	Immunohistology, RT-PCR, ELISA
CYFRA21.1	Protein	Urine	ELISA
Methylation	DNA/gene	Urine sediment—exfoliated cells	PCR
BLCA4	Protein	Urine, exfoliated cells	ELISA
HA	Glycosaminoglycan	Urine	ELISA
Lewis X	Antigen	Urine, exfoliated cells	ELISA, RT-PCR
TNF	DNA/gene	Blood	ELISA, RT-PCR
FGFR3	Protein	Urine sediment	SSCP
VEGF	Protein	Urine, tissue	Immunohistology
EGFR	Protein	Tissue	Immunoassay
CXCL1	Protein	Urine	ELISA
TATI	Antigen	Urine	Immunofluorometric assay
Survivin	Protein	Urine	ELISA, RT-PCR

Note: TRAP, Telomerase repeat amplification protocol.

inflammation, and hematuria, and cystoscopy can cause a false-positive reading. *NMP22* has, however, not gained widespread use in routine urology practice for several reasons. First, reluctance may stem from the high false-positive rate, and the absence of large-scale testing to confirm that *NMP22* improves prediction of disease recurrence/progression in patients with bladder cancer (Shariat and Kattan, 2008). Another method suitable for neoplasia of bladder cancer from voided urine and blood is microsatellite (MI) analysis. MIs are highly polymorphic DNA repeats that can undergo mutations, leading to loss of heterogeneity and thus can be used as markers of neoplasia from (van Rhijn et al., 2001).

21.2.2 Markers from Exfoliated Cells in Urine

The most of recently used markers belong to this group. ImmunoCyt detects cellular markers for bladder cancer in exfoliated urothelial cells using three fluorescent monoclonal antibodies to pinpoint a high molecular weight form of carcinoembryonic antigen and two bladder tumor cell-associated mucins. This test may prove useful as an adjunct to cytology, but currently it requires further testing to define its role in the management of bladder cancer (Vriesema et al., 2001). Multiple chromosomes, such as 1, 3, 4, 7, 8, 9, 11, and 17, are altered in urothelial tumors (Junker et al., 2003). These chromosomal alterations can be easily detected with fluorescence in situ hybridization (FISH) assay (UroVysion). Regardless of its high sensitivity, FISH depends on the presence of adequate numbers of exfoliated abnormal cells in the urine specimen. UBC™, a point-of-care test that qualitatively measures cytokeratins 8 and 18 in the urine (Heicappell et al., 2000). *BLCA 1* is a nuclear transcription factor present in the tumor area of the bladder, but not in adjacent benign tissue or nonmalignant bladder. *BLCA-1* levels are increased in bladder cancer exfoliated cells with higher tumor stage. *BLCA-4* is present in both the tumor and adjacent benign areas of the bladder but not in benign bladders (Konety et al., 2000a). *BLCA-1* and *BLCA-4* seem to be promising markers for bladder cancer, with a high sensitivity and specificity. The Lewis X antigen is expressed in epithelium from urothelial carcinoma, regardless of the tumor grade or stage, detectable in exfoliated cells (Friedrich et al., 2002). Survivin is a novel member of the inhibitor of apoptosis gene family that counteracts cell death, controls mitotic progression, and induces changes in gene expression that are associated with tumor cell invasiveness (Altieri, 2003). It is undetectable or expressed at low levels in most differentiated normal adult tissues and is overexpressed in human cancers. Survivin is detectable in exfoliated cells. Malignant neoplasms, including bladder cancer, have been shown to produce telomerase and thus to regenerate telomeres and prevent cell death (Muller, 2002). The standard technique to measure telomerase activity is the telomerase repeat amplification protocol assay (TRAP assay) from exfoliated cells (Eissa et al., 2007b). However, because many bladder cancer patients have other urological and nonurological comorbidities, the clinical applicability of the telomerase assay could be limited (Shariat and Kattan, 2008).

21.2.3 Markers from Tissue

These markers are detectable in the later phases of bladder cancer after the occurrence of others symptoms like blood in urine. First of them is epidermal growth factor receptor (*EGFR*). It is involved in various forms of cancers and serves as prognostic markers or therapeutic targets (Rotterud et al., 2005). High *EFGR* was associated with nonpapillary, high-grade, and invasive tumors, can be detected from tissue, and also may help select patients with urinary cancer for more aggressive therapy (Kassouf et al., 2008). Another important marker could be vascular endothelial growth factor (*VEGF*). It is a positive regulator of angiogenesis and shows a high expression in almost all known tumors including urinary cancers (Das et al., 2007). Its expression can be detected from tumor tissue.

21.3 Markers Based on Type

21.3.1 Genetic Markers

21.3.1.1 Telomeres and Telomerase

Telomeres are repetitious sequences at the end of chromosomes that protect genetic stability during DNA replication. There is loss of telomeres during each cell division, which causes chromosomal instability and cellular senescence. Bladder cancer cells express telomerase, an enzyme that regenerates telomeres at the end of each DNA replication and therefore sets the cellular clock to immortality. Three major subunits comprising the human telomerase complex have been identified: a ribosomal RNA component that serves as a template for telomere repeat synthesis, a protein component responsible for enzymatic activity of telomerase enzyme, and finally telomerase enzyme associated with proteins with an unclear function (Muller, 2002). The standard technique to measure telomerase activity is the TRAP assay (Kim et al., 2005). Another telomerase-based assay detects the catalytic subunit of telomerase, human telomerase reverse transcriptase, using polymerase chain reaction (PCR).

When compared with TRAP, human telomerase reverse transcriptase PCR has higher sensitivity than the TRAP assay, ranging between 75% and 100% (Mellissourgos et al., 2003). Overall sensitivity and specificity of the telomerase assay, as reported by Lokeshaw et al. (2005), were 70%–100% and 60%–70%, respectively (Lokeshwar et al., 2005b). In a systematic review Glas et al. (2003) showed that telomerase had the best sensitivity (75%) compared to the other markers, including cytology. Specificity, however, was lower than cytology (Glas et al., 2003). A more recently conducted case-control study on 218 men showed an overall sensitivity of 90% and specificity of 88%, which increased to 94% for individuals younger than 75 years of age (Sanchini et al., 2005). The same phenomenon was noted by Bravaccini et al. (2007), in a case-control study conducted in 212 women, sensitivity was 87% and specificity 66%. A breakdown analysis as a function of age showed a higher assay accuracy in women younger than 75 years (sensitivity 91% and specificity 69%) compared to older women (sensitivity 64% and specificity 59%) (Bravaccini et al., 2007). The authors noted that a possible explanation for this effect is the higher number of viable and telomerase-positive nonurothelial cells, such as epithelial cells from the lower genital tract or inflammatory elements in urine of the elderly. In a study by Eissa et al. (2007b), 200 patients were included that had been diagnosed with bladder carcinoma. They did not specify whether these were primary or recurrent tumors. Eighty-five individuals with benign bladder lesions and 30 healthy individuals served as the control group. All were tested for relative telomerase activity in urothelial cells from voided urine. The sensitivity and the specificity of human telomerase reverse transcriptase for detecting bladder cancer was 96%. They concluded that detection of human telomerase reverse transcriptase in urine by real-time PCR improves sensitivity and specificity for the diagnosis of bladder cancer (Eissa et al., 2007b).

In conclusion, the clinical applicability of the telomerase assay may be limited, because many UCB patients have other urological and nonurological comorbidities. Another possible limitation of this test is the potential for inactivation of the telomerase enzyme in urine, leading to extremely low sensitivity (7% in the study of Muller et al. [1998]) (Muller et al., 1996). An ideal bladder cancer screening and monitoring test would be noninvasive, rapid, objective, and easy to perform and interpret and have high sensitivity and specificity (Shariat and Kattan, 2008). Ideal samples for the earlier detection occur in urine or extrafoliated cells (urine sediment). Moreover, test results can be influenced by inflammation and age. These disadvantages make it a suboptimal test for detection of bladder cancer.

21.3.1.2 Microsatellite Analysis

MSIs are highly polymorphic short-tandem DNA repeats found in the human genome. Two types of MSI alterations can be found in many cancers: loss of heterozygosity (LOH), and an allelic deletion and somatic alteration of MSI repeat length (Mao et al., 1996). In bladder cancer, most mutations are in the form of LOH (Turyn et al., 2006). LOH can be identified by comparing the peak ratio of the two alleles from tumor or urine DNA with that from blood. A multitude of different loci of alterations have been identified in bladder cancer. MSI alterations in exfoliated urine are detected by a PCR using DNA primers for a panel of known MSI markers (van Tilborg et al., 2012).

Most LOH were found with the marker for chromosome 9. They found a relatively low sensitivity of 58% and a specificity of 73%. A potential limitation of their study is that their main analysis is based on the combined data from the two arms. Separate analysis of the patients in the MSI arm showed an improved sensitivity (70%) of the MSI analysis test. A number of different MSIs are used dispersed over a number of chromosomes to improve the accuracy of detection. Up to 20 different MSI markers have usually been analyzed for each sample. This number and the need to compare allele ratios with normal (blood) DNA make the method difficult to carry out. Recently, Bartoletti introduced a method in which 10 markers were combined in 3 multiplex PCRs (van Rhijn et al., 2001). This improved analysis has a median sensitivity of 82% and a median specificity of 89% (Amira et al., 2002). In contrast to conventional cytology, it appears that MSA has the ability to detect low-grade and low-stage disease as accurately as high-grade and high-stage disease (Little et al., 2005). Frigerio et al. (2007) found that the combined use of cytology and LOH analysis had high sensitivity for identifying primary tumors and had the ability to detect almost all recurrent diseases in voided urine. They found that the sensitivity for Grade 1–2 tumors was 72% and that for Grade 3 tumors was 96% (Frigerio et al., 2007).

In conclusion, MSI analysis has good overall sensitivity and specificity, but this test is complex, expensive, and together with the fact that voided urine samples are currently not sufficiently sensitive promotes this test not suitable for daily clinical practice.

21.3.1.3 Methylation

CpG dinucleotides are clustered in the promoters of many genes and these so-called CpG islands are generally unmethylated in order to allow gene expression. Alteration of methylation of CpGs is a frequent phenomenon in cancer (Collings et al., 2013). Methylation usually shuts down gene expression, and when the promoter in question belongs to a tumor suppressor gene, this can contribute to cancer development. Methylation of specific promoters can quite easily be detected by many different techniques (Laird, 2005). The first report on methylation of the promoter of the *p16/CDKN2A* gene in bladder carcinoma appeared already over a decade ago and several papers have appeared since (Gonzalgo et al., 2007).

Recently, methylation detection techniques have also been used in order to detect bladder tumor cells in urinary sediment (Knowles, 2007). So far, no publications have appeared that report sensitivity of these techniques for the detection of recurrent bladder cancer in more than 50 patients under surveillance. Hoque et al. (2006) describe in a recent paper that sensitivity in the detection of non-muscle-invasive cancer (including urine from patients with a primary tumor) is 75%. This is a promising result, and a further study on this approach for surveillance is eagerly awaited. Although the study of Roupret et al. (2008) included only 40 patients, they were able to detect 13 out of 15 recurrent tumors (86%) with a panel of 11 promoter regions. However, of the 25 patients with no evidence of recurrent disease, only 2 had no aberrant methylation of any promoter site (specificity 8%). The finding that methylation was also found in normal urothelium and seems to increase with advanced age is a serious drawback for this type of assay (Yates et al., 2006). This emphasizes the need for a thorough selection of gene promoters in order to design an optimal panel for surveillance studies. Scher et al. (2012) were monitoring DNA methylation of genes *BCL2*, *CDKN2A*, and *NID2* and found that using these genes they were able to differentiate bladder cancer from other urogenital malignancies and nonmalignant conditions with a sensitivity of 80.9% and a specificity of 86.4%. Another study of Chung et al. (2011) selected five novel candidate genes (*MYO3A, CA10, SOX11, NKX6-2, PENK*, and *DBC1*) from the most frequently hypermethylated genes detected by DNA microarray and bisulfite pyrosequencing of bladder cancers and applied them to detect bladder cancer in urine sediments. A panel of these genes had 85% sensitivity and 95% specificity for detection of bladder cancer (area under curve = 0.939). By analyzing the data by cancer invasiveness, detection rate was 47 of 58 (81%) in nonmuscle-invasive tumors. Lin et al. (2010) observed that also promoter hypermethylation in four genes (*E-cadherin, p16, p14,* and *RASSF1A*) is suitable for identification reliable biomarkers for bladder cancer diagnosis in primary tumor DNA and urine sediment. Diagnostic sensitivity was 75% for combining *RASSF1A* and *p14* and 83% for *RASSF1A, p14,* and *E-cadherin*. Importantly, hypermethylation was detected in the urine DNA of 90% superficial tumors with negative or atypia cytology.

21.3.2 Mutation or Polymorphism Markers

21.3.2.1 Fibroblast Growth Factor Receptor 3

Fibroblast growth factors (*FGF*) represent a large family of polypeptides that are potent regulators of cell proliferation, migration, and differentiation. FGF receptors (*FGFR*) belong to the family of tyrosine kinases, an enzyme that plays an important role in activation of several different intracellular signaling pathways.

Specific point mutations that constitutively activate the tyrosine kinase activity of *FGFR3* are found in 50%–60% of primary bladder tumors. The role of these mutations in the carcinogenesis is not exactly known yet. These mutations are most prominent in the pTa category with a mutation percentage of 80% (van Rhijn et al., 2003). This would make the detection of *FGFR3* mutations in urine an excellent assay for the follow-up of patients presenting with a lower risk *FGFR3*-mutant tumor. Although several studies have been able to show a correlation between *FGFR3* status and prognosis, these studies were all carried out on DNA isolated from the original tumor (Burger et al., 2007; van Oers et al., 2009). It has been shown that these mutations can also be detected in urine using single-strand conformation polymorphism analysis (SSCP). SSCP is a very laborious assay and does not detect mutations with high efficiency. Recently, an easy-to-use Snapshot assay has been developed in which 11 of the most frequent point mutations can be assessed in 1 multiplex reaction (van Oers et al., 2005). This technique is able to detect a mutant *FGFR3* allele in an excess of wild-type DNA, making the assay suitable for sensitive detection of mutant tumor cells in urine (van Oers et al., 2005). Currently, a longitudinal study is underway to determine the sensitivity of this assay for the urine-based detection of recurrent bladder cancer in patients with an *FGFR3*-mutant primary tumor. In a study by Rieger et al. (2003) they took urine sediment DNA samples from 192 patients, of whom 72 had undergone TURB of mainly Ta lesions and 120 had undergone cystectomy. The patients in the cystectomy group had more advanced tumors than those in the TURB group. They found that 67% of patients in the TURB group and 28% of patients in the cystectomy group displayed *FGFR3* mutations. In 122 cases comparative analysis of cytology was performed and *FGFR3* analysis identified change in 68% of urine sediment DNA, whereas cytology recorded the presence of tumor cells in 32% of the DNA samples. But more importantly it seems that *FGFR3* is expressed in low-grade and low-stage disease (Rieger-Christ et al., 2003). This was confirmed by Gomez et al. (2005) who used a microarray to evaluate *FGFR3* messenger RNA (mRNA) expression in urinary carcinomas at different stages. They also showed a marked overexpression of both *FGFR3* mRNA and protein in urinary cancer with a greater expression that was observed in Stages pTa and pT1 (Goméz-Román et al., 2005). van Oers et al. (2007) examined four markers (*Ki-67, TP53, CK20*, and *FGFR3*). In this study an *FGFR3* mutation analysis was performed in a group of 255 unselected patients with a primary urinary cancer. Mutations in the *FGFR3* gene were detected in 47% of 208 bladder tumors, of which 61% occurred in pTa and pT1 tumors. *FGFR3* mutations were predominantly present in tumors of Stage pTa (73%) and Grade 1 (82%) (van Oers et al., 2007). Almost all *FGFR3* mutations occurred in tumors without adjacent CIS, only 1% concurrence. Because of this observation, they state that *FGFR3* mutations and CIS must be considered as exclusive events, and *FGFR3* mutations are associated with favorable histopathological characteristics. The authors concluded with regard to *FGFR3* that it is a useful marker to identify superficial tumors with low malignant potential but that grade and stage are still better predictors.

In conclusion, *FGFR3* plays an important role in the development of low-grade and non-muscle-invasive urinary cancer. Used as a molecular marker, it is diagnostic for low grade/low stage, and *FGFR3* mutations seem to be associated with favorable tumor characteristics. This development gives a lot of information about molecular pathways that occur in the development of urinary cancer.

21.3.3 Insertions and Deletions

21.3.3.1 Fluorescence In Situ Hybridization

FISH with four multitarget probes to the centromeres of chromosomes 3, 7, and 17 and to the 9p21 band forms the FISH UroVysion assay. Polysomy or (homozygous) 9p21 loss indicates the presence of cancer cells. Loss of 9p21, the locus of the *p16* tumor suppressor gene, is one of the earliest and most frequent genetic aberrations in bladder cancer (Vrooman et al., 2009).

This test has been approved by the FDA both for monitoring patients with a history of UCB and for detection in patients with hematuria. The FISH test combines assessment of the morphologic changes of conventional cytology with molecular DNA changes. Each probe is a fluorescently labeled, single-stranded DNA fragment (nucleic acid sequence) complementary to specific target sequences of cellular DNA that are denatured to allow hybridization with the probe. Fluorescence microscopy allows visualization of the hybridized, labeled probe. The kit contains a mixture of unlabeled blocking DNA to suppress sequences contained within the target loci that are common to other chromosomes. A minimum of 25 morphologically abnormal cells is viewed. If four or more cells exhibit polysomy, the case is considered positive for tumor (Chade et al., 2009). Combining morphology with FISH may prove an alternative modality of cancer detection (Daniely et al., 2005, 2007). The combination of morphology and FISH resulted in 100% sensitivity and 65% specificity (Lotan et al., 2008). Atypical findings are problematic because they raise concerns with the patient and the physician about the possible presence of cancer. One of the possible applications of FISH is to clarify the therapeutic dilemma associated with an atypical cytological result (Bergman et al., 2008).

In various case-control studies, as recently summarized by Lokeshwar et al. (2005b), the sensitivity of FISH varies between 69% and 87%. All studies reported a low sensitivity of FISH to detect low-grade (36%–57%) and low-stage (62%–65%) tumors, but FISH has high sensitivity to detect high-grade and high-stage tumors (83%–97%). The detection of CIS is close to 100%. The specificity of FISH is high (89%–96%) and is comparable to cytology. The limited performance of FISH in low-grade or low-stage tumors is not consistent. Jones (2006) also reviewed published reports on the role of FISH in bladder cancer surveillance. He concluded that FISH outperformed conventional cytology across all stages and grades in all published reports. Notably, cytology detected only 67% of CIS versus 100% detection by FISH. Marin-Aguilera et al. (2007) found in their study higher overall sensitivity for FISH versus cytology (70.3% vs. 35.1%). In this study the significant difference was maintained when non-muscle-invasive UC detection was broken down into low-grade and high-grade tumors. In contrast with these two studies, Moonen et al. (2007) found no improvement of FISH over cytology in the diagnosis of recurrent nonmuscle-invasive bladder cancer (NMIBC) in a study including 64 patients with biopsy-proven UC. Sensitivity and specificity were, respectively, 39.1% and 89.7% for FISH and 40.6% and 89.7% for cytology. A potential advantage of FISH is its ability to detect occult diseases not visible on urethrocystoscopy. Many authors note that a false-positive FISH test can predict future recurrence within 3–12 months in 41%–89% of patients (Sarosdy et al., 2002; Skacel et al., 2003). Veeramachaneni et al. (2003) concluded in a cohort study that a positive FISH test may indicate frank neoplastic urothelial transformation or it may merely be an indicator of unstable urothelium. Specificity of FISH, therefore, may be underestimated because of this phenomenon and explains why FISH performs different in different patient populations, for example, less in surveillance compared to detection of primary tumors.

In conclusion, several limitations have precluded a wider use of this test by urologists: the high cost and the necessity of large urine volume and/or tumor burden as well as exfoliation of tumor cells. Bladder washing may help increase the number of cells available for inspection with FISH, thereby increasing the diagnostic yield (Bergman et al., 2008). Finally, another limitation is that the FISH assay does not detect diploid cells without 9p21 deletions. However, most authors agree that FISH is better than cytology, although the test might have limited sensitivity to detect low-grade tumors. The fairly high false-positive rate is explained by some to reflect the potential of the FISH test to predict future recurrences (Kipp et al., 2005).

21.3.3.2 Tumor Necrosis Factor

Tumor necrosis factor (TNF) α and *TNF*-β are structurally related cytokines that are secreted by macrophages and lymphocytes, respectively (Beutler and Cerami, 1986). The *TNF* genes contain a relatively large number of polymorphisms, possibly associated with a susceptibility to bladder cancer and prognosis. Nonomura et al. (2006) looked at a possible correlation between polymorphism in the *TNF*-β and *TNF*-α gene, and clinical features of bladder cancer in a group of 141 Japanese patients with bladder cancer and 173 Japanese controls with benign disease. Genotyping was done through PCR of blood samples. They could not find a correlation between *TNF*-α polymorphisms and clinicopathological parameters. In the *TNF*-β group, however, there was a significant difference in the genotype distribution between the bladder cancer patients and the controls. Patients with the β1/2 genotype showed a 1.71-fold increased risk of bladder cancer compared with the β2/2 genotype (Nonomura et al., 2006). In contrast, Kim et al. (2005) performed PCR of blood samples of 153 patients with primary bladder cancer and 153 control subjects in an earlier study and found a significant increase of the *TNF*-α genotype and cancer stage. They concluded that these data suggest that these genetic polymorphisms may be useful as prognostic markers for bladder cancer in the clinical setting. A possible explanation for these differences is given by Nonomura et al. (2006): the frequency of *TNF*-α polymorphisms appears to differ among ethnic groups.

In conclusion, *TNF* can have prognostic value, but the polymorphisms can differ between ethnic groups. More clinical studies are necessary to define the place of *TNF* as a marker of progression.

21.3.4 Protein Markers

21.3.4.1 The Nuclear Matrix Protein 22

The *NMP22* test detects a nuclear mitotic apparatus protein that is a component of the nuclear matrix. NMPs make up the framework of a cell's nucleus and play an important role in gene expression (Gordon et al., 1993). *NMP22* is a protein that localizes to the spindle poles during mitosis and thus regulates chromatid and daughter cell separation (Compton and Cleveland, 1993). However, because this protein is released from dead and dying urothelial cells, many nonmalignant conditions of the urinary tract, such as stones, infection, inflammation, and hematuria, as well as instrumentation (i.e., cystoscopy), can cause a false-positive test result (Shelfo et al., 2005).

The first *NMP22* test was a quantitative enzyme-linked immunosorbent assay (ELISA) test. The newer *NMP22* "BladderChek" is a point-of-care assay using monoclonal antibodies in a lateral flow strip, detecting the *NMP22* with a cutoff value of 10 U/mL. Grossman et al. (2005) investigated the capability of this test in detecting malignancy in 1331 patients with risk factors of bladder cancer. They found sensitivity of 55.7% and specificity of 85% for *NMP22* as compared to 15.8% and 99.2% for cytology (Grossman et al., 2006). Miyanaga et al. (1999) published a paper on the detection of recurrent tumors with *NMP22*. Sensitivity was 19% and specificity 85% at a cutoff of 10 U/mL. With a cutoff of 5 U/mL, sensitivity increased to 49%, but specificity dropped to 66% (Miyanaga et al., 1999). Shariat et al. (2006) analyzed *NMP22* in 302 patients at risk for recurrence, and 180 of these indeed had bladder cancer. Sensitivity and specificity were 66% and 73% at the 6.5 U/mL cutoff levels that were preferred by the authors (Shariat et al., 2006). However, a relatively large group of 80 patients had pT1 and muscle-invasive recurrences and 63 tumors were Grade 3. The high percentage of patients with a recurrence, and the considerable number of >T1 stages (28%), suggests that this patient population was not limited to patients under surveillance for superficial bladder cancer but also patients awaiting treatment for invasive disease. This might therefore have increased sensitivity. In a second paper by this group, 2871 patients were included in an international follow-up cohort (Grosman et al., 2006). One thousand forty-five patients had a recurrence at the moment of urine sampling. At 6.5 U/mL cutoff, sensitivity was 68% and specificity 67%. There was variability in the performance of the assay between different laboratories, which made it impossible to define a clear cutoff value for the assay.

In conclusion, the current *NMP22* point-of-care test is easy to perform, with sensitivity better than cytology and a reasonable specificity. However, its sensitivity seems to be hampered by benign conditions (Trischler et al., 2007).

21.3.4.2 Cytokeratins

Cytokeratins are intermediate filaments; their main function is to enable cells to withstand mechanical stress. In humans 20 different cytokeratin isotypes have been identified. Cytokeratins 8, 18, 19, and 20 have been associated with bladder cancer (Southgate et al., 1999). The urinary bladder cancer (UBC) test detects cytokeratins 8 and 18 fragments in urine. Sensitivity of the UBC test varies from 35% to 79% and depends on tumor grade and Stage 2, but UBC tests were inferior to voided cytology in test quality (Hakenberg et al., 2004). *CYFRA 21-1* is a soluble fragment of cytokeratin 19 and is analyzed with ELISA. It is measurable in serum and urine. Abnormal serum levels of *CYFRA 21-1* in patients with bladder cancer were only seen in patients with metastatic disease (Pariente et al., 2000). Abnormal *CYFRA 21-1* levels also showed a significantly worse overall median survival and correlated with response to systemic treatment (Andreadis et al., 2005).

21.3.4.2.1 Urinary Bladder Cancer Test

The UBC test is an ELISA that detects the presence of fragments of cytokeratins 8 and 18 in the urine. Cytokeratins 8 and 18 are part of the normal cell structure and therefore present in normal bladder epithelium, especially the umbrella cells. Increased expression and modification have been found in transitional cell carcinoma, especially in high-grade tumors (Wiener et al., 1998). A recent study by Babjuk et al. (2008) followed 88 patients with NMIBC for the presence of recurrent tumors. The sensitivity of the assay was 54%, the specificity 97%. They concluded that quantitative UBC tests have a low sensitivity in the detection of bladder cancer recurrence and cannot be used routinely to reduce the number of cystoscopies during follow-up (Babjuk et al., 2008).

21.3.4.2.2 Cytokeratin 20 (CK20)

Cytokeratins are intermediate filament proteins specific for epithelial cells. Cytokeratin 20 is selectively expressed in bladder and gastrointestinal epithelia (Moll et al., 1992). It is detectable in normal cells, but upregulated in carcinoma (Christoph et al., 2004).

In two older studies, the *CK20* test had a median sensitivity of 85% and a median specificity of 76% (Golijanin et al., 2000; Rotem et al., 2000). *CK20* expression can be determined with reverse transcription-polymerase chain reaction (RT-PCR) or an immunohistochemical staining. In a newer small study,

Bhatia et al. (2007) looked at the utility of *CK20* immunostaining in identifying malignant cells in urine cytology smears. Fourteen cases, each with an unequivocal diagnosis of UC, were collected. Fourteen cases of benign urinary cytology and five cases with a diagnosis of atypical cells were also subjected to immunohistochemistry. Twelve cases in the UC group stained positive with *CK20*, indicating high sensitivity (86%). All cases with benign cytology were negative, indicating a high specificity (100%). Also other authors, such as van Oers et al. (2007), found that 65% of pTa tumors revealed an abnormal *CK20* pattern, which implies that deregulation of *CK20* is an early event in the development of UC.

In conclusion, *CK20* seems to be a good marker for prognostication in which normal *CK20* is associated with low-grade tumors (van Oers et al., 2007).

21.3.4.2.3 CYFRA21.1

The test for *CYFRA21.1* expression is an ELISA-based assay that detects fragments of cytokeratin 19 with the help of two monoclonal antibodies (BM19.21 and KS19.1). Fernandez-Gomez et al. (2007) recently evaluated the *CYFRA21.1* test on 446 patients in follow-up for pTa or pT1 bladder cancer (Fernandez-Gomez et al., 2007). The total number of recurrent tumors was 125. Sensitivity and specificity for detection were 43% and 68% at a cutoff level of 4 ng/mL. With this cutoff level, none of the 12 pTa recurrent tumors were detected. Lowering the cutoff point to 1.5 ng/mL increased detection of pTa recurrences to 73% but decreased specificity to 43%. The authors concluded that *CYFRA21.1* is not a useful marker for follow-up of bladder cancer patients. This is disappointing because in three previous studies from two institutes, a median sensitivity of 85% and median specificity of 82% were reported for this test (Sanchez-Carbayo et al., 2001; Nisman et al., 2002). Whether combination with a molecular test is useful remains to be evaluated.

In conclusion, *CYFRA 21-1* shows a disappointing performance in low-stage bladder cancer, and *CYFRA21-1* levels are strongly influenced by benign urological diseases and intravesical instillations.

21.3.4.2.4 BLCA Proteins

There are six NMPs identified that are specifically expressed in bladder cancer, and these proteins were termed as the *BLCA* proteins. Two main of them are *BLCA-1* and *BLCA-4*. Overexpression of *BLCA-4* seems to increase the growth rate in cells and also causes cells to express a more tumorigenic phenotype (Meyers-Irvin et al., 2005). Both *BLCA-1* and *BLCA-4* are nuclear transcription factors present in UCB. *BLCA-1* is not expressed in nonmalignant urothelium (Meyers-Irvin et al., 2005), while *BLCA-4* is expressed in both the tumor and adjacent benign areas of the bladder, but not in noncancerous bladders (Konety et al., 2000b). *BCLA-4* is measured in the urine using an ELISA assay; its sensitivity ranges from 89% to 96% and its specificity reaches 100% (Van Le et al., 2004). Similarly, in a small study, *BLCA-1* demonstrated good performance with 80% sensitivity and 87% specificity (Van Le et al., 2005). Tumor grade did not seem to affect the expression of these markers. *BLCA-4* has been suggested as an NMP and a member of the ETS transcription factor family, a group of proteins shown to have deregulated expression and activity in cancer (Myers-Irvin et al., 2005). An indirect immunoassay using *BLCA-4* antibodies detected *BLCA-4* in precipitated urine samples from patients with bladder cancer, but not in samples from healthy individuals. On the basis of a prospectively defined cutoff, the indirect *BLCA-4* immunoassay demonstrated a sensitivity of 96.4% and specificity of 100% for detecting bladder cancer (Konety et al., 2000b). Van Le et al. (2000) used a sandwich-based assay on 75 urine samples of patients with primary bladder cancer and showed a sensitivity of 89% and a specificity of 95% (Van Le et al., 2004). *BLCA-4* is analyzed with ELISA and has a reported sensitivity of 89%–96.4% and its specificity ranges between 95% and 100% (Myers-Irvin et al., 2005). A large multicenter trial is currently being performed. *BLCA-1*, another NMP expressed in bladder cancer, shows a sensitivity of 80% and a specificity of 87% in a study involving 25 patients with bladder cancer and 46 controls. A limitation of this study was the small number of low-grade tumors (Van Le et al., 2005).

In conclusion, *BLCA-4* seems to have good sensitivity and specificity for detecting bladder cancer, but a larger trial is needed to confirm this. There is as yet not much evidence about the performance of *BLCA-1* in detecting bladder cancer.

21.3.4.3 ImmunoCyt

The ImmunoCyt test uses three fluorescent monoclonal antibodies directed against a mucin-like antigen (M344 and LDQ10) and a high molecular weight glycosylated form of carcinoembryonic antigen (*19A211*). Cell surface mucins are complex glycoproteins expressed on the apical membrane surface of all mucosal epithelial cells. In malignant epithelial cells, including bladder cancer, they are thought to influence cell adhesion and are clinical targets for tumor immunotherapy and serum tumor marker assays (Olsson and Zackrisson, 2001).

Sensitivity varies between 38.5% and 100% (Vriesema et al., 2001). ImmunoCyt shows specificity between 73% and 84.2% (Mian et al., 1999). A prospective study in which 942 patients were enrolled showed 298 patients with histopathologically proven bladder cancer. The results were encouraging: sensitivity for Grade 1 tumors was 79.3%, 84.1% for Grade 2, and 92.1% for Grade 3. Specificity was 72.5% (Pfister et al., 2003). Schmitz-Dräger et al. (2007) found high sensitivity and good specificity in a population of 189 patients with microhematuria. They found bladder cancer in eight patients, and only one tumor of low malignant potential was missed. They concluded that the high sensitivity and good specificity in a population with low disease prevalence could have prevented 154 costly and invasive diagnostic procedures. A prospective study, also by Schmitz-Dräger et al. (2008) in which the role of immunocytology in patients with gross hematuria was assessed, showed that the combination of cystoscopy and immunocytology gave 100% sensitivity, while combining cystoscopy and cytology marginally improved the sensitivity of cystoscopy alone. In this study they included 61 consecutive patients with a first episode of painless gross hematuria, but no previous UC. Sensitivity for cystoscopy, immunocytology, and cytology were 76%, 88%, and 47% and specificity was 100%, 77%, and 95%, respectively. The most important observation was that the combination of cystoscopy and immunocytology gave 100% sensitivity.

In conclusion, sensitivity of ImmunoCyt is good, but it fails in comparison to conventional cytology with regard to specificity. Another aspect is the high inter-observer variability and the need for constant quality control. Other disadvantages are the large number of exfoliated cells necessary to perform an accurate test and its high cost (Greene et al., 2006). Its advantage may be an improved sensitivity when compared to cytology, especially in low-grade tumors (Mian et al., 2006).

21.3.4.4 Soluble Fas

The Fas signaling pathway is involved in apoptosis, and Fas ligands (*FasL*) induce apoptosis when bound to its transmembrane receptor *Fas*. Alternative splicing of Fas mRNA can generate soluble forms of Fas (*sFas*) that have a deletion or disruption of the membrane-spanning domain. Levels of *sFas* are elevated in tissue and serum of cancer patients. Moreover, greater tissue and/or blood levels of *sFas* have been associated with adverse pathologic characteristics and poor clinical outcomes in various cancers. *sFas* encoding mRNAs are increased in bladder cancer when compared with normal urothelium.

These data prompted Svatek et al. (2006) to investigate whether an ELISA test for *sFas* would be of use for the detection of recurrent bladder cancer (Svatek et al., 2006). In this study *sFas* was compared with *NMP22* and *sFas* had a slightly higher AUC (area under the curve) than *NMP22*. With sensitivity for both tests of about 75% as interpreted from the receiver operating curves, the specificity was only 50%. Furthermore, it was remarked that the *sFas* assay used showed a relatively high inter-assay and intra-assay variability.

In conclusion, sFas can be an important advantage over other urinary markers, since false-positive results are a main concern for clinical use. Nevertheless, further assay improvements are needed in addition to external validation in large studies.

21.3.4.5 Survivin

Survivin is a member of the family of proteins that regulates cell death, the so-called inhibitor of apoptosis family. Its overexpression inhibits extrinsic and intrinsic pathways of apoptosis (Moussa et al., 2006). This mechanism is shown in Figure 21.2. It is expressed in the G2/M phase of the cell cycle and has been shown to be involved in the regulation of chromosome alignment and segregation. Survivin is expressed

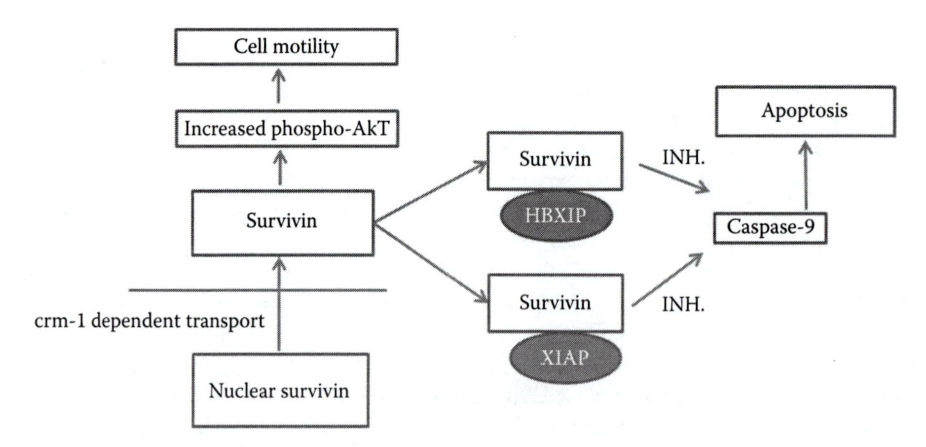

FIGURE 21.2 Mechanism of survivin inhibition of extrinsic and intrinsic pathways of apoptosis. (According to Kanwar, R.K. et al., *Curr. Med. Chem.*, 17(15), 1509, 2010.)

during fetal development, but is not expressed in terminally differentiated adult tissues (Dabrowski et al., 2004); however, it is one of the most commonly overexpressed genes in cancer (Black et al., 2006). In bladder cancer there is expression of survivin in urine, and its expression is associated with disease recurrence, stage, progression, and mortality (Shariat et al., 2007). RT-PCR provides a diagnostic tool to detect survivin mRNA in urine.

In recent published reports, sensitivity and specificity from 64% to 94% and 93% to 100%, respectively, have been noted (Shariat et al., 2004). Schultz et al. (2007) looked at the mRNA expression of 23 genes in 44 primary pTa tumors (Schultz et al., 2007), and survivin mRNA expression helped to distinguish between long or short recurrence-free intervals in patients with primary Ta UC. Survivin identified 71.4% and 69.6% of the patients with long or short recurrence-free periods, respectively. Chen et al. (2008) studied the use of survivin and Ki-67 as potential markers for grading non-muscle-invasive UC. In this study 51 bladder biopsies were graded blindly by five experienced pathologists. The protein and mRNA expression profiles of survivin and Ki67 were analyzed using immunohistochemistry and RT-PCR. Survivin outperformed Ki67 in separating the high-grade group from the low-grade group and showed a significantly higher predictive accuracy for high-grade recurrence than the histological grade (Chen et al., 2008).

Another study reported that survivin mRNA copy number (obtained from bladder washings) correlated with recurrence-free survival (Schultz et al., 2004). Similarly, survivin mRNA was detected in urine from 24 of 35 (68%) patients with UCB (Weikert et al., 2005). None of the 33 healthy patients had detectable urinary survivin mRNA. The authors reported a sensitivity of 68.6% and a specificity of 100% for urinary survivin mRNA, compared to 31.4% and 97.1%, respectively, for voided cytology.

In conclusion, survivin is a very promising marker with good sensitivity and very good specificity and also deserves further study. Survivin seems predictive for recurrence and can be helpful in preventing unnecessary urethrocystoscopies.

21.3.4.6 Epidermal Growth Factor Receptor

Members of the *EGFR* family, a type I tyrosine kinase growth factor receptor, are involved in various forms of cancers and serve as prognostic markers or therapeutic targets (Rotterud et al., 2005). Activation of *EGFR* leads to a wide variety of biological responses such as proliferation, differentiation, migration, modulation of apoptosis, invasion, and metastasis, leading to the progression of many tumors, including urinary cancer (Villares et al., 2007).

Kassouf et al. (2008) found that *EGFR* expression predicts disease progression. In this study the authors did a urinary cancer tissue array from 248 archival paraffin blocks. High *EFGR* was associated with nonpapillary, high-grade, and invasive tumors and may help select patients with urinary cancer for more aggressive therapy (Kassouf et al., 2008). A study with archival tissue by Litlekalsoy et al. (2007) showed a time-dependent pattern of biological features in urinary cancer. In the 1930s these tumors tended to have a high proportion of high molecular weight cytokeratin and *EGFR*-positive cases, combined with more metastases and shorter life span. Seventy years later there is a tendency for the opposite pattern indicating the different environmental and carcinogenic influences that account for the development of bladder cancer.

In conclusion, the usage of growth factors bears promise, but it is mainly study-based and prognostic. No large trials have been conducted yet; therefore, no clinically usable urinary markers have been identified.

21.3.4.7 CXCL1

CXCL1 is a member of the *CXC* chemokine family that functions as chemoattractants for neutrophils and potent angiogenic factors. The concentration of *CXCL1* in the urine was examined by ELISA in 67 patients with bladder cancer (Kawanishi et al., 2008). They did not specify whether these were primary or recurrent tumors. A significant difference was observed between noninvasive and invasive tumors ($P = 0.0028$). These results suggested that the corrected *CXCL1* level in the urine would predict the existence of both noninvasive and invasive bladder tumors. Measurement of the urine *CXCL1* level had a sensitivity of 70.1% and a specificity of 80.6%. Also *CXCL1* has not been tested during follow-up.

21.3.4.8 Tumor-Associated Trypsin Inhibitor

Tumor-associated trypsin inhibitor (*TATI*) is a low molecular-weight (6 kDa) trypsin inhibitor that has been used as a marker for bladder cancer. The role of trypsin as a proteolytic enzyme in cancer is not known. The expression of *TATI* in urine is determined with an immunofluorometric assay.

Recently, Gkialas et al. (2008) was able to use *TATI* for the detection of primary bladder cancer in 80 patients with a sensitivity of 85.7% and a specificity of 76%. No data exist yet on its performance during follow-up.

21.3.4.9 Vascular Endothelial Growth Factor

Angiogenesis or the development of new blood vessels from the surrounding vasculature is essential for the growth and progression of solid tumors. *VEGF*, a positive regulator of angiogenesis, plays a pivotal role in tumor angiogenesis and shows a high expression in almost all known tumors including urinary cancers (Das et al., 2007). The induction of antiapoptotic signaling and promotion of enhanced proliferation are shown in Figure 21.3.

Yang et al. (2004) studied the expression of *VEGF* in urinary cancer. Tissue samples from 161 patients were examined with immunohistochemical staining for the expression of the *VEGF* gene. The expression rate was compared to 32 normal bladder mucosal samples obtained from transurethral surgery from noncancer patients. The *VEGF* gene was expressed in none of the 32 normal bladder mucosal samples (0%), while in the cancer group, 88 out of 161 samples (54.7%) showed positive expression. They found that expression of *VEGF* was associated with both locally confined and invasive tumors indicating that *VEGF* expression might be a predictive marker for the degree of invasiveness and thus can be of prognostic value (Yang et al., 2004). Brian and Xu (2007) found a sensitivity of *VEGF* expression in urinary samples of 69% and a specificity of 88% for detection of urinary cancer (Brian and Xu, 2007). Eissa et al. (2007a) conducted a study in which urinary samples were taken from 120 patients with bladder cancer, 54 patients with benign urological disorders, and 55 healthy volunteers. The study revealed a sensitivity of 76.7% and a specificity of 61.5% for *VEGF* in the detection of urinary cancer (Eissa et al., 2007a).

In conclusion, *VEGF* seems to play an important role in tumor progression, and the identification of *VEGF* in urinary samples is mainly of prognostic value.

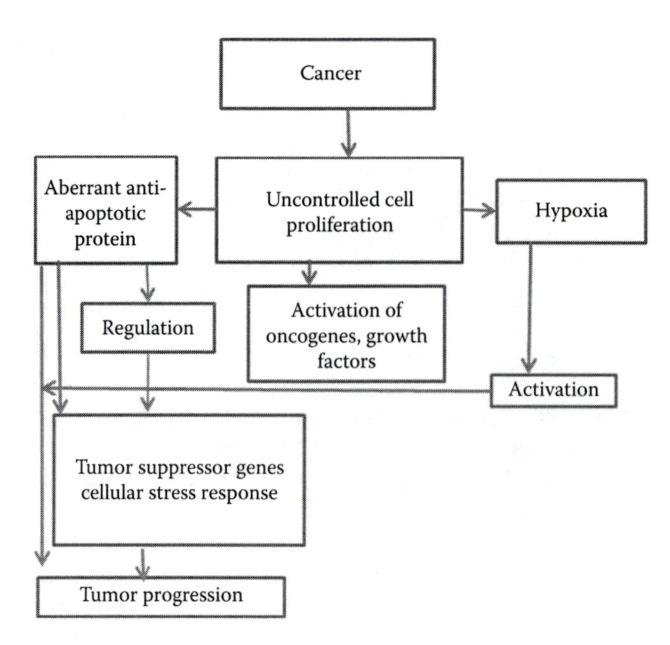

FIGURE 21.3 General mechanism of the induction of antiapoptotic signaling and promotion of enhanced proliferation. (According to Grossman, H.B. et al., *JAMA*, 293, 810, 2005.)

21.3.5 Antigen Markers

21.3.5.1 Bladder Tumor Antigen Tests

The term BTA describes at least three distinct tests. The original BTA (Bard Diagnostic Sciences, Inc., Redmond, WA) had lower specificity than, and equivalent sensitivity to, urine cytology and was therefore taken off the market (Heicappell et al., 1999). Subsequently, the BTA stat and BTA TRAK (Polymedco Inc., Cortlandt Manor, New York) tests were introduced. The BTA stat is a qualitative point-of-care test with an immediate result, whereas BTA TRAK is a quantitative test that requires trained personnel and a reference laboratory. These assays detect human complement factor H-related protein (as well as complement factor H), which is present in the urine of patients with UCB (Kinders et al., 1998). It is believed that complement factor H production by tumor cells may prevent tumor cell lysis by immune cells.

The overall sensitivity and specificity for the BTA stat test are 57%–83% (Wiener et al., 1998) and 60%–92% (Takashi et al., 1999), respectively. The reported specificity, however, must be assessed critically. Many of the studies excluded patients who had other commonly occurring genitourinary problems, such as renal stones, infection, and hematuria. In healthy persons without genitourinary signs or symptoms, the specificity is 97%, but in patients with benign genitourinary conditions, the specificity is only 46% (Leyh et al., 1999). When patients without UCB present with hematuria for other causes, the blood in the urine also contains complement factor H, which can react with the antibody in the test and lead to a false-positive result (Oge et al., 2002). In a recent prospective, multicenter trial of over 500 patients, the reported sensitivity of BTA stat to monitor for bladder cancer recurrence, was greater than that of cytology, particularly in Grade 1 lesions (47.9% vs. 12.5%) (Raitanen, 2008). However, prior intravesical treatment, benign prostatic hyperplasia, kidney stones, and urinary tract infections caused a high false-positive rate, and the BTA stat test by itself would have missed 46.6% of tumors detected on cystoscopy. The BTA TRAK test is a quantitative sandwich immunoassay that is performed in a reference laboratory (Malkowicz, 2000). The cutoff limit of human complement factor H-related protein to detect bladder cancer is 14 U/mL as recommended by the manufacturer (Thomas et al., 1999). When this cutoff is used, the reported overall sensitivity is 62%–91% (Mahnert et al., 1999). However, with a set sensitivity of 90%, the specificity of BTA TRAK was only 24.8% (Sharma et al., 1999). As with the BTA stat test, benign genitourinary conditions, particularly noncancerous related hematuria, may yield false-positive results (Irani et al., 1999). Both tests have sensitivities comparable to that of cytology for high-grade tumors and better than cytology for low-grade tumors. These tests are approved by the US Food and Drug Administration (FDA) only in combination with cystoscopy for monitoring of bladder cancer.

In conclusion, because of their high false-positive rate, they are not sufficiently accurate to be used for screening, early detection, or surveillance without cystoscopy of urothelial carcinoma, particularly in patients with other genitourinary symptoms.

21.3.5.2 Lewis X Antigen

Lewis-related antigens are cell surface molecules divided into four subclasses, of which only the Lewis X group is associated with UCB (Pode et al., 1998). Lewis X antigen is normally absent from urothelial cells, except for umbrella cells. Enhanced expression was found in urothelial carcinoma independent of the secretor status, grade, and stage of the tumor.

In three older studies investigating the usefulness of this marker in surveillance, the Lewis X antigen had a median sensitivity of 75% and a median specificity of 85% (Segerman et al., 1994). Overall, the sensitivity ranges from approximately 80% to 94% with a specificity of approximately 83% (Friedrich et al., 2002). The sensitivity increases when two consecutive urine samples are examined. Nonetheless, further studies are necessary before recommending this test for clinical care.

In conclusion, it is still unknown whether this biomarker has sufficient sensitivity and specificity to be used in a study protocol to reduce the cystoscopy frequency. New techniques linking Lewis antigen expression in urine to Lewis genotypes in blood determined by PCR need further evaluation in proper sample sets (Nagao et al., 2007).

21.3.6 Glycosaminoglycan Markers

21.3.6.1 Hyaluronic Acid and Hyaluronidase

Hyaluronic acid (HA) is a glycosaminoglycan and a normal component of tissue matrices and body fluids. Tumor-associated HA and its degrading enzyme hyaluronidase (HAase) are associated with angiogenesis of bladder tumors and are secreted in urine (Lokeshwar and Block, 2000). Three *HAase* genes have been identified and bladder tumor-derived HAase was shown to be the HYAL1 type. HAase levels are elevated in bladder tumor tissue, and an increase is correlated with tumor grade (Pham et al., 1997). With the HA–HAase urine test, the level of HA and HAase are measured in an ELISA-like test or with an RT-PCR test. A potential problem is that HA is also increased in patients with cystitis and because bladder cancer patients often have leukocyturia this may lead to false-positive results (Lokeshwar, 2006).

In a study by Lokeshwar et al. (2005a) it was shown that blocking *HYAL1* expression in a bladder cancer cell line results in a fourfold decrease in cell growth rate, suggesting that HYAL1 expression by tumor cells is required for cell proliferation. They also mentioned that *HYAL1* plays a role in promoting the invasive potential of bladder tumor cells and is not elevated in low-grade tumors (Lokeshwar et al., 2005a). The HA test detects bladder cancer regardless of tumor grade and, as mentioned previously, the HAase test preferentially detects Grades 2 and 3 bladder tumors. Sensitivity of the combined HA–HAase test varies between 83% and 94% (Lokeshwar et al., 2002). The overall specificity varies between 77% and 93.4% (Eissa et al., 2005). A study by Passerotti et al. (2006) in which urine samples were taken from 83 patients (22 controls and 61 diagnosed positive for bladder cancer) showed sensitivity of 92.9% and specificity of 83% (Passerotti et al., 2006).

In conclusion: HA–HAase is a very promising marker that deserves further study. The test has high sensitivity to detect both low- and high-grade/stage tumors.

21.4 Concluding Remarks and Future Perspective

Noninvasive tests for transitional cell carcinoma (UCC) have many potential applications including the diagnosis of recurrent UCC. High grade tumors should be detected early and the percentage of tumors missed should be as low as possible. Therefore, the optimal approach for these patients will continue to include both frequent urethrocystoscopy (UCS) and cytology as an adjunct to detect invisible disease. In this chapter we described commonly used detection techniques such as MSI analysis, *CYFRA21-1*, and LewisX, which are the most promising non-FDA-approved urine markers while ImmunoCyt, *NMP22*, and FISH are the best FDA-approved ones for surveillance. These markers were based mainly on sensitivity and specificity. Future studies for urine markers should use these assays in combination with a novel methodics based on biomolecular and biochemical markers, regarding the optimal costs to prolong patients life and increase survival rate even in later stages of bladder cancer.

References

Alexandroff, AB., Jackson, A., O'Donnell, MA., and James, K. 1999. BCG immunotherapy of bladder cancer: 20 years on. *Lancet* 353(9165):1689–1694.

Altieri, DC. 2003. Survivin, versatile modulation of cell division and apoptosis in cancer. *Oncogene* 22:8581–8589.

Amira, N., Mourah, S., Rozet, F. et al. 2002. Non-invasive molecular detection of bladder cancer recurrence. *Int. J. Cancer* 101:293–297.

Andreadis, C., Touloupidis, S., Galaktidou, G., Kortsaris, A., Boutis, A., Mouratidou, D. 2005. Serum CYFRA21-1 in patients with invasive bladder cancer and its relevance as a tumor marker during chemotherapy. *J. Urol.* 174:1771–1776.

American Urological Association. 2010. Guideline for the management of nonmuscle invasive bladder cancer (stages Ta, T1, and Tis). http://www.auanet.org/education/guidelines/prostate-cancer-detection.cfm

Babjuk, M., Oosterlinck, W., Sylvester, R. et al. 2011. EAU guidelines on non-muscle-invasive urothelial carcinoma of the bladder, the 2011 update. *Eur. Urol.* 59:997–1008.

Babjuk, M., Soukup, V., Pesl, M. et al. 2008. Urinary cytology and quantitative BTA and UBC tests in surveillance of patients with pTapT1 bladder urothelial carcinoma. *Urology* 71(4):718–772.

Bergman, J., Reznichek, R., and Rajfer, J. 2008. Surveillance of patients with bladder carcinoma using fluorescent in-situ hybridization on bladder washings. *BJU Int.* 101(1):26–29.

Beutler, B. and Cerami, A. 1986. Cachectin and tumour necrosis factor as two sides of the same biological coin. *Nature* 320:584–588.

Bhatia, A., Dey, P., Kumar, Y. et al. 2007. Expression of cytokeratin 20 in urine cytology smears: A potential marker for the detection of urothelial carcinoma. *Cytopathology* 18:84–86.

Black, P., Brown, G., and Dinney, C. 2006. Molecular markers of urothelial cancer and their use in the monitoring of superficial urothelial cancer. *J. Clin. Oncol.* 35:5528–5534.

Bravaccini, S. Sanchini, M., Granato, A. et al. 2007. Urine telomerase activity for the detection of bladder cancer in females. *J. Urol.* 178:57–61.

Brian, W. and Xu, Z. 2007. Combined assay of CYFRA21-1, telomerase and endothelial growth factor in the detection of bladder transitional cell carcinoma. *Int. J. Urol.* 14:108–111.

Burger, M., van der Aan, MN., van Oers, JM. et al. 2007. Prediction of progression of non-muscle-invasive bladder cancer by WHO 973 and 2004 grading and by *FGFR3* mutation status: A prospective study. *Eur. Urol.* 54:843–844.

Chade, DC., Shariat, SF., Godoy, G. et al. 2009. Critical review of biomarkers for the early detection and surveillance of bladder cancer. *J. Mens Health* 6:368–382.

Chen, YB., Tu, J., Kao, J., Zhou, K., and Chen, YT. 2008. Survivin as a useful adjunct marker for the grading of papillary urothelial carcinoma. *Arch. Pathol. Lab. Med.* 132:224–231.

Christoph, F., Muller, M., Schostak, M., Soong, R., Tabiti, K., and Miller, K. 2004. Quantitative detection of cytokeratin 20 mRNA expression in bladder carcinoma by real-time reverse transcriptase-polymerase chain reaction. *Urology* 64:157–161.

Chung, W., Bondaruk, J., Jelinek, J., Lotan, Y., Liang, S., Czerniak, B., and Issa, JP. 2011. Detection of bladder cancer using novel DNA methylation biomarkers in urine sediments. *Cancer Epidemiol. Biomarkers Prev.* 20:1483–1491.

Cliff, AM., Heatherwick, B., Scoble, J., and Parr, N. 2000. The effect of fasting or desmopressin before treatment on the concentration of mitomycin C during intravesical administration. *BJU Int.* 86:644–647.

Collings, CK., Waddell, PJ., and Anderson, JN. 2013. Effects of DNA methylation on nucleosome stability. *Nucleic Acids Res.* 41:2918–2931.

Compton, DA. and Cleveland, DW. 1993. NuMA is required for the proper completion of mitosis. *J. Cell Biol.* 120:947–957.

Dabrowski, A., Filip, A., and Zgodzinski, W. 2004. Assessment of prognostic significance of cytoplasmic survivin expression in advanced oesophageal cancer. *Folia Histochem. Cytobiol.* 42:169–172.

Daniely, M., Rona, R., Kaplan, T., Olsfanger, S., Elboim, L., Freiberger, A. et al. 2007. Combined morphologic and fluorescence in situ hybridization analysis of voided urine samples for the detection and follow-up of bladder cancer in patients with benign urine cytology. *Cancer* 111(6):517–524.

Daniely, M., Rona, R., Kaplan, T., Olsfanger, S., Elboim, L., Zilberstien, Y. et al. 2005. Combined analysis of morphology and fluorescence in situ hybridization significantly increases accuracy of bladder cancer detection in voided urine samples. *Urology* 66(6):1354–1359.

Das, K., Zhao, Y., Sugiono, M., Lau, W., Tan, PH., Cheng, C. 2007. Differential expression of vascular endothelial growth factor165b in transitional cell carcinoma of the bladder. *Urol. Oncol.* 25:317–321.

Eissa, S., Kassim, S., Labib, R. et al. 2005. Detection of bladder carcinoma by combined testing of urine for hyaluronidase and cytokeratin 20 RNAs. *Cancer* 103:1356.

Eissa, S., Salem, AM., Zohny, SF., and Hegazy, MG. 2007a. The diagnostic efficacy of urinary TGF-beta1 and VEGF in bladder cancer: Comparison with voided urine cytology. *Cancer Biomark.* 3:275–285.

Eissa, S., Swellam, M., Ali-Labib, R., Mansour, A., El-Malt, O., and Tash, FM. 2007b. Detection of telomerase in urine by 3 methods: Evaluation of diagnostic accuracy for bladder cancer. *J. Urol.* 17(1):1068–1072.

Fernandez-Gomez, J., Rodriguez-Martinez, J., Escaf Barma-dah, S. et al. 2007. Urinary CYFRA 21.1 is not a useful marker for the detection of recurrences in the follow-up of superficial bladder cancer. *Eur. Urol.* 51:1267–1274.

Friedrich, MG., Hellstern, A., Hautmann, SH., Graefen, M., Conrad, S., Huland, E. et al. 2002. Clinical use of urinary markers for the detection and prognosis of bladder carcinoma: A comparison of immunocytology with monoclonal antibodies against Lewis X and 486p3/12 with the BTA STAT and NMP22 tests. *J. Urol.* 168(2):470–474.

Frigerio, S., Padberg, B., Strebel, R. et al. 2007. Improved detection of bladder carcinoma cells in voided urine by standardized microsatellite analysis. *Int. J. Cancer* 121:329–338.

Fritsche, HA., Grossman, HB., Lerner, SP., and Sawczuk, I. 2006. National academy of clinical biochemistry guidelines for the use of tumor markers in bladder cancer. Online: http://www.aacc.org/SiteCollectionDocuments/NACB/LMPG/tumor/chp3h_bladder.pdf

Gaya, JM., Palou, J., Cosentino, M. et al. 2012. A second transurethral resection could be not necessary in all high grade non-muscle-invasive bladder tumours. *Actas Urol. Esp.* 36:539–544.

Gkialas, I., Papadopoulos, G., Iordanidou, L., Stathouros, G., Tzavara, C., Gregorakis, A., and Lykourinas, M. 2008. Evaluation of urine tumor-associated trypsin inhibitor, CYFRA 21-1, and urinary bladder cancer antigen for detection of high-grade bladder carcinoma. *Urology* 72(5):1159–1163.

Glas, A., Roos, D., Deutekom, M., Zwinderman, A., Bossuyt, PM., and Kurth, KH. 2003. Tumor markers in the diagnosis of primary bladder cancer. A systematic review. *J. Urol.* 169:1975–1982.

Golijanin, D., Shapiro, A., and Pode, D. 2000. Immunostaining of cytokeratin 20 in cells from voided urine for detection of bladder cancer. *J. Urol.* 164:1922–1925.

Gómez-Román, JJ., Saenz, P., Molina, M. et al. 2005. Fibroblast growth factor receptor 3 is overexpressed in urinary tract carcinomas and modulates the neoplastic cell growth. *Clin. Cancer Res.* 11:459–465.

Gonzalgo, ML., Datar, RH., Schoenberg, MP., and Cote, RJ. 2007. The role of deoxyribonucleic acid methylation in development, diagnosis, and prognosis of bladder cancer. *Urol. Oncol.* 25:228–235.

Gordon, JN., Shu, WP., Schlussel, RN., Droller, MJ., and Liu, BS. 1993. Altered extracellular matrices influence cellular processes and nuclear matrix organisations of overlying human bladder urothelial cells. *Cancer Res.* 53:4971–4977.

Greene, KL., Berry, A., and Konety, BR. 2006. Diagnostic utility of the ImmunoCyt/uCyt+ test in bladder cancer. *Rev. Urol.* 8(4):190–197.

Grossman, HB., Messing, E., Soloway, M. et al. 2005. Detection of bladder cancer using a point-of-care proteomic assay. *JAMA* 293:810–816.

Grossman, HB., Soloway, M., Messing, E. et al. 2006. Surveillance for recurrent bladder cancer using a point-of-care proteomic assay. *JAMA* 295:299–305.

Hajdinjak, T. 2008. UroVysion FISH test for detecting urothelial cancers: Meta-analysis of diagnostic accuracy and comparison with urinary cytology testing. *Urol. Oncol.* 26:646–651.

Hakenberg, O., Fuessel, S., Richter, K. et al. 2004. Qualitative and quantitative assessment of urinary cytokeratin 8 and 18 fragments compared with voided urine cytology in diagnosis of bladder carcinoma. *Urology* 64:1121–1126.

Heicappell, R., Schostak, M., Muller, M., and Miller, K. 2000. Evaluation of urinary bladder cancer antigen as a marker for diagnosis of transitional cell carcinoma of the urinary bladder. *Scand. J. Clin. Lab. Invest.* 60:275–282.

Heicappell, R., Wettig, IC., Schostak, M., Muller, M., Steiner, U., Sauter, T. et al. 1999. Quantitative detection of human complement factor H-related protein in transitional cell carcinoma of the urinary bladder. *Eur. Urol.* 35(1):81–87.

Hoque, MO., Begum, S., Topaloglu, O. et al. 2006. Quantitation of promoter methylation of multiple genes in urine DNA and bladder cancer detection. *J. Natl. Cancer Inst.* 98:996–1004.

Irani, J., Desgrandchamps, F., Millet, C., Toubert, ME., Bon, D., Aubert, J. et al. 1999. BTA stat and BTA TRAK: A comparative evaluation of urine testing for the diagnosis of transitional cell carcinoma of the bladder. *Eur. Urol.* 35(2):89–92.

Jahnson, S., Wiklund, F., Duchek, M. et al. 2005. Results of second-look resection after primary resection of T1 tumour of the urinary bladder. *Scand. J. Urol. Nephrol.* 39:206–210.

Jemal, A., Siegel, R., Xu, J., and Ward, E. 2010. Cancer statistics. *CA Cancer J. Clin.* 60:277–300.

Jones, JDN. 2006. A-based molecular cytology for bladder cancer surveillance. *Urology* 67(3):35–45.

Junker, K., Boerner. D., Schulze, W. et al. 2003. Analysis of genetic alterations in normal bladder urothelium. *Urology* 62:1134–1138.

Kanwar, RK., Cheung, CH., Chang, JY., and Kanwar, JR. 2010. Recent advances in anti-survivin treatments for cancer. *Curr. Med. Chem.* 17(15):1509–1515.

Kassouf, W., Black, PC., Tuziak, T. et al. 2008. Distinctive expression pattern of ErbB family receptors signifies an aggressive variant of bladder cancer. *J. Urol.* 179:353–358.

Kawanishi, H., Matsui, Y., Ito, M., Watanabe, J., Takahashi, T., Nishizawa, K. et al. 2008. Secreted CXCL1 is a potential mediator and marker of the tumor invasion of bladder cancer. *Clin. Cancer Res.* 14(9):2579–2587.

Kim, EJ., Jeong, P., Quan, C., Kim, J., Bae, SC. et al. 2005. Genotypes of TNF-alpha, VEGF, hOGG1, GSTM1, and GSTT1: Useful determinants for clinical outcome of bladder cancer. *Urology* 65(1):70–75.

Kim, NW., Piatyszek, MA., Prowse, KR., Harley, CB., West, MD., Ho, PL. et al. 2011. Specific association of human telomerase activity with immortal cells and cancer. *Science* 266:2011–2015.

Kinders, R., Jones, T., Root, R., Bruce, C., Murchison, H., Corey, M. et al. 1998. Complement factor H or a related protein is a marker for transitional cell cancer of the bladder. *Clin. Cancer Res.* 4(10):2511–2520.

Kipp, B., Karnes, R., and Brankley, S. 2005. Monitoring intravesical therapy for superficial bladder cancer using fluorescence in situ hybridization. *J. Urol.* 173:401–404.

Knowles, MA. 2007. Tumor suppressor loci in bladder cancer. *Front. Biosci.* 12:2233–2251.

Konety, BR., Nguyen, TS., Brenes, G. et al. 2000a. Clinical usefulness of the novel marker *BLCA-4* for the detection of bladder cancer. *J. Urol.* 164(1):634–639.

Konety, BR., Nguyen, TS., Dhir, R., Day, RS., Becich, MJ., Stadler, WM. et al. 2000b. Detection of bladder cancer using a novel nuclear matrix protein, *BLCA-4. Clin. Cancer Res.* 6(7):2618–2625.

Laird, PW. 2005. Cancer epigenetics. *Hum. Mol. Genet.* 14:R65–R76.

Lamm, D. and Torti F. 1996. Bladder cancer. *CA Cancer J. Clin.* 49:93–112.

Lamm, DL., Blumenstein, BA., Crissman, JD. et al. 2000. Maintenance bacillus Calmette-Guerin immunotherapy for recurrent TA, T1 and carcinoma in situ transitional cell carcinoma of the bladder: A randomized Southwest Oncology Group Study. *J. Urol.* 163:1124–1129.

Leliveld, AM., Bastiaannet, E., Doornweerd, BH., Schaapveld, M., and de Jong, IJ. 2011. High risk bladder cancer: Current management and survival. *Int. Braz. J. Urol.* 37:203–210.

Leyh, H., Marberger, M., Conort, P., Sternberg, C., Pansadoro, V., Pagano, F. et al. 1999. Comparison of the BTA stat test with voided urine cytology and bladder wash cytology in the diagnosis and monitoring of bladder cancer. *Eur. Urol.* 35(1):52–56.

Lin H.H., Ke HL., Huang SP., Wu WJ., Chen YK., and Chang LL. 2010. Increase sensitivity in detecting superficial, low grade bladder cancer by combination analysis of hypermethylation of E-cadherin, p16, p14, RASSF1A genes in urine. *Urol. Oncol.* 28:597–602.

Litlekalsoy, J., Vatne, V., Hostmark, J., and Laerum, O. 2007. Immunohistochemical markers in urinary bladder carcinomas from parafin-embedded archiva tissue after storage for 5–70 years. *BJU Int.* 99:1013–1019.

Little, B., Hughes, A., Young, M., and O'Brien, A. 2005. Use of polymerase chain reaction analysis of urine DNA to detect bladder carcinoma. *Urol. Oncol.* 23:102–107.

Lokeshwar, V., Cerwinka, W., and Lokeshwar, B. 2005a. HYAL1 Hyaluronidase: A molecular determinant of bladder tumor growth and invasion. *Cancer Res.* 65:2243–2250.

Lokeshwar, V., Schroeder, G., Selzer, M. et al. 2002. Bladder tumor markers for monitoring recurrence and screening comparison of hyaluronic acid-hyaluronidase and BTA-Stat tests. *Cancer* 95:61–72.

Lokeshwar, VB. 2006. Are there molecular signatures for predicting bladder cancer prognosis? *J. Urol.* 176(1):2347–2348.

Lokeshwar, VB. and Block, NL. 2000. HA-HAase urine test. A sensitive and specific method for detecting bladder cancer and evaluating its grade. *Urol. Clin. North Am.* 27:53–61.

Lokeshwar, VB., Habuchi, T., and Grossman, B. 2005b. Bladder tumor markers beyond cytology: International consensus on bladder tumor markers. *Urology* 66(1):35–63.

Lokeshwar, VB., Obek, C., Pham, HT. et al. 2000. Urinary hyaluronic acid and hyaluronidase: Markers for bladder cancer detection and evaluation of grade. *J. Urol.* 163:348–356.

Lotan, Y., Bensalah, K., Ruddell, T., Shariat, SF., Sagalowsky, AI., and Ashfaq, R. 2008. Prospective evaluation of the clinical usefulness of reflex fluorescence in situ hybridization assay in patients with atypical cytology for the detection of urothelial carcinoma of the bladder. *J. Urol.* 179(6):2164–2169.

Lotan, Y., Shariat, SF., Schmitz-Drager, B. et al. 2010. Considerations on implementing diagnostic markers into clinical decision making in bladder cancer. *Urol. Oncol.* 28:441–448.

Mahnert, B., Tauber, S., Kriegmair M., Schmitt, UM., Hasholzner, U., Reiter, W. et al. 1999. BTATRAK—A useful diagnostic tool in urinary bladder cancer? *Anticancer Res.* 19(4):2615–2619.

Malik, S. and Murphy, W. 1999. Monitoring patients for bladder neoplasms: What can be expected of urinary cytology consultations in clinical practice. *Urology* 54:64–70.

Malkowicz, SB. 2000. The application of human complement factor H-related protein (BTA TRAK) in monitoring patients with bladder cancer. *Urol. Clin. North Am.* 27(1):63–73.

Malmstrom, PU., Sylvester, RJ., Crawford, DE. et al. 2009. An individual patient data meta-analysis of the long-term outcome of randomised studies comparing intravesical mitomycin C versus bacillus Calmette-Guerin for non-muscle-invasive bladder cancer. *Eur Urol.* 56:247–256.

Mao, L., Schoenberg, M., Scicchiatano, M. et al. 1996. Molecular detection of primary bladder cancer by microsatellite analysis. *Science* 271:659–662.

Marin-Aguilera, M., Mengual, L., Ribal, MJ. et al. 2007. Utility of a multiprobe fluorescence in situ hybridization assay in the detection of superficial urothelial bladder cancer. *Cancer Genet. Cytogenet.* 173:131–135.

Meijer, RP., van Onna, IE., Kok, ET. et al. 2011. The risk profiles of three clinical types of carcinoma in situ of the bladder. *BJU Int.* 108:839–843.

Melissourgos, N., Kastrinakis, NG., Davilas, I., Foukas, P., Farmakis, A., and Lykourinas, M. 2003. Detection of human telomerase reverse transcriptase mRNA in urine of patients with bladder cancer: Evaluation of an emerging tumor marker. *Urology* 62(2):362–367.

Meyers-Irvin, J., Van Le, T., and Gertzenberg, R. 2005. Mechanistic analysis of the role of *BLCA-4* in bladder cancer pathobiology. *Cancer Res.* 65:7145–7150.

Mian, C., Chautard, D., and Devonec, M. 1999. Immunocyt: A new tool for detecting transitional cell cancer of the urinary tract. *J. Urol.* 161:1486.

Mian, C., Maier, K., Comploj, E. et al. 2006. uCyt+/ImmunoCyt in the detection of recurrent urothelial carcinoma: An update on 1991 analyses. *Cancer* 108:60–65.

Miyanaga, N., Akaza, H., Tsukamoto, T., Ishikawa, S., Noguchi, R., Ohtani, M. et al. 1999. Urinary nuclear matrix protein 22 as a new marker for the screening of urothelial cancer in patients with microscopic hematuria. *Int. J. Urol.* 6(4):173–177.

Moll, R., Lowe, A., Laufer, J., and Franke, W. 1992. Cytokeratin 20 in human carcinomas. A new histodiagnostic marker detected by monoclonal antibodies. *Am. J. Pathol.* 140:427–447.

Moonen, P., Merkx, G., Peelen, P., Karthaus, H., Smeets, D., and Witjes, J. 2007. Urovysion compared with cytology and quantitative cytology in the surveillance of non-muscle-invasive bladder cancer. *Eur. Urol.* 51:1275–1280.

Moussa, O., Abol-Enein, H., Bissada, N., Keane, T., Ghoneim, M., and Watson, D. 2006. Evaluation of survivin reverse transcriptase-polymerase chain reaction for noninvasive detection of bladder cancer. *J. Urol.* 175:2312–2316.

Mowatt, G., Zhu, S., Kilonzo, M. et al. 2010. Systematic review of the clinical effectiveness and cost-effectiveness of photodynamic diagnosis and urine biomarkers (FISH, ImmunoCyt, NMP22) and cytology for the detection and follow-up of bladder cancer. *Health Technol. Assess.* 14:1–33.

Müller, M. 2002. Telomerase: Its clinical relevance in the diagnosis of bladder cancer. *Oncogene* 21:650–655.

Muller, M., Krause, H., Heicappell, R., Tischendorf, J., Shay, JW., and Miller, K. 1998. Comparison of human telomerase RNA and telomerase activity in urine for diagnosis of bladder cancer. *Clin. Cancer Res.* 4(8):1949–1954.

Myers-Irvin, JM., Landsittel, D., and Getzenberg, RH. 2005. Use of the novel marker BLCA-1 for the detection of bladder cancer. *J. Urol.* 174(1):64–68.

Nagao, K., Itoh, Y., Fujita, K., and Fujime, M. 2007. Evaluation of urinary CA19-9 levels in bladder cancer patients classified according to the combinations of Lewis and Secretor blood group genotypes. *Int. J. Urol.* 14:795–799.

Nagele, U., Kugler, M., Nicklas, A. et al. 2011. Waterjet hydrodissection: First experiences and short-term outcomes of a novel approach to bladder tumor resection. *World J. Urol.* 29:423–427.

Nieder, AM., Brausi, M., Lamm, D. et al. 2005. Management of stage T1 tumours of the bladder: International consensus panel. *Urology* 66:108–125.

Nisman, B., Barak, V., Shapiro, A., Golijanin, D., Peretz, T., and Pode, D. 2002. Evaluation of urine CYFRA 21-1 for the detection of primary and recurrent bladder carcinoma. *Cancer* 94:2914–2922.

Nonomura, N., Tokizane, T., Nakayama, M. et al. 2006. Possible correlation between polymorphism in the tumor necrosis factor-beta gene and the clinicopathological features of bladder cancer in Japanese patients. *Int. J. Urol.* 13:971–976.

Oge, O., Kozaci, D., and Gemalmaz, H. 2002. The BTA stat test is nonspecific for hematuria: An experimental hematuria model. *J. Urol.* 167(3):1318–1319.

Olsson, H. and Zackrisson, B. 2001. ImmunoCyt a useful method in the follow-up protocol for patients with urinary bladder carcinoma. *Scand. J. Urol. Nephrol.* 35:280–282.

Pariente, J., Bordenave, L., Jacob, F. et al. 2000. Analytical and prospective evaluation of urinary cytokeratin 19 fragment in bladder cancer. *J. Urol.* 163:1116–1119.

Passerotti, C., Bonfim, A., Martins, J. et al. 2006. Urinary hyaluronan as a marker for the presence of residual transitional cell carcinoma of the urinary bladder. *Eur. Urol.* 49:71–75.

Pfister, C., Chautard, D., Devonec, M. et al. 2003. Immunocyt test improves the diagnostic accuracy of urinary cytology: Results of a French multicenter study. *J. Urol.* 169:921–924.

Pham, H., Block, N., and Lokeshwar, V. 1997. Tumor-derived hyaluronidase: A diagnostic urine marker for high-grade bladder cancer. *Cancer Res.* 57:778–783.

Ploeg, M., Aben, K., and Kiemeney, LA. 2009. The present and future burden of urinary bladder cancer in the world. *World J. Urol.* 27:289–292.

Pode, D., Golijanin, D., Sherman, Y., Lebensart, P., and Shapiro, A. 1998. Immunostaining of Lewis X in cells from voided urine, cytopathology and ultrasound for noninvasive detection of bladder tumours. *J. Urol.* 159(2):389–392.

Raitanen, MP. 2008. The role of BTA stat test in follow-up of patients with bladder cancer: Results from FinnBladder studies. *World J. Urol.* 26(1):45–50.

Rieger-Christ, KM., Mourtzinos, A., Lee, PJ. et al. 2003. Identification of fibroblast growth factor receptor 3 mutations in urine sediment DNA samples complements cytology in bladder tumor detection. *Cancer* 98:737–744.

Rigaud, J., Karam, G., Braud, G. et al. 2002. T1 bladder tumours: Value of a second endoscopic resection. *Prog. Urol.* 12:27–30.

Rotem, D., Cassel, A., Lindenfeld, N. et al. 2000. Urinary cytokeratin 20 as a marker for transitional cell carcinoma. *Eur. Urol.* 37:601–604.

Rotterud, R., Nesland, J., Berner, A., and Fossa, S. 2005. Expression of the epidermal growth factor receptor family in normal and malignant urothelium. *BJU Int.* 95:1344–1350.

Roupret, M., Hupertan, V., Yates, DR. et al. 2008. A comparison of the performance of microsatellite and methylation urine analysis for predicting the recurrence of urothelial cell carcinoma, and definition of a set of markers by Bayesian network analysis. *BJU Int.* 101:1448–1453.

Sagerman, PM., Saigo, PE., Sheinfeld, J., Charitonowics, E., and Cordon-Cardo C. 1994. Enhanced detection of bladder cancer in urine cytology with Lewis X, M344 and 19A211 antigens. *Acta Cytol.* 38:517–523.

Sanchez-Carbayo, M., Urrutia, M., Gonzalez de Buitrago, JM., and Navajo, JA. 2001. Utility of serial urinary tumor markers to individualize intervals between cystoscopies in the monitoring of patients with bladder carcinoma. *Cancer* 92:2820–2828.

Sanchini, M., Gunelli, R., Nanni, O. et al. 2005. Relevance of urine telomerase in the diagnosis of bladder cancer. *JAMA* 294:2052–2056.

Sarosdy, M., Schellhammer, P., Bobinsky, G. et al. 2002. Clinical evaluation of a multi-target fluorescent in situ hybridization assay for detection of bladder cancer. *J. Urol.* 168:1950–1954.

Schenkman, E. and Lamm, DL. 2004. Superficial bladder cancer therapy. *Sci. World J.* 1(Suppl):387–399.

Scher, MB., Elbaum, MB., Mogilevkin, Y., Hilbert, DW., Mydlo JH., Sidi, AA., Adelson, ME., Mordechai, E., and Trama, JP. 2012. Detecting DNA methylation of the BCL2, CDKN2A and NID2 genes in urine using a nested methylation specific polymerase chain reaction assay to predict bladder cancer. *J. Urol.* 188:2101–2107.

Schips, L., Augustin, H., Zigeuner, RE. et al. 2002. Is repeated transurethral resection justified in patients with newly diagnosed superficial bladder cancer? *Urology* 59:220–223.

Schmitz-Drager, B., Beiche, B., Tirsar, L., Schmitz-Drager, C., Bismarck, E., and Ebert, T. 2007. Immunocytology in the assessment of patients with asymptomatic microhaematuria. *Eur. Urol.* 51:1582–1588.

Schmitz-Drager, B., Tirsar, LA., Schmitz-Dräger, C., Dörsam, J., Bismarck, E., and Ebert, T. 2008. Immunocytology in the assessment of patients with painless gross haematuria. *BJU Int.* 101(4):455–458.

Schultz, I., Wester, K., Straatman, H. et al. 2007. Gene expression analysis for the prediction of recurrence in patients with primary Ta urothelial cell carcinoma. *Eur. Urol.* 51:416–423.

Schultz, IJ., Kiemeney, LA., Karthaus, HF., Witjes, JA., Willems, JL., Swinkels, DW., Gunnewiek, JM., and de Kok, JB. 2004. Survivin mRNA copy number in bladder washings predicts tumor recurrence in patients with superficial urothelial cell carcinomas. *Clin. Chem.* 50(8):1425–1428.

Shariat, S., Ashfaq, R., Karakiewicz, P., Saeedi, O., Sagalowsky, A., and Lotan, Y. 2007. Survivin expression is associated with bladder cancer presence, stage, progression, and mortality. *Cancer* 109:1106–1113.

Shariat, S., Casella, R., Khoddami, S. et al. 2004. Urine detection of survivin is a sensitive marker for the non-invasive diagnosis of bladder cancer. *J. Urol.* 171:626–630.

Shariat, S. and Kattan, M. 2008. Risk assessment in prostate cancers. In: *Textbook of Prostate Cancer*. Tewari, A. (ed.). Springer Verlag, Germany.

Shariat, SF., Karam, JA., Lotan, Y., and Karakiewizc, PI. 2008. Critical evaluation of urinary markers for bladder cancer detection and monitoring. *Rev. Urol.* 10(2):120–135.

Shariat, SF., Marberger, MJ., Lotan, Y. et al. 2006. Variability in the performance of nuclear matrix protein 22 for the detection of bladder cancer. *J. Urol.* 176:919–926.

Sharma, S., Zippe, CD., Pandrangi, L., Nelson, D., and Agarwal, A. 1999. Exclusion criteria enhance the specificity and positive predictive value of NMP22 and BTA stat. *J. Urol.* 162(1):53–57.

Shelfo, SW. and Soloway, MS. 1997. The role of nuclear matrix protein 22 in the detection of persistent or recurrent transitional-cell cancer of the bladder. *World J. Urol.* 15:107–111.

Shirodkar, SP. and Lokeshwar, VB. 2009. Potential new urinary markers in the early detection of bladder cancer. *Curr. Opin. Urol.* 19:488–493.

Siegel, R., Naishadham, D., and Jemal, A. 2012. Cancer statistics. *CA Cancer J. Clin.* 62:10.

Skacel, M., Fahmy, M., Brainard, J. et al. 2003. Multitarget fluorescence in situ hybridization assay detects transitional cell carcinoma in the majority of patients with bladder cancer and atypical or negative urine cytology. *J. Urol.* 169:2101–2105.

Southgate, J., Harnden, P., and Trejdosiewicz, LK. 1999. Cytokeratin expression patterns in normal and malignant urothelium: A review of the biological and diagnostic implications. *Histol. Histopathol.* 14:657–664.

Svatek, RS., Herman, MP., Lotan, Y., Casella, R., Hsieh, JT., Sagalowsky, AI. et al. 2006. Soluble Fas—A promising novel urinary marker for the detection of recurrent superficial bladder cancer. *Cancer* 106(8):1701–1707.

Takashi, M., Schenck, U., Kissel, K., Leyh, H., and Treiber, U. 1999. Use of diagnostic categories in urinary cytology in comparison with the bladder tumour antigen (BTA) test in bladder cancer patients. *Int. Urol. Nephrol.* 31(2):189–196.

Thomas, L., Leyh, H., Marberger, M., Bombardieri, E., Bassi, P., Pagano, F. et al. 1999. Multicenter trial of the quantitative BTA TRAK assay in the detection of bladder cancer. *Clin. Chem.* 45(4):472–477.

Tritschler, S., Scharf, S., Karl, A. et al. 2007. Validation of the diagnostic value of NMP22 BladderChek test as a marker for bladder cancer by photodynamic diagnosis. *Eur. Urol.* 51:403–407.

Turyn, J., Matuszewski, M., and Schlichtholtz, B. 2006. Genomic instability analysis of urine sediment versus tumor tissue in transitional cell carcinoma of the urinary bladder. *Oncol. Rep.* 15:259–265.

van der Poel, HG and Debruyne, FM. 2001. Can biological markers replace cystoscopy? An update. *Curr. Opin. Urol.* 11:503–509.

Van Le, T., Miller, R., Barder, T., Babjuk, M., Potter, D., and Gertzenberg, R. 2005. Highly specific urine-based marker of bladder cancer. *Urology* 66:1256–1260.

Van Le, TS., Myers, J., Konety, BR., Barder, T., Getzenberg, RH. et al. 2004. Functional characterization of the bladder cancer marker, *BLCA-4. Clin. Cancer Res.* 10:1384–1391.

van Oers, JM., Lurkin, I., van Exsel, AJ. et al. 2005. A simple and fast method for the simultaneous detection of nine fibroblast growth factor receptor 3m mutations in bladder cancer and voided urine. *Clin. Cancer Res.* 11:7743–7748.

van Oers, JM., Wild, PJ., Burger, M. et al. 2007. 3 mutations and a normal CK20 staining pattern define low-grade noninvasive urothelial bladder tumours. *Eur. Urol.* 52:760–768.

van Oers, JM., Zwarthoff, EC., Rehman, I. et al. 2009. *FGFR3* mutations indicate better survival in invasive upper urinary tract and bladder tumours. *Eur. Urol.* 55:650–658.

van Rhijn, BW., Lurkin, I., Kirkels, WJ. et al. 2001. Microsatellite analysis–DNA test in urine competes with cystoscopy in follow-up of superficial bladder carcinoma: A phase II trial. *Cancer* 92:768–775.

van Rhijn, BW., Vis, AN., van der Kwast, TH. et al. 2003. Molecular grading of nurothelial cell carcinoma with fibroblast growth factor receptor 3 and MIB-1 is superior to pathologic grade for the prediction of clinical outcome. *J. Clin. Oncol.* 21:1912–1921.

van Tilborg, AA., Kompier, LC., Lurkin, I., Poort, R., El Bouazzaoui, S., van der Keur, K. et al. 2012. Selection of microsatellite markers for bladder cancer diagnosis without the need for corresponding blood. *PLoS One* 7:e43345.

Veeramachaneni, R., Nordberg, M., Shi, R., Herrera, G., and Turbat-Herrera, E. 2003. Evaluation of fluorescence in situ hybridization as an ancillary tool to urine cytology in diagnosing urothelial carcinoma. *Diagn. Cytopathol.* 28:301–307.

Villares, GJ., Zigler, M., Blehm, K. et al. 2007. Targeting EGFR in bladder cancer. *World J. Urol.* 25:573–579.

Vriesema, J., Atsma, F., Kiemeney, L., Peelen, W., Witjes, J., and Schalken J. 2001. Diagnostic efficacy of the ImmunoCyt test to detect superficial bladder cancer recurrence. *Urology* 58:367–371.

Vrooman, OP. and Witjes, JA. 2008. Urinary markers in bladder cancer. *Eur. Urol.* 53:909–916.

Vrooman, OP. and Witjes, JA. 2009. Molecular markers for detection, surveillance and prognostication of bladder cancer. *Int. J. Urol.* 16(3):234–243.

Weikert, S., Christoph, F., Schrader, M., Krause, H., Miller, K., Mülle, RM. 2005. Quantitative analysis of survivin mRNA expression in urine and tumor tissue of bladder cancer patients and its potential relevance for disease detection and prognosis. *Int. J. Cancer* 116(1):100–104.

Wiener, HG., Mian, C., Haitel, A., Pycha, A., Schatzl, G., and Marberger, M. 1998. Can urine bound diagnostic tests replace cystoscopy in the management of bladder cancer? *J. Urol.* 159(6):1876–1880.

Wolters, M., Kramer, MW., Becker, JU. et al. 2011. Tm:YAG laser en bloc mucosectomy for accurate staging of primary bladder cancer: Early experience. *World J. Urol.* 29:429–432.

Yang, CC., Chu, KC., and Yeh, WM. 2004. The expression of vascular endothelial growth factor in transitional cell carcinoma of urinary bladder is correlated with cancer progression. *Urol. Oncol.* 22:1–6.

Yates, DR., Rehman, I., Meuth, M., Cross, SS., Hamdy, FC., and Catto, JW. 2006. Methylational urinalysis: A prospective study of bladder cancer patients and age stratified benign controls. *Oncogene* 25:1984–1988.

22

Screening for Prostate Cancer: New Markers and Future Aspects

Nigel P. Murray

CONTENTS

ABSTRACT Total PSA, although imperfect, remains the first line test for prostate cancer screening: the sequential use of complementary tests may improve the diagnostic accuracy, not only in detecting prostate cancer but also in detecting significant tumors that are likely to cause illness during the patient's life. In modern health economics, the cost of new tests is important, especially in the public health system, and thus is a parameter that needs to be considered. Prostate biopsy is not a test without side effects, and thus, biomarkers that reduce the necessity of prostate biopsies are necessary.

22.1 Introduction

With the changing demographics of the world population and increasing life expectancy, prostate cancer has become the most common non-skin cancer in the developed countries. In the United Kingdom, it is the most common cancer in men, representing 24% of all new cancer cases, 37,051 cases in 2008 with a lifetime risk of 1 in 9 (Office for National Statistics, Cancer Statistics Registrations, United Kingdom, 2008). In the United States, an estimated 218,890 men were newly diagnosed with prostate cancer in 2007 with a lifetime risk of 1 in 6 (National Cancer Institute Surveillance Epidemiology

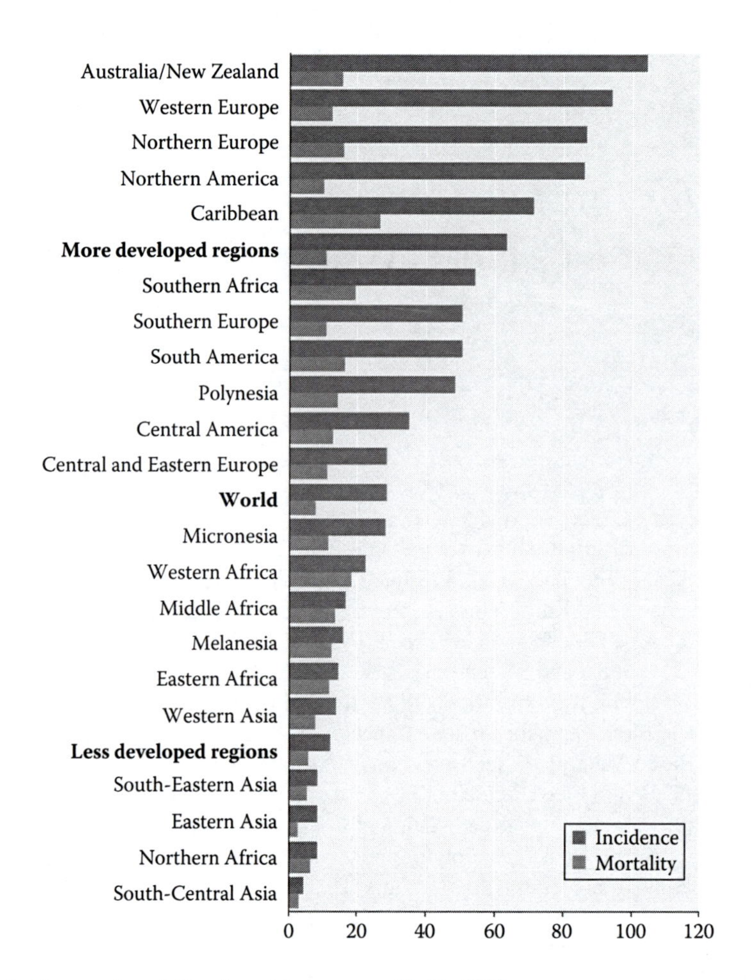

FIGURE 22.1 Incidence and mortality of prostate cancer worldwide, 2008.

and End Results (SEER) Program, Cancer Stat Fact Sheets—Cancer of Prostate 2006). Worldwide, an estimated 899,000 men were diagnosed with prostate cancer in 2008, and more than two-thirds are diagnosed in developed countries (Ferlay et al., 2008). The highest rates of prostate cancer are in Australia/New Zealand, Western, Northern Europe, and North America, largely because prostate-specific antigen (PSA) testing of the prostate and subsequent biopsy have become widespread in these regions (Figure 22.1, Table 22.1).

Within the United States, there are significant differences between racial groups, the incidence of prostate cancer being 50% higher in Afro-Americans than for white Americans, while rates for Asian Americans are 40% lower than for white Americans; the 2001–2005 age standardized incidences being 249/100,000, 157/100,000, and 94/100,000 for Afro-, white, and Asian Americans (Ries, 2005).

The risk of prostate cancer rises steeply with age, with the highest rates occurring in the 75–79-year-old age group. In the United Kingdom, the incidence is 155/100,00 men aged 55–59 years, 510/100,000 for the group 65–69 years, and 751/100,000 by 75–79 years (Office for National Statistics, Cancer Statistics Registrations, United Kingdom, 2010) (Figure 22.2). In the United States, the median age at diagnosis for prostate cancer is 67 years, 0.6% of cases between 35 and 44 years, 9.1% between 45 and 54 years, 30.7% between 55 and 64 years, 35.3% between 65 and 74 years, 19.9% between 75 and 84 years, and 4.4% 85+ years of age (National Cancer Institute SEER Program, Cancer Stat Fact Sheets—Cancer of Prostate, 2006).

However, studies published using postmortem data have shown that approximately half of all men in their fifties have histological evidence of prostate cancer, which in men over 80 rises to 80% (Sakr et al., 1996;

TABLE 22.1

Estimated Number of Newly Diagnosed Cases of Prostate Cancer Worldwide in Thousands

Estimated Numbers (Thousands)	Cases	Deaths
World	899	258
More developed regions	644	136
Less developed regions	255	121
WHO Africa region (AFRO)	34	24
WHO Americas region (PAHO)	334	76
WHO East Mediterranean region (EMRO)	12	9
WHO Europe region (EURO)	379	94
WHO Southeast Asia region (SEARO)	28	19
WHO Western Pacific region (WPRO)	109	33
IARC membership (22 countries)	611	128
United States of America	186	28
China	33	14
India	14	10
European Union (EU-27)	323	71

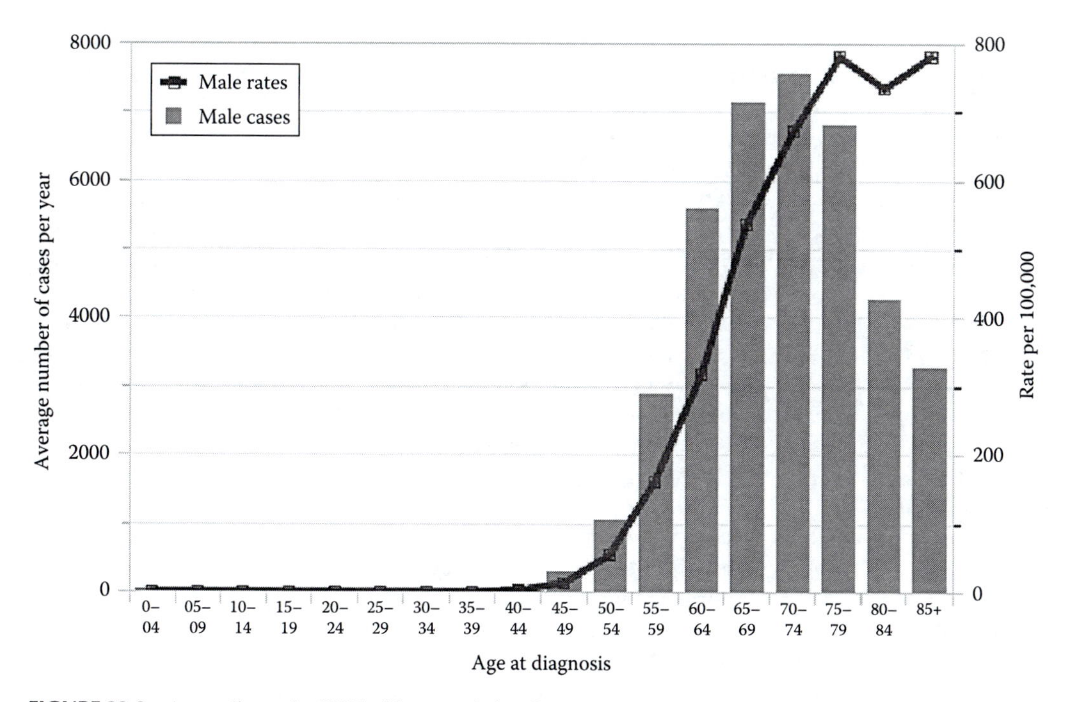

FIGURE 22.2 Age at diagnosis. (UK incidence statistics: Cancer Research.)

Burford et al., 2008), but only 1 in 26 men (3.8%) will die from this cancer. This means that more men will die with their prostate cancer than from it, of importance when considering population screening of asymptomatic men (Selly et al., 1997; Frankel et al., 2003). Statistics from the SEER database (Table 22.2) are concordant with thc UK statistics.

Thus, whatever screening test used to detect men with prostate cancer has to differentiate between the mere presence of prostate cancer on biopsy and clinically significant prostate cancer.

TABLE 22.2

Incidence and Mortality Rates by Race in the United States

	Incidence Rate by Race per 100,000 Men	Date Rate by Race per 100,000 Men
All races	156.0	24.4
White	149.5	22.4
Afro-American	233.8	54.9
Asian/Pacific Islander	88.3	10.5
American Indian/Alaska Native	75.3	20.7
Hispanic	129.0	18.5

Source: National Cancer Institute, SEER data base 2004–2008, Bethseda, MD.

22.2 PSA Controversy for Prostate Cancer Screening

PSA is a glycoprotein produced almost exclusively by the epithelial of the prostate gland. Serum levels may be elevated due to increased PSA production or architectural distortions in the prostate gland that allow greater PSA access to the circulation. Only approximately 30% of men with a serum PSA >4.0 ng mL, a standard cutoff point to determine the need for a prostate biopsy, have cancer confirmed on biopsy; many false positives are attributed to benign prostatic hyperplasia or to subclinical prostatic inflammation (Nadler et al., 1995). It has been published that the cutoff value of 4.0 ng/mL has a sensitivity of 46% with respect to the identification of cases of prostate cancer than would occur over a 10-year period. However, the specificity of 91% in this population with a mean age of 63 years fell to 54% in men over 80 years as a result in the increase of benign prostatic hyperplasia (Gann et al., 1995). Moreover, two studies have shown that biopsies taken from men with serum PSA values of 2.5–4.0 ng/mL detected cancer in 12%–23% of cases (Catalona et al., 1997; Babaian et al., 2001). Thus, there is no cutoff point for PSA that determines if there is or is no prostate cancer.

To confound matters, the benefits of screening are controversial; a screening test should ideally detect clinically significant cancer that if not treated would increase mortality and/or morbidity and not detect those cancers that clinically would not cause harm to the patient. Two large-scale studies designed to address this question from the United States and Europe reported conflicting results. The US study reported by Andriole et al. (2009) compared a screening group with annual serum and digital rectal examination (DRE) and a group of usual care that sometimes included screening; in this control group at the sixth year, 52% of patients underwent screening tests. They concluded that there was a 22% increase in the rate of prostate cancer diagnosis in the screening group as compared with the control group; however, there were no reduction in prostate cancer mortality during the first 7 years of the trial.

In men with an increased serum PSA, detected as part of a screening program, a prostate biopsy is recommended. A prostate biopsy is not without risks; Rietbergen et al. (1997), in a study of 5802 patients undergoing transrectal prostate biopsy, reported an incidence of complications of 0.5% hospitalizations, 2.1% rectal hemorrhage, 2.3% fever, and 7.2% persistent hematuria. Of further concern is that not all detected prostate cancers need treatment, and active observation is an option for small, low-grade tumors. Treatment options include radical prostatectomy or radiotherapy, both of which are associated with long-term complications, such as incontinence, erectile dysfunction, and radiation proctitis. Thus, overtreatment in men in whom prostate cancer would not have been detected in their lifetime may be associated with significant morbidity and mortality without concurrent benefits.

In contrast, the European study showed a reduction of 20% in the rate of death from prostate cancer among men between the ages of 55 and 69 years at study entry (Schroder et al., 2009).

Thus, whatever new screening test developed to detect prostate cancer has to improve on the standard serum PSA test, in other words, detect clinically significant prostate cancer and not indolent cancer.

22.3 Use of Biomarkers in Blood to Detect Prostate Cancer

22.3.1 PSA Variants and Kallikreins

PSA is synthesized by the prostate epithelial cells with a 17 amino acid leader sequence, denominated preproPSA; this is cleaved cotranslationally to form an inactive 244 amino acid precursor protein, proPSA, which is secreted into the lumen of the prostate glands (Lundwall and Lilja, 1987). Cleavage of seven amino acids from the N-terminal results in proPSA; this cleavage normally occurs between the amino acid arginine at position 7 and the isoleucine at position 8. ProPSA is inactive but is activated by the trypsin-like enzyme hK2 that is found in the prostate secretary epithelium and also by other prostate kallikreins such as prostase (hK4) (Takayama et al., 1997, 2001). Approximately 30% of the PSA in seminal plasma is the active enzyme; the rest is inactive due to cleavage of the protein. These PSA isoforms have been termed benign PSA as they are increased in benign prostatic hypertrophy (Mikolajczyk et al., 2000) and decreased in prostate cancer (Mikolajczyk et al., 2000a). Other forms of PSA have been found in prostate cancer tissue; these truncated forms of proPSA have extra amino acids relative to the active mature PSA and are both inactive and are resistant to cleavage by trypsin and kH2 (Mikolajczyk et al., 1997). This isoform, termed [−2]pPSA, forms part of the free PSA component in plasma. Further truncated forms, [−1], [−4], and [−5]pPSA, have been identified (Mikolajczyk et al., 1997, 2000b).

22.3.1.1 Free PSA and Percent Free PSA

Total serum PSA refers to all the immunologically detectable forms of PSA; the major form of PSA is complexed with alpha-1-antichymotrypsin (PSA-ACT); about 10%–30% of total serum PSA is unbound, free PSA (Stephan et al., 2000); and its proportion is higher in normal men than those with prostate cancer (Djava et al., 2002). Retrospective studies have reported percent free PSA cutoff values ranging from 14% to 25%, with a sensitivity of 90%–100% and an increased specificity ranging from 20% to 40% (Catalona et al., 1995; Luderer et al., 1995; Partin et al., 1996). Prospective studies using percent free PSA have shown that while maintaining a sensitivity of over 90%, the optimum reflex range of total PSA values of between 4.0 and 10.0 ng/mL for the clinical utility of percent free PSA only affects 56% of cases (Stenman et al., 1991). A single cutoff point of 25% free PSA demonstrated a specificity of 95% and could eliminate 20% of prostate biopsies for men with a total PSA of between 4.0 and 10.0 ng/mL (Partin et al., 1998). However, complexed PSA added very little value to the clinical utility of total PSA for early detection of prostate cancer. In addition, the level of free PSA is affected by many factors, including age, prostate volume, prostate manipulation, sample handling and type of assay used (Han et al., 2000), and race, being lower in Chinese men (Zhang et al., 2008); it is negatively associated with glomerular filtration rates (Joseph et al., 2010), and there is an intraindividual variability of between 12% and 16% (Kobayashi et al., 2005). As such, although in the range of total PSA between 4.0 and 10.0 ng/mL, it appears that percent free PSA increases the specificity for prostate cancer detection; there is no current agreement on its use outside of these ranges and of which cutoff point is considered to be most appropriate.

22.3.1.2 ProPSA and Percent ProPSA

Proenzyme PSA (proPSA) is a cancer-associated form of free PSA found primarily in the peripheral zone of the prostate as well as in the circulation (Mikolajczyk et al., 2000, 2001). The (−2) proPSA is a stable form, resistant to activation to mature PSA for which there is an automated assay for its detection, and is approved by the European Union regulatory body for prostate cancer detection. There is less consensus on the utility of measuring (−7) proPSA or (−5, −7) proPSA either individually or summed to form total proPSA (Bangma et al., 2004; Stephan et al., 2009). Median PSA concentrations and percent (−2) proPSA are significantly higher in men with cancer than those with benign diseases, but areas under the curve were similar for PSA, percent free PSA, and percent (−2) proPSA (Sokoll et al., 2010); in the PSA range 4.0–10.0 ng/mL, the same authors concluded that statistical significance was not achieved between percent free PSA and percent (−2) proPSA. The use of combination of the sum proPSA, total PSA, and percent free PSA at a 90% sensitivity achieved a specificity of 44% in the detection of prostate cancer, whereas individually achieved a specificity of 23% for total PSA, 33% free PSA, and 13% sum proPSA in the 4.0–10.0 ng/mL range (Khan et al., 2003). In a study by Jansen et al. (2010), the addition of (−2) proPSA increased the specificity of total PSA from 8% to 24% and percent free PSA from 7% to 23% at a specificity of 95%. In men with a percent free PSA of <15%, the ratio of proPSA and benign PSA may improve the sensitivity of the diagnostic test (Khan et al., 2004.)

However, the great drawback of these PSA isoforms either alone or in combination is that although statistically the specificity is increased, in the clinical practice it has not greatly helped as some 40%–50% of clinical patients remain in the gray area, which is probably benign or probably cancer. Thus, a large number of men still undergo prostate biopsy for benign diseases. Apart from increasing the costs of detection, there is no consensus if these tests be used together as a standard package or in sequence after a total PSA of >4.0 ng/mL is detected or for standard cutoff points for each isoform. To further complicate the picture, the isoforms equally undergo an intrapatient variability as does total PSA.

22.3.1.3 Serum Kallikrein-Related Peptidase 2 (hK2)

Another member of the same kallikrein gene family of secreted serine proteases as PSA is the human kallikrein-related peptidase 2 (hK2). Like PSA (hK3), hK2 shows greatest abundance in the prostate tissues (Yousef and Demandis, 2001); it is overexpressed in prostate cancer (Darson et al., 1997). hK2 levels can be measured in serum samples (Becker et al., 2000; Haese et al., 2001). Some studies have found that hK2 may be useful in predicting, preoperatively, disease that is non-organ confined and the risk of biochemical recurrence (Recker et al., 2000; Haese et al., 2001). However, other studies (Kurek et al., 2004) have not found hK2 to be more beneficial than PSA for prognostic prediction preoperatively. The ratio of hk2 to fPSA has been shown to be a useful tool in prostate cancer detection in patients within the 2–10 ng/mL PSA range (Magklara et al., 1999; Partin et al., 1999). Vickers et al. (2010), using 4 PSA markers plus hK2, showed that a model incorporating them all, with an estimated extra cost/patient of $100 per patient, improved the prediction of prostate cancer detection in men with a PSA of 4.0–10.0 ng/mL. They suggest that this combined method would decrease the number of unnecessary biopsies without missing high-grade cancers.

22.4 Novel Diagnostic Biomarkers for Prostate Cancer

A biomarker must be shown to correlate with an interested outcome, in this case, the detection of clinically significant prostate cancer. The selection of a biomarker should have a biological or therapeutic basis or at least indicate a reliable correlation with the presence of prostate cancer. An ideal biomarker should be quick, consistent, economical, and quantifiable in an accessible biological fluid or clinical sample, for example, plasma, urine, or prostatic fluid and that is readily interpretable by the treating physician, that is, should the patient undergo prostate biopsy. Its expression should be increased (or decreased) in the related disease condition and no overlap should exist in the levels of biomarker between healthy controls and untreated patients. In the case of prostate cancer detection, the biomarker should be prostate specific and able to differentiate between normal, benign hyperplasia, prostatic intraepithelial dysplasia, and prostatic cancer. Thus, the ideal marker will indicate the presence of an early cancer or that cancer will occur with nearly 100% certainty within a very short time interval.

Biomarkers for the detection of prostate cancer can be divided into three groups: DNA-based markers, RNA-based markers and protein markers, and, more recently, circulating tumor cells (CTCs).

22.4.1 DNA-Based Markers for the Detection of Prostate Cancer

22.4.1.1 Serum Free Circulating DNA

The presence of circulating cell-free nucleic acids in cancer patients has been well documented, and the correlation between elevated levels of free circulating DNA (fDNA) in cancer patients as compared with healthy subjects was reported by Leon et al. in 1977. Further studies showed elevated levels of circulating serum or plasma DNA in patients with malignant tumors as compared with benign controls (Allen et al., 2004; Boddy et al., 2005). It has been shown to distinguish between patients with prostate cancer and healthy controls and correlates with pathological stage (Altimari et al., 2008) and independent of the established clinical variables such as age and total PSA (Chun et al., 2006). However, contrary results have also been published, showing that fDNA levels are higher in benign prostatic hypertrophy as compared with men with prostate cancer (Jung et al., 2004; Boddy et al., 2005). The results are very dependent on the primer used to detect cell-free DNA; in a prospective study using a cohort of patients suspected of having prostate cancer, based on DRE and a total PSA >4.0 ng/mL, the authors used real-time PCR for glutathione S-transferase P1 (GSTP1). Median fDNA has been found to vary across different studies, being attributed to the source of fDNA, variations in the methodology of sample processing, and fDNA quantitation. A critical factor for determining a standard fDNA cutoff value is to establish uniform methodologies for sample collection, processing, DNA extraction, and fDNA quantitation and analysis (Xue et al., 2009). Cell lysis and apoptosis have been postulated to be the predominant mechanism of release of DNA into the circulation (Jahr et al., 2001; Wu et al., 2002). Further concern about the application of free DNA is the occurrence of false positives, particularly in patients with autoimmune, inflammatory diseases and a recent history of trauma or surgical procedures (Holdenrieder et al., 2001; Taback and Hoon, 2004). Furthermore, GSPT-1 is not specific for prostate cancer, and thus, its use in a general screening population is doubtful.

To address this problem, the use of specific loss of heterozygosity of free plasma DNA in blood and bone marrow samples has been reported to overcome this difficulty of false positivity (Chun et al., 2006; Schwarzenbach et al., 2007) (Figure 22.3).

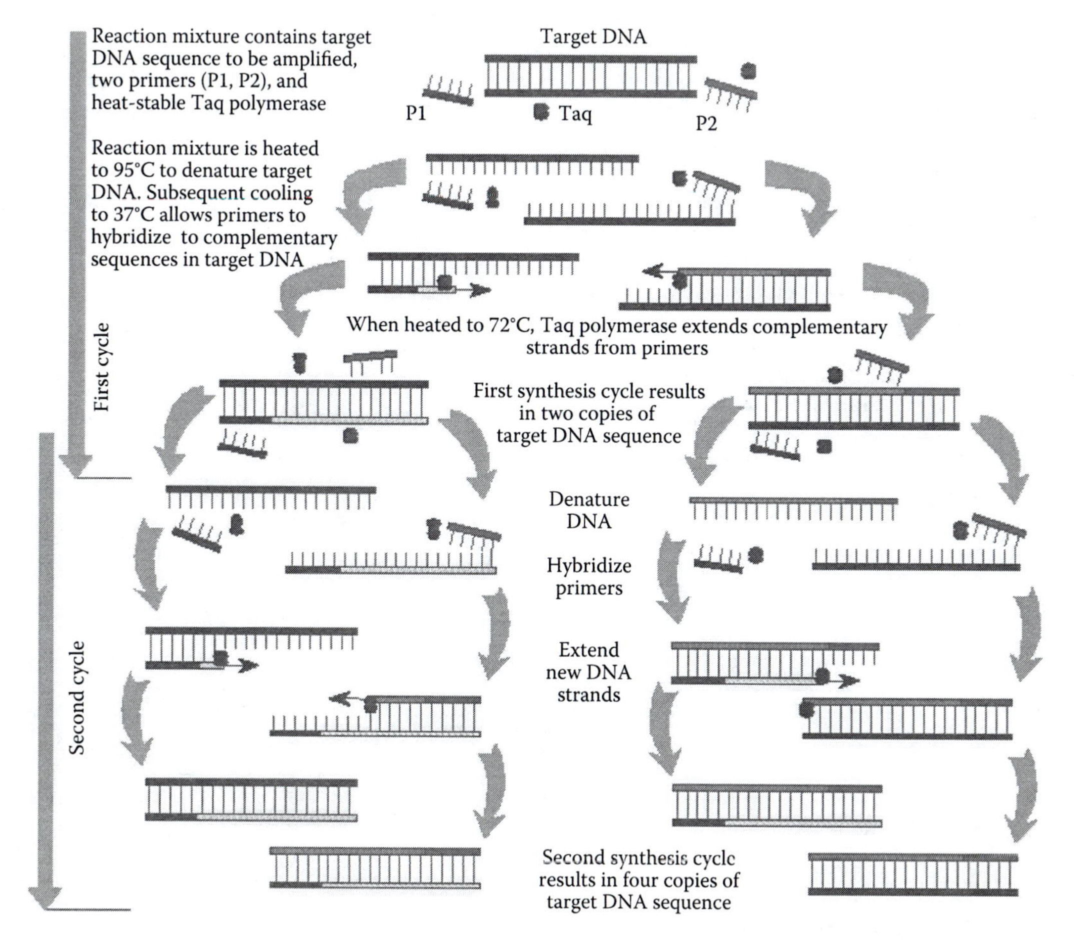

FIGURE 22.3 DNA amplification using polymerase chain reaction. (DNA Science, see Fig 13.)

22.4.1.2 Promoter Hypermethylation of Cell-Free Plasma DNA

Promoter hypermethylation is a common epigenetic alteration affecting normal and cancer-related genes. Specific methylation changes are being tested as promising markers for early tumor detection (Jerónimo et al., 2004) In particular, hypermethylation of the *GSTP1* is the most common epigenetic alteration in CaP, and its detection by means of methylation-specific polymerase chain reaction (MSP) discriminates between normal and neoplastic status in prostate tissues and body fluids with high sensitivity and specificity (Harden et al., 2003; Henrique and Jerónimo, 2004).

Epigenetic alterations, including hypermethylation of CpG islands in the gene promoters, are believed to be early events in neoplastic progression (Hanahan and Weinberg, 2000; Strathdee and Brown, 2002; Lund and Lohuizen, 2004; Ducasse and Brown, 2006; Shelton BP et al., 2008; Schulz and Hoffmann, 2009). However, recent findings in prostate carcinogenesis provide evidence that DNA hypomethylation changes occur subsequent to CpG island hypermethylation in later stages of carcinogenesis (Yegnasubramanian et al., 2008).

Hypermethylation of tumor suppressor gene promoters contributes to their silencing during the neoplastic process (Jones and Baylin, 2002). Thus, methylated gene promoters can serve as markers for the detection of cancer from clinical specimens such as tissue biopsies or body fluids (Hoque , 2009). Compared to tests that measure cancer-related proteins or RNAs, tests that measure gene alterations at the DNA level have several advantages for the early detection of cancer. DNA is stable in many of the conditions under which clinical specimens are collected and stored. Many DNA modifications can be reliably detected by PCR-based techniques (Sidransky, 1997; Cairns , 2007), meaning that very small amounts of DNA are needed for such tests. PCR amplification-based tests also allow detection of as few as one cancer cell (or genome copy) in a background of thousands of normal cells, thereby permitting detection of a cancer before it can be visualized by imaging or traditional pathology. Moreover, DNA alterations can be measured qualitatively, as well as quantitatively. Finally, assays based on the DNA alterations can be both diagnostic and prognostic. Therefore, methylated DNA sequences can form the basis of a sensitive and specific, robust, and informative test for the detection of cancer (Cairns, 2007).

DNA methylation refers to the covalent binding of a methyl group specifically to the carbon-5 position of cytosine residues of the dinucleotide CpG and catalyzed by a family of enzymes, the DNA methyltransferases (DNMTs) (Figure 22.4).

DNMT transfers methyl group from S-adenosyl methionine (SAM-CH3) to cytosine yielding S-adenosyl homocysteine (SAH) and 5-methylcytosine.

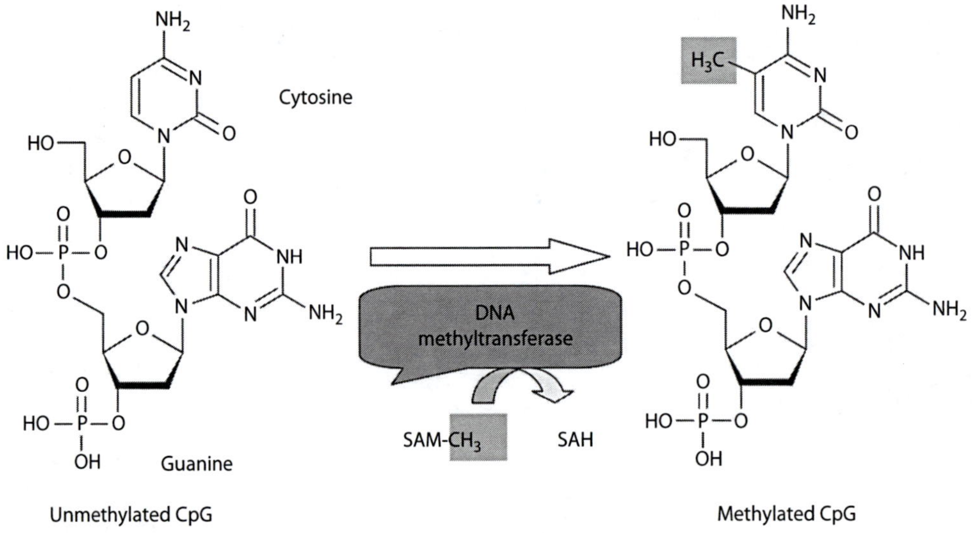

FIGURE 22.4 DNA methylation catalyzed by DNA methyltransferase.

Hypermethylation of CpG islands in the promoter regions of tumor suppressor and other regulatory genes that are normally unmethylated is found in cancer cells. The promoter regions of these genes may be inactivated by methylation, which silences their expression. However, differential methylation is not a general mechanism for regulating gene expression, because most inactive promoter remains unmethylated (Weber et al., 2007) (Figure 22.5).

It has been suggested that hypermethylation plays an important role in the process of carcinogenesis, with the inactivation of many well-characterized tumor suppressor genes and inactivation of DNA repair genes, resulting in increased levels of genetic damage; GSTP-1 is one such example. In prostate cancer, a large number of genes (e.g., DNA damage repair genes, tumor suppressors, cell cycle control genes, cell adhesion molecules, and signal transduction genes) contribute to initiation and progression of the disease, and expression of these genes is correlated with the pathological grade (Hoque, 2009; Schulzand Hoffman, 2009). Hypermethylation can be detected using MSP and is the most commonly used method (details in Hoque [2009]). In prostate cancer, *GSTP1* is silenced by promoter methylation (Cairns et al., 2001; Cairns, 2007; Meiers et al., 2007) and has been detected in cancerous as well as prostatic intraepithelial neoplasia (PIN) lesions, whereas it has been rarely detected in normal prostate or BPH tissues (Jerónimo et al., 2001; Nakayama et al., 2003). Hypermethylation of *GSTP1* was also found in a subset of proliferative inflammatory atrophy (PIA) lesions, which are believed to be preneoplastic (Nakayama et al., 2003).

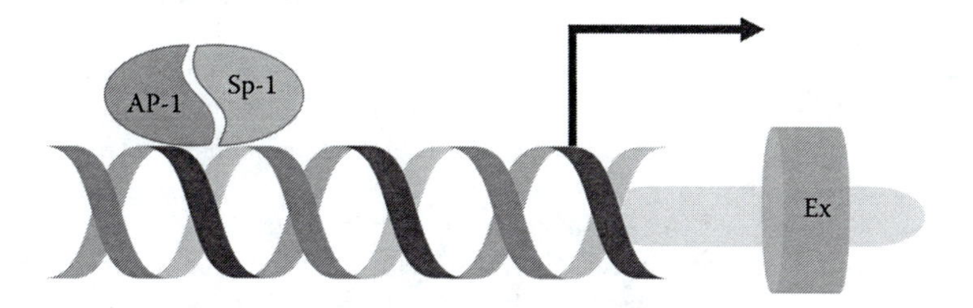

(a) Unmethylated CpG in the promoter: active

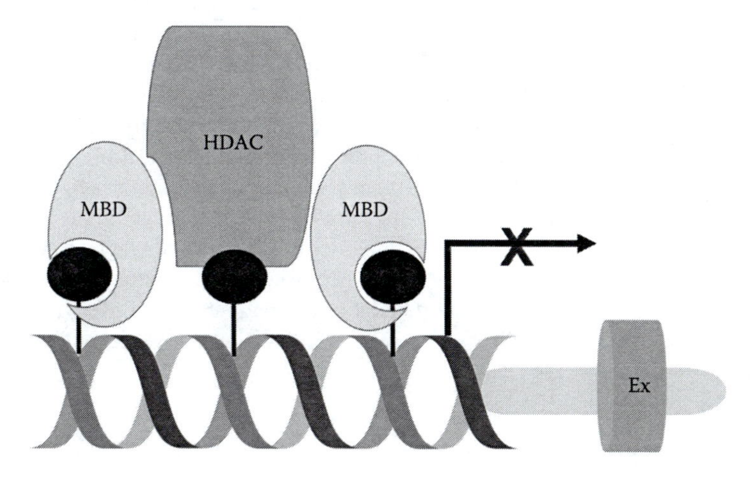

(b) Methylated CpG in the promoter: inactive

FIGURE 22.5 Simplified diagram showing (a) gene transcription by unmethylated promoter and (b) gene silencing by the methylated promoter. (a) In normal prostate and pituitary tissues, tumor suppressor promoter is unmethylated and accessible to binding to the transcription factors such as AP-1 and Sp-1 for stimulation of gal3 transcription. (b) In prostate cancer, promoters of several genes such as tumor suppressor, DNA repair gene, and gal3 are methylated and therefore bound by the methyl-binding proteins (MBD) and histone deacetylase (HDAC). Thus, the methylated promoter is not accessible to binding to the transcription factors and inactive.

Although many genes are methylated in prostate cancer, some have insufficient methylation to be sufficiently sensitive, while others are present in benign hyperplasia. GSTP-1 hypermethylation appears to be the most ideal DNA marker as it is present in 90% of prostate cancers, two-thirds of HG-PIN, and rarely found in benign hyperplasia. The first study using plasma samples of prostate cancer patients for the detection of methylated GSTP-1 found that the promoter was methylated in 72% of patients with prostate cancer and none of the patients with benign hyperplasia (Goessl et al., 2001). Using a 4-gene assay to measure hypermethylation, the genes GSTP-1, TIG1, PTGS2, and reprimo had a higher methylation frequency of 42.3%, 9.55%, 2.4%, and 1.2%, respectively, than in men with benign hyperplasia, 7.7%, 0%, 0%, and 0%, respectively, whereas in all healthy controls, hypermethylation was not detected (Ellinger et al., 2008). Using only GSTP-1 and comparing men with prostate cancer to those with benign hyperplasia, the test was highly specific 92% but less sensitive 42%–47%.

However, it should be emphasized that most published studies have been in small scale. Large-scale studies will be necessary before any of these assays can be considered clinically useful. In addition to clinical validation, assays for methylated genes must be robust, simple, sensitive, specific, and made available at affordable costs. Regarding specificity of the assay, the most important consideration is to select a gene or genes whose promoter methylation is specific to prostate cancer. For example, *GSTP1* is methylated in 90% of prostate cancer, 30% of breast cancer, 25% of hepatic cancer, and less than 10% in bladder and renal cancers. Given that prostate cancer is a disease of males and that hepatic cancer is relatively rare in the Western world, methylation analysis of *GSTP1* from male specimens would provide specificity to prostate cancer around 90%.

In terms of sensitivity, most studies of single genes or combinations of multiple genes did not reach a sensitivity of more than 75%, and most importantly, these markers failed to detect early stages of prostate cancer (Tokumaru et al., 2004; Vener et al., 2008). Therefore, a reliable marker for early detection (stage I, II) of prostate cancer is yet to be identified.

Altimari et al. (2008), using cell-free plasma DNA, obtained a sensitivity of 80% and specificity of 82% to detect patients with prostate cancer. Not all patients with prostate cancer reached the cutoff point for a positive test. The authors considered this not to be related to low DNA amplification capability of their PCR assay but a defect of free DNA release from some tumors. They highlighted the fact that at present it remains unclear whether free DNA is just released, actively secreted by the primary tumor, or derives from the rupture of CTCs. What is important is that healthy donors and >95% of men with benign hyperplasia did not have GSTP1 methylation in the plasma. Methylation in the promoter region of the GSTP1 gene is an early epigenetic alteration in prostate cancer and is detected in approximately 90% of prostate cancer tissue samples. However, the detection rate of *GSTP1* methylation in one series was 25% in the plasma and 94% in the corresponding paraffin-embedded CaP tissue samples; in other words, not all men with GSTP1 methylation in biopsy samples have positive plasma samples. This corresponds to 75% of men with biopsy-proven prostate cancer having a negative plasma test. In the plasma of patients with CaP, the detection rates of *GSTP1* methylation range between 13% and 72% according to different reports (see review by Henrique and Jerónimo). This variability has been explained by the enrollment of different populations of patients with CaP (which also included subjects with disseminated neoplastic disease) or by the use of a quantitative rather than a conventional MSP procedure.

22.4.1.3 Single Nucleotide Polymorphisms

Several single nucleotide polymorphisms (SNPs) have been evaluated with regard to the risk of prostate cancer, such as polymorphisms of the androgen receptor (Giovannucci et al., 1997), vitamin D receptor (Ingles et al., 1997), 5-alpha reductase enzyme (Nam et al., 2001), CYP17 (Gsur et al., 2000), and CYP3A4 genes (Rebbeck et al., 1998). These have been associated with the presence of prostate cancer in one or more case-control studies.

However, to date, no genetic test is used in clinical practice to evaluate prostate cancer risk. Associations are often not reproducible and the lack of correlation between SNPs and the protein expression or activity has been noted of concern to some authors. One possible candidate for SNP screening is an SNP for the kH2 gene, which consists of a nucleotide change from cytosine to thymine on exon 5 (Herrala et al., 1997). Whether this mutation is associated with a functional change or a quantitative change in the kH2 gene product is not known as yet. In vitro, the two alleles code for an active and an inactive gene product, the common allele codes for Arg^{226}–hK2 that has a trypsin-like activity, and the mutated form, Trp^{226}–hK2, is inactive (Herrala et al., 1997). Nam et al. (2003) analyzed men with an altered PSA value or abnormal rectal examination referred for prostate biopsy; they evaluated whether the SNP for hK2 predicted serum levels of hK2 and prostate cancer risk. In a study of 1437 unselected men who presented for prostate cancer screening, they found a positive association between the hK2 gene, hK2 serum level, and prostate cancer risk; both the gene expression and serum protein levels were independently associated with prostate cancer risk. They reported that the probability of having prostate cancer detected at the first biopsy was 31.5%, 38.7%, and 47.1% for the common–common, common–mutated, and mutated–mutated phenotypes, for a positive predictive value of 53% in patients with an SNP positive for the mutation.

Although several studies have shown that patients with prostate cancer have significantly higher serum levels of hK2 than those without prostate cancer, there is no established standardized cutoff point for serum levels, and the distribution of hK2 serum levels varies widely between studies. Thus, the SNP mutation may be more clinically useful in that it gives a yes/no type of result for the treating physician. However, one disadvantage is that the SNP mutation has only a 53% specificity, although an improvement on the 30% for total serum PSA levels in the range 4.0–10.0 ng/mL, which still leaves 47% of patients having a negative biopsy for cancer.

22.4.2 Circulating Tumor Cells

In men with prostate cancer, there is an early dissemination of cancer cells, first to the neurovascular structures and then into the circulation (Moreno et al., 1992). Although the number of these cells is small, they can be detected by methods of reverse transcription polymerase chain reaction (RT-PCR) and/or immunocytochemistry. PSA is not specific for prostate cancer; circulating prostate cells (CPCs) have been detected in cases of prostatitis (Murray et al., 2010); thus, PSA-expressing cells detected in blood may not represent malignancy but benign cells that have escaped into the blood due to acute inflammation of the prostate gland. There it is important that the biomarker or combination of biomarkers used to detect CPCs can distinguish between benign and malignant CPCs.

The "seed and soil hypothesis" proposed by Stephen Paget in 1889 states that specialized subpopulations of cancer cells within the primary tumor are endowed with specific properties, which enable them to detach from the primary tumor, migrate to the adjacent tissues, adhere to the wall of the lymph and/or blood capillaries, enter into the vessels, and disseminate through the systemic vasculature. They avoid the shear forces in the circulation and are anchorage independent, ultimately arresting in specific tissues where they implant, extravasculate, and eventually may proliferate in a permissive organ. The cancer cells may be protected from undergoing apoptosis by the loss of cell anchorage dependence (anoikis), surviving in the circulation through acquired phenotypic and genetic alterations. One hypothesis supports the view that most invasive cancer cells, although representing a small fraction of the original tumor, undergo epithelial to mesenchymal transition and adopt a phenotype with increased cell motility and invasiveness that allows them to infiltrate adjacent tissues and cross endothelial barriers (Bates and Mercurio, 2005; Thompson et al., 2005; Yang et al., 2006). This transition is thought to be a highly conserved and fundamental process that achieves morphogenetic transformation that leads to tumor dissemination and metastatic spread. It is thought to be characterized by a decrease in epithelial markers, for example, cytokeratins and EpCAM; a poor histological differentiation; and an increase in mesenchymal markers, for example, vimentin (Lang et al., 2002; Willipinski-Stapelfeldt et al., 2005). Once the target tissue is reached, these mesenchymal cells may need to reverse to an epithelial identity via a mesenchymal–epithelial transition in order to regain their ability to proliferate (Christiansen and Rajasekaran, 2006).

This may have important implications, firstly, the possible loss of tumor cells during immunomagnetic separation used in the CellSearch® system, the most aggressive cancer cell population due to the loss or reduction in expression of epithelial markers during the epithelial to mesenchymal transition (Yang et al., 2006), and in the cancer cell marker chosen to identify tumor cells (Panteleakou et al., 2009).

22.4.2.1 Use of RT-PCR to Detect CPCs

Peripheral blood is the source for mRNA; the detection of prostate-specific mRNAs in the blood implies the existence of prostate epithelial cells and therefore tumor spread (Katz, 1994; Ghossein and Bhattacharya, 2000). RT-PCR is more sensitive than immunocytochemical detection of tumor cells; however, a number of critical parameters have been identified that determine the effectiveness of this method. The most crucial is the choice of the target marker; its expression should be limited to prostatic cells and have no or minimal expression in other cell types. However, in the real world, the ultrasensitivity of RT-PCR can give rise to false-positive results due to illegitimate transcription (Chelly et al., 1989), with an estimated expression level of 1 tumor marker gene for every 500–1000 noncancer cells, that is, these genes, although detected, are not expressed at the protein level (Zieglschmid et al., 2005). In clinical terms, this presents the problem of determining a cutoff point (as with the CellSearch system discussed later) of what number of CTCs has clinical relevance (Lembessis et al., 2007).

The expression of PSA has been considered to be specific for prostate tissue and has been used as a marker for RT-PCR detection protocols for prostate cancer patients. However, PSA mRNA has been detected in nonprostatic cell lines and in blood from healthy males and females (Smith et al., 1995; Henke et al., 1997; Gala et al., 1998). The use of prostate membrane-specific antigen, also thought to be prostate specific and highly expressed in metastatic prostate cancer, has been found to be expressed in leukocytes from healthy donors (Gala et al., 1998). The primer selected should span an intron/exon boundary and should avoid pseudogenes, which lack introns. Hara et al. (2001) suggested that prostate biopsy may release prostate cells into the circulation and therefore the timing of RT-PCR-based detection should be at least 4 weeks post biopsy. In patients with acute bacterial prostatitis, cells may also be detected in the circulation (Dumas et al., 1997). To avoid contamination by epithelial and/or endothelial cells, it is recommended that the first few milliliters of blood are discarded.

With regards to prostate cancer detection, studies have shown that the use of RT-PCR for PSA mRNA can differentiate patients with extracapsular extension for those with localized prostate-confined disease with a sensitivity of 64% and specificity of 84% (Katz et al., 1994; Cama et al., 1995). However, Patel et al. (2004) failed to detect a difference between healthy patients and patients with localized prostate cancer. In patients with localized prostate cancer, levels of PSA mRNA expression were low and no different from those identified in blood samples from healthy volunteers.

Their result is in contrast to other studies using conventional nonquantitative RT-PCR or quantitative real-time RT-PCR (Gelmini et al., 2001; Straub et al., 2001). However, previous studies have not compared levels in patient samples with those from healthy volunteers. They suggest that the discordant results most likely reflect the increased discriminatory power of the real-time quantitative method and definition of what constitutes a positive result. Using the highly sensitive quantitative real-time RT-PCR, they confirmed the presence of low-level expression of PSA by monocytes in blood samples from healthy volunteers. Thus, compensation for the low-level signal due to illegitimate transcription of the target gene is important if the true clinical utility of RT-PCR is to be realized.

Some have sought to achieve this by either selecting out the monocyte population (CD34 + cells) before RNA extraction or RT-PCR (Fava et al., 2001), although this risks losing CTCs during the isolation process and requires additional sample manipulation. Alternatively, some have suggested reducing the amount of total RNA or cDNA analyzed by the RT-PCR (Lopez-Guerrero et al., 1997; Fava et al., 2001), which may improve specificity but will reduce the overall sensitivity of detection of CTCs. Therefore, a robust definition for contamination of a blood sample with a prostate cancer cell based on the PSA mRNA level compared with that in blood samples from healthy controls needs to be established. A further study by Thiounn et al. (1997) reported 8.5% of men with benign prostatic hypertrophy, 17.6% with nonprostatic disease, and 22% of men with T1–T2 prostate cancer had PSA-positive cells detected by RT-PCR. Although the difference in PSA-positive cell was significantly different between men with cancer and men with benign hyperplasia, they concluded that the method is highly unspecific and its clinical utility low.

Prostate-specific membrane antigen (PMSA) is a folate gamma glutamyl carboxypeptidase that is found in the membrane of normal and prostate cancer cells and is located on the short arm of chromosome 11. It is a highly specific marker of the prostate gland and has been used as a marker gene, indicating dissemination to the circulation in men with prostate cancer. It is also highly expressed in the endothelium of tumor-associated neovasculature of nonprostatic solid tumors but not expressed in that of normal tissue. Nonprostatic tissues express lower amounts of PMSA, such as small intestine, proximal tubules of the kidney, salivary gland, and muscle (Fair et al., 1997). Its expression, as detected by immunohistochemistry, increases from normal, benign, precancerous PIN, adenocarcinoma, and metastatic tissue, being highest in high-grade tumors (Bostwick et al., 1998).

However, studies using PMSA RT-PCR have encountered the same problems as with PSA RT-PCR; Llanes et al. (2002) found that nested PCR detected 38% positivity in a group of healthy men and women. In contrast, Loric et al. (1995) suggested that the detection of PMSA-expressing cells in blood may predict the development of cancer in patients without clinically apparent prostate cancer. However, Sokoloff et al. (1996) found that such cells were only identified in advanced cancer.

A further possible candidate is the prostate stem cell antigen (PSCA), a cell surface antigen that is predominantly prostate specific but is also expressed at lower levels in placenta, kidney, and small intestine (Reiter et al., 1998). Located on chromosome 8q24.2, it is often amplified in metastatic and recurrent prostate cancer and considered to indicate a poor prognosis. However, its role in localized prostate cancer and therefore in screening tests is in doubt and its expression correlated with extraprostatic tumor extension, being positive in 47% of cases, whereas all organ-confined tumors were negative (Hara et al., 2002).

At present, there are no studies published using RT-PCR as a screening test for prostate cancer.

22.4.2.2 Use of Immunocytochemistry to Detect CPCs

22.4.2.2.1 CellSearch®

The CellSearch system (Veridex) is intended for the enumeration of CTCs of epithelial origin (CD45−, EpCAM+, and cytokeratins 8, 18+, and/or 19+) in whole blood. It is approved by the Federal Drug Administration for research purposes in metastatic breast, prostate, and colon cancer. It uses ferro-immunomagnetic separation for enrichment and isolation of CTCs. Iron nanoparticles of 120–200 nm have anti-EpCAM or anti-cytokeratin 8/18 or 19 and are the basis of the enrichment process. A 7.5 mL blood sample is taken in commercially available tubes (CellSearch); the plasma is removed after centrifugation and the ferrofluid added with buffer. There is an incubation, the anti-EpCAM or anti-cytokeratin-coated iron nanoparticles binding to epithelial cells but not to leukocytes, using magnetic field cells bound to the nanoparticles that are withheld in the system, and the aspirate containing leukocytes is removed. Thus, after removing the magnets, the bound epithelial cells are washed and identified using a biotin–streptavidin-based system, which is automated. Analytic data showed a 93% recovery of spiked epithelial cells and the ability to detect one cell per 7.5 mL of blood; the automated system showed that the detection was linear over the reported range of 0–1238 tumor cells detected.

Miller et al. (2010) published the results of the CellSearch system in normal controls, benign disease, and metastatic breast colon and prostate cancer (see Table 22.3). In normal or patients with benign disease up to 7.5% may have one circulating cell detected.

The frequency of CTC in 7.5 mL of blood from normal donors: patients with benign disease and metastatic breast, colorectal, and prostate cancer before initiation of a new therapy is shown in Table 22.3.

TABLE 22.3

Frequency of CTCs Detected using Cell-Search® System

		Percentage of Patients with CTC above Threshold						
	# pat	≥1	≥5	≥10	≥50	≥100	≥500	≥1000
Normal	295	3.4	0.0	0.0	0.0	0.0	0.0	0.0
Benign	255	7.5	0.4	0.4	0.0	0.0	0.0	0.0
Breast	177	70.6	49.7	38.4	20.9	15.8	3.4	2.8
Colorectal	413	47.5	18.2	11.6	2.4	1.0	0.0	0.0
Prostate	218	77.5	57.3	45.0	20.6	13.8	3.7	2.3

Source: Miller, M.C. et al., *J. Oncol.*, 2010, 61742, 2010.

In studies of localized prostate cancer, Davis et al. (2008) evaluated the CellSearch system in 97 men with localized cancer and compared the results with 25 men with an increased serum PSA and biopsy negative for cancer. CTCs were detected in 21% of cancer patients as compared with 20% of controls. In terms of the number of CTCs detected, only 3% of cancer patients and 8% of controls had ≥3 cells/22.5 mL of blood (3 CellSearch tubes). This figure increased to 42% in patients with localized cancer in a second study by Stott et al. (2010). Fizazi et al. (2007), using anti-BerEP-4 epithelial antigen combined with telomerase activity, detected primary CPCs in 79% of patients with localized cancer. One possible reason for the wide discrepancy of results is the technology used. Regardless of the system used for isolation or enrichment, detection almost always relies on staining for cytokeratin or EpCAM and, in the case of CellSearch, enrichment or isolation of CTCs using a cytokeratin- or EpCAM-based system. The widely accepted concept that all cytokeratin- and/or EpCAM-positive, CD45-negative cells with a nucleus in cancer patients are CTCs has imposed a clear bias on the study of CTCs. The failure to include tumor cells that have reduced or absent cytokeratin and/or EpCAM expression and the failure to identify such cell types limits investigations into additional tumor types. EpCAM is expressed in most but not all tumors (Went et al., 2004); there is downregulation with cancer progression and metastasis; cytokeratins are heterogeneously expressed in tumor cells and also may be downregulated during disease progression or in poorly differentiated tumors. During the progression of epithelial to mesenchymal transition, both markers are downregulated (Paterlini-Brechot and Benali, 2007); EpCAM may be downregulated to allow epithelial cell dissociation from the tumor and cytokeratin downregulated to facilitate cell plasticity and migration (Raimondi et al., 2011). The finding of CTCs that express EpCAM is not in question, but there is concern over false negatives in the failure to detect CTCs that do not express EpCAM. Furthermore, one possible explication of the high number of positive controls is that CTCs can be found in men with prostatitis.

At present, while in patients with metastatic prostate cancer the CellSearch system is approved by the FDA, the few studies in men with localized cancer have produced varying frequencies of positive patients and no significant differences with the control groups. There are at present no studies published of its use in the detection of prostate cancer.

22.4.2.2.2 Epispot®

Differing from the CellSearch System, the Epispot system detects proteins secreted by viable tumor cells. In contrast to the common concept that cytokeratins are released in fragmented forms only by epithelial cells (e.g., as a result of apoptosis), there is evidence for a release of full-length CK19 by viable epithelial tumor cells, as a result of an active process and not as a result of apoptosis. Using a membrane coated with anti-total PSA, it was possible to detect PSA-secreting cells. In patients without prostate cancer, no PSA-SCs were detected in the blood of 27 patients with BPH, 4 patients with AP (Table 22.2 of the online Data Supplement), and 35 with NPD (Table 22.3 of the online Data Supplement) or in 6 healthy controls (data not shown), although most had abnormally increased serum PSA. Among 12 PCa patients tested before treatment, 5 (42%) had detectable PSA-SCs (Alix-Panabières et al., 2005).

The method (see figure) is that the nitrocellulose membranes of ELISPOT® plates are coated with an antibody against a specific protein marker, in this case total PSA. Cells are seeded in each well and cultured for 48 h. During this incubation step, the specific secreted proteins are directly captured on the antibody-coated membrane. Cells are then washed off and the specific protein marker is detected by a second antibody. Immunospots were counted by video camera imaging and computer-assisted analysis (KS ELISPOT, Carl Zeiss Vision). One immunospot corresponds to one viable marker protein-secreting cell. As previously shown, viable cells are needed to accumulate a sufficient amount of the released marker proteins and dying cells are therefore not detected (Czerkinski et al., 1983; Alix-Panabières et al., 2005). Using the method, Alix-Panabières et al. (2007) detected cells in 83% of men with metastatic prostate cancer, 65% of men with nonmetastatic prostatic cancer, and none of the controls in men with benign disease or healthy controls. The method requires a cell culture facility, and the protein used to identify a CTC must be actively secreted, shed, or released outside these cells.

To date there are no published studies of the methods used to detect prostate cancer in a screening population, although there are ongoing studies comparing Epispot with CellSearch® in breast cancer patients (Figure 22.6).

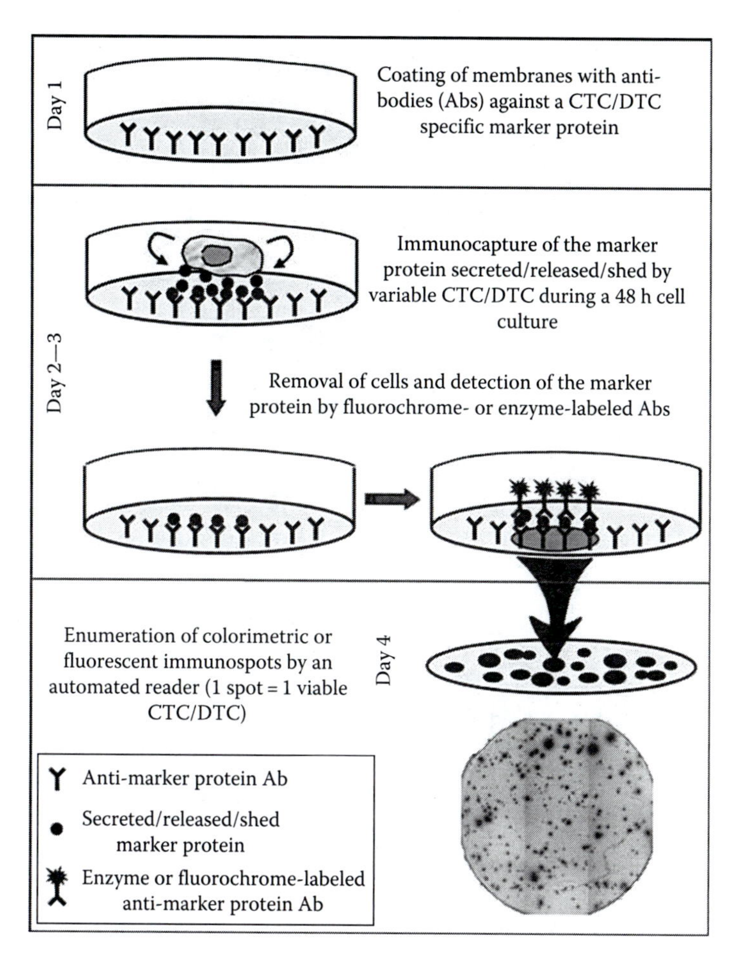

FIGURE 22.6 Epispot® method of CTC detection.

22.4.2.2.3 ProTECT®

Using standard immunocytochemical methods, a Chilean group has published two studies on the use of CPCs for the detection of prostate cancer. Blood samples were collected from a general population and compared with the serum PSA and in the second with the results of the prostate biopsy (Murray et al., 2010, 2011). Mononuclear cells were obtained using standard differential gel centrifugation and detected using standard double immunocytochemistry. Monoclonal antibodies directed against PSA were used to identify CPCs and positive samples underwent a second process using anti-P504S. A CPC was defined according to the criteria of the International Society of Hematotherapy and Genetic Engineering (ISHAGE) (Borgen et al., 1999) and the expression of P504S according to the Consensus of the American Association of Pathologists (Rubin et al., 2002). A malignant CPC was defined as a cell that expressed PSA and P504S; a benign cell could express PSA but not P504S and leukocytes could be P504S positive or negative but did not express PSA. The concentration of CPCs detected was determined as the number of cells detected/mL blood, and they considered a test as positive when at least one cell was detected (Figure 22.7).

Differing from other studies, the double immunocytochemistry allowed the definition of benign CPCs, which had previously been shown to be present in some patients with prostatitis and which were not considered to be associated with prostate cancer. The use of the biomarker P504S, although not prostate specific (Zhou et al., 2002), has facilitated the differentiation between normal, dysplastic, and malignant tissues in prostate biopsy samples. Normal or benign cells do not express P504S, whereas cells arising from PIN or cancer are positive (Beach et al., 2002). Although not scientifically proven, the assumption

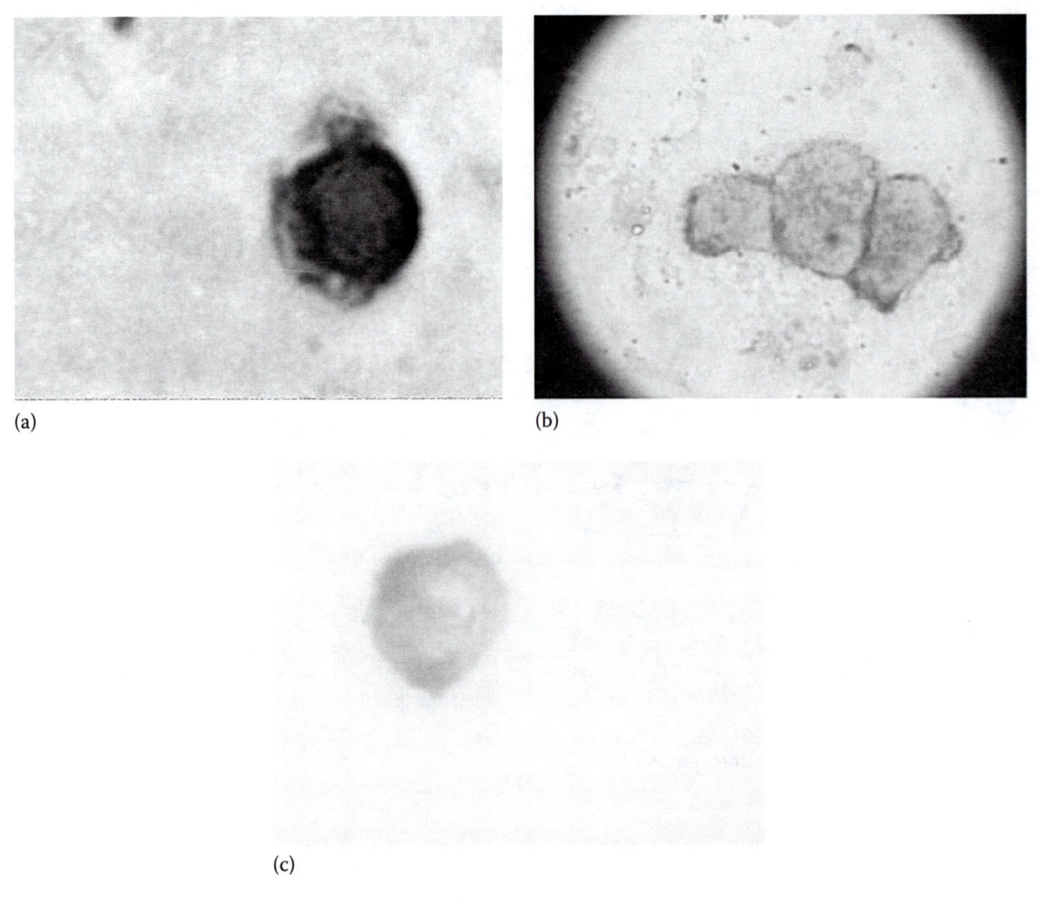

FIGURE 22.7 (See color insert.) (a) Malignant CPC PSA (+) red and P504S (+) black. (b) Benign CPC PSA (+) red and P504S (–). (c) Leukocyte PSA (–) P504S (–).

is that cells arising from PIN do not disseminate, which implies that CPCs expressing P504S are therefore malignant. For this reason, it is essential that double immunolabeling is used to detect mCPCs. Double immune marcation is the sequential use of two monoclonal antibodies and two differing systems of detection, thus labeling cells as positive or negative for two different biomarkers. Only cells positive for the two biomarkers are considered as positive.

The first study published in 2010 showed that there was no cutoff point for the detection of malignant CPCs; men with a serum PSA of <2.0 ng/mL had malignant CPCs detected in X% of cases. The second study published in 2011, was a prospective blinded study using malignant CPC detection as a sequential test in men with an increased serum PSA or abnormal rectal examination. In the population of 228 men, they found a cancer prevalence of 28.5% (CI 22.7–34.8); a sensibility of 86.2% (CI 75.3–93.5); a specificity of 90.8% (CI 85.3–94.8), for a positive predictive value of 78.9% (CI 67.6–87.7); and a negative predictive value of 94.3% (CI 89.4–97.3). The patients with a cancer detected on biopsy but negative for malignant CPCs had low-grade low-volume tumors, the type recommended for active surveillance. They further published the cost benefit of the system (Murray et al., 2013) whereby the incorporation of the test in men with suspicion of state cancer saved the hospital system €32,068 in a population of 263 patients, by excluding 70% of prostate biopsies. This was the first type of study to look at men prebiopsy and not comparing men with localized prostate cancer with men without prostate cancer. The use of a test with a positive or negative result simplified clinical decisions; the incorporation of the number of cells detected/mL increased the specificity by 8% but significantly reduced the sensibility. The use of this simple standard immunocytochemistry method meant that it could be incorporated in the routine laboratory without the initial high setup costs or running costs, although with a manual method, interobserver variation is higher than in automated systems.

22.4.2.3 Use of Biomarkers in Urine to Detect Prostate Cancer

22.4.2.3.1 Prostate Cancer Antigen 3 Gene

A number of genes have been identified that are specifically expressed in the human prostate, and one such gene is prostate cancer antigen 3 (PCA3) (formerly DD3). Described in 1999 by Bussemakers and coworkers, using differential display analysis of tumor tissue and adjacent nonneoplastic tissue of radical prostatectomy specimens, they identified a cDNA PCA3, which was highly overexpressed in almost all prostatic tumors and metastatic lesions studied. Using RT-PCR, they did not detect PCA3 expression in normal tissue, other human tumor tissue types, or tumor-derived cell lines. This overexpression of PCA3 in prostate cancer as opposed to normal prostate or benign hypertrophy tissues made it candidate for its use as a diagnostic or prognostic biomarker. Evidence suggests that the PCA3 gene is a member of a unique class of noncoding RNAs and that the RNA is the final and functional product of the gene. It is thought to be expressed by prostate and not stromal cells, because it is highly expressed in adenocarcinoma that is derived from epithelial cells (Bussemakers et al., 1999). The gene encoding PCA3 is located on chromosome 9, 9q21–22, a region that has not previously been shown to be frequently affected in prostate cancer, and its expression is regulated by a unique prostate cancer–specific transcriptional mechanism that is normally suppressed (Verhaegh et al., 2000).

The detection of PCA3 mRNA in urine has been used as a biomarker to detect prostate cancer. The method uses patient urine obtained after prostate stimulation (massage), three strokes of each prostate lobe. After centrifugation of the urine sample, the sediment is used to detect the PCA3 mRNA using fluorescent RT-PCR.

One of the first studies to use PCA3 detection in men with a serum PSA ≥2.5 ng/mL and a previous biopsy negative for cancer showed that using a PCA3 threshold of 35, calculated as urinary PCA3 mRNA to PSA mRNA × 1000, showed a sensitivity of 58% and specificity of 72% (Marks et al., 2007). While only 12% of men with a PCA3 score of <5 had a positive biopsy, compared with 50% of those with a PCA3 score of >100. More recently, Roobol et al. (2010) evaluated previously screened men from the Rotterdam section of the European Randomized Study of Screening for Prostate Cancer. The study included 721 patients, of whom 122 (16.9%) had prostate cancer detected. A PSA cutoff value of 3.0 ng/mL had a 35.2% sensitivity and 69.0% specificity of detecting prostate cancer; in comparison the PCA3 test with a score of >10 had a 69.7% sensitivity and 47% specificity for cancer detection; using a score of >35, this had a sensitivity of 68.0% and specificity of 55.7%. Of the prostate cancers detected, 19 (15.5%) were classified as >T2a and/or Gleason ≥4. Using a PSA cutoff of 3.0 ng/mL would have missed 79 out of 122 cancers of which 11 were classified as needing treatment. PCA3 cutoffs of >10 and >35 would have missed 4 (3.3%) and 39 (32%) of cancers, respectively, including 0 and 5 meeting the aforementioned criteria for "serious" tumors. However, 32 (4.4%) and 373 (51.7%) of biopsies would have been spared using a PCA3 cutoff of >10 and >35, respectively. Notwithstanding it must be noted that this population had undergone multiple rounds of PSA screening, whereby the predictive power of PSA may have been expended during earlier screening rounds.

In the last 2 years, there have been further publications on the use of PCA3 for the detection of prostate cancer, which have shed further light on this biomarker and may in fact show the same drawbacks as serum PSA. Firstly, the level of PCA3 is age related, and Klatte et al. (2012) reported that the strongest impact on the PCA3 score was age, with a 4.77-fold difference, using an age-specific range of PCA3; a score over the age-specific limit was associated with a 4.17-fold increased odds of being diagnosed with prostate cancer. They concluded that age-specific PCA3 scores were superior to total PSA, continuous PCA3 score, and a PCA3 >35 in predicting the initial biopsy outcome. A Swedish study in a mixed population of patients failed to show that PCA3 and total PSA performed equally well as diagnostic markers and concluded that PCA3 did not have a role in replacing total PSA in prostate cancer detection (Nyberg et al., 2010). An Italian study looked at the use of PCA3 in initial and repeat biopsies in a study population of 1246 men (Bollito et al., 2012). They reported that a cutoff of >39 had the highest accuracy in the repeat biopsy group; a cutoff score of 39 would have avoided 51.9% of repeat biopsies, missing 7.8% of all cancers (all low risk); however, a cutoff score of 50 would have avoided 56.5% of repeat biopsies, missing 10.3% of tumors of which 5 were aggressive. In the initial biopsy, the PCA3 score performed poorly and was not superior to total PSA.

There is a commercial kit available for PCA3 detection, PROGENSA®, approved in Europe for the evaluation of PCA3 expression. In a prospective European study on 516 men, the positive biopsy rate was 40%; the mean PC3 score was higher in men with cancer as was the median score. A cutoff PCA3 value of 35 had a sensitivity of 64% and specificity of 76% (de la Taille et al., 2011). In a French study of 245 men, using a cutoff PCA3 score of 38, the median PCA3 score was higher in men with positive biopsies; notwithstanding the PCA3 test had a 59% sensitivity and a 72% specificity for prostate cancer detection, compared with a 66% sensitivity and 32% specificity for total PSA (threshold 4 ng/mL) and 81% sensitivity and 32% specificity for free/total PSA ratio (threshold 25%). Thus, although significantly more specific, it was less sensitive in detecting prostate cancer (Vlaeminck-Guillem et al., 2011). Finally, a South African study of men, with a positive biopsy incidence of 42.9%, reported a positive predictive value of 54% with a cutoff score of 35 and a positive predictive value of 60% with a cutoff score of 60; however, the PSA level performed better than the PCA3 score (Adam et al., 2011).

Thus, a significant drawback on the pCA3 assay is the cutoff point to decide a positive or negative test and if the use of age-specific levels should be used. In initial biopsies, it appears that total PSA is equivalent or superior to PCA3 assay. The Progensa PCA3 test for prostate cancer detection is licensed for use in repeat biopsy; the higher the score, the higher the likelihood of a positive biopsy; the score increases linearly with tumor volume and is higher in men with grade of cancer detected and is independent of prostate volume. A meta-analysis by Ruiz-Aragon (2010) concluded that the specificity was in the range 56%–89% and sensitivity 48%–82%, with a negative predictive value of >60% but a positive predictive value of <39%. The results were limited, according to the authors, by a series of factors; the type of prostate biopsy was not the same in all studies, lack of blinding, lack of explanation of patient loss, and variable cutoff score.

22.5 Comparing Sensitivity and Sensibility of the Various Biomarkers

Using the gold standard of prostate biopsy and the total PSA as the reference point, we analyze the differing sensitivities, specificities, positive, and negative predictive values of the differing tests for the detection of prostate cancer. Considering only those studies in which the test is used for the initial biopsy, the men had clinical parameters that indicated a prostate biopsy, that is, total PSA >4.0 ng/mL and/or an abnormal rectal examination. The results are shown in Table 22.4.

TABLE 22.4

Comparison of Sensitivity and Specificity of Biomarkers to Detect Prostate Cancer

	Sensitivity (%)	Specificity (%)	PPV (%)	PPN (%)
Total PSA >4.0 ng/mL	90–100	20–40		
Free PSA ratio	90–100	20–40		
ProPSA	90	44		
Serum DNA	80	82		
SNP	31–47	53		
ProTECT-CPC®	86	90.8	78.9	94.3
PCA3	59–69	47–75	39–69	60

22.6 Cost

The only cost-benefit analysis published is that of ProTECT from the Chilean group (Murray et al., 2011), whereby a cost analysis of using total PSA versus CPC detection in 228 patients has a cost saving of €30,000, including follow-up costs. No other test has analyzed the cost impact of incorporating the new biomarkers.

The CellSearch system has a cost of US$700–1000, the PCA3 Progensa has a cost of US$500, the ProTECT has a cost of US$56, total PSA has a cost of US$14, and free PSA ratio has a cost of US$14, and the other tests that are not commercially available have not been priced.

Acknowledgments

My wife, Ana Maria Palazuelos, for her help and patience in the writing of this chapter.

References

Adam A, Engelbrecht MJ, Bornman MS et al. The role of the PCA3 assay in predicting prostate biopsy outcome in a South African setting. *BJU Int* 2011; 108:1728–1733.

Alix-Panabieres C, Rebillard X, Brouillet JP et al. Detection of circulating prostate-specific antigen-secreting cells in prostate cancer patients. *Clin Chem* 2005; 51:1538–1541.

Alix-Panabieres C, Vendrell JP, Pelle O et al. Detection and characterization of putative metastatic precursor cells in cancer patients. *Clin Chem* 2007; 53:537–539.

Allen D, Butt A, Cahill D et al. Role of cell free plasma DNA as a diagnostic marker for prostate cancer. *Ann NY Acad Sci* 2004; 1022:76–80.

Altimari A, Grigioni AD, Benedettini E et al. Diagnostic role of circulating free plasma DNA detection in patients with localized prostate cancer. *Am J Clin Pathol* 2008; 129:756–762.

Andriole GL, Grubb RL, Buys SS et al. Mortality results from a randomized prostate cancer screening trial. *N Eng J Med* 2009; 360:1310–1319.

Babaian RJ, Johnston DA, Naccarato W et al. The incidence of prostate cancer in a screening population with a serum PSA between 2.5 and 4.0 ng/ml. *J Urol* 2001; 165:757–760.

Bangma CH, Wildhagen MF, Yurdakul G et al. The value of (-7, -5) pro PSA and human kallikrein-2 as serum markers for grading prostate cancer. *BJU Int* 2004; 93:720–724.

Bates RC and Mercurio AM. The epithelial-mesenchymal transition and colorectal cancer progression. *Cancer Biol Ther* 2005; 4:365–370.

Beach R, Gown AM, Peralta-Venturina MN et al. P504S immunohistochemical detection in 405 prostatic specimens including 376 18-gauge needle biopsies. *Am J Surg Pathol* 2002; 26:1588–1596.

Becker C, Piironen T, Pettersson K et al. Clinical value of human glandular kallikrein 2 and free and total prostate-specific antigen in serum from a population of men with prostate-specific antigen levels 3.0 ng/mL or greater. *Urology* 2000; 55(5):694–699.

Boddy JL, Gal S, Malone PR et al. Prospective study of quantitation of plasma DNA levels in the diagnosis of malignant versus benign prostate disease. *Clin Cancer Res* 2005; 11:1394–1399.

Bollito E, De Luca S, Cicilano M et al. PCA3 gene urine assay cutoff in diagnosis of prostate cancer: A validation study on an Italian patient population undergoing first and repeat biopsy. *Anal Quant Cytol Histol* 2012; 34:96–104.

Borgen E, Naume B, Nesland JM et al. Standardization of the immunocitochemical detection of cancer cells in bone marrow and blood: Establishment of objective criteria for the evaluation of immunostained cells. *ISHAGE Cytotherapy* 1999; 5:377–388.

Bostwick DG, Pacelli A, Blute M et al. PMSA expression in prostatic intraepithelial neoplasia and adenocarcinoma: A study of 184 cases. *Cancer* 1998; 82:2256–2261.

Burford DC, Kirby M, and Austoker J. Prostate Cancer Risk Management Programme information for Primary Care; PSA testing for a symptomatic men. 2008, NHS Cancer Screening Programmes: Sheffield, South Yorkshire, U.K.

Bussemakers MJ, van Bokhoven A, Verhaegh GW et al. DD3: A new prostate specific gene, highly over-expressed in prostate cancer. *Cancer Res* 1999; 59:5975–5979.

Cairns P. Gene methylation and early detection of genitourinary cancer: The road ahead. *Nat Rev Cancer* 2007; 7:531–543.

Cairns P, Esteller M, Herman JG et al. Molecular detection of prostate cancer in urine by *GSTP1* hypermethylation. *Clin Cancer Res* 2001; 7:2727–2730.

Cama C, Olsson CA, Raffo AJ et al. Molecular staging of prostate cancer. II A comparison of the application of an enhanced RT-PCR assay for PSA versus PSMA. *J Urol* 1995; 153:1373–1378.

Catalona WJ et al. Evaluation of percentage free serum PSA to improve specificity of prostate cancer screening. *JAMA* 1995; 274:1214–1220.

Catalona WJ, Smith DS, and Ornstein DK. Prostate cancer detection in men with serum PSA concentrations of 2.6–4.0 ng/ml and benign prostate examination: Enhancement with free PSA measurements. *JAMA* 1997; 277:1452–1455.

Chelley J, Concordet JP, Kaplan JC et al. Illegitimate transcription: Transcription of any gene in any cell type. *Proc Natl Acad Sci USA* 1989; 86:2617–2621.

Christiansen JJ and Rajasekaran AK. Reassessing epithelial to mesenchymal transition as a prerequisite for carcinoma invasion and metastasis. *Cancer Res* 2006; 66:8319–8326.

Chun FK, Muller I, Lange I et al. Circulating tumor associated plasma DNA represents an independent and informative predictor of prostate cancer. *BJU Int* 2006; 98:544–548.

Czerkinski C, Nilsson LA, Nygren H et al. A solid-phase enzyme-linked immunospot (ELISPOT) assay for enumeration of specific antibody-secreting cells. *J Immunol Methods* 1983; 65:109–121.

Darson M, Pacelli A, Roche P et al. Human glandular kallikrein 2 (hK2) expression in prostatic intraepithelial neoplasia and adenocarcinoma: A novel prostate cancer marker. *Urology* 1997; 49(6):857–862.

Davis JW, Nakanishi H, Kumar VS et al. Circulating tumor cells in peripheral blood samples from patients with increased serum prostate specific antigen: Initial results in early prostate cancer. *J Urol* 2008; 179:2187–2191.

De la Taille A, Irani J, Graefen M et al. Clinical evaluation of the PCA3 assay in guiding initial biopsy decisions. *J Urol* 2011; 185:2119–2125.

Djava B, Remzi M, Zlotta A et al. Complexed PSA, complexed PSA density of total and transition zone, complexed/total PSA ratio, free to total PSA ratio, density of total and transition zone PSA: Results of the prospective multicenter European trial. *Urology* 2002; 60:4–9.

Ducasse M and Brown MA. Epigenetic aberrations and cancer. *Mol Cancer* 2006; 5:60.

Dumas F, Eschwege P, and Loric S. Acute bacterial prostatitis induces hematogenous dissemination of prostate epithelial cells. *Clin Chem* 1997; 43:2007–2008.

Ellinger J, Haan K, Heukamp LC et al. CpG island hypermethylation in cell-free serum DNA identifies patients with localized prostate cancer. *Prostate* 2008; 68:42–49.

Fair WR, Israeli RS, and Heston WD. PSMA. *Prostate* 1997; 32:140–148.

Fava TA, Desnoyers R, Schulz S et al. Ectopic expression of guanylyl cyclase C in CD34 progenitor cells in peripheral blood. *J Clin Oncol* 2001; 19:3951–3959.

Ferlay J, Shin HR, Bray F et al. GLOBOCAN 2008 v1.2. Cancer incidence and mortality worldwide: IARC Cancerbase Nl 10, International Agency for Research on Cancer 2010: Lyon, France. www.globocan.iarc.fr

Fizazi K, Morat L, Chauveinc L et al. High detection rate of circulating tumor cells in blood of patients with prostate cancer using telomerase activity. *Ann Oncol* 2007; 18:518–521.

Frankel, S et al. Screening for prostate cancer. *Lancet* 2003; 361(9363):1122–1128.

Gala JL, Heusterspreute M, Loric S et al. Expression of PSA and PSMA transcripts in blood cells: Implications for the detection of hematogenous prostate cells and standardization. *Clin Chem* 1998; 44:472–481.

Gann PH, Hennekens CH, and Stampfer MJ. A prospective evaluation of plasma PSA for detection of prostate cancer. *JAMA* 1995; 273:289–294.

Gelmini S, Tricarico C, Vona G et al. Real-time quantitative reverse transcriptase-polymerase chain reaction (RT-PCR) for the measurement of prostate-specific antigen mRNA in the peripheral blood of patients with prostate carcinoma using the TaqMan™ detection system. *Clin Chem Lab Med* 2001; 39:385–391.

Ghossein RA and Bhattacharya S. Molecular detection and characterisation of circulating tumor cells and micrometastasis in solid tumors. *Eur J Cancer* 2000; 36:1681–1694.

Giovannucci E, Stampfer MJ, Krithvas K et al. The CAG repeat within the androgen receptor gene and its relationship to prostate cancer. *Proc Natl Acad Sci USA* 1997; 94:3320–3323.

Goessl C, Müller M, Heicappell R et al. DNA-based detection of prostate cancer in blood, urine, and ejaculates. *Ann N Y Acad Sci* 2001; 945:51–58.

Gsur A, Bemhofer G, Hinterregger S et al. A polymorphism in the CYP17 gene is associated with prostate cancer risk. *Int J Cancer* 2000; 87:434–437.

Haese A, Graefen M, Steuber T et al. Human glandular kallikrein 2 levels in serum for discrimination of pathologically organ-confined from locally-advanced prostate cancer in total PSA levels below 10 ng/ml. *Prostate* 2001; 49(2):101–109.

Han M, Potter SR, and Partin AW. The role of free PSA in prostate cancer detection. *Curr Urol Rep* 2000; 1:78–82.

Hanahan D and Weinberg RA. The hallmarks of cancer. *Cell* 2000; 100:57–70.

Hara N, Kasahara T, Kawasaki T et al. Frequency of PSA mRNA bearing cells in the peripheral blood of patients after prostate biopsy. *Br J Cancer* 2001; 85:557–562.

Hara N, Kasahara T, Kawasaki T et al. RT-PCR detection of PSA, PMSA and PSCA in 1 ml of peripheral blood: Value for the staging of prostate cancer. *Clin Cancer Res* 2002; 8:1794–1799.

Harden SV, Sanderson H, Goodman SN et al. Quantitative GSTP1 methylation and the detection of prostate adenocarcinoma in sextant biopsies. *J Natl Cancer Inst* 2003; 95:1634–1637.

Henke W, Jung M, Jung K et al. Increased analytical sensitivity of RT-PCR of PSA mRNA decreases diagnostic specificity of detection of prostatic cells in blood. *Int J Cancer* 1997; 70:52–56.

Henrique R and Jerónimo C. Molecular detection of prostate cancer: A role for GSTP1 hypermethylation. *Eur Urol* 2004; 46:660–669.

Herrala A, Kurkela R, Porvari K et al. human prostate specific glandular kallikrein is expressed as an active and an inactive protein. *Clin Chem* 1997; 43:279–284.

Holdenrieder S, Stieber P, Bodenmüller H et al. Nucleosomes in serum of patients with benign and malignant diseases. *Int J Cancer* 2001; 95:114–120.

Hoque MO. DNA methylation changes in prostate cancer: Current developments and future clinical implementation. *Expert Rev Mol Diagn* 2009; 9:243–257.

Ingles SA, Ross RK, Yu MC et al. Association of prostate cancer risk with genetic polymorphisms in vitamin D receptor and androgen receptor. *J Natl Cancer Inst* 1997; 89:166–170.

Jahr S, Hentze H, Englisch S et al. DNA fragments in blood plasma of cancer patients: Quantitations and evidence for their origin from apoptotic and necrotic cells. *Cancer Res* 2001; 61:1659–1665.

Jansen FH, van Schaik RH, Kurstjens J et al. PSA isoform (-2)proPSA in combination with total PSA and free PSA improves diagnostic accuracy in prostate cancer detection. *Eur Urol* 2010; 57:921–927.

Jerónimo C, Henrique R, Hoque MO et al. A quantitative promoter methylation profile of prostate cancer. *Clin Cancer Res* 2004; 10:8472–8478.

Jerónimo C, Usadel H, Henrique R et al. Quantitation of *GSTP1* methylation in non-neoplastic prostatic tissue and organ-confined prostate adenocarcinoma. *J Natl Cancer Inst* 2001; 93:1747–1752.

Jones PA and Baylin SB. The fundamental role of epigenetic events in cancer. *Nat Rev Genet* 2002; 3:415–428.

Joseph DA, Thompson T, Saraiya M, and Werny DM. Association between GFR, free, total and percent free PSA. *Urology* 2010; 76:1042–1046.

Jung K, Stephan C, Lewandowski M et al. Increased cell free DNA in plasma of patients with metastatic spread in prostate cancer. *Cancer Lett* 2004; 205:173–180.

Katz AE, Olsson CA, Raffo AJ et al. Molecular staging of prostate cancer with the use of an enhanced RT-PCR assay. *Urology* 1994; 43:765–775.

Khan MA, Partin AW, Rittenhouse HG et al. Evaluation of proPSA for early detection of prostate cancer in men with total PSA range of 4.0–10.0 ng/ml. *J Urol* 2003; 170:723–726.

Khan MA, Sokoll LJ, Chan DW et al. Clinical utility of proPSA and "benign" PSA when percent free PSA is less than 15%. *Urology* 2004; 64:1160–1164.

Klatte T, Waldert M, de Martino M et al. Age specific PCA3 score reference values for diagnosis of prostate cancer. *World J Urol* 2012; 30:405–410.

Kobayashi M, Kurokawa S, and Tokue A. Intraindividual variation in total and percent free PSA in prostate cancer suspects. *Urol Int* 2005; 74:198–202.

Kurek R, Nunez G, Tselis N et al. Prognostic value of combined "triple"-reverse transcription-PCR analysis for *prostate-specific antigen, human kallikrein 2,* and *prostate-specific membrane antigen* mRNA in peripheral blood and lymph nodes of prostate cancer patients. *Clin Cancer Res* 2004; 10(17):5808–5814.

Lang SH, Hyde C, Reid IN et al. Enhanced expression of vimentin in motile prostate cell lines and in poorly differentiated and metastatic prostate carcinoma. *Prostate* 2002; 52:253–263.

Lembessis P, Msaouel P, Halpas A et al. Combined androgen blockade therapy can convert RT-PCR detection of PSA and PSMA transcripts from positive to negative in the peripheral blood of patients with clinically localized prostate cancer and increase biochemical failure free survival after curative therapy. *Clin Chem Lab Med* 2007; 45:1488–1494.

Leon SA, Shapiro B, Skiaroff DM et al. Free DNA in the serum of cancer patients and the effect of therapy. *Cancer Res* 1977; 37:646–650.

Llanes L, Ferruelo A, Pérez A et al. The clinical utility of PSMA RT-PCR to detect circulating prostate cells: An analysis in healthy men and women. *BJU Int* 2002; 89:882–885.

Lopez-Guerrero JA, Bolufer-Gilabert P, Sanz-Alonso MB et al. Minimal illegitimate levels of cytokeratin K19 expression in mononucleated blood cells detected by a reverse transcription PCR method (RT-PCR). *Clin Chim Acta* 1997; 263:105–116.

Loric S, Dumas F, Eschwege P et al. Enhanced detection of hematogenous circulating prostate cells in patients with prostate adenocarcinoma by using nested RT-PCR assay based on PMSA. *Clin Chem* 1995; 41:1698–1704.

Luderer AA et al. Measurement of the proportion of free to total PSA improves diagnostic performance of PSA. *Urology* 1995; 146:187–194.

Lund AH and van Lohuizen M. Epigenetics and cancer. *Genes Develop* 2004; 18:2315–2335.

Lundwall A and Lilja H. Molecular cloning of human prostate specific antigen cDNA. *FEBS Lett* 1987; 214:317–322.

Magklara A, Scorilas A, Catalona W, and Diamandis E. The combination of human glandular kallikrein and free prostate specific antigen (PSA) enhances discrimination between prostate cancer and benign prostatic hyperplasia in patients with moderately increased total PSA. *Clin Chem* 1999; 45(11):1960–1966.

Marks LS, Fradet Y, Deras IL et al. PCA3 molecular urine assay for prostate cancer in men undergoing repeat biopsy. *J Urol* 2007; 69:532–535.

Meiers I, Shanks JH, and Bostwick DG. Glutathione S-transferase pi (*GSTP1*) hypermethylation in prostate cancer: Review. *Pathology* 2007; 39:299–304.

Mikolajczyk SD, Grauer LS, Millar LS et al. A precursor form of PSA (pPSA) is a component of the free PSA in prostate cancer serum. *Urology* 1997; 50:710–714.

Mikolajczyk SD, Marker KM, Miller LS, Kumar A, Saedi MS, Paune JK et al. A truncated precursor form of PSA is a more specific serum marker for prostate cancer. *Cancer Res* 2001; 61:6958–6963.

Mikolajczyk SD, Millar LS, Marker KM et al. Seminal plasma contains "BPSA," a molecular form of prostate-specific antigen that is associated with benign prostatic hyperplasia. *Prostate* 2000a; 45:271–276.

Mikolajczyk SD, Millar LS, Wang TJ et al. "BPSA," a specific molecular form of free prostate-specific antigen, is found predominantly in the transition zone of patients with nodular benign prostatic hyperplasia. *Urology* 2000b; 55:41–45.

Mikolajczyk SD, Millar LS, Wang TJ et al. A precursor form of prostate-specific antigen is more highly elevated in prostate cancer compared with benign transition zone prostate tissue. *Cancer Res* 2000c; 60:756–759.

Miller MC, Doyle GV, and Terstappen LW. Significance of circulating tumor cells detected by the cell search system in patients with metastatic breast colorectal and prostate cancer. *J Oncol* 2010; 2010:61742 Epub 2009.

Moreno JG, Croce CM, Fischer R et al. Detection of hematogenous micrometastasis in patients with prostate cancer. *Cancer Res* 1992; 52:6110–6112.

Murray NP, Calaf GM, Badinez L et al. P504S expressing circulating prostate cells as a marker for prostate cancer. *Oncol Rep* 2010; 24:687–692.

Murray NP, Reyes E, Orellana N, and Tapia P. Cost-benefit analysis of the use of circulating prostate cell detection in prostate cancer screening. *Arch Esp Urol* 2013; 66:277–286.

Murray NP, Reyes E, Tapia P, Orellana N, Duenas R, Fuentealba C et al. Diagnostic yield of the detection of circulating prostate cells from the detection of prostate cáncer: A comparison with results of the prostate biopsy. *Arch Esp Urol* 2011; 64:953–963.

Nadler RB, Humphrey PA, Smith DS et al. Effect of inflammation and benign prostatic hyperplasia on elevated serum PSA levels. *J Urol* 1995; 154:407–413.

Nakayama M, Bennett CJ, Hicks JL et al. Hypermethylation of the human glutathione S-transferase- pi gene (*GSTP1*) CpG island is present in a subset of proliferative inflammatory atrophy lesions but not in normal or hyperplastic epithelium of the prostate: a detailed study using laser-capture microdissection. *Am J Pathol* 2003; 163:923–933.

Nam RK, Toi, A, Vesprini D et al. V89L polymorphism of type-2 5-alpha reductase enzyme gene predicts prostate cancer presence and progression. *Urology* 2001; 57:199–204.

Nam RK, Zhang WW, Trachtenberg J et al. SNP of the human kallikrein-2 gene highly correlates with serum human kallikrein-2 levels and in combination enhances prostate cancer detection. *J Clin Oncol* 2003; 21:2312–2319.

National Cancer Institute, SEER data base 2004–2008, Bethseda, MD.

National Cancer Institute Surveillance Epidemiology and End Results Program. Cancer Stat Fact Sheets-Cancer of Prostate 2006. Accessed at www.seer.cancer.gov/statfacts/html/prost.html

Nyberg M, Ulmert D, Lindgren A et al. PCA3 as a diagnostic marker for prostate cancer: A validation study on a Swedish patient population. *Scand J Urol Nephrol* 2010; 44:378–383.

Office for National Statistics. Cancer Statistics registrations: Registrations of cancer diagnosed in 2008, England. Series MB1 No.39 2010. London, U.K.: National Statistics.

Panteleakou Z, Lembessis P, Sourla A et al. Detection of circulating tumor cells in prostate cancer patients: Methodological pitfalls and clinical relevance. *Mol Med* 2009; 15:101–114.

Partin AW et al. Analysis of percent free PSA for prostate cancer detection: Influence of total PSA, prostate volume and age. *Urology* 1996; 48:55–61.

Partin AW, Brawer MK, Subong ENP et al. Prospective evaluation of percent free PSA and complexed PSA for early detection of prostate cancer. *Prostate Cancer P D*1998; 1:197–203.

Partin AW, Catalona W, Finlay J et al. Use of human glandular kallikrein 2 for the detection of prostate cancer: Preliminary analysis. *Urology* 1999; 54(5):839–845.

Patel K, Whelan PJ, Prescott S, Brownhill SC, Johnston CF, Selby PJ et al. The use of real time RT-PCR for PSA mRNA to discriminate between healthy volunteers and from patients with metastatic prostate cancer. *Clin Cancer Res* 2004; 10:7511–7519.

Paterlini-Brechot P and Benali NL. Circulating tumor cells detection: Clinical impact and future directions. *Cancer Lett* 2007; 2:180–204.

Raimondi C, Gradilone A, Naso G et al. Epithelial-mesenchymal transition and stemness features in circulating tumor cells from breast cancer patients. *Breast Cancer Res Treat* Feb 5, 2011; 130:449–455.

Rebbeck TR, Jaffe JM, Walker AH et al. Modification of clinical presentation of prostate tumors by a novel genetic variant in CYP3A4. *J Natl Cancer Inst* 1998; 90:1225–1229.

Recker F, Kwiatkowski M, Piironen T et al. Human glandular kallikrein as a tool to improve discrimination of poorly differentiated and non-organ-confined prostate cancer compared with prostate-specific antigen. *Urology* 2000; 55(4):481–485.

Reiter RE, Gu Z, Watabe T et al. PSCA: A cell surface marker over-expressed in prostate cancer. *Proc Natl Acad Sci USA* 1998; 95:1735–1740.

Ries LAG. *SEER Cancer Statistics Review* 1975–2002. 2005 NCI: Bethesda, MD.

Rietbergen JB, Kruger AE, Kranse R, and Schroder F. Complications of transrectal ultrasound guided systematic sextant biopsies of the prostate: Evaluation of complication rates and risk factors within a population based screening program. *Urology* 1997; 49:875–880.

Roobol MJ, Schroader FH, van Leeuwen P et al. Performance of the pCA3 gene and PSA in prescreened men: Exploring the value of PCA3 for a first line diagnostic test. *Eur Urol* 2010; 58:475–481.

Rubin MA, Zhou M, and Dhanasekaran SM. Alpha-methylacyl coenzyme A racemase as a tissue biomarker for prostate cancer. *JAMA* 2002; 287:1662–1670.

Ruiz-Aragón J and Márquez-Peláez S. Assessment of the PCA3 test for prostate cancer diagnosis: A systemic review and meta-analysis. *Actas Urológicas Esapañolas* 2010; 34:346–355.

Sakr WA et al. Age and racial distribution of prostatic intraepithelial neoplasia. *Eur Urol* 1996; 30(2):138–144.

Schroder FH, Hugosson J, Roobol MJ et al. Screening and prostate cancer mortality in a randomized European study. *N Eng J Med* 2009; 360:1320–1328.

Schulz WA and Hoffmann MJ. Epigenetic mechanisms in the biology of prostate cancer. *Semin Cancer Biol* 2009; 19:172–180.

Schwarzenbach H, Chun FK, Lange I et al. Detection of tumor-specific DNA in blood and bone marrow plasma from patients with prostate cancer. *Int J Cancer* 2007; 120:1465–1471.

Selley S et al. Diagnosis, management and screening of early localized prostate cancer. *Health Technol Assess* 1997; 1(2):1–96.

Shelton BP, Misso NL, Shaw OM et al. Epigenetic regulation of human epithelial cell cancers. *Curr Opin Mol Ther* 2008; 10:568–578.

Sidransky D. Nucleic acid-based methods for the detection of cancer. *Science* 1997; 278:1054–1058.

Smith MR, Biggar S, and Hussain M. PSA mRNA is expressed in non-prostate cells: Implications for the detection of micrometastasis. *Cancer Res* 1995; 55:2640–2644.

Sokoll LJ, Sanda MG, Eng Z et al. A prospective multicentre, National Cancer Institute early detection research network study of (-2) proPSA: Improving prostate cancer detection and correlating with cancer aggressiveness. *Cancer Epidemiol Biomark Prev* 2010; 19:1192–1200.

Sokoloff MH, Tso CL, Kaboo R et al. Quantitative PCR does not improve preoperative prostate cancer staging: A clinicopathological molecular analysis of 121 patients. *J Urol* 1996; 156:1560–1566.

Stenman VH et al. A complex between PSA and alpha-1-antichymotrypsin is the major form of pSA in serum of patients with prostate cancer. Assay of the complex improves clinical sensitivity for cancer. *Cancer Res* 1991; 51:222.

Stephan C, Kahrs AM, Cammann H et al. (-2) proPSA based artificial neural network significantly improves differentiation between prostate cancer and benign prostatic diseases. *Prostate* 2009; 69:198–207.

Stephan C, Lein M, Jung K et al. The influence of prostate volume on the ratio of free to total PSA in serum of patients with prostate carcinoma and benign prostate hyperplasia. *Cancer* 2000; 79:104–109.

Stott SL, Lee RJ, Nagrath S et al. Isolation and characterization of circulating tumor cell from patients with localized and metastatic prostate cancer. *Sci Transl Med* 2010; 25:25.

Strathdee G and Brown R. Aberrant DNA methylation in cancer: Potential clinical interventions. *Expert Rev Mol Med* 2002; 4:1–17.

Straub B, Muller M, Krause H et al. Detection of prostate-specific antigen RNA before and after radical retropubic prostatectomy and transurethral resection of the prostate using 'Light-cycler'-based quantitative real-time polymerase chain reaction. *Urology* 2001; 58:815–820.

Taback B and Hoon DSB. Circulating nucleic acids and proteomics of plasma/serum: Clinical utility. *Ann N Y Acad Sci* 2004; 1022:1–8.

Takayama TK, Fujikawa K, and Davie EW. Characterization of the precursor of prostate-specific antigen. Activation by trypsin and by human glandular kallikrein. *J Biol Chem* 1997; 272:21582–21588.

Takayama TK, McMullen BA, Nelson PS et al. Characterization of prostate specific antigen (proPSA) and single-chain urokinase-type plasminogen activator and degradation of prostatic acid phosphatase. *Biochemistry* 2001; 40:15341–15348.

Thiounn N, Saporta F, Flam TA et al. Positive PSA circulating cells detected by RT-PCR does not imply the presence of micrometastasis. *Urology* 1997; 50:245–250.

Thompson EW, Newgreen DF, and Tarin D. Carcinoma invasion and metastasis: A role for epithelial mesenchymal transition? *Cancer Res* 2005; 65:5991–5995.

Tokumaru Y, Harden SV, Sun DI et al. Optimal use of a panel of methylation markers with *GSTP1* hypermethylation in the diagnosis of prostate adenocarcinoma. *Clin Cancer Res* 2004; 10:5518–5522.

Vener T, Derecho C, Baden J et al. Development of a multiplexed urine assay for prostate cancer diagnosis. *Clin Chem* 2008; 54:874–882.

Verhaegh GW, van Bokhoven A, Smit F et al. Isolation and characterization of the promoter of the human cancer specific DD3 gene. *J Biol Chem* 2000; 275:37496–37503.

Vickers A, Cronin A, Roobol M et al. Reducing unnecessary biopsy during prostate cancer screening using a four-kallikrein panel: An independent replication. *J Clin Oncol* 2010; 15:2493–2498.

Vlaeminck-Guillem V, Campos-Fernandez JL, Champetier D et al. Value of PCA3 urinary test for prostate biopsy decision: The Lyon-Sud University Hospital experience. *Ann Biol Clin (Paris)* 2011; 69:31–39.

Weber M, Hellmann I, Stadler MB et al. Distribution, silencing potential and evolutionary impact of promoter DNA methylation in the human genome. *Nat Genet* 2007; 39:457–466.

Went PT, Lugli A, Meier S et al. Frequent EpCam protein expression in human carcinomas. *Hum Pathol* 2004; 1:122–128.

Willipinski-Stapelfeldt B, Riethdorf S et al. Changes in cytoskeletal protein composition indicative of an epithelial-mesenchymal transition in human micrometastatic and primary breast carcinoma cells. *Clin Cancer Res* 2005; 11:8006–8014.

Wu TL, Zhang D, Chia Jl et al. Cell free DNA measurement in various carcinomas and establishment of normal reference ranges. *Clin Chim Acta* 2002; 321:77–87.

Xue X, Teare MD, Holen I et al. Optimizing the yield and utility of circulating cell free DNA from plasma and serum. *Clin Chim Acta* 2009; 404:100–104.

Yang J, Mani SA, and Weinberg R. Exploring a new twist on tumor metastasis. *Cancer Res* 2006; 66:4549–4552.

Yegnasubramanian S, Haffner MC, Zhang Y et al. DNA hypomethylation arises later in prostate cancer progression than CpG island hypermethylation and contributes to metastatic tumor heterogeneity. *Cancer Res* 2008; 68:8954–8967.

Yousef G and Diamandis E. The new human tissue kallikrein gene family: Structure, function, and association to disease. *Endocr Rev* 2001; 22(2):184–204.

Zhang P, Wang ZM, Zhong T, and Zhao LH. Analysis of the results of percent free PSA detection among men without prostate diseases in Xi'an. *Nan Fang Yi Ke Da Xue Xue Bao* 2008; 28:269–271.

Zieglschmid V, Hollmann C, and Bicher O. Detection of disseminated tumor cells in peripheral blood. *Crit Rev Clin Lab Sci* 2005; 42:155–196.

Zhou M, Chinnaiyan AM, Lleer CG et al. Alpha-methylacyl-CoA racemase: A novel tumor marker over-expressed in several human cancers and their precursor lesions. *Am J Surg Pathol* 2002; 26:926–931.

Part VI

Gynecological and Endocrine Cancers

23

Early Biomarkers in Breast Cancer

Ruchika Kaul-Ghanekar, Snehal Suryavanshi, and Prerna Raina

CONTENTS

ABSTRACT Breast cancer is one of the leading causes of cancer deaths in women worldwide. However, over the last few decades, there has been a steady decline in mortality rates due to increasingly effective adjuvant medical treatments. Mammography screening programs have increased the diagnosis of early-stage breast cancer with better prognosis. Moreover, the discovery of specific prognostic and predictive biomarkers in the past few years has enormously helped in the early detection and treatment of breast cancer. With the advent of high-throughput technologies, more and more biomarkers based on either genomics or proteomics are being explored for early detection as well as better prognosis of the breast cancer. This chapter focuses on the traditional as well as novel biomarkers that are being used or proposed to use for early prognosis, diagnosis, as well as treatment of the breast cancer to reduce morbidity as well as mortality.

KEY WORDS: *breast cancer, diagnosis, invasive and noninvasive biomarkers, prognosis, therapy*

Outline

Breast cancer is the most commonly diagnosed cancer and the leading cause of death in women worldwide (National NCI program database; Patnaik et al., 2011). It accounts for about 23% (1.38 million) of the total cancer cases and 14% (458,400) of the total cancer-related deaths (Jemal et al., 2011). The incidence rates are higher in Western and Northern Europe, Australia/New Zealand, and North America; moderate in South America, the Caribbean, and Northern Africa; and lower in sub-Saharan Africa and Asia (Jemal et al., 2011). However, 60% of the breast cancer-related deaths have been found to occur in economically developing countries.

Breast cancer is a clinically heterogeneous disease with multifactorial etiology (Jensen et al., 2008). Age, hormonal, genetic and environmental factors, molecular oncogenic aberrations in DNA repair, cell cycle control, and cell survival are some of the factors that may contribute towards the development of the breast cancer (Perou et al., 2000; King et al., 2003; Nguyen et al., 2008; Boyd et al., 2011). Increased lifetime exposure to endogenous or exogenous hormones has been recognized as one of the major risk factors in the development of the disease (Kurian et al., 2009; Crooke et al., 2011). Besides these, socioeconomic status (SES) has also been found to determine the risk of breast cancer. Unlike other cancers, the risk of breast cancer development has been shown to be positively associated with the higher SES (Heck et al., 1997; Robert et al., 2004; Inumaru et al., 2012). The socioeconomic factors that affect the breast cancer risk include reproductive, lifestyle, and behavioral factors that involve age, parity, age at first childbirth, body mass index (BMI), alcohol consumption, age at menarche, and hormonal imbalance (Adami et al., 2002; Braaten et al., 2004; Butt et al., 2012).

Breast cancer has been categorized into various major classes by different research groups based on molecular characterization such as gene expression profiling or immunohistochemical characteristics (Cakir et al., 2012). Some studies divide the breast cancer into five major classes such as normal breast-like, luminal A, luminal B, basal-like, and human epidermal growth factor receptor 2 (HER2) positive (Perou et al., 2000; Sørlie et al., 2001). Other studies categorize it into three major classes such as HER2+/ER+, ER−/HER2−, and HER2+ breast cancers based on ER/PR and Her2 expression (Onitilo et al., 2009). Such type of heterogeneity in breast cancer subtypes poses a great challenge in the early detection of the disease, thereby inviting attention towards identification of more biomarkers that are differentially expressed during carcinogenesis. Even though routine mammography screening programs have led to an increase in early diagnosis of the breast cancer (Sakorafas et al., 2008; Wiechmann et al., 2008), but due to its suboptimal accuracy, discovery of more specific diagnostic markers is needed.

Biomarkers are powerful tools that would help in identification of high-risk subjects and timely regulation of the cancer (Weigel et al., 2010). The discovery of biomarkers has increased the early diagnosis, prognosis, and therapeutics of breast cancer (Sotiriou et al., 2003). This chapter focuses on traditional and new biomarkers that are being used or have potential to be used for early detection of breast cancer that would help in the management of the disease.

23.1 Introduction

23.1.1 Why Is It Important?

Breast cancer, reported to date back to 3000 BC, is the most threatening socioeconomic burden in the world that affects not only the patients but also their families (Donegan et al., 1995; Ferlay et al., 2010). Despite advanced diagnosis and therapeutics, management of breast cancer is a major clinical challenge due to its heterogeneity, complexity, and aggressiveness (Harnett et al., 2009). The treatment strategies available are linked with enormous side effects (Shapiro et al., 2001). Besides this, inadequate access to the screening programs, social and cultural barriers, lack of awareness, financial problems, and certain taboos are some of the important barriers in the prognosis and diagnosis of the disease, particularly in developing and underdeveloped nations (Parsa et al., 2006). Contrarily, in the developed countries, such problems are rare because of the high SES as well as awareness of the advanced health-care system that includes screening and treatment modalities (Jemal et al., 2010). However, the limitations associated with the diagnosis and imaging of breast cancer have focused the global attention towards the use of biomarkers that would help in early diagnosis of the disease, thereby leading to timely intervention strategies (Bhatt et al., 2010).

23.1.2 Epidemiology

Despite the availability of advanced diagnostics and therapeutic interventions, breast cancer remains a leading cause of cancer death worldwide in the women aged between 35 and 55 years (American Cancer

Society, 2012). Table 23.1 elucidates the incidence and mortality of breast cancer, depicting a wide geographical distribution all over the world. Breast cancer is most frequent among women in both the developed and the developing regions with almost similar incidence rates; however, the mortality rates vary between 189.5×10^3 and 269×10^3 in more developed and underdeveloped regions, respectively (GLOBOCAN, 2008). The rate of occurrence is on the rise in urban areas compared to the rural ones with widespread incidence in the women of higher SES (Hausauer et al., 2009). According to the recent reports, the mortality rate in females has been estimated to be around 130,000/year (Tyczynski et al., 2002). The chance that breast cancer would be responsible for a woman's death has been reported to be around 1 in 35 (about 3%) wherein the incidence of developing invasive breast cancer is approximately 1 in 9 (American Cancer Society, 2012). In the recent years, substantial progress has been made in understanding the genetics and molecular biology of the disease (Eroles et al., 2012). Various factors such as environmental, hormonal, dietary, lifestyle and genetic factors, radiation, as well as age, race, ethnicity, gender, and family history are considered to be involved in the development of the disease (Figure 23.1) (MacMahon et al., 2006).

All these factors may disturb the cellular signaling pathways resulting into altered molecular mechanisms leading to carcinogenesis (Nguyen et al., 2008; Marotta et al., 2011). Exposure to radiations and mutagenic agents (Ronckers et al., 2005), use of oral contraceptives, postmenopausal hormone therapy (PHT), hormone replacement therapy (HRT), and menopausal hormone therapy (MHT) are some of the reasons that may be responsible for the rise in breast cancer incidence rates (Norman et al., 2003). Alcohol consumption and cigarette smoking are some other life style factors that may also increase the

TABLE 23.1

World Key Statistics of Breast Cancer

	Incidence			Mortality		
Regions	**Cases (1000)**	**ASR[a] per (100,000)**	**Cum. Risk[a] (%) (Age 0–74)**	**Cases (1000)**	**ASR[a] per (100,000)**	**Cum. Risk[a] (%) (Age 0–74)**
World	1383.5	39	4.1	458.4	12.5	1.3
More developed regions	692.2	66.4	7.1	189.5	15.3	1.7
Less developed regions	691.3	27.3	2.8	269	10.8	1.2
Eastern Africa	17.9	19.3	2.1	10	11.4	1.3
Middle Africa	8.3	21.3	2.1	4.7	13.1	1.4
Northern Africa	28	32.7	3.2	14.6	17.8	1.8
Southern Africa	9	38.1	4.2	4.5	19.3	2.1
Western Africa	29.4	31.8	3.4	16.3	19	2.1
Caribbean	9	39.1	4.3	3.4	14.2	1.6
Central America	17.5	26	2.8	6.5	9.6	1
South America	88.4	44.3	4.8	27.1	13.2	1.4
Northern America	205.5	76.7	8.4	45.6	14.8	1.6
Eastern Asia	240.3	25.3	2.6	61.7	6.3	0.7
Southeastern Asia	87	31	3.2	36.8	13.4	1.4
South Central Asia	173	24	2.5	82.6	12	1.3
Western Asia	28.5	32.5	3.4	12.3	14.3	1.5
Central and Eastern Europe	114.6	45.3	5	47.5	17	1.9
Northern Europe	69.5	84	9	18.3	17.8	1.9
Southern Europe	91.3	69	7.4	25.6	15.3	1.7
Western Europe	149.4	90	9.6	37.3	17.5	1.9
Australia/New Zealand	16.1	85.5	9.4	3.4	15.4	1.7
Melanesia	0.6	22.8	2.4	0.3	13.2	1.4
Micronesia/Polynesia	0.3	58	6.1	0.1	13.2	1.5
India	115	22.9	—	53	11.1	—

Source: The data have been gathered from GLOBOCAN 2008.

[a] ASR, age-standardized rates; Cum. Risk, cumulative risk.

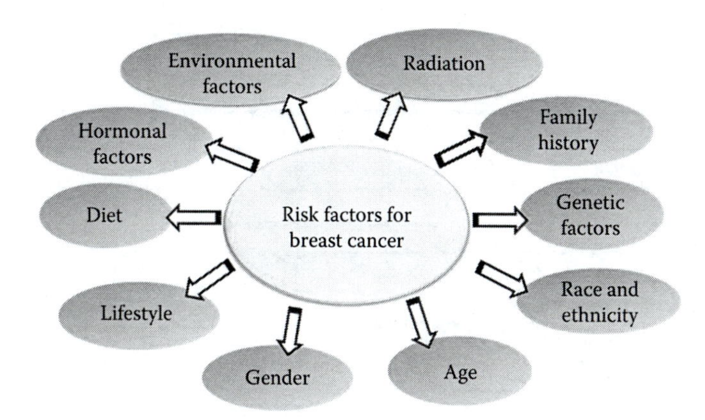

FIGURE 23.1 Risk factors for breast cancer development: several factors are involved in breast cancer development that include environmental, hormonal, dietary, lifestyle, and genetic factors, exposure to the ionizing radiation, as well as age, race, ethnicity, gender, and family history.

cancer risk (Chen et al., 2011). Obesity is also considered to be one of the main risk factors and is positively associated with postmenopausal women (Sinicrope et al., 2011) as it may raise the estrogen levels. Besides the previously mentioned factors, around 5%–10% of breast cancer cases have been attributed to genetic mutations (Stoppa-Lyonnet et al., 2009). For example, inherited mutations in BRCA1 and BRCA2 genes are the most common hereditary cause of breast cancer (Pijpe et al., 2012). Older age has also been linked to the cancer development wherein 1 out of 8 invasive breast cancers are found in women younger than 45, while about 2 out of 3 invasive breast cancers are found in women around 55 years of age or older (Harrison et al., 2010). Breast cancer has been reported to be common in American-African women than in Asian, Hispanic, and Native American women (Chen et al., 2011). Incidences are more prevalent in women than men; women having a family history are at a greater risk (Metcalfe et al., 2010).

23.1.3 Types of Breast Cancer

Breast cancer may be invasive or noninvasive depending upon the type and the stage of the disease (Souzaki et al., 2011) (Figure 23.2). It has been divided into ductal carcinoma in situ (DCIS), invasive ductal carcinoma (IDC), noninvasive lobular carcinoma (lobular carcinoma in situ [LCIS]), and invasive lobular carcinoma (ILC) (Hanby et al., 2008; Muggerud et al., 2010) (Figure 23.3). DCIS, representing around 1 in 5 cases, is the noninvasive type wherein the cancer cells are present inside the ducts and do not invade the surrounding breast tissue (Suryadevara et al., 2010). IDC starts in the milk duct of the breast wherein the cancer cells break all the way through the wall of the duct into the fatty tissue of the breast followed by metastasis to other parts of the body. These represent around 8 out of 10 cancer cases and are further divided into various subtypes such as adenocystic, adenosquamous, medullary, mucinous, papillary, micropapillary, tubular, and metaplastic carcinoma (Suryadevara et al., 2010; Kapp et al., 2006). LCIS is generally not regarded as a true cancer wherein the cells remain confined to the lobules (Foster et al., 2004). ILC represents around 1 out of 10 invasive cases and starts in the milk-producing glands (lobules) wherein the cancer cells undergo metastasis (Suryadevara et al., 2010).

Besides the earlier, there are additional types that include inflammatory breast cancer (IBC), phyllodes tumor, angiosarcoma, Paget's disease of the nipple, and triple-negative breast cancer (Dalberg et al., 2007; Glazebrook et al., 2008; Yang et al., 2009). IBC is the invasive form wherein the breast looks red and its skin becomes thick and pitted. Phyllodes tumor develops in the stroma of the breast and is usually benign that may become malignant only in rare cases (Kapali et al., 2010). Angiosarcoma, rarely found in the breast, usually occurs in cells that line the blood or lymph vessels (Desbiens et al., 2011; Heiko, 2000). It can also be found in the patients with lymphedema that may be caused due to lymph node surgery or radiation therapy (Tahir et al., 2006). These cancers have the tendency to grow and metastasize rapidly. Paget's disease is the rarest form that arises from the breast ducts, affecting the skin of the nipple and areola showing crusted, scaly, and reddish appearance with areas of bleeding or oozing (Dalberg et al., 2008). In triple-negative

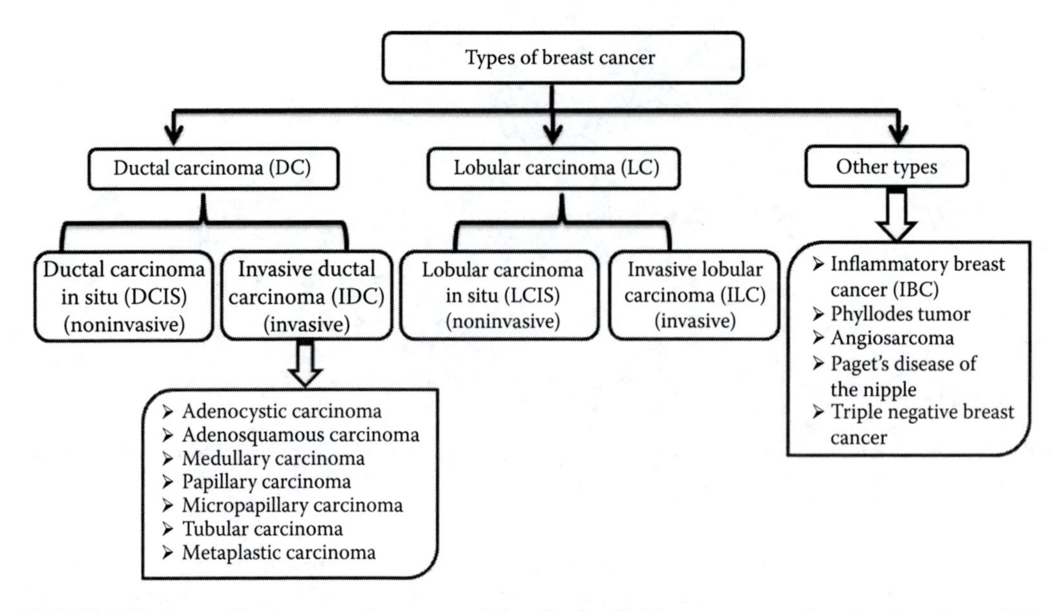

FIGURE 23.2 Types of breast cancer. Breast cancer is broadly classified into two types such as ductal carcinoma (DC) and lobular carcinoma (LC). DC is divided into DCIS (noninvasive) and IDC, the latter being divided into adenocystic, adenosquamous, medullary, mucinous, papillary, micropapillary, tubular, and metaplastic carcinoma. LC is further grouped into noninvasive or LCIS and ILC. However, there are some other types that include IBC, phyllodes tumor, angiosarcoma, Paget's disease of the nipple, and triple-negative breast cancer.

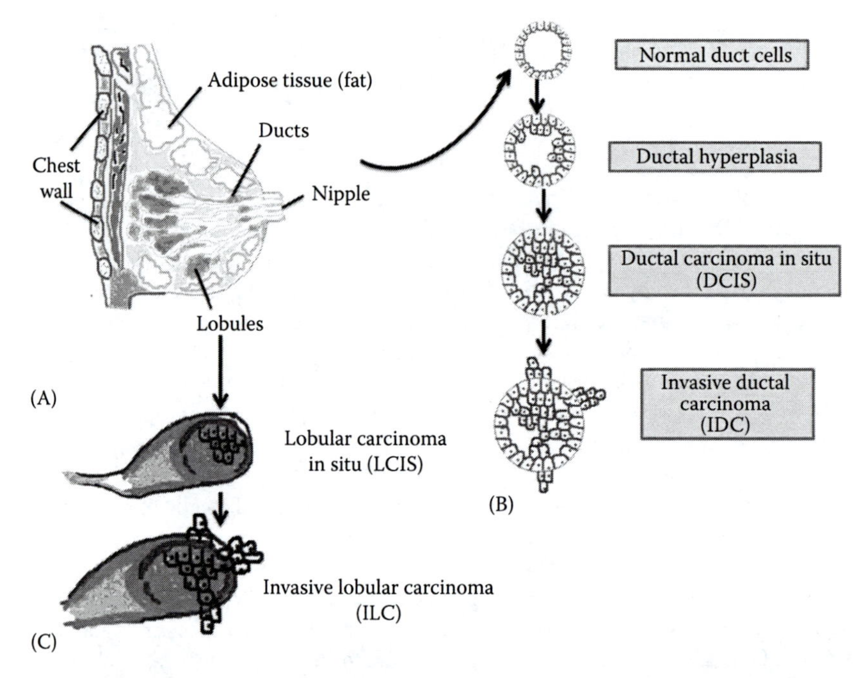

FIGURE 23.3 Anatomy of normal breast along with different types of breast cancer: (A) anatomy of normal breast. Anatomy of breast showing ducts, lobules, nipple, adipose tissue, and chest wall. (B) Development of DC. Hyperplasia is a precancerous condition that describes an accumulation of abnormal cells in a normal breast duct and is associated with an increased risk of developing cancer. In atypical hyperplasia (AH), cells keep dividing and become more abnormal, then the condition may be reclassified as noninvasive breast cancer (DCIS). When the abnormal cells tend to outgrow and start migrating to the nearby organs, the condition may be classified as IDC. (C) Development of LC. If the cells start proliferating abnormally and tend to accumulate inside the lobules, but do not spread to the other tissues, the condition is known as LCIS. If LCIS cells tend to outgrow and metastasize to the nearby organs, then the condition is known as ILC.

breast cancer, the cells lack estrogen, progesterone, and HER2 receptors on their surfaces and such cancers tend to grow and metastasize more quickly (William et al., 2010; Roberti et al., 2012; Foulkes et al., 2010).

The staging of any cancer describes upon the extent of its spread in the body and helps in better prognosis and treatment, thereby increasing the chances of survival in the patients. Stages can be decided by the tumor size (less than 2 cm, or between 2 and 5 cm or, more than 5 cm), by lymph node involvement, as well as by invasive or noninvasiveness of the tumor (Abeloff et al., 2008).

The American Joint Committee on Cancer (AJCC) has designated the TNM system ("T" stands for tumor, "N" for node, and "M" for metastasis) for staging the cancer and has categorized the breast tumors into stages 0, I, IIA, IIB, IIIA, IIIB, and IV (Table 23.2) (Singletary et al., 2002). Stage 0 is noninvasive, whereas I–IV are the invasive stages of the breast cancer. In stage 0, the cancer has not spread to the lymph nodes or to the distant sites. Around 30% of the breast cancers are detected at stage 0 with 99% of the 5-year survival rate (Lee et al., 2007). It includes DCIS, LCIS, and Paget's disease of the nipple (Atoum et al., 2010). Stage I tumor is less than or equal to 2 cm in size and has not spread to the lymph nodes (N0) or distant sites (M0). Stage II is divided into IIA and IIB. The tumors that are less than 2 cm with micrometastases in axillary lymph nodes or tumors between 2 and 5 cm without axillary lymph node involvement are grouped into stage IIA. Tumors between 2 and 5 cm with micrometastases in 1–3 axillary lymph nodes or the tumors larger than 5 cm that do not grow into the chest wall or skin and have not spread to the lymph nodes are included in stage IIB. Stage III is also divided into IIIA and IIIB. Stage IIIA, also called as local spread of breast cancer, includes tumor of any size that has spread to 4–9 axillary lymph nodes or to internal mammary nodes, as well as tumors larger than 5 cm with micrometastases in 1–3 axillary lymph nodes. Stage IIIB tumors are of any size (T0–T4) that extend to the chest wall or the skin with any member of lymph node involvement (N0–N4). Stage IV is the most aggressive stage wherein the tumor, irrespective of its size, has spread to other organs of the body with nodal involvement and is always associated with poor survival (Carey et al., 2005; Weigel et al., 2010).

TABLE 23.2

Breast Cancer Stages

Stage	TNM	Description	5-Year Survival (%)
0	Tis N0 M0	No tumor in regional lymph nodes; no distant metastases	99
I	T1 N0 M0	Tumor is less than or equal to 2 cm; no spread of tumor to regional lymph nodes; no distant metastases	92
IIA	T0 N1 M0	Tumor is smaller than 2 cm with micrometastases in 1–3 axillary lymph nodes; no distant metastases	82
	T1 N1 M0	Tumor is less than or equal to 2 cm; metastases to movable ipsilateral nodes; no distant metastases	
	T2 N0 M0	Tumor is between 2 and 5 cm; no tumor is regional lymph nodes; no distant metastases	
IIB	T2 N1 M0	Tumor is between 2 and 5 cm; metastases to movable ipsilateral nodes; no distant metastases	65
	T3 N0 M0	Tumor is over 5 cm; no tumor is regional lymph nodes; no distant metastases	
IIIA	T0 N2 M0	Tumor is less than or equal to 2 cm; metastases to 4–9 axillary lymph nodes; no distant metastases	47
	T1 N2 M0	Tumor is between 2 and 5 cm; metastases to 4–9 axillary lymph nodes; no distant metastases	
	T2 N2 M0	Tumor is over 5 cm; metastases to movable ipsilateral nodes; no distant metastases	
	T3N2M0	Tumor is over 5 cm; metastases to 4–9 axillary lymph nodes; no distant metastases	
IIIB	T4 any N M0	Tumor of any size growing into the chest wall or skin; any nodal involvement; no distant metastases	44
	Any T N3 M0	Any primary tumor involvement; metastases to more than 10 axillary lymph nodes; no distant metastases	
IV	Any T Any N M1	Any primary tumor involvement; any nodal involvement; distant metastases	14

23.1.4 Current Methods for Early Diagnosis, Prognosis, and Therapy

Detection of breast cancer at an early stage would not only help to cure the disease (by providing an opportunity for treatment) but would also improve the survival rates. Early detection has become easy with advances in screening techniques that include routine mammography programs and/or palpation (either self-examination or by physician or nurse practitioner), digital mammography, sonogram, thermography, transillumination, xeromammography, CT scan, magnetic resonance imaging (MRI), biopsy, as well as genetic testing (Lehtimaki et al., 2011; Vaughan et al., 2012). In the latter, detection of *BRCA1* and *BRCA2* gene mutations is recommended, usually for women having a strong family history of breast or ovarian cancer (Deng and Brodie, 2000). It is also tested in women who have been detected earlier with DCIS and LCIS or whose biopsies have tested positive for precancerous lesions (Nelson et al., 2005; Palma et al., 2006; Mackay et al., 2010). Breast cancers detected by screening mammography have more favorable prognostic characteristics than cancers detected by other methods (McCann et al., 2002; Kobeissi et al., 2011; Gunsoy et al., 2012). Despite the available screening facilities, diagnosis of the breast cancer remains inadequate due to the low sensitivity/specificity, relative complexity, and high cost-to-benefit ratio (Prasad et al., 2007; Schoder et al., 2007).

During the past few years, biomarkers have gained significant importance in the diagnosis of many diseases. Prognostic and predictive biomarkers such as ER, PR, HER2, p53, and BRCA1/2 are currently being used for the early diagnosis of breast cancer that would help in determining the risk of the disease (Cianfrocca et al., 2004). The biomarkers can be measured more quickly and have high sensitivity and specificity, thereby making them promising candidates for breast cancer detection. Table 23.3 enlists various imaging methods that are being used in the breast cancer detection along with their sensitivity, specificity, as well as advantages and disadvantages.

23.1.5 Test Providers and Popular Tests with Cost Involved

Mammogram and MRI are the two commonly used tests for breast cancer screening (Lehman et al., 2005; Vaughan et al., 2012). These can be performed by clinicians (doctor or nurse). A mammogram is an x-ray of the breast that may help in finding tumors that are too small to be palpable (Kobeissi et al., 2012). It can detect DCIS as well as abnormal cells in the lining of a breast duct, which may become invasive in some women. The sensitivity of a mammogram depends on the size of the tumor as well as on the density of the breast tissue. The cost for mammography in developed countries such as the United States is around 150–200 USD, whereas in developing countries such as India, the cost is around 54 USD. MRI is more sensitive than mammography and may be used to detect lumps in the breast that may have been left behind even after surgery or radiation therapy. It helps to study breast lumps or enlarged lymph nodes suspected during a clinical breast exam (CBE) or a breast self-exam (BSE) as well as in presurgical planning of patients with detected breast cancer. The cost for MRI screening in developed countries such as the United States is around 1080 USD, whereas in developing countries such as India, the cost is around 216 USD.

The National Breast and Cervical Cancer Early Detection Program (NBCCEDP) as well as the Indiana Breast and Cervical Cancer Program (BCCP) are among the leading programs for the breast cancer prevention (Howard et al., 2010). The NBCCEDP is unique in being the first and the only national cancer screening program in the United States (American Cancer Society, 2012). It aims to provide access to breast cancer screening services to the underprivileged women, emphasizes on rescreening of women at recommended time intervals, and invests resources on rescreening (Eheman et al., 2006). The BCCP offers breast cancer screening, diagnostic testing, as well as treatment to women with non-privileged or underprivileged status. It offers free treatment to the needy women and provides free services for breast cancer screening as well as diagnostic tests that include liquid-based cytology tests, CBEs, mammograms (screening and diagnostic), and diagnostic breast ultrasounds (BCCP Website: http://public.health.oregon.gov/DiseasesConditions/ChronicDisease/Cancer/Documents/2010/bhtf/breastguide.pdf). At the National Cancer Institute (NCI), National Institutes of Health (NIH), the Early Detection Research Network (EDRN) is a program where biomarkers for early detection of cancer are identified and validated clinically (http://edrn.nci.nih.gov/biomarkers).

TABLE 23.3

List of Imaging Tools along with Their Sensitivity, Specificity, as well as Advantages and Disadvantages

Imaging Tools	Sensitivity (%)	Specificity (%)	Advantages	Disadvantages	References
Screening mammography by x-ray	90	75	Mortality reduction; improved treatment of early disease; low cost; minimal discomfort	Radiation risk and other risks; risk of false alarm	Gotzsche et al. (2011)
Ultrasound by sound waves	89	78	Ultrasound pictures may show whether a lump is solid or filled with fluid; useful for detecting cancer in women at higher risk	Associated with false-positive and false-negative results; not widely available or routinely used	Ingram et al. (2012)
Scan by CT	—	—	Best way to image internal mammary nodes and to evaluate the chest and axilla after mastectomy	Radiation exposure in CT scan can accumulate and can increase the risk of developing cancer; risk of allergic reaction due to dye administration	Pettrigre et al. (2009)
PET scan by radioactive material	75	92.3	Diagnose disease even before the structural changes are visible; provides both an anatomical and functional view of the suspected cells	It does not reliably detect tumors smaller than 5–10 mm	Stephan (2010)
MRI by magnetic fields	90	72	MRI is more sensitive; identifies the primary site of cancer in the breast; high sensitivity; noninvasive; usually painless medical test	False-positive results; more expensive than mammography	Houssami et al. (2009)

23.2 Treatment Strategy, Targeted Therapy, Drug Targets, and Pharmacogenomics for Breast Cancer

23.2.1 Treatment Strategy

Treatment options for the breast cancer vary with the stage and the type, certain characteristics of the cancer cells, menopausal status, as well as the general health of the patient (Naeim et al., 2010; Patnaik et al., 2011). The currently available treatment options include surgery, radiation therapy, chemotherapy, hormone therapy, and targeted therapy.

In surgery, the affected part of the breast is removed. It involves various options such as lumpectomy, quadrantectomy, total or simple mastectomy, modified radical mastectomy, and sentinel lymph node biopsy (SLNB). In lumpectomy, only the breast lump is removed, whereas quadrantectomy involves removal of one-quarter of the breast (Fisher et al., 2002). Both the surgical procedures are followed by chemotherapy and/or radiotherapy (Bassiouny et al., 2005). In total or simple mastectomy, the entire breast is removed along with other nearby tissues, whereas in modified radical mastectomy, the whole breast along with some lymph nodes is removed (Veronesi et al., 2002). In SLNB, the sentinel lymph node is removed during the surgery whose presence is often associated with metastatic breast disease (Weaver et al., 2010).

TABLE 23.4

FDA-Approved Drug Combinations Used in Breast Cancer

Abbreviations	Commonly Used Drug Combinations
AC	Doxorubicin hydrochloride (Adriamycin) + cyclophosphamide
AC-T	Doxorubicin hydrochloride (Adriamycin) + cyclophosphamide + paclitaxel (Taxol)
CAF	Cyclophosphamide + doxorubicin hydrochloride (Adriamycin) + fluorouracil
CMF	Cyclophosphamide + methotrexate + fluorouracil
FEC	Fluorouracil + epirubicin hydrochloride + cyclophosphamide

Note: The data have been gathered from the American Cancer Society 2012.

Radiation therapy is also used to treat the cancer that has metastasized to the other parts of the body, for example, to the bones or brain. It uses high-energy x-rays to shrink the tumors as well as to kill the cancer cells. Radiation therapy can be used in the form of either external beam or brachytherapy. In the former, an external source of radiation is directed at the tumor site from outside the body, whereas in brachytherapy, the radiation source is placed inside or next to the area requiring the treatment (Fisher et al., 2002; Smith et al., 2012).

Chemotherapy involves the use of drugs to damage or kill the cancer cells. It can be given either as an adjuvant or a neoadjuvant chemotherapy wherein the former is given to the patient after the surgery and the latter is given to the patient before the surgery. Adjuvant chemotherapy has been reported to reduce the risk of relapse and death (Fornier et al., 2005). Neoadjuvant chemotherapy may shrink the size of large tumors so that they are small enough to be removed with less extensive surgery (Schott et al., 2012). Table 23.4 mentions various Food and Drug Administration (FDA)-approved drug combinations that are being given to breast cancer patients.

Chemotherapy is usually associated with several side effects that include hair loss, mouth sores, loss of appetite or increased appetite, nausea and vomiting, low blood cell counts, neuropathy, cardiotoxicity, increased risk of leukemia, increased chances of infections, easy bruising or bleeding, as well as fatigue (Tchen et al., 2003; Hermelink et al., 2007; Lemieux et al., 2008; Azim et al., 2011). However, these side effects are outweighed by potential benefits of chemotherapy in terms of decreasing the mortality rates and increasing the patient survival. Chemotherapy kills both invasive and noninvasive cancer cells, thereby reducing the likelihood of recurrence or death after adjuvant therapy (Cianfrocca et al., 2005). It can shrink the large tumors to operable size and thus make surgery less invasive. Chemotherapy can also help in increasing the effectiveness of radiation therapy (Schott et al., 2012).

Besides the previously mentioned treatments, hormone therapy is used to block the female hormones (estrogen and progesterone) that might promote the growth of any cancer cells that may have remained even after surgery (Lea et al., 2004). This may be done either by using drugs that block the action of hormones such as tamoxifen or an aromatase inhibitor or by surgical removal of hormone making organs, such as the ovaries. Hormone therapy does not help patients having ER- and PR-negative tumors.

23.2.2 Targeted Therapy

Targeted therapy uses drugs to identify and attack specific markers on cancer cells. It may interfere with the molecules involved in the malignant cell signal transduction, cell invasion, metastasis, apoptosis, cell cycle, and angiogenesis (Suter et al., 2007; Munagala et al., 2011). Targeted therapy mainly focuses on inhibition of HER2, estrogen, insulin-like growth factor, PARP, and PI3K/Akt/mTOR signaling pathways (Martelli et al., 2010; Sachdev et al., 2010; Higgins et al., 2011; Nielsen, 2013). Some targeted therapies use the monoclonal antibodies that work like the natural antibodies synthesized by our immune system to target cancer cells (Bernard-Marty et al., 2006). These therapies are new and are sometimes called as immune-targeted therapies.

The first molecular target for breast cancer treatment was the cellular receptor for the female sex hormone, estrogen (Hanstein et al., 2004; Suter et al., 2007). The binding of estrogen to the estrogen receptor (ER) in cells activates the hormone–receptor complex, which in turn activates the genes involved in cell growth and proliferation (Lindberg et al., 2011). Interference with estrogen ability to stimulate

TABLE 23.5

List of FDA-Approved Drugs for the Treatment of Breast Cancer

FDA-Approved Drugs for Breast Cancer	Key Targets
Tamoxifen, raloxifene, toremifene, fulvestrant	Selective ER modulators
Anastrozole, exemestane, letrozole	Aromatase inhibitors
Cetuximab, lapatinib, gefitinib, erlotinib	EGFR (HER1) inhibitors
Trastuzumab, pertuzumab, lapatinib	HER2 inhibitors
Rapamycin (also called sirolimus), temsirolimus, everolimus	mTOR inhibitors
Perifosine	Akt inhibitors

Note: The data have been gathered from the American Cancer Society 2012.

the growth of breast cancer cells (ER-positive breast cancer cells) could serve as an effective treatment approach (Kumar et al., 2008). Several drugs have been approved by the FDA for the treatment of ER-positive breast cancers. Drugs such as Herceptin (trastuzumab) kill the breast cancer cells having high levels of HER2 protein, whereas tamoxifen and toremifene (Fareston®) bind to the ER and prevent estrogen binding (Verma et al., 2010). Another drug, fulvestrant (Faslodex®) binds to the ER and promotes its destruction, thereby reducing ER levels inside the cells (Lynn et al., 2004). In Table 23.5, the list of FDA-approved drugs for the treatment of breast cancer has been mentioned.

23.2.3 Pharmacogenomics in Breast Cancer

The field of pharmacogenomics (PG) involves studying the influence of an individual's genetic variations on drug response (Yiannakopoulou, 2012). The efficacy and toxicity of drugs in an individual depends upon genetic polymorphisms in drug-metabolizing enzymes, transporters, receptors, and other drug targets (Wajapeyee et al., 2004). This relatively new field combines pharmaceutical sciences with molecular biology, high-throughput biotechnology, and bioinformatics to develop effective, safe, and customized drug treatment regimens for a particular individual or patient population (Rofaiel et al., 2010; Wang, 2010).

Several factors such as genetics of an individual, environmental factors, diet, age, lifestyle, and state of health of a patient can influence an individual's response to medicines (Wajapeyee et al., 2004). PG determines how genetic variations would influence the drug response in an individual and thus provides personalized therapy based on individual genetic variability (Evans, 2003). This in turn helps not only in maximizing the efficacy of the drug but also in reducing the drug-associated side effects. The advantages of PG include improved therapeutic index as well as dose regimen and selection of optimal drug (Ingle, 2008). For example, tamoxifen is an anticancer drug that is used for treating breast cancer patients having ER+ tumors. The pharmacological activity of tamoxifen depends on cytochrome P450 2D6 (CYP2D6) enzyme that converts tamoxifen to its active metabolite, endoxifen (Rofaiel et al., 2010). Patients with reduced CYP2D6 activity (owing to genetic polymorphisms in the cytochrome p450 gene) produce little endoxifen and, thus, get partial therapeutic benefit from tamoxifen (Holmes et al., 2005). Thus, PG would help in selection of optimal drugs for the patients who are genetically resistant to the specific drugs.

The study of the PG of chemotherapy response mainly examines metabolizing enzymes such as cytochrome P450, UDP-glucuronosyltransferase (UGT), and drug transporters such as ATP-binding cassette (ABC) (Fajac et al., 2010). The field of PG offers personalized medicine compared to the traditional "one-drug-fits-all" approach. FDA (US) has approved two commercially available pharmacogenomic tests that detect variations in the genes coding for enzymes involved in drug metabolism. These include cytochrome P450 CYP2C19 and CYP2D6 (Roche AmpliChip, http://www.roche.com/products/product-details.htm?type=product&id=17) and UGT (Invader UGT1AI Molecular Assay; Third Wave Technologies, http://www.twt.com/) (Swen et al., 2007). However, the usage of these tests remains limited in routine clinical practice because of many challenges that may include analytic, ethical, and technological issues involved in generation and management of large drug response data sets (Williams-Jones et al., 2003; Bansal et al., 2005).

However, implementation of PG in routine clinical practice presents significant challenges. These include identifying candidate genes and pathways involved in variable drug response, correlating disease genes with drug response genes, describing drug response phenotypes, selection of clinically relevant tests that could also predict the outcome of drug treatment, cost-effective and wide availability of tests, and focusing on analytic, ethical, and technological issues involved in generation and management of large data sets (Williams-Jones et al., 2003; Roden et al., 2006; Swen et al., 2007). By overcoming such challenges and by generating strong scientific evidence, PG can help in safe and more effective usage of drugs through personalized therapy (Swen et al., 2007). Moreover, regulatory agencies should recommend the use of PG-based tests prior to drug prescriptions and pharma companies as well as patient groups should advocate the use of such tests, which would gear up its use in clinical practice (Swen et al., 2007).

23.3 Invasive and Noninvasive Biomarkers: Advantages and Disadvantages

A biomarker is a signature molecule used as an indicator of biological state that may be either secreted by a tumor in body fluids or it can be a specific response of the body to the presence of cancer (Falasca et al., 2012). Biomarkers include nucleic acids, proteins, sugars, lipids, small metabolites, cytogenetic and cytokinetic parameters, as well as whole tumor cells found in the body fluid whose expression may be altered in tumors (Bhatt et al., 2010). Some of the clinicopathological features of the tumor that are routinely used as biomarkers include tumor size, histological type, cellular and nuclear characteristics, mitotic index, lymphovascular invasion, hormonal receptors, lymph node metastases, and axillary lymph node status (Sarkar et al., 2008). However, these parameters are not sufficient to predict the course of cancer (Weigel et al., 2010). Thus, massive efforts have been put together to identify and validate specific prognostic and predictive biomarkers of breast cancer that would reduce the mortality through early detection, risk stratification, prediction, and better prognosis (Weigel et al., 2010).

Depending upon sampling method, biomarkers could be either invasive or noninvasive (Song et al., 2012). Invasive biomarkers involve invasive surgical procedures that require penetration into body through incision or cut. For example, immunohistochemical analysis of ER, PR, HER2, Ki-67, and p53 requires biopsy samples or tissue samples that could be obtained by surgery. Invasive biomarkers are specific, sensitive, and widely used for rapid and accurate diagnosis and prognosis of the disease. However, invasive surgical procedures are associated with anxiety, prolonged recovery time, and high follow-up costs that cause discomfort to the patients.

Noninvasive biomarkers are proteins, enzymes, hormones, tumor cells or cell-free DNAs, and nucleic acids produced and released either by tumor cells or by host cells and would be easily detected in the body fluids such as serum, nipple aspiratory fluid, tear, urine, or saliva. Biomarkers that have been used clinically for breast cancer detection are mostly noninvasive (Zhau et al., 2010). For example, the development of novel methylation-based biomarkers (obtained noninvasively from patient) as well as serum microRNAs (miRNAs or miRs) helps in early detection of the disease. Noninvasive biomarkers are more sensitive, specific, and easily detectable than invasive biomarkers. They are more valuable in prognosis and diagnosis and in making therapeutic decisions. They are associated with the less anxiety and discomfort to the patients (Madu et al., 2010; Misek et al., 2011; Robertson et al., 2011). However, limited availability of a sufficient number of good quality samples for evaluation of biomarkers is one of the drawbacks of noninvasive biomarkers (Richard Mayeux, 2004). Both invasive and noninvasive biomarkers in panels may provide higher predictive potential resulting in improved clinical outcomes (Zhu et al., 2011).

23.4 Different Invasive Biomarkers Currently Used and under Development

23.4.1 Currently Used Invasive Biomarkers in Breast Cancer Detection

23.4.1.1 Estrogen Receptors (ERα, ERβ)

The steroid hormone estrogen plays a central role in the etiology of breast cancer (Baglietto et al., 2010). It mediates its biologic effects through ERs that are expressed in around 70% of human breast cancers. ER is a ligand-inducible transcription factor that belongs to the nuclear receptor NR3B subfamily. It is the most powerful predictive and prognostic biomarker in breast cancer that provides the index for sensitivity to endocrine treatment (Giguère et al., 1988).

ER has two different isoforms, namely, ERα and ERβ, that are encoded on different chromosomes and act as hormone-dependent transcriptional regulators. ERα, located on chromosome 6q (Menasce et al., 1993), is a 66 kDa protein (Kong et al., 2003), while ERβ, located on chromosome 14q (Gosden et al., 1986), is a 59 kDa protein (Ogawa et al., 1998). ERα acts as a tumor promoter, whereas ERβ is a tumor suppressor. The presence of ERβ in breast tumors is associated with better prognosis and longer disease-free survival (Chen et al., 2008). ERα is an important functional modulator of the estrogen signaling pathway and is more frequently expressed than ERβ. ERα expression is a useful clinical biomarker of breast tumor progression and thereby an effective therapeutic target. ERα-positive breast cancers have long been considered relatively resistant to traditional chemotherapeutic drugs (Allegra et al., 1978). These are characterized by slow growth, high degree of differentiation, and increase of the relapse-free survival (Schiff et al., 2005). It has been reported that the patients with ER-positive tumors have a significantly higher response rate to antiestrogens such as tamoxifen than patients with ER-poor/ER-negative tumors (Lee and Dutta, 2007).

23.4.1.2 Progesterone Receptor

The progesterone receptor (PR) is a member of the nuclear receptor superfamily, which specifically regulates the expression of target genes in response to the hormonal stimulus (Yin et al., 2012). PR exists in two isoforms, namely, PR-A (94 kDa protein) and PR-B (116 kDa protein), wherein the latter activates transcription of target genes and PR-A represses transcription of PR-B as well as few other nuclear receptors (Dressing et al., 2009; Pathiraja et al., 2011). Xiao-Dong Fu et al. showed that PR enhances breast cancer cell motility and invasion through activation of focal adhesion kinase (Fu et al., 2010b). The ratio of PR-A to PR-B expression controls the PR signaling and any imbalance between the two isoforms may lead to alterations in PR signaling (Viale et al., 2007). PR is an important biomarker for predicting the outcome in breast cancer patients. Several clinical studies have reported ER-/PR-negative breast cancer patients at a high risk of mortality than ER-/PR-positive ones as the latter responds better to endocrine therapies (Varghese et al., 2007).

23.4.1.3 HER-2

HER-2/neu/c-ErbB-2 proto-oncogene is located on chromosome 17q12 and encodes for a 185 kDa transmembrane glycoprotein belonging to the epidermal growth factor receptor (EGFR) family (Ross et al., 2004a). Other members of the EGFR family include EGFR (HER-1 or erbB1), HER-2, HER-3 (erbB3), and HER-4 (erbB4). HER-2 is found to be amplified in about 10%–35% of human breast carcinomas and is considered as a key prognostic factor in early stages of the disease (Bofin et al., 2004). Amplification of HER-2/neu is an established predictive and prognostic factor in aggressive breast cancer (Davis et al., 2007). Studies have also reported that the overexpression of HER-2 may influence the sensitivity of breast carcinoma to chemotherapy (Zhang et al., 2008). Van de Vijver et al. reported for the first time the overexpression of HER-2/neu oncogene in 189 samples of breast cancer patients by using immunohistochemistry (Van de Vijver et al., 1988). Berger et al. determined HER-2/neu protein overexpression associated with lymph node status and breast cancer tumor grade (Berger et al., 1988). Slamon et al. found that the overexpression of HER2/neu gene is associated with a more aggressive phenotype and poor prognosis (Slamon et al., 1988; Paik et al., 1990). The humanized monoclonal antibody trastuzumab has been reported to have high affinity for the extracellular domain of HER-2 and is, thus, used against HER2-positive early breast cancer (Vogel et al., 2002). Recent prospective randomized trials of adjuvant trastuzumab therapies have demonstrated the reduced risk of recurrence and mortality in patients with HER-2 positive early stage breast cancer (Smith et al., 2007).

23.4.1.4 Ki-67

Proliferation is a key feature of the tumor progression and it has a major impact on the risk of recurrence. Breast cancers expressing high levels of Ki-67, a nuclear marker of cell proliferation, are associated with worse outcomes (Miglietta et al., 2010). Studies have confirmed that Ki-67 is an important predictive and prognostic factor in early breast cancer. It is a non-histone nuclear antigen, universally expressed in the cells during the proliferative phases of the cell cycle (mid-G1, S, G2, and M phase) and is absent in G0 phase (Lopez et al., 1991; Jung et al., 2009). The prognostic and predictive value of Ki-67 is independent of age, nodal and hormonal status, as well as ERs and is, thus, associated with poor prognosis (Cheang et al., 2009). Patients having tumors overexpressing Ki-67 in more than 50% of the cells are at a high risk of developing the recurrent disease. Increased expression of Ki-67 in breast cancer is associated with poor prognosis and better response to chemotherapy (Jung et al., 2007; Jones et al., 2010; Keam et al., 2011). Many studies have shown that Ki-67 expression gets progressively increased from benign to DCIS and to invasive breast cancer, thereby leading to worse clinical outcomes (Kim et al., 2011).

23.4.1.5 p53

p53 is a short-lived transcription factor located on 17 p13.1 chromosome that acts as a "guardian of the genome" and is also known as a master tumor suppressor protein (Wang et al., 2010). Several studies have established the role of p53 in tumor suppression, regulation of genes involved in cell adhesion, cell cycle, apoptosis, control of genome stability, neuronal growth, angiogenesis, metastasis, oxidative stress, cell fate, and cytoskeleton organization (Qin et al., 2007; Wang et al., 2009a). Oxidative stress and exposure to mutagenic agents involved in DNA damage result into the activation of p53 that in turn further activates p21 (a cell cycle regulator) and proapoptotic proteins, resulting into regulation of the cell proliferation and apoptosis (Figure 23.4).

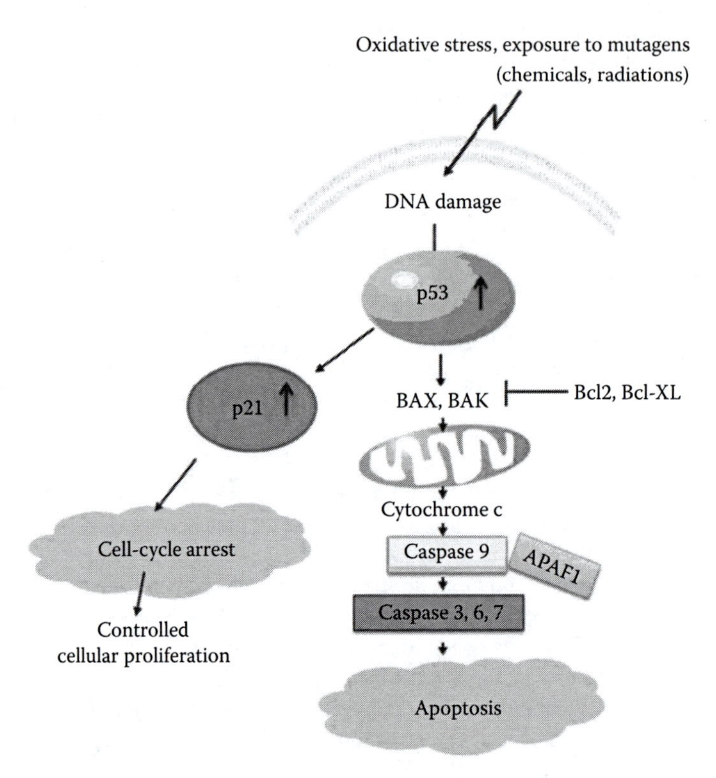

FIGURE 23.4 p53 signaling pathway. p53 plays an important role in regulation of cell proliferation and apoptosis. Oxidative stress as well as exposure to mutagens (chemicals, radiations) leads to DNA damage, resulting into the activation of tumor suppressor protein p53 that results into transcriptional activation of proapoptotic proteins BAX and BAK and repression of antiapoptotic Bcl2 and Bcl-XL proteins. BAX and BAK help in the activation of procaspase-9 by the release of cytochrome c from the mitochondria as well as the cleavage of caspase 9 into caspase 3, 6, and 7 resulting into the apoptosis. Activation of p53 also causes the transcriptional induction of p21 (a cell cycle regulator), which in turn inhibits CDK–cyclin activity and arrests the cell cycle leading to the regulation of cell proliferation.

TABLE 23.6
Role of Breast Cancer Invasive Biomarkers with Their Testing Methods

Proteins	Testing Methods	Role in Breast Cancer
ER	Immunohistochemistry	Stimulates proliferation of mammary cells; involved in cell division and DNA replication
PR	Immunohistochemistry	Involved in metastatic disease; predicting outcome in cancer patients
HER-2	Immunohistochemistry Fluorescence in situ hybridization (FISH)	Strongly associated with increased disease recurrence; prognostic factor in early stages of the disease
Ki-67	Immunohistochemistry Antibody labeling	Prognosis and prediction of cell proliferation
p53	Antibody labeling	Potential prognostic and predictive biomarker of breast cancer involved in apoptosis, cell proliferation, metastasis

p53 mutation has gained attention as a potential prognostic and predictive marker of breast cancer. It is estimated that almost one-third of breast cancers have altered p53, which is associated with more aggressive phenotype (Miller et al., 2005). Results by several groups have shown that p53 mutation status is a useful predictive marker that is linked with a two–three fold increased risk of recurrence and death (Bull et al., 2004; Bourdon et al., 2011). Recent immunohistochemical studies suggest that p53 mutation is associated with several other adverse prognostic factors such as high tumor grade, high proliferation rate, and ER^-/PR^- status. Olivier et al. studied the prognostic value of mutant p53 gene in 1794 patients with breast cancer wherein they found that patients with mutated p53 have worse prognosis. They also found that p53 mutations were more frequent in aggressive tumors and node-positive cases and in women <60 years old (Olivier et al., 2006). Gonzalez-Angulo et al. found the altered expression of p53 in majority of patients with IBC (Gonzalez-Angulo et al., 2004). Thus, p53 is a useful biomarker for predicting prognosis and patient's response to therapy (Stoklosa et al., 2005). Table 23.6 enlists currently used invasive molecular biomarkers along with their regulatory role in breast cancer.

23.4.2 Different Invasive Molecular Biomarkers Currently under Development for This Cancer

23.4.2.1 SMAR1

Scaffold/matrix attachment region binding protein 1(SMAR1) (Chattopadhoy, Genomics, 2000) is a matrix-associated region (MAR) binding protein, whose tumor suppressor function was first reported by Kaul et al. (2003). SMAR1 gene is located on 16q24.3 chromosome and its expression has been reported to be downregulated in several breast cancer cell lines and tissues (Kaul et al., 2003; Kamini et al., 2007). SMAR1 has been shown to regulate the cell proliferation by arresting the cells at G2/M phase through direct interaction and activation of tumor suppressor p53 (Kaul et al., 2003; Jalota et al., 2005). Rampalli et al. reported that SMAR1 represses cyclin D1 (CCND1) expression by recruiting HDAC1–mSin3A corepressor complex at CCND1 promoter locus (Rampalli et al., 2005). Moreover, SMAR1 has been reported to downregulate the metastasis of breast cancer through transforming growth factor (TGF)-β pathway (Kamini et al., 2007). It has also been shown to regulate T-cell receptor beta enhancer activity through interaction with CDP/CUX, a positive regulator of cell cycle (Kaul-Ghanekar et al., 2004). Kamini Singh et al. performed SMAR1 expression analysis in 30 fibroadenoma benign cases and 30 malignant breast cancer patients including grade I, II, and III, wherein they found that SMAR1 is downregulated during the advanced stages and the decreased SMAR1 expression correlated with defective p53 subcellular localization (Singh et al., 2007). Kamini Singh et al. showed that SMAR1 inhibited TNF-α-induced induction of NF-κB, thereby suggesting that SMAR1 regulated tumorigenesis through modulation of NF-κB target genes (Singh et al., 2009). Kaul-Ghanekar et al. have shown by atomic force microscopy studies that SMAR1 expression correlated with cell surface smoothness in different cancer cell lines, in different grades of human breast cancer tissues,

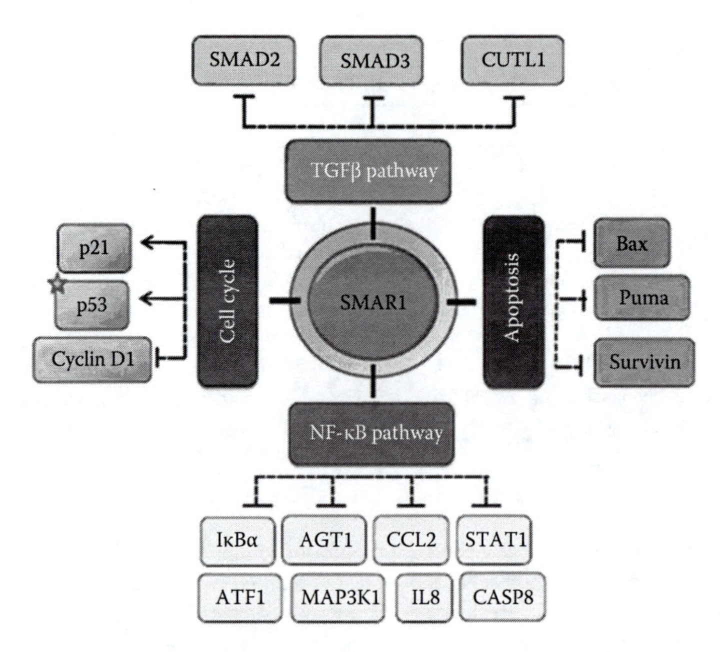

FIGURE 23.5 Different molecular targets and pathways regulated by SMAR1. The figure shows the role of SMAR1 in cell cycle regulation, apoptosis, as well as TGFβ and NF-κB signaling pathways. (From Malonia SK et al., *BBA Rev. Can.*, 1815, 1, 2011.)

as well as in mouse tumor sections (Ghanekar et al., 2009). They found that human breast cancer tissues showing lower expression of SMAR1 exhibited increased surface roughness compared to the normal breast tissue. Based on their findings, the authors indicated that the tumor suppressor protein SMAR1 might be used as a phenotypic differentiation marker between cancerous and noncancerous cells (Kaul-Ghanekar et al., 2009). Figure 23.5 depicts the different molecular targets and pathways regulated by SMAR1.

23.4.2.2 CDP/Cux

The CCAAT-displacement protein/cut homeobox (CDP/Cux) is a MARBP as well as a transcriptional activator that has been reported to regulate mammary-specific gene transcription as well as breast tumorigenesis (Zhu et al., 2004). It has been found to be overexpressed in breast cancer (Michl et al., 2006). Cux/CDP/CUTL1 is involved in higher-order chromatin organization and may be able to target certain regulatory loci to specific regions of the nucleus (Truscott et al., 2003). Cux is known to regulate transcription of developmental genes and plays an important role in cell proliferation and differentiation (Nepveu, 2001; Goulet et al., 2007). Studies have reported that CDP/Cux represses a large number of genes, particularly those expressed in precursor cells prior to terminal differentiation (Vadnais et al., 2012). Michl et al. have shown that increased expression of Cux enhances tumor metastasis (Michl et al., 2005). In transgenic mice, both CDP/Cux isoforms, p75 and p110, were shown to cause malignancies in several organs and cell types including breast cancer (Cadieux et al., 2006).

23.4.2.3 SATB1

Special AT-rich sequence binding protein 1 (SATB1) is a genome organizer that regulates chromatin structure, histone modification, and nucleosomal positioning (Galande et al., 2007; Han et al., 2008; Fessing et al., 2011). It is one of the key proteins involved in the development and progression of breast cancer (Iorns et al., 2010; Hanker et al., 2011). SATB1 expression is upregulated in aggressive rather than nonaggressive breast cancer cells. In highly aggressive breast cancer, SATB1 overexpression has been reported to be associated with metastasis, whereas its downregulation has been reported to overturn the metastatic and tumorigenic characteristics of cells. Several studies have reported SATB1 as a prognostic marker for breast cancer (Patani et al., 2009; Chen et al., 2011).

23.4.2.4 BRCA1

Breast cancer type 1 susceptibility protein (BRCA1) gene is a tumor suppressor located on 17q21 chromosome that encodes a 220 kDa nuclear phosphoprotein (Suter et al., 2007). It plays an important role in regulating genome integrity, cell cycle checkpoint proteins, key mitotic or cell division steps, cell proliferation, apoptosis, as well as chromatin remodeling (Deng et al., 2006). Around 5%–10% of breast carcinomas are hereditary and BRCA1 plays a major role in the hereditary susceptibility for the cancer (Christopoulou et al., 2006). Women with BRCA1 germ line mutations have more than three times the risk of developing breast cancer (Christopoulou et al., 2006; Mackay et al., 2010). Studies have shown that there is a cumulative lifetime risk of 50%–85% of developing breast cancer in women having a germ line mutation in BRCA1 (King et al., 2003). Majority of breast cancers having BRCA1 mutations are ER negative (ER^-) (Tung et al., 2010). BRCA1-mutated tumors occur at an early age and are ER, PR, and HER2/neu negative (Xu et al., 2012; Anna et al., 2004). Such tumors are poorly differentiated and have worst prognosis (James, 2007).

23.4.2.5 BTG3/ANA/APRO4

BTG3/ANA/APRO4 is a member of the antiproliferative B-cell translocation gene (BTG)/Tob (transducer of ErbB2) gene family (Matsuda et al., 2001). The BTG family of antiproliferative gene products has been shown to play a significant role in the negative control of the cell cycle (Ou et al., 2007). BTG3 is a negative regulator of SRC tyrosine kinase and it inhibits the activity of the E2F1 transcription factor (Yu et al., 2008). Latest reports show that BTG3 is a p53 target and provides evidence for its DNA damage response and explains its anticancer potential through inhibition of E2F1 transcription factor (Ou et al., 2001). Some reports suggest that promoter region of the BTG3 gene is hypermethylated in breast cancer, thereby implicating its potential as a possible biomarker (Yu et al., 2008).

23.4.2.6 Cyclin D1

CCND1 gene, located on chromosome 11q13, has been reported to regulate G1/S phase during the cell cycle (Kim, 2009; Saha et al., 2011). It activates cdk 4/6 and plays an important role in sequestering cdk inhibitors in the G1/S phase (Alao, 2007). CCND1 has been found to promote cell proliferation and differentiation by shortening the G1/S transition in many human tumors including breast cancer (Colozza et al., 2005). It is a key factor amplified in 15% breast cancer patients and overexpressed at genetic and protein level in over 50% of breast cancer cases (Ormandy et al., 2003; Zelivianski et al., 2010). Overexpression of CCND1 in both in situ ductal and lobular subtypes suggests its possible role as a biomarker in the early detection of breast cancer (Rennstam et al., 2001). Several studies have shown a strong positive correlation of CCND1 with ER and PR expression levels, wherein overexpression in ER-positive breast cancer patients has been found to be associated with relapse-free survival (Tobin et al., 2011). Table 23.7 enlists various invasive molecular biomarkers that are currently under development and their regulatory role in breast cancer.

TABLE 23.7

Different Invasive Biomarkers Having the Potential for Prognostic Markers

Protein	Role in Breast Cancer
SMAR1	Regulates the cell proliferation, cell cycle, chromatin modulator
SATB1	Proliferation marker that regulate histone modification, nucleosomal positioning
BRCA1	Regulates cell proliferation, apoptosis, chromatin remodeling
BTG3/ANA/APRO4	It has antiproliferative activity, act as chromatin modulator
Cyclin D1	It is a proliferation marker and plays a regulatory role in cell cycle regulation

23.5 Different Noninvasive Biomarkers Currently Used and under Development

23.5.1 Noninvasive Biomarkers Currently Used in Breast Cancer

23.5.1.1 Nipple Aspirate Fluid or Ductal Lavage Fluid Biomarkers

Nipple aspiration is a noninvasive and low-cost procedure used for obtaining breast fluids from the duct openings of the nipple for the evaluation of abnormalities associated with breast cancer (Fabian et al., 2005). Nipple fluid may provide a better source of ductal epithelial cells, cell-free nucleic acids (DNA, RNA, miRNA), and proteins released from the tumors (Dooley et al., 2001; Suijkerbuijk et al., 2008; Fabian and Kimler, 2001). Breast fluid provides a rich and superior source of biomarkers for breast cancer because the proteins present are specifically released from the breast tissue (Li et al., 2005). In combination with high-throughput novel proteomic profiling technology, specific biomarkers of nipple fluid have been discovered and validated (He et al., 2007; Celis Julio et al., 2004). ER Sauter et al. collected nipple aspirate fluid (NAF) from 177 subjects using a modified breast pump; and out of that, samples from 144 subjects were analyzed to evaluate promising cellular biomarkers (epithelial cells obtained from NAF). They analyzed cytology by computerized image analysis of NAF epithelial cells and observed that DNA index as well as percentage of cells in G2/M phase or with hypertetraploidy increased with abnormal cytology that correlated with increased breast cancer risk. All these results suggest that biomarkers from NAF may prove useful either as an adjunct to currently accepted breast cancer screening methods or to evaluate response to chemopreventive agents (Sauter et al., 1997).

Zhao analyzed carcinoembryonic antigen (CEA) and prostate-specific antigen (PSA) in NAF samples from 44 women with newly diagnosed invasive breast cancers, 67 women with proliferative breast lesions (DCIS and LCIS as well as atypical ductal hyperplasia), and 277 controls without these lesions. They found elevated levels of nipple fluid CEAs in breast cancer patients compared to the healthy controls. However, nipple fluid PSA levels were similar in breast cancer patients as well as healthy control women. Their results suggested that nipple fluid CEA could be a potent biomarker for early breast cancer detection (Zhao et al., 2001).

Pawlik et al. collected NAF samples from both the breasts from 18 women with stage I or II unilateral invasive breast carcinoma and 4 healthy volunteers by handheld suction cup. The samples were analyzed using isotope-coded affinity tag (ICAT) labeling, sodium dodecyl sulfate-polyacrylamide gel (SDS-PAGE), liquid chromatography (LC), and MS to quantify and identify differential expression of tumor-specific proteins in NAF. They identified around 353 peptides and found that five proteins were differentially expressed in the NAF samples from cancer patients compared to that from healthy controls. Alpha2-HS-glycoprotein (heavy–light [H:L] ratio 0.63) was downregulated, while lipophilin B (H:L ratio 1.42), beta-globin (H:L ratio 1.98), hemopexin (H:L ratio 1.73), and vitamin D-binding protein precursor (H:L ratio 1.82) were overexpressed in NAF from cancer patients. Thus, proteomic-based techniques could be used to find markers for diagnosis of breast cancer (Pawlik et al., 2006; Laronga and Drake, 2007).

He et al. analyzed NAF samples from 76 different women, including 63 samples from noncancerous breasts and 38 samples from breasts with invasive cancer by surface-enhanced laser desorption/ionization coupled to time-of-flight mass spectrometry (SELDI-TOF MS) technique to identify protein biomarkers. A set of eight markers were identified that include albumin, apolipoprotein A–I, apolipoprotein D, hemoglobin-ß, hemoglobin-α, lactotransferrin, prolactin-induced protein, and α-1-antitrypsin that collectively gave 63% sensitivity, 89% specificity, and 76% accuracy for distinguishing cancerous cases from noncancerous one (He et al., 2007).

Aberrantly methylated genes found in breast epithelial cells of NAF can be used as promising candidates for the early detection of breast cancer (Krassenstein et al., 2004). Methylation markers in NAF can be detected by various techniques that include methylation-specific PCR (MSP), quantitative multiplex methylation-specific PCR (QM-MSP), and sodium bisulfite treatment-based nested quantitative assay (Suijkerbuijk et al., 2010). Krassenstein et al. analyzed methylation status of GSTP1 (glutathione S-transferase P), RARB (retinoic acid receptor beta), p16INK4a, p14^{ARF} (p14 alternate reading frame), RASSF1A (Ras association domain-containing protein 1A), and DAPK (death-associated protein kinase 1) from matched specimens of tumor and normal tissue as well NAF from 22 breast cancer patients. They found hypermethylation of one or more genes in 82% of NAF DNAs in breast cancer patients compared to the normal controls (Krassenstein et al., 2004). Besides these, methylation of cyclin D2, HIN1, RAR-b2, CCND2 (cyclin D2), cyclin-dependent kinase inhibitor 2A (CDKN2A), RARB, RASSF1, twist-related protein 1 (TWIST1), BRCA1/2, secretoglobin 3A1 (SCGB3A1), and APC (adenomatous polyposis coli) genes in NAF samples has been reported in other studies to predict the breast cancer risk (Lewis et al., 2005; Euhus et al., 2007; Locke et al., 2007).

23.5.1.2 Serum Biomarkers

23.5.1.2.1 MUC-1

Mucins are large glycoproteins with high carbohydrate content (50%–90% by weight) and are divided into seven structurally identifiable families (MUC1–MUC7) (Rose and Voynow, 2006). These are normally expressed at the apical surface of polarized epithelial cells of normal mammary glands. However, in cancer, transformation and disruption of polarity leads to their release into the bloodstream of patients.

The MUC1 gene product is a transmembrane glycoprotein that is frequently overexpressed in malignant glandular cell surfaces and leads to increased serum levels of MUC-1 that could be measured as an important predictive marker of breast cancer (Rakha et al., 2005). It is a high molecular weight (250–1000 kDa) protein that can activate membrane receptors for growth factors, reduce E-cadherin-mediated cell adhesion, and diminish cell–cell and cell–extracellular matrix interactions, thereby promoting cell migration and invasion. It can also reduce the cellular apoptotic response to oxidative stress (Hudson et al., 2001; Costa et al., 2011). Detection of high levels of these mucins in breast cancer patients correlates with increasing tumor burden and poor prognosis (Mukhopadhyay et al., 2011; Treon et al., 2000). Members of the MUC-1 family include CA15.3, BR27.29, MCA, and CA549 that are the most commonly implicated serum tumor markers in breast cancer.

23.5.1.2.1.1 CA15-3 and CA 27.29 (Also Known as BR 27.29) Cancer antigen 15-3 (CA15-3), is a mucin-like transmembrane glycoprotein with a molecular weight of 290 kDa that is shed from the tumor cells into the bloodstream (Nicolini et al., 2006). It is overexpressed in more than 90% of breast carcinomas and is used in the diagnosis, treatment, and clinical management of the disease (Senapati et al., 2010). It is a useful marker in evaluating recurrence of the disease as well as response to the treatment (Al-azawi et al., 2006). The potential uses of CA 15-3 in clinical practice lead to improved diagnosis and cost-effectiveness (Prabasheela et al., 2011). CA 15-3 is the most sensitive test in detecting metastatic breast cancer (Kruit et al., 2010).

Cancer antigen 27.29 (CA27.29) is a soluble form of the glycoprotein MUC1 (Cen et al., 2008) and can be detected by the monoclonal antibody B27.29 (Steven et al., 2000). It is overexpressed in variety of cancers including breast cancer (Handy, 2009). Elevated serum CA 27.29 protein levels are highly associated with progression of breast cancer (Harris et al., 2007) and have been reported in approximately one-third of women with early-stage (stage I or II) and two-thirds of women with late-stage breast cancer (stage III or IV) (Hussain et al., 2006). It is highly specific and sensitive in detecting metastatic disease (Duffy, 2006). The US FDA has approved CA 27.29 as a biomarker for monitoring breast cancer (Kurian et al., 2008).

CA 15-3 and CA 27.29 are useful markers in monitoring the response to either endocrine or cytotoxic therapy. Both are well-characterized serum biomarkers that allow the detection of circulating MUC-1 antigen in the peripheral blood. Several studies have reported CA 15-3 and CA 27.29 as the predictive markers for breast cancer detection (Kumpulainen et al., 2002; Molina et al., 2010; Van der Auwera et al., 2010). Mahindocht Keyhani et al. in their study have measured CA15-3 levels in 54 patients with benign lesions, 43 with malignant lesions, and 39 normal controls before and after mastectomy. They tried to find out the correlation between serum levels of CA15-3 and age, clinical stage, as well as the number of lymph nodes involved. They found elevated levels of CA 15-3 in 10% of patients with stage I, 20% with stage II, 40% with stage III, and 75% with stage IV breast cancer (Keyhani et al., 2005).

23.5.1.2.1.2 MCA, MSA, and CA 549 Mucin like carcinoma-associated antigen (MCA) is a macromolecular glycoprotein belonging to the heterogeneous family of mucins (Ogawa et al., 2000). It has a molecular weight of 35 kDa and has been tested for breast cancer detection, although it is not widely used as a biomarker (Seregni et al., 2008).

Mammary serum antigen (MSA) is a mucin-like glycoprotein of molecular weight of 30 kDa (Stacker et al., 1988). It is defined by the antibody 3EL.2 and is an important biomarker in breast cancer detection (Smart et al., 1990; Nicolini et al., 2006).

Cancer antigen 549 (CA549) is an acidic glycoprotein of molecular weight of around 400–512 kDa (Chan et al., 1988). It is a serum antigen defined by the monoclonal antibody BC4E 549 and belongs to the polymorphic epithelium mucins (PEMs) (Dnistrian et al., 1991). Elevated levels of CA 549 have been reported in serum of breast cancer patients by using sensitive immunoassays. However, these assays have high sensitivity and specificity for advanced breast cancer than the early-stage breast cancer (Malati, 2007).

Gion et al. evaluated serum levels of CA549, CA15.3, and MCA markers from 184 healthy women and 237 patients with primary breast cancer by using immunometric assay technique. All these three markers significantly associated with tumor size and lymph node status and thus could be effective indicators of the tumor (Gion et al., 1994).

Nicolini et al. evaluated MCA, CEA, CA15.3, and tissue polypeptide antigen (TPA) markers in serum samples of 289 breast cancer patients aged between 27 and 80 years (Ikeda et al., 2004). In this study, they compared sensitivity and specificity of MCA with that of CEA, CA15.3, and TPA for early detection of relapse. Moreover, they compared the diagnostic accuracy and predictive value of the MCA–CA15.3 association to that of CEA–TPA–CA15.3 panel. MCA sensitivity was higher than that of CEA or TPA or CA15.3, while specificity of MCA was similar to TPA and lower than that of CEA and CA15.3. MCA–CA15.3 association showed higher sensitivity but lower specificity, accuracy, and positive predictive value than CEA–TPA–CA15.3 panel. These findings concluded that CEA–TPA–CA15.3 panel is more accurate than MCA–CA15.3 association and can detect early relapsed patients with limited metastatic disease, thereby suggesting more favorable prognosis (Nicolini et al., 2006).

Verring et al. in their study analyzed serum levels of CA 549, MCA, and CA 15-3 from 56 healthy women, 63 primary breast cancer patients, and 232 breast cancer patients with different stages. They reported elevated serum levels of CA 549, MCA, and CA 15-3 markers in the patients with breast cancer, thereby suggesting them as good indicators for predicting the disease extent as well as prognosis (Verring et al., 2011).

23.5.1.2.2 Carcinoembryonic Antigen

CEA is a serum glycoprotein of 200 kDa and belongs to the immunoglobulin gene superfamily (Schumann et al., 2004). It is expressed in normal mucosal cells and is found to be overexpressed in a variety of malignancies including breast cancer (Park et al., 2008b). It is detected in the serum of cancer patients by using radioimmunoassay or enzyme-linked immunosorbent assay (ELISA) and can also be determined by immunohistochemical analysis of biopsy samples (Ikeda et al., 1994). In breast tumors, CEA is more prevalent in ductal compared to the lobular carcinomas. Since it has been found in patients with DCIS, CEA could be used as an early marker of the tumorigenic process. High levels of CA15-3 and/or CEA in breast cancer patients is an indicative of metastatic disease (Molina et al., 2010). Recent reports suggested that CEA and CA15-3 are the markers used for early detection of recurrent of the disease (Ghasabeh and Keyhanian, 2013).

23.5.1.2.3 Cytokeratins

Fragments of cytokeratin 8, 18, and 19 are proposed as serum markers for early-stage breast cancer (Giovanella et al., 2002; Olofsson et al., 2007; Cîmpean et al., 2008; Habets et al., 1988).

23.5.1.2.3.1 Cytokeratin 19/CYFRA21-1 Cytokeratin 19 fragment (CK19), also known as CYFRA21-1, is an acidic cytoplasmic protein that has been reported in the serum of cancer patients (Marrakchi et al., 2008; Kosacka and Jankowska, 2009). It is a member of the intermediate filament group of proteins with a molecular weight of 40 kDa and is the most widely studied biomarker in the early detection of breast cancer (Oremek et al., 2007; Chang et al., 2009). Serum CYFRA 21-1 levels have a prognostic and predictive value for detecting disease relapse as well as the treatment efficacy (Nakata et al., 2004; Xenidis et al., 2009; Saloustros et al., 2011). Stathopoulou et al. were the first to detect the presence of CK-19 mRNA in the peripheral blood of patients with stages I and II breast cancer before initiation of adjuvant therapy (Stathopoulou et al., 2002).

Xenidis et al. evaluated the clinical relevance of CK-19 mRNA-positive circulating tumor cells (CTCs) in a total of 437 patients who had received adjuvant chemotherapy for stage I–III cancer by using a quantitative real-time (RT)-PCR assay. CK-19 mRNA-positive CTCs were detected in 179 patients before chemotherapy (41.0%). Around 51% patients with CK-19 mRNA-positive disease turned negative after adjuvant chemotherapy and around 22% of patients with initial CK-19 mRNA-negative disease became positive. These findings suggest that the detection of CK-19 mRNA-positive CTCs in the blood after adjuvant chemotherapy is an independent risk factor indicating the presence of chemotherapy-resistant residual disease (Xenidis et al., 2009; Danila et al., 2007).

The prognostic value of CK-19 mRNA-positive CTCs has been found to be associated with the hormone receptor status (Saloustros et al., 2011). Ignatiadis et al. observed that detection of CK-19 mRNA-positive CTCs before adjuvant chemotherapy in early stages was related to the status of ER and HER2. The poor clinical outcome was observed in patients with ER-negative, triple-negative, and HER 2-positive early-stage cancer (Ignatiadis et al., 2007). Gaforio et al. found that CK-19 mRNA-positive CTCs correlated with ER status in a positive manner, thereby indicating poor clinical outcome (Gaforio et al., 2003; Lianidou and Markou, 2011).

23.5.1.2.3.2 TPA and TPS TPA is a circulating complex of polypeptide fragments of low molecular weight (LMW) cytokeratins 8, 18, and 19 (Barak et al., 2004). These three cytokeratins are characteristic of internal epithelium and are widely distributed in normal tissues and in tumors derived from them. These fragments are shed into the bloodstream during necrosis and lysis of the carcinoma cells (Śliwowska et al., 2006). TPA has been reported as a marker of cell proliferation and its elevated levels in serum have been found in a variety of cancers including breast, lung, gastrointestinal, urological, and gynecological cancers (Sugita et al., 2002; Barak et al., 2004). It is used in the early diagnosis, treatment planning, as well as follow-up of breast cancer. It is known to be a sensitive but nonspecific tumor marker; however, along with other serum markers (Beverly, 2009), TPA helps in monitoring the disease (Malati, 2007).

Tissue polypeptide-specific antigen (TPS) is a specific epitope structure of a peptide in serum associated with human cytokeratin 18 (Gonzalez-Quintela et al., 2006). It is associated with the proliferative activity of breast tumors (Liska et al., 2007; Paulin-Levasseur et al., 2011) and its presence indicates poor disease-free survival (Ahn et al., 2013).

Śliwowska et al. analyzed serum levels of CA 15-3, TPA, and TPS in 90 female breast cancer patients at various stages of the disease. They found a positive association between the percentage of women with increased levels of all the three markers and the advanced stage of the disease. Their results suggested that the serum levels of CA 15-3, TPA, and TPS may be useful markers to establish the stage of the disease and would help in deciding the treatment options (Śliwowska et al., 2006).

23.5.1.2.4 HER-2

C-erbB-2/HER2/neu is the most frequently used and best-known biomarker (Fritz et al., 2005) that is overexpressed in 20%–30% of patients with breast cancer (Fiszman and Jasnis, 2011). This oncoprotein is cell membrane bound but its extracellular domain is shed into circulation; thus, it becomes a potent serum biomarker (Carney, 2007). Elevated c-erbB-2/HER2/neu protein levels have been found in the serum of patients with breast carcinoma and have been associated with poor clinical outcome (Lipton et al., 2002). It is a key biomarker that is useful to detect therapy response as well as recurrence in patients with diagnosed breast carcinoma (Misek and Kim, 2011).

23.5.1.2.5 Mammaglobin

Mammaglobin is a member of the secretoglobin family, mapped on to the human chromosome 11q13, that is overexpressed in around 70%–80% of primary and metastatic breast cancer tissues (Bhargava et al., 2007; Rehman et al., 2010).

Zehentner et al. studied peripheral blood samples from 147 breast cancer patients and 50 healthy controls. The samples were tested for mammaglobin gene expression by a multigene RT-PCR assay and for serum mammaglobin protein by a sandwich ELISA assay. Mammaglobin expression was detected in 61% of blood samples from women with confirmed breast cancer and was not found in 50 healthy controls. Circulating

TABLE 23.8

Serum Biomarkers for Early Detection of Breast Cancer

Markers	Structure	Function	References
CA 15-3	Glycoprotein	Mucins	Chourb et al. (2011)
CA27.29	Glycoprotein	Mucins	Klee et al. (2004)
MCA	Glycoprotein	Mucins	Ogawa et al. (2000)
CA549	Glycoprotein	Mucins	Beveridge et al. (1988)
CEA	Glycoprotein	Cell–cell interaction	Bidard et al. (2011)
CK19	Protein	Cytokeratin	Molina et al. (2006)
TPA	Protein	Cytokeratin	Nolen et al. (2008)
TPS	Protein	Tumor-associated antigen	Duffy (2006)
HER-2 (shed form)	Protein	Cell proliferation	Carney (2007)
Mammaglobin	Immunoglobulin	Cell signaling	Brown et al. (2006)
RS/DJ-1	Protein	Circulating tumor antigen	Naour F et al. (2001)

mammaglobin protein was detected in 70% of the samples of the breast cancer sera. The RT-PCR assay and the ELISA for mammaglobin produced a combined sensitivity of 84% and specificity of 97% suggesting that these are valuable tools in diagnosis and prognosis of breast cancer (Zehentner et al., 2004).

Bernstein et al. performed an ELISA-based study to identify the expression of mammaglobin in a sera from 56 healthy control and 26 metastatic breast cancer patients. The level of mammaglobin was significantly high in diseased group as compared to the healthy controls. Thus, mammaglobin protein is an important serum marker for breast cancer diagnosis (Bernstein et al., 2005).

Chen et al. investigated CK19, human mammaglobin, and CEA-positive CTCs from peripheral blood of 50 patients with early-stage breast cancer (Van der Auwera et al., 2008). The study was carried before giving any systemic adjuvant therapy, and it suggested that CK19, mammaglobin, and CEA markers have important predictive and prognostic value in detection of the disease (Chen et al., 2010). In Table 23.8, different serum biomarkers along with their structure and function have been mentioned that could be used in early detection.

23.5.1.2.6 Autoantibody Biomarkers

Serum and other body fluids of the cancer patients are rich sources of antigens, glycoproteins, CTCs, and autoantibodies that could be used as biomarkers for the early detection (Zhong et al., 2008). These autoantibodies are stable, highly specific, and easily purified from serum and are readily detected with well-validated secondary reagents (Anderson et al., 2011). Detection of serum antibodies against tumor antigens may provide reliable serum markers for cancer diagnosis and prognosis (Macdonald et al., 2012). Chapman et al. detected the presence of autoantibodies against the known tumor-associated proteins such as p53, c-myc, HER2, NY-ESO-1 (cancer/testis antigen), BRCA1, BRCA2, and MUC1 antigens from serum samples of 94 normal controls, 97 primary breast cancer patients, and 40 patients with DCIS by ELISA. Elevated levels of antibodies in serum samples against one or more of these tumor-associated antigens were observed in 64% of the primary breast cancer patient sera and 45% of patients with DCIS at a specificity of 85%. These findings concluded that autoantibody assays against a panel of antigens could be used as biomarkers in the detection and diagnosis of early breast cancer (Chapman et al., 2007).

23.5.1.2.7 Circulating Tumor Cell Biomarkers

CTCs are the key predictive markers in breast cancer (Bidard et al., 2012; Cohen et al., 2008) and their detection is useful in prognosis, diagnosis, prediction of response to therapy, as well as treatment of primary or metastatic disease (Swaby and Cristofanilli, 2011; Danila et al., 2007; Cohen et al., 2008). Wiedswang et al. observed that isolated tumor cells present in bone marrow from stage I and II breast cancer patients predict unfavorable clinical outcome (Wiedswang et al., 2004). Similar findings were observed by Braun et al. wherein they analyzed bone marrow micrometastasis in breast cancer patients of stage I, II, and III, indicating reduced disease-free and overall survival (Braun et al., 2005). There are multiple approaches to detect CTCs in the blood that include immunocytochemical methods, cell search system, and RT-qPCR (Auwera et al., 2010). Among these, multi-marker qRT-PCR is one of the most sensitive and specific method utilized for the molecular detection of circulating cancer cells in blood (Mario Giuliano et al., 2011; Nadal et al., 2012). Circulating tumor markers such as HER2/neu; p53 autoantibodies; cytokeratin-positive cells; autoantibodies to nucleophosmin (NPM); serum soluble vascular cell adhesion molecules (VCAMs) such as intracellular adhesion molecule-1 (ICAM-1), VCAM-1, and E-selectin; and CK-19 mRNA-positive cells are some of the interesting and mostly studied biomarkers that can predict progression-free and overall survival of the patients (Nicolini et al., 2011).

23.5.2 Noninvasive Biomarkers under Development in Breast Cancer

23.5.2.1 Tear Fluid Biomarkers

Tear fluid offers a potential noninvasive source of biomarkers (Mann and Tighe, 2007). It is composed of a complex mixture of mucins, glycoproteins, unglycosylated proteins, peptides, lipids, lysozyme, lactoferrin, secretory immunoglobulin A (sIgA), lipocalin, and lipophilin (Li, 2010). Tear biomolecules have been presumed to act as biomarkers for local eye diseases, autoimmune diseases (Sjogren's syndrome), ocular bacterial infections (trachoma), diabetes, as well as different cancers (Wu and Zhang, 2007; Lebrecht et al., 2009; Zhou et al., 2009; Csősz et al., 2012). The global interest is rising in using tear biomarkers for prognosis as well as diagnosis of breast cancer because the collection of tears is relatively simple, safe, noninvasive, inexpensive, and repetitive with minimal discomfort to the patients (Li, 2010; Böhm et al., 2012; Yong, 2010). However, tear fluid biomarkers have not been clinically assessed due to few hurdles such as low throughput, lack of automation potential, and the requirement of large sample volume (Kelly et al., 2011). Another challenge is the need for highly sensitive and reliable techniques for analysis of small amount of tear samples to ensure reproducible and quantifiable results (Li, 2010; Karns and Herr, 2011).

Lebrecht et al. had established protein biomarker profile from tear fluid samples of 50 breast cancer patients and 50 healthy women by using SELDI-TOF MS technique (Kann, 2007). They generated a panel of 20 tear biomarkers that differentiate the breast cancer patients from healthy controls with 70.94% accuracy and approximately 70% specificity and sensitivity. The study suggested that the proteomic pattern of tear fluid may be useful in the diagnosis as well as high-throughput biomarker discovery (Lebrecht et al., 2009; Ou et al., 2001). The hurdles in tear fluid biomarker discovery highlight the need for standard sampling procedure as well as very sensitive techniques for detection.

23.5.2.2 Salivary Biomarkers

Over the past decade, considerable efforts have been expended to discover and validate the salivary biomarkers for the noninvasive detection of breast cancer by using transcriptomic and proteomic approaches (Al-Tarawneh et al., 2011). Several studies have been conducted to detect putative salivary biomarkers for early detection of breast cancer wherein the potential use of salivary proteins such as c-erbB-2, VEGF, EGF, and CEA has been implicated (Brooks et al., 2008; Zhang et al., 2010; Streckfus et al., 2012).

23.5.2.3 Heat Shock Proteins

Heat shock proteins (HSPs) are a family of highly conserved proteins that play an important role in the regulation of apoptosis (Gupta and Knowlton, 2005). Desmetz et al. showed that HSP60 could be considered as a relevant tumor-associated antigen for early-stage DCIS detection (Desmetz et al., 2008; Hamrita et al., 2010).

23.6 Genetic Biomarkers

Cancer involves deregulation of gene expression profiles and disruption of molecular networks (Bhatt et al., 2010). Various genetic alterations that have been found to be associated with cancer include nonrandom mutations and single-nucleotide polymorphisms (SNPs), insertions, deletions, and translocations/rearrangements within the regulatory region of the gene (Sadikovic et al., 2008). Copy number variations as well as microsatellite instability (MSI) are also known to play a significant role in breast tumorigenesis (Sadikovic et al., 2008; Lee et al., 2001; Ana et al., 2012). Recent advances in high-throughput genomics as well as application of integrative approaches have resulted in the discovery of promising candidate biomarkers that would help in diagnosis and better prognosis of the disease (Hicks et al., 2011; Van der Akker, 2011).

23.6.1 Genetic Variations

23.6.1.1 Mutations and SNPs in Breast Cancer

Genomic instability refers to an increased rate of genomic alteration that plays an important role in cancer development (Kwei et al., 2010). Germ line mutations in several genes, due to an abnormal number of centrosomes, inefficient DNA repair, and unwanted telomere maintenance, confer a high risk in developing breast cancer (Antoniou et al., 2008). Several genes have been shown to exhibit germ line mutations in breast cancer that include TP53, core-binding factor subunit beta (CBFB), phosphatidylinositol-4,5-bisphosphate 3-kinase (PIK3CA), v-akt murine thymoma viral oncogene homolog 1 (AKT1), GATA3, mitogen-activated protein kinase kinase kinase 1 (MAP3K1), and v-erb-b2 erythroblastic leukemia viral oncogene homolog 2 (ERBB2) (Usary et al., 2004; Ralhan et al., 2007; Lim et al., 2009; Kancha et al., 2011; Banerji et al., 2012). Germ line mutations in BRCA1 and BRCA2 genes have been linked to the development of hereditary breast cancers (Mote et al., 2004). Telomere dysfunction has also been regarded as one of the possible mechanisms responsible for genomic instability (Artandi and DePinho, 2000). It has been reported to play an imperative role in situ progression of breast cancer from ductal hyperplasia to DCIS (Chin et al., 2004).

Besides the earlier mutations, SNPs have been reported as the primary cause of genetic disorders in humans and may be used as therapeutic markers in determining the individual's risk of developing breast cancer (Gobbi et al., 2006; Onay et al., 2006). SNPs refer to single-nucleotide variation in an individual's genome that may occur within the coding sequences of genes, noncoding regions of genes, or in the intergenic regions (Onay et al., 2006; Schmid et al., 2012). SNPs are divided into normal and abnormal type wherein the former polymorphisms occur in the DNA sequence that does not alter the normal protein structure. In abnormal SNPs, polymorphisms occur in the DNA sequence that encodes for the structural or functional domains of the protein. Abnormal SNPs have been found to be involved in the development of breast cancer (Huang et al., 2010). Approximately 500,000 noncoding, 200,000 silent coding, and 200,000 replacement coding SNPs are likely to occur in the human genome (Halushka et al., 1999).

Onay et al. in their study have reported a cross talk among genes/SNPs from DNA repair, cell cycle, immune system, and cancer metabolism pathways. Recently it has been shown that breast cancer-associated SNPs are enriched in the cistromes (set of cis-acting targets for a transacting factor) of forkhead box protein A1 (FOXA1), ESR1, and the epigenome of histone H3 lysine 4 monomethylation (H3K4me1) (Cowper-SalLari et al., 2012). FOXA1 is highly correlated with ERα^+ and PR$^+$ protein expression as well as endocrine signaling in breast cancer (Badve et al., 2007; Albergaria et al., 2009). FOXA1 acts as a marker to identify ERα^+ cancers that are resistant to endocrine therapy. In ERα^- breast cancer, the expression of FOXA1 is highly correlated with improved disease-free survival. Overexpression of neurogenic locus notch homolog protein 2 (NOTCH2) has been reported in the patients with rs11249433 SNP, which has been reported to promote the development of ER+ luminal tumors (Fu et al., 2010a). Table 23.9 enlists the different mutated genes, type of mutations involved, and their role in breast cancer.

23.6.1.2 Insertions, Deletions, Translocations

Chromosome rearrangements such as translocations, inversions, and deletions have been frequently reported in breast cancer (Hanahan and Weinberg, 2000; Albertson et al., 2003). The aberrant function of the genes may result from naturally occurring DNA polymorphisms that include gene amplification or duplication, deletion, or insertion in coding regions and splice sites, chromosomal translocation, as well as inversion (Futreal et al., 2004; Kolusayin et al., 2005). Such aberrations may lead to changes in genome copy number, chromosome structure, as well as epigenetic modifications that may have been reported to suppress the expression of tumor suppressor genes or activate the oncogenes leading to breast cancer development (Feinberg Tycko, 2004; Mitelman et al., 2004; Ushijima, 2005). For example,

TABLE 23.9

List of Mutated Genes, Type of Mutation, and Their Role in Breast Cancer

Mutated Genes	Full Form	Type of Cancer	Type of Mutation	Role in Breast Cancer
BRCA1 and BRCA2	Breast cancer type 1 susceptibility protein	Hereditary breast cancer	Somatic/point mutations	• Uncontrolled cell proliferation
CBFB	Core-binding factor subunit beta	ER-positive breast cancer	Recurrent mutations	• Involved in metastasis
TP53	Tumor protein 53	Node-positive breast cancer	Somatic mutations	• Controls cell fate in response to DNA damage • It has a specific role in blocking homologous recombination between divergent sequences.
PIK3CA	Phosphatidylinositol-4, 5-bisphosphate 3-kinase	ER-positive breast cancer	Hot-spot mutations	• Activate the PI3K pathway
AKT1	V-akt murine thymoma viral oncogene homolog	ER-positive breast cancer	Somatic mutations	
GATA3	Trans-acting T-cell-specific transcription factor	ER-positive breast cancer	Somatic mutations	• Involved in metastasis, aggressive tumor development • Deletion of GATA3 in the mammary epithelium is involved in morphogenesis and differentiation of luminal epithelial cells
MAP3K1	Mitogen-activated protein kinase kinase kinase 1	ER-positive breast cancer and luminal-type breast cancer	Somatic mutations	• *MAP3K1* encodes serine/threonine protein kinases that play a major role in the activation of JUN signaling pathway.
ERBB2	v-erb -b2 erythroblastic leukemia viral oncogene homolog 2	Her2-enriched and luminal B subtypes, typically have ERBB2 amplification	Point mutations	• ErbB2 overexpression leads to increased chemoresistance. • It is also associated with increased metastasis.
MAGI3–AKT3 fusion gene	Membrane-associated guanylate kinase-3-v-aktmurinethymomaviraloncogenehomolog3	Triple-negative breast cancer	Somatic mutations	• MAGI3–AKT3 translocation and deletion results in loss of function of a tumor suppressor gene PTEN and activation of an oncogene AKT3.

BRCA1-deficient tumors have been reported to exhibit gross mutations (inversions, deletions) at the locus of tumor suppressor gene PTEN resulting into its dysfunction (Heikkinen et al., 2011).

23.6.1.3 Copy Number Variations

Several studies have demonstrated the role of DNA copy number variation (CNV) in normal development and disease (Krepischi et al., 2012). CNV deletions have been reported in almost 30% of genes involved in breast cancer development that include BRCA1, BRCA2, APC, SMAD4, tumor protein p53 (TP53), as well as mismatch repair genes human mutL homolog 1 (hMLH1) and human mutS homolog 2 (hMSH2) (Krepischi et al., 2012; Ana et al., 2002).

23.6.1.4 Microsatellite Instability

Microsatellites/short tandem repeats (STRs) are simple sequence repeats of 2–6 base pairs in the human genome (Turnpenny and Ellard, 2005). These are genetic markers having biological functions, according to their location, such as affecting protein coding (in coding regions) or regulating gene expression (in regulatory regions) (Gemayel et al., 2010; Lacroix-Triki et al., 2010). They are involved in genetic mapping, forensic analysis, and bone marrow engraftment monitoring (Gymrek et al., 2012). MSI results from defects in DNA mismatch repair, leading to mutations at simple sequence repeats (microsatellites) (Siah et al., 2000). The reported incidence of MSI in breast cancers is 5%–30% (Lee et al., 2001; Kamat et al., 2012; Fernando et al., 2005). Microsatellites in the ER (ESR1, ESR2) and androgen receptor (AR) genes have been hypothesized to be predisposing factors for breast cancer. Over the last decade, various studies have been conducted to test the relationship between these three microsatellites and breast cancer risk in men and women (Zheng et al., 2012).

MSI, a type of genetic instability involving frequent errors during the replication of short nucleotide repeats, is mostly due to a defective DNA mismatch repair gene such as hMSH2, hMLH1, hPMS2, and hMSH6 (Anghel et al., 2006; Lin et al., 2007; Stacey et al., 2010; Huo et al., 2012). Two MSI phenotypes have been described in cancer that include MSI-high (MSI-H) cancers, resulting from defective mismatch repair, and MSI-low (MSI-L) tumors, having lower levels of MSI but are not associated with defective mismatch repair (Calvo et al., 2000; Cox et al., 2006). Murata et al. in their study have investigated the MSI, protein expression of hMSH2 and hMLH1, as well as genetic and epigenetic modifications of these genes in sporadic breast tumors. They revealed the association of MSI with reduced expression of hMLH1 and hMSH2 genes in the patients with sporadic breast tumors. They have also shown that the tumors with MSI contain both genetic and epigenetic modifications of these mismatch repair genes (Murata et al., 2002; Fonseca et al., 2005). MSI has been reported in a number of breast cancer-related genes such as BAT25, BAT-26, BAT-40, D17S250, D5S346, D2S123, D18S55, D18S58, mutation frequency decline-28 (MFD-28), mutation frequency decline-41 (MFD-41), and tumor protein p53ALU repeat polymorphism (TP53ALU) (Luqmani and Matthew, 2004; Fonseca et al., 2005; Lee et al., 2010; Kamat et al., 2012). MSI, thus, plays a chief role in the genomic instability and tumorigenesis in sporadic breast cancer and can serve as a therapeutic target in future.

23.7 Epigenetic Biomarkers

Epigenetics refers to the study of heritable changes in gene expression with no change in the gene sequence (Sadikovic et al., 2008). DNA methylation, histone tail modifications, posttranslational modifications, as well as alterations in miRNA expression profiles are the most important epigenetic changes associated with the cancer (Veeck and Esteller, 2010).

23.7.1 Methylation Biomarkers in Breast Cancer

DNA methylation plays an important role in chromatin organization, silencing of transposable elements, X chromosome inactivation, tissue-specific expression, and genetic imprinting (Miranda and Jones, 2007; Levenson and Melniko, 2012). Methylation has been reported as one of the imperative factors in tumor development and thus may serve as a valuable biomarker in breast cancer early detection (Kornegoor et al., 2012). During the process of tumorigenesis, hypermethylation at tumor suppressor genes leads to silencing of transcription, cancer initiation, as well as progression (Brook et al., 2009). It has been found that around 600–10,000 genes show aberrant methylation in a single tumor (Ushijima and Asada, 2010). Within these genes, some are important in cancer development, whereas some code for important miRNAs (Costello et al., 2000; Momparler, 2003; Jones and Baylin, 2007; Esteller, 2008; Novak et al., 2009). Moreover, not only the malignant cells but the surrounding tissue also shows defective methylation pattern (Yan et al., 2006).

23.7.1.1 Methylation Markers in Nipple Fluid

Nipple aspiration is a noninvasive procedure and the aspirate fluid is known to contain breast epithelial cells (Fabian et al., 2005). Methylation of *GSTP1,* RARB, CDKN2A/p16INK4a, p14^{ARF}, RASSF1A, and DAPK genes has been reported in breast cancer by a number of studies (Suijkerbuijik et al., 2010). Genes such as CDKN2A, CCND2 (cyclin D2), APC, SCGB3A1, RASSF1, TWIST1, or RARB have been shown to be associated with the history of breast cancer (Suijkerbuijik et al., 2010).

23.7.1.2 Methylation Markers in Blood

Methylation has been found to be rarely detectable in serum or plasma of healthy individuals than that of the patients with breast cancer. Matuschek et al. in their study collected serum samples from 85 breast cancer patients and 22 healthy controls and analyzed the methylation status of APC, RASSF1A, ESR1, CDKN2A/p16, and GSTP1 genes. They observed the hypermethylation of APC, RASSF1A, GSTP1, and ESR1 in 29%, 26%, 18%, and 38% of breast cancer patients, respectively (Jin et al., 2008). On the other hand, hypermethylation of ESR1 and RASSF1A, APC, and GSTP1 was found to be around 23%, 9%, and 6% in healthy controls, respectively. They also found a strong correlation between the hypermethylation of GSTP1 and ESR1 with Her2/neu-status of cancer patients (Matuschek et al., 2010).

Sebova et al. analyzed the DNA methylation levels of RASSF1A and CDH1 genes in blood samples collected from 92 breast cancer patients and 50 healthy controls. They observed methylation of RASSF1A in 82.6% and CDH1 in 21.7% of breast cancer patients. However, no methylation of these genes was found in healthy controls. A positive correlation was observed between the elevated levels of RASSF1A methylation with the tumor size, lymph node status, as well as TNM stage (Zeinab et al., 2012). Thus RASSF1A and CDH1 genes could be useful methylation markers for breast cancer detection (Sebova et al., 2011).

Barekati et al. investigated the methylation profiles of cancer-related genes APC, bridging integrator 1 (BIN1), bone morphogenetic protein 6 (BMP6), BRCA1, cystatin E/M (CST6), ESR-b, GSTP1, p14/ARF, p16/CDKN2A, p21/CDKN1A, PTEN, and TIMP3, in the axillary lymph node metastasis in breast cancer. They reported a higher rate of methylation of genes APC, BMP6, BRCA1, and p16 genes in the lymph node metastasis than in the normal tissue, thereby suggesting them to be useful for screening metastasis (Barekati et al., 2012). In Table 23.10, the methylation markers found in the blood of breast cancer patients have been enlisted.

23.7.2 miRNAs as Biomarkers

miRNAs or miRs are a major class of small endogenous noncoding RNA molecules, 22 nucleotides long, and were described in 1993 by Lee et al. (1993). Many miRNAs have been found to be involved in several human cancers, including breast cancer (Farazi et al., 2011). The loss of several tumor suppressor miRNAs (miR-206, miR-17-5p, miR-125a, miR-125b, miR-200, let-7, miR-34a miR-335, miR-27b, miR-126, miR-101, miR-145, miR-146a/b, miR-205, miR-31) and the overexpression of certain oncogenic miRNAs (miR-21, miR-155, miR-10b, miR-373, miR-520c, miR-27a, miR-221/222) have been observed in many breast cancers (Heneghan et al., 2010; Day et al., 2010). The gene networks implicated by these miRNAs are still largely unknown, although their key targets have been identified (Thomas et al., 2010). Measurement of the miRs in plasma or serum from the cancer patients is a promising approach for the prognosis, diagnosis, and theragnosis of breast and other cancers (Heneghan et al., 2011). Lawrie et al. first identified serum miRNAs in patients with diffuse large B-cell lymphoma (Lawrie et al., 2008). In a study done by Schrauder et al. in 2012, microarray-based miRNA profiling on whole blood of 48 early-stage breast cancer patients was performed and 57 healthy individuals were kept as control. They found that 59 miRNAs were differentially expressed in whole blood of the early-stage patients compared to the healthy controls, out of which 13 were upregulated and 46 were downregulated. These results suggested that breast cancer is associated with changes in the expression of multiple miRNAs (Schrauder et al., 2012) that may disturb the functioning of network of genes in normal cell signaling pathways. Table 23.9 enlists various early-stage miRNAs that may function as tumor suppressors or activators in breast cancer.

TABLE 23.10

Methylation Markers in Blood, Their Chromosomal Location, and Their Role

Methylation Markers	Full Forms	Chromosome Location	Role	References
CDKN2A/p16^{Ink4A}	Cyclin-dependent kinase inhibitor 2A	9p21	Acts as a tumor suppressor; negative regulator of CDKs and p14(ARF1); an activator of TP53	Rao et al. (2004)
CDH1	Cadherin-1	16q22.1	Acts as a tumor suppressor gene; plays an important role in cell adhesion, thus may keep cancer cells from metastasizing	Rao et al. (2004)
RASSF1	Ras association domain-containing protein 1	3p21.31	Acts as a tumor suppressor	Suijkerbuijk et al. (2010); Voyatzi et al. (2010)
APC	Adenomatous polyposis coli	5q21	Acts as a tumor suppressor; plays an important role in cell attachment and signaling	Rao et al. (2004)
DAPK1	Death-associated protein kinase 1	9q21.33	Acts as a tumor suppressor gene; plays an important role in cell growth, apoptosis	Suijkerbuijk et al. (2010)
RARβ	Retinoic acid receptor beta	3p24	Steroid receptor; antiproliferative	Piperi et al. (2010); Voyatzi et al. (2010)
MGMT	O-6-methylguanine-DNA methyltransferase	10q26	Involving recognition and repair of damaged DNA and subsequent synthesis of new DNA	Piperi et al. (2010)
TMS1	Target of methylation-induced silencing	16p11.2–12	Apoptosis; inflammation	Gordian et al. (2009)
BRCA1	Breast cancer type 1	17q21	Tumor suppressor; DNA damage sensor; signal transducers proliferation; apoptosis; chromatin remodeling	Stefansson et al. (2011); Snell et al. (2008)
ESR1	Estrogen receptor 1	6q25.1	DNA-binding transcription factor; plays an important role in cell division and DNA replication	Martínez-Galán et al. (2008)
pRB	Retinoblastoma protein	13q14.2	Steroid receptor; tumor suppressors; plays an important role in cell growth by inhibiting cell cycle progression	Stefansson et al. (2011)
CCND2	Cyclin D2	12p13.3	Regulator of CDKs whose activity is required for cell cycle G1/S transition	Suijkerbuijk et al. (2010)
CDKN2A	Cyclin-dependent kinase inhibitor 2A	9p21	Negative regulator of CDKs	Debniak et al. (2005)
p16	—	9p21	Acts as a tumor suppressor; regulating the cell cycle	HU et al. (2003)
p14	—	9p21	Acts as a tumor suppressor; stabilizes nuclear p53	Barekat et al. (2012)
SLIT2	Slit homolog 2 protein	4p15.3	Antiproliferative; antimetastasis	Dallol et al. (2002)

TABLE 23.10 (continued)

Methylation Markers in Blood, Their Chromosomal Location, and Their Role

Methylation Markers	Full Forms	Chromosome Location	Role	References
14-3-3σ	Stratifin	1p36.11	G2 checkpoint	Martínez-Galán et al. (2008)
RUNX3	Runt-related transcription factor 3	1p36	Acts as a tumor suppressor; antiproliferative	Fan et al. (2011)
TWIST1	Twist homolog 1	7p21.2	Cancerous cell dissemination	Swift-Scanlan et al. (2011)
SCGB3A1	Secretoglobin 3A1	5q35	Cell growth, cell migration, invasion	Suijkerbuijk et al. (2010)
ATM	Ataxia telangiectasia mutated	11q22-q23	Role in cell division and DNA repair	Brennan et al. (2012)
HSD17β4	Type 4 17-beta-hydroxysteroid dehydrogenase	17q21.2	Steroid hormone receptor	Christensen et al. (2010)

23.7.2.1 Tumor Suppressor miRNAs Involved in Breast Cancer

23.7.2.1.1 miR-206

miR-206 plays an important role in regulation of the ER gene *ERα* (*ESR1*) (Day et al., 2010). It has been shown to be upregulated in ERα-negative breast cancers indicating its possible role in the regulation of *ESR1* (Adams et al., 2007). ERα agonists have been shown to be involved in repressing the expression of miR-206, whereas ERβ agonist have not been found to possess any inhibitory effect on the expression of miR-206 (Adams et al., 2007).

23.7.2.1.2 miR-17-5p

miR-17-5p, also known as miR-91, has been reported to be involved in the regulation of cell proliferation in breast cancer (Eiriksdottir et al., 1998). It has been reported to repress the expression of *AIB1* (oncogene amplified in breast cancer), thereby inhibiting the function of E2F1 and ERα. This further results into inhibition of estrogen-stimulated as well as estrogen-/ER-independent proliferation of breast cancer cells through downregulation of *AIB1* (Hossain et al., 2006; Quin et al., 2008). The gene *CCND1*, which is involved in the proliferation, has also been identified as a direct target of miR-17-5p (Day et al., 2010).

23.7.2.1.3 miR-125a and miR-125b

miR-125a and miR-125b are downregulated in HER2-overexpressing breast cancers (Mattie et al., 2006). In SKBR3 cells (a HER2-dependent human breast cancer cell line), they have been reported to reduce the anchorage dependence, growth, cell motility, and invasive potential (Scott et al., 2007).

23.7.2.1.4 miR-200 Family

miR-200 family of miRNAs include miR-200c and miR-141 (located on chromosome 12) as well as miR-200a/b and miR-429 (located on chromosome 1) (Park et al., 2008a). miR-200 family plays an important role in regulating the tumor progression and metastasis in breast cancer (Korpal and Kang, 2008). It has been reported to suppress "epithelial–mesenchymal transition" (EMT) through downregulation of zinc finger E-box-binding homeobox 1 and 2 (2ZEB1 and ZEB2), which are repressors of the cell–cell contact protein, E-cadherin (Spaderna et al., 2008; Gonzalez-Angulo et al., 2013). EMT is responsible for the malignant transformation of many human cancers by allowing detachment of cells, thereby increasing tumor cell mobility and metastasis (Day et al., 2010). Downregulation of miR-200 has been shown to increase the tumor metastasis in breast cancer (Day et al., 2010). The functional pathway for miR-200 is TGF-β signaling. Gregory et al. found that TGF-β-induced EMT in human Madin–Darby canine kidney (MDCK) epithelial cells resulted into the downregulation of miR-200 (Gregory et al., 2008).

23.7.2.1.5 let-7 Family

The miRNA let-7 (lethal-7) is widely studied tumor suppressor whose expression is downregulated in many cancers including breast cancer. let-7 family miRNAs are critical regulators of proliferation, cell differentiation, self-renewal, as well as tumorigenicity of breast cancer cells (Yu et al., 2007). Reports suggest that let-7 represses the expression of Harvey rat sarcoma viral oncogene (*H-RAS*), high-mobility group AT-hook 2 (*HMGA2*), *LIN28/*zinc finger CCHC domain-containing protein 1, and phosphatidylethanolamine-binding protein 1(*PEBP*) oncogenes involved in tumorigenesis (Lee et al., 2007; Yu et al., 2007). Recently let-7 and HMGA2 have also been reported to be associated with the Raf kinase inhibitory protein (RKIP)-mediated inhibition of invasion and metastasis in breast cancer (Dangi-Garimella et al., 2010). Zhao et al. performed microarray screening of RNA samples obtained from formalin-fixed paraffin-embedded (FFPE) breast tissues of 13 benign, 16 DCIS, and 15 IDC. They found that expression of let-7 family miRNAs was significantly downregulated in DCIS and IDC breast tissues compared to benign tissues. There was an inverse correlation between ER-α expression and several members of let-7 family in the FFPE tissues. The results suggest that let-7 family miRNAs regulate ER alpha signaling in ER-positive breast cancer.

23.7.2.1.6 miR-34a

miR-34a plays an important role in regulation of DNA damage and cellular proliferation in breast cancer (Kato et al., 2009). It has been reported as a direct transcriptional target of p53 and has been found to be downregulated in a number of cancers, including breast cancer (Calin and Croce, 2006; Chang et al., 2007). miR-34a downregulates the expression of CCND1, *cyclin-dependent kinase 6* (CDK6), E2F transcription factor 3 (E2F3), and V-myc myelocytomatosis viral oncogene (MYC), thereby inducing cell cycle arrest in cancer (Sun et al., 2008). Low expression of miR-34a has been found in the cell lines derived from ER/PR/HER2-negative tumors (Kato et al., 2009). Studies have shown the role of miR-34 in governing the expression of genes such as CDK4, CDK6, and BCL2 that are involved in the regulation of cell cycle, proliferation, and survival in breast cancer (Zuoren et al., 2010).

23.7.2.1.7 miR-31

miR-31 is expressed in normal breast cells and has been shown to inhibit the metastasis by repressing the expression of prometastatic breast cancer genes (Zhu et al., 2007; Day et al., 2010). It is moderately decreased in nonmetastatic breast cancer cell lines and is barely detectable in metastatic breast cancer cell lines (Valastyan et al., 2009). The reported target prometastatic genes that are downregulated by miR-31 are frizzled3 (*Fzd3*), integrin α-5 (*ITGA5*), myosin phosphatase Rho-interacting protein (*M-RIP*), matrix metallopeptidase 16 (*MMP16*), radixin (*RDX*), and the ras homolog gene family member A (*RhoA*) (Baranwal and Alahari, 2010). Expression of *ITGA5, RDX,* and RhoA in the breast cancer cells has been shown to abolish the functions mediated by miR-31 such as inhibition of motility and invasion as well as induction of apoptosis (Day et al., 2010). Thus, miR-31 may prove as an attractive therapeutic target for breast cancer.

23.7.2.2 Oncogenic miRNAs Involved in Breast Cancer

23.7.2.2.1 miR-21

miR-21 functions as an oncogene and is one of the most studied miRNAs in cancer (Iorio et al., 2006; Volinia et al., 2006). It regulates the tumor suppressor genes *BCL-2*, tumor suppressor protein tropomyosin 1 (TPM1), programmed cell death protein 4 (*PDCD4*), phosphatase and tensin homolog (*PTEN*), and mammary serine protease inhibitor (*MASPIN*). In breast cancer cell line MCF-7, inhibition of miR-21 has been reported to sensitize the tumor cells to anticancer agents. Overexpression of miR-21 in breast cancer has been correlated to advanced tumor stage, lymph node metastasis, and poor survival of the patient (Yan et al., 2008).

23.7.2.2.2 miR-155

miR-155 expression is elevated in a number of human malignancies including breast cancer (Iorio et al., 2005; Volinia et al., 2006). It has been reported to inhibit the expression of *RhoA*, a gene that plays an important role in many cellular processes such as cell adhesion, motility, polarity, cell junction formation,

TABLE 23.11
List of miRNAs and Their Role in Breast Cancer

Role	Tumor Suppressor miRs	Tumor Activator miRs
Regulation of cell proliferation	miR-17-5p, Let-7, miR-34a	—
Regulation of cell signaling	miR-206, miR-200c	miR-155
Regulation of cell cycle progression	miR-126	miR-27a
Regulation of metastasis and cell invasion	miR-31, miR-335, miR-101 miR-145, miR-27b, miR-126, miR-146a/b, miR-205	miR-10b, miR-373/520c

as well as stability (Boureux et al., 2007; Dagan et al., 2012). It has also been shown to mediate TGF-β-induced EMT and cell invasion in various cells by disrupting the tight junction formation and promoting cell migration and invasion (Kong et al., 2008). Oncogenic role of miR-155 in breast cancer progression has recently been described (Mattiske et al., 2012).

23.7.2.2.3 miR-10b

miR-10b is overexpressed in metastatic cancer cells (Ma et al., 2007). It promotes cell invasion through RhoC–AKT signaling pathway by downregulating the homeobox D10 (HOXD10) gene. Downregulation of HOXD10 activates the pro-metastatic gene ras homologue gene family member C (RHOC) that is involved in cell migration and invasion in breast cancer (Liu et al., 2012).

23.7.2.2.4 miR-373/520c

miR-373/520c promotes tumor invasion and metastasis and its reported target gene is *CD44* (Huang et al., 2008; Keklikoglou et al., 2012). Huang et al., in their study, have reported the role of miR-373 and miR-520c in metastasis and invasion of breast cancer cells. In the study, a nonmetastatic, human breast tumor cell line was transduced with a miRNA expression library and subjected to a trans-well migration assay. The study demonstrated that the ectopic expression of human miR-373 and miR-520c in the cancer cells stimulated the migratory and invasive phenotype (Huang et al., 2008). Table 23.11 enlists different tumor suppressor and activator miRNAs along with their putative role in breast cancer.

23.8 Proteomic Biomarkers of Breast Cancer

Proteomics can be defined as the identification, characterization, and quantification of the proteins in a wide variety of biological samples such as tissues or body fluids (Bantscheff et al., 2007). The analysis of proteins in early-stage cancers has provided new insights into the changes that occur during tumorigenesis (Wulfkuhle et al., 2003; Roy and Shukla, 2008). Proteomics is the choice for discovery of biomarkers as it can bridge the gap between the genetic alterations underlying cancer and cellular physiology (Gast et al., 2009). The recent comprehensive technologies that include protein microarrays, MS such as matrix-assisted laser desorption/ionization time-of-flight mass spectrometry (MALDI-TOF MS) as well as its variant SELDI-TOF MS, and capillary zone electrophoresis (CZE) for proteome analysis have led to the identification of biomarkers that can be specifically applied in clinical diagnosis (Aebersold and Mann, 2003; Simpson and Smith, 2005; Neubauer et al., 2007). A hierarchical cluster analysis of protein profiles in normal and malignant breast tissues has shown the ability of the proteomic biomarkers to differentiate between normal, benign, and different stages of breast cancer (Bertucci et al., 2006).

Tumor tissues as well as their microenvironment are the richest source of potential biomarkers. ER, PR, HER-2, BRCA1, Ki-67, and p53 are well-established invasive protein biomarkers that are in routine use (Ross et al., 2004b). Investigational biomarkers under development include SMAR1, CUX, SATB1, CCND1, BTG3, mitosin, HSPs, adhesion molecules, insulin-like growth factors, and plasminogen activators and inhibitors. Recent studies have identified and validated some more proteomic biomarkers for breast cancer. Elevated levels of galectin-3-binding protein, ALDH1A1, CK19, transferrin, transketolase, thymosin β4 and β10, enolase, vimentin, peroxiredoxin 5, Hsp 70, periostin precursor, RhoA, cathepsin D, and annexin have been reported in breast cancer patients (He et al., 2011). These could serve as promising candidates in guiding tumor classification and predicting response. Ou et al. identified and validated four novel, differentially expressed breast cancer biomarkers ANX1, CRAB, 6-phosphogluconolactonase (6PGL), and CAZ2 by integrative proteomic and gene expression mapping. Despite valuable sample source, there are limitations in tissue sampling due to high invasive procedures involved. This invites attention towards the protein profiling of body fluids (noninvasive procedures involved) to identify more specific biomarkers.

Circulating protein markers are widely accepted because they are easy to sample, readily accessible, reproducible, and sensitive than other markers (Van De Voorde et al., 2012). These include autoantibodies, tumor antigens, cytokeratins, tumor-secreted proteins, normal tissue, and plasma proteins digested by tumor proteases that are found in the serum and plasma (Malati, 2007; Abhilash, 2009). The circulating biomarkers that have been validated by protein profiling include RS/DJ-1, HSPs, MUC1, CA 15-3, CEA, CA 27.29, MCA, MSA and CA 549, cytokeratins, HER-2/neu, p53, α1-acid glycoprotein 2, monocyte differentiation antigen CD14, biotinidase (BTD), glutathione peroxidase 3, HSP27, 14-3-3 sigma, afamin, apolipoprotein E, isoform 1 of inter-alpha-trypsin inhibitor heavy chain H4 (ITIH4), alpha-2-macroglobulin, and ceruloplasmin (Perkins et al., 2003). NAF and ductal lavage fluid (DLF) are traditionally used biological samples for diagnosis of the breast cancer (Misek et al., 2011). However, proteomic profiling of breast NAF and DLF biomarkers could help in identifying specific proteins as potential diagnostic or prognostic markers of breast cancer (Li et al., 2005). Currently available NAF and DLF biomarkers include GCDFP-15, apolipoprotein D (apoD), alpha1-acid glycoprotein (AAG), α-2-HS -glycoprotein, lipophilin b, beta-globin, hemopexin, and vitamin D-binding protein (Alexander et al., 2004; Teng et al., 2010). A panel of protein markers can reflect breast cancer complexity, thereby yielding improved sensitivity and specificity in early detection of the disease.

23.9 Glycobiomarkers

Glycosylation is one of the most important modifications of proteins and lipids and plays an important role in the regulation of many cellular events such as cell–cell and cell–substrate interactions, bacterial adhesion, membrane organization, cell immunogenicity, and protein targeting (Li and d'Anjou, 2009; Zhang et al., 2011b). For example, sialyl-Lewisx (sLex) antigens are the ligands for selectins and are involved in the recruitment of leukocytes to lymphoid tissues and inflammation sites (Varki, 1994; Cazet et al., 2010).

Alteration in glycosylation is a common phenotypic change observed in cancer cells that mainly affects the outer part of glycans, leading to the expression of tumor-associated carbohydrate antigens (TACAs) (Wang, 2005; Cazet et al., 2010). For example, increased β1, 6-branching or increase in sLe^x or sialyl-$Lewis^a$ (sLe^a) antigens or increased sialylation has been observed in *N*-linked and *O*-linked glycans present on cancer cells. These are usually associated with grade, invasion, metastasis, and poor prognosis (Wang et al., 2005). Alteration of glycosylation has been observed in a variety of cancers (Varki et al., 2009; Cazet et al., 2010). These modified glycoforms including glycoproteins, proteoglycans, and glycolipids may serve as the potential glycobiomarkers for the early detection of the disease (Kim et al., 2009). The altered expression of glycoforms on cell surface or in the circulation has highlighted their role in cancer research (Drake et al., 2010). Currently, CA 15-3, CEA, and CA 27.29 are the most common serum glycoproteins with altered glycan profiles that are used as biomarkers for breast cancer (Meany and Chan, 2011). Alterations in the expression of glycosyltransferase (GT) genes result into change in glycosylation pattern that lead to overexpression of tumor-associated antigens sLe^x, s-Le^a, and sialyl-Thomsen-nouvelle (sTn) on the surface of breast cancer cells (Ura et al., 1992;

Narita et al., 1993; Soares et al., 1996). These are usually associated with poor prognosis and reduced overall survival of the patients (Miles et al., 1994).

Nakagoe et al. analyzed the expression of ABH/Lewis-related antigens immunohistochemically from breast cancer tissue samples as an independent prognostic factor of survival without clinicopathological features of the primary tumor (Nakagoe et al., 2002). Raval et al. evaluated alterations in serum levels of sialic acid forms, sialyltransferase, and sialoproteins from 225 breast carcinoma patients to investigate the potential clinical utility of these markers in diagnosis, prognosis, and treatment of breast carcinoma (Raval et al., 2003).

Saldova et al. observed that the high levels of specific serum N-glycans containing sLe^x epitopes (A2F1G1, A3F1G1, A4F1G1, and A4F2G2) from sera of 51 breast cancer patients were associated with CTCs that could provide a new noninvasive approach for prognosis and prediction. Moreover, glycobiomarkers are more stable, thereby making them more suitable for wide population screening (Saldova et al., 2010). Glycan profiling of human sera, blood, and tissue samples by MALDI FT-ICR, MALDI-TOF, electrospray ionization (ESI), and liquid chromatography–mass spectrometry (LC-MS)/MS techniques is an important approach in the emerging potential field of glycobiomarkers (Neubauer et al., 2007; Dunna et al., 2008).

23.10 Lipid Biomarkers

Lipids are the important components of our body and regulate various biological functions including energy metabolism and various signal transduction mechanisms (Simons and Toomre, 2000; Watkins et al., 2002). They have been reported to participate in many human diseases including cancer (Chajès et al., 2011). Various studies have shown a direct association between lipids and incidence of breast cancer. Since altered lipid metabolism and profiling has shown a significant correlation with breast cancer risk, disease status, recurrence, and treatment outcome, lipidomics provides an opportunity to identify reliable lipid markers associated with breast cancer (McGrowder et al., 2011). Lipid profiling of cell extracts, body fluids, and biopsy specimens by using isotope labeling, thin-layer chromatography (TLC), high-performance LC (HPLC), MS technology, MALDI, and ESI techniques has helped in isolation of lipid biomarkers for breast cancer (Wenk, 2005; Hou et al., 2008).

Lipid rafts are cholesterol-enriched, highly dynamic, heterogeneous microdomains of the cell membrane that regulate cell adhesion and membrane signaling through proteins located within these rafts (Simons and Toomre, 2000; Simons and Sampaio, 2011). Recent studies have shown the critical role of lipid rafts in cancer cell adhesion and migration. The lipid molecules include fatty acids, triglycerides, cholesterol, phosphoglycerides, sphingomyelins, glycosphingolipids, ceramide, sphingosine, phosphate phosphatidylcholine (PC), phosphatidylethanolamine (PE), as well as lipoproteins including high-density lipoprotein (HDL), low-density lipoprotein (LDL), and very-low-density lipoprotein (VLDL). These could be used as potential biomarkers for prognosis, diagnosis, as well as treatment of cancer.

Franky Dhaval Shah et al. analyzed plasma lipid profile including cholesterol, HDL, LDL, VLDL, and triglycerides of 70 healthy controls, 30 patients with benign breast disease (BBD), 125 untreated breast cancer patients, and 93 posttreatment follow-up samples by highly sensitive and specific spectrophotometric methods. They found a positive correlation between altered lipid profile levels and breast cancer risk (Shah et al., 2008).

OWiredu et al. investigated lipid profile in 100 breast cancer patients and 100 healthy controls. There was a significant increase in total cholesterol, triglyceride, and LDL cholesterol in the breast cancer patients compared to the controls, thereby suggesting that the alterations in lipid profile are associated with risk of developing breast cancer (Owiredu et al., 2009).

Analysis of breast tissue samples by immunohistochemistry, ultraperformance LC/MS, and other techniques are routinely used for the analysis of invasive lipid biomarkers. Hilvo et al. analyzed the global lipid profiles in 267 human breast cancer tissues. They observed the increased expression of palmitate-containing phosphatidylcholines in breast ER-negative and grade three tumors that was associated with cancer progression and patient survival (Hilvo et al., 2011). Immunohistochemical analyses of lipid metabolism regulating genes acetyl-CoA carboxylase α (ACACA), elongation of very long chain fatty acid-like 1 (ELOVL1), fatty acid synthase (FASN), insulin-induced gene 1x (insulin-induced gene 1), sterol regulatory element-binding protein cleavage-activating protein (SCAP), stearoyl-CoA desaturase (SCD), and thyroid hormone-responsive protein (THRSP) showed that they are highly expressed in clinical breast cancer samples (Hilvo et al., 2011). These findings suggest the diagnostic potential of these lipid makers that could provide early therapeutic options.

Borrelli et al. compared the serum concentrations of cholesterol, HDL cholesterol, triglycerides, and total lipids of women having breast cancer with the patients having BBD. The higher serum concentration of HDL cholesterol was observed in breast cancer patients as compared to benign patients, whereas there was no difference observed in the serum concentration of total cholesterol, triglycerides, and total lipids between the two groups. Their results suggest that high serum HDL cholesterol could be a biochemical index of increased breast cancer risk. They have also shown that the changes in the lipid profile could be associated with increased estrogen activity that is involved in the development of breast cancer (Borrelli et al., 1993). Thus, lipid profile is a promising biomarker for the early detection of breast cancer.

23.11 Metabolomic Biomarkers

Metabolomics includes profiling of the endogenous metabolites present in biological cells and tissues or shed into the body fluids such as serum, plasma, urine, cerebrospinal fluid, tears, saliva, and NAF (Jordan et al., 2009; Serkova and Glunde, 2009). It may play an important role in identification of new prognostic and predictive markers associated with breast cancer progression (Denkert et al., 2012). The altered metabolic activities of cancer cells may generate wide range of metabolites that may help in distinguishing them from their healthy counterparts (Locasale et al., 2010). The analytical platforms used for metabolomic studies are based on nuclear magnetic resonance spectroscopy (NMR), mass spectroscopy or LC-MS, Fourier transform infrared (FTIR) spectrometry, and ultraperformance LC combined with mass spectroscopy (UPLC-MS) (Griffin and Shockcor, 2004).

Nam et al. proposed a systematic computational method for the identification of metabolic biomarkers in urine samples by selecting candidate biomarkers from altered genome-wide gene expression signatures of cancer cells. They have analyzed gene expression profiles in cancer cells and urine samples of 50 breast cancer patients and 50 healthy controls by this method. From the gene expression profiles, they found that nine metabolic pathways (pyrimidine, purine metabolism, valine, leucine and isoleucine, tyrosine metabolism, arachidonic acid metabolism, metabolism of xenobiotics, butanoate metabolism, tryptophan metabolism, and fatty acid metabolism) were altered. Out of these, four metabolic biomarkers that include homovanillate, 4-hydroxyphenylacetate, 5-hydroxy indoleacetate, and urea were found to be altered in breast cancer patients compared to their normal counterparts (Nam et al., 2009). Thus, metabolic markers from urine samples of cancer patients could help not only in discriminating them from their healthy control subjects but also in detecting the early stage of the disease.

Silva et al. studied the urinary metabolomic profile of 26 breast cancer patients and 21 healthy individuals with the aim of investigating the volatile organic metabolites (VOMs) as biomarkers in early diagnosis. They detected the presence of 79 VOMs, belonging to distinct chemical classes, in control as well as breast cancer groups. They observed a significant increase in the levels of (-)-4-carene, 3-heptanone, 1,2,4-trimethylbenzene, 2-methoxythiophene, and phenol in VOMs of cancer patients compared to that of controls. They also identified the presence of dimethyl disulfide in lower amounts in cancer patients. Their study, thus, provided an evidence for the use of VOMs as valuable biomarkers for breast cancer detection (Silva et al., 2012).

23.12 Imaging Biomarkers

Imaging biomarkers play a key role in evaluating the efficacy, activity, and response of new candidate drugs and/or innovative therapeutic regimens that would improve clinical outcome (Silberman et al., 2012). Imaging biomarkers have the ability to assess the molecular events at an early stage and hence in predicting the treatment outcome (Moffat et al., 2006). Anatomic imaging modalities include mammography, planar x-ray, ultrasounds, computed tomography (CT), and MRI (Herranz and Ruibal, 2012). Evidences have suggested that diffusion-weighted (DW) and dynamic contrast-enhanced (DCE) MRI are reliable and quantitative measures implemented in clinical research to noninvasively predict the response in patients with breast cancer following neoadjuvant chemotherapy (Whitcher and Schmid, 2011). Xing et al. have proposed, quantified, and tested two MRI imaging biomarkers such as parenchyma volume and parenchyma enhancement for their ability to assess the breast cancer risk (Xing et al., 2008). MRI has also been shown to improve the detection of early breast cancers in patients with hereditary BRCA mutations (Saslow et al., 2007). However, a few disadvantages of these biomarkers include low specificity, limited sensitivity in detecting DCIS, association with false-positive results, and their inability to determine accurate response to drugs.

Valuable contribution has been made by noninvasive molecular imaging techniques in clinical evaluation and targeted therapeutic interventions (Shankar, 2012). They help to visualize and quantify cellular and physiologic processes in vivo for accurate tumor staging, design individually suited therapies, and assess the drug response and early detection of disease recurrence (Pouliot et al., 2009). Positron emission tomography (PET), scintimammography (SMM), electrical impedance tomography (EIT), T-scan electrical impedance imaging, and galactography are the recent noninvasive molecular imaging tools. Among these, PET molecular imaging gained widespread acceptance for the diagnosis, staging, as well as management of a variety of malignancies, including breast cancer. Molecules related to tumor microenvironment, angiogenesis, hypoxia, metabolisms, apoptosis, proliferation, tumor receptors, and transport proteins are the PET imaging molecular biomarkers (Penuelas et al., 2012).

Fluorodeoxyglucose (FDG)-PET is a primary PET radioactive tracer that includes glucose analogs (FDG) as biomarkers for initial diagnosis and staging of primary breast cancer (Rosen et al., 2007). It accurately differentiates cancerous tissue from its benign counterpart based on the glycolysis rate and glucose avidity of malignant cells (Quon and Gambir, 2005). FDG-PET along with CT is another biomarker that contributes in defining the extent of the disease with improved sensitivity, early assessment of therapeutic response, as well as relapse in patients with advanced tumors (Rosen et al., 2007).

3′-Deoxy-3′-[18F] fluorothymidine (18FLT-PET) is a clinically used biomarker for in vivo imaging of cell proliferation that could predict lesion response with good sensitivity after initiating chemotherapy. Studies have shown that 18FLT-PET positively correlates with Ki67, a proliferation marker in cancer tissues (Vesselle et al., 2002; Shah et al., 2009; Richard et al., 2011).

Apoptosis imaging marker [F-18]-labeled annexin V is a widely studied agent for in vivo study to assess apoptosis. Studies have shown the potential applications of [F-18]-labeled annexin V as an imaging marker for early response to therapy in cancer, acute cerebral and myocardial ischemic injury and infarction, immune-mediated inflammatory disease, and transplant rejection (Toretsky et al., 2004; Li et al., 2008; Oremek et al., 2007).

16α-[18F]-fluoro-17β-estradiol (18 F-FES-PET) is a biomarker that noninvasively assesses the molecular information of ER expression in both primary and tumor metastasis cases and helps in the therapeutic management and prognostic evaluation (Tsuchida et al., 2007).

Imaging biomarker [18F] fluoromisonidazole (18 FMISO-PET) is used to image hypoxia generated by the tumors, thereby improving the diagnostic understanding as well as providing information regarding antiangiogenic therapy in breast cancer patients (Penuelas et al., 2012).

N-[11C] methyl-choline (11C-choline) imaging biomarker has been used to assess the altered choline metabolism in breast cancer (Contractor et al., 2011). 11C/99m Tc-methionine amino acid-based

TABLE 23.12

Imaging Biomarkers for Breast Cancer

Imaging Biomarker	Uses	References
FDG-PET	Initial diagnosis of primary breast cancer and the staging of axillary lymph nodes	Rosen et al. (2007)
18FLT-PET	In vivo imaging of cell proliferation	Shah et al. (2009)
[F-18]-labeled annexin V	Apoptosis imaging marker	Li et al. (2008)
18F-FES-PET	Detection of ER expression in primary and metastasis breast cancer	Tsuchida et al. (2007)
18 FMISO-PET	Imaging biomarker for angiogenesis	Yoo et al. (2005)

radiotracer is used to detect breast cancer (Sharma et al., 2009). ^{99m}Tc-NC100692 and ^{18}F-galacto-RGD are radiolabeled RGD peptides (peptide sequence that consists of arginine–glycine–aspartic acid) that are used for the breast cancer imaging (Axelsson et al., 2010). Apart from these, some other radioactive tracers that are used for the breast cancer imaging include ^{99m}Tc-methylene diphosphonate, ^{99m}Tc-pentavalent DMSA, ^{18}F-fluoride, ^{18}F-fluciclatide, and Tc-99m sestamibi, which offer great promise in breast cancer patients (Massardo et al., 2005; Doot et al., 2010; Tomasi et al., 2011). Table 23.12 enlists various imaging biomarkers used for breast cancer detection.

23.13 Integrative Omics-Based Molecular Markers for Early Diagnosis, Prognosis, and Therapy

Genomics, transcriptomics, proteomics, epigenomics, lipidomics, metabolomics, PG, and bioinformatics are the platforms for identification of novel cancer biomarkers (Sikaroodi et al., 2010; Borgan et al. 2010) (Figure 23.6). All these approaches play an important role in oncology research with differing strengths and limitations. Integration of all these "omics-based approaches" would lead to a better

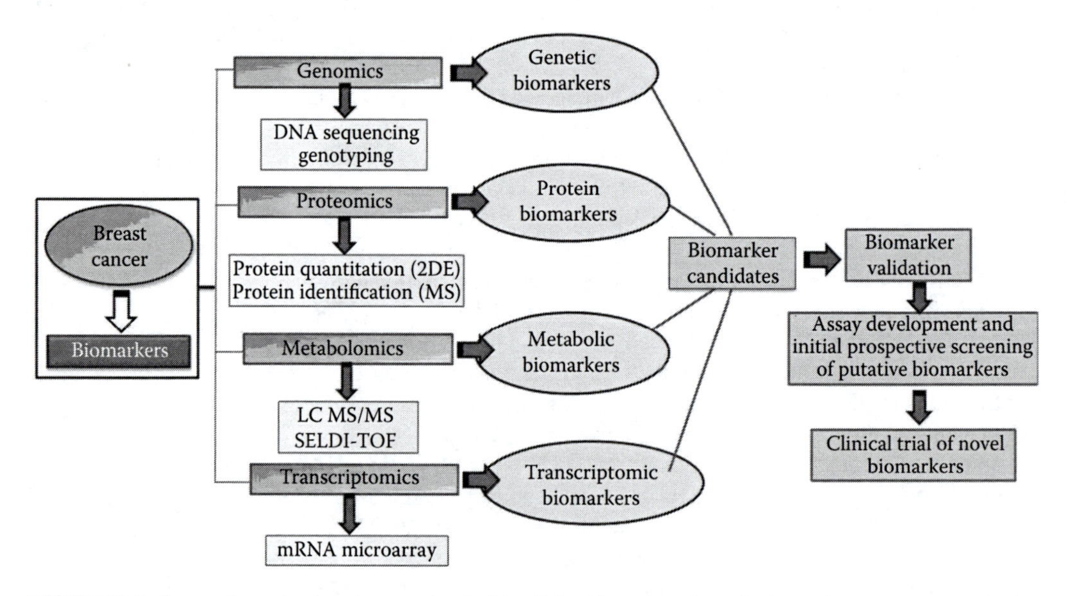

FIGURE 23.6 Integrative omics-based approaches for identifying biomarkers for early diagnosis of breast cancer. Omics-based approaches include genomics, proteomics, metabolomics, and transcriptomics that are platforms for identification of novel and breast cancer-specific biomarker.

understanding of the disease and would help in discovery and initial characterization of candidate biomarkers for cancer staging, prediction of recurrence, prognosis, as well as treatment selection (Palsson and Zengler, 2010).

Cancer is now recognized as systems dysfunction of cellular regulatory pathways caused due to the combination of environmental/lifestyle-related factors and genetic defects such as somatic or germ line mutations, SNPs, copy number alternations, and epigenetic modifications (Shimokawa et al., 2010). Recent developments in high-throughput omics-based technologies have shifted the focus from identification of genes and proteins to mapping the networks of interactions that take place among them (Zhang and Chen, 2011; Pei et al., 2009). Thus, detailed clinical/environmental information together with the molecular networks is required to elucidate the process of carcinogenesis (Abba et al., 2004). Recently, the field of systems biology is gaining significance in elucidation of complex molecular interactions within a cell by combining computational, engineering, and physical analysis along with biological and medical inputs (Wang et al., 2010). The effectiveness of such network-based approaches in the identification of multiple disease markers has been demonstrated in human breast cancer (Pujana et al., 2007). Pujana et al. have identified genes through network modeling strategy that could be potentially associated with higher risk of developing breast cancer. They started with four known tumor suppressor genes of breast cancer (ATM, BRCA1, BRCA2, CHEK2), and by combining gene expression profiles with functional genomic and proteomic data from various species, they could generate a network containing 118 genes linked by 866 potential functional associations (Pujana et al., 2007; Roy and Shukla, 2008). Barh et al. have recently shown the presence of more than one cross talking signaling pathways and targets in most of the breast cancer cases by combining various omics data for breast cancer with integrative bioinformatics approach. They have shown the association between various transcription factors, miRNAs, fetal oncogenes, and pluripotent stem cell factors in the regulation of tumorigenesis (Clarke and Fuller, 2006). The identified transcription factors and miRNAs are differentially expressed in breast cancer and thus have been proposed to be used as early diagnostic and prognostic markers (Barh et al., 2012).

Various open-access as well as commercial tools such as Georgetown Database of Cancer (G-DOC), Oncomine, ArrayExpress, the Stanford Microarray Database, the Gene Expression Omnibus, Integrated Clinical Omics Database (iCOD), International Cancer Genome Consortium (ICGC), and the Cancer Genome Atlas (TCGA) have been developed for storage, analysis, and interpretation of omics-based data. G-DOC is an open-access tool that allows physicians, scientists, and translational researchers to mine and analyze a variety of "omics" data (Madhavan et al., 2011). This would help basic and clinical research through integration of patient characteristics and clinical outcome data with various high-throughput research data. It mainly provides data related to mRNA and miRNA expression, CNVs, and metabolite MS (Madhavan et al., 2011). At present, G-DOC contains data from 24 different studies that include more than 3600 breast cancer patients and around 4400 biospecimens (Georegetown, Lombardi Comprehensive Cancer Center 2013). Oncomine is another microarray database and web-based data mining platform that provides data related to differentially expressed genes across multiple microarray experiments from various cancers (Rhodes et al., 2007). Unlike G-DOC, Oncomine provides only transcriptome data, of which majority of data sets are not openly accessible. ArrayExpress, the Stanford Microarray Database, and the Gene Expression Omnibus repositories provide cancer microarray data but do not allow the user to efficiently mine and analyze the data (Sherlock et al., 2001; Edgar et al., 2002; Rocca-Serra et al., 2003). The other two agencies, ICGC and TCGA, contain omics (genomic) data that are openly accessible and allow us to understand the molecular mechanisms underlying cancer (Zhang et al., 2011a). The iCOD not only includes molecular omics data such as comparative genomic hybridization (CGH) and gene expression profiles but also consists clinical information that include clinical manifestations, medical images (CT, x-ray, ultrasounds, etc), laboratory tests, drug history, pathological findings, and even lifestyle/environmental information (Shimokawa et al., 2010).

23.13.1 Challenges in Translation of Cancer Omics Findings

The increased availability of omics data poses new challenges both for the data management and analysis (Zhang et al., 2012). The major challenge, at bioinformatics level, for example, arises during integration of a transcriptomic data set with a proteomic data set wherein it becomes difficult to map transcript identifiers to protein identifiers (Wang et al., 2009b). For example, the integration of transcriptional and translational data in prokaryotic and some lower eukaryotic organisms becomes easier as per one gene one protein hypothesis. However, in higher eukaryotes, it becomes difficult to integrate the two data sets because the one gene–one protein hypothesis doesn't stand true. In them, a single gene encodes multiple transcripts by means of alternative splicing, transcripts can be translated into multiple protein isoforms, and posttranslational modifications are also involved. The problem becomes even more complex when one tries to integrate a transcriptomic or proteomic data set with a metabolomic, glycomic, or lipidomic data set (Choi and Pavelka, 2011). However, such challenges could be overcome by mapping the enzymes responsible for synthesis or chemical conversion of metabolites with the help of metabolic networks as provided by Kyoto Encyclopedia of Genes and Genomes (KEGG) (Kanehisa and Goto, 2000) or Reactome (Joshi-Tope et al., 2005). Besides, the systems biology markup language (SBML) is one of the successful efforts to develop a unified language to represent complex models of interacting biological molecules (Hucka et al., 2003). However, only few genes encode metabolic enzymes, the rest being structural, regulatory, or signal transduction proteins (Choi and Pavelka, 2011). Thus, it becomes a challenge for the integrative omics data analysis methods to deal with molecules that cannot be directly mapped between the two types of data sets.

Lack of well-defined data standards and standardized nomenclature across different data repositories makes the retrieval and assembly of integrated data sets difficult. Semantic web technologies offer an immediate integration of data, which can be easily queried across different databases (Choi and Pavelka, 2011). They also allow a precise characterization of the "semantics" of the data, that is, the integration between represented entities and their relations. However, use of such technology depends upon the implementation by developers of primary omics databases.

Due to complexity of the available models from multilayered omics data, statistical analysis becomes a big challenge (Ideker et al., 2011). Thus, the models should be established in a way that would ensure highly sensitive, specific, and reproducible results. Other practical challenges include lack of availability of well-defined, clinically characterized cohorts for biomarker evaluation along with information related to collection, handling, and storage of specimens. These challenges can be efficiently overcome by integrative computational methods that include the development of new designs for databases, new software and workflows for integration of heterogeneously distributed data, well-defined mathematical and statistical tools, and analytical methods to identify complex signals in different data sets and upgradation of standards for generating, maintaining, and sharing data. This would ultimately help in identification of authentic omics-based biomarkers that would help in early diagnosis and prognosis of breast cancer.

23.14 Ethnic Group Specific Markers with Specificity, Sensitivitly, and Techniques

Human kallikreins hK2 and hK3, the members of human kallikrein family, are the serine proteases that are downregulated in breast cancer (Borgoño et al., 2004). hK3 is also known as PSA and is a marker of breast as well as prostate cancer (Becker et al., 2001). hK2 and hK3 share significant homology at both DNA and protein level and hK2 may also regulate the activity of hK3 (Yousef and Diamandis, 2001). Studies have shown that systemic progesterone levels, which appear to upregulate hK3, are significantly influenced by ethnicity (Sauter et al., 2002; Carla et al., 2004). Thus, Sauter et al. analyzed the expression of hK2/hK3 in NAF collected from 285 (244 white and 41 black) women who were categorized into risk groups, with no risk factors, having a history of first-degree relative with breast cancer, history of cancer in the breast contralateral to that being studied, biopsy-proven atypical hyperplasia (AH), biopsy-proven LCIS, biopsy-proven DCIS, or biopsy-proven invasive carcinoma (Clegg et al., 2002). They found that the expression of hK2, hK3, and the ratio hK2/hK3 were lower in breast cancer patients than normal subjects. Moreover, the expression of hK2 and hK3 was significantly lower in black than in white population and was higher in pre- than in postmenopausal whites. hK3 level was lower in postmenopausal women with breast cancer, regardless of ethnicity (Sauter et al., 2002).

A recent study by Liang et al. evaluated the ethnic-specific expression of 10 differentially expressed hydrophobic proteins from breast cancer patients of three different ethnicities, that is, Chinese, Malay, and Indian. They found significantly elevated expression levels of 4 hydrophobic proteins that include peroxiredoxin-2, HSP60, protein disulfide isomerase, and calreticulin in cancerous tissues as compared to the normal controls. They concluded that these four hydrophobic proteins may serve as ethnic-related potential markers for Chinese, Malay, and Indian cohorts (Liang et al., 2011).

23.15 Authors' with Awards in Breast Cancer Research

The authors who have won awards in the field of breast cancer research along with their significant contributions have been mentioned in Table 23.13.

TABLE 23.13

List of Scientists Who Have Won Awards in Breast Cancer Research

Author's Name	Won Research in This Field	Award Presented By	Year
Douglas Easton	• Establishment of the breast cancer lineage consortium • Elucidated the genetic epidemiology of BRCA1 and BRCA2, which has provided definitive evidence for the localization of a breast cancer susceptibility locus on BRCA1 and provided the first estimates of the breast and ovarian cancer risks in BRCA1 mutation carriers	Outstanding investigator award in breast cancer research funded by Komen for the Cure	2008
Dr. Joan Massague	• Defined the mechanisms by which signals initiated by TGF-b are conveyed from their receptors on the cell membrane to the nucleus to affect cell proliferation, differentiation, and cancer • In his studies, he identified genes that define metastatic tissue tropism, providing a firm genetic basis for understanding the ability of breast cancer cells to colonize either the lung or bone	AACR distinguished lectureship in breast cancer research	2009
Elizabeth H. Blackburn	• Discovered how chromosomes are protected by telomeres and the enzyme telomerase • Blackburn codiscovered telomerase, the enzyme that replenishes the telomere	Nobel Prize in physiology or medicine	2009
Charles M. Perou	• His seminal work has shown that breast cancer is not a single disease but instead represents a series of diseases that include the more favorable prognosis luminal A subtype and multiple worse prognosis subtypes including the luminal B, HER2-positive (HER2+), basal-like, and claudin-low groups	AACR outstanding investigator award for breast cancer	2009
Klaus Pantel	• The pioneer work of Prof. Pantel in the field of cancer micometastasis and CTCs is reflected by more than 300 publications in excellent high-ranking biomedical and scientific journals (incl. NEJM, Lancet, Nature Journals, PNAS, JCO, JNCI, Cancer Res.) and has been awarded recently	AACR outstanding investigator award 2010, German cancer award 2010, ERC advanced investigator grant 2011	2010
Ramon E. Parsons	• Dr. Parsons has made the seminal discovery of the PTEN tumor suppressor and showed that PTEN was inactivated by mutation in a wide variety of human malignancies including breast cancer and in the rare breast cancer predisposition syndrome, Cowden disease	AACR outstanding investigator award for breast cancer research	2011

TABLE 23.14

Various Test Panels Commercially Available with Specificity and Sensitivity

Name	Description	Specificity (%)	Sensitivity (%)	References
Oncotype Dx	It is used to diagnose the patients with early-stage (stage I or II), node-negative, ER-positive (ER+), invasive breast cancer	68–93	48–73	Cronin et al. (2007)
Theros H/I^{SM} and MGI^{SM}	This molecular diagnostic test is a combination of two gene indexes, Theros H/I^{SM} and Theros MGI^{SM}, that measures the ratio of HOXB13/IL17BR gene expression as a predictor of clinical outcome for breast cancer patients treated with tamoxifen Theros MGI^{SM} is an additional test that uses a five-gene expression index to stratify ER$^+$ breast cancer patients into high or low risk of recurrence by reclassifying tumors and also provides information about the tumor grade, proliferative status, sensitivity, or resistance to chemotherapy	67	63	Ma et al. (2008)
Breast Bioclassifier™	It is a 55-gene qRT-PCR assay that provides information about the biological subtype (luminal A, luminal B, HER2, and basal) of tumor and provides a risk score that enables physicians to make treatment decisions for the patients	79–64	44	Perreard et al. (2006)
Celera Metastatic Score™	It is a 14-gene multiplex RT-PCR test that provides information about the tumor grade and quantifies the risk for metastasis for variable time periods in breast cancer patients	94	88	Garber (2004)
CellSearch™	It is a simple blood test that captures and assesses CTCs to determine the prognosis of patients with metastatic disease	93–99	27–57	Riethdorf et al. (2007)
eXagen™	It is a prognostic assay proposed for ER-/PR-positive (ER/PR$^+$) and ER/PR$^-$ patients	92	87	Ross (2008)
Mammostrat	The assay is used for calculating risk index score for breast cancer patients. The higher the risk index score, the more likely is the cancer recurrence	93	48	Bartlett et al. (2012)
ProEXTMBr	Score ≥2 associated with disease relapse in LN− and LN+ breast cancer patients	—	—	Whitehead et al. (2004)
MammaPrint	It is a molecular diagnostic tool of 70-gene signature that is used for risk assessment in patients with node-negative breast cancer It is recommended for patients up to 60 years with stage 1 or 2, lymph node-negative, invasive breast cancer	73	91	Buyse et al. (2006)

TABLE 23.14 (continued)

Various Test Panels Commercially Available with Specificity and Sensitivity

Name	Description	Specificity (%)	Sensitivity (%)	References
MapQuant Dx™	It is a gene expression assay used to diagnose the patients with ER-positive, grade II breast cancer. The test provides information about tumor grade and tumor aggressiveness	42–50	68–90	Sotiriou et al. (2006)
BLN Assay	The assay detects the presence of breast tumor metastasis in lymph nodes by detection of gene expression markers present in breast tissue but not in the nodal tissue	71.4–83.9	80–98.1	Mansel et al. (2009)
Invasive Gene Signature	Risk prediction for death and metastasis in breast cancer	100	96	Liu et al. (2007)
Wound Response Indicator	Here the set of genes represent the wound healing response and provides improved risk prediction for death and metastasis	48	93	Chang et al. (2005)
DirectHit™	It provides information about the presence of certain proteins in the tumor that helps to prescribe the most effective drug treatment for both hormonal and chemotherapeutic drugs	87–91[a]		http://directhittest.com/patients.html
Rotterdam Signature 76-Gene Panel	The kit is used to evaluate ER-positive as well as ER-negative samples	48	93	Oakman et al. (2009); Pusztai (2008)
HERmark™ assay	Measures total HER2 expression and HER2 homodimers	—	—	Larson JS et al., 2010
OncoVue® Test	Combines the SNP patterns of 117 genes and personal history to predict breast cancer risk	99.9[a]		Ralph et al. (2007) http://www.intergenetics.com/cms/technologyandproducts/whatisoncovue/testresults
GeneSearch™ BLN	Detection of gene expression markers mammaglobin and CK19 via qRT-PCR. Detects breast tumor cell metastasis in lymph nodes	97.4	88.9	Viale et al. (2005); Sun et al. (2011)
DiaGenic BCtect®	Analyzes gene expression signatures from peripheral blood	73	72	Imbeaud et al. (2005); Tobin et al. (2007)

[a] Accuracy—combined values of specificity and sensitivity.

23.16 Various Test Panels Commercially Available with High Specificity and Sensitivity

Biomarkers can promise outstanding prediction efficiency for the early detection of breast cancer, thereby enabling better patient therapy (Bhatt et al., 2010). A wide number of breast cancer diagnostic kits are readily available in the market, most of which rely on the gene expression profiles of the prognostic biomarkers (Ross, 2008). Some of the multigenic tests developed for breast cancer detection include Oncotype Dx, Theros Breast Cancer Index, Breast Bioclassifier, Celera Metastatic Score, eXagen, Mammostrat, ProEXTMBr, MammaPrint, MapQuant Dx, Breast Lymph Node (BLN) Assay, Invasive Gene Signature, Wound Response Indicator, Breast Cancer Gene Expression Ratio, 2-gene ratio, H/I or HOXB13/IL17BR, and Rotterdam Signature 76-Gene Panel (Jansen et al., 2007) (Table 23.14). Of the previously mentioned tests, the Oncotype DX assay is the most widely used (Cronin et al., 2007). More than 135,000 tests have been performed by using this kit (Genomic Health Annual Report, 2009, http://www.genomichealth.com/OncotypeDX.aspx#.UhXSMKw04xE). Besides the previously mentioned tests, the test called "DirectHit™" is a pharmacodiagnostic test that helps to determine the tumor sensitivity or resistance to drug regimens recommended for the treatment of breast cancer. It provides information about the presence of certain proteins in the tumor that helps to prescribe the most effective drug treatment. The presence of these proteins may be related to the mechanism of action of particular drugs. DirectHit™ is the only test of its kind that may be used to recommend effective treatment for both hormonal and chemotherapeutic drugs (http://directhittest.com/patients.html).

23.17 Recommended Tests/Panels in Combination with/without Imaging for Early Diagnosis of Breast Cancer

The American Cancer Society recommends the use of mammograms, MRI, CBEs, and BSE for early detection that may help in reduction of mortality. Table 23.15 describes various tests alone or in combination along with rationale that are used in early breast cancer detection.

TABLE 23.15

Recommended Tests/Panels in Combination along with Their Rationale

Categories of Women at Risk	Age (Year)	Test[a]	Screening Intervals	Rationale
Women at average risk	20	BSE	Monthly	The chance of breast cancer occurrence is very low for women in their 20s and gradually increases with age
	20–30	CBE and mammography	Every 3 years	The chance of breast cancer occurrence is very low for women in their 20s and gradually increases with age
	40	Mammography	Annually	Significant reduction in mortality due to mammography screening
Women at high risk				
>20% lifetime risk	45–55	MRI and mammography	Annually	MRI is more sensitive than mammograms but may miss some cancers that a mammogram would detect
Women at moderately increased risk				
15%–20% lifetime risk	<40	Mammography and/or MRI	Annually	MRI may miss some cancers that a mammogram would detect
Women at low risk				
<15% lifetime risk	>60	Mammography	Annually	Significant reduction in mortality due to mammography screening

Note: American Cancer Society Last Revised: 30/08/2012.

[a] BSE—breast self-examination; CBE—clinical breast exam; MRI—magnetic resonance imaging.

23.18 Advantages and Challenges in Developing Molecular Biomarkers for Early Detection, Prognosis, and Therapy

Biomarkers provide a dynamic and powerful approach for understanding the biology of cancer. They are widely used in the risk assessment, diagnosis, prognosis, and monitoring of cancer progression and may contribute in understanding of the pathophysiology of the disease (Bhatt et al., 2010). Biomarkers play an important role in predicting the response of the patients to treatment, to guess the efficacy and safety of novel therapeutic agents, in determining the drug doses and in the development of more effective and disease-specific chemotherapeutic drugs with minimal undesired systemic toxicity (Morey et al., 2012). A panel of biomarkers may provide higher predictive power and may improve the statistical performance compared to individual biomarkers (Tesch et al., 2010). They help in accurate detection of the presence of cancer, thereby resulting in fewer false-positive and false-negative tests (Mayeux, 2004). They are powerful tools for identification of potential drug targets and adapting therapies for individual needs by allowing the selection of patients who are most likely to respond or react adversely to a particular treatment (Tesch et al., 2010). Biomarker discovery is a boon for the medical and pharmaceutical communities as well as for the oncology researchers (Mayeux, 2004).

Despite all the potential benefits of biomarkers in cancer diagnosis, prognosis, and therapy, several biological as well as economical challenges are faced by the research and medical communities in the development of new biomarkers. Biological challenges such as cancer progression, natural history, heterogeneity of the disease, and biomarker performance are the barriers in biomarker development (Bensalah et al., 2007). One of the major challenges of biomarker development in clinical domain is the translation of the knowledge gained through animal studies to humans (Marrer et al., 2007). Although a number of biomarkers are available for cancer diagnosis and detection, none of them have been found to achieve 100% sensitivity and specificity (Bensalah et al., 2007). Moreover, development and validation of biomarkers through clinical evidence is time-consuming, labor intensive, and financially challenging (Tesch et al., 2010). Another major drawback for the development of biomarkers is the limited availability of sufficient number of good quality samples for evaluation. Besides, the normal clinical range of these biomarkers is difficult to establish and is possibly associated with laboratory errors (Tworoger and Hankinson, 2006; Kotsopoulos, 2010). Some other drawbacks include nonuniform preparation and storage of sample, sample heterogeneity, as well as cost of analysis (Camillo et al., 2012).

23.19 Market and Market Players of the Molecular Biomarkers for Early Diagnosis, Prognosis, and Therapy

The worldwide market of biomarkers is increasing with several new companies coming into the scenario. The popularity and wide use of biomarkers in drug discovery, for example, used in medical areas such as cancer research, is highly increasing its demand. Moreover, the understanding of the importance of biomarkers in the early detection as well as treatment of cancer has boosted the growth of this market to a large extent. Table 23.16 enlists various market players as well as the gene signature kits commercially available and under development for breast cancer.

23.20 Patent Information of Molecular Markers/Tests for Invasive, Noninvasive, Early Diagnostic, Prognostic, and Therapeutic Aspects

The list of the patents of molecular markers/tests and methods for early diagnostic, prognostic and therapeutics for breast cancer have been elaborated in Table 23.17.

TABLE 23.16

Market and Market Players of the Molecular Biomarkers

Company	Kit Name	Available	Sample[a]	Technique[b]	Diagnostic Aim
Genomic health	Oncotype Dx	USA	FFP	q-RT-PCR	Prognosis, recurrence after tamoxifen therapy
Biotheranostics	Theros breast cancer index	USA	FFP	q-RT-PCR	Prognosis, recurrence after endocrine therapy
ARUP	Breast bioclassifier	USA	FFP	RT-PCR	Prognosis
Applera	Celera Metastatic score	USA	FFP	RT-PCR	Prognosis, recurrence after tamoxifen therapy
eXagen diagnostics	eXagenBC	USA	FFP	FISH	Prognosis
Applied genomics	Mammostrat	USA	—	IHC	Prognosis
TriPath	ProEXTMBr	USA	—	IHC	Prognosis
Agendia	MammaPrint	USA	F/F	Microarray	Prognosis in patients over 61 years
Ipsoggen	MapQuant Dx	EU	F/F	Microarray	Prognosis
GeneSearch Veridex	BLN Assay	UK	F/F	Microarray	Intraoperative metastasis Identification
bioTheranostics	HOXB13/IL17BR (H/I) ratio	USA	FFP	IHC	Prognosis and diagnosis
Veridex	CellSearch™	USA	Blood	IS/IF	Risk stratification
OncoMed Pharmaceuticals	Invasive Gene Signature	CA	F/F	Microarray	Prognosis
Not commercialized	Wound Response Indicator	—	F/F	Microarray	Prognosis
Veridex	Rotterdam Signature 76-Gene Panel	USA	F/F	Microarray	To predict prognosis of breast cancer recurrence
Nuvera Biosciences	NuvoSelect™	USA	F/F	Microarray	Prognosis and response to therapy
In development	ARUP Bioclassifier	—	FFPE	RT-PCR	Multigene predictors for breast cancer
Not commercialized	Sørlie–Perou Classifier	—	F/F	Microarray	Breast cancer prediction
Roche Diagnostics/ Merck	Roche AmpliChip (cytochrome P450 CYP2D6)	USA	F/F	Microarray	To study the response of tamoxifen in breast cancer patients
Medco/Lab					

[a] F/F, fresh/frozen; FFP, formalin-fixed paraffin-embedded.

[b] IHC, immunohistochemistry; FISH, fluorescent in situ hybridization; IS/IF, immunostaining/immunofluorescence; q-RT-PCR, quantitative real-time polymerase chain reaction; RT-PCR, reverse transcriptase polymerase chain reaction.

TABLE 23.17

List of the Patents of Molecular Markers/Tests and Methods for Early Diagnostic, Prognostic, and Therapeutics for Breast Cancer

Year	Application No.	Title of the Patent	Inventors	Description
2002	US 0137064	Id-1 and Id-2 genes and products as diagnostic and prognostic markers and therapeutic targets for treatment of breast cancer and other types of carcinoma	Pierreyves et al.	Concerns with the use of Id-1 and/or Id-2 genes or Id-1 and/or Id-2 products as diagnostic markers for diagnosis, prognosis, and treatment of breast cancer and other types of cancers.
2003	EP 0785216	Chromosome 13-linked breast cancer susceptibility gene BRCA2	Sean et al.	This invention relates to germ line mutations in the BRCA2 gene, which can be used in the diagnosis of predisposition to breast cancer.
2004	US 6762020	Methods of diagnosing breast cancer	David et al.	The invention relates to the identification of expression profiles and the nucleic acids and their use in diagnosis and prognosis of breast cancer. The invention further relates to methods for identifying and using candidate agents and/or targets that modulate breast cancer.
2004	US 6737040	Method and antibody for imaging breast cancer	Yongming et al.	This invention relates, in part, to newly developed assays for detecting, diagnosing, monitoring, staging, prognosticating, imaging, and treating cancers, particularly breast cancer.
2004	US 6730477	Method of diagnosing, monitoring, and staging breast cancer	Yongming et al.	This invention relates to newly developed assays for detecting, diagnosing, monitoring, staging, prognosticating, imaging, and treating breast cancer.
2004	US 6780586	Methods of diagnosing breast cancer	Kurt et al.	The invention relates to the identification of expression profiles and the nucleic acids involved in breast cancer and their use in diagnosis and prognosis of breast cancer.
2005	WO 083429	Breast cancer prognostics	Yixin	This invention relates to breast cancer patient prognosis based on the gene expression profiles of patient biological samples.
2006	WO 015312	Prognosis of breast cancer patients	Hongyue et al.	Present invention relates to the identification of marker genes useful in the diagnosis and prognosis of breast cancer.
2007	US 7306910	Breast cancer prognostics	Yixin	Invention is a method of assessing the recurrence or metastasis of breast cancer in a patient diagnosed with or treated for breast cancer.
2007	US 0054271	Gene expression in breast cancer	Kornelia et al.	The invention features nucleic acids encoding proteins that are expressed at a higher or a lower level in breast cancer cells. This invention relates to methods of diagnosing and treating breast cancers of various grades and stages.

(continued)

TABLE 23.17 (continued)

List of the Patents of Molecular Markers/Tests and Methods for Early Diagnostic, Prognostic, and Therapeutics for Breast Cancer

Year	Application No.	Title of the Patent	Inventors	Description
2007	US 7229770	YKL-40 as a marker and prognostic indicator for cancers	Paul et al.	This invention is directed to assays for the detection and quantitation of molecules and fragments of YKL-40 whereby serum levels of YKL-40 are indicative of the presence and/or prognosis of cancer including breast cancer.
2008	US 7419785	Methods and compositions in breast cancer diagnosis and therapeutics	Suzanne et al.	The present invention is directed to the determination of susceptibility to breast cancer and the diagnosis of invasive breast cancer.
2008	WO 132167	Diagnostic, prognostic, and/or predictive indicators of breast cancer	O'driscoll et al.	The invention relates to a novel panel of mRNAs that have potential as diagnostic, prognostic, and/or predictive indicators and novel therapeutic targets of breast cancer.
2009	WO 074364	Novel prognostic breast cancer marker	Edgar et al.	This invention relates to the epigenetic silencing of the DKK3 gene in breast cancers, and the uses of this marker in the prognosis, diagnosis, and selection of appropriate treatments against breast cancer.
2009	US 0239763	Markers for breast cancer	Cox et al.	Methods of diagnosing, prognosing, and treating breast cancer are provided.
2009	WO 138130	Breast cancer prognostics	Stocksund et al.	The present invention generally relates to breast cancer prognostics, and in particular to molecular markers having prognostic value and uses thereof.
2009	US 7504214	Predicting outcome with tamoxifen in breast cancer	Mark et al.	The invention relates to the identification and use of gene expression profiles, or patterns, with clinical relevance to the treatment of breast cancer using tamoxifen.
2009	WO 108917	Markers for improved detection of breast cancer	Herman et al.	The present invention relates to the identification of a cell proliferative disorder of breast by determining aberrant DNA methylation patterns of particular genes in breast cancer and precancer.
2009	US 0092973	Grading of breast cancer	Mark et al.	The invention relates to the identification and use of gene expression profiles or patterns used to identify different grades of breast cancer within and between stages thereof.
2010	US 7642050	Method for predicting responsiveness of breast cancer to antiestrogen therapy	Nevalainen et al.	The application relates to the use of activated Stat5 for diagnosing and monitoring cancer and predicting the prognosis of breast cancer patients and the outcome of cancer therapies.

TABLE 23.17 (continued)

List of the Patents of Molecular Markers/Tests and Methods for Early Diagnostic, Prognostic, and Therapeutics for Breast Cancer

Year	Application No.	Title of the Patent	Inventors	Description
2010	US 7695915	Molecular prognostic signature for predicting breast cancer distant metastasis, and uses thereof	Lau et al.	The present invention relates to a unique 14-gene molecular prognostic signature for prognosis of breast cancer metastasis.
2010	US 0105087	LMW peptides as early biomarkers for breast cancer	Petricoin et al.	The LMW peptides have been discovered that are useful in detecting breast cancer during its early stages.
2011	US 0015092	Markers for breast cancer	Cox et al.	The present invention provided the methods and systems and kits for diagnosing, prognosis, and treating breast cancer.
2011	US 0307427	Molecular markers predicting response to adjuvant therapy or disease progression, in breast cancer	Linke et al.	The present invention concerns a method for the prediction of response to adjuvant therapy or disease progression in breast cancer and a kit consisting of a panel of antibodies, the binding of which with breast cancer tumor samples has been correlated with breast cancer treatment outcome or patient prognosis.
2011	US 0251082	Biomarkers for breast cancer	Hong-lin Chou et al.	The present invention uses 2D differential gel electrophoresis gel (2D-DIGE) and MS techniques to identify breast cancer biomarkers from various stages of breast cancer. The invention aids in developing proteins identified as useful diagnostic and therapeutic candidates on breast cancer research.
2011	US 0144198	Breast cancer prognostics	Uhlén et al.	The present invention provides new methods, uses, and means for breast cancer prognostics.
2011	US 7879614	Methods for detection of breast cancer	Krepinsky et al.	The invention relates to a simple screening test for neoplasia or breast cancer to detect breast cancer marker in breast fluid.
2011	US 0217297	Methods for classifying and treating breast cancers	Kao et al.	The present invention relates to a method of treating breast cancer in a subject, comprised of determining the molecular subtype of the breast cancer in the subject and administering to the subject a therapy that is effective for treating the molecular subtype of the breast cancer.
2011	US 7955848	miRNA biomarkers for human breast and lung cancer	Dmitrovsky et al.	The present invention relates to novel molecular markers for diagnosis and classification of human breast cancer and lung cancer.
2011	WO 133770	Salivary protein markers for detection of breast cancer	Streckfus et al.	This invention relates to a method of diagnosing a patient's risk of breast cancer and comprises of measuring the protein marker from the saliva sample of the patient.

(continued)

TABLE 23.17 (continued)

List of the Patents of Molecular Markers/Tests and Methods for Early Diagnostic, Prognostic, and Therapeutics for Breast Cancer

Year	Application No.	Title of the Patent	Inventors	Description
2012	US 8101352	Detection of ESR1 amplification in breast cancer	Sauter et al.	This invention provides an in vitro method of identifying an individual with a non-cancerous proliferative breast disease who is at risk of developing breast cancer.
2012	WO 021887	Biomarkers for the early detection of breast cancer	Labaer et al.	The present invention provides reagents and methods for breast cancer detection.
2012	US 0184560	Molecular diagnostic methods for predicting brain metastasis of breast cancer	Wong et al.	This invention provides the methods for predicting brain metastasis of breast cancer, as well as methods for drug repositioning to identify existing and new therapeutics for use in developing individualized, patient-specific treatment regimens for improving diagnoses and patient outcomes in individuals at risk for brain metastasis of breast cancer.
2012	US 8097423	MN/CA IX and breast cancer therapy	Harris et al.	This invention concerns methods of detecting and quantitating MN antigen and/or MN gene expression in tumors, tumor samples, or body fluids of ER-positive breast cancer patients, which would help in predicting patient resistance to endocrine therapy for breast cancer and for making clinical decisions concerning cancer treatment.
2012	WO 060760	Molecular marker for cancer	Parris et al.	The present invention relates to the assessment of a gene in the 8p11–p12 chromosomal region and gene products thereof, and their use as powerful molecular markers in decisions related to the diagnosis and/or prognosis of cancer, in particular breast cancer.
2012	US 8187889	Protein markers for the diagnosis and prognosis of ovarian and breast cancer	Lomnytska et al.	The present invention is directed to new protein markers and their use in diagnosing and monitoring ovarian and breast cancer.

23.21 Conclusions and Possible Future Directions

The global burden of the breast cancer continues to increase despite of advances in therapeutics and clinical research. Thus, early detection would not only reduce the suffering but also the associated cost. Despite efficient screening modalities available to diagnose breast cancer, there is an urgent need for most efficient, sensitive, as well as cost-effective methodologies for early screening. Biomarkers are the useful tools that can help not only in diagnosis and detection but also in deciding treatment option at an early stage that would reduce the associated mortality as well as morbidity. Promising developments in integrative omics approaches have led to the discovery of novel, specific, sensitive, easily measurable, reliable, cost-effective, and less complex biomarkers (both invasive and noninvasive) for the detection of breast cancer. Noninvasive biomarkers have more potential for the detection of disease at an early stage due to their easy access as well as potential for repeated sampling. Among these, circulating biomarkers present in the peripheral blood and bone marrow are the promising candidates for population-based screening that facilitate easy detection (Ramona and Massimo, 2011). No single biomarker is likely to have perfect predictive accuracy; however, biomarkers in panels may provide higher predictive power and thus provide a promising potential in clinical research.

Current proteomic-based approaches help in characterizing molecular alterations that could help in early cancer detection, subclassification, and accurate prognosis. Advanced platforms such as Orbitrap MS, Fourier transform ion cyclotron resonance MS, and protein microarrays combined with advanced bioinformatics are currently being used to identify molecular signatures of individual tumors that may be amplified by using emerging nanotechnology strategies (Pusztai and Hess, 2004). However, DNA methylation-based biomarkers are probably the most attractive analytes for development because epigenetic changes in genome are considered as an early event in the process of carcinogenesis. Moreover, current reports suggest that abnormal DNA methylation occur in asymptomatic patients before the appearance of the early symptoms of cancer, so the detection of methylated genes would help in the accurate early detection. Thus, epigenetic biomarkers may provide one of the best promising platforms to develop reliable, specific, and sensitive screening tests for early breast cancer detection. Besides, metabolomic-based markers may also play an essential role in early identification of breast cancer as it may help to identify metabolites that may be released in the early stages of the disease. Thus, the management of breast cancer would lie in the potency and efficacy of the biomarkers to identify the symptomatic and asymptomatic disease condition. The accumulated knowledge about the correlative biomarkers would not only overcome the challenge of early detection and clinical diagnosis but would also provide appropriate therapeutic alternatives that would benefit the patients.

Acknowledgments

We thank our Director, Dr PK Ranjekar as well as IRSHA for supporting this work. We also thank Mr Amit S Choudhari, CSIR-SRF, for helping us in the editing of the manuscript.

References

Abba MC, Drake JA, Hawkins KA et al. (2004) Transcriptomic changes in human breast cancer progression as determined by serial analysis of gene expression. *Breast Cancer Res* 6:R499–R513.

Abhilash M. (2009) Applications of proteomics. *Int J Gen Prot* 4(1), ISSN: 1540–2630.

Adami HO, Hunter D, and Trichopoulos D. (2002) *Textbook of Cancer Epidemiology*. New York: Oxford University Press, Inc.

Adams BD, Furneaux H, and White BA. (2007) The micro-ribonucleic acid (miRNA) miR-206 targets the human estrogen receptor-alpha (ERalpha) and represses ERalpha messenger RNA and protein expression in breast cancer cell lines. *Mol Endocrinol* 21:1132–1147.

Aebersold R and Mann M. (2003) Mass spectrometry-based proteomics. *Nature* 422(6928):198–207.

Ahn SK, Moon HG, Ko E et al. (2013) Preoperative serum tissue polypeptide-specific antigen is a valuable prognostic marker in breast cancer. *Int J Cancer* 132(4):875–881.

Alao JP. (2007) The regulation of cyclin D1 degradation: Roles in cancer development and the potential for therapeutic invention. *Mol Cancer* 6:24.

Al-azawi D, Kelly G, Myers E et al. (2006) CA15-3 is predictive of response and disease recurrence following treatment in locally advanced breast cancer. *BMC Cancer* 6:220.

Albergaria A, Paredes J, Sousa B et al. (2009) Expression of FOXA1 and GATA-3 in breast cancer: The prognostic significance in hormone receptor-negative tumours. *Breast Cancer Res* 11(3):R4.

Albertson DG, Collins C, McCormick F, and Gray JW. 2003. Chromosome aberrations in solid tumors. *Nat Gen* 34(4):369–376.

Alexander H, Stegner AL, Wagner-Mann C et al. (2004) Proteomic analysis to identify breast cancer biomarkers in nipple aspirate fluid. *Clin Cancer Res* 10(22):7500–7510.

Allegra JC and Lippman ME (1978) Growth of a human breast cancer cell line in serum-free hormone-supplemented medium. *Cancer Res* 38:3823–3829.

Al-Tarawneh SK, Border MB, Dibble CF et al. (2011) Defining salivary biomarkers using mass spectrometry-based proteomics: A systematic review. *OMICS* 15(6):353–361.

Ana KCV, Achatz MIW, Santos EMM et al. (2012) Germline DNA copy number variation in familial and early-onset breast cancer. *Breast Cancer Res* 14:R24.

Anderson KS, Sibani S, Wallstrom G et al. (2011) Protein microarray signature of autoantibody biomarkers for the early detection of breast cancer. *J Proteome Res* 10(1):85–96.

Anghel A, Raica M, Marian C et al. (2006) Combined profile of the tandem repeats CAG, TA and CA of the androgen and estrogen receptor genes in breast cancer. *J Cancer Res Clin Oncol* 132:727–733.

Anna MB, Borgny Y, and Cara M. (2004) Detection and quantitation of HER-2 Gene amplification and protein expression in breast carcinoma. *Am J Clin Pathol* 122:110–119.

Antoniou AC, Spurdle AB, Sinilnikova OM et al. (2008) Common breast cancer-predisposition alleles are associated with breast cancer risk in BRCA1 and BRCA2 mutation carriers. *Am J Hum Genet* 82(4):937–948.

Artandi SE and DePinho RA. (2000) A critical role for telomeres in suppressing and facilitating carcinogenesis. *Curr Opin Genet Dev* 10:39–46.

Atoum MF, Hourani HM, Shoter A et al. (2010) TNM staging and classification (familial and non familial) of breast cancer in Jordanian females. *Indian J Cancer* 47(2):194–198.

Axelsson R, Bach-Gansmo T, Castell-Conesa J et al. (2010) An open-label, multicenter, phase 2a study to assess the feasibility of imaging metastases in late-stage cancer patients with the alpha v beta 3-selective angiogenesis imaging agent 99mTc-NC100692. *Acta Radio* 151(1):40–46.

Badve S, Turbin D, and Thorat MA. (2007) FOXA1 expression in breast cancer—Correlation with luminal subtype A and survival. *Clin Cancer Res* 13:4415–4421.

Baglietto L, Severi G, English DR et al. (2010) Circulating steroid hormone levels and risk of breast cancer for postmenopausal women. *Cancer Epidemiol Biomarkers Prev* 19(2):492–502.

Banerji S, Cibulskis K, Rangel-Escareno C et al. (2012) Sequence analysis of mutations and translocations across breast cancer subtypes. *Nature* 486(7403):405–409.

Bansal V, Kumar V, and Medhi B (2005) Future challenges of pharmacogenomics in clinical practice. *JK Sci* 7(3):176–179.

Bantscheff M, Chirle M, Sweetman G et al. (2007) Quantitative mass spectrometry in proteomics: A critical review. *Anal Bioanal Chem* 389:1017–1031.

Barak V, Goike H, Panaretakis KW et al. (2004) Clinical utility of cytokeratins as tumor markers. *Clin Biochem* 37(7):529–540.

Baranwal S and Alahari (2010). miRNA control of tumor cell invasion and metastasis. *Int J Cancer* 126(6):1283–1290.

Barekati Z, Radpour R, Lu Q et al. (2012) Methylation signature of lymph node metastases in breast cancer patients. *BMC Cancer* 12:244.

Bartlett JM, Bloom KJ, Piper T et al. (2012) Mammostrat as an immunohistochemical multigene assay for prediction of early relapse risk in the tamoxifen versus exemestane adjuvant multicenter trial pathology study. *J Clin Oncol.* 30(36):4477–4484.

Bartlett JM, Thomas J, Ross DT et al. (2010) Mammostrat as a tool to stratify breast cancer patients at risk of recurrence during endocrine therapy. *Breast Cancer Res* 12(4):R47.

Bassiouny M, El-Marakby HH, Saber N et al. (2005) Quadrantectomy and nipple saving mastectomy in treatment of early breast cancer: Feasibility and aesthetic results of adjunctive latissmus dorsi breast reconstruction. *J Egypt Natl Canc Inst* 17(3):149–157.

Becker C, Noldus J, Diamandis E, and Lilja H. (2001) The role of molecular forms of prostate-specific antigen (PSA or hK3) and of human glandular kallikrein 2 (hK2) in the diagnosis and monitoring of prostate cancer and in extra-prostatic disease. *Crit Rev Clin Lab Sci.* 38(5):357–399.

Bensalah K, Montorsi F, and Shariat SF. (2007) Challenges of cancer biomarker profiling. *Eur Urol* 52(6):1601–1609.

Berger MS, Locher GW, Saurer S et al. (1988) Correlation of c-erb B2 gene amplification and protein expression in human breast carcinoma with nodal status and nuclear grading. *Cancer Res* 48:1238–1243.

Bernard-Marty C, Lebrun F, Awada A et al. (2006) Monoclonal antibody-based targeted therapy in breast cancer: Current status and future directions. *Drugs* 66(12):1577–1579.

Bernstein JL, Godbold JH, Raptis G et al. (2005) Identification of mammaglobin as a novel serum marker for breast cancer. *Clin Cancer Res* 11(18):6528–6535.

Bertucci F, Birnbaum D, and Goncalves A. (2006) Proteomics of breast cancer: Principles and potential clinical applications. *Mol Cell Proteomics* 5(10):1772–1786.

Beverly H. (2009) The clinical utility of tumor markers. *Labmedicine* 40(2):99–103.

Bhargava R, Beriwal S, and Dabbs DJ. (2007) An immunohistologic validation survey for sensitivity and specificity. *Am J Clin Pathol* 127:103–113.

Bhatt AN, Mathur R, Farooque A et al. (2010) Cancer biomarkers—Current perspectives. *Indian J Med Res* 132:129–149.

Bidard FC, Hajage D, and Bachelot T. (2012) Assessment of circulating tumor cells and serum markers for progression-free survival prediction in metastatic breast cancer: A prospective observational study. *Breast Cancer Res* 14:R29.

Bohm D, Keller K, Pieter J et al. (2012) Comparison of tear protein levels in breast cancer patients and healthy controls using a de novoproteomic approach. *Oncol Rep* 28:429–438.

Borgan E, Sitter B, Lingjaerde OC et al. (2010) Merging transcriptomics and metabolomics—Advances in breast cancer profiling. *BMC Cancer* 10:628.

Borrelli R, del Sordo G, De Filippo E et al. (1993) High serum HDL-cholesterol in pre-and post-menopausal women with breast cancer in southern Italy. *Adv Exp Med Biol* 348:149–153.

Bourdon JC, Khoury MP, Diot A et al. (2011) p53 mutant breast cancer patients expressing p53γ have as good a prognosis as wild-type p53 breast cancer patients. *Breast Cancer Res*13:R7.

Boureux A, Vignal E, Faure S et al. (2007) Evolution of the Rho family of ras-like GTPases in eukaryotes. *Mol Biol Evol* 24(1):203–216.

Boyd NF, Melnichouk O, Martin LJ et al. (2011) Mammographic density, response to hormones, and breast cancer risk. *J Clin Oncol* 2985–2992.

Braaten T, Weiderpass E, Kumle M, Adami HO, and Lund E. (2004) Education and risk of breast cancer in the Norwegian-Swedish women's lifestyle and health cohort study. *Int J Cancer* 110(4):579–583.

Braun S, Vogl FD, Naume B et al. (2005) A pooled analysis of bone marrow micrometastasis in breast cancer. *N Engl J Med* 353(8):793–802.

Breast and Cervical Cancer Program (BCCP) Website: http://public.health.oregon.gov/DiseasesConditions/ChronicDisease/Cancer/Documents/2010/bhtf/breastguide.pdf

Brooks J, Cairns P, and Zeleniuch-Jacquotte. (2009) A promoter methylation and the detection of breast cancer. *Cancer Causes Control* 20(9):1539–1550.

Brooks MN, Wang J, Li Y et al. (2008) Salivary protein factors are elevated in breast cancer patients. *Mol Med Report* 1(3):375–378.

Bull SB et al. (2004) The combination of p53 mutation and neu/erbB-2 amplification is associated with poor survival in node-negative breast cancer. *J Clin Oncol* 22:86–96.

Butt S, Harlid S, Borgquist S et al. (2012) Genetic predisposition, parity, age at first childbirth and risk for breast cancer. *BMC Res Notes* 5:414.

Buyse M, Loi S, van 't Veer L et al. (2006) Validation and clinical utility of a 70-gene prognostic signature for women with node-negative breast cancer. *J Natl Cancer Inst* 98(17):1183–1192.

Cadieux C, Fournier S, Peterson AC et al. (2006) Transgenic mice expressing the p75 CCAAT-displacement protein/Cut homeobox isoform develop a myeloproliferative disease-like myeloid leukemia. *Cancer Res* 66(19):9492–9501.

Cakir A, Gonul II, and Uluoglu O. (2012) A comprehensive morphological study for basal-like breast carcinomas with comparison to non basal-like carcinomas. *Diagn Pathol* 7:145.

Calin GA and Croce CM. (2006) MicroRNA signatures in human cancers. *Nat Rev Cancer* 6:857–866.

Calvo RM, Asuncion M, Sancho J et al. (2000) The role of the CAG repeat polymorphism in the androgen receptor gene and of skewed X-chromosome inactivation, in the pathogenesis of hirsutism. *J Clin Endocrinol Metab* 85:1735–1740.

Carey LA, Metzger R, Dees EC et al. (2005) American Joint Committee on Cancer tumor-node-metastasis stage after neo adjuvant chemotherapy and breast cancer outcome. *J Natl Cancer Inst* 97(15):1137–1142.

Carla AB, Iacovos PM, and Eleftherios PD. (2004) Human tissue kallikreins: Physiologic roles and applications in cancer. *Mol Cancer Res* 5:257–280.

Carney WP. (2007) Circulating oncoproteins HER2/neu, EGFR and CAIX (MN) as novel cancer biomarkers. *Expert Rev Mol Diagn* 7(3):309–319.

Cavazzana-Calvo M, Bagnis C, Mannoni P et al. (1999) Peripheral stem cells in bone marrow transplantation. Peripheral blood stem cell and gene therapy. *Baillieres Best Pract Res Clin Haematol* 12(1–2):129–138.

Cazet A, Julien S, Bobowski M et al. (2010) Tumour-associated carbohydrate antigens in breast cancer. *Breast Cancer Res* 12:204.

Celis Julio E, Gromov P, Cabezón T et al. (2004) Proteomic characterization of the interstitial fluid perfusing the breast tumor microenvironment: A novel resource for biomarker and therapeutic target discovery. *Mol Cell Proteomics* 3:327–344.

Cen P, Duvic M, Cohen PR et al. (2008) Increased cancer antigen 27.29 (CA27.29) level in patients with mycosis fungoides. *J Am Acad Dermatol* 58(3):382–386.

Chan DW, Beveridge RA, Bruzek DJ et al. (1988) Monitoring breast cancer with CA 549. *Clin Chem* 34(10):2000–2004.

Chang CC, Yang SH, Chien CC et al. (2009) Clinical meaning of age-related expression of fecal cytokeratin 19 in colorectal malignancy. *BMC Cancer* 22(9):376.

Chang HY, Nuyten DS, Sneddon JB et al. (2005) Robustness, scalability, and integration of a wound-response gene expression signature in predicting breast cancer survival. *Proc Natl Acad Sci USA* 102:3738–3743.

Chang TC, Wentzel EA, and Kent OA. (2007) Transactivation of miR-34a by p53 broadly influences gene expression and promotes apoptosis. *Mol Cell* 26(5):745–752.

Chapman C, Murray A, Chakrabarti J et al. (2007) Autoantibodies in breast cancer: Their use as an aid to early diagnosis. *Ann Oncol* 18(5):868–873.

Charles L, Shapiro MD, and Abram Recht MD. (2001) Side effects of adjuvant treatment of breast cancer. *N Engl J Med* 344:1997–2008.

Chattopadhyay S, Kaul R, Charest A et al. (2000) SMAR1, a novel, alternatively spliced gene product, binds the Scaffold/Matrix-associated region at the T cell receptor beta locus. *Genomics* 68(1):93–96.

Chen F, Chen GK, Millikan RC et al. (2011) Fine-mapping of breast cancer susceptibility loci characterizes genetic risk in African Americans. *Hum Mol Genet* 20(22):4491–4503.

Chen H, Takahara M, Oba J et al. (2011) Clinicopathologic and prognostic significance of SATB1 in cutaneous malignant melanoma. *J Dermatol Sci* 64(1):39–44.

Chen HW, Huang CH, Lin YS et al. (2008) Breast cancer comparison and identification of estrogen-receptor related gene expression profiles in breast cancer of different ethnic origins. *Breast Cancer (Auckl.)* 1:35–49.

Chen WY, Rosner B, Hankinson SE et al. (2011) Moderate alcohol consumption during adult life, drinking patterns, and breast cancer risk. *JAMA* 306(17):1884–1890.

Chen Y, Zou TN, Wu ZP et al. (2010) Detection of cytokeratin 19, human mammaglobin, and carcinoembryonic antigen-positive circulating tumor cells by three-marker reverse transcription-PCR assay and its relation to clinical outcome in early breast cancer. *Int J Biol Markers* 25(2):59–68.

Chin K, deSolorzano CO, Knowles D et al. (2004) in situ analyses of genome instability in breast cancer. *Nat Genet* 36(9):984–988.

Choi H and Pavelka N. (2011) When one and one gives more than two: Challenges and opportunities of integrative omics. *Front Genet* 2:105.

Christensen BC, Kelsey KT, Zheng S et al. (2010) Breast cancer DNA methylation profiles are associated with tumor size and alcohol and folate intake. *PLoS Genet* 6(7):e1001043.

Christopoulou A and Spiliotis J. (2006) The role of BRCA1 AND BRCA2 in hereditary breast cancer. *Gene Ther Mol Biol* 10:95–100.

Cianfrocca M and Goldstein LJ. (2004) Prognostic and predictive factors in early-stage breast cancer. *Oncologist* 9(6):606–616.

Cîmpean AM, Suciu C, Ceauşu R et al. (2008) Relevance of the immunohistochemical expression of cytokeratin 8/18 for the diagnosis and classification of breast cancer. *Roman J Morphol Embryol* 49(4):479–483.

Clarke MF and Fuller M. (2006) Stem cells and cancer: Two faces of eve. *Cell* 124:1111–1115.

Clegg LX, Li FP, Hankey BF et al. (2002) Cancer survival among US whites and minorities: A SEER (Surveillance, Epidemiology, and End Results) program population-based study. *Arch Intern Med* 162:1985–1993.

Cohen SJ, Punt CJA, Iannotti N et al. (2008) Relationship of circulating tumor cells to tumor response, progression-free survival, and overall survival in patients with metastatic colorectal cancer. *J Clin Oncol* 26(19):3213–3221.

Colozza M, Azambuja E, and Cardoso F. (2005) Proliferative markers as prognostic and predictive tools in early breast cancer: Where are we now? *Ann Oncol* 16:1723–1739.

Contractor KB, Kenny LM, Stebbing J et al. (2011) 18F-3deoxy-3-fluorothymidine positron emission tomography and breast cancer response to docetaxel. *Clin Cancer Res* 17(24):7664–7672.

Costa NR, Paulo P, Caffrey T et al. (2011) Impact of MUC1 mucin downregulation in the phenotypic characteristics of MKN45 gastric carcinoma cell line. *PLoS One* 6(11):e26970.

Costello JF, Fruhwald MC, and Smiraglia DJ. (2000) Aberrant CpG-island methylation has non-random and tumour-type-specific patterns. *Nat Genet* 24(2):132–138.

Cowper-SalLari R, Zhang X, Wright JB et al. (2012) Breast cancer risk-associated SNPs modulate the affinity of chromatin for FOXA1 and alter gene expression. *Nat Genet.* 44(11):1191–1198.
Cox DG, Tamimi RM, and Hunter DJ. (2006) Gene x Gene interaction between MnSOD and GPX-1 and breast cancer risk: A nested case-control study. *BMC Cancer* 6:217.
Cronin M, Sangli C, Liu M et al. (2007) Analytical validation of the oncotype DX genomic diagnostic test for recurrence prognosis and therapeutic response prediction in node-negative, estrogen receptor–positive breast cancer. *Clin Chem* 53(6):1084–1091.
Crooke PS, Justenhoven C, Brauch H et al. (2011) Estrogen metabolism and exposure in a genotypic–phenotypic model for breast cancer risk prediction. *Cancer Epidemiol Biomarkers Prev* 20:1502–1515.
Csősz É, Boross P, Csutak A et al. (2012) Quantitative analysis of proteins in the tear fluid of patients with diabetic retinopathy. *J Proteomics* 75(7):2196–2204.
Dagan LN, Jiang X, Bhatt S et al. (2012) miR-155 regulates HGAL expression and increases lymphoma cell motility. *Blood* 119(2):513–520.
Dalberg K, Hellborg H, and Wärnberg F. (2007) Paget's disease of the nipple in a population based cohort. *Breast Cancer Res Treat* 111(2):313–319.
Dallol A, DaSilva NF, Viacava P et al. (2002) SLIT2, a human homologue of the Drosophila Slit2 gene, has tumor suppressor activity and is frequently inactivated in lung and breast cancers. *Cancer Res* 62(20):5874–5880.
Dangi-Garimella S, Strouch MJ, Grippo PJ, Bentrem DJ, and Munshi HG. (2010) Collagen regulation of let-7 in pancreatic cancer involves TGF-β1-mediated membrane type1-matrix metallo proteinase expression. *Oncogene* 30(8):1002–1008. Published Online First September 13, 2011; doi: 10.1158/0008-5472.CAN-11-1035
Dangi-Garimella S, Yun J, Eva ves ME et al. (2009) Raf kinase inhibitory protein suppresses a metastasis signalling cascade involving LIN28 and let-7. *EMBO J* 28(4):347–358.
Danila DC, Heller G, Gignac GA et al. (2007) Circulating tumor cell number and prognosis in progressive 17. Castration-resistant prostate cancer. *Clin Cancer Res* 13(23):7053–7058.
Davis LM, Harris C, Tang L et al. (2007) Amplification patterns of three genomic regions predict distant recurrence in breast carcinoma. *J Mol Diagn* 9(3):327–336.
De̦bniak T, GoÁrski B, Huzarski T et al. (2005) A common variant of CDKN2A (p16) predisposes to breast cancer. *J Med Genet* 42:763–765.
Deng CX. (2006) BRCA1: Cell cycle checkpoint, genetic instability, DNA damage response and cancer evolution. *Nucl Acids Res* 34(5):1416–1426.
Deng CX and Brodie SG. (2000) Roles of BRCA1 and its interacting proteins. *Bio Essays* 22:728–737.
Denkert C, Bucher E, Hilvo M et al. (2012) Metabolomics of human breast cancer: New approaches for tumor typing and biomarker discovery. *Genome Med* 4(4):37.
Desbiens C, Hogue JC, and Lévesque Y. (2011) Primary breast angiosarcoma: Avoiding a common trap. *Case Rep Oncol Med* 5 pages.
Desmetz C, Bibeau F, Boissière F et al. (2008) Proteomics-based identification of HSP60 as a tumor-associated antigen in early stage breast cancer and ductal carcinoma in situ. *J Proteome Res* 7(9):3830–3837.
Di Camillo B, Sanavia T, Martini M, Jurman G, Sambo F et al. (2012) Effect of size and heterogeneity of samples on biomarker discovery: Synthetic and real data assessment. *PLoS ONE* 7(3):e32200.
Dnistrian AM, Schwartz MK, and Greenberg EJ. (1991) CA 549 as a marker in breast cancer. *Int J Biol Mark* 6:139–143.
Donegan WL and Spratt JS. (1995) Introduction to the history of breast cancer. In: Donegan S. (ed.) *Cancer of the Breast*. WB Saunders, New York, pp. 1–14.
Dooley WC, Ljung BM, Veronesi U et al. (2001) Ductal lavage for detection of cellular atypia in women at high risk for breast cancer. *J Natl Cancer Inst* 93:1624–1632.
Doot RK, Muzi M, Peterson LM et al. (2010) Kinetic analysis of 18F-fluoride PET images of breast cancer bone metastases. *J Nucl Med* 51(4):521–527.
Drake PM, Cho W, Li B et al. (2010) Sweetening the pot: Adding glycosylation to the biomarker discovery equation. *Clin Chem* 56:223–236.
Dressing GE and Lange CA. (2009) Integrated actions of progesterone receptor and cell cycle machinery regulate breast cancer cell proliferation. *Steroids* 74:573–576.
Duffy MJ. (2006) Serum tumor markers in breast cancer: Are they of clinical value? *Clin Chem* 52(3):345–351.

Dunna WB, Broadhurst D, Brown M et al. (2008) Metabolic profiling of serum using ultra performance liquid chromatography and the LTQ-orbitrap mass spectrometry system. *J Chromatogr B* 871:288–298.

Edgar R, Domrachev M, and Lash AE. (2002) Gene expression omnibus: NCBI gene expression and hybridization array data repository. *Nucl Acids Res* 30:207–210.

Eheman CR, Benard VB, Blackman D et al. (2006) Breast cancer screening among low-income or uninsured women: Results from the National Breast and Cervical Cancer Early Detection Program, July 1995 to March 2002 (United States). *Cancer Causes Cont* 17:29–38.

Eiriksdottir G, Johannesdottir G, Ingvarsson S et al. (1998) Mapping loss of heterozygosity at chromosome 13q: Loss at 13q12-q13 is associated with breast tumour progression and poor prognosis. *Eur J Cancer* 34:2076–2081.

Eroles P, Bosch A, Pérez-Fidalgo JA et al. (2012) Molecular biology in breast cancer: Intrinsic subtypes and signaling pathways. *Cancer Treat Rev* 38(6):698–707.

Esteller M (2008). Epigenetics in cancer. *N Engl J Med* 358(11):1148–1159.

Evans WE. (2003) Pharmacogenomics: Marshalling the human genome to individualise drug therapy. *Gut.* 52:ii10–ii18.

Fabian CJ and Kimler BF. (2001) Breast cancer risk prediction: Should nipple aspiration fluid cytology be incorporated into clinical practice? *J Natl Cancer Inst* 93(23):1762–1763.

Fabian CJ, Kimler BF, and Mayo MS. (2005) Breast-tissue sampling for risk assessment and prevention. *Endocr Relat Cancer* 12(2):185–213.

Fajac A, Gligorov J, Rezai K et al. (2010) Effect of ABCB1 C3435T polymorphism on docetaxel pharmacokinetics according to menopausal status in breast cancer patients. *Br J Cancer* 103(4):560–566.

Falasca M (2012) Cancer biomarkers: The future challenge of cancer. *J Mol Biomark Diagn* S2:e001.

Farazi TA, Horlings HM, TenHoeve JJ et al. (2011) MicroRNA sequence and expression analysis in breast tumors by deep sequencing. *Cancer Res* 71(13):4443–4453.

Feinberg AP and Tycko B. (2004) The history of cancer epigenetics. *Nat Rev Cancer* 4:143–153.

Ferlay J, Héry C, Autier P et al. (2010) Global burden of breast cancer. *Breast Cancer Epidemiol*:1–19.

Fernando LA, Aleksandra VL, Sant A et al. (2005) Systemic chemotherapy induces microsatellite instability in the peripheral blood mononuclear cells of breast cancer patients. *Breast Cancer Res* 7(1):R28–R32.

Fessing MY, Mardaryev AN, Gdula MR et al. (2011) p63 regulates Satb1 to control tissue-specific chromatin remodeling during development of the epidermis. *J Cell Biol* 194(6):825–839.

Fisher B, Anderson S, Bryant J et al. (2002) Twenty-year follow-up of a randomized trial comparing total mastectomy, lumpectomy, and lumpectomy plus irradiation for the treatment of invasive breast cancer. *N Engl J Med* 347(16):1233–1241.

Fiszman GL and Jasnis MA. (2011) Molecular mechanisms of trastuzumab resistance in HER2 overexpressing breast cancer. *Int J Breast Cancer* 60:295–299.

Fonseca FL, SantAna AV, Bendit I et al. (2005) Systemic chemotherapy induces microsatellite instability in the peripheral blood mononuclear cells of breast cancer patients. *Breast Cancer Res* 7(1):R28–R32.

Fornier M and Norton L. (2005) Dose-dense adjuvant chemotherapy for primary breast cancer. *Breast Cancer Res* 7(2):64–69.

Foster MC, Helvie MA, Gregory NE et al. (2004) Lobular carcinoma in situ or atypical lobular hyperplasia at core-needle biopsy: Is excisional biopsy necessary. *Radiology* 231:813–819.

Foulkes WD, Smith IE, and Reis-Filho JS. (2010) Triple-negative breast cancer. *N Engl J Med* 363:1938–1948.

Fritz P, Cabrera CM, Dippon J et al. (2005) c-erbB2 and topoisomerase IIα protein expression independently predict poor survival in primary human breast cancer: A retrospective study. *Breast Cancer Res* 7:R374–R384.

Fu XD, Goglia L, Sanchez AM et al. (2010b) Progesterone receptor enhances breast cancer cell motility and invasion via extranuclear activation of focal adhesion kinase. *Endocr Relat Cancer* 17(2):431–443.

Fu YP, Edvardsen H, Kaushiva A et al. (2010a) NOTCH2 in breast cancer: Association of SNP rs11249433 with gene expression in ER-positive breast tumors without TP53 mutations. *Mol Cancer* 9:113.

Futreal PA, Coin L, Marshall M et al. (2004) A census of human cancer genes. *Nat Rev Cancer* 4:177–183.

Gaforio JJ, Serrano MJ, Sánchez-Rovira P et al. (2003) Detection of breast cancer cells in the peripheral blood is positively correlated with estrogen-receptor status and predicts for poor prognosis. *Int J Cancer* 107:984–990.

Galande S, Purbey PK, Notani D et al. (2007) The third dimension of gene regulation: Organization of dynamic chromatin loopscape by SATB1. *Curr Opin Genet Dev* 17(5):408–414.

Garber K. (2004) Genomic medicine. Gene expression tests foretell breast cancer's future. *Science* 303:1754–1755.

Gast MC, Schellens JH, and Beijnen JH. (2009) Clinical proteomics in breast cancer: A review. *Breast Cancer Res Treat* 116(1):17–29.

Gemayel R, Vinces MD, Legendre M et al. (2010) Variable tandem repeats accelerate evolution of coding and regulatory sequences. *Annu Rev Genet* 44:445–477.

Genomic Health Annual Report, 2009, http://www.genomichealth.com/OncotypeDX.aspx#.UhXSMKw04xE

Ghasabeh HR and Keyhanian S. (2013) Relationship between tumor markers CEA and CA15–3 and recurrence breast cancer. *J Paramed Sci* (JPS) 4(1):16–20.

Giguère V, Yang N, Segui P et al. (1988) Identification of a new class of steroid hormone receptors. *Nature* 331:91–94.

Gion M, Plebani M, Mione R et al. (1994) Serum CA549 in primary breast cancer: Comparison with CA15.3 and MCA. *Br J Cancer* 69(4):721–775.

Giovanella L, Ceriani L, Giardina G et al. (2002) Serum cytokeratin fragment 21.1 (CYFRA 21.1) as tumour marker for breast cancer: Comparison with carbohydrate antigen 15.3 (CA 15.3) and carcinoembryonic antigen (CEA). *Clin Chem Lab Med* 40(3):298–303.

Giuliano M, Giordano A, Jackson S et al. (2011) Circulating tumor cells as prognostic and predictive markers in metastatic breast cancer patients receiving first-line systemic treatment. *Breast Cancer Res* 13:R67.

Glazebrook KN, Magut MJ, and Reynolds C. (2008) Angiosarcoma of the breast. *AJR* 190(2):533–538.

Gobbi MD, Viprakasit V, and Hughes JR. (2006) A regulatory SNP causes a human genetic disease by creating a new transcriptional promoter. *Science* 312(5777):1215–1217.

Gonzalez-Angulo AM, Chen H, Karuturi MS et al. (2013) Frequency of mesenchymal-epithelial transition factor gene (MET) and the catalytic subunit of phosphoinositide-3-kinase (PIK3CA) copy number elevation and correlation with outcome in patients with early stage breast cancer. *Cancer* 119(1):7–15.

Gonzalez-Quintela A, Mallo N, Mella C et al. (2006) Serum levels of cytokeratin-18 (tissue polypeptide-specific antigen) in liver diseases. *Liver Int* 26(10):1217–1224.

Gordian E, Ramachandran K, and Singal R. (2009) Methylation mediated silencing of TMS1 in breast cancer and its potential contribution to docetaxel cytotoxicity. *Anticancer Res* 29:3207–3210.

Gosden JR, Middleton PG, and Rout D. (1986) Localization of the human oestrogen receptor gene to chromosome 6q24—q27 by in situ hybridization. *Cytogenet Cell Genet* 43(3–4):218–220.

Goulet B, Sansregret L, Leduy L et al. (2007) Increased expression and activity of nuclear cathepsin L in cancer cells suggests a novel mechanism of cell transformation. *Mol Cancer Res* 5(9):899–907.

Gregory PA, Bert AG, Paterson EL et al. (2008a) Themi R-200 family and miR-205 regulate epithelial to mesenchymal transition by targeting ZEB1 and SIP1. *Nat Cell Biol* 10(5):593–601.

Griffin JL and Shockcor JP. (2004) Metabolic profiles of cancer cells. *Nat Rev Cancer* 4(7):551–561.

Gunsoy NB, Garcia-Closas M, and Moss SM. (2012) Modelling the over diagnosis of breast cancer due to mammography screening in women aged 40–49 in the United Kingdom. *Breast Cancer Res* 14 (6):R152.

Gupta S and Knowlton AA. (2005) HSP60, bax, apoptosis and the heart. *J Cell Mol Med* 9(1):51–58.

Gymrek M, Golan D, Rosset S et al. (2012) lobSTR: A short tandem repeat profiler for personal genomes. *Genome Res* 22(6):1154–1162.

Habets JM, Tank B, Vuzevski VD et al. (1988) Absence of cytokeratin 8 and inconsistent expression of cytokeratins 7 and 19 in human basal cell carcinoma. *Anticancer Res* 8(4):611–616.

Halushka MK, Fan JB, Bentley K et al. (1999) Patterns of single-nucleotide polymorphisms in candidate genes for blood-pressure homeostasis. *Nat Genet* 22(3):239–247.

Hamrita B, Nasr HB, Chahed K et al. (2010) Proteomic analysis of human breast cancer: New technologies and clinical applications for biomarker profiling. *J Proteomics Bioinform* 3:091–098.

Han HJ, Russo J, Kohwi Y et al. 2008 SATB1 reprogrammes gene expression to promote breast tumour growth and metastasis. *Nature* 452(7184):187–193.

Hanahan D and Weinberg RA. (2000) The hallmarks of cancer. *Cell* 100:57–70.

Hanby AM and Hughes TA. (2008) In situ and invasive lobular neoplasia of the breast. *Histopathology* 52(1):58–66.

Hanker LC, Karn T, Mavrova-Risteska L et al. (2011) SATB1 gene expression and breast cancer prognosis. *Breast* 20(4):309–313.

Hanstein B, Djahansouzi S, Dall P et al. (2004) Insights into the molecular biology of the estrogen receptor define novel therapeutic targets for breast cancer. *Euro J Endocrinol* 150:243–255.

Harnett A, Smallwood J, Titshall V et al. (2009) Diagnosis and treatment of early breast cancer, including locally advanced disease—Summary of NICE guidance. *BMJ* 338:b438.

Harris L, Fritsche H, Mennel R et al. (2007) American society of clinical oncology 2007 update of recommendations for the use of tumor markers in breast cancer. *JCO* 25(33):5287–5312.

Hausauer AK, Keegan TH, Chang ET et al. (2009) Recent trends in breast cancer incidence in US white women by county-level urban/rural and poverty status. *BMC Med* 7:31.

He J, Gornbein J, Shen D et al. (2007) Detection of breast cancer biomarkers in nipple aspirate fluid by SELDI-TOF and their identification by combined liquid chromatography-tandem mass spectrometry. *Int J Oncol* 30:145–154.

He J, Whelan SA, Lu M et al. (2011) Proteomic-based biosignatures in breast cancer classification and prediction of therapeutic response. *Int J Proteomics* 2011:16.

Heck KE and Pamuk ER. (1997) Explaining the relation between education and postmenopausal breast cancer. *Am J Epidemiol* 145:366–372.

Heikkinen T, Greco D, Pelttari LM et al. (2011) Variants on the promoter region of PTEN affect breast cancer progression and patient survival. *Breast Cancer Res* 13:R130.

Heiko S. (2009) Molecular imaging of cancer: Receptors, angiogenesis, and gene. *Exp Curr Clin Oncol* 107–114.

Heneghan HM, Miller N, and Kerin MJ. (2010) Role of microRNAs in obesity and the metabolic syndrome. *Obesity Rev*11(5):354–361.

Heneghan HM, Miller N, McAnena OJ et al. (2011) Differential miRNA expression in omental adipose tissue and in the circulation of obese patients identifies novel metabolic biomarkers. *J Clin Endocrinol Metab* 96(5):E846–E850.

Hermelink K, Untch M, Lux MP et al. (2007) Cognitive function during neoadjuvant chemotherapy for breast cancer. *Cancer* 109:1905–1913.

Herranz M and Ruibal A. (2012) Optical imaging in breast cancer diagnosis: The next evolution, *J Oncol*, 2012:10.

Hicks C, Asfour R, Pannuti A et al. (2011) An integrative genomics approach to biomarker discovery in breast cancer. *Cancer Inform* 11(10):185–204.

Higgins MJ and Baselga J. (2011) Targeted therapies for breast cancer. *J Clin Invest* 121(10):3797–3803.

Hilvo M, Denkert C, Lehtinen L et al. (2011) Novel theranostic opportunities offered by characterization of altered membrane lipid metabolism in breast cancer progression. *Cancer Res* 71(9):3236–3245.

Holmes FA and Liticker JD. (2005) Pharmacogenomics of tamoxifen in a nutshell—And who broke the nutcracker? *J Oncol Pract* 1(4):155–159.

Hossain A, Kuo MT, and Saunders GF. (2006) Mir-17–5p regulates breast cancer cell proliferation by inhibiting translation of AIB1 mRNA. *Mol Cell Biol* 26:8191–8201.

Hou W, Zhou H, Elisma F et al. (2008) Technological developments in lipidomics. *Brief Funct Gen Proteomics* 7:395–409.

Howard DH, Ekwueme DU, Gardner JG et al. (2010) The impact of a national program to provide free mammograms to low-income, uninsured women on breast cancer mortality rates. *Cancer* 116:4456–4462.

http://edrn.nci.nih.gov/biomarkers

http://www.roche.com/products/product-details.htm?type=product&id=17

http://directhittest.com/patients.html

http://www.intergenetics.com/cms/technologyandproducts/whatisoncovue/testresults

Hu XC, Wong IH, and Chow LW. (2003) Tumor-derived aberrant methylation in plasma of invasive ductal breast cancer patients: Clinical implications. *Oncol Rep* 10(6):1811–1815.

Huang Q, Gumireddy K, Schrier M et al. (2008) The microRNAs miR-373 and miR-520c promote tumour invasion and metastasis. *Nat Cell Biol* 10(2):202–210.

Huang Y, Hinds DA, Qi L et al. (2010) Pooled versus individual genotyping in a breast cancer genome-wide association study. *Genet Epidemiol* 34(6):603–612.

Hucka M, Finney A, Sauro HM et al. (2003) The systems biology markup language (SBML): A medium for representation and exchange of biochemical network models. *Bioinformatics* 19(4):524–531.

Hudson MJ, Stamp GW, Chaudhary KS et al. (2001) Human MUC1 mucin: A potent glandular morphogen. *J Pathol* 194(3):373–383.

Huo D, Zheng Y, Ogundiran TO et al. (2012) Evaluation of susceptibility loci of breast cancer in women of African ancestry. *Carcinogenesis* 33:835–840.

Hussain R, Lodhi FB, and Ali M. (2006) Serum tumor markers. *Professional Med J* 13(1):1–10.

Ideker T., Dutkowski J., and Hood L. (2011) Boosting signal-to-noise in complex biology: Prior knowledge is power. *Cell* 144:860–863.

Ignatiadis M, Xenidis N, Perraki M et al. (2007) Different prognostic value of cytokeratin-19 mRNA positive circulating tumor cells according to estrogen receptor and HER2 status in early-stage breast cancer. *J Clin Oncol* 25(33):5194–5202.

Ikeda Y, Kuwano H, Ikebe M et al. (1994) Immunohistochemical detection of CEA, CA19–9, and DF3 in esophageal carcinoma limited to the submucosal layer. *J Surg Oncol* 56(1):7–12.

Imbeaud S, Graudens E, Boulanger V et al. (2005) Towards standardization of RNA quality assessment using user-independent classifiers of microcapillary electrophoresis traces. *Nucleic Acids Res* 33(6):e56.

Ingle JN. (2008) Pharmacogenomics of tamoxifen and aromatase inhibitors. *Cancer* 112(3):695–699.

Iorio MV, Ferracin M, Liu CG et al. (2005) Micro RNA gene expression deregulation in human breast cancer. *Cancer Res* 65(16):7065–7070.

Iorio MV, Ferracin M, Liu CG et al. (2006) A microRNA expression signature of human solid tumors defines cancer gene targets. *Proc Natl Acad Sci* 103:2257–2261.

Iorns E, Hnatyszyn HJ, Seo P et al. (2010) The role of SATB1 in breast cancer pathogenesis. *J Nat Cancer Inst* 102(16):1284–1296.

Jalota A, Singh K, Pavithra L et al. 2005. Tumor suppressor SMAR1 activates and stabilizes p53 through its arginine-serine-rich motif. *J Biol Chem* 280:16019–16029.

James CR, Quinn JE, Mullan PB et al. (2007) BRCA1, a potential predictive biomarker in the treatment of breast cancer. *Oncologist* 12(2):142–150.

Jansen MP, Sieuwerts AM, Look MP et al. (2007) HOXB13-to-IL17BR expression ratio is related with tumor aggressiveness and response to tamoxifen of recurrent breast cancer: A retrospective study. *J Clin Oncol* 25(6):662–668.

Jemal A, Bray F, Center MM et al. (2011) Global cancer statistics. *CA Cancer J Clin* 61:69–90.

Jemal A, Center MM, Santis CD et al. (2010) Global patterns of cancer incidence and mortality rates and trends. *Cancer Epidemiol Biomarkers Prev* 19:1893.

Jensen A, Sharif H, Olsen JH et al. (2008) Risk of breast cancer and gynecologic cancers in a large population of nearly 50,000 infertile danish women. *Am J Epidemiol* 168(1):49–57.

Jin Z, Cheng Y, Olaru A. (2008) Promoter hypermethylation of CDH13 is a common, early event in human esophageal adenocarcinogenesis and correlates with clinical risk factors. *Int J Cancer* 123:2331–2336.

Jones PA and Baylin SB. (2007) The epigenomics of cancer. *Cell* 128(4):683–692.

Jordan KW, Nordenstam J, Lauwers GY et al. (2009) Metabolomic characterization of human rectal adenocarcinoma with intact tissue magnetic resonance spectroscopy. *Dis Colon Rectum* 52(3):520–525.

Joshi-Tope G, Gillespie M, Vastrik I et al. (2005) Reactome: A knowledgebase of biological pathways. *Nucl Acids Res* 33:D428–D432.

Jung SY, Han W, Lee JW et al. (2009) Ki-67 expression gives additional prognostic information on St. Gallen 2007 and Adjuvant! Online risk categories in early breast cancer. *Ann Surg Oncol* 16(5):1112–1121.

Kamat N, Khidhir MA, Jaloudi M et al. (2012) High incidence of microsatellite instability and loss of heterozygosity in three loci in breast cancer patients receiving chemotherapy: A prospective study. *BMC Cancer* 12:373.

Kancha RK, von Bubnoff N, Bartosch N et al. (2011) Differential sensitivity of ERBB2 kinase domain mutations towards lapatinib. *PLoS One* 6(10):e26760.

Kanehisa M and Goto S. (2000) KEGG: Kyoto encyclopedia of genes and genomes. *Nucl Acids Res* 28:27–30.

Kann MG. (2007) Protein interactions and disease: Computational approaches to uncover the etiology of diseases. *Brief Bioinform* 8:333–346.

Kapali AS, Singh M, Deo SVS et al. (2010) Aggressive palliative surgery in metastatic phyllodes tumor: Impact on quality of life. *Indian J Palliat Care* 16:101–104.

Kapp A, Jeffrey S, Langerød A et al. (2006) Discovery and validation of breast cancer subtypes. *BMC Gen* 7:231.

Karns K and Herr AE. (2011) Human tear protein analysis enabled by an alkaline microfluidic homogeneous immunoassay. *Anal Chem* 83(21):8115–8122.

Kato M, Paranjape T, Müller RU et al. (2009) The mir-34 microRNA is required for the DNA damage response in vivo in *C. elegans* and in vitro in human breast cancer cells. *Oncogene* 28:2419–2424.

Kaul R, Mukherjee S, Ahmed F et al. (2003) Direct interaction with and activation of p53 by SMAR1 retards cell-cycle progression at G2/M phase and delays tumor growth in mice. *Int J Cancer* 103(5):606–615.

Kaul-Ghanekar R, Jalota A, Pavithra L et al. (2004) SMAR1 and Cux/CDP modulate chromatin and act as negative regulators of the TCRbeta enhancer (Ebeta). *Nucl Acids Res* 32(16):4862–4875.

Kaul-Ghanekar R, Singhet S, Hitesh M et al. (2009) Tumor suppressor protein SMAR1 modulates the roughness of cell surface: Combined AFM and SEM study. *BMC Cancer* 9:350.

Keam B, Im SA, Lee KH et al. (2011) Ki-67 can be used for further classification of triple negative breast cancer into two subtypes with different response and prognosis. *Breast Cancer Res* 13:R22.

Keklikoglou I, Koerner C, Schmidt C et al. (2012) MicroRNA-520/373 family functions as a tumor suppressor in estrogen receptor negative breast cancer by targeting NF-κBand TGF-β signaling pathways. *Oncogene* 31(37):4150–4163.

Kelly K and Amy EH. (2011) Ophthalmologist-on-a-chip: Fully integrated icrofluidic tear osmolarity and protein biomarker quantification for dry eye stratification. *15th International Conference on Miniaturized Systems for Chemistry and Life Sciences*, Seattle, WA, pp. 21–23.

Keyhani M, Nasizadeh S, and Ardeshir D. (2005) Serum CA15-3 measurement in breast cancer patients before and after mastectomy. *Arch Iranian Med* 8(4):263–266.

Kim JK, Jung KH, Noh JH et al. (2009) Targeted disruption of S100P suppresses tumor cell growth by down-regulation of cyclinD1 and CDK2 in human hepatocellular carcinoma. *Int J Oncol* 35(6):1257–1264.

Kim YS, Yoo HS, and Ko JH. (2009) Implication of aberrant glycosylation in cancer and use of lectin for cancer biomarker discovery. *Protein Pept Lett* 16(5):499–507.

King MC, Marks JH, and Mandell JB. (2003) Breast and ovarian cancer risks due to inherited mutations in BRCA1 and BRCA2. *Science* 643–646.

Kobeissi L, Hamra R, Samari G et al. (2012) The 2009 lebanese national mammography campaign: Results and assessment using a survey design. *Epidemiology* 2:1.

Köhrmann A, Kammerer U, Kapp M et al. (2009) Expression of matrix metalloproteinases (MMPs) in primary human breast cancer and breast cancer cell lines: New findings and review of the literature. *BMC Cancer* 9:188.

Kolusayin Ozar MO and Orta T. (2005) The use of chromosome aberrations in predicting breast cancer risk. *J Exp Clin Cancer Res* 24(2):217–222.

Kong EH, Pike AC, and Hubbard RE. (2003) Structure and mechanism of the oestrogen receptor. *Biochem Soc Trans* 31:56–59.

Kong W, Yang H, He L et al. (2008) MicroRNA-155 is regulated by the transforming growth factor beta/Smad pathway and contributes to epithelial cell plasticity by targeting RhoA. *Mol Cell Biol* 28:6773–6784.

Kornegoor R, Moelans CB, and Verschuur-Maes AHJ. (2012) Promoter hypermethylation in male breast cancer: Analysis by multiplex ligation-dependent probe amplification. *Breast Cancer Res* 14:R101.

Korpal M and Kang Y. (2008) The emerging role of miR-200 family of microRNAs in epithelial-mesenchymal transition and cancer metastasis. *RNA Biol* 5(3):115–119.

Kosacka M and Jankowska R. (2009) Comparison of cytokeratin 19 expression in tumor tissue and serum CYFRA 21-1 levels in non-small cell lung cancer. *Pol Arch Med Wewn* 119(1–2):33–37.

Kotsopoulos J, Tworoger SS, Campos H et al. (2010) Reproducibility of plasma and urine biomarkers among premenopausal and postmenopausal women from the Nurses' Health Studies. *Cancer Epidemiol Biomarkers Prev* 19(4):938–946.

Krassenstein R, Sauter E, Dulaimi E et al. (2004) Detection of breast cancer in nipple aspirate fluid by CpG island hypermethylation. *Clin Cancer Res* 10(1):28–32.

Kruit A, Gerritsen WB, Pot N et al. (2010) CA 15-3 as an alternative marker for KL-6 in fibrotic lung diseases. *Sarcoidosis Vasc Diffuse Lung Dis* 27(2):138–146.

Kumar KS and Kumar MMJ. (2008) Antiestrogen therapy for breast cancer: An overview. *Cancer Ther* 6:655–664.

Kumpulainen EJ, Keskikuru R, and Johansson RT. (2002) Serum tumor marker CA 15.3 and stage are the two most important predictors of survival in primary breast cancer. *Breast Cancer Res Treat* 76:95–102.

Kurian AW, McClure LA, John EM et al. (2009) Second primary breast cancer occurrence according to hormone receptor status. *J Natl Cancer Inst* 101:1058–1065.

Kurian S, Khan M, and Grant M. (2008) CA 27–29 in patients with breast cancer with pulmonary fibrosis. *Clin Breast Cancer* 8(6):538–540.

Kwei KA, Kung Y, Salari K et al. (2010) Genomic instability in breast cancer: Pathogenesis and clinical implications. *Mol Oncol* 4(3):255–266.

Lacroix-Triki M, Lambros MB, Geyer FC et al. (2010) Absence of microsatellite instability in mucinous carcinomas of the breast. *Int J Clin Exp Pathol* 4(1):22–31.

Laronga C and Drake RR. (2007) Proteomic approach to breast cancer. *Cancer Cont* 14(4):360–368.

Larson JS, Goodman LJ, Tan Y. et al. (2010) Analytical validation of a highly sensitive, accurate, and reproducible assay (HERmark) for the measurement of HER2 total protein and HER2 homodimers in FFPE breast cancer tumor specimens. *Pathol Res* 814176.

Lawrie CH, Gal S, Dunlop HM et al. (2008) Detection of elevated levels of tumour-associated microRNAs in serum of patients with diffuse large B-cell lymphoma. *Br J Haematol* 141(5):672–675.

Lea R, Bannister E, Case A et al. (2004) Use of hormonal replacement therapy after treatment of breast cancer. *J Obstet Gynaecol Can* 26(1):49–60.

Lebrecht A, Boehm D, Schmidt M et al. (2009) Diagnosis of breast cancer by tear proteomic pattern. *Cancer Gen Proteomics* 6(3):177–182.

Lee MC, Patel-Parekh L, Bland KI et al. (2007) Increased frequency of estrogen receptor (ER) negative and aneuploid breast cancer in African American women at all stages of disease: First analysis of the National Cancer Data Base. Program and abstracts of the 2007 Breast Cancer Symposium; San Francisco, CA. Abstract 121.

Lee RC, Feinbaum RL, and Ambros V (1993) The C. elegans heterochronic gene lin-4 encodes small RNAs with antisense complementarity to lin-14. *Cell* 75:843–854.

Lee SC, Berg KD, Sherman M et al. (2001) Microsatellite instability is infrequent in medullary breast cancer. *Am J Clin Pathol* 115:823–827.

Lee YS and Dutta A. (2007) The tumor suppressor microRNA let-7 represses the HMGA2 oncogene. *Genes Dev* 21(9):1025–1030.

Lehman CD, DePeri ER, Peacock S et al. (2005) Clinical experience with MRI-guided vacuum-assisted breast biopsy. *AJR* 184:1782–1787.

Lehtimäki T, Lundin M, Linder N et al. (2011) Long-term prognosis of breast cancer detected by mammography screening or other methods. *Breast Cancer Res* 13(6):R134.

Lemieux J, Maunsell E, and Provencher L. (2008) Chemotherapy-induced alopecia and effects on quality of life among women with breast cancer: A literature review. *Psycho-Oncol* 17:317–328.

Levenson VV and Melniko AA. (2012) DNA methylation as clinically useful biomarkers—Light at the end of the tunnel. *Pharmaceuticals* 5:94–113.

Lewis CM, Cler LR, Bu DW et al. (2005) Promoter hypermethylation in benign breast epithelium in relation to predicted breast cancer risk. *Clin Cancer Res* 11:166–172.

Li H and d'Anjou M. (2009) Pharmacological significance of glycosylation in therapeutic proteins. *Curr Opin Biotechnol* 20:678–684.

Li J, Zhao J, Yu X et al. (2005) Identification of biomarkers for breast cancer in nipple aspiration and ductal lavage fluid. *Clin Cancer Res* 11:8312–8320.

Li X, Link JM, Stekhova S et al. (2008) Site-specific labeling of Annexin V with F-18 for apoptosis imaging. *Bioconjug Chem* 19(8):1684–1688.

Li Y. (2010) The detection of tear biomarkers for future prostate cancer diagnosis. *Open Biomark J* 3:26–29.

Liang S, Singh M, and Gam LH. (2011) Potential hydrophobic protein markers of breast cancer in Malaysian Chinese, Malay and Indian patients. *Cancer Biomark* 8(6):319–330.

Lianidou ES and Markou A. (2011) Circulating tumor cells as emerging tumor biomarkers in breast cancer. *Clin Chem Lab Med* 49:1579–1590.

Lim LY, Vidnovic N, Ellisen LW et al. (2009) Mutant p53 mediates survival of breast cancer cells. *Br J Cancer* 101:1606–1612.

Lin PI, Vance JM, Pericak-Vance MA et al. (2007) No gene is an island: The flip-flop phenomenon. *Am J Hum Genet* 80:531–538.

Lindberg K, Helguero LA, Omoto Y et al. (2011) Estrogen receptor β represses Akt signaling in breast cancer cells via downregulation of HER2/HER3 and upregulation of PTEN: Implications for tamoxifen sensitivity. *Breast Cancer Res* 13:R43.

Lipton A, Ali SM, Leitzel K et al. (2002) Elevated Serum HER-2/neu level predicts decreased response to hormone therapy in metastatic breast cancer. *J Clin Oncol* 20(6):1467–1472.

Liska V, Holubec L, Treska V et al. (2007) Tumor markers as useful predictors of survival rate after exploratory laparotomy for liver malignancies. *Anticancer Res* 27:1887–1892.

Liu R, Wang X, Chen GY et al. (2007) The prognostic role of a gene signature from tumorigenic breast-cancer cells. *N Engl J Med* 356(3):217–226.

Liu Z, Zhu J, Cao H et al. (2012) miR-10b promotes cell invasion through RhoC-AKT signaling pathway by targeting HOXD10 in gastric cancer. *Int J Oncol* 40(5):1553–1560.

Locasale JW and Cantley LC. (2010) Altered metabolism in cancer. *BMC Biol* 8:88.

Locke I, Kote-Jarai Z, Fackler MJ et al. Gene promoter hypermethylation in ductal lavage fluid from healthy BRCA gene mutation carriers and mutation-negative controls. *Breast Cancer Res* 9:R20.

Lopez F, Belloc F, Lacombe F et al. (1991) Modalities of synthesis of Ki67 antigen during the stimulation of lymphocytes. *Cytometry* 12(1):42–49.

Luqmani YA and Mathew M. (2004) Allelic variation of BAT-25 and BAT-26 mononucleotide repeat loci in tumours from a group of young women with breast cancer. *Int J Oncol* 25(3):771–775.

Lynn J. (2004) Fulvestrant ('Faslodex')-a new hormonal treatment for advanced breast cancer. *Eur J Oncol Nurs* 8(Suppl 2):S83–S88.

Ma L, Teruya-Feldstein J, and Weinberg RA. (2007) Tumour invasion and metastasis initiated by microRNA-10b in breast cancer. *Nature* 449:682–688.

Ma XJ, Salunga R, Dahiya S et al. (2008) A five-gene molecular grade index and HOXB13: IL17BR are complementary prognostic factors in early stage breast cancer. *Clin Cancer Res* 14(9):2601–2608.

Macdonald IK, Allen J, Murray A et al. (2012) Development and validation of a high throughput system for discovery of antigens for autoantibody detection. *PLoS One* 7(7):e40759.

Mackay J and Szecsei CM. (2010) Genetic counselling for hereditary predisposition to ovarian and breast cancer. *Ann Oncol* 21(7):334–338.

MacMahon B. (2006) Epidemiology and the causes of breast cancer. *Int J Cancer* 118(10):2373–2378.

Madhavan S, Gusev Y, Harris M et al. (2011) G-DOC: A systems medicine platform for personalized oncology. *Neoplasia* 13(9):771–783.

Madu CO and Lu Y. (2010) Novel diagnostic biomarkers for prostate cancer. *J Cancer* 1:150–177.

Malati T. (2007) Tumour markers: An overview. *Ind J Clin Biochem* 22(2):17–31.

Malonia SK, Sinha S, Pavithra L et al. (2011) Gene regulation by SMAR1 and its role as candidate tumor suppressor. *BBA Rev Can* 1815(1):1–12 (IF:12).

Mann AM and Tighe BJ. (2007) Tear analysis and lens-tear interactions: Part I. Protein fingerprinting with microfluidic technology. *Cont Lens Anterior Eye* 30(3):163–173.

Mansel RE, Goyal A, Douglas-Jones A et al. (2009) Detection of breast cancer metastasis in sentinel lymph nodes using intra-operative real time gene search BLN assay in the operating room: Results of the Cardiff study. *Breast Cancer Res Treat* 115(3):595–600.

Marotta LL, Almendro V, and Marusyk A. (2011) The JAK2/STAT3 signaling pathway is required for growth of $CD44^{+}CD24^{-}$ stem cell-like breast cancer cells in human tumors. *J Clin Invest* 121(7):2723–2735.

Marrakchi R, Ouerhani S, Benammar S et al. (2008) Detection of cytokeratin 19 mRNA and CYFRA 21-1 (cytokeratin 19 fragments) in blood of Tunisian women with breast cancer. *Int J Biol Markers* 23(4):238–243.

Martelli AM, Evangelisti C, Chiarini F et al. (2010) The phosphatidylinositol 3-kinase/Akt/mTOR signaling network as a therapeutic target in acute myelogenous leukemia patients. *Oncotarget* 1(2):89–103.

Martínez-Galán J, Torres B, Del MR et al. (2008) Quantitative detection of methylated ESR1 and 14-3-3-sigma gene promoters in serum as candidate biomarkers for diagnosis of breast cancer and evaluation of treatment efficacy. *Cancer Biol Ther* 7(6):958–965.

Massardo T, Alonso O, Llamas-Ollier A et al. (2005) Planar Tc99m—Sestamibi scintimammography should be considered cautiously in the axillary evaluation of breast cancer protocols: Results of an international multicenter trial. *BMC Nucl Med* 5:4.

Matsuda S, Rouault J, Magaud J et al. (2001) In search of a function for the TIS21/PC3/BTG1/TOB family. *FEBS Lett* 497(2–3):67–72.

Mattie MD, Benz CC, Bowers J et al. (2006) Optimized high-throughput microRNAs expression profiling provides novel biomarker assessment of clinical prostate and breast cancer biopsies. *Mol Cancer* 5:24.

Mattiske S, Suetani RJ, and Neilsen PM. (2012) Theoncogenicroleofmi R-155inbreastcancer. *Cancer Epidemiol Biomarkers Prev* 21(8):1236–1243.

Matuschek C, Bölke E, and Lammering G. (2010) Methylated APC and GSTP1 genes in serum DNA correlate with the presence of circulating blood tumor cells and are associated with a more aggressive and advanced breast cancer disease. *Eur J Med Res* 15:277–286.

Mayeux R. (2004) Biomarkers: Potential uses and limitations. *NeuroRx* 1(2):182–188.
McGrowder D, Riley C, Y St A Morrison E et al. (2011) The role of high-density lipoproteins in reducing the risk of vascular diseases, neurogenerative disorders, and cancer. *Cholesterol* 1–9. University of Toronto, Toronto, Ontario, Canada.
Meany DL and Chan DW (2011) Aberrant glycosylation associated with enzymes as cancer biomarkers. *Clin Proteomics* 8:7.
Menasce LP, White GR, and Harrison CJ. (1993) Localisation of the estrogen receptor locus (ESR) to chromosome 6q25.1 by FISH and a simple post-FISH banding technique. *Genomics* 17:263–265.
Metcalfe K, Lubinski J, Lynch HT et al. (2010) Hereditary Breast Cancer Clinical Study Group. Family history of cancer and cancer risks in women with BRCA1 or BRCA2 mutations. *J Natl Cancer Inst* 102(24):1874–1878.
Michl P and Downward J. (2006) CUTL1: A key mediator of TGFbeta-induced tumor invasion. *Cell Cycle* 5(2):132–134.
Michl P, Ramjaun AR, and Pardo OE. (2005) CUTL1 is a target of TGF (beta) signaling that enhances cancer cell motility and invasiveness. *Cancer Cell* 7(6):521–532.
Miglietta L, Vanella P, Canobbio L, Naso C et al. (2010) Prognostic value of estrogen receptor and Ki-67 index after neoadjuvant chemotherapy in locally advanced breast cancer expressing high levels of proliferation at diagnosis. *Oncology* 79(3–4):255–261.
Miles DW, Happerfield LC, Smith P et al. (1994) Expression of sialyl-Tn predicts the effect of adjuvant chemotherapy in node-positive breast cancer. *Br J Cancer* 70:1272–1275.
Miller LD, Smeds J, George J et al. (2005) An expression signature for p53 status in human breast cancer predicts mutation status, transcriptional effects, and patient survival. *Proc Natl Acad Sci* 102:13550–13555.
Miranda BT and Jones PA. (2007) DNA methylation: The nuts and bolts of repression. *J Cell Physiol* 213:384–390.
Misek DE and Kim EH. (2011) Protein biomarkers for the early detection of breast cancer. *Int J Proteomics* 9:343582.
Misek DE, Kondo T, and Duncan MW. (2011) Proteomics-based disease biomarkers. *Int J Proteomics* 2011:894618.
Mitelman F, Johansson B, and Mertens F. Fusion genes and rearranged genes as a linear function of chromosome aberrations in cancer. *Nat Genet* 36:331–334.
Moffat BA, Chenevert TL, Meyer CR et al. (2006) The functional diffusion map: An imaging biomarker for the early prediction of cancer treatment outcome. *Neoplasia* 8(4):259–267.
Molina R, Auge JM, Farrus B et al. (2010) Prospective evaluation of carcinoembryonic antigen (CEA) and carbohydrate antigen 15.3 (CA15.3) in patients with primary locoregional breast cancer. *Clin Chem* 56(7):1148–1157.
Momparler RL. (2003) Cancer epigenetics. *Oncogene* 22(42):6479–6483.
Morey P, Jadhav SM, Karpe M et al. (2012) Biomarkers in oncology. *J Appl Pharm Sci* 2(3):182–191.
Mote PA, Leary JA, Avery KA et al. (2004) Germ-line mutations in BRCA1 or BRCA2 in the normal breast are associated with altered expression of estrogen-responsive proteins and the predominance of progesterone receptor A. *Gen Chromosomes Cancer* 39(3):236–248.
Muggerud AA, Rønneberg JA, Wärnberg F et al. (2010) Frequent aberrant DNA methylation of ABCB1, FOXC1, PPP2R2B and PTEN in ductal carcinoma in situ and early invasive breast cancer. *Breast Cancer Res* 12(1):R3.
Mukhopadhyay P, Chakraborty S, Ponnusamy MP et al. (2011) Mucins in the pathogenesis of breast cancer: Implications in diagnosis, prognosis and therapy. *Biochim Biophys Acta* 1815(2):224–240.
Munagala R, Aqil F, and Gupta RC. (2011) Promising molecular targeted therapies in breast cancer. *Ind J Pharmacol* 43(3):236–245.
Murata H, Khattar NH, Kang Y et al. (2002) Genetic and epigenetic modification of mismatch repair genes hMSH2 and hMLH1 in sporadic breast cancer with microsatellite instability. *Oncogene* 21(37):5696–5703.
Nadal R, Fernandez A, Sanchez-Rovira P et al. (2012) Biomarkers characterization of circulating tumour cells in breast cancer patients. *Breast Cancer Res* 14:R71.
Naeim A, Wong FL, Pal SK et al. (2010) Oncologists' recommendations for adjuvant therapy in hormone receptor-positive breast cancer patients of varying age and health status. *Clin Breast Cancer* 10(2):136–143.
Nakagoe T, Itoyanagi T, Ikuta Y et al. (2002) Preoperative serum levels of sialyl lewisa, sialyl lewisx, and carcinoembryonic antigens as prognostic factors after resection for primary breast cancer. *Acta Med Nagasaki* 47:37–41.

Nakata B, Ogawa TY, Ishikawa T et al. (2004) Serum CYFRA 21–1 (cytokeratin-19 fragments) is a useful tumour marker for detecting disease relapse and assessing treatment efficacy in breast cancer. *Brit J Cancer* 91:873–878.

Nam H, Chung BC, Kim Y et al. (2009) Combining tissue transcriptomics and urine metabolomics for breast cancer biomarker identification. *Bioinformatics* 25(23):3151–3157.

Narita T, Funahashi H, Satoh Y et al. (1993) Association of expression of blood group-related carbohydrate antigens with prognosis in breast cancer. *Cancer* 71:3044–3053.

National Cancer Institute, Surveillance, Epidemiology and End results program database.

Nelson HD, Huffman LH, Fu R et al. (2005) Genetic risk assessment and BRCA mutation testing for breast and ovarian cancer susceptibility: Systematic evidence review for the US Preventive Services Task Force. *Ann Intern Med* 143:355–361.

Nepveu A. (2001) Role of the multifunctional CDP/Cut/Cux homeodomain transcription factor in regulating differentiation, cell growth and development. *Gene* 270(1–2):1–15.

Neubauer H, Fehm T, Schütz C et al. (2007) Proteomic expression profiling of breast cancer. *Recent Results Cancer Res* 176:89–120.

Nguyen PL, Taghian AG, Katz MS et al. (2008) Breast cancer subtype approximated by estrogen receptor, progesterone receptor, and HER-2 is associated with local and distant recurrence after breast-conserving therapy. *J Clin Oncol* 26(14):2373–2378.

Nicolini A, Carpi A, and Tarro G. (2006) Biomolecular markers of breast cancer. *Front Biosci* 11:1818–1843.

Nielsen DL, Kümler I, Palshof JA et al. (2013) Efficacy of HER2-targeted therapy in metastatic breast cancer. Monoclonal antibodies and tyrosine kinase inhibitors. *Breast* 22(1):1–12.

Norman SA, Berlin JA, Weber AL et al. (2003) Combined effect of oral contraceptive use and hormone replacement therapy on breast cancer risk in postmenopausal women. *Cancer Cause Control* 14(10):933–943.

Novak P, Jensen TJ, Garbe JC et al. (2009) Stepwise DNA methylation changes are linked to escape from defined proliferation barriers and mammary epithelial cell immortalization. *Cancer Res* 69(12):5251–5258.

Oakman C, Bessi S, Zafarana E et al. (2009) Recent advances in systemic therapy. New diagnostics and biological predictors of outcome in early breast cancer. *Breast Cancer Res* 11:205.

O'Day E and Lal A. (2010) MicroRNAs and their target gene networks in breast cancer. *Breast Cancer Res.* 12(2):201.

Ogawa S, Inoue S, Watanabe T et al. (1998) The complete primary structure of human estrogen receptor beta (hER beta) and its heterodimerization with ER alpha in vivo and in vitro. *Biochem Biophys Res Commun* 243(1):122–126.

Ogawa Y, Ishikawa T, Ikeda K et al. (2000) Evaluation of serum KL-6, a mucin-like glycoprotein, as a tumor marker for Breast Cancer. *Clin Cancer Res* 6:4069–4072.

Olivier M, Langerød A, Carrieri P et al. (2006) The clinical value of somatic TP53 gene mutations in 1,794 patients with breast cancer. *Clin Cancer Res* 12, 1157–1167.

Olofsson MH, Ueno T, Pan Y et al. (2007) Cytokeratin-18 is a useful serum biomarker for early determination of response of breast carcinomas to chemotherapy. *Clin Cancer Res* 13(11):3198–3206.

Onay VU, Briollais L, Julia A et al. (2006) SNP-SNP interactions in breast cancer susceptibility. *BMC Cancer* 6:114.

Onitilo AA, Engel JM, Greenlee RT et al. (2009) Breast cancer subtypes based on ER/PR and Her2 expression: Comparison of clinicopathologic features and survival. *Clin Med Res* 7(1–2):4–13.

Oremek GM, Sauer-Eppel H, Bruzdziak TH. (2007) Value of tumour and inflammatory markers in lung cancer. *Anticancer Res* 27:1911–1916.

Ormandy CJ, Musgrove EA, Hui R et al. (2003) Cyclin D1, EMS1 and 11q13 amplification in breast cancer. *Breast Cancer Res Treat* 78(3):323–335.

Ou K, Seow TK, Liang RC et al. (2001) Proteome analysis of a human hepatocellular carcinoma cell line, HCC-M: An update. *Electrophoresis* 22(13):2804–2811.

Ou YH, Chung PH, and Hsu FF. (2007) The candidate tumor suppressor BTG3 is a transcriptional target of p53 that inhibits E2F1. *EMBO J* 26(17):3968–3980.

Owiredu WK, Donkor S, Addai BW et al. (2009) Serum lipid profile of breast cancer patients. *Pak J Biol Sci* 12(4):332–338.

Paik S, Hazan R, Fisher ER et al. (1990) Pathologic findings from the nations' surgical adjuvant breast and bowel project: Prognostic significance of erb B2 protein overexpression in primary breast cancer. *J Clin Oncol* 8:103–112.

Palma M, Ristori E, Ricevuto E et al. (2006) BRCA1 and BRCA2: The genetic testing and the current management options for mutation carriers. *Crit Rev Oncol/Hematol* 57(1):1–23.

Palsson B and Zengler K. (2010) The challenges of integrating multi-omic data sets. *Nat Chem Biol* 11:787–789.

Park BW, Oh JW, Kim JH et al. (2008b) Preoperative CA 15–3 and CEA serum levels as predictor for breast cancer outcomes. *Ann Oncol* 19(4):675–681.

Park SM, Gaur AB, Lengyel E et al. (2008a) The miR-200 family determines the epithelial phenotype of cancer cells by targeting the E-cadherin repressors ZEB1 and ZEB2. *Gene Dev* 22(7):894–907.

Parsa P, Kandiah M, and Rahman HA. (2006) Barriers for breast cancer screening among Asian women: A mini literature review. *Asian Pacific J Cancer Prev* 7:509–514.

Patani N, Jiang W, Mansel R et al. (2009) The mRNA expression of SATB1 and SATB2 in human breast cancer. *Cancer Cell Int* 9:18.

Pathiraja TN, Shetty PB, Jelinek J et al. (2011) Progesterone receptor isoform-specific promoter methylation: Association of PRA promoter methylation with worse outcome in breast cancer patients. *Clin Cancer Res* 17:4177–4186.

Patnaik JL, Byers T, DiGuiseppi C et al. (2011) Cardiovascular disease competes with breast cancer as the leading cause of death for older females diagnosed with breast cancer. *Breast Cancer Res* 13(3):64.

Paulin-Levasseur M and Julien M. (1992) Expression of intermediate filament proteins in TPA-induced MPC-11 and HL-60 cells. *Exp Cell Res* 2:363–372.

Pawlik TM, Hawke DH, Liu Y et al. (2006) Proteomic analysis of nipple aspirate fluid from women with early-stage breast cancer using isotope-coded affinity tags and tandem mass spectrometry reveals differential expression of vitamin D binding protein. *BMC Cancer* 6:68.

Pei Y, Zhang T, Renault V et al. (2009) An overview of hepatocellular carcinoma study by omics-based methods. *Acta Biochim Biophys Sin* 41(1):1–15.

Penuelas I, Domınguez-Prado I, Garcıa-Velloso MJ et al. (2012) PET tracers for clinical imaging of breast cancer. *J Oncol* 9 pages.

Perkins GL, Slater ED, Sanders GK et al. (2003) Serum tumor markers. *Am Fam Phys* 68(6):1075–1082.

Perou CM, Sørlie T, Eisen MB et al. (2000) Molecular portraits of human breast tumours. *Nature* 406(6797):747–752.

Perreard L, Fan C, Quackenbush JF et al. (2006) Classification and risk stratification of invasive breast carcinomas using a real-time quantitative RT-PCR assay. *Breast Cancer Res* 8:R23.

Pijpe A, Andrieu N, Easton DF et al. (2012) Exposure to diagnostic radiation and risk of breast cancer among carriers of BRCA1/2 mutations: Retrospective cohort study (GENE-RAD-RISK). *BMJ* 345:e5660.

Piperi C, Themistocleous MS, and Papavassiliou GA. (2010) High incidence of MGMT and RARβ promoter methylation in primary glioblastomas: Association with histopathological characteristics, inflammatory mediators and clinical outcome. *Mol Med* 16(1–2):1–9.

Pouliot F, Johnson M, and Wu L. (2009) Non-invasive molecular imaging of prostate cancer lymph node metastasis. *Trends Mol Med* 15(6):254–262.

Prabasheela B and Arivazhagan R. (2011) CA-15–3 and breast cancer. *Int J Pharma and Bio Sci* 2(2):B34–B38.

Prasad SN and Houserkova D. (2007) A comparison of mammography and ultrasonography in the evaluation of breast masses. *Biomed Pap Med Fac Univ Palacky Olomouc Czech Repub* 151(2):315–322.

Pujana MA, Han JD, Starita LM et al. (2007) Network modeling links breast cancer susceptibility and centrosome dysfunction. *Nat Genet* 39:1338–1349.

Pusztai L. (2008) Current status of prognostic profiling in breast cancer. *Oncologist* 13:350–360.

Pusztai L and Hess K. (2004) Clinical trial design for microarray predictive marker discovery and assessment. *Ann Oncol* 15:1731–1737.

Qin H, Yu T, Qing T et al. (2007) Regulation of apoptosis and differentiation by p53 in human embryonic stem cells. *J Biol Chem* 282(8):5842–5852.

Quon A and Gambhir SS. (2005) FDG-PET and beyond: Molecular breast cancer imaging. *JCO* 23(8):1664–1673.

Radpour R, Barekati Z, Kohler C et al. (2011) Integrated epigenetics of human breast cancer: Synoptic investigation of targeted genes, micrornas and proteins upon demethylation treatment. *PLoS One* 6(11):e27355.

Rakha EA, Boyce RW, Abd El-Rehim D et al. (2005) Expression of mucins (MUC1, MUC2, MUC3, MUC4, MUC5AC and MUC6) and their prognostic significance in human breast cancer. *Mod Pathol* 18(10):1295–1304.

Ralhan R, Kaur J, Kreienberg R et al. (2007) Links between DNA double strand break repair and breast cancer: Accumulating evidence from both familial and nonfamilial cases. *Cancer Lett* 248:1–17.

Ralph DA, Zhao LP, Aston CE et al. (2007) Age-specific association of steroid hormone pathway gene polymorphisms with breast cancer risk. *Cancer* 109(10):1940–1948.

Ramona FS and Massimo C. (2011) Circulating tumor cells in breast cancer: A tool whose time has come of age. *BMC Med* 9:43.

Rampalli S, Pavithra L, Bhatt A et al. (2005) Tumor suppressor SMAR1 mediates cyclin D1 repression by recruitment of the SIN3/histone deacetylase 1 complex. *Mol Cell Biol* 25(19):8415–8429.

Raval GN, Patel DD, Parekh LJ et al. (2003) Evaluation of serum sialic acid, sialyltransferase and sialoproteins in oral cavity cancer. *Oral Dis* 9(3):119–128.

Rehman F, Nagi AH, and Hussain M. (2010) Immunohistochemical expression and correlation of mammaglobin with the grading system of breast carcinoma. *Ind J Pathol Microbiol* 53:619–623.

Rennstam K, Baldetorp B, Kytölä S et al. (2001) Chromosomal rearrangements and oncogene amplification precede aneuploidization in the genetic evolution of breast cancer. *Cancer Res* 61(3):1214–1219.

Rhodes DR, Kalyana-Sundaram S, Mahavisno V et al. (2007) Oncomine 3.0: Genes, pathways, and networks in a collection of 18,000 cancer gene expression profiles. *Neoplasia* 9:166–180.

Richard SD, Bencherif B, Edwards RP et al. (2011) Noninvasive assessment of cell proliferation in ovarian cancer using [18F] 3′deoxy-3 fluorothymidine positron emission tomography/computed tomography imaging. *Nucl Med Biol* 38(4):485–491.

Riethdorf S, Fritsche H, Müller V et al. (2007) Detection of circulating tumor cells in peripheral blood of 15. Patients with metastatic breast cancer: A validation study of the cellsearch system. *Clin Cancer Res* 13(3):920–928.

Robert SA, Strombom IA, Trentham-Dietz A et al. (2004) Socioeconomic risk factors for breast cancer: Distinguishing individual-and community-level effects. *Epidemiology* 15:442–450.

Roberti MP, Arriaga JM, Bianchini M et al. (2012) Protein expression changes during human triple negative breast cancer cell line progression to lymph node metastasis in xenografted model in nude mice. *Cancer Biol Ther* 13(11):1123–1140.

Robertson DG, Watkins PB, and Reily MD. (2011) Metabolomics in toxicology: Preclinical and clinical applications. *Toxicol Sci* 120(S1):S146–S170.

Rocca-Serra P, Brazma A, Parkinson H et al. (2003) Array express: A public database of gene expression data at EBI. *Current Res Biol* 326:1075–1078.

Roden DM, Altman RB, Benowitz NL et al. (2006) Pharmacogenomics: Challenges and opportunities. *Ann Intern Med* 145(10):749–757.

Rofaiel S, Muo EN, and Mousa SA. (2010) Pharmacogenetics in breast cancer: Steps toward personalized medicine in breast cancer management. *Pharmacogenomics Pers Med* 3:129–143.

Ronckers CM, Erdmann CA, and Land CE. (2005) Radiation and breast cancer: A review of current evidence http://www.ncbi.nlm.nih.gov/pubmed/14750532. *Breast Cancer Res* 7:21–32.

Rose MC and Voynow JA. (2006) Respiratory tract mucin genes and mucin glycoproteins in health and disease. *Physiol Rev* 86(1):245–278.

Rosen EL, Eubank WB, and Mankoff DA. (2007) FDG PET, PET/CT, and breast cancer imaging. *Radiographics* 27(1):S215–S229.

Ross JS. (2008) Multigene predictors in early-stage breast cancer: Moving in or moving out? *Expert Rev Mol Diagn* 8(2):129–135.

Ross JS, Fletcher JA, and Bloom KJ (2004a) Targeted therapy in breast cancer: The HER-2/neu gene and protein. *Mol Cell Proteomics* 3(4):379–398.

Ross JS, Hatzis C., Symmans WF et al. (2008) Commercialized multigene predictors of clinical outcome for breast cancer. *Oncologist* 13:477–493.

Ross JS, Linette GP, Stec J et al. (2004b) Breast cancer biomarkers and molecular medicine: Part II. *Expert Rev Mol Diagn* 4(2):169–188.

Roy P and Shukla Y. (2008) Applications of proteomic techniques in cancer research. *Cancer Ther* 6:841–856.

Sachdev D. (2010) Targeting the type I insulin-like growth factor system for breast cancer therapy. *Curr Drug Targets* 11(9):1121–1132.

Sadikovic B, Al-Romaih K, Squire JA et al. (2008) Cause and consequences of genetic and epigenetic alterations in human cancer. *Curr Genomics* 9(6):394–408.

Saha A, Halder S, Upadhyay SK et al. Epstein-Barr virus nuclear antigen 3C facilitates G1-S transition by stabilizing and enhancing the function of cyclin D1. *PLoS Pathog* 7(2):e1001275.

Sakorafas GH, Farley DR, and Peros G. (2008) Recent advances and current controversies in the management of DCIS of the breast. *Cancer Treat Rev* 34:483–497.

Saldova R, Rueben JM, Abd Hamid et al. (2010) Levels of specific serum N-glycans identify breast cancer patients with higher circulating tumor cell counts. *Ann Oncol* 22(5):1113–1119.

Saloustros E, Perraki M, and Apostolaki S. (2011) Cytokeratin-19 mRNA-positive circulating tumor cells during follow-up of patients with operable breast cancer: Prognostic relevance for late relapse. *Breast Cancer Res* 13:R60.

Sarkar DK, Lahiri S, Kar RG et al. (2008) Utility of prognostic markers in management of breast cancer. *Int J Surg* 17(1).

Saslow D, Boetes C, Burke W et al. (2007) American Cancer Society guidelines for breast screening with MRI as an adjunct to mammography. *CA Cancer J Clin* 57:75–89.

Sauter E, Welch T, Magklara A et al. (2002) Ethnic variation in kallikrein expression in nipple Aspirate fluid. *Int J Cancer* 100:678–682.

Sauter ER, Ross E, Daly M et al. (1997) Nipple aspirate fluid: A promising non-invasive method to identify cellular markers of breast cancer risk. *Brit J Cancer* 76(4):494–501.

Schiff R, Massarweh SA, Shou J et al. (2005) Advanced concepts in estrogen receptor biology and breast cancer endocrine resistance: Implicated role of growth factor signaling and estrogen receptor coregulators. *Cancer Chemother Pharmacol* 56(l):10–20.

Schmid F, Burock S, Klockmeier K et al. (2012) SNPs in the coding region of the metastasis-inducing gene MACC1 and clinical outcome in colorectal cancer. *Mol Cancer* 11:49.

Schott AF and Hayes DF. (2012) Defining the benefits of neoadjuvant chemotherapy for breast cancer. *J Clin Oncol* 30(15):1747–1749.

Schrauder MG, Strick R, Schulz-Wendtland R et al. (2012) Circulating micro-RNAs as potential blood-based markers for early stage breast cancer detection. *PLoS One* 7(1):e29770.

Schumann D, Huang J, Clarke PE et al. (2004) Characterization of recombinant soluble carcinoembryonic antigen cell adhesion molecule. *Biochem Biophys Res Commun* 318:227–233.

Scott GK, Goga A, Bhaumik D et al. 2007 Coordinate suppression of ERBB2 and ERBB3 by enforced expression of micro-RNA miR-125a or miR-125b. *J Biol Chem* 282:1479–1486.

Sebova K, Zmetakova I, Bella V et al. (2011–2012) RASSF1A and CDH1 hypermethylation as potential epimarkers in breast cancer. *Cancer Biomark* 10(1):13–26.

Senapati S, Das S, and Batra SK. (2010) Mucin interacting proteins: From function to therapeutics. *Trend Biochem Sci* 35:236–245.

Seregni E, Coli A, and Mazzucca N. (2004) Circulating tumour markers in breast cancer. *Eur J Nucl Med Mol Imaging* 31(Suppl)1:S15–S22.

Serkova NJ and Glunde K. (2009) Metabolomics of cancer. *Method Mol Biol* 520:273–295.

Shah C, Miller TW, Wyatt SK et al. (2009) Therapy in preclinical models of breast cancer imaging biomarkers predict response to anti-HER2 (ErbB2). *Clin Cancer Res* 15:4712–4721.

Shah FD, Shukla SN, Shah PM et al. (2008) Significance of alterations in plasma lipid profile levels in breast cancer. *Integr Cancer Ther* 7(1):33–41.

Shankar LK. (2012) The clinical evaluation of novel imaging methods for cancer management. *Nat Rev Clin Oncol* 9:738–744.

Sharma R, Tripathi M, Panwar P et al. (2009) 99mTc-methionine scintimammography in the evaluation of breast cancer. *Nucl Med Commun* 30(5):338–342.

Sherlock G, Hernandez-Boussard T, Kasarskis A et al. (2001) The stanford microarray database. *Nucl Acids Res* 29:152–155.

Shimokawa K, Mogushi K, Shoji S et al. (2010) iCOD: An integrated clinical omics database based on the systems-pathology view of disease. *BMC Gen* (4):S19.

Siah SP, Quinn DM, Graeme DB et al. (2000) Microsatellite instability markers in breast cancer: A review and study showing MSI was not detected at 'BAT 25' and 'BAT 26' microsatellite markers in early-onset breast cancer. *Breast Cancer Res Treat* 60(2):135–142.

Sikaroodi M, Galachiantz Y, and Baranova A. (2010) Tumor markers: The potential of "Omics" approach. *Curr Mol Med* 10:249–257.

Silberman S, Breitfeld P, and Butzbach A. (2012) Imaging biomarkers in oncology drug development. *J Clin Stud* 4(3):22–24.

Silva CL, Passos M, and Câmara JS. (2012) Solid phase microextraction, mass spectrometry and metabolomic approaches for detection of potential urinary cancer biomarkers—A powerful strategy for breast cancer diagnosis. *Talanta* 89:360–368.

Simons K and Sampaio JL. (2011) Membrane organization and lipid rafts. *Cold Spring Harb Perspect Biol* 3:a004697.

Simons K and Toomre D. (2000) Lipid rafts and signal transduction. *Nat Rev Mol Cell Biol* 1(1):31–39.

Simpson DC and Smith RD. (2005) Combining capillary electrophoresis with mass spectrometry for applications in proteomics. *Electrophoresis* 26(7–8):1291–1305.

Singh K et al. (2009) Tumor suppressor SMAR1 represses IkappaBalpha expression and inhibits p65 transactivation through matrix attachment regions. *J Biol Chem* 284(2):1267–1278.

Singh K, Mogare D, Giridharagopalan RO et al. (2007) p53 target gene SMAR1 Is dysregulated in breast cancer: Its role in cancer cell migration and invasion. *PLoS One* 2(8):e660.

Singletary SE, Allred C, Ashley P et al. (2002) Revision of the American joint committee on cancer staging system for breast cancer. *J Clin Oncol* 20:3628–3636.

Sinicrope FA and Dannenberg AJ (2011) Obesity and breast cancer prognosis: Weight of the evidence. *J Clin Oncol* 29(1):4–7.

Slamon DJ and Clark GM (1988) Amplification of C-ERB-B2 and aggressive breast tumors? *Science* 240:1795–1798.

Śliwowska I, Kopczyñski Z, and Grodecka-Gazdecka S. (2006) Diagnostic value of measuring serum CA 15–3, TPA, and TPS in women with breast cancer. *Postepy Hig Med Dosw* 60:295–299.

Smart YC, Stewart JF, Bartlett LD et al. (1990) Mammary serum antigen (MSA) in advanced breast cancer. *Breast Cancer Res Treat* 16(1):23–28.

Smith GL, Xu Y, Buchholz TA et al. (2012) Association between treatment with brachytherapy vs whole-breast irradiation and subsequent mastectomy, complications, and survival among older women with invasive breast cancer. *JAMA* 307(17):1827–1837.

Smith I, Procter M, Gelber RD et al. (2007) 2-year follow-up of trastuzumab after adjuvant chemotherapy in HER2-positive breast cancer: A randomized controlled trial. *Lancet* 369(9555):29–36.

Snell C, Krypuy M, Wong EM et al. (2008) BRCA1 promoter methylation in peripheral blood DNA of mutation negative familial breast cancer patients with a BRCA1 tumour phenotype. *Breast Cancer Res* 10:R12.

Soares R, Marinho A, and Schmitt F. (1996) Expression of sialyl-Tn in breast cancer. Correlation with prognostic parameters. *Pathol Res Pract* 192:1181–1186.

Song M, Pan K, Su H et al. (2012) Identification of serum micrornas as novel non-invasive biomarkers for early detection of gastric cancer. *PLoS One* 7(3):e33608.

Sørlie T, Perou CM, Tibshirani R et al. (2001) Gene expression patterns of breast carcinomas distinguish tumor sub-classes with clinical implications. *Proc Natl Acad Sci USA* 98(19):10869–10874.

Sotiriou C, Neo SY, McShane LM et al. (2003) Breast cancer classification and prognosis based on gene expression profiles from a population-based study. *Proc Natl Acad Sci USA* 100(18):10393–10398.

Sotiriou C, Wirapati P, Loi S et al. (2006) Gene expression pro-filing in breast cancer: Understanding the molecular basis of histologic grade to improve prognosis. *J Natl Cancer Inst* 98(4):262–272.

Souzaki M, Kubo M, Kai M et al. (2011) Hedgehog signaling pathway mediates the progression of non-invasive breast cancer to invasive breast cancer. *Cancer Sci* 102(2):373–381.

Spaderna S, Schmalhofer O, Wahlbuhl M et al. (2008) The transcriptional repressor ZEB1 promotes metastasis and loss of cell polarity in cancer. *Cancer Res* 68:537–544.

Stacey SN, Sulem P, Zanon C et al. (2010) Ancestry-shift refinement mapping of the C6orf97-ESR1 breast cancer susceptibility locus. *PLoS Genet* 6:e1001029.

Stacker SA, Thompson CH, Sacks NPM et al. (1988) Cancer patients using monoclonal antibody 3e1.2 detection of mammary serum antigen in sera from breast. *Cancer Res* 48:7060–7066.

Stathopoulou A, Vlachonikolis I, Mavroudis D et al. (2002) Molecular detection of cytokeratin-19 –positive cells in the peripheral blood of patients with operable breast cancer: Evaluation of their prognostic significance. *J Clin Oncol* 20(16):3404–3412.

Stefansson OA, Jonasson JG, Olafsdottir K et al. (2011) CpG island hypermethylation of BRCA1 and loss of pRb as co-occurring events in basal/triple-negative breast cancer. *Epigenetics* 6(5):638–649.

Stokłosa T and Gołąb J. (2005) Prospects for p53-based cancer therapy. *Acta Biochimica Polonica* 52(2):321–328.

Stoppa-Lyonnet D, Buecher B, Houdayer C et al. (2009) Implications of genetic risk factors in breast cancer: Culprit genes and associated malignancies. *Bull Acad Natl Med* 193(9):2063–2083.

Streckfus CF, Arreola D, Edwards C et al. (2012) Salivary protein profiles among HER2/neu-receptor-positive and -negative breast cancer patients: Support for using salivary protein profiles for modeling breast cancer progression. *J Oncol* 9 pages.

Sugita M, Geraci M, Gao B et al. (2002) Combined use of oligonucleotide and tissue microarrays identifies cancer/testis antigens as biomarkers in lung carcinoma. *Cancer Res* 62(14):3971–3979.

Suijkerbuijk KP, van Diest PJ, and van der Wall E (2010) Improving early breast cancer detection: Focus on methylation. *Ann Oncol* 22(1):24–29.

Suijkerbuijk KPM, Wall E, Vooijs M et al. (2008) Molecular analysis of nipple fluid for breast cancer screening. *Pathobiology* 75:149–152.

Sun F, Fu H, Liu Q et al. (2008) Down regulation of CCND1 and CDK6 by miR-34 a induces cell cycle arrest. *FEBS Lett* 582(10):1564–1568.

Sun X, Liu JJ, Wang YS et al. (2011) Using intra-operative gene searchTM breast lymph node assay to detect breast cancer metastases in sentinel lymph nodes: Results from a single institute in China. *Chin Med J (Engl)* 124(7):973–977.

Suryadevara A, Paruchuri LP, Banisaeed N et al. (2010) The clinical behavior of mixed ductal/lobular carcinoma of the breast: A clinicopathologic analysis. *World J Surg Oncol* 8:51.

Suter R and Marcum JA. (2007) The molecular genetics of breast cancer and targeted therapy. *Biologics* 1(3):241–258.

Swaby RF and Cristofanilli M. (2011) Circulating tumor cells in breast cancer: A tool whose time has come of age. *BMC Med* 9:43.

Swen JJ, Huizinga TW, Gelderblom H et al. (2007) Translating pharmacogenomics: Challenges on the road to the clinic. *PLoS Med* 4(8):e209.

Swift-Scanlan T, Vang R, Blackford A, Fackler MJ, and Sukumar S. (2011) Methylated genes in breast cancer: Associations with clinical and histopathological features in a familial breast cancer cohort. *Cancer Biol Ther* 11(10):853–865.

Tahir M, Hendry P, Baird L et al. (2006) Radiation induced angiosarcoma a sequela of radiotherapy for breast cancer following conservative surgery. *Int Semin Surg Oncol* 3:26.

Tchen N, Juffs HG, Downie FP et al. (2003) Cognitive function, fatigue, and menopausal symptoms in women receiving adjuvant chemotherapy for breast cancer. *J Clin Oncol* 21:4175–4183.

Teng P, Bateman NW, Hood BL et al. (2010) Conrads advances in proximal fluid proteomics for disease biomarker discovery. *J Proteome Res* 9(12):6091–6100.

Tesch GH. (2010) Review: Serum and urine biomarkers of kidney disease: A pathophysiological perspective. *Nephrology* 15(6):609–616.

Thomas M, Lieberman J, and Lal A. Desperately seeking microRNA targets. *Nat Struct Mol Biol* 17(10):1169–1174.

Tobin D, Lindahl T, Hagen N et al. (2007) Employing a blood based gene expression signature to detect early stage breast cancer. *J Clin Oncol* 25(18S):21117.

Tobin NP, Sims AH, Lundgren KL et al. (2011) Cyclin D1, Id1 and EMT in breast cancer. *BMC Cancer* 11:417.

Tomasi G, Kenny L, Mauri F et al. (2011) Quantification of receptor-ligand binding with [18F]fluciclatide in metastatic breast cancer patients. *Eur J Nucl Med Mol Imaging* 38:2186–2197.

Toretsky J, Levenson A, Weinberg IN et al. (2004) Preparation of F-18 labeled annexin V: A potential PET radiopharmaceutical for imaging cell death. *Nucl Med Biol* 31(6):747–752.

Treon SP., Maimonis P, Bua D et al. (2000) Elevated soluble MUC1 levels and decreased anti-MUC1 antibody levels in patients with multiple myeloma. *Blood* 96:3147–3153.

Truscott M, Raynal L, Premdas P et al. (2003) CDP/Cux stimulates transcription from the DNA polymerase alpha gene promoter. *Mol Cell Biol* 23(8):3013–3028.

Tsuchida T, Okazawa H, Mori T et al. (2007) In vivo imaging of estrogen receptor concentration in the endometrium and myometrium using 18F-FES PET—Influence of menstrual cycle and endogenous estrogen level. *Nucl Med Biol* 34(2):205–210.

Tung N, Miron A, Schnitt SJ et al. (2010) Prevalence and predictors of loss of wild type BRCA 1 in estrogen receptor positive and negative BRCA1-associated breast cancers. *Breast Cancer Res* 12(6):R95.

Turnpenny P and Ellard S. (2005) *Emery's Elements of Medical Genetics*, 12th edn. Elsevier, London, U.K.

Tworoger SS and Hankinson SE. (2006) Use of biomarkers in epidemiologic studies: Minimizing the influence of measurement error in the study design and analysis. *Cancer Causes Control* 17(7):889–899.

Tyczynski JE, Bray F, and Parkin DM (2002) Breast cancer in Europe. ENCR Cancer Fact Sheets, Vol. 2.

Ura Y, Dion AS, Williams CJ et al. (1992) Quantitative dot blot analyses of blood-group-related antigens in paired normal and malignant human breast tissues. *Int J Cancer* 50:57–63.

Usary J, Llaca V, Karaca G et al. (2004) Mutation of GATA3 in human breast tumors. *Oncogene* 23(46):7669–7678.

Ushijima T. (2005) Detection and interpretation of altered methylation patterns in cancer cells. *Nat Rev Cancer* 5:223–231.

Ushijima T and Asada K. (2010) Aberrant DNA methylation in contrast with mutations. *Cancer Sci* 101(2):300–305.

Vadnais C, Davoudi S, Afshin M et al. (2012) CUX1 transcription factor is required for optimal ATM/ATR-mediated responses to DNA damage. *Nucl Acid Res* 40(10):4483–4495.

Valastyan S, Reinhardt F, Benaich N et al. (2009) A pleiotropically acting microRNA, miR-31, inhibits breast cancer metastasis. *Cell* 137:1032–1046.

Van den Akker EB, Verbruggen B, Heijmans BT et al. (2011) Integrating protein-protein interaction networks with gene-gene co-expression networks improves gene signatures for classifying breast cancer metastasis. *J Integr Bioinform* 8(2):188.

Van de Vivjer MJ, Peterse JL, Mooi WJ et al. (1988) Neu-protein overexpression in breast cancer. *N Engl J Med* 319:1239–1245.

Van DeVoorde L, Speeckaert R, VanGestel D et al. (2012) DNA methylation-based biomarkers in serum of patients with breast cancer. *Mutat Res* 751(2):304–325.

Van der Auwera I, Peeters D, Benoy IH et al. (2010) Circulating tumour cell detection: A direct comparison between the CellSearch System, the AdnaTest and CK-19/mammaglobin RT–PCR in patients with metastatic breast cancer. *Br J Cancer* 102(2):276–284.

Van der Auwera I, Van Laere SJ, Van den Bosch SM et al. (2008) Aberrant methylation of the Adenomatous Polyposis Coli (APC) gene promoter is associated with the inflammatory breast cancer phenotype. *Br J Cancer* 99:1735–1742.

Varghese C. (2007) The significance of oestrogen and progesterone receptors in breast cancer. *J Clin Diagn Res* 1:198–203.

Varki A. (1994) Selectin ligands. *Proc Natl Acad Sci USA* 91:7390–7397.

Varki A, Cummings RD, Esko JD et al. (2009) *Essentials of Glycobiology*. 2nd edn. Cold Spring Harbor Laboratory Press, New York.

Vaughan CL. (2012) New developments in medical imaging to detect breast cancer. *Contin Med Edu* 30(1):122–125.

Veeck J and Esteller M. (2010) Breast cancer epigenetics: From DNA methylation to microRNAs. *J Mammary Gland Biol Neoplasia* 15(1):5–17.

Verma S, Lavasani S, Mackey J et al. (2010) Optimizing the management of her2-positive early breast cancer: The clinical reality. *Curr Oncol* 17(4):20–33.

Verma S, Miles D, Gianni L et al. (2012) Trastuzumab emtansine for HER2-positive advanced breast cancer. *N Engl J Med* 367(19):1783–1791.

Verring A, Clouth A, Ziolkowski P et al. (2011) Clinical usefulness of cancer markers in primary breast cancer. *Pathology* 4 pages.

Vesselle H, Grierson J, Muzi M et al. (2002) In vivo Validation of 3′deoxy-3′-[18F]fluorothymidine ([18F] FLT) as a proliferation imaging tracer in humans: Correlation of [18F]FLT uptake by positron emission tomography with Ki-67 immunohistochemistry and flow cytometry in human lung tumors. *Clin Cancer Res* 8(11):3315–3323.

Viale G, Maiorano E, Pruneri G et al. (2005) Predicting the risk for additional axillary metastases in patients with breast carcinoma and positive sentinel lymph node biopsy. *Ann Surg* 241(2):319–325.

Viale G, Regan MM, Maiorano E et al. (2007) Prognostic and predictive value of centrally reviewed expression of estrogen and progesterone receptors in a randomized trial comparing letrozole and tamoxifen adjuvant therapy for postmenopausal early breast cancer: BIG1-98. *J Clin Oncol* 25(25):3846–3852.

Vogel CL, Cobleigh MA, Tripathy D. (2002) Efficacy and safety of trastuzumab as a single agent in first-line treatment of HER2-overexpressing metastatic breast cancer. *J Clin Oncol* 20(3):719–726.

Volinia S, Calin GA, Liu CG et al. (2006) A microRNA expression signature of human solid tumors defines cancer gene targets. *Proc Natl Acad Sci* 103(7):2257–2261.

Voyatzi S, Desiris K, Paikos DA et al. (2010) Promoter methylation of $p16^{INK4A}$, RASSF1A, and RAR2b genes in tumor DNA from patients with breast cancer (BC) in correlation with clinical recurrence. *J Clin Oncol* 28:15.

Wajapeyee N and Somasundaram K. (2004) Pharmacogenomics in breast cancer: Current trends and future directions. *Curr Opin Mol Ther* 6(3):296–301.

Wang K, Lee I, Carlson G et al. (2010) Systems biology and the discovery of diagnostic biomarkers. *Dis Markers* 28:199–207.

Wang L. (2010) Pharmacogenomics: A systems approach. *Wiley Interdiscip Rev Syst Biol Med* 2(1):3–22.

Wang PH. (2005) Altered glycosylation in cancer: Sialic acids and sialyltransferases. *J Cancer Mole* 1(2):73–81.

Wang SP, Wang WL, Chang YL et al. (2009) p53 controls cancer cell invasion by inducing the MDM2-mediated degradation of Slug. *Nat Cell Biol* 11:694–704.

Wang Z, Gerstein M, and Snyder M. (2009) RNA-Seq: A revolutionary tool for transcriptomics. *Nat Rev Genet* 10:57–63.

Watkins SM, Reifsnyder PR, Pan HJ et al. (2002) Lipid metabolome-wide effects of the PPARγ agonist rosiglitazone. *J Lipid Res* 43:1809–1817.

Weaver DL. (2010) Pathology evaluation of sentinel lymph nodes in breast cancer: Protocol recommendations and rationale. *Mod Pathol* 23(Suppl 2):S26–S32.

Weigel MT and Dowsett M. (2010) Current and emerging biomarkers in breast cancer: Prognosis and prediction. *Endocr Relat Cancer* 17(4):R245–R262.

Weigel MT and Dowsett M. (2010) Current and emerging biomarkers in breast cancer: Prognosis and prediction. *Endocr Relat Cancer* 17R245–17R262.

Wenk MR. (2005) The emerging field of lipidomics. *Nat Rev Drug Discov* 4(7):594–610.

Whitcher B and Schmid VJ. (2011) Quantitative analysis of dynamic contrast-enhanced and diffusion-weighted magnetic resonance imaging for oncology in R. *J Stat Software* 44:5.

Whitehead CM, Nelson R, Hudson P et al. (2004) Selection and optimization of a panel of early stage breast cancer prognostic molecular markers. *Mod Pathol* 17:50A.

Wiechmann L and Kuerer HM. (2008) The molecular journey from ductal carcinoma in situ to invasive breast cancer. *Cancer* 112(10):2130–2142.

Wiedswang G, Borgen E, Kåresen R et al. (2004) Isolated tumor cells in bone marrow three years after diagnosis in disease-free breast cancer patients predict unfavorable clinical outcome. *Clin Cancer Res* 10(16):5342–5348.

Williams-Jones B and Carriyan OP. (2003) Rheotoric and type: Where's the ethics in pharmacogenomics? *Am J Pharmacogenomics* 3(6):375–383.

Wu K and Zhang Y. (2007) Clinical application of tear proteomics: Present and future prospects. *PROTEO–Clin Appl* 1(9):972–982.

Wulfkuhle JD, Paweletz CP, Steeg PS et al. (2003) Proteomic approaches to the diagnosis, treatment, and monitoring of cancer. *Adv Exp Med Biol* 532:59–68.

Xenidis N, Ignatiadis M, Apostolaki S et al. (2009) Cytokeratin-19 mRNA-positive circulating tumor cells after adjuvant chemotherapy in patients with early breast cancer. *JCO* 27(13):2177–2184.

Xiao-yuan F, Xin-lei H, Tie-mei H et al. (2011) Association between RUNX3 promoter methylation and gastric cancer: A meta-analysis. *BMC Gastroenterol* 11:92.

Xing Y, Xue Z, Englander S et al. (2008) Improving parenchyma segmentation by simultaneous estimation of tissue property T1 map and group-wise registration of inversion recovery MR breast images. *Med Image Comput Comput Assist Interv* 11(1):342–350.

Xu J, Wang B, and Zhang Y. (2012) Clinical implications for BRCA gene mutation in breast cancer. *Mol Biol Rep* 39(3):3097–3102.

Yan LX, Huang XF, Shao Q et al. (2008) MicroRNA miR-21 overexpression in human breast cancer is associated with advanced clinical stage, lymph node metastasis and patient poor prognosis. *RNA* 14(11):2348–2360.

Yan PS, Venkataramu C, Ibrahim A et al. (2006) Mapping geographic zones of cancer risk with epigenetic biomarkers in normal breast tissue. *Clin Cancer Res* 12(22):6626–6636.

Yang R, Cheung MC, Hurley J et al. (2009) A comprehensive evaluation of outcomes for inflammatory breast cancer. *Breast Cancer Res Treat* 117(3):631–641.

Yiannakopoulou EC. (2012) Pharmacogenomics of breast cancer targeted therapy: Focus on recent patents. *Recent Pat DNA Gene Seq* 6:33–46.

Yin P, Roqueiro D, Huang L et al. (2012) Genome-wide progesterone receptor binding: Cell type-specific and shared mechanisms in T47D. Breast cancer cells and primary leiomyoma cells. *PLoS One* 7(1):e29021.

Yong L. (2010) The detection of tear biomarkers for future prostate cancer diagnosis. *Open Biomark J* 3:26–29.

Yousef GM and Diamandis EP. (2001) The new human tissue Kallikrein gene family: Structure, function, and association to disease. *Endocrine Rev* 22(2):184–204.

Yu F, Yao H, Zhu P et al. (2007) Let-7 regulates self renewal and tumorigenicity of breast cancer cells. *Cell* 131(6):1109–1123.

Yu J, Zhang Y, and Qi Z. (2008) Methylation-mediated downregulation of the B-cell translocation gene 3 (BTG3) in breast cancer cells. *Gene Expr* 14(3):173–182.

Zehentner BK, Persing DH, Deme A et al. (2004) Mammaglobin as a novel breast cancer biomarker: Multigene reverse transcription-PCR assay and sandwich ELISA. *Clin Chem* 50(11):2069–2076.

Zeinab B, Ramin R, Qing L et al. (2012) Methylation signature of lymph node metastases in breast cancer patients. *BMC Cancer* 12:244.

Zelivianski S, Cooley A, Kall R et al. (2010) Cyclin-dependent kinase 4-mediated phosphorylation inhibits Smad3 activity in cyclin D-overexpressing breast cancer cells. *Mol Cancer Res* 8(10):1375–1387.

Zhang F and Chen JY. (2011) Data mining methods in Omics-based biomarker discovery. *Methods Mol Biol* 719:511–526.

Zhang J, Baran J, Cros A et al. (2011a) International Cancer Genome Consortium Data Portal—A one-stop shop for cancer genomics data. Database (Oxford). 19;2011:bar026.

Zhang J, Bowers J, Liu L, Wei S et al. (2012) Esophageal cancer metabolite biomarkers detected by LC-MS and NMR methods. *PLoS ONE* 7(1):e30181.

Zhang J and Liu YJ. (2008) HER2 over-expression and response to different chemotherapy regimens in breast cancer. *Zhejiang Univ Sci B* 9(1):5–9.

Zhang L, Kelly G, and Hagen T. (2011b) The cellular microenvironment and cell adhesion: A role for o-glycosylation. *Biochem Soc Trans* 39(1):378–382.

Zhang L, Xiao H, Karlan S et al. (2010) Discovery and preclinical validation of salivary transcriptomic and proteomic biomarkers for the non-invasive detection of breast cancer. *PLoS One* 5(12):e15573.

Zhang S, Liu C, Li W et al. (2012) Discovery of multi-dimensional modules by integrative analysis of cancer genomic data. *Nucl Acid Res* 1–13.

Zhao H, Shen J, Medico L et al. (2010) A pilot study of circulating miRNAs as potential biomarkers of early stage breast cancer. *PLoS One* 5(10):e13735.

Zhao Y, Deng C, Wang J, Xiao J, Gatalica Z, Recker RR, and Xiao GG. (2010) Let-7 family miRNAs regulate estrogen receptor alpha signaling in estrogen receptor positive breast cancer. *Breast Cancer Res Treat* 127(1):69–80.

Zhao Y, Verselis SJ, Klar N et al. (2001) Nipple fluid carcinoembryonic antigen and prostate-specific antigen in cancer-bearing and tumor-free breasts. *J Clin Oncol* 19(5):1462–1467.

Zheng Y, Huo D, Zhang J et al. (2012) Microsatellites in the Estrogen Receptor (ESR1, ESR2) and Androgen Receptor (AR) genes and breast cancer risk in African American and Nigerian women. *PLoS One* 7(7):e40494.

Zhong Li, Ge Kun, Zu Jin-chi et al. (2008) Autoantibodies as potential biomarkers for breast cancer. *Breast Cancer Res* 10:R40.

Zhou L, Beuerman RW, Chan CM et al. (2009) Identification of tear fluid biomarkers in dry eye syndrome using iTRAQ quantitative proteomics. *J Proteome Res* 8(11):4889–4905.

Zhu CS, Pinsky PF, Cramer DW et al. (2011) A framework for evaluating biomarkers for early detection: Validation of biomarker panels for ovarian cancer. *Cancer Prev Res* 4(3):375–383.

Zhu S, Si M, Wu H et al. (2007) MicroRNA-21 targets the tumor suppressor gene tropomyosin 1 (TPM1). *J Biol Chem* 282:14328–14336.

Zhu W, Qin W, Sauter ER. (2004) Large-scale mitochondrial DNA deletion mutations and nuclear genome instability in human breast cancer. *Cancer Detect Prev* 28(2):119–126.

Zuoren Y, Renato B, Lide C et al. (2010) microRNA, cell cycle, and human breast cancer. *Am J Pathol* 176(3):1058–1064.

24

Noninvasive Biomarkers in Ovarian Cancer

Sharon A. O'Toole, Eugen Ancuta, Ream Langhe, Dolores J. Cahill, Mairead Murphy, Cara Martin, Lynda McEvoy, Cathy Spillane, Orla Sheils, Emmanuel Petricoin, Lance Liotta, and John J. O'Leary

CONTENTS

ABSTRACT One of the major challenges in cancer research is the identification of stable biomarkers, which can be routinely measured noninvasively in easily accessible samples. Ovarian cancer is one such disease that would benefit from improved diagnostic markers.

Ovarian cancer is the leading cause of death from gynecological malignancy in the western world. The vast majority of patients present with advanced-stage disease, and this is due to lack of a reliable screening test and the absence of symptoms. Improved early detection of ovarian cancer is likely to have substantial effects on overall ovarian cancer survival and quality of life, since the disease demonstrates excellent survival with currently available therapies when diagnosed at an early stage. One way to facilitate early detection of ovarian cancer is through screening, but currently available diagnostic tools, including ovarian cancer biomarkers and clinical imaging, lack sufficient specificity and sensitivity for implementation in a population-based screening program.

This chapter reviews currently available noninvasive biomarkers for the early detection of ovarian cancer and provides an outlook on the potential improvements in these noninvasive diagnostic tools that may lead to improved diagnosis of ovarian cancer. The utility of novel technologies to identify noninvasive biomarkers in ovarian cancer is discussed, such as miRNA detection, autoantibody profiling, and circulating tumor cell enumeration.

The ability to sensitively and specifically predict the presence of early disease and its status, stage, and associated therapeutic efficacy has the potential to revolutionize ovarian cancer detection and treatment and to greatly improve the quality of life and survival rates of ovarian cancer patients.

KEY WORDS: *ovarian cancer, noninvasive, diagnosis, biomarker, early detection.*

24.1 Introduction: Ovarian Cancer Background

Ovarian cancer is the leading cause of death from gynecological malignancy in the western world. The worldwide distribution of incidence and mortality are depicted in Figures 24.1 and 24.2 (Globocan 2008; http://globocan.iarc.fr). Ovarian cancer has remained the most challenging of gynecological malignancies for two reasons: First, early-stage disease cannot be detected easily. Second, standard chemotherapy often fails and patients develop chemoresistant disease.

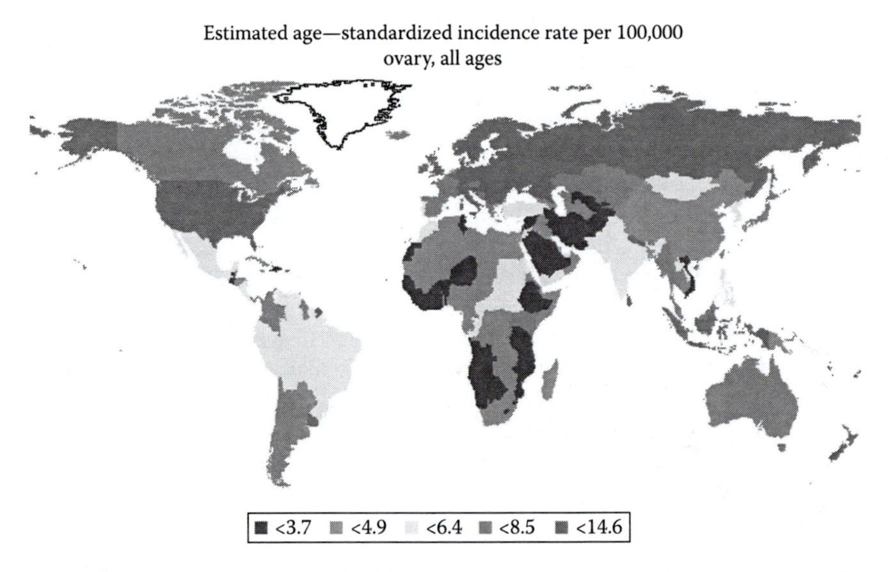

FIGURE 24.1 Estimated age standardized worldwide incidence rate of ovarian cancer. (From Ferlay, J. et al., GLOBOCAN 2008, Cancer Incidence and Mortality Worldwide: IARC CancerBase No. 10 [Internet]. Lyon, France: International Agency for Research on Cancer, 2010.)

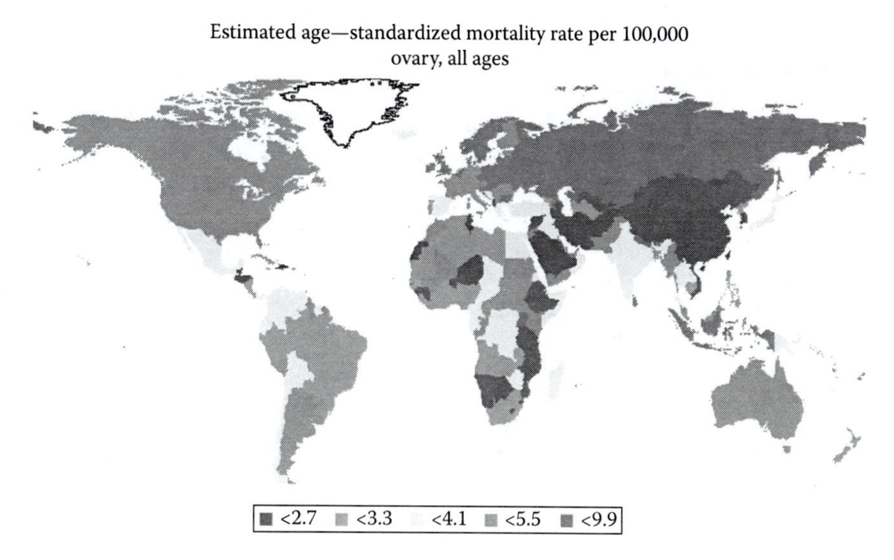

FIGURE 24.2 Estimated age standardized worldwide mortality rate of ovarian cancer. (From Ferlay, J. et al., GLOBOCAN 2008, Cancer Incidence and Mortality Worldwide: IARC CancerBase No. 10 [Internet]. Lyon, France: International Agency for Research on Cancer, 2010.)

Incidence of disease rises dramatically after onset of menopause. Genetic alterations in the breast cancer susceptibility 1 (*BRCA1*) and 2 (*BRCA2*) genes are associated with an increased lifetime risk for ovarian cancer (Hensley et al., 2002). Ovarian cancer risk tends to be reduced by factors that interrupt ovulation (Sueblinvong and Carney, 2009).

The vast majority of ovarian cancers are epithelial tumors that are then subdivided into a number of histological categories that differ in many respects including epidemiology, genetics, responsiveness to chemotherapy, and expression of tumor markers (Bast et al., 2009). Generally, epithelial ovarian tumors can be categorized into type I and type II (Bell, 2005). Type I tumors are slow growing, while type II tumors are high grade and rapidly metastasize.

Schorge et al. (2010) describe a number of hypotheses regarding ovarian cancer etiology that can be related to the risk factors identified, for example, incessant ovulation. Generally, it is thought that ovarian cancer occurs as a result of transformation of the surface epithelium (Landen et al., 2008); however, more recent studies of ovarian cancer have postulated that it may have developed in the fallopian tube and metastasized (Crum et al., 2007; Kurman and Shih, 2010).

24.1.1 Symptoms and Treatment of Ovarian Cancer

The symptoms of ovarian cancer are nonspecific and often occur when the disease is already spread throughout the abdominal cavity. Early-stage ovarian cancer has up to a 90% 5-year overall survival rate, whereas late-stage cancers have less than a 30% 5-year survival rate.

The accepted standard of care treatment is debulking surgery and carboplatin/paclitaxel chemotherapy. While many women respond well to chemotherapy, the disease usually recurs and patients develop chemoresistant disease. New targeted biologic agents, particularly those involved in anti-angiogenesis (e.g., bevacizumab) and those targeting the poly(ADP-ribose) polymerase (PARP) enzyme, hold the most promise for improving outcome of ovarian cancer.

24.1.2 Current Diagnostic Approaches

Currently, there are no established national ovarian cancer screening programs in place. Current detection strategies include ultrasound and cancer antigen-125 (CA-125); however, both have their drawbacks resulting in the lack of a reliable, sensitive screening test for ovarian cancer. Recently, the Prostate, Lung, Colorectal, and Ovarian (PLCO) Cancer Screening Trial in the United States reported

TABLE 24.1

Noninvasive Diagnostic Markers for Ovarian Cancer

Marker	Source	Details	Marker Type	Sensitivity (%)	Specificity (%)	Reference
CA-125	Serum	Cell surface glycoprotein	Protein	89	72	Moss et al. (2005)
HE4 (ROMA)	Serum	HE4 used in conjunction with CA-125	Protein	83	90	Wu et al. (2012)
				94.3	75	Moore (2010)
OVA1	Serum	CA-125 II, transthyretin (prealbumin), apolipoprotein A1, b2-microglobulin, and transferrin	Protein	93	43	Abraham (2010); Muller (2010)
RMI	Serum, imaging, and menopausal status	Ultrasound, menopausal status, and CA125	Protein and imaging and menopausal status	71–88	74–97	
				84.6	75	Moore (2010)
Ultrasound	Imaging	Morphologic (gray scale) ultrasound	Imaging	88–100	39–87	Webb (2007)
FDG-PET	Imaging		Imaging	92	60	Fenchel et al. (2002)
FDG-PET, MRI, and ultrasound	Imaging	Combination of three imaging modalities	Imaging	92	85	Fenchel et al. (2002)

no mortality benefit for annual screening with CA-125 and transvaginal ultrasound (Buys et al., 2011). However, results are awaited from the UK Collaborative Trial of Ovarian Cancer Screening (UKCTOCS) (http://www.ukctocs.org.uk/) that will report in 2014 on the effectiveness of ultrasound and CA-125 for screening. The trial uses a calculation called the "risk of ovarian cancer algorithm" (ROCA). Rather than just looking at the results of a single CA-125 test, they look for changes in CA-125 over time to try to predict the woman's risk of having the disease (Menon et al., 2012). In contrast, PLCO used a single cutoff for CA-125.

Other markers used routinely include CA 19-9 (a monosialoganglioside antigen widely used in gastrointestinal adenocarcinoma diagnostics) that is elevated in 68%–83% of mucinous ovarian cancers but in only 28%–29% of non-mucinous types, providing a differential diagnostic tool for non-mucinous versus mucinous subtypes. Serum CA 15-3, CA 72-4, and CEA levels are often measured as the can be elevated in, respectively, 50%–56%, 63%–71%, and 25%–50% of ovarian cancer patients (Kobayashi et al., 2012). These markers assist in the management of tumors that do not express CA-125 and may assist in distinguishing tumors of non-ovarian origin. Details on the most common currently used noninvasive biomarkers are listed in Table 24.1.

24.2 Invasive and Noninvasive Diagnostic Biomarkers

The National Institutes of Health defines a biomarker as "a characteristic that is objectively measured and evaluated as an indicator of normal biological processes, pathogenic processes, or pharmacologic responses to a therapeutic intervention" (Biomarkers Definitions Working Group, 2001). The ability to diagnose or treat a disease by measuring a biological molecule from a noninvasive source, such as blood or urine, has a significant advantage over traditional pathological techniques because direct access to diseased tissue is not required. Invasive procedures particularly in obtaining ovarian tissue carry significant risk for the patient but also involve a more prolonged hospital visit, specialist consultants, and significantly higher costs.

While bodily fluids are one of the more attractive noninvasive procedures for biomarker discovery, it also has disadvantages in the degree of heterogeneity seen between patients, and as previously mentioned, there are many ovarian cancer subtypes. Blood is a complex body fluid with fluid and cellular components, and this complexity can influence biomarker discovery. The manner in which blood is collected and stored can, for some assay formats, also impact on the results. The large dynamic range of proteins in the blood, serum, plasma, or other body fluids can also add to the complexity (Anderson and Anderson, 2002). Imaging is also a popular choice for non-invasive cancer diagnostics, but it has not proven sensitive enough to date; however, the evolution of molecular imaging holds a lot of promise in this area.

24.3 Brief Description on Invasive Biomarkers

Recent research publications about invasive and noninvasive biomarkers for ovarian cancer are widely available, focusing on their role in diagnosis, clinical prognosis, treatment efficacy, and monitoring (Coticchia et al., 2008; Suh et al., 2010). To date, a large panel of putative invasive biomarkers are described in ovarian cancer, the most important being listed in Table 24.2 (Suh et al., 2010).

According to their role in specific diagnosis, ovarian cancer biomarkers can be classified as (1) *stage nonspecific biomarkers* including hK6 and hK7, hepatocyte nuclear factor (HNF)-1β, and WT-1; (2) *early tumor stage* including CBK; and (3) *late-tumor-stage biomarkers* such as TP, chloride intracellular channel 4 (CLIC4), and VSGP/F-spondin (Suh et al., 2010). Moreover, in relation to their prognostic value, candidate invasive biomarkers for ovarian cancer can be subdivided as

TABLE 24.2

List of Invasive Biomarkers for Ovarian Cancer Diagnosis and Prognosis

Ovarian Cancer Invasive Biomarkers
• Kallikreins: hK6, hK7, hK11, hK13
• HNF-1β (hepatocyte nuclear factor)
• WT-1 (Wilms' tumor 1)
• CKB[a] (creatine kinase, brain)
• TP[a] (thymidine phosphorylase)
• CLIC4 (chloride intracellular channel 4)
• VSGP/F-spondin (vascular smooth muscle growth-promoting factor)
• PR (progesterone receptor)
• Integrins: $\alpha_5\beta_6$ intregrin, α-V integrin
• β III tubulin
• CD24
• c-Ets1
• EMMPRIN (extracellular matrix metalloproteinase inducer)
• GEP (granulin–epithelin precursor)
• Indoleamine 2,3-dioxygenase
• M-CAM
• p-glycoprotein
• Topoisomerase II
• ATP7B

[a] Biomarkers identified in both tissue and serum.

(1) *favorable-prognostic biomarkers* such as progesterone receptor (PR), hK11, and hK13 and (2) *unfavorable-prognostic biomarkers* consisting of integrins, WT-1, CD24, M-CAM, c-Ets1, β III tubulin, extracellular matrix metalloproteinase inducer (EMMPRIN), granulin–epithelin precursor (GEP), p-glycoprotein, and topoisomerase II (Suh et al., 2010). Several reports on prognostic biomarkers focus on global prognostic value as well as on specific subtypes and different stages of ovarian cancer reflected in survival analysis.

Some of the interesting biomarkers are discussed in more detail as follows. Vascular smooth muscle growth-promoting factor (VSGP)/F-spondin is overexpressed in patients with advanced ovarian cancer (Pyle-Chenault et al., 2005) and is implicated in exonal guidance and differentiation of nerve cells (Attur et al., 2009). Its role in disease progression monitoring, treatment efficacy, and prognosis remains uncertain (Suh et al., 2010). TP (thymidine phosphorylase) is used to detect late-stage ovarian cancer; the level and activity significantly correlates with malignant and advanced-stage tumors, as well as with high-grade disease (Miszczak-Zaborska et al., 2004). Based on its role in pathologic cancer pathways (tumor growth, neoangiogenesis, metastasis), TP has diagnostic value, but also has potential as a prognostic and efficacy biomarker (Bronckaers et al., 2009). CLIC4 may have a dual role in the diagnosis and prognosis of advanced-stage ovarian tumors. Increased cellular expression and mislocalization in subcellular compartments are commonly reported (Suh et al., 2007). Kallikreins present with both diagnostic and prognostic function in ovarian cancer and are discussed in more detail later. Although overexpression of hK8, hK11, and hK13 is considered "protective" being associated with better survival and reduced risk of recurrence (Borgoño et al., 2003; Scorilas et al., 2004; Borgoño et al., 2006; McIntosh et al., 2007), hK6, hK7, and hK10 are well-known indicators of advanced ovarian cancer and progressive disease (Hoffman et al., 2002; Luo et al., 2003; Psyrri et al., 2008). Moreover, a combination of different members of the kallikrein family and other non-kallikrein markers offers prognostic potential in ovarian cancer (Shan et al., 2007). Wilms' tumor (WT)-1 protein is a specific diagnostic and a prognostic invasive biomarker for the serous subtype of ovarian carcinoma (Hwang et al., 2004). HNF-1β expression is upregulated in patients with clear cell ovarian carcinoma as a specific diagnostic marker, being also detected in peritoneal fluid (Tsuchiya et al., 2003; Kato et al., 2007).

The search for novel biomarkers in tissue and ascites material continues using technologies such as whole genome analysis, transcription profiling, microRNA (miRNA) profiling, and proteomic profiling. The ultimate goal is to translate these biomarkers into early diagnostic markers.

24.4 Noninvasive Biomarkers for Ovarian Cancer Diagnosis

24.4.1 FDA-Approved Biomarkers of Ovarian Cancer

24.4.1.1 CA-125

To date CA-125 is the most widely used biomarker for ovarian cancer. CA-125 is a cell surface glycoprotein that is encoded by the MUC16 gene. The protein has a single transmembrane domain and provides a protective mucosal barrier against foreign particles and infectious agents on the surface of epithelial cells on the surface of the female reproductive tract (Singh et al., 2008). The CA-125 antigen can be secreted into the circulation following phosphorylation by epidermal growth factor (Verheijen et al., 1999). Its serum levels are elevated in 90% of patients with late-stage ovarian cancer, yet CA-125 levels are only elevated in approximately 50% of early-stage ovarian cancers, thus limiting its use for early diagnosis. An additional limitation of CA-125 is its elevation in a variety of cancers other than ovarian such as pancreatic, breast, and lung cancer and in noncancerous conditions such as endometriosis, fibroids, pelvic inflammatory disease, benign cysts, pregnancy, and liver disease (Nossov et al., 2008). The sensitivity and specificity for CA-125 are 89% and 72%, respectively (Moss et al., 2005); it is raised in approximately only 50% of early-stage epithelial ovarian cancers (EOCs) and in 75%–90% of patients with advanced disease (Moss et al., 2005; Gupta and Lis, 2009). CA-125 screening combined with transvaginal ultrasonography (TVU) increases sensitivity and specificity to 89.4% and 99.8%, respectively (Menon et al., 2009).

24.4.1.2 HE4

Human epididymis protein 4 (HE4) is a low molecular weight glycoprotein that is expressed predominantly in epithelial cells of the epididymis and other tissues throughout the body including breast and the female genital tract (Drapkin et al., 2005; Holcomb et al., 2011). HE4 is encoded by the WFDC2 gene and contains two whey acid proteins and a four-disulphide core made up of eight cysteine residues (Gao et al., 2011). HE4 was initially predicted to be a protease inhibitor involved in the process of sperm maturation (Kirchhoff, 1998; Bingle et al., 2002; Clauss et al., 2005); however, the physiological functions of HE4 have, as yet, not been fully identified. It has been reported to be overexpressed in early and recurrent ovarian cancers; pulmonary, endometrial, and breast adenocarcinomas; mesotheliomas; and less frequently in renal, gastrointestinal, and transitional cell carcinomas (Bingle et al., 2002; Drapkin et al., 2005; Galgano et al., 2006; Anastasi et al., 2010).

24.4.1.2.1 Serum/Plasma HE4

The diagnostic and prognostic potential of serum/plasma HE4 levels has been examined in numerous ovarian cancer studies. HE4 has been detected at high concentrations in serum of patients with ovarian cancer, particularly women with serous and endometrioid adenocarcinoma, and furthermore, it was found to be increased in more than half of the ovarian cancers, which do not express CA-125 (Drapkin et al., 2005; Bouchard et al., 2006; Moore et al., 2008; Van Gorp et al., 2011; Kalapotharakos et al., 2012). In addition, HE4 is not overexpressed as often in endometriosis or in many benign gynecological diseases (Hellstrom et al., 2003; Moore et al., 2012).

HE4 has been approved by the Food and Drug Administration (FDA) for monitoring recurrence and progression in patients with EOC (Andersen et al., 2010; Montagnana et al., 2011) and more recently as part in the multiassay algorithm ROMA™ to aid the estimate of the risk of malignancy in premenopausal and postmenopausal women presenting with an adnexal mass who will undergo surgical intervention (Moore et al., 2009, 2011). Several studies showed that HE4 could predict the recurrence of the disease earlier than CA-125 (Anastasi et al., 2010; Schummer et al., 2012). In addition, HE4 has been reported recently as a novel biomarker that has the highest sensitivity either alone or in combination with CA-125 for detecting ovarian cancer particularly in the early stages (Moore et al., 2008). Moreover, HE4 was shown to have a higher specificity and comparable sensitivity to CA-125 (HE4 sensitivity of 88.9% and specificity of 91.8% compared to CA-125 sensitivity of 83.3% and specificity of 59.5%) for detection of ovarian cancer in premenopausal women with adnexal masses, thus reducing the number of unnecessary surgeries for benign disease (Holcomb et al., 2011).

High preoperative HE4 measurements were found to be associated with advanced-stage disease and poor prognosis in patients with ovarian cancer (Paek et al., 2011; Kalapotharakos et al., 2012; Kong et al., 2012), and HE4 is a marker for aggressiveness of the disease and a predictor of overall survival (Trudel et al., 2012). High levels of preoperative HE4 have been suggested in a retrospective study to be correlated with shorter progression-free survival in multivariate analysis (Paek et al., 2011). Another study found that increasing levels of HE4 before initiating first-line chemotherapy were associated with poor prognosis in EOC (Steffensen et al., 2011). Therefore, serum HE4 may be useful as an independent prognostic marker in patients with ovarian cancer.

A meta-analysis, which reviewed 9 studies involving 1807 women, showed that the pooled sensitivity and specificity for HE4 for diagnosis of ovarian cancer (where the control group was healthy women) were 83% and 90%, respectively. When the control group was made up of women with benign disease, the pooled sensitivity and specificity for HE4 were 74% and 90%, respectively (Wu et al., 2012).

HE4 has also been assessed in a multianalyte assay, named the Risk of Ovarian Malignancy Algorithm (ROMA) to predict malignancy and facilitate further management planning in women who present with ovarian masses (Moore et al., 2009, 2011). This assay combines the result of HE4 and CA-125 as well as the menopausal status into a numerical score. ROMA has been validated for the following combinations: HE4 enzyme immunoassay (EIA) + CA-125 EIA, HE4 EIA + CA-125 Architect, HE4 Architect + CA-125 Architect, and HE4 Elecsys + CA-125 Elecsys. At 75% specificity, ROMA has demonstrated 93%–94% sensitivity with a negative predictive value of 93%–98%. ROMA has been shown to be more sensitive (94%) than the risk of malignancy index (RMI) (75%) at 75% specificity (Moore et al., 2011).

A recent meta-analysis found that ROMA had a higher sensitivity to predict advanced EOC than early-stage EOC and was more accurate in postmenopausal women compared to premenopausal women (Li et al., 2012). Furthermore, ROMA is less specific, but more sensitive, than HE4, and both ROMA and HE4 are more specific than CA-125 for EOC prediction (Li et al., 2012), but CA-125 had better diagnostic accuracy. ROMA has potential in the clinic in distinguishing EOC from benign pelvic mass (Chan et al., 2012; Li et al., 2012), but further work needs to be done especially is assessing its potential in early-stage disease.

24.4.1.2.2 Urinary HE4

Measuring HE4 in urine can provide a less invasive way of detecting and monitoring ovarian cancer. Hellstrom et al. (2010) detected HE4 in urine at a specificity of 94.4%. The area under the curve (AUC) for early cases was 0.969, while for late cases, the AUC was 0.964 (Hellstrom et al., 2010). In a limited study, this mode of ovarian cancer diagnosis has been investigated as a point-of-care device and shows promising results (Wang et al., 2011).

24.4.1.3 OVA1

OVA1 (Vermillion, Quest Diagnostics) is the first FDA-approved blood test that assists the clinician to determine if an ovarian adnexal mass is malignant or benign prior to planned surgery. The test is FDA approved for women older than age 18 with an ovarian adnexal mass for which surgery is planned and who are not yet referred to gynecological oncologists, as an aid to further assess the likelihood that malignancy is present when the physician's independent clinical and radiological evaluation does not indicate malignancy. The test is not approved as a screening or stand-alone diagnostic test. The test measures the levels of five different proteins in patient serum, CA-125-II, transthyretin (prealbumin), apolipoprotein A1, beta-2-microglobulin, and transferrin (ova-1.com). The levels of these proteins are interpreted by proprietary software to determine a single numerical OVA1 score. The software algorithm determines a score based on menopausal status, differentiating patients either into a low- or high-risk group (Rein et al., 2011). The software generates a score between 0 and 10, 0 indicating high probability of a benign growth and 10 indicating high probability of malignancy. This test is used to determine which patients are at highest risk of malignancy and hence are most suitable to be referred to a gynecological oncologist. Surgery performed by a gynecological oncologist on malignant ovarian adnexal mass results in improved patient survival compared with surgery performed by less specialized surgeons (Engelen et al., 2006). OVA1 is claimed to have a sensitivity of 92.5% and a specificity of 42.8%, with a positive predictive value (PPV) of 42.3% and a negative predictive value of 92.7% (Muller, 2010). However, OVA1 has not been tested in screening patients for early-stage disease (Rein et al., 2011). There are also limitations to the use of this test due to assay interference as a result of triglyceride levels and rheumatoid factor levels (Muller, 2010).

24.4.2 Proteomics

The discovery of new biomarkers in biofluids such as blood, urine, and saliva can help to develop more sensitive and specific diagnostic and prognostic tests that will permit the early detection and treatment of patients with ovarian cancers, early detection of recurrence, treatment monitoring, and discrimination of benign pelvic masses. Proteomics, together with the innovative high-throughput technologies, might be a highly promising way to identify new biomarkers for both detection and tailoring therapy. Some new recent advances in proteomics combined with upfront sample enrichment nanotechnologies are producing powerful biomarker discovery workflows that are able to detect proteins at ultralow levels of detection (Fredolini et al., 2010). These new proteomic pipelines provide an accelerated opportunity to extend beyond the initial broadscale profiling efforts that indicated an untapped biomarker archive was present for early-stage ovarian cancer detection (Petricoin et al., 2002). As the proteomic field is rapidly advancing in the technical analytical precision, sensitivity, and accuracy of the tools and platforms used as the engines for biomarker discovery and measurement, significant challenges remain (Liotta and Petricoin, 2012) for facile biomarker discovery efforts. Such impediments include sample processing and biobanking issues, biofluid collection methodologies, and lack of biological tie-in of the marker to disease pathophysiology that result in overall slow rates of rigorous validation in large clinical trials. Despite these roadblocks, the field has produced a series of candidate biomarkers that appear to be very promising and that together may represent future panels of assays that could demonstrate the high sensitivity and specificity required for clinical implementation in the ovarian cancer field. Some of the interesting biomarkers in this area are discussed in more detail later.

24.4.2.1 Osteopontin

Ye et al. (2006) identified osteopontin fragments in urine as a marker for ovarian cancer. The marker provides an example of the information content of low molecular weight proteins/peptides in urine and their posttranslational modifications. Ye et al. collected urine samples preoperatively from postmenopausal women with ovarian cancer and benign conditions, and from nonsurgical controls, these were analyzed by surface-enhanced laser desorption/ionization mass spectrometry and 2D gel electrophoresis. Selected proteins from mass profiles were purified by chromatography and followed by liquid chromatography tandem mass spectrometry sequence analysis. Specific antibodies were generated for further characterization, including immunoprecipitation and glycosylation. Enzyme-linked immunosorbent assays (ELISAs) were employed for preliminary validation in patients of 128 ovarian cancer, 52 benign conditions, 44 other cancers, and 188 healthy controls. A protein ($m/z \sim 17{,}400$) with higher peak intensities in cancer patients than in benign conditions and controls was identified and subsequently defined as eosinophil-derived neurotoxin (EDN). A glycosylated form of EDN was specifically elevated in ovarian cancer patients. A cluster of COOH-terminal osteopontin was identified from 2D gels of urine from cancer patients. Modified form EDN and osteopontin fragments were elevated in early-stage ovarian cancers and a combination of both resulted to 93% specificity and 72% sensitivity. Specific elevated posttranslationally modified urinary EDN and osteopontin COOH-terminal fragments in ovarian cancer might lead to potential noninvasive screening tests for early diagnosis. Urine is a promising noninvasive body fluid for measurement novel biomarkers.

24.4.2.2 Kallikreins

Kallikrein-related peptidases are secreted serine proteases that exert stimulatory or inhibitory effects on tumor progression. A recent study by Bandiera et al. (2009) demonstrated that kallikrein-related peptidase 5 (KLK5) is elevated in serum of patients with ovarian carcinoma. Bandiera et al. examined KLK5 levels and antibody (IgG and IgM) response to KLK5 in the serum of 50 healthy women, 50 patients with benign pelvic masses, 17 patients with ovarian borderline tumors, and 50 patients with ovarian carcinomas, using ELISA. At 95% specificity for healthy controls, 52% of patients with ovarian carcinoma showed high serum KLK5 (sKLK5) levels, whereas patients with benign pathological lesions or borderline tumors showed low or undetectable sKLK5 levels. sKLK5 levels were positively associated to ovarian cancer stage categories (International Federation of Gynecologists and Obstetricians [FIGO]), implying a possible role of sKLK5 in ovarian cancer progression. Elevated levels of KLK5-specific antibodies were noted in 20% of patients with benign masses, 26% of patients with borderline tumors, and 36% of patients with ovarian carcinomas when compared with healthy controls. The authors reported that KLK5 antibodies were also found in patients with undetectable sKLK5 levels. Based on this study KLK5 is a potential new biomarker that could be used in combination with other biomarkers for ovarian cancer detection. The existence of KLK5 antibodies in ovarian cancer suggests that KLK5 might represent a possible target for immune-based therapies. Kallikreins are a subgroup of serine proteases with diverse physiological functions. The human kallikrein gene family has now been fully characterized and includes 15 members tandemly located on chromosome 19q13.4. Strong experimental evidence supports a link between kallikreins and endocrine malignancies and especially ovarian cancer (Yousef and Diamandis, 2002). Three new kallikreins have been shown to be potential diagnostic and prognostic markers for ovarian cancer. Many other kallikreins are also differentially expressed in ovarian cancer, and preliminary reports underline their possible prognostic value. The mechanism by which kallikreins could be involved in ovarian cancer pathology is not known. A likely link could be their regulation through the steroid hormone receptor pathway.

24.4.2.3 Mesothelin

Mesothelin (MSLN) is a 40 kDa glycosylphosphatidylinositol-linked glycoprotein. In normal tissues, the expression of MSLN has subsequently been shown to be largely restricted to mesothelial cells, although immunoreactivity has also been reported in epithelial cells of the trachea, tonsil, fallopian tube, and kidney. MSLN has been shown to be overexpressed in pancreatic carcinomas, gastric carcinoma, and ovarian carcinoma cell lines. MSLN is overexpressed in ovarian cancer tissues with a poor clinical outcome and has been previously identified to activate phosphoinositide 3-kinase (PI3K)/Akt signaling and inhibit paclitaxel-induced apoptosis. Chang et al. (2012) investigated the correlation between MSLN and matrix metalloproteinase (MMP)-7 in the progression of ovarian cancer and the mechanism of MSLN in enhancing ovarian cancer invasion. The expression of MSLN correlated with MMP-7 expression in human ovarian cancer tissues. Overexpressing MSLN or ovarian cancer cells treated with MSLN showed enhanced migration and invasion of cancer cells through the induction of MMP-7. MSLN regulated the expression of MMP-7 through the extracellular-signal-regulated kinase (ERK) 1/2, Akt, and JNK c-Jun N-terminal kinase (JNK) pathways. The expression of MMP-7 and the migrating ability of MSLN-treated ovarian cancer cells were suppressed by ERK1/2- or JNK-specific inhibitors or a decoy activator protein 1 (AP-1) oligonucleotide in in vitro experiments, whereas in vivo animal experiments also demonstrated that mice treated with mitogen-activated protein kinase (MAPK)/ERK- or JNK-specific inhibitors decreased intratumor MMP-7 expression, delayed tumor growth, and extended the survival of mice. MSLN enhances ovarian cancer invasion by MMP-7 expression through the MAPK/ERK and JNK signal transduction pathways. Blocking the MSLN-related pathway could be a potential strategy for inhibiting the growth of ovarian cancer.

It has been also recently reported (Luborsky et al., 2011) that women with prematurely reduced ovarian function, such as with *ovulatory dysfunction*, *ovarian failure*, and unexplained infertility, have significantly more MSLN antibodies (59%, 44%, and 25%, respectively) compared with a control group. This is in contrast to women with endometriosis who did not have the MSLN antibodies, although they are also at higher risk of ovarian cancer. The results of this study support the suggestion that infertility in women is linked to increased risk of ovarian cancer, which also has similar characteristics in women who have an autoimmune disease of the ovary. The study involved 109 women with infertility, 28 women with ovarian cancer, 24 women with benign ovarian tumors (BOTs) or cysts, and 152 healthy women. Among those categorized as infertile, they were 25 women with the risk of premature ovarian failure, 23 women with endometriosis, 17 women with ovulatory dysfunction, and 44 women with unexplained infertility. Overall, compared with healthy women, the MSLN antigen levels in infertility women and those with ovarian cancer and BOTs or cysts are higher.

24.4.2.4 Matrix Metalloproteinases

Recent reports (Kamat et al., 2006; Zhang et al., 2011) describe that increased expression of (MMP)-2, MMP-9, and the urokinase-type plasminogen activator (uPA) is associated with progression from benign to advanced ovarian cancer. Proteases have been linked to the malignant phenotype of cancer. Gelatinolytic activity and protein expression of MMP-2 and MMP-9 were analyzed in tissue extracts of 19 cystadenomas and 18 low-malignant-potential (LMP) tumors, as well as 41 primary tumors of advanced ovarian cancer stage International Federation of Gynecology and Obstetrics IIIc/IV and their corresponding omentum metastases by quantitative gelatin zymography and Western blot. In the same tissue extracts, antigen levels of uPA and its inhibitor PAI-1 were determined by ELISA. Protein expression of pro-MMP-2 (72 kDa) and pro-MMP-9 (92 kDa) and antigen levels of uPA and PAI-1 were low in BOTs but increased significantly from LMP tumors to advanced ovarian cancers. The highest values of all of the proteolytic factors were detected in omentum metastases. Active MMP-2 enzyme (62 kDa) was detected only in ovarian cancer (66%) and corresponding metastases (93%) but never in benign or LMP tumors. The activation rate of MMP-2 to its active isoform was higher in the metastases. Comparing both proteolytic systems, higher PAI-1 concentrations were consistently found in cancers with high pro-MMP-9 expression. These data indicate that members of the plasminogen activator system, as well as the metalloproteinases MMP-2/9, increase with growing malignant potential of ovarian tumors. Zhang et al. (2011) reported significantly higher serum levels of MMP-9 in malignant ovarian cancer patients compared to benign and normal controls. Elevated MMP-9 correlated with FIGO staging, tumor grade, and peritoneal metastasis. In addition, Laios et al. (2013) have reported similar finding and have also shown that chemosensitivity can be restored when resistant ovarian cancer cells are treated with an MMP-9 inhibitor. These findings are of particular relevance to the development of protease inhibitors as new therapeutic approaches in ovarian cancer.

24.4.3 Molecular Approaches

Many of the molecular approaches to date including comparative genomic hybridization and transcription profiling have being performed on tumor tissue and are briefly discussed in the previous invasive section. However, some molecular approaches have shown promise in the noninvasive diagnosis of ovarian cancer using blood, serum, plasma, urine, and saliva as sources of genetic material.

24.4.3.1 Transcriptome

24.4.3.1.1 Blood

Whole blood RNA expression profiles offer potential, but it is not possible to discriminate the signature from the blood components versus the tumor cells unless the circulating tumor cells (CTCs) are isolated directly; this is discussed in more detail later. Studies examining whole blood RNA expression profiles have interrogated genes that are differentially expressed in patients to determine prognosis as opposed to diagnosis but may offer potential in the preoperative setting in relation to tumor biology and optimization of treatment. A signature of genes involved in metastasis, invasion, and inflammation was found to be significantly downregulated in native unstimulated blood leukocytes from ovarian cancer patients with a poor prognosis (Isaksson et al., 2012).

24.4.3.1.2 Saliva

A recent study has examined the potential of using transcriptome analysis of saliva to detect ovarian cancer. A panel of five biomarkers (AGPAT1, B2M, BASP2, IER3, and IL1B) had the potential to discriminate ovarian cancer patients from healthy controls in a study of 56 women with a sensitivity of 85.7% and a specificity of 91.4% (Lee et al., 2012). This approach offers potential and warrants validation in a large trial.

24.4.3.2 MicroRNAs

miRNAs are endogenous noncoding RNA sequences of about 22 nucleotides (Lagos-Quintana et al., 2001). miRNAs inhibit gene expression by inducing degradation or repressing translation of mRNAs when the nucleotide sequences of miRNAs are entirely or partially complementary to the 3′-untranslated regions (UTRs) of targeted mRNAs (Miska, 2005; Esquela-Kerscher and Slack, 2006). Several studies report that miRNAs are aberrantly expressed in human cancer (Calin and Croce, 2006; Esquela-Kerscher and Slack, 2006), which indicate that such miRNAs may function as oncogenes or tumor suppressor genes (Calin et al., 2002; Takamizawa et al., 2004; Chan et al., 2005; He et al., 2005; Iorio et al., 2005; Lu et al., 2005; Zhang et al., 2006). An accumulating body of evidence shows that expression patterns of miRNAs might be beneficial in diagnosis of cancer and prediction of outcome (Dahiya and Morin, 2010).

miRNAs have been interrogated in many ovarian cancer studies and have demonstrated prognostic capabilities, but many of these studies involved analysis of tumor tissue (Flavin et al., 2008; Merritt et al., 2008). Other studies showed that the deregulated miRNAs seen in ovarian cancer are associated with histological type, tumor stage/grade, BRCA mutated/epigenetically changed, primary or recurrent tumors, and survival (Iorio et al., 2007; Laios et al., 2008; Nam et al., 2008; Zhang et al., 2008; Eitan et al., 2009; Gallagher et al., 2009; Lee et al., 2009; Wyman et al., 2009; van Jaarsveld et al., 2010).

Recent studies have demonstrated that miRNAs are circulating freely in serum and other body fluids in a highly stable, cell-free form (Chen et al., 2008; Chim et al., 2008; Gilad et al., 2008; Hunter et al., 2008; Lawrie et al., 2008; Mitchell et al., 2008; Taylor and Gercel-Taylor, 2008). In addition, miRNAs have been shown to be released into the circulation from tumor cells (Mitchell et al., 2008). Profiles of miRNAs in serum and plasma were found to be changed in cancer and other diseases compared to normal healthy controls (Chen et al., 2008; Lawrie et al., 2008; Mitchell et al., 2008; Taylor and Gercel-Taylor, 2008). This indicates the feasibility of using miRNAs as novel noninvasive diagnostic and prognostic biomarker. The first study that reported miRNAs in serum was in 2008 and showed that serum level of miR-21 was associated with relapse-free survival in patients diagnosed with diffuse large B-cell lymphoma (Lawrie et al., 2008).

The feasibility of profiling miRNAs from serum of ovarian cancer patients was described in one study (Resnick et al., 2009). In this study three overexpressed miRNAs were identified as potential oncomirs: miR-21, miR-92, and miR-93, with miR-92 being the most consistent overexpressed miRNA in serum. High expression levels of miR-93 were associated with shorter progression-free and overall survival in ovarian cancer patients. Furthermore, miR-127, miR-155, and miR-99b were underexpressed in the serum of ovarian cancer patients (Resnick et al., 2009). Interestingly, miR-127 was identified previously as a potent tumor suppressor in ovarian cell lines (Zhang et al., 2008), which supports the underexpression seen in this study.

Overexpressed miRNAs were also identified from tumor releasing exosomes of patients with ovarian cancer. These structures are endosome-derived organelles that are actively secreted through an exocytosis pathway (Iero et al., 2008). One study showed that the level of circulating tumor-derived exosomes in serum of women with invasive ovarian cancer was higher than their level in women with benign ovarian disease and normal controls. In addition to that the level of the exosomes was significantly greater in women with advanced disease. These results suggest that profiling of miRNAs from circulating tumor exosomes could be used as a potential diagnostic marker for screening of asymptomatic women and monitoring of the disease recurrence (Taylor and Gercel-Taylor, 2008).

Profiling of whole blood miRNAs in ovarian cancer patients was examined in one study; however, the pattern of profiling was not sensitive enough to be used for screening or monitoring of progression of ovarian cancer (Hausler et al., 2010). Profiling of peripheral blood miRNA could be combined with other serum biomarkers such as CA-125 and transvaginal ultrasound to improve the overall screening of ovarian cancer (Hausler et al., 2010).

In addition to miRNAs, small nucleolar RNAs (snoRNAs) that guide chemical modifications of other RNAs have received attention recently. Liao et al. (2010) have described how differential expression of snoRNA species may be detected in plasma samples from patients with non-small cell lung cancer. This approach holds much promise for application in the ovarian cancer field as distinct repertoires of snoRNAs are ascribed to particular ovarian neoplasms.

24.4.4 Metabolomics

In the search for more sensitive and specific biomarkers for cancer, metabolomics has offered great promise as a noninvasive diagnostic method for diagnosis (Griffin and Shockcor, 2004).

24.4.4.1 Blood

In ovarian cancer, Zhang et al. (2012) have used metabolomics to discriminate between EOC and BOT. They confirmed four metabolomic biomarkers (L-tryptophan, LysoPC(18:3), LysoPC(14:0), and 2-piperidinone) as having discriminatory ability. Recently, Chen et al. (2011) developed an ultra performance liquid chromatography tandem mass spectrometry analytical method according to FDA guidance to obtain reproducible, sensitive, and abundant metabolic information for ovarian cancer. 27-nor-5β-cholestane-3,7,12,24,25 pentol glucuronide (CPG) was verified as a potential biomarker for EOC. Furthermore, CPG was proven to have an elevated concentration level in ovarian cancer tissues compared to benign ovarian tumor tissues.

24.4.4.2 Urine

Slupsky et al. (2010) have successfully used urine metabolite analysis for detecting early-stage breast and ovarian cancer. They discovered differences in 67 metabolite concentrations measured in urine from a cohort of apparently healthy female subjects compared to subjects with ovarian cancer. The urinary metabolite changes revealed many metabolites decreased in relative concentration with a cancer (both EOC and breast) phenotype when compared with healthy samples.

24.4.5 Autoantibody Profiling

Autoantibody (AAb) profiling of ovarian cancer patient serum to identify biomarkers has received a lot of interest, and recently a number of studies have interrogated the AAb profile associated with ovarian cancer (Hudson et al., 2007; Gagnon et al., 2008; Taylor et al., 2009; Gnjatic et al., 2010; Murphy et al., 2012a). The method by which the tumor-associated AAb response is generated is an area of increasing interest and has recently been reviewed (Murphy et al., 2012b). There is a known humoral immune response to malignancy (a proposed model of generation is outlined in Figure 24.3). AAbs as biomarker entities have advantages over other markers as they are present in serum, preventing more invasive biopsy procedures, and the AAb can remain for months and even years. Antibodies are also stable entities with a long half-life (t ½ = 21 days). A further advantage in terms of bioassay development is that as the serum AAbs bind the protein biomarker, even if a panel of different proteins are used in the assay, only one labeled secondary antibody, which detects the Fc region of the primary antibody (e.g., antihuman IgG), is required for detection (Murphy et al., 2012b). In terms of ovarian cancer, histotype, grading, and staging are the most important parameters relating to the AAb profile. The serous papillary histotype has a strong correlation with the presence of p53 AAbs (Murphy et al., 2012a).

The best characterized autoantigen/AAb relationship is the tumor suppressor protein p53. AAbs to p53 have been identified in the serum of patients with many different cancers (Soussi, 2000) and are also found in approximately 25% of ovarian cancer patients (Vogl et al., 2000; Li et al., 2008; Murphy et al., 2012a). There is a high association of p53 mutation with type II tumors, meaning that anti-p53 AAbs are predominantly associated with high-grade ovarian cancers (Tsai-Turton et al., 2009). Up to 80% of type II

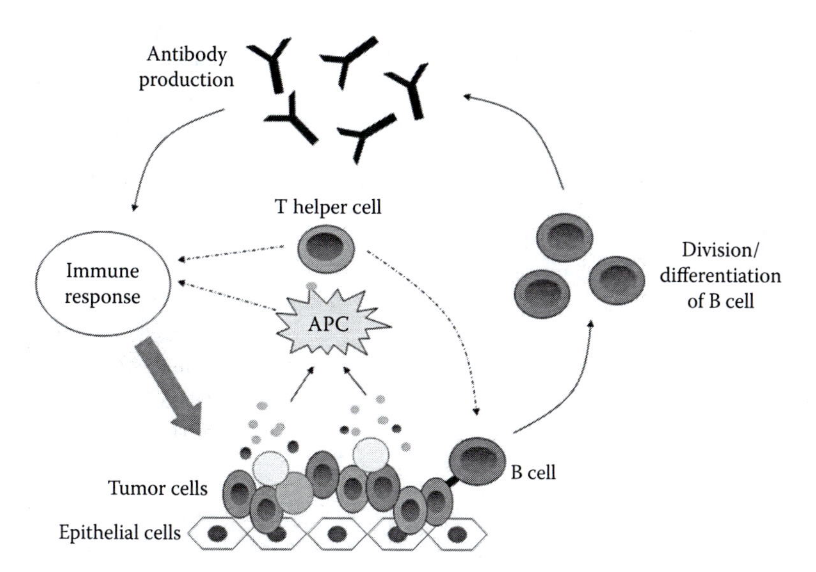

FIGURE 24.3 Model proposing the generation of circulating AAbs in cancer patients. At the site of tumor development, tissue damage leads to the release of proteins and cellular debris. The antigen-presenting cells (APCs) then present these proteins to the immune response, ultimately resulting in B-cell proliferation and antibody production.

tumors exhibit mutated p53; however, it is still unclear and there is ongoing investigation into why just a subset (20%–40%) of these cases generate anti-p53 antibodies (Piura and Piura, 2009).

AAbs to MSLN have relatively recently been characterized and are being interrogated for their usefulness in the clinic. Some studies have identified AAbs to MSLN to be OC specific (Ho et al., 2005); however, other studies have also identified MSLN AAbs in healthy women (Hellstrom et al., 2008).

AAbs to NY-ESO-1 have been identified in many studies that have interrogated the AAb profile of ovarian cancer patients (Stockert et al., 1998; Odunsi et al., 2003; Milne et al., 2008; Piura and Piura, 2009). Similarly to p53 AAbs, AAbs to NY-ESO-1 have been suggested to be associated with type II tumors (Lu et al., 2011). However, AAbs to NY-ESO-1 have also been identified in other cancers, such as melanoma (Stockert et al., 1998) and breast cancer (Piura and Piura, 2010).

AAbs to heat shock protein 90 (HSP90) have been implicated in the pathogenesis of autoimmune diseases (Faulds et al., 1995; Hayem et al., 1999) and also in malignancies such as osteocarcinoma (Trieb et al., 2000) and ovarian cancer (Vidal et al., 2004). Vidal et al. have postulated that AAbs to HSP90 are tumor-associated and stage specific (Vidal et al., 2004). Anti-HSP90 AAbs of the IgA class have also been linked to ovarian cancer (Korneeva et al., 2000).

AAbs to survivin have also been identified in two studies of ovarian cancer patient sera; however, these antibodies are not specific to OC (Taylor et al., 2009). AAbs to survivin are not specific to ovarian cancer; however, they may be of use in an AAb biomarker panel, perhaps in ovarian cancer staging.

Although AAbs identify a great hope for cancer diagnosis, including early diagnosis, for example, the EarlyCDT-Lung™, a test offered by Oncimmune (United States), may aid in the early detection of lung cancer in high-risk populations (Chapman et al., 2012). However, AAb diagnostic tests for cancers, including ovarian, have yet to be fully translated in the clinic/materialize in the hands of clinicians.

24.4.6 Circulating DNA and Epigenetic Changes

Cell-free tumor DNA can exist in the circulation of a patient with cancer that can carry information on mutations and tumor burden. Individual mutations have been assessed but recently a method for tagged-amplicon deep sequencing (TAm-Seq) has been developed and used to identify mutations in ovarian cancer patients. Mutations were identified in *TP53* in circulating DNA from 46 plasma samples of advanced ovarian cancer patients. This low-cost, high-throughput method offers potential for future diagnostics and personalized medicine approaches (Forshew et al., 2012).

As sequencing technologies develop, this area will become a hot topic for the future. Shotgun DNA sequencing has also shown promise in the area of ovarian cancer diagnostics (Chan et al., 2013) by obtaining a noninvasive, genome-wide view of cancer-associated copy number variations and mutations in DNA in plasma. These technologies require further validation and while costly at present, sequencing costs continue to fall as the technology develops.

Various epigenetic changes including CpG island methylation and histone modification have been identified in ovarian cancer. These aberrations are associated with distinct disease subtypes and may be both present and detectable in circulating serum of ovarian cancer patients. Several epigenetic changes have shown promise for their diagnostic, prognostic, and predictive capacity but still need further validation (Seeber and van Diest, 2012).

24.4.7 Circulating Tumor Cells

Hematogenous dissemination of tumor cells, referred to as CTCs, from a primary tumor, is a necessary step for the establishment of metastases at secondary sites in the body. CTCs circulate in the peripheral blood of cancer patients and are extremely rare in healthy people; thus their detection and isolation can provide significant clinical insight into disease diagnosis and prognosis. Indeed, CTCs have been demonstrated to be of predictive and prognostic value among patients with prostate, breast, and colorectal cancers (Allard et al., 2004; Cristofanilli et al., 2004; Paterlini-Brechot and Benali, 2007; de Bono et al., 2008).

These findings have lead to speculation that CTCs may hold potential as novel diagnostic and prognostic biomarkers for other solid tumors, including ovarian cancer.

While distant metastasis is a late complication of ovarian cancer and historically ovarian cancer was thought to spread primarily by direct extension into the abdominal cavity, multiple studies have established the presence of tumorlike epithelial cells in the peripheral blood of ovarian cancer patients (Marth et al., 2002; Judson et al., 2003; Wimberger et al., 2007; Fan et al., 2009; Aktas et al., 2011; Poveda et al., 2011; Obermayr et al., 2013). However, although there is a strong consensus in the literature that CTCs are present in a subset of women with ovarian malignancy, no clear consensus has been reached on the clinical relevance of these CTCs. Initial studies seemed to indicate that there was no prognostic value in the detection of CTCs in the peripheral blood of ovarian cancer patients (Marth et al., 2002; Judson et al., 2003; Wimberger et al., 2007). However, more recent studies have suggested that CTC positivity (Fan et al., 2009; Aktas et al., 2011) or elevated levels of CTCs (Poveda et al., 2011) can significantly correlate with disease-free survival. The discrepancies observed within the literature are probably due to differing study design, study population, sample size, and follow-up periods.

In addition to a growing body of evidence of the prognostic utility of CTCs in ovarian malignancies, a recent study by Obermayr et al. (2013) demonstrated the potential of CTCs to inform treatment regimes. This study described a novel panel of ovarian CTC markers, which were used to interrogate the peripheral blood of ovarian cancer patient for the presence of CTCs. Overall in this study CTCs were detected in 24.5% of baseline samples and 20.4% of follow-up samples; of the 68 CTC positive samples, 69% were identified by the overexpression of cyclophilin C (PPIC). Moreover, the detection of PPIC positive CTCs in patients 6 months after completion of adjuvant chemotherapy was observed to be significantly overrepresented in platinum-resistant patients and also predicative of poor outcome. This demonstrates that enumeration and characterization of CTCs may offer an improved method for early detection of aggressive disease coupled with assessment of treatment efficacy and/or inform treatment regime.

Several technologies have been used for isolation of CTCs from patients (Yu et al., 2011), and one promising technology is the ScreenCell device (Desitter et al., 2011) that is a simple and innovative noninvasive technology for isolating circulating rare cells from whole blood. It provides easy access to fixed or live CTCs and circulating tumor microemboli, allowing a full range access to phenotypical, genotypical, and functional characterization of these cells. An example of CTCs isolated from an ovarian cancer patient with this device is shown in Figure 24.4.

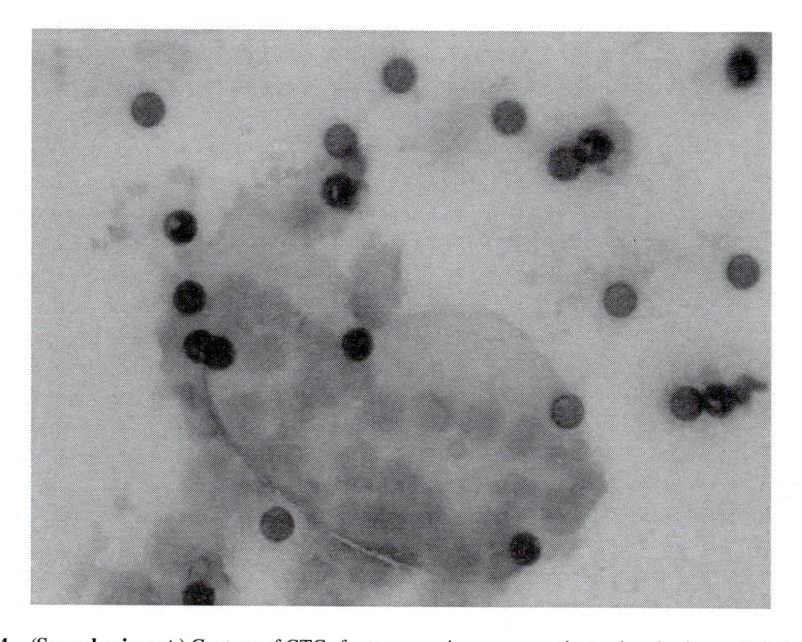

FIGURE 24.4 **(See color insert.)** Capture of CTCs from an ovarian cancer patient using the ScreenCell device.

24.5 Imaging

Imaging plays an integral role in the diagnosis and management of ovarian cancer patients; examples of imaging technologies are displayed in Figure 24.5. Ovarian masses or cysts are commonly detected by noninvasive imaging in patients with pelvic symptoms or in patients being screened for ovarian cancer. The majority of these masses are benign, particularly in premenopausal women. Thin-walled, unilocular, cystic structures smaller than 5 cm in diameter are likely to be benign and can be followed with imaging. However, cysts may be very complex in appearance, and differentiation from ovarian malignancy may not be possible using standard imaging techniques alone, resulting in patients undergoing surgical exploration. The mainstay of ovarian imaging is transvaginal grayscale ultrasound (TVS). Structural features of ovarian cysts (size, septa, solid projections) may be correlated with likelihood of malignancy. The presence of ascites or peritoneal nodules is also suggestive of malignancy. While there are many benefits to ultrasound, the main limitations include cost and difficulty in tracking progression and location of the tumor, given that it is felt the majority of ovarian cancers spread rapidly (Rein et al., 2011). TVS augmented by color Doppler mapping of vessel distribution has recently been shown to improve detection of adnexal malignancies when compared to grayscale imaging (Guerriero et al., 2002). Computed axial tomography (CT) is of limited value in assessing ovarian masses but will detect metastatic disease. It is most widely used for disease staging, selection of patients for cytoreductive surgery, assessment of treatment response, and the detection of recurrence. Preoperative CT is also important in identifying unusual disease patterns that may suggest nonovarian origin. Magnetic resonance imaging (MRI) provides structural information (Okamoto et al., 2007) and is of value in further characterizing masses that are indeterminate in the United States or where clinical circumstances dictate. Evaluating different MRI sequences allows recognition of blood products and fat and fibrous tissues and, therefore, enables accurate diagnosis of benign lesions such as endometriomas, ovarian dermoids, and fibromas that can appear complex in the United States. MRI has been shown to be as accurate as CT in the evaluation of disease extent in advanced ovarian cancer (Tempany et al., 2000); however, it is not widely used as a staging tool due to its expense and limited availability. ^{18}Fluoro-deoxy-glucose positron emission tomography [FDG-PET] scanning has emerged as a useful technique in the management of ovarian tumors (Picchio et al., 2003; Yoshida et al., 2004). FDG-PET does not play a significant additional role in diagnosis; however, the role of combined PET/CT modality has recently begun to be reexplored for initial disease staging, particularly because PET/CT can pick up small unsuspected lesions and, thereby, provide a better disease assessment of the whole body in a single examination. Castellucci et al. (2007) have shown that the PPV (100%) and accuracy (92%) of FDG-PET imaging for malignant ovarian disease were higher than the PPV (80%) and accuracy (80%) of TVUS. Fenchel et al. (2002) evaluated the utility of FDG-PET in the

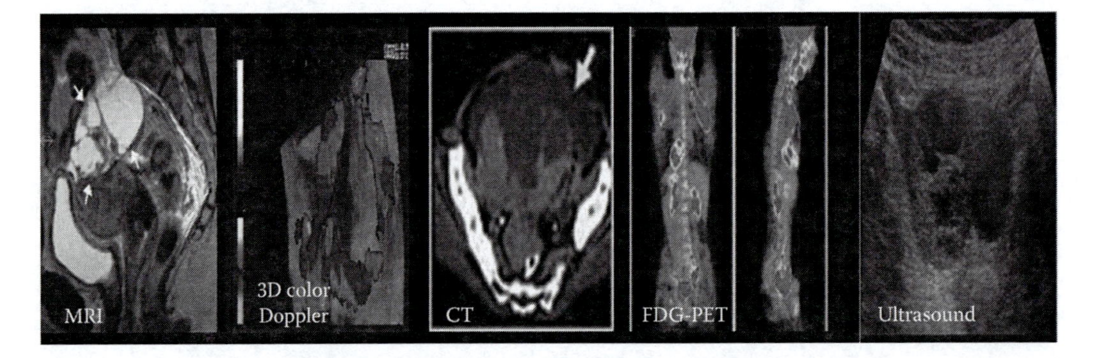

FIGURE 24.5 (See color insert.) Different imaging methodologies used in ovarian cancer diagnosis and monitoring: MRI, 3D color Doppler, CT, FDG-PET, and ultrasound. The arrows in CT and MRI point to presumed tumor. The color Doppler shows blood flow: red for arterial and blue for venous. In the FDG-PET image, the red is activity, presumed tumor. The ultrasound shows what appears to be a normal right ovary and queries pelvic fluid/mass on the left.

characterization of asymptomatic adnexal masses in a series of 101 preoperative patients and showed a sensitivity of 58% and specificity of 76%. This was compared with MRI and ultrasound and the overall sensitivities and specificities are outlined in Table 24.1. When FDG-PET is analyzed jointly with US and MRI findings, the three modalities had a sensitivity of 92% and specificity of 85%. However, this is similar to using US and MRI together, and there is no reported advantage in adding FDG-PET for characterization of adnexal lesions.

24.6 Genetic Testing and Ethnic Group Markers for Ovarian Cancer

As alluded to the previous discussion, mutations in the *BRCA1* and *BRCA2* genes are associated with an increased lifetime risk for development of ovarian cancer (Hensley et al., 2002). These mutations are present in about 10%–15% of ovarian cancer patients. Ovarian cancer risk differs by gene, with *BRCA1* associated with a 36%–63% lifetime risk and *BRCA2* mutation carriers having a 10%–27% lifetime risk (Anglian breast cancer study group, 2000; Chen and Parmigiani, 2007). Prophylactic salpingo-oophorectomy significantly reduces cancer risk and mortality in these women (Rebbeck et al., 2002; Domchek et al., 2006).

People of Ashkenazi Jewish heritage are more likely to harbor mutations in the *BRCA* genes than the general population. Three common mutations have been identified in Ashkenazi Jewish *BRCA1/2* mutation carriers: c.68_69delAG (185delAG or 187delAG) and c.5266dupC (5382insC or 5385insC) in *BRCA1* and c.5946delT (6174delT) in *BRCA2* (Struewing et al., 1995; Neuhausen et al., 1996; Oddoux et al., 1996). The high frequency of these mutations has led to the development of panel testing for the three common Jewish mutations.

24.7 Innovative Technologies in Ovarian Cancer Diagnosis

The development of point-of-care devices that have revolutionized the medical world has also entered the field of ovarian cancer diagnosis with point-of-care devices being developed for CA-125 (Raamanthan et al., 2012; Wang et al., 2012) and HE4 (Wang et al., 2011). Technologies range from bio-nano-chip systems to 3D electrochemical devices to microchip ELISA-based detection modules that employ a portable detection system, that is, a cell phone/charge-coupled device. Such technologies have the potential to influence survival outcome from ovarian cancer by allowing access to rapid, low-cost screening tools. In addition, the ability to multiplex and perform highly sensitive assays is crucial for future validation of biomarker panels, and many of these emerging technologies offer this potential.

24.8 Recommended Tests/Panels in Combination with/without Imaging for Early Diagnosis

Any test panel or algorithm for ovarian cancer diagnosis involves CA-125 and has been developed to increase the accuracy of CA-125. The RMI uses ultrasound, menopausal status and CA-125 and has been utilized in the United Kingdom for two decades, providing sensitivity that has ranged from 71% to 88% and specificity from 74% to 97% for identifying patients with malignant disease. The ROMA has been used in combination with CA-125 to increase sensitivity. Although not routinely used in the clinic, ROMA has recently been approved by the FDA for ovarian cancer diagnosis in patients presenting with a pelvic mass. This algorithm combines serum levels of CA-125 and HE4 along with menopausal status in a logistic regression model to identify a patient as low risk or high risk for having ovarian carcinoma. The OVA1 panel previously described also utilizes CA-125. CA-125 screening combined with TVU increases sensitivity and specificity to 89.4% and 99.8%, respectively (Menon et al., 2009). The UKCTOCS trial uses a calculation called the ROCA. Rather than just looking at the results of a single CA-125 test, they look for changes in CA-125 over time, to try to predict the woman's risk of having the disease. This is used in conjunction with ultrasound and takes into account age-specific risk. Results are awaited from this trial that will report in 2014.

24.9 Advantages and Challenges in Developing Molecular Biomarkers for Early Detection

The advantages of developing early detection markers for ovarian cancer are clear from the statistics, as diagnosis when the disease is confined to the ovary (stage I) can result in greater than 90% cure (Engel et al., 2002). As previously mentioned the challenges in achieving this are numerous, as early-stage disease may have no symptoms or nonspecific symptoms, which is why ovarian cancer is often referred to as the "silent killer." Early-stage diagnosis that accounts for about 25% of cases is often an incidental finding and often is identified when the patient is undergoing routine examination or being investigated for a non-gynecological condition. In addition, effective screening tools are currently not available, in particular for early-stage disease. Owing to the rather low incidence of the disease in the general population, potential screening tests must provide very high specificity to avoid unnecessary interventions in false-positive cases (Bast, 2003). Another major challenge for researchers in this area is the lack of availability of blood samples from early-stage cancer patients that is necessary for the validation of any potential early diagnostic marker. Biobanks from the ovarian cancer and other cancer screening trials have assisted in overcoming this challenge, but such samples may be limited, may not have ethical approval to be used in other studies, and are very precious indicating the need for well-curated biobanks on an international scale.

24.10 Market Players in Ovarian Cancer

The past year has seen major changes in the global ovarian cancer therapeutic market that is expected to achieve threefold growth by 2020, reaching $2352 m (http://www.reportlinker.com/p0843058-summary/Ovarian-Cancer-Therapeutics-Global-Drug-Forecasts-and-Treatment-Analysis.html [Feb 2012]). This high growth rate is expected due to the strength of the pipeline candidates, which are anticipated to change the treatment paradigm of ovarian cancer when launched. Bevacizumab (Avastin), a VEGF inhibitor, is leading the way in new biological drugs for ovarian cancer, and ongoing randomized trials will help identify which patients should receive bevacizumab in first line rather than in the relapsed setting, the optimal duration of bevacizumab therapy, and how it should be combined with alternative treatment strategies. The major players in the therapeutic market include F. Hoffmann-La Roche Ltd, GlaxoSmithKline PLC, Amgen Inc, AstraZeneca PLC, and Boehringer Ingelheim GmbH. The key classes of mechanism of action include microtubule stabilizers, vascular endothelial growth factor receptor (VEGFR) inhibitors, immunomodulators, folate receptor inhibitors, PARP inhibitors, topoisomerase inhibitors, interleukins, mammalian target of rapamycin (mTOR) inhibitors, and phosphatidylinositol-3-kinase (PI3K) inhibitors.

The diagnostic arena has also seen some advances; Vermillion Inc., a molecular diagnostics company, developed OVA1, with support from Quest Diagnostics. OVA1 is only available through Quest Diagnostics. Abbott, Fujirebio, and F. Hoffmann-La Roche Ltd all play major roles in ovarian cancer diagnostics, and with FDA approval for HE4 and ROMA, this area will grow in the future. Molecular diagnostics is a rapidly advancing area of research and medicine, with new technologies and applications being continually added that will transform the ovarian cancer diagnostic and therapeutic markets in the years ahead.

24.11 Patents for Ovarian Cancer Diagnosis

A patent search on http://www.patentlens.net/for ovarian cancer diagnosis reveals 192 entries, either granted or applied for. These vary in technology with some of the recent patents focusing on miRNA profiles and proteomics. Others focus on combined panels for breast and ovarian cancer and consist of mRNA gene signature profiles. Many of the patents contain work performed on tissue specimens so may not be suitable for noninvasive diagnosis. A list of granted patents from 2010 to 2012 is given in Table 24.3.

TABLE 24.3

Summary of Patents Granted for Ovarian Cancer Diagnosis from 2011 to 2012

Patent No	Title	Date	Marker	Technology
US 8187889	Protein markers for the diagnosis and prognosis of ovarian and breast cancer	May 29, 2012	Truncated forms of cytosolic serine hydroxymethyl transferase (cSHMT), T-box transcription factor 3 (Tbx3), and utrophin	2D gel electrophoresis and MALDI TOF mass spectrometry
US 8088390	Methods for the early diagnosis of ovarian cancer	Jan 3, 2012	Stratum corneum chymotryptic enzyme	mRNA (tissue)
US 8030060	Gene signature for diagnosis and prognosis of breast cancer and ovarian cancer	Oct 4, 2011	28 Gene signature for prognosis in ovarian cancer	mRNA (tissue)
US 7985843	Compositions and methods for the therapy and diagnosis of ovarian cancer	Jul 26, 2011	Antibody or antigen-binding fragment	Immunoassay
US 7935531	Methods for the early diagnosis of ovarian cancer	May 3, 2011	Hepsin protease	Polymerase chain reaction (PCR) (tissue)
US 792818	Antigen polypeptide for the diagnosis and/or treatment of ovarian cancer	Apr 19, 2011	OVTA	ELISA
US 7906635	Nucleotide and amino acid sequences and assays and methods of use thereof for diagnosis of ovarian cancer	Mar 15, 2011	Novel nucleotide and amino acid sequences	Sequencing
US 7795211	Methods for the early diagnosis of ovarian cancer	Sep 14, 2010	Hepsin	PCR (Tissue)
US 7785841	Methods for the early diagnosis of ovarian cancer	Aug 31, 2010	PUMP-1 protease (MMP-7)	PCR and immunohistochemistry (tissue)

24.12 Concluding Remarks and Future Perspective

While the future looks bright for ovarian cancer treatment with the introduction of new drugs, the diagnosis of ovarian cancer clearly needs more research to identify novel epidemiologic, genetic, or blood-based markers of ovarian cancer risk. A combination of improved imaging techniques, potentially incorporating molecular markers, may improve diagnostic capability. As ovarian cancer is quite a heterogenous disease, it is likely that one single biomarker will not be sufficient for diagnosis but a panel of biomarkers may be more appropriate. In the emerging era of personalized medicine, these biomarkers may also be useful in determining the most suitable treatment for ovarian cancer patients. As regards screening, the medical and scientific field awaits the results of the UKCTOCS trial that are due in 2014. This will determine if screening for ovarian cancer using ultrasound and CA-125 can improve the overall mortality from this disease. In conclusion, research must continue to develop a reliable and sensitive diagnostic test for ovarian cancer.

This review was inspired by research gratefully funded by the Ovarian Cancer Charity, the Emer Casey Foundation (www.emercaseyfoundation.com).

References

Abraham, J. 2010. OVA1 test for preoperative assessment of ovarian cancer. *Community Translations* 7:249–250.

Aktas, B. Kasimir-Bauer, S. Heubner, M. Kimmig, R. Wimberger, P. 2011. Molecular profiling and prognostic relevance of circulating tumor cells in the blood of ovarian cancer patients at primary diagnosis and after platinum-based chemotherapy. *International Journal of Gynecological Cancer* 21:822–830.

Allard, WJ. Matera, J. Miller, MC. Repollet, M. Connelly, MC. Rao, C. Tibbe, AG. Uhr, JW. Terstappen, LW. 2004. Tumor cells circulate in the peripheral blood of all major carcinomas but not in healthy subjects or patients with non-malignant diseases. *Clinical Cancer Research* 10:6897–6904.

Anastasi, E. Marchei, GG. Viggiani, V. Gennarini, G. Frati, L. Reale, MG. 2010. HE4: A new potential early biomarker for the recurrence of ovarian cancer. *Tumour Biology* 31:113–119.

Andersen, MR. Goff, BA. Lowe, KA. Scholler, N. Bergan, L. Drescher, CW. Paley, P. Urban, N. 2010. Use of a Symptom Index, CA125, and HE4 to predict ovarian cancer. *Gynecologic Oncology* 116:378–383.

Anderson, NL. Anderson, NG. 2002. The human plasma proteome: History, character, and diagnostic prospects. *Molecular Cell Proteomics* 1:845–867.

Anglian Breast Cancer Study Group. 2000. Prevalence and penetrance of BRCA1 and BRCA2 mutations in a population-based series of breast cancer cases. *British Journal of Cancer* 83:1301–1308.

Attur, MG. Palmer, GD. Al-Mussawir, HE. Dave, M. Teixeira, CC. Rifkin, DB. Appleton, CT. Beier, F. Abramson, SB. 2009. F-spondin, a neuroregulatory protein, is up-regulated in osteoarthritis and regulates cartilage metabolism via TGF-beta activation. *FASEB Journal* 23:79–89.

Bandiera, E. Zanotti, L. Bignotti, E. Romani, C. Tassi, R. Todeschini, P. Tognon, G. et al. 2009. Human kallikrein 5: An interesting novel biomarker in ovarian cancer patients that elicits humoral response. *International Journal of Gynecological Cancer* 19:1015–1021.

Bast, RC Jr. 2003. Status of tumor markers in ovarian cancer screening. *Journal of Clinical Oncology* 21:200s–205s.

Bast, RC Jr. Hennessy, B. Mills, GB. 2009. The biology of ovarian cancer: New opportunities for translation. *Nature Reviews Cancer* 9:415–428.

Bell, DA. 2005. Origins and molecular pathology of ovarian cancer. *Modern Pathology* 18(Suppl 2):S19–S32.

Bingle, L. Singleton, V. Bingle, CD. 2002. The putative ovarian tumour marker gene HE4 (WFDC2) is expressed in normal tissues and undergoes complex alternative splicing to yield multiple protein isoforms. *Oncogene* 21:2768–2773.

Biomarkers Definitions Working Group. 2001. Biomarkers and surrogate endpoints: Preferred definitions and conceptual framework. *Clinical Pharmacology and Therapeutics* 69:89–95.

Borgoño, CA. Fracchioli, S. Yousef, GM. Rigault de la Longrais, IA. Luo, LY. Soosaipillai, A. Puopolo, M. et al. 2003. Favorable prognostic value of tissue human kallikrein 11 (hK11) in patients with ovarian carcinoma. *International Journal of Cancer* 106:605–610.

Borgoño, CA. Kishi, T. Scorilas, A. Harbeck, N. Dorn, J. Schmalfeldt, B. Schmitt, M. Diamandis, EP. 2006. Human kallikrein 8 protein is a favorable prognostic marker in ovarian cancer. *Clinical Cancer Research* 12:1487–1493.

Bouchard, D. Morisset, D. Bourbonnais, Y. Tremblay, GM. 2006. Proteins with whey-acidic-protein motifs and cancer. *The Lancet Oncology* 7:167–174.

Bronckaers, A. Gago, F. Balzarini, J. Liekens, S. 2009. The dual role of thymidine phosphorylase in cancer development and chemotherapy. *Medicinal Research Reviews* 29:903–953.

Buys, SS. Partridge, E. Black, A. Johnson, CC. Lamerato, L. Isaacs, C. Reding, DJ. et al. PLCO Project Team. 2011. Effect of screening on ovarian cancer mortality: The Prostate, Lung, Colorectal and Ovarian (PLCO) cancer screening randomized controlled trial. *The Journal of the American Medical Association* 305:2295–2303.

Calin, GA. Croce, CM. 2006. MicroRNA signatures in human cancers. *Nature Reviews Cancer* 6:857–866.

Calin, GA. Dumitru, CD. Shimizu, M. Bichi, R. Zupo, S. Noch, E. Aldler, H. et al. 2002. Frequent deletions and down-regulation of micro- RNA genes miR15 and miR16 at 13q14 in chronic lymphocytic leukemia. *Proceedings of the National Academy of Sciences of the United States of America* 99:15524–15529.

Castellucci, P. Perrone, AM. Picchio, M. Ghi, T. Farsad, M. Nanni, C. Messa, C. et al. 2007. Diagnostic accuracy of 18F-FDG PET/CT in characterizing ovarian lesions and staging ovarian cancer: Correlation with transvaginal ultrasonography, computed tomography, and histology. *Nuclear Medicine Communications* 28:589–595.

Chan, JA. Krichevsky, AM. Kosik, KS. 2005. MicroRNA-21 is an antiapoptotic factor in human glioblastoma cells. *Cancer Research* 65:6029–6033.

Chan, KC. Jiang, P. Zheng, YW. Liao, GJ. Sun, H. Wong, J. Siu, SS. et al. 2013. Cancer genome scanning in plasma: Detection of tumor-associated copy number aberrations, single-nucleotide variants, and tumoral heterogeneity by massively parallel sequencing. *Clinical Chemistry* 59:211–224.

Chan, KK. Chen, CA. Nam, JH. Ochiai, K. Wilailak, S. Choon, AT. Sabaratnam, S. et al. 2012. The use of HE4 in the prediction of ovarian cancer in Asian women with a pelvic mass. *Gynecologic Oncology.* doi 10.1016/j.ygyno.2012.09.034.

Chang, MC. Chen, CA. Chen, PJ. Chiang, YC. Chen, YL. Mao, TL. Lin, HW. Lin Chiang, WH. Cheng, WF. 2012. Mesothelin enhances invasion of ovarian cancer by inducing MMP-7 through MAPK/ERK and JNK pathways. *Biochemical Journal* 442:293–302.

Chapman, CJ. Healey, GF. Murray, A. Boyle, P. Robertson, C. Peek, LJ. Allen, J. et al. 2012. EarlyCDT®-Lung test: Improved clinical utility through additional autoantibody assays. *Tumour Biology* 33:1319–1326.

Chen, J. Zhang, X. Cao, R. Lu, X. Zhao, S. Fekete, A. Huang, Q. et al. 2011. Serum 27-nor-5β-cholestane-3,7,12,24,25 pentol glucuronide discovered by metabolomics as potential diagnostic biomarker for epithelium ovarian cancer. *Journal of Proteome Research* 10:2625–2632.

Chen, S. Parmigiani, G. 2007. Meta-analysis of BRCA1 and BRCA2 penetrance. *Journal of Clinical Oncology* 25:1329–1333.

Chen, X. Ba, Y. Ma, L. Cai, X. Yin, Y. Wang, K. Guo, J. et al. 2008. Characterization of microRNAs in serum: A novel class of biomarkers for diagnosis of cancer and other diseases. *Cell Research* 18:997–1006.

Chim, SS. Shing, TK. Hung, EC. Leung, TY. Lau, TK. Chiu, RW. Lo, YM. 2008. Detection and characterization of placental microRNAs in maternal plasma. *Clinical Chemistry* 54:482–490.

Clauss, A. Lilja, H. Lundwall, A. 2005. The evolution of a genetic locus encoding small serine proteinase inhibitors. *Biochemical and Biophysical Research Communications* 333:383–389.

Coticchia, CM. Yang, J. Moses, MA. 2008. Ovarian cancer biomarkers: Current options and future promise. *Journal of the National Comprehensive Cancer Network* 6:795–802.

Cristofanilli, M. Budd, GT. Ellis, MJ. Stopeck, A. Matera, J. Miller, MC. Reuben, JM. et al. 2004. Circulating tumor cells, disease progression, and survival in metastatic breast cancer. *The New England Journal of Medicine* 351:781–791.

Crum, CP. Drapkin, R. Miron, A. Ince, TA. Muto, M. Kindelberger, DW. Lee, Y. 2007. The distal fallopian tube: A new model for pelvic serous carcinogenesis. *Current Opinion in Obstetrics & Gynecology* 19:3–9.

Dahiya, N. Morin, PJ. 2010. MicroRNAs in ovarian carcinomas. *Endocrine-Related Cancer* 17:F77–F89.

de Bono, JS. Scher, HI. Montgomery, RB. Parker, C. Miller, MC. Tissing, H. Doyle, GV. et al. 2008. Circulating tumor cells predict survival benefit from treatment in metastatic castration-resistant prostate cancer. *Clinical Cancer Research* 14:6302–6309.

Desitter, I. Guerrouahen, BS. Benali-Furet, N. Wechsler, J. Jänne, PA. Kuang, Y. Yanagita, M. et al. 2011. A new device for rapid isolation by size and characterization of rare circulating tumor cells. *Anticancer Research* 31:427–441.

Domchek, SM. Friebel, TM. Neuhausen, SL. Wagner, T. Evans, G. Isaacs, C. Garber, JE. et al. 2006. Mortality after bilateral salpingo-oophorectomy in BRCA1 and BRCA2 mutation carriers: A prospective cohort study. *The Lancet Oncology* 7:223–229.

Drapkin, R. von Horsten, HH. Lin, Y. Mok, SC. Crum, CP. Welsh, WR. Hecht, JL. 2005. Human epididymis protein 4 (HE4) is a secreted glycoprotein that is overexpressed by serous and endometrioid ovarian carcinomas. *Cancer Research* 65:2162–2169.

Eitan, R. Kushnir, M. Lithwick-Yanai, G. David, MB. Hoshen, M. Glezerman, M. Hod, M. et al. 2009. Tumor microRNA expression patterns associated with resistance to platinum based chemotherapy and survival in ovarian cancer patients. *Gynecologic Oncology* 114:253–259.

Engel, J. Eckel, R. Schubert-Fritschle, G. Kerr, J. Kuhn, W. Diebold, J. Kimmig, R. Rehbock, J. Hölzel, D. 2002. Moderate progress for ovarian cancer in the last 20 years: Prolongation of survival, but no improvement in the cure rate. *European Journal of Cancer* 38:2435–2445.

Engelen, MJ. Kos, HE. Willemse, PH. Aalders, JG. de Vries, EG. Schaapveld, M. Otter, R. van der Zee, AG. 2006. Surgery by consultant gynecologic oncologists improves survival in patients with ovarian carcinoma. *Cancer* 106:589–598.

Esquela-Kerscher, A. Slack, FJ. 2006. Oncomirs—MicroRNAs with a role in cancer. *Nature Reviews Cancer* 6:259–269.

Fan, T. Zhao, Q. Chen, JJ. Chen, WT. Pearl, ML. 2009. Clinical significance of circulating tumor cells detected by an invasion assay in peripheral blood of patients with ovarian cancer. *Gynecologic Oncology* 112:185–191.

Faulds, G. Conroy, S. Madaio, M. Isenberg, D. Latchman, D. 1995. Increased levels of antibodies to heat shock proteins with increasing age in Mrl/Mp-lpr/lpr mice. *British Journal of Rheumatology* 34:610–615.

Fenchel, S. Grab, D. Nuessle, K. Kotzerke, J. Rieber, A. Kreienberg, R. Brambs, HJ. Reske, SN. 2002. Asymptomatic adnexal masses: Correlation of FDG PET and histopathologic findings. *Radiology* 223:780–788.

Ferlay, J. Shin, HR. Bray, F. Forman, D. Mathers, C. Parkin, DM. 2010. GLOBOCAN 2008, Cancer Incidence and Mortality Worldwide: IARC CancerBase No. 10 [Internet]. Lyon, France: International Agency for Research on Cancer.

Flavin, RJ. Smyth, PC. Finn, SP. Laios, A. O'Toole, SA. Barrett, C. Ring, M. et al. 2008. Altered eIF6 and Dicer expression is associated with clinicopathological features in ovarian serous carcinoma patients. *Modern Pathology* 21:676–684.

Forshew, T. Murtaza, M. Parkinson, C. Gale, D. Tsui, DW. Kaper, F. Dawson, SJ. et al. 2012. Noninvasive identification and monitoring of cancer mutations by targeted deep sequencing of plasma DNA. *Science Translational Medicine* 4:136ra68.

Fredolini, C. Meani, F. Luchini, A. Zhou, W. Russo, P. Ross, M. Patanarut, A. et al. 2010. Investigation of the ovarian and prostate cancer peptidome for candidate early detection markers using a novel nanoparticle biomarker capture technology. *American Association of Pharmaceutical Scientists Journal* 12:504–518.

Gagnon, A. Kim, JH. Schorge, JO. Ye, B. Liu, B. Hasselblatt, K. Welch, WR. Bandera, CA. Mok, SC. 2008. Use of a combination of approaches to identify and validate relevant tumor-associated antigens and their corresponding autoantibodies in ovarian cancer patients. *Clinical Cancer Research* 14:764–771.

Galgano, MT. Hampton, GM. Frierson, HF Jr. 2006. Comprehensive analysis of HE4 expression in normal and malignant human tissues. *Modern Pathology* 19:847–853.

Gallagher, MF. Flavin, RJ. Elbaruni, SA. McInerney, JK. Smyth, PC. Salley, YM. Vencken, SF. et al. 2009. Regulation of microRNA biosynthesis and expression in 2102Ep embryonal carcinoma stem cells is mirrored in ovarian serous adenocarcinoma patients. *Journal of Ovarian Research* 2:19.

Gao, L. Cheng, HY. Dong, L. Ye, X. Liu, YN. Chang, XH. Cheng, YX et al. 2011. The role of HE4 in ovarian cancer: Inhibiting tumour cell proliferation and metastasis. *The Journal of International Medical Research* 39:1645–1660.

Gilad, S. Meiri, E. Yogev, Y. Benjamin, S. Lebanony, D. Yerushalmi, N. Benjamin, H. et al. 2008. Serum microRNAs are promising novel biomarkers. *PLoS One* 3:e3148.

Gnjatic, S. Ritter, E. Buchler, MW. Giese, NA. Brors, B. Frei, C. Murray, A. et al. 2010. Seromic profiling of ovarian and pancreatic cancer. *Proceedings of the National Academy of Sciences of the United States of America* 107:5088–5093.

Griffin, JL. Shockcor, JP. 2004. Metabolic profiles of cancer cells. *Nature Reviews Cancer* 4:551–561.

Guerriero, S. Alcazar, JL. Coccia, ME. Ajossa, S. Scarselli, G. Boi, M. Gerada, M. Melis, GB. 2002. Complex pelvic mass as a target of evaluation of vessel distribution by color doppler sonography for the diagnosis of adnexal malignancies: Results of a multicenter European study. *Journal of Ultrasound in Medicine* 21:1105–1111.

Gupta, D. Lis, CG. 2009. Role of CA125 in predicting ovarian cancer survival—A review of the epidemiological literature. *Journal of Ovarian Research* 2:13.

Hausler, SF. Keller, A. Chandran, PA. Ziegler, K. Zipp, K. Heuer, S. Krockenberger, M. et al. 2010. Whole blood-derived miRNA profiles as potential new tools for ovarian cancer screening. *British Journal of Cancer* 103:693–700.

Hayem, G. De Bandt, M. Palazzo, E. Roux, S. Combe, B. Eliaou, JF. Sany, J. Kahn, MF. Meyer, O. 1999. Anti-heat shock protein 70 kDa and 90 kDa antibodies in serum of patients with rheumatoid arthritis. *Annals of the Rheumatic Diseases* 58:291–296.

He, H. Jazdzewski, K. Li, W. Liyanarachchi, S. Nagy, R. Volinia, S. Calin, GA. et al. 2005. The role of microRNA genes in papillary thyroid carcinoma. *Proceedings of the National Academy of Sciences of the United States of America* 102:19075–19080.

Hellstrom, I. Friedman, E. Verch, T. Yang, Y. Korach, J. Jaffar, J. Swisher, E. et al. 2008. Anti-mesothelin antibodies and circulating mesothelin relate to the clinical state in ovarian cancer patients. *Cancer Epidemiology, Biomarkers & Prevention* 17:1520–1526.

Hellstrom, I. Heagerty, PJ. Swisher, EM. Liu, P. Jaffar, J. Agnew, K. Hellstrom, KE. 2010. Detection of the HE4 protein in urine as a biomarker for ovarian neoplasms. *Cancer Letters* 296:43–48.

Hellström, I. Raycraft, J. Hayden-Ledbetter, M. Ledbetter, JA. Schummer, M. McIntosh, M. Drescher, C. Urban, N. Hellström, KE. 2003. The HE4 (WFDC2) protein is a biomarker for ovarian carcinoma. *Cancer Research* 63:3695–3700.

Hensley, M. Alektiar, D. Chi, D. 2002. Ovarian and fallopian-tube cancer. In: Barakat, R. Bevers, M. Gershenson, D. Hoskins, W. (eds.). *Handbook of Gynecologic Oncology*. London, U.K.: Martin Dunitz.

Ho, M. Hassan, R. Zhang, J. Wang, QC. Onda, M. Bera, T. Pastan, I. 2005. Humoral immune response to mesothelin in mesothelioma and ovarian cancer patients. *Clinical Cancer Research* 11:3814–3820.

Hoffman, BR. Katsaros, D. Scorilas, A. Diamandis, P. Fracchioli, S. Rigault de la Longrais, IA. Colgan, T. et al. 2002. Immunofluorometric quantification and histochemical localisation of kallikrein 6 protein in ovarian cancer tissue: A new independent unfavourable prognostic biomarker. *British Journal of Cancer* 87:763–771.

Holcomb, K. Vucetic, Z. Craig Miller, M. Knapp, RC. 2011. Human epididymis protein 4 offers superior specificity in the differentiation of benign and malignant adnexal masses in premenopausal women. *American Journal of Obstetrics and Gynecology* 205:358 e1–358 e6.

Hudson, ME. Pozdnyakova, I. Haines, K. Mor, G. Snyder, M. 2007. Identification of differentially expressed proteins in ovarian cancer using high-density protein microarrays. *Proceedings of the National Academy of Sciences of the United States of America* 104:17494–17499.

Hunter, MP. Ismail, N. Zhang, X. Aguda, BD. Lee, EJ. Yu, L. Xiao, T. et al. 2008. Detection of microRNA expression in human peripheral blood microvesicles. *PLoS One* 3:e3694.

Hwang, H. Quenneville, L. Yaziji, H. Gown, AM. 2004. Wilms tumor gene product: Sensitive and contextually specific marker of serous carcinomas of ovarian surface epithelial origin. *Applied Immunohistochemistry & Molecular Morphology* 12:122–126.

Iero, M. Valenti, R. Huber, V. Filipazzi, P. Parmiani, G. Fais, S. Rivoltini, L. 2008. Tumour-released exosomes and their implications in cancer immunity. *Cell Death and Differentiation* 15:80–88.

Iorio, MV. Ferracin, M. Liu, CG. Veronese, A. Spizzo, R. Sabbioni, S. Magri, E. et al. 2005. MicroRNA gene expression deregulation in human breast cancer. *Cancer Research* 65:7065–7070.

Iorio, MV. Visone, R. Di Leva, G. Donati, V. Petrocca, F. Casalini, P. Taccioli, C. et al. 2007. MicroRNA signatures in human ovarian cancer. *Cancer Research* 67:8699–8707.

Isaksson, HS. Sorbe, B. Nilsson, TK. 2012. Whole blood RNA expression profiles in ovarian cancer patients with or without residual tumors after primary cytoreductive surgery. *Oncology Reports* 27:1331–1335.

Judson, PL. Geller, MA. Bliss, RL. Boente, MP. Downs, LS. Argenta, PA. Carson, LF. 2003. Preoperative detection of peripherally circulating cancer cells and its prognostic significance in ovarian cancer. *Gynecologic Oncology* 91:389–394.

Kalapotharakos, G. Asciutto, C. Henic, E. Casslen, B. Borgfeldt, C. 2012. High preoperative blood levels of HE4 predicts poor prognosis in patients with ovarian cancer. *Journal of Ovarian Research* 5:20.

Kamat, AA. Fletcher, M. Gruman, LM. Mueller, P. Lopez, A. Landen, CN Jr. Han, L. Gershenson, DM. Sood, AK. 2006. The clinical relevance of stromal matrix metalloproteinase expression in ovarian cancer. *Clinical Cancer Research* 12:1707–1714.

Kato, N. Toukairin, M. Asanuma, I. Motoyama, T. 2007. Immunocytochemistry for hepatocyte nuclear factor-1b (HNF-1b): A marker for ovarian clear cell carcinoma. *Diagnostic Cytopathology* 35:193–197.

Kirchhoff, C. 1998. Molecular characterization of epididymal proteins. *Reviews of Reproduction* 3:86–95.

Kobayashi, E. Ueda, Y. Matsuzaki, S. Yokoyama, T. Kimura, T. Yoshino, K. Fujita, M. Kimura, T. Enomoto, T. 2012. Biomarkers for screening, diagnosis, and monitoring of ovarian cancer. *Cancer Epidemiology, Biomarkers & Prevention* 21:1902–1912.

Kong, SY. Han, MH. Yoo, HJ. Hwang, JH. Lim, MC. Seo, SS. Yoo, CW. et al. 2012. Serum HE4 level is an independent prognostic factor in epithelial ovarian cancer. *Annals of Surgical Oncology* 19:1707–1712.

Korneeva, I. Bongiovanni, AM. Girotra, M. Caputo, TA. Witkin, SS. 2000. IgA antibodies to the 27-kDa heat-shock protein in the genital tracts of women with gynecologic cancers. *International Journal of Cancer* 87:824–828.

Kurman, RJ. Shih, IeM. 2010. The origin and pathogenesis of epithelial ovarian cancer: A proposed unifying theory. *The American Journal of Surgical Pathology* 34:433–443.

Lagos-Quintana, M. Rauhut, R. Lendeckel, W. Tuschl, T. 2001. Identification of novel genes coding for small expressed RNAs. *Science* 294:853–858.

Laios, A. Mohamed, BM. Kelly, L. Flavin, R. Finn, S. McEvoy, L. Gallagher, M. et al. 2013. Pre-treatment of platinum resistant ovarian cancer cells with an MMP-9/MMP-2 inhibitor prior to cisplatin enhances cytotoxicity as determined by high content screening. *International Journal of Molecular Sciences* 14:2085–2103.

Laios, A. O'Toole, S. Flavin, R. Martin, C. Kelly, L. Ring, M. Finn, SP. et al. 2008. Potential role of miR-9 and miR-223 in recurrent ovarian cancer. *Molecular Cancer* 7:35.

Landen, CN. Birrer, MJ. Sood, AK. 2008. Early events in the pathogenesis of epithelial ovarian cancer. *Journal of Clinical Oncology* 26:995–1005.

Lawrie, CH. Gal, S. Dunlop, HM. Pushkaran, B. Liggins, AP. Pulford, K. Banham, AH. et al. 2008. Detection of elevated levels of tumour-associated microRNAs in serum of patients with diffuse large B-cell lymphoma. *British Journal of Haematology* 141:672–675.

Lee, CH. Subramanian, S. Beck, AH. Espinosa, I. Senz, J. Zhu, SX, Huntsman, D. van de Rijn, M. Gilks, CB. 2009. MicroRNA profiling of BRCA1/2 mutation-carrying and non-mutation-carrying high-grade serous carcinomas of ovary. *PLoS One* 4:e7314.

Lee, YH. Kim, JH. Zhou, H. Kim, BW. Wong, DT. 2012. Salivary transcriptomic biomarkers for detection of ovarian cancer: For serous papillary adenocarcinoma. *Journal of Molecular Medicine* 90:427–434.

Li, F. Tie, R. Chang, K. Wang, F. Deng, S. Lu, W. Yu, L. Chen, M. 2012. Does risk for ovarian malignancy algorithm excel human epididymis protein 4 and CA125 in predicting epithelial ovarian cancer: A meta-analysis. *BMC Cancer* 12:258.

Li, L. Wang, K. Dai, L. Wang, P. Peng, XX. Zhang, JY. 2008. Detection of autoantibodies to multiple tumor-associated antigens in the immunodiagnosis of ovarian cancer. *Molecular Medicine Reports* 1:589–594.

Liao, J. Yu, L. Mei, Y. Guarnera, M. Shen, J. Li, R. Liu, Z. Jiang, F. 2010. Small nucleolar RNA signatures as biomarkers for non-small-cell lung cancer. *Molecular Cancer* 9:198.

Liotta, LA. Petricoin, EF 3rd. 2012. Omics and cancer biomarkers: Link to the biological truth or bear the consequences. *Cancer Epidemiology, Biomarkers & Prevention* 21:1229–1235.

Lu, D. Kuhn, E. Bristow, RE. Giuntoli, RL 2nd. Kjaer, SK. Shih, IeM. Roden, RB. 2011. Comparison of candidate serologic markers for type I and type II ovarian cancer. *Gynecologic Oncology* 122:560–566.

Lu, J. Getz, G. Miska, EA. Alvarez-Saavedra, E. Lamb, J. Peck, D. Sweet-Cordero, A. et al. 2005. MicroRNA expression profiles classify human cancers. *Nature* 435:834–838.

Luborsky, JL. Yu, Y. Edassery, SL. Jaffar, J. Yip, YY. Liu, P. Hellstrom, KE. Hellstrom, I. 2011. Autoantibodies to mesothelin in infertility. *Cancer Epidemiology, Biomarkers & Prevention* 20:1970–1978.

Luo, LY. Katsaros, D. Scorilas, A. Fracchioli, S. Bellino, R. van Gramberen, M. de Bruijn, H et al. 2003. The serum concentration of human kallikrein 10 represents a novel biomarker for ovarian cancer diagnosis and prognosis. *Cancer Research* 63:807–811.

Marth, C. Kisic, J. Kaern, J. Trope, C. Fodstad, O. 2002. Circulating tumor cells in the peripheral blood and bone marrow of patients with ovarian carcinoma do not predict prognosis. *Cancer* 94:707–712.

McIntosh, MW. Liu, Y. Drescher, C. Urban, N. Diamandis, EP. 2007. Validation and characterization of human kallikrein 11 as a serum marker for diagnosis of ovarian carcinoma. *Clinical Cancer Research* 13:4422–4428.

Menon, U. Gentry-Maharaj, A. Hallett, R. Ryan, A. Burnell, M. Sharma, A. Lewis, S. et al. 2009. Sensitivity and specificity of multimodal and ultrasound screening for ovarian cancer, and stage distribution of detected cancers: Results of the prevalence screen of the UK collaborative trial of ovarian cancer screening (UKCTOCS). *The Lancet Oncology* 10:327–340.

Menon, U. Kalsi, J. Jacobs, I. 2012. The UKCTOCS experience—Reasons for hope? *International Journal of Gynecological Cancer* 22:S18–S20.

Merritt, WM. Lin, YG. Han, LY. Kamat, AA. Spannuth, WA. Schmandt, R. Urbauer, D. et al. 2008. Dicer, Drosha, and outcomes in patients with ovarian cancer. *The New England Journal of Medicine* 359:2641–2650.

Milne, K. Barnes, RO. Girardin, A. Mawer, MA. Nesslinger, NJ. Ng, A. Nielsen, JS. et al. 2008. Tumor-infiltrating T cells correlate with NY-ESO-1-specific autoantibodies in ovarian cancer. *PLoS One* 3:e3409.

Miska, EA. 2005. How microRNAs control cell division, differentiation and death. *Current Opinion in Genetics & Development* 15:563–568.

Miszczak-Zaborska, E. WójcikKrowiranda, K. Kubiak, R. Bieñkiewicz, A. Bartkowiak, J. 2004. The activity of thymidine phosphorylase as a new ovarian tumor marker. *Gynecologic Oncology* 94:86–92.

Mitchell, PS. Parkin, RK. Kroh, EM. Fritz, BR. Wyman, SK. Pogosova-Agadjanyan, EL. Peterson, A. et al. 2008. Circulating microRNAs as stable blood-based markers for cancer detection. *Proceedings of the National Academy of Sciences of the United States of America* 105:10513–10518.

Montagnana, M. Danese, E. Giudici, S. Franchi, M. Guidi, GC. Plebani, M. Lippi, G. 2011. HE4 in ovarian cancer: From discovery to clinical application. *Advances in Clinical Chemistry* 55:1–20.

Moore, RG. Brown, AK. Miller, MC. Skates, S. Allard, WJ. Verch, T. Steinhoff, M. et al. 2008. The use of multiple novel tumor biomarkers for the detection of ovarian carcinoma in patients with a pelvic mass. *Gynecologic Oncology* 108:402–408.

Moore, RG. Jabre-Raughley, M. Brown, AK. Robison, KM. Miller, MC. Allard WJ, Kurman, RJ. et al. 2010. Comparison of a novel multiple marker assay vs the Risk of Malignancy Index for the prediction of epithelial ovarian cancer in patients with a pelvic mass. *American Journal of Obstetrics and Gynecology* 203:228.e1–228.e6.

Moore, RG. McMeekin, DS. Brown, AK. DiSilvestro, P. Miller, MC. Allard, WJ. Gajewski, W. et al. 2009. A novel multiple marker bioassay utilizing HE4 and CA125 for the prediction of ovarian cancer in patients with a pelvic mass. *Gynecologic Oncology* 112:40–46.

Moore, RG. Miller, MC. Disilvestro, P. Landrum, LM. Gajewski, W. Ball, JJ. Skates, SJ. 2011. Evaluation of the diagnostic accuracy of the risk of ovarian malignancy algorithm in women with a pelvic mass. *Obstetrics Gynecology* 118:280–288.

Moore, RG. Miller, MC. Steinhoff, MM. Skates, SJ. Lu, KH. Lambert-Messerlian, G. Bast, RC Jr. 2012. Serum HE4 levels are less frequently elevated than CA125 in women with benign gynecologic disorders. *American Journal of Obstetrics and Gynecology* 206:351.e1–351.e8.

Moss, EL. Hollingworth, J. Reynolds, TM. 2005. The role of CA125 in clinical practice. *Journal of Clinical Pathology* 58:308–312.

Muller, CY. 2010. Doctor, should I get this new ovarian cancer test-ova1? *Obstetrics and Gynecology* 116:246–247.

Murphy, MA. O'Connell, DJ. O'Kane, SL. O'Brien, JK. O'Toole, S. Martin, C. Sheils, O. O'Leary, JJ. Cahill, DJ. 2012a. Epitope presentation is an important determinant of the utility of antigens identified from protein arrays in the development of autoantibody diagnostic assays. *Journal of Proteomics* 75:4668–4675.

Murphy, MA. O'Leary, JJ. Cahill, DJ. 2012b. Assessment of the humoral immune response to cancer. *Journal of Proteomics* 7515:4573–4579.

Nam, EJ. Yoon, H. Kim, SW. Kim, H. Kim, YT. Kim, JH. Kim, JW. Kim, S. 2008. MicroRNA expression profiles in serous ovarian carcinoma. *Clinical Cancer Research* 14:2690–2695.

Neuhausen, SL. Mazoyer, S. Friedman, L. Stratton, M. Offit, K. Caligo, A. Tomlinson, G. et al. 1996. Haplotype and phenotype analysis of six recurrent BRCA1 mutations in 61 families: Results of an international study. *American Journal of Human Genetics* 58:271–280.

Nossov, V. Amneus, M. Su, F. Lang, J. Janco, JM. Reddy, ST. Farias-Eisner, R. 2008. The early detection of ovarian cancer: From traditional methods to proteomics. Can we really do better than serum CA-125? *American Journal of Obstetrics and Gynecology* 199:215–223.

Obermayr, E. Castillo-Tong, DC. Pils, D. Speiser, P. Braicu, I. Van Gorp, T. Mahner, S. et al. 2013. Molecular characterization of circulating tumor cells in patients with ovarian cancer improves their prognostic significance—A study of the OVCAD consortium. *Gynecologic Oncology* 128:15–21.

Oddoux, C. Struewing, JP. Clayton, CM. Neuhausen, S. Brody, LC. Kaback, M. Haas, B. et al. 1996. The carrier frequency of the BRCA2 6174delT mutation among Ashkenazi Jewish individuals is approximately 1%. *Nature Genetics* 14:188–190.

Odunsi, K. Jungbluth, AA. Stockert, E. Qian, F. Gnjatic, S. Tammela, J. Intengan, M. et al. 2003. NY-ESO-1 and LAGE-1 cancer-testis antigens are potential targets for immunotherapy in epithelial ovarian cancer. *Cancer Research* 63:6076–6083.

Okamoto, Y. Tanaka, YO. Tsunoda, H. Yoshikawa, H. Minami, M. 2007. Malignant or borderline mucinous cystic neoplasms have a larger number of loculi than mucinous cystadenoma: A retrospective study with MR. *Journal of Magnetic Resonance Imaging* 26:94–99.

Paek, J. Lee, S.-H. Yim, G.-W. Lee, M. Kim, Y.-J. Nam, E.-J. 2011. Prognostic significance of human epididymis protein 4 in epithelial ovarian cancer. *European Journal of Obstetrics, Gynecology, and Reproductive Biology* 158:338–342.

Paterlini-Brechot, P. Benali, NL. 2007. Circulating tumor cells (CTC) detection: Clinical impact and future directions. *Cancer Letters* 253:180–204.

Petricoin, EF. Ardekani, AM. Hitt, BA. Levine, PJ. Fusaro, VA. Steinberg, SM. Mills, GB. et al. 2002. Use of proteomic patterns in serum to identify ovarian cancer. *Lancet* 359:572–577.

Picchio, M. Sironi, S. Messa, C. Mangili, G. Landoni, C. Gianolli, L. Zangheri, B. et al. 2003. Advanced ovarian carcinoma: Usefulness of [(18)F]FDG-PET in combination with CT for lesion detection after primary treatment. *The Quarterly Journal of Nuclear Medicine* 47:77–84.

Piura, B. Piura, E. 2009. Autoantibodies to tumor-associated antigens in epithelial ovarian carcinoma. *Journal of Oncology* 2009:581939.

Piura, E. Piura, B. 2010. Autoantibodies to tumor-associated antigens in breast carcinoma. *Journal of Oncology* 2010:264926.

Poveda, A. Kaye, SB. McCormack, R. Wang, S. Parekh, T. Ricci, D. Lebedinsky, CA. et al. 2011. Circulating tumor cells predict progression free survival and overall survival in patients with relapsed/recurrent advanced ovarian cancer. *Gynecologic Oncology* 122:567–572.

Psyrri, A. Kountourakis, P. Scorilas, A. Markakis, S. Camp, R. Kowalski, D. Diamandis, EP. Dimopoulos, MA. 2008. Human tissue kallikrein 7, a novel biomarker for advanced ovarian carcinoma using a novel in situ quantitative method of protein expression. *Annals of Oncology* 19:1271–1277.

Pyle-Chenault, RA. Stolk, JA. Molesh, DA. Boyle-Harlan, D. McNeill, PD. Repasky, EA. Jiang, Z. Fanger, GR. Xu, J. 2005. VSGP/F-spondin: A new ovarian cancer marker. *Tumour Biology* 26:245–257.

Raamanathan, A. Simmons, GW. Christodoulides, N. Floriano, PN. Furmaga, WB. Redding, SW. Lu, KH. Bast, RC Jr. McDevitt, JT. 2012. Programmable bio-nano-chip systems for serum CA125 quantification: Toward ovarian cancer diagnostics at the point-of-care. *Cancer Prevention Research* 5:706–716.

Rebbeck, TR. Lynch, HT. Neuhausen, SL. Narod, SA. Van't Veer, L. Garber, JE. Evans, G. et al. 2002. Prevention and Observation of Surgical End Points Study Group. Prophylactic oophorectomy in carriers of BRCA1 or BRCA2 mutations. *The New England Journal of Medicine* 346:1616–1622.

Rein, BJD. Gupta, S. Dada, R. Safi, J. Michener, C. Agarwal, A. 2011. Potential markers for detection and monitoring of ovarian cancer. *Journal of Oncology* 2011:475983.

Resnick, KE. Alder, H. Hagan, JP. Richardson, DL. Croce, CM. Cohn, DE. 2009. The detection of differentially expressed microRNAs from the serum of ovarian cancer patients using a novel real-time PCR platform. *Gynecologic Oncology* 112:55–59.

Schorge, JO. Modesitt, SC. Coleman, RL. Cohn, DE. Kauff, ND. Duska, LR. Herzog, TJ. 2010. SGO White Paper on ovarian cancer: Etiology, screening and surveillance. *Gynecologic Oncology* 119:7–17.

Schummer, M. Drescher, C. Forrest, R. Gough, S. Thorpe, J. Hellstrom, I. Hellstrom, KE. Urban, N. 2012. Evaluation of ovarian cancer remission markers HE4, MMP7 and Mesothelin by comparison to the established marker CA125. *Gynecologic Oncology* 125:65–69.

Scorilas, A. Borgoño, CA. Harbeck, N. Dorn, J. Schmalfeldt, B. Schmitt, M. Diamandis, EP. 2004. Human kallikrein 13 protein in ovarian cancer cytosols: A new favorable prognostic marker. *Journal of Clinical Oncology* 22:678–685.

Seeber, LM. van Diest, PJ. 2012. Epigenetics in ovarian cancer. *Methods in Molecular Biology* 863:253–269.

Shan, SJ. Scorilas, A. Katsaros, D. Diamandis, EP. 2007. Transcriptional upregulation of human tissue kallikrein 6 in ovarian cancer: Clinical and mechanistic aspects. *British Journal of Cancer* 96:362–372.

Singh, AP. Senapati, S. Ponnusamy, MP. Jain, M. Lele, SM. Davis, JS. Remmenga, S. Batra, SK. 2008. Clinical potential of mucins in diagnosis, prognosis, and therapy of ovarian cancer. *The Lancet Oncology* 9:1076–1085.

Slupsky, CM. Steed, H. Wells, TH. Dabbs, K. Schepansky, A. Capstick, V. Faught, W. Sawyer, MB. 2010. Urine metabolite analysis offers potential early diagnosis of ovarian and breast cancers. *Clinical Cancer Research* 16:5835–5841.

Soussi, T. 2000. p53 Antibodies in the sera of patients with various types of cancer: A review. *Cancer Research* 60:1777–1788.

Steffensen, KD. Waldstrom, M. Brandslund, I. Jakobsen, A. 2011. Prognostic impact of prechemotherapy serum levels of HER2, CA125, and HE4 in ovarian cancer patients. *International Journal of Gynecological Cancer* 21:1040–1047.

Stockert, E. Jager, E. Chen, YT. Scanlan, MJ. Gout, I. Karbach, J. Arand, M. Knuth, A. Old, LJ. 1998. A survey of the humoral immune response of cancer patients to a panel of human tumor antigens. *The Journal of Experimental Medicine* 187:1349–1354.

Struewing, JP. Abeliovich, D. Peretz, T. Avishai, N. Kaback, MM. Collins, FS. Brody, LC. 1995. The carrier frequency of the BRCA1 185delAG mutation is approximately 1 percent in Ashkenazi Jewish individuals. *Nature Genetics* 11:198–200.

Sueblinvong, T. Carney, ME. 2009. Current understanding of risk factors for ovarian cancer. *Current Treatment Options in Oncology* 10:67–81.

Suh, KS. Crutchley, JM. Koochek, A. Ryscavage, A. Bhat, K. Tanaka, T. Oshima, A. Fitzgerald, P. Yuspa, SH. 2007. Reciprocal modifications of CLIC4 in tumor epithelium and stroma mark malignant progression of multiple human cancers. *Clinical Cancer Research* 13:121–131.

Suh, KS. Park, WS. Castro, A. Patel, H. Blake, P. Liang, M. Goy, A. 2010. Ovarian cancer biomarkers for molecular biosensors and translational medicine. *Expert Review of Molecular Diagnostics* 10:1069–1083.

Takamizawa, J. Konishi, H. Yanagisawa, K. Tomida, S. Osada, H. Endoh, H. Harano, T. et al. 2004. Reduced expression of the let-7 microRNAs in human lung cancers in association with shortened postoperative survival. *Cancer Research* 64:3753–3756.

Taylor, DD. Gercel-Taylor, C. 2008. MicroRNA signatures of tumor-derived exosomes as diagnostic biomarkers of ovarian cancer. *Gynecologic Oncology* 110:13–21.

Taylor, DD. Gercel-Taylor, C. Parker, LP. 2009. Patient-derived tumor reactive antibodies as diagnostic markers for ovarian cancer. *Gynecologic Oncology* 115:112–120.

Tempany, CM. Zou, KH. Silverman, SG. Brown, DL. Kurtz, AB. McNeil, BJ. 2000. Staging of advanced ovarian cancer: Comparison of imaging modalities—Report from the Radiological Diagnostic Oncology Group. *Radiology* 215:761–767.

Trieb, K. Gerth, R. Holzer, G. Grohs, JG. Berger, P. Kotz, R. 2000. Antibodies to heat shock protein 90 in osteosarcoma patients correlate with response to neoadjuvant chemotherapy. *British Journal of Cancer* 82:85–87.

Trudel, D. Tetu, B. Gregoire, J. Plante, M. Renaud, M.-C. Bachvarov, D. Douville, P. Bairati, I. 2012. Human epididymis protein 4 (HE4) and ovarian cancer prognosis. *Gynecologic Oncology* 127:511–515.

Tsai-Turton, M. Santillan, A. Lu, D. Bristow, RE. Chan, KC. Shih, IeM. Roden, RB. 2009. p53 autoantibodies, cytokine levels and ovarian carcinogenesis. *Gynecologic Oncology* 114:12–17.

Tsuchiya, A. Sakamoto, M. Yasuda, J. Chuma, M. Ohta, T. Ohki, M. Yasugi, T. Taketani, Y. Hirohashi, S. 2003. Expression profiling in ovarian clear cell carcinoma: Identification of hepatocyte nuclear factor-1 beta as a molecular marker and a possible molecular target for therapy of ovarian clear cell carcinoma. *The American Journal of Pathology* 163:2503–2512.

Van Gorp, T. Cadron, I. Despierre, E. 2011. HE4 and CA125 as a diagnostic test in ovarian cancer: Prospective validation of the Risk of Ovarian Malignancy Algorithm. *British Journal of Cancer* 104:863–870.

Van Jaarsveld, MT. Helleman, J. Berns, EM. Wiemer, EA. 2010. MicroRNAs in ovarian cancer biology and therapy resistance. *The International Journal of Biochemistry & Cell Biology* 42:1282–1290.

Verheijen, RH. von Mensdorff-Pouilly, S. van Kamp, GJ. Kenemans, P. 1999. CA 125: Fundamental and clinical aspects. *Seminars in Cancer Biology* 9:117–124.

Vidal, CI. Mintz, PJ. Lu, K. Ellis, LM. Manenti, L. Giavazzi, R. Gershenson, DM. et al. 2004. An HSP90-mimic peptide revealed by fingerprinting the pool of antibodies from ovarian cancer patients. *Oncogene* 23:8859–8867.

Vogl, FD. Frey, M. Kreienberg, R. Runnebaum, IB. 2000. Autoimmunity against p53 predicts invasive cancer with poor survival in patients with an ovarian mass. *British Journal of Cancer* 83:1338–1343.

Wang, P. Ge, L. Yan, M. Song, X. Ge, S. Yu, J. 2012. Paper-based three-dimensional electrochemical immunodevice based on multi-walled carbon nanotubes functionalized paper for sensitive point-of-care testing. *Biosensors and Bioelectronics* 32:238–243.

Wang, S. Zhao, X. Khimji, I. Akbas, R. Qiu, W. Edwards, D. Cramer, DW. Ye, B. Demirci, U. 2011. Integration of cell phone imaging with microchip ELISA to detect ovarian cancer HE4 biomarker in urine at the point-of-care. *Lab on a Chip* 11:3411–3418.

Webb, J. 2007. Ultrasound in ovarian carcinoma. In: Reznek, RH, ed. *Cancer of the Ovary*. Cambridge: Cambridge University Press, pp. 94–111.

Wimberger, P. Heubner, M. Otterbach, F. Fehm, T. Kimmig, R. Kasimir-Bauer, S. 2007. Influence of platinum-based chemotherapy on disseminated tumor cells in blood and bone marrow of patients with ovarian cancer. *Gynecologic Oncology* 107:331–338.

Wu, L. Dai, ZY. Qian, YH. Shi, Y. Liu, FJ. Yang, C. 2012. Diagnostic value of serum human epididymis protein 4 (HE4) in ovarian carcinoma: A systematic review and meta-analysis. *International Journal of Gynecological Cancer* 22:1106–1112.

Wyman, SK. Parkin, RK. Mitchell, PS. Fritz, BR. O'Briant, K. Godwin, AK. Urban, N. et al. 2009. Repertoire of microRNAs in epithelial ovarian cancer as determined by next generation sequencing of small RNA cDNA libraries. *PLoS One* 4:e5311.

Ye, B. Skates, S. Mok, SC. Horick, NK. Rosenberg, HF. Vitonis, A. Edwards, D. et al. 2006. Proteomic-based discovery and characterization of glycosylated eosinophil-derived neurotoxin and COOH-terminal osteopontin fragments for ovarian cancer in urine. *Clinical Cancer Research* 12:432–441.

Yoshida, Y. Kurokawa, T. Kawahara, K. Tsuchida, T. Okazawa, H. Fujibayashi, Y. Yonekura, Y. Kotsuji, F. 2004. Incremental benefits of FDG positron emission tomography over CT alone for the preoperative staging of ovarian cancer. *AJR American Journal of Roentgenology* 182:227–233.

Yousef, GM. Diamandis, EP. 2002. Kallikreins, steroid hormones and ovarian cancer: Is there a link? *Minerva Endocrinology* 27:157–166.

Yu, M. Stott, S. Toner, M. Maheswaran, S. Haber, DA. 2011. Circulating tumor cells: Approaches to isolation and characterization. *The Journal of Cell Biology* 192:373–382.

Zhang, L. Huang, J. Yang, N. Greshock, J. Megraw, MS. Giannakakis, A. Liang, S. et al. 2006. microRNAs exhibit high frequency genomic alterations in human cancer. *Proceedings of the National Academy of Sciences of the United States of America* 103:9136–9141.

Zhang, L. Volinia, S. Bonome, T. Calin, GA. Greshock, J. Yang, N. Liu, CG. et al. 2008. Genomic and epigenetic alterations deregulate microRNA expression in human epithelial ovarian cancer. *Proceedings of the National Academy of Sciences of the United States of America* 105:7004–7009.

Zhang, T. Wu, X. Yin, M. Fan, L. Zhang, H. Zhao, F. Zhang, W. et al. 2012. Discrimination between malignant and benign ovarian tumors by plasma metabolomic profiling using ultra performance liquid chromatography/mass spectrometry. *Clinica Chimica Acta* 413:861–868.

Zhang, W. Yang, HC. Wang, Q. Yang, ZJ. Chen, H. Wang, SM. Pan, ZM. et al. 2011. Clinical value of combined detection of serum matrix metalloproteinase-9, heparanase, and cathepsin for determining ovarian cancer invasion and metastasis. *Anticancer Research* 31:3423–3428.

25

Early Markers for Neoplastic Lesions of the Uterine Cervix

Pablo Conesa-Zamora

CONTENTS

ABSTRACT Cervical cancer (CC) is one of the most common cancers in women worldwide and is caused by a persistent infection of certain human papillomavirus (HPV) genotypes. Although cytological examination using the Papanicolaou (Pap) test is considered the most cost-effective test for reducing CC mortality, a considerable number of high-grade precursor lesions of CC could pass unnoticed with the Pap. The addition of high-risk HPV genotype detection in cervical cytology has improved the sensitivity, but due to its low specificity, further biomarkers of malignancy have been searched for. The oncogenic role of HPV is exerted primary by affecting cell cycle control, and thus, most of the useful biomarkers of HPV-related uterine lesions are cell cycle proteins, being p16 and Ki-67 the most widely used. More recently, molecular profiling and marker combination tests have identified the utility of antibody cocktails such as p16/Ki-67 dual and ProEx C, which detect both TOP2A and MCM2 cell cycle proteins. In this work we revise the rationale for the use of the most common biomarkers in cervical neoplasia and their clinical utility drawing attention to novel biomarkers and how HPV vaccination could influence their use.

KEY WORDS: *squamous intraepithelial lesion, cervical carcinoma; human papillomavirus; diagnostic marker, prognostic marker, immunohistochemistry.*

25.1 Introduction

25.1.1 Why It Is Important

Cervical cancer (CC) is a problem of worldwide magnitude; it is the second most incident and the third most mortal cancer in women worldwide being especially relevant in less developed countries where CC is the second cancer in mortality (Ferlay et al., 2010). Infection by human papillomavirus (HPV) is a necessary but not sufficient factor for CC appearance. Fortunately, CC is developed through a well-established series of precursor lesions termed squamous intraepithelial lesions (SILs) that can be detected in cytological specimens taken from the uterine cervix. The knowledge of the molecular processes involved in HPV-induced cervical carcinogenesis is well characterized, and therefore, several biomarkers have proven their utility for CC precursor lesion management.

25.1.2 Epidemiology

The GLOBOCAN project indicates that CC is the second most common cancer in women and accounts for the third cause of cancer death in females, with an estimated 530,000 new cases in 2008. More than 85% of the global burden occurs in developing countries, where it accounts for 13% of all female cancers. High-risk regions are Eastern and Western Africa (age standardized rate [ASR] greater than 30 per 100,000), Southern Africa (26.8 per 100,000), South–Central Asia (24.6 per 100,000), and South America and Middle Africa (ASRs 23.9 and 23.0 per 100,000, respectively). Rates are lowest in Western Asia,

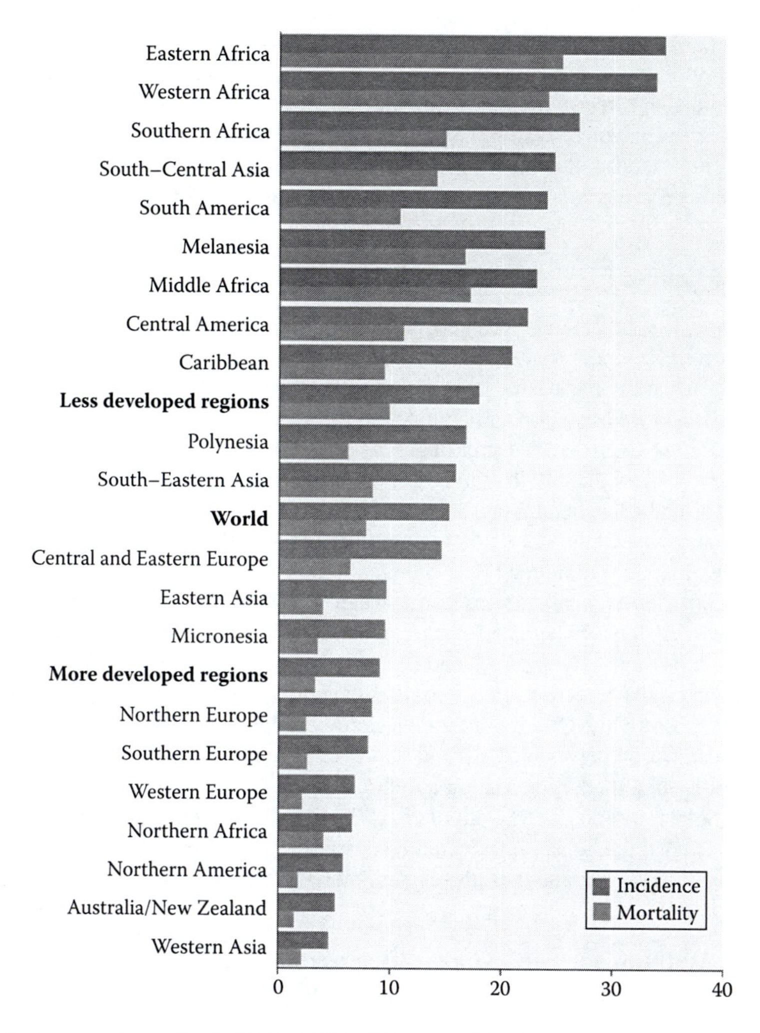

FIGURE 25.1 Incidence and mortality for 2008 of CC in different world regions. (From Globocan, International Agency for Research on Cancer [IARC], 2008, http://globocan.iarc.fr/)

Northern America, and Australia/New Zealand (ASRs less than 6 per 100,000). CC remains the most common cancer in women only in Eastern Africa, South–Central Asia, and Melanesia. Overall, the mortality incidence ratio is 52%, and CC is responsible for 275,000 deaths in 2008, about 88% of which occur in developing countries: 53,000 in Africa, 31,700 in Latin America and the Caribbean, and 159,800 in Asia (Ferlay et al., 2010). Figure 25.1 represents the incidence and mortality associated with CC in different geographic locations (Ferlay et al., 2010).

That geographical difference is mostly due to the suboptimal application, in less developed countries, of screening measures for SIL and CC that consist on the cytological identification of SIL and CC and the adequate clinical and surgical management of patients according to the risk or presence of malignancy (Muñoz et al., 2003). Besides, the HPV genotypes found in different regions of the world vary both in type and relative incidence. There is also evidence of the prevalence of specific variants of defined genotypes in certain ethnic groups (Arias-Pulido et al., 2005; Calleja-Macías et al., 2005; Prado et al., 2005). In fact, some HPV variants correlate with human migration flows (Calleja-Macías et al., 2004), suggesting a degree of genotype fixation in certain populations. These differences modify the overall incidence of CC worldwide as even among the so-called high-risk HPVs (HR-HPV), the oncogenic potential of each genotype also differs (Muñoz et al., 2003).

The incidence of HR-HPV infection decreases with women age because most infection resolved or is controlled by the host immune system. Most women infected with a certain HPV genotype do not show evidence of this infection after 18 months (Xi et al., 1995). Therefore, the development of high-grade cervical neoplasia arises in women who cannot resolve their infection and who maintain persistent active infection for years or decades following initial exposure. For this reason, CC occurs in women less than 50 years old, but it is very uncommon in women younger than 20 (Chhabra et al., 2010).

25.1.3 Types of Cancer

The most common CC type is squamous cell carcinoma (SCC) accounting for 80% of invasive CC (ICC) and arising from squamous (flattened) epithelial cells that line the cervix. The second in incidence and mortality is adenocarcinoma arising from glandular epithelial cells. Traditionally, adenocarcinoma accounts for 5%–15% of invasive cervical carcinomas. However, its incidence is increasing in United States, now up to 25% of CCs, due to decreasing rates of SCC and difficulty in diagnosis using current screening methods (Wang et al., 2004b). Other less frequent CC types are adenosquamous (presenting features of both SCC and adenocarcinoma) and undifferentiated CC (Wells et al., 2003).

Cervical carcinoma, especially SCC, is developed through a well-established sequence of precursor lesions termed SILs that can subdivided into low- and high-grade SIL (LSIL and HSIL, respectively). According to the 2001 Bethesda guidelines (Solomon et al., 2002), LSIL comprises two types of lesions: condyloma and cervical intraepithelial neoplasia (CIN 1). The development of high-grade neoplasia (termed HSIL encompassing CIN grades 2 and 3) arises in women who cannot resolve their infection maintaining sustained active infection after years after the initial exposure. The term SIL is often referred to a cytological diagnosis, while CIN is used for a histological diagnosis. However, current evidence has point out that the distinction between CIN 2 and CIN 3 (carcinoma in situ) is subjective because of the lack of reproducibility in CIN 2, representing a mixture of true CIN 1/LSIL and true precancer/CIN 3 (Park et al., 1998; Solomon et al., 2002; Wells et al., 2003; Baak et al., 2009). Furthermore, the use of the term "neoplasia" included in CIN acronym could be misunderstood as many of these lesions, especially CIN 1, spontaneously regressed, and thus, the expression CIN is being substituted by SIL.

25.1.4 Current Methods for Early Diagnosis, Prognosis, and Therapy with Specificity, Sensitivity, Advantages, and Disadvantages

25.1.4.1 Early Diagnosis

As previously commented, CC is developed through a pathological *continuum* of precursor lesions (termed SILs), and therefore, most common methods for CC early diagnosis are based on the identification of SILs. The most widely used test for abnormal cytological identification is the Papanicolaou (Pap) test, considered to be as the most effective screening tool for cancer prevention ever devised (Boronow, 1998). However, Pap test is subjected to a high proportion (up to 30%) of false-negative and false-positive results. To prevent this, colposcopy/biopsy is recommended by the 2001 Bethesda guidelines (Solomon et al., 2002) for a confident LSIL and HSIL diagnosis (DeMay, 1996). Other techniques such as visual inspection with acetic acid (VIS) and Lugol's iodine (VILI) are being used for increasing Pap sensitivity reaching values of 45.8%–72.4% for VIS and 62.2%–85.9% for VILI. Besides, these tests are especially suitable for developing countries given their low cost and simplicity (Surendra et al., 2005).

For this reason a great effort has been made during the last two decades to obtain useful markers that can be used in clinical practice for a proper identification and follow-up of preneoplastic CC lesions. Given that SIL and thus CC are HPV-driven lesions, cytological HPV genotyping is being used to increase the sensitivity of Pap test. The problem encountered then has been the high frequency of HPV infections inducing asymptomatic lesions and regressing spontaneously, especially in younger females. Molecular studies have demonstrated that the HPV disturbance effect on the cell cycle control of the cervical keratinocyte is the main mechanism for the HPV oncogenic action. Consequently, most of the biomarkers used to increase the specificity of HPV genotyping for SIL detection are proteins involved in the control of cell cycle.

It is well known which are the main etiological agents, the molecular alterations, and the sequence of lesions leading to an invasive cancer in cervical carcinogenesis. Excellent reviews have addressed the molecular pathogenesis of HPV in SIL and CC (zur Hausen, 2002; Doorbar, 2006), and some other interesting reviews have revised specific issues (Tindle, 2002; Woodman et al., 2007). In order to understand the role and utility of biomarkers, we will briefly describe some essential aspects of cervical carcinogenesis. Infection by HPV is a necessary cause for CC as HPV genome can be detected in virtually all ICCs. Infection by HPV requires that virus particles get access to the basal layer of cervical epithelium through micro-lesions. HPV has no enzymatic machinery for DNA replication, and for this reason, the basal layer cell is the target of the virus since this is the cell that undertakes the epithelial renewal. This infection leads to the establishment of the HPV genome as stable episomes in these cells (Figure 25.2). For an effective viral cycle, the HPV needs the differentiation process of the keratinocytes from the basal to the exfoliating cells to express the viral proteins in a very well-concerted order. In this way, E6 and E7 viral proteins are expressed to induce cell cycle activity in suprabasal cells, thus allowing HPV genome replication. Only in the upper layers, when the cells become exfoliated, HPV expresses L1 and L2 proteins that assemble to construct the viral capsid that, in turn, permits the packaging of the replicated genomes, thus allowing viral spread into the cervical lumen. As we will comment later, HR-HPV genotypes (more prevalently HPV16 and HPV18) can initially exert an alteration in cell cycle control of the keratinocytes that can be evidenced morphologically by cytological changes called LSILs (Figure 25.2). In women with HSIL there is a continuous activation of proliferation by E7, coupled with an increase in chromosomal instability driven by E6 inhibition of p53 protein. Approximately 20% of CIN 1 will progress to CIN 2, and 30% of these lesions will progress to CIN 3 that, in 40% of the cases, will develop to ICC (Peto et al., 2004).

Most of cervical neoplasia arises in the cervical transformation zone where the columnar cells of the endocervix meet the stratified squamous epithelial cells of the ectocervix because the basal cells from this zone are more accessible to HPV particles than those protected by a permanent stratified epithelial layer (Bosch and SanJosé, 2003). HSIL has a more extensive proliferating phase than LSIL as the viral genome amplification occurs closer to the epithelial surface. This is mainly caused by the changes in the levels of E6 and E7 expression that occur following the integration of the viral genome into the host cell chromosome (Figure 25.2). Integrated HPV DNA is detected in most ICC and in a subset of HSIL (Klaes et al., 1999).

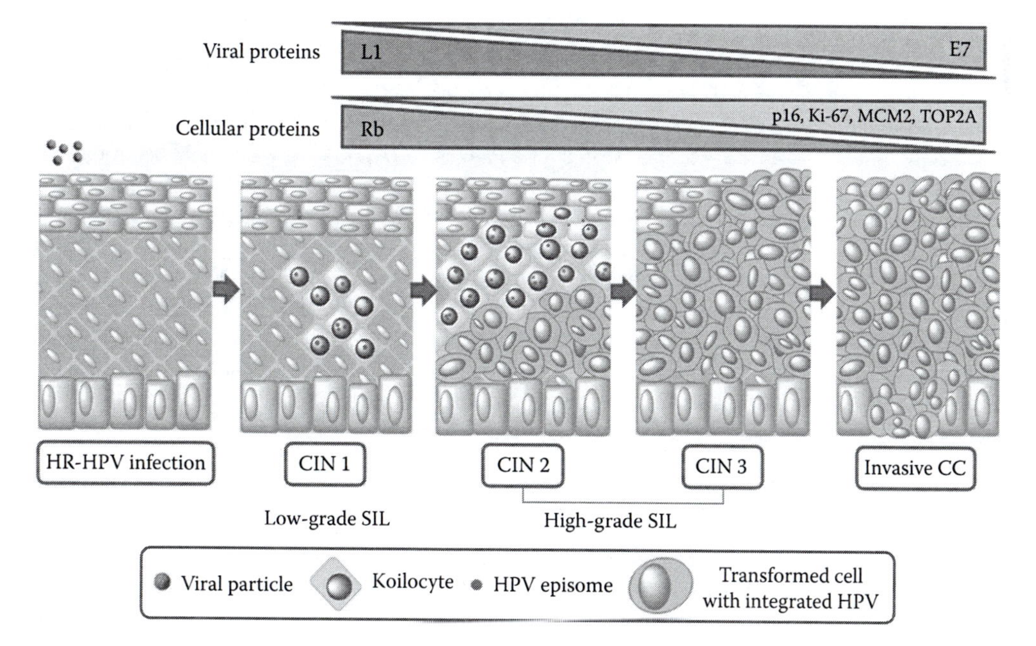

FIGURE 25.2 Model of cervical carcinogenesis. Differences in viral and cellular protein activities and in epithelium morphology during the cervical carcinogenesis sequence induced by HR-HPV infection. CIN, Cervical intraepithelial neoplasia; HR-HPV, High-risk human papillomavirus; SIL, squamous intraepithelial lesion.

ICC can be divided in two major histological types: SCC and adenocarcinoma. In terms of percentages, 80%–85% of ICC cases are SCC, 10% are adenocarcinoma that is mainly caused by HPV18 infection, and 3% are adenosquamous carcinoma and other rare tumors (Trinh et al., 2004).

25.1.4.2 Prognosis

The Classification of Malignant Tumours (TNM) and International Federation of Gynecology and Obstetrics (FIGO) are the most commonly used staging systems for establishing CC prognosis. The TNM for CC is currently used by the American Joint Committee on Cancer (AJCC) and is based on the size and extension of the primary tumor, its lymphatic involvement, and the presence of metastases. The FIGO has developed the current staging score for CC. FIGO I is used for describing a CC confined to the uterine cervix area and has a 5-year survival rate of 80%–93%. In FIGO II stage, CC has developed beyond the cervix but affecting less than one-third of the vagina and has 58%–63% of 5-year survival. FIGO III represents a stage in which CC extends to the pelvic wall and the 5-year survival decreases to 32%–35%. Finally, in FIGO IV stage CC is spread also outside the pelvis affecting bladder mucosa or rectum and even distant organs and the associated survival ranged between 15% and 16%. CC in this stage is generally treated with surgery, chemotherapy, and/or radiation although the chances of cure are small (Pecorelli et al., 2009; American Cancer Society, 2012). Table 25.1 represents the correlation between the TNM categories and FIGO stages for CC.

25.1.4.3 Therapies

Combined therapies including surgery, chemotherapy, and radiotherapy are commonly used in advanced stages of CC. The treatment of choice will depend on both tumor (size, location, and stage) and patient (age, general health status) parameters. Since the outcome of locally advanced disease is still unsatisfactory as the standard treatment (cisplatin-based chemoradiation) fails to cure at least 15%–45% of bulky FIGO IB to IIIB patients and the addition of radiotherapy does not substantially increase the cure rate (Dueñas-González et al., 2003), most of therapeutic strategies tend to focus on earlier stages of the disease when CC is not still invasive. Among these, surgical interventions such as cone biopsy and loop electrosurgical excision procedure (LEEP) are very useful to treat and cure HSIL/CIN 3 (cervical carcinoma in situ) stages.

25.1.5 Test Providers and Popular Tests with Cost

The type of test and its associated cost will be highly dependent on the target population (screening versus outpatient populations), the amount of determinations, and the grade of development of the country where they are going to be performed. Whereas the cost of a Pap test, VIA, or VIA/VILI could be around $1–3 (Goldhaber-Fiebert et al., 2006), estimating the cost of HPV testing is much more difficult since there are several kinds of tests providing diverse degrees of information, some differentiating between HR-HPV and low-risk HPV (LR-HPV) or HPV16/HPV18 from other HR-HPVs such as hybrid capture II or COBAS platforms and others specifically identifying individual genotypes, such as the CLART 2 system. Prices can vary from $10 to $25 for the former and $30 to $45 for the latter. Similarly, the cost immunohistochemistry (IHC), which is performed on cytological and biopsy specimens, will depend not only on the type of antibody (Ki-67 is cheaper than p16) but also on the number of antibodies analyzed per slide (p16/Ki-67 dual is obviously more expensive than p16 IHC alone). In general, the IHC cost is around $10–$20 per slide, while antibody cocktails (e.g., p16/Ki-67 dual or ProEx C) used to be more expensive.

25.2 Treatment Strategy, Drug Targets, Targeted Therapy, and Pharmacogenomics

25.2.1 Treatment Strategy

As previously mentioned, CC can be cured if treated in early stages. The surgical strategies used comprise cryosurgery, laser treatment, and excision. Cryosurgery consists on freezing abnormal cervical tissue and

TABLE 25.1

TNM and FIGO Classifications for CC

Primary Tumor (T)		
TNM	**FIGO**	**Surgical–Pathological Findings**
Categories	Stages	
TX		Primary tumor cannot be assessed
T0		No evidence of primary tumor
Tis		Carcinoma in situ (preinvasive carcinoma)
T1	I	Cervical carcinoma confined to the cervix (disregard extension to the corpus)
T1a	IA	Invasive carcinoma diagnosed only by microscopy; stromal invasion with a maximum depth of 5.0 mm measured from the base of the epithelium and a horizontal spread of 7.0 mm or less; vascular space involvement, venous or lymphatic, does not affect classification
T1a1	IA1	Measured stromal invasion ≤3.0 mm in depth and ≤7.0 mm in horizontal spread
T1a2	IA2	Measured stromal invasion >3.0 mm and ≤5.0 mm with a horizontal spread ≤7.0 mm
T1b	IB	Clinically visible lesion confined to the cervix or microscopic lesion greater than T1a/IA2
T1b1	IB1	Clinically visible lesion ≤4.0 cm in greatest dimension
T1b2	IB2	Clinically visible lesion >4.0 cm in greatest dimension
T2	II	Cervical carcinoma invades beyond uterus but not to pelvic wall or to lower third of vagina
T2a	IIA	Tumor without parametrial invasion
T2a1	IIA1	Clinically visible lesion ≤4.0 cm in greatest dimension
T2a2	IIA2	Clinically visible lesion >4.0 cm in greatest dimension
T2b	IIB	Tumor with parametrial invasion
T3	III	Tumor extends to pelvic wall and/or involves lower third of vagina and/or causes hydronephrosis or nonfunctional kidney
T3a	IIIA	Tumor involves lower third of vagina, no extension to pelvic wall
T3b	IIIB	Tumor extends to pelvic wall and/or causes hydronephrosis or nonfunctional kidney
T4	IV	Tumor invades mucosa of bladder or rectum and/or extends beyond true pelvis (bullous edema is not sufficient to classify a tumor as T4)
T4a	IVA	Tumor invades mucosa of bladder or rectum (bullous edema is not sufficient to classify a tumor as T4)
T4b	IVB	Tumor extends beyond true pelvis
Regional lymph nodes (N)		
NX	Regional lymph nodes cannot be assessed	
N0	No regional lymph node metastasis	
N1	Regional lymph node metastasis	
Distant metastasis (M)		
M0	No distant metastasis	
M1	Distant metastasis (including peritoneal spread, involvement of supraclavicular, mediastinal, or para-aortic lymph nodes, and lung, liver, or bone)	

constitutes a safe treatment option for noninvasive lesions. On the other hand, it is not possible to obtain tissue sample for subsequent evaluation (Jacob et al., 2005). In case of locally advanced CC, neoadjuvant therapy using cisplatin is usually applied. The use of chemotherapy before surgery or radiotherapy has proven its utility as radiotherapy alone usually fails to control the CC progression (Yin et al., 2011).

25.2.2 Targeted Therapy

Advanced (stage IVB) and recurrent cervical carcinomas have poor prognosis and treatment at this stage is palliative. In this context, targeted therapies have been proposed as interesting drugs that could be used in this group of patients in addition to standard chemotherapy regimens. Abnormal activity of epidermal growth factor receptor (EGFR) and vascular endothelial growth (VEGF) has been implicated in CC progression, and thus, these two proteins have been investigated in clinical trials as potential molecular targets (Gerber, 2008). Although anti-EGFR-targeted therapy is currently in use for several types of cancer including non-small cell lung cancer and colorectal cancer, to date, only the anti-VEGF agent bevacizumab has shown positive outcomes warranting further trials (Monk et al., 2009).

25.2.3 Pharmacogenetics

The study of genetic variation in drug response is an emerging area of research with interesting applications in clinical practice for an efficient and tailored design of pharmacological treatments. The genes frequently studied in pharmacogenetics are those coding for enzymes involved in drug metabolism or those that are related with the molecular target. To date, there is no genetic marker of response to chemotherapy to be determined in the clinical management of CC patients. However, it is important to highlight the interesting potential of this area, and possibly, already described polymorphisms in several genes (GSTs, TMPT, XRCC1, GGH) associated with differences in cisplatin response and adverse effect occurrence (Kim et al., 2008; McWhinney et al., 2009; Mukherjea and Rybak, 2011; Silva et al., 2013) could be determined in the near future prior to the election of chemotherapy regimens in CC.

25.3 Relevance of Biomarkers in Uterine Lesions

As briefly commented before, CC incidence and mortality can be controlled as long as its precursor lesions, which constitute a pathological *continuum*, can be correctly identified. The current triage option for LSIL is either cytological surveillance or immediate referral to colposcopy, or finally triage with HR-HPV test. Each of these options has its limitations such as the default of follow-up in women under cytological surveillance, the presence of high-grade lesions in 28% of women with cytological LSIL (Cox et al., 2003), and the risk of overtreatment with potential adverse pregnancy outcomes in women referred immediately to colposcopy. Concerning HSIL management, women with biopsy-confirmed CIN 2–3 should undergo an excisional treatment that though efficacious has also been associated with pregnancy complications, such as cervical stenosis or incompetence, especially in younger women (Guo et al., 2011). For these reasons, the use of biomarkers is crucial to identify not only SIL from normal or benign conditions of the uterine cervix but also among SIL to select those with higher likelihood of progression in order to provide appropriate follow-up and to avoid unnecessary treatment. This is especially paradigmatic for LSIL where most of them regressed spontaneously.

Prior to the biomarker evaluation, it is crucial to take into account two important considerations: first, which are the pros and cons of each type of specimen we can obtain from cervical epithelium, and second, what kind of lesions can mimic SIL because in these circumstances the biomarker performance could be critical.

25.3.1 Invasive and Noninvasive Markers: Advantages and Disadvantages

It is important to mention that in this chapter we have considered as invasive technique any medical procedure in which a part of the body is entered, as by puncture or incision. Therefore, we have included as invasive markers those obtained from colposcopy-driven biopsy. On the other hand, we have considered as noninvasive markers those obtained from serum, urine, and cytological specimens.

25.3.1.1 Cytology versus Histology

It is important to highlight that HPV and its preinvasive cervical-induced lesions remain localized in the uterine cervix, and thus, the optimal specimen for biomarker assessment comes from this location. Therefore, there are two main types of samples: the noninvasive cytology collected with cytobrush and the invasive colposcopy-driven biopsy. It is essential to understand which are the advantages and disadvantages of these two kinds of specimens for biomarkers assessment. A cervical cytological specimen has the advantage of being obtained through a minimal invasive, simple, and cost-effective technique and is perfectly suitable for screening purposes. Besides, it provides fresh material for molecular techniques such as HPV genotyping, whereas histology specimens are generally paraffin-embedded and the DNA quality is often worse. On the other hand, cytology does not reflect the histological architecture and it is subjected to sampling errors. Technical improvements of the Pap test such as the liquid-based cytology (LBC) have now been shown to improve sensitivity or specificity for detection of high-grade CIN compared to the conventional cytology (Arbyn et al., 2008), thus reducing the unsatisfactory sample rate and allowing the use of the residual fluid for ancillary techniques, such as HPV genotyping (Ronco et al., 2007). Histology specimens are procured through colposcopy, an invasive procedure, and have the advantage of allowing the evaluation of the tissue architecture and the assessment of the extension of the dysplastic cells or biomarker expression within the epithelial layers. In fact, histology diagnosis is considered as the gold standard for any cervical lesion. These specimens comprise biopsy, conization, and hysterectomy. While the first one is only for diagnostic purposes, the other two are also therapeutic.

25.3.1.2 Controversial Cervical Lesions and SIL Mimics

One interesting topic is that a plethora of nonmalignant lesions or lesion without a clear malignant potential could be diagnosed as SIL. Cervical epithelium is subjected not only to self-renewal as previously commented, but it can also be affected by non-HPV infections and hormone-induced cycles that, ultimately, could induce morphological epithelial changes. Thus, the ideal marker must identify the precursor lesion of CC from SIL mimics such as cervicitis and menstruation-associated and metaplastic morphological changes such as atypical immature squamous metaplasia (AIM). The most frequent controversial squamous lesion is probably the atypical squamous cell of undetermined significance (ASCUS). This is a cytological diagnosis that may reflect an exuberant benign change or a potentially serious lesion that cannot be unequivocally classified (Duggan, 2000). Follow-up cytological–histological correlations have not found a histological ASCUS counterpart. MA Duggan revised 12 published studies reporting the histopathology of the ASCUS, finding a median overall SIL rate of 37.2% and a median HSIL rate of 11.5%. Those studies qualifying the ASCUS reported a median of reactive changes in 30.3% of cases (Duggan, 2000). The 2001 Bethesda System for reporting results of cervical cytology modified the category of ASC added the term "atypical squamous cells cannot exclude high-grade squamous intraepithelial lesion" (ASC-H) indicating that atypical Pap smears are associated with either a true HSIL or its undetermined imitators (Solomon et al., 2002). Cervicitis is mainly caused by infection by *Chlamydia trachomatis* and *Neisseria gonorrhoeae* that induce an inflammatory response in the cervical epithelium that could resemble cytological changes produced by HPV. In cytological specimens cervicitis can be diagnosed as ASCUS, although the absence of atypical nuclei and the inflammatory response used to be sufficient for a clear diagnosis. AIM is a loosely defined cervical lesion characterized by immature metaplastic cells displaying cytological atypia. It is associated with abnormal Pap smears and with a colposcopically visible abnormality (Crum et al., 1983). While the role of AIM as a precursor lesion of cervical carcinoma shares some histological features with condyloma and SIL, it still remains mostly uncertain (Geng et al., 1999; Duggan et al., 2006; Iaconis et al., 2007). Because the age at presentation is similar to LSIL and HPV, it is frequently detected. It was concluded that AIM represents an HPV infection of immature, metaplastic squamous epithelium. Although in histology AIM resembles CIN 3, the average Ki-67 index (Duggan, 2000) and p16 expression (Conesa-Zamora et al., 2009a) of AIM makes it more similar to LSIL. Papillary immature metaplasia (PIM) is a lesion of the proximal part of the transformation zone characterized by a variable koilocytosis, a high presence of HPV (83%–70%), and it is infrequently associated with LSIL or HSIL. The Pap smear associated with PIN is often diagnosed as ASCUS or LSIL (Mosher et al., 1998), and the morphological appearance and HPV DNA data suggest that PIM is an LSIL variant (Duggan, 2000). The appearance of hyperchromatic crowed groups in Pap tests from women during menstruation can be a diagnostic pitfall due to morphological similarities with significant cervical lesions (Ge et al., 2012). In addition, in peri- or postmenopausal women, it is a frequent and incidental finding the observation of the transitional cell metaplasia (TCM) that is a benign condition of the transformation zone endocervical glands and that histologically can be confused with HSIL (Duggan, 2000).

25.4 Invasive Molecular Biomarkers

The invasive procedures for biomarkers assessment in cervical carcinoma precursor lesions are biopsy, conization, and hysterectomy. However, the evaluation of markers in these specimens is not common in early detection of cervical neoplasia since the cells of origin form the uterine cervix are easily accessible by means of cervical scrapping. Therefore, the use of biopsy samples is indicated to confirm a given morphological or immunostaining feature observed in a cytological specimen. The pros and cons of cytological versus histological samples have previously been commented. Any maker determined cytological (noninvasive) can be also identified samples in biopsy, conization, or hysterectomy.

25.4.1 Histological Protein Biomarkers: Effect of HPV on Cell Cycle Control

In-depth knowledge of the HPV-driven alteration of cell cycle in the female keratinocyte has been obtained from invasive specimens, mainly biopsy and conization. This information has allowed the application of these histological markers to cytological specimens that can be procured through a noninvasive procedure. In this section we will revise this evidence. The assessment of the particular pattern of protein expression in histological uterine lesions is generally performed by IHC. As commented earlier, HPV infection is a very common and frequently transient infection and the development of HSIL constitutes a failure of the HPV infective process. In fact, recent developments showed that cellular biomarkers related with HR-HPV lesions could be of use in identifying LSIL cases harboring high-grade disease, thus compensating the low specificity of HR-HPV tests. Considering these facts, one could argue that for a better marker discovery, it would be more reasonable to explore the molecular effects of HPV on the keratinocyte than the HPV itself. These markers would be especially useful to identify the 3%–7% of cases with normal Pap smear and HR-HPV positive where there is an underlying HSIL (Petry et al., 2003; Thrall et al., 2010).

As cell cycle activation is not exclusive of neoplastic cells, cell cycle markers assessment should consider also the cell morphology and the distribution of protein expression in the epithelial layers. However, some cell cycle markers offer some grade of specificity for neoplastic and not just proliferating activity. In-depth knowledge of molecular mechanism underlying cervical carcinogenesis has allowed the discovery of proteins such as p16 with a certain specificity for HPV-induced neoplastic lesions.

In uninfected epithelium, the expression of proteins necessary for cell cycle activation is controlled by Rb protein, which in quiescent cells associates with members of the E2F transcription factors. In the presence of growth factors, the cyclin D/Cdk6/6 protein complex is activated, leading to Rb phosphorylation and the release of E2F, which ultimately, induces the expression of proteins involved in the progression to DNA synthesis phase (S phase) (Figure 25.3). p16 then regulates the levels of active cyclin D/Cdk in the cell, providing a feedback mechanism that controls the levels of minichromosome maintenance (MCM) proteins, proliferating-cell nuclear antigen (PCNA), and cyclin E. Although many HPV types can infect the cervix, only HR-HPVs are associated with CC because of the specific oncogenic activity of their E6 and E7 proteins. In cervical epithelium infected by HR-HPV, progression through the cell cycle is not dependent on external growth factors, but it is stimulated by E7, which binds Rb and allows the expression of E2F-dependent S phase proteins. Although p16 increases its expression, normal feedback is

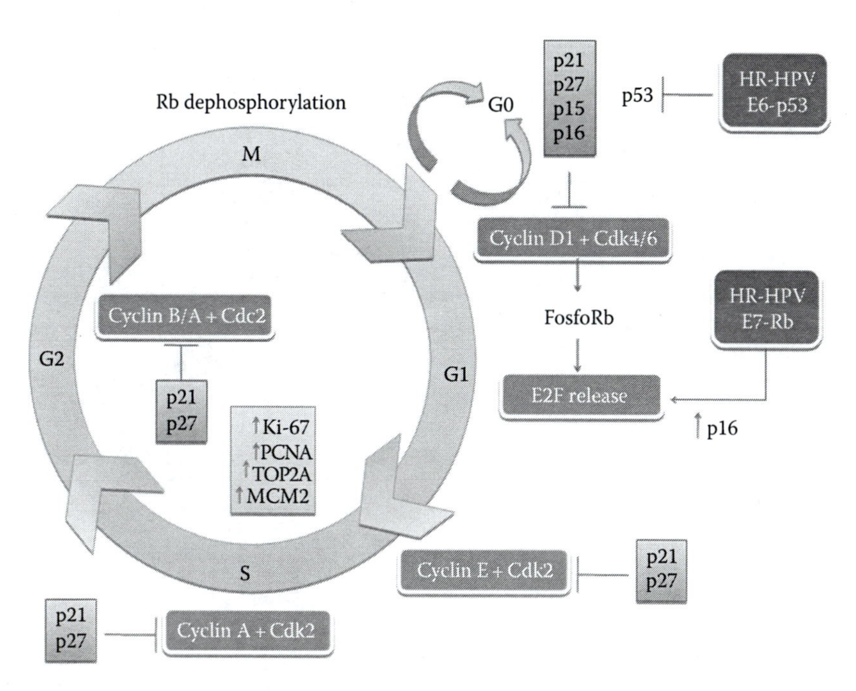

FIGURE 25.3 Molecular control of cell cycle. Proteins in intermediate gray squares indicate cell cycle positive regulators, whereas those in boxes showing gray gradations are cell cycle repressors. Inductor mechanisms of HPV are represented in dark gray boxes. Proliferation markers are in the light gray box. HR-HPV, high-risk human papillomavirus; M, cell mitosis; S, DNA synthesis; G, growth phase; G0, quiescent phase.

bypassed since HPV-induced proliferation is not dependent on cyclin D/Cdk. E6, in turn, associates with E6AP ubiquitin ligase to stimulate p53 degradation, thus inhibiting cell cycle arrest, DNA repair, and apoptosis and creating a permissive state for the appearance of novel mutations and genomic instability.

Functional alteration of cell cycle regulators in CC is, therefore, paradigmatic and seems to have a major role in CC pathogenesis. Consequently, much effort has been expended in attempts to identify useful cell cycle marker to monitor the progression of SILs to CC. In addition to p53 and pRb as targets of E6 and E7 HPV oncoproteins, cyclins such as cyclin D1 and cyclin inhibitors such as p16 are key proteins in the study of the molecular alterations that characterize cervical carcinoma (Figure 25.3). In the following sections we will present the molecular basis for the use of each of these cell cycle markers, the situations in which they are useful, their pros and cons, and what we could expect from them in the future.

25.4.2 Cell Cycle Markers

25.4.2.1 p16

As previously discussed, p16 is a tumor suppressor protein belonging to the family of INK4 cyclin-dependent kinase inhibitors. There are several mechanisms for p16 dysfunction in cancer comprising p16 promoter hypermethylation, p16 inactivating mutation, and gene copy number alteration. Mutation, gene deletion of p16, or promoter methylation is not common in cervical carcinogenesis (Tsuda et al., 2003; Bahnassy et al., 2007).

In the particular case of HPV-induced lesions, p16 aberrant expression seems mainly to be the result of the negative feedback induced by p16 on Rb inactivation by HPV E7 (zur Hausen, 1994). Not surprisingly, the expression of p16 has been associated with HPV-infected dysplastic and neoplastic epithelium of the cervix (Sano et al., 1998; Klaes et al., 1999; Murphy et al., 2005; Nam et al., 2007) and considered as an independent predictor of HR-HPV (Branca et al., 2008). This characteristic makes p16 a very interesting marker for detecting precursor lesions of ICC. In fact, Sano et al. reported that the status of p16 immunoreactivity allows differentiation between infection with LR-HPV and HR-HPV (Sano et al., 1998). As commented earlier, what makes oncogenic a given HPV genotype is the capacity of its E6 and E7

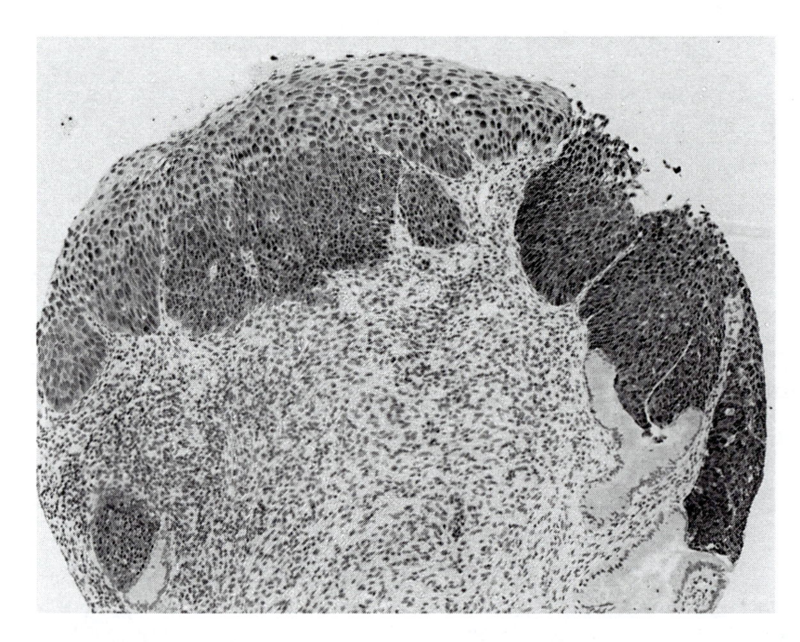

FIGURE 25.4 **(See color insert.)** Tissue microarray core showing cellular localization of p16 in HSIL. Note predominant cytoplasmic staining in the lower third of the epithelium and main nuclear stain in the upper layers (H&E counterstain, ×10).

proteins to alter the cell cycle and genome stability of cervical keratinocytes. Therefore, an HR-HPV E7 is more able to downregulate Rb, and so, the increase in p16 would also be more prominent than for an LR-HPV E7.

p16 immunohistochemical expression is positively associated with the grade of dysplasia seen in cervical squamous epithelium (Klaes et al., 1999; Wang et al., 2004a; Lambert et al., 2006; Nam et al., 2007; Conesa-Zamora et al., 2009a). Furthermore, when comparing the interval for disease progression from initial biopsy to CIN 3 or ICC, p16 positive expression was associated with shorter time to progression compared to p16 negative (Wang et al., 2004a), and p16 expression has also been reported as a predictive factor of lymph node metastasis and poor prognosis in ICC (Huang and Lee, 2012b).

With regard to AIM, p16 has demonstrated to distinguish this entity, where p16 was frequently negative, from CIN 3 (Regauer and Reich, 2007).

One interesting issue is the possible useful information given by the epithelial distribution and by the cell compartment of p16 expression. Diffuse p16 overexpression in basal and parabasal cells is indicative of HPV-mediated transformation, whereas focal p16 is occasionally observed in non-dysplastic epithelium possibly reflecting the necessary p16 expression to exert cell cycle arrest. In fact, Reuschenbach et al. demonstrated that diffuse p16 staining was associated with Ki-67 expression, whereas metaplastic lesions showed focal p16 and negative Ki-67 expressions (Reuschenbach et al., 2012).

Cytoplasmic predominant localization of p16 seems to be related to the increasing cell-layer level of staining (Figure 25.4), to the histological grade of cervical lesion (Conesa-Zamora et al., 2009a), and with HR-HPV infection in cervical lesions (Liang et al., 2010). Although a cytoplasmic overexpression pattern of p16 has been related with progression in some other cancer (Emig et al., 1998; Zhao et al., 2006), further studies will be needed to confirm this association with a higher grade of lesion in cervical neoplasia.

25.4.2.2 p53

The tumor suppressor p53, among its many functions, exerts its control on the cell cycle through the activation of p21, an inhibitor of cyclin and cyclin-dependent kinase complexes. Although in many human cancers p53 appears to be downregulated by point mutations or loss of heterozygosity (LOH), in CC, the HPV oncoprotein E6 binds p53 and causes its degradation by the cellular ubiquitin proteolysis system

(Vogelstein et al., 2000). It was recently shown that RITA, a small molecule, is able to rescue p53 function by blocking E6-mediated degradation (Zhao et al., 2010).

Conflicting results are obtained on the association of p53 expression with increase grade of dysplasia: some studies showed a significant correlation of p53 expression with CIN 3 or ICC compared with normal cervix or LSIL (Grace et al., 2003; Silva-Filho et al., 2004; Bahnassy et al., 2007), whereas others showed no significant association (Ngan et al., 1999; Hiller et al., 2006; Conesa-Zamora et al., 2009a). The probable relationship between positive p53 and poor disease outcome in ICC is also a matter of contradiction; some authors reported this association, although not as an independent prognostic factor (Huang et al., 2001; Jain et al., 2003), while others did not find such correlation (Ebara et al., 1996; Hunt et al., 1996; Kainz et al., 1995). The possible reasons for these inconsistencies could be that although at not very high frequencies, point mutations (Giarnieri et al., 2000; Bahnassy et al., 2007) and LOH (Kim et al., 1997) also occur in cervical carcinogenesis as well as E6-induced degradation. These circumstances may hamper the correct evaluation of p53 immunohistochemical analysis in HPV-induced cervical lesions.

Moreover, different groups have observed that depending on the HPV genotype, the p53 expression pattern is different. Thus, an association between higher p53 expression and no HPV infection or infection with LR-HPV (Kurvinen et al., 1996; Giannoudis and Herrington, 2000; Tsuda et al., 2003) has been reported. As suggested elsewhere the detectable p53 expression could occur as a result of the stabilization of p53 by either E6 protein binding produced by LR-HPV types in which p53 degradation does not occur (Giannoudis and Herrington, 2000). In this context, Hiller et al. (2006) and Zehbe et al. (2009) reported that in cell cultures that HPV16 E6 and HPV18 E6 induce higher p53 degradation than other less oncogenic HPVs. Others have suggested that a polymorphism (Pro > Arg) in codon 72 of p53 gene could influence the susceptibility of p53 degradation by E6 since Arg72 carriers had seven times higher risk for HPV-associated cancers (Storey et al., 1998), although later studies reported conflicting results on this issue (Hu et al., 2010a; Ueda et al., 2010). All these findings suggest that the different forms of p53 dysfunction in cervical carcinogenesis could disguise the real status of p53 functionality in these lesions and therefore complicate its utility as a diagnostic or prognostic marker.

25.4.2.3 Ki-67

Ki-67 is a nonhistone protein expressed in the nucleus during the whole cell cycle, except in the G0 and G1 early phases that can be detected with the MIB-1 antibody. Therefore, it constitutes an efficient marker of proliferating cells and has been associated with an increasing degree of cervical dysplasia (Silva-Filho et al., 2004; Qiao et al., 2005; Sarian et al., 2006; Bahnassy et al., 2007; Conesa-Zamora et al., 2009a). Ki-67 is also useful in distinguishing nondiagnostic atypia from SIL (Wells et al., 2003). Moreover, it has been reported as an additional prognostic marker of CC (Silva-Filho et al., 2004). Its expression has been associated with ASCUS showing HPV positivity (Longatto Filho et al., 2005). On the other hand, it is expressed also in nonneoplastic proliferating lesions, its function remains largely unknown, and there is evidence that the molecule is not essential for cell proliferation (Verheijen et al., 1989).

25.4.2.4 Cyclin D1

Cyclin D1 forms a complex with cyclin-dependent kinase 4 or 6 to carry out the phosphorylation of pRb that, as previously commented, release E2F to induce the S phase of the cell cycle.

The relationship between cyclin D1 positive expression and an increasing degree of dysplasia has been observed in several studies (Nichols et al., 1996; Cheung et al., 2001a; Bahnassy et al., 2007; Conesa-Zamora, 2009a). Reports on the reduced expression of cyclin D1 in cases of HSIL compared with normal cervix are rare (Bae et al., 2001; Vijayalakshmi et al., 2007). However, in both of these studies, an increase in cyclin D1 expression was observed from CIN 3 to invasive carcinoma (Bae et al., 2001; Vijayalakshmi et al., 2007), which means that finding higher expression in N/B or LSIL cases compared with HSIL cases would be unlikely. The inability of overexpressed p16 to inactivate Cdk4/6, the partner of cyclin D1, may lend support to a molecular basis for the increased immunohistochemical expression of cyclin D1 in CC progression. We reported a considerable proportion of the N/B cases showing cyclin D1 expression, but this was restricted to the lower third layer. Therefore, it seems that normal or benign epithelium retains some degree of cyclin D1 expression in this cell layer that could explain the positivity observed in previous studies, suggesting that evaluation of abnormal cyclin D1 must be considered only when expression occurs beyond this level. When this is taken into account, the relationship between cyclin D1 expression and diagnosis becomes statistically significant (Conesa-Zamora et al., 2009a). Using logistic regression analysis, cyclin D1 has been found to be an independent predictor of SIL diagnosis as well as p16 and ProEx C (Conesa-Zamora et al., 2012).

As commented for p16, cyclin D1 can also be detected by IHC as a cytoplasmic or nuclear stain. We and some other authors (Carreras et al., 2007; Conesa-Zamora et al., 2009a) observed a significant increase in the cytoplasmic staining associated with an increasing degree of dysplasia (Images 2C and 2D). Taking into account the dynamic behavior of CIN, we observed that when cyclin D1 is expressed beyond the lower third of the epithelium, cytoplasmic staining is more noticeable in the basal and parabasal layers, suggesting a recently acquired alteration directly related to a high-grade dysplasia phenotype and the progression of the disease. Possible explanations for this transition from nuclear to cytoplasmic cyclin D1 localization have been provided by Carreras et al. (2007) and Baldin et al. (1993). Briefly, cyclin D1 is located in the nucleus in the G1 phase; thereafter, it undergoes phosphorylation and ubiquitination and is carried to the cytoplasm in the S phase. The increase in grade of lesion is, therefore, related to the number of cells in the S phase when cyclin D1 is located in the cytoplasm. Furthermore, overexpression of cyclin D1 has been found to be an independent factor associated with a poor prognosis in cervical carcinoma (Bae et al., 2001).

Cyclin D1 distribution in the lower third of the epithelium was the best marker for distinguishing AIM from normal epithelium. Further evidence indicating low oncogenic potential of these lesions is the predominant nuclear staining seen for cyclin D1 (Conesa-Zamora et al., 2009a).

25.4.2.5 Other Cell Cycle Markers

Other cyclins and cell cycle inhibitors have been studied for its utility in SIL identification and ICC risk. The expression of cyclin A and p21 (the p53 downstream effector on cell cycle arrest) has been found at increased levels in HSIL and ICC (Southern et al., 1998; Bae et al., 2001; Cheung et al., 2001b; Van de Putte et al., 2004; Santopietro et al., 2006) being cyclin A a predictor of CIN 3 and more significantly expressed in HR-HPV-positive than HR-HPV-negative lesions (Santopietro et al., 2006). Bahnassy et al. (2007) showed that p27 (a cyclin-dependent kinase inhibitor) was negatively associated and identified as an independent marker of reduced overall survival, whereas cyclin E and Rb were positively associated with increasing grade of lesion from negative for intraepithelial lesion or malignancy (NILM) to ICC. Nonetheless, Tsuda et al. (2003) did not find a significant relationship between Rb expression and the grade of lesions. Considering that Rb is one of the main targets of E7 HPV oncoprotein, one can propose the possible utility of Rb expression as an adjunct to SIL diagnosis. However, the main mechanism of Rb regulation is through different grades of phosphorylation and this circumstance cannot be detected by common IHC. PCNA is a marker similar to Ki-67 that has been found to increase its expression in SIL and ICC compared to normal or inflamed cervix (Wang et al., 2004a). A score based on PCNA and proapoptotic molecule Bcl2 has been patented (ref: RU2310197) for its utility in discerning that CIN 1s are more likely to develop to high-grade lesions.

Despite all these findings there is no consistent evidence for their use in routine practice and no significant advantages over the most used and robust markers such as p16 and Ki-67.

25.5 Noninvasive Molecular Biomarkers

The majority of useful noninvasive markers for cervical neoplasia management is performed upon cytological specimens and will be commented in the following section. The HPV infection and its induction of neoplastic lesions are highly constrained to the cervical epithelium; for this reason it is not unexpected that other sources of specimens such as sputum or saliva have not given useful biomarkers, whereas only few markers have been studied in urine and serum biomarkers and have their utility when the cervical carcinoma has already been established.

25.5.1 Urine Biomarkers

Some reports have demonstrated that HPV genotypes can be detected in urine samples of male partners of women with CIN and VIH women (Brinkman et al., 2002; Guiliano et al., 2007; Martín-Ezquerra et al., 2012).

Previous evidences have focus on the study of metabolic markers in urine samples from CC females. Lee et al. (2003) observed that the combination of cortisol metabolites 16α-OH E1/-OG E1 and THF/5α-THF may discriminate benign cervical diseases from CC. Early studies reported the relevance of urine levels of cyclic guanosine monophosphate (cGMP) and cyclic adenosine monophosphate (cAMP) being a higher cGMP/cAMP ratio suggestive of cervical cytological abnormalities (Duttagupta et al., 1982), whereas other authors showed that cGMP urine level could be a valuable tool in the follow-up of patients with CC (Orbo et al., 1998). More recently, this latter group demonstrated that early changes in cGMP predict long-term prognosis in CC with higher cGMP urine concentration associated with relapse (Orbo et al., 2007).

However, none of these studies have been replicated in large cohorts.

25.5.2 Serum Biomarkers

25.5.2.1 Serum Genetic Markers

Circulating tumor DNA (ctDNA) is an emerging marker of tumor dynamics that can be detected in serum. HPV DNA can be found in the blood of women infected, and some authors support its value for monitoring therapeutic response and disease progression and metastasis in CC (Mutirangura, 2001; Pornthanakasem et al., 2001; Yang et al., 2004). However, there is no current use in clinical practice. As pointed out previously, HPV genome becomes integrated into host cellular genome as the CC progresses. To determine whether the sequence of the cell–viral junction could be used in routine analysis as a specific marker of ctDNA, Campitelli et al. (2012) studied a series of CC patient serums and found that ctDNA concentration was related to tumor dynamics suggesting that HPV mutation insertion can constitute a new molecular surrogate of minimal residual disease and of subclinical relapse in HPV-associated tumors.

Quantification of mRNA expression of HPV oncogenes has also been proposed as a useful maker. Tseng et al. (1999) observed that patients who were positive for peripheral-blood HPVE6 gene mRNA had a significantly higher risk of recurrence than those who were negative. There was also a statistically significant association of peripheral-blood HPVE6 gene mRNA positivity with distant metastasis.

25.5.2.2 Serum Protein Markers

Early studies have highlighted the importance of protein serum markers such as carcinoma antigen 125 (CA-125) and especially squamous cell carcinoma antigen (SCCA) as increased with disease stage (Pectasides et al., 1994; Sproston et al., 1995) being CA-125 a significant independent predictor of treatment outcome (Sproston et al., 1995). SCCA is a subfraction of the glycoprotein TA-4 expressed by SCC cervical tissues and is the most common serum marker for monitoring early recurrence of SCC after treatment (Yoon et al., 2010). Esajas et al. (2001) estimated the sensitivity of SCCA for this detection in 75%. In order to increase this sensitivity, additional markers such as CYFRA 21.1 and IGF II have been studied, although rendering conflicting results (Molina et al., 2005). In this line, the pretreatment levels of carcinoembryonic antigen (CEA) higher than 10 ng/mL were reported as an additional risk factor of para-aortic lymph node relapse following definitive concurrent chemoradiotherapy for SCC of the uterine cervix in patients with pretreatment SCCA levels less than 10 ng/mL, thus complementing the value of SCCA (Huang et al., 2012a). Very recently, the study by Siegel et al. (2012) showed that women with the highest ferritin levels in serum were less likely to clear incident oncogenic and HPV-16 infections than women with low ferritin.

The National Academy of Clinical Biochemistry (NACB) from the United States presented the guidelines for use of tumor markers in CC and reported only SCCA, CA-125, and CEA as potentially useful serum markers (Sturgeon et al., 2008). Table 25.2 shows the proposed use and the phase of development for each of these markers. Of note, most markers need further evaluation and only SCCA shows correlation with the grade of lesion. This committee recommended that the SCCA is useful for pretreatment

TABLE 25.2

NACB Recommendations for the Use of Serum Markers in CC

Cancer Marker	Proposed Use	Phase of Development	References
SCC	Pretreatment identification of high-risk group with lymph node metastases in SCC	Needs further evaluation for clinical usefulness	Avall-Lundqvist et al. (1992)
	Pretreatment prediction of prognosis in SCC	Independent prognostic value, not validated for individualizing treatment	Avall-Lundqvist et al. (1992)
	Prediction of response to treatment in SCC	Needs further evaluation	Bae et al. (1997)
	Monitoring disease and detecting recurrent disease in SCC	Strong correlation with course of disease	Ngan et al. (1994)
CA 125	Pretreatment prediction of prognosis, in particular in CA	Needs further evaluation	Avall-Lundqvist et al. (1992)
	Preoperative prediction of the presence of lymph node metastases, in particular in CA	Needs further evaluation	Avall-Lundqvist et al. (1992)
	Monitoring disease, in particular in CA	Needs further evaluation	Ngan et al. (1998)
CEA	Pretreatment prediction of prognosis	Needs further evaluation, conflicting results	Avall-Lundqvist et al. (1992); Bae et al. (1997)
	Preoperative prediction of the presence of lymph		
	Node metastases, in particular in CA	Needs further evaluation	Avall-Lundqvist et al. (1992)
	Pretreatment prediction of clinical response to neoadjuvant chemotherapy	Needs further evaluation	Bae et al. (1997)
Cytokeratins (TPA, TPS, CYFRA, 21–1)	Pretreatment prediction of prognosis	Needs further evaluation, conflicting results	Avall-Lundqvist et al. (1992); Ngan et al. (1994)
	Monitoring disease after primary treatment	Needs further evaluation, conflicting results	Ngan et al. (1998)

Source: Sturgeon, C.M. et al., *Clin. Chem.*, 54, e11, 2008.
Note: NACB, National Academy of Clinical Biochemistry; SCC, squamous cell cervical carcinoma; CA, cervical adenocarcinoma.

identification of patients at risk of positive lymph node metastasis, for predicting prognosis, and for disease monitoring, but not for screening and diagnosis (Sturgeon et al., 2008).

25.5.3 Cervical Genetic Biomarkers

As commented earlier, the HPV infection and SIL development are confined in the cervical epithelium, and thus, most useful biomarkers in CC management are determined in cervical specimens of either cytological or histological nature.

25.5.3.1 HPV-Related Markers

The use of HPV markers is obvious as HPV is implicated in virtually all ICC cases and plays an active and well-characterized role along the cervical carcinogenesis sequence. There are several types of HPV markers, being HPV genotyping the most useful to date, especially in ASCUS because it allows the detection of the HPV-related origin of an abnormal cytology. There are several types of commercial kits for cervical HPV detection and genotyping that have been recently revised (Poljak and Kocjan, 2010), and the most common types are shown in Table 25.3. These assays can

TABLE 25.3

Different Commercially Available Assays for HPV Detection and Genotyping

DNA-based HR-HPV amplification screening assays

- Hybrid capture 2 HPV DNA test[a]
- Cervista HPV HR test[a]
- Amplicor HPV test
- CareHPV test
- HPV4A ACE screening CE and HPV/STD4 ACE screening CE assays

DNA-based HR-HPV amplification screening assays with concurrent or reflex HPV16 and HPV18 genotyping

- HR-HPV DlttNA-based screening assays with concurrent individual genotyping for HPV16 and HPV18
  - Real-time HR-HPV test
  - Cobas 4800 HPV test
- HR-HPV DNA-based screening assays with reflex genotyping for HPV16 and HPV18
  - Cervista HPV16/HPV18 test[a]
  - HR-HPV16/HPV18/HPV45 probe set test

HPV DNA-based genotyping assays

- Reverse line-blot hybridization-based HPV genotyping assays
  - INNO-LiPA HPV genotyping
  - Linear array HPV genotyping test
  - Digene HPV genotyping RH test RUO
  - EasyChip HPV blot kit
  - REBA-HPV-ID
- Microarray-based HPV genotyping assays
  - PapilloCheck HPV-screening test
  - Clart HPV 2—papillomavirus clinical arrays
  - HPV GenoArray test kit
  - GeneTrack HPV DNA chip
  - GeneSQUARE HPV microarray
  - Infiniti HPV assays
  - PANArray HPV genotyping chip
  - HPVDNA chip
  - GG HPV chip
- Suspension array (xMAP, Luminex)-based HPV genotyping assays
  - Multiplex HPV genotyping kit
  - Digene HPV genotyping LQ test RUO
- Gel electrophoresis-based HPV genotyping assays
  - BIOTYPAP kit

HR-HPV E6/E7 mRNA-based screening assays

- PreTect HPV-proofer
- NucliSENS EasyQ HPV
- APTIMA HPV assay

ISH

- INFORM HPV
- GenPoint HPV biotinylated DNA probe
- ZytoFast HPV probes
- HPV OncoTect test kit

Source: Poljak, M. and Kocjan, B.J., *Expert Rev. Anti. Infect. Ther.,* 8, 1139, 2010.
Note: HPV, Human papillomavirus; HR, High risk.
[a] US FDA-approved assays.

TABLE 25.4

Performance Characteristics of HPV Detection and Genotyping Techniques for CIN2 + (HSIL) Assessment

Test Type	Test Name	Purveyor	SN (%)	SP (%)	PPV (%)	Reference
DNA-based detection	Hybrid capture 2	Qiagen	96.3	19.5	37.4	Szarewski et al. (2012)
	Cobas	Roche	95.2	24	37.6	Szarewski et al. (2012)
	Real-time PCR	Abbott	93.3	27.3	38.2	Szarewski et al. (2012)
	HPV test	BD	95	24.2	37.8	Szarewski et al. (2012)
DNA-based genotyping	Linear array	Roche	98.2	32.8	37.7	Szarewski et al. (2008)
	Clinical arrays	Genomica	80.9	37.1	33	Szarewski et al. (2008)
mRNA-based detection	Aptima	Gen-Probe	95.3	28.8	39.3	Szarewski et al. (2012)
	PreTect HPV-Proofer	NorChip	74.1	70.8	55.4	Szarewski et al. (2012)

Note: SN, sensitivity; SP, specificity; PPV, positive predictive value.

be grouped in four different techniques: DNA-based HPV amplification systems based on real-time PCR, DNA-based HPV genotyping based on reverse hybridization, RNA-based HPV detection based on real-time PCR, and in situ hybridization (ISH). Szarewski et al. (2008, 2012) have carried out comparison studies of the most common commercially available kits for HPV detection and genotyping. Sensitivity, specificity, and positive predictive value (PPV) of these kits for detection of HSIL in females with abnormal cytology are shown in Table 25.4. Similar performance characteristics were observed for DNA-based detection systems, whereas mRNA-based showed higher specificity. DNA-based genotyping assays, in general, render slightly lower sensitivity with higher specificities compared to DNA-based detection systems. In turn, ISH techniques have less sensitivity than PCR amplification assays (Biedermann et al., 2004).

Due to its sensitivity, HPV testing has been proposed for early detection of patients at increased disease recurrence and progression after being treated with conization for a SIL (Costa et al., 2003). However, there are important concerns about this test. First, asymptomatic HPV infections that induce lesions regressing spontaneously are very common. In fact, the prevalence of HR-HPV infection among young women (25 mean age) has a cumulative incidence over 5 years of 60% in some populations (Woodman et al., 2001), and it is estimated that HR-HPV infection can be detected in 3.8%–21.5% women with normal cytology (Woodman et al., 2001; Kulasingam et al., 2002). Therefore, the general use of HPV genotyping in young females could lead to unnecessary follow-up or overtreatment with the consequent costs for healthcare services. For this reason the specificity of a positive HR-HPV test for HSIL is very low (Schiffman et al., 2005). Besides, HPV detection has not generally proven to be useful for the triage of SIL patients. The ALTS trial (ASCUS/LSIL Triage Study) found that 83% of LSIL cases were positive for HPV, although no more than 25% of these cases would be expected to have CIN 2–3 by colposcopic biopsy (Schiffman et al., 2005).

Second, it is important to stress that the distinction between HR-HPV and LR-HPV genotype, alone, may not be sufficient nowadays because even among the high risks there are considerable differences in the oncogenic risk. In their seminal epidemiologic study, Muñoz et al. reported that females infected with HPV16 have a 434.5-fold higher risk of developing squamous CC than HPV-negative patients, whereas this risk decreases to 73.8 for genotype 35 (Muñoz et al., 2003). Moreover, taking into account that the persistent infection is one of the most important risk factors associated with SIL progression (Woodman et al., 2007), it is critical to distinguish when an infection is produced by a different or by the same genotype detected in the previous cytology. Moreover, HPV vaccines against HPV16 and HPV18 will modify the genotype-associated risks, and it is important to know which HPV genotypes will be the most oncogenic ones in a given area when HPV16 and HPV18 be removed. In this context it would also be advisable to know the specific genotypes in the case of coinfection by several HPV types (Conesa-Zamora et al., 2009c).

For all these reasons other HPV markers more related with the changes of the viral genome during the carcinogenic process are being evaluated, Among them, HPV genome integration test (either by real-time PCR or by ISH) and HPV viral load could be of use in clinical practice in the next future, although currently they still present methodological and standardization problems. Apparently, the HPV ISH probes are seen as diffuse signals when the HPV genome is episomal and as punctuate when it is integrated into the cellular genome (Samana et al., 2008; De Marchi Tiglia et al., 2009). As the transition from episomic to integrated status is associated with the LSIL to HSIL progression, some reports have demonstrated that punctuate signals in the basal cells identify CIN 1 with potentially aggressive behavior (De Marchi Triglia et al., 2009). Some evidence against the utility of these markers would be that HPV genome, which depending on the genotype, was not always found integrated in CC cases. Besides, the number of copies of HPV genome is lower when the genome is integrated than when it is in its episomic form, thus complicating the utility of viral load (Woodman et al., 2007). Probably, the combination of both tests in conjunction with the HPV genotype could be a promising biomarker for SIL management.

Finally, mRNA quantification of HPV E6 and HPV E7 expression has also demonstrated to be more specific than Pap test in post-colposcopy follow-up of women with negative cervical biopsy showing 98.1% sensitivity and 92.5% specificity for detecting HSIL (Sorbye et al., 2011). Moreover, compared with HPV DNA detection, the presence of E6/E7 mRNA transcripts was less sensitive, but more specific for the detection of disease and follow-up (Cuschieri et al., 2004).

25.5.3.2 Cellular-Related Markers

Several studies have evaluated in cytological and histological specimens the role of cytogenetic and point mutation abnormalities in cervical carcinogenesis. Chromosomal instability during CC development is exerted to a major extent by E6 HPV oncoprotein and can be evidenced by cytogenetic gains and losses of cellular chromosomal material (Duensing et al., 2008; Korzeniewski et al., 2011). The most studied chromosomal alteration in CC is the gain in chromosome arm 3q, which results in increased copy numbers of the human telomerase gene (*hTERC*). The transition from LSIL to HSIL is characterized by increased *hTERC*, and the use of fluorescence in situ hybridization (FISH) to assess *hTERC* has proven to be useful in predicting LSIL with progression potential in Pap smears (Heselmeyer-Haddad et al., 2005).

Constitutive activation of human oncogene is mainly caused by somatic point mutations. In cervical carcinogenesis several somatic mutations have been associated with disease progression such as those in *LKB1* (Wingo et al., 2009), *PIK3CA* (Cui et al., 2009), and β-catenin (Shinohara et al., 2001) genes. Interestingly, important mutations for their therapeutic implications such as those in *EGFR* or *p53* genes are not frequently found in cervical lesions (Busby-Earle et al., 1994; Denk et al., 2001; Arias-Pulido et al., 2008).

25.5.4 Cervical Epigenetic Biomarkers

25.5.4.1 Methylation of HPV Genome

The long control region (LCR) of the HPV genome controls the expression of viral oncoproteins E6 and E7. DNA methylation of the HPV16 LCR is one mechanism by which E6 and E7 are down-regulated (Hong et al., 2008; Ding et al., 2009). The LCR is also where E2 binding sites are located and contains CpG sites for potential methylation resulting in inhibition of E2 function. Several reports have found that CpG hypermethylation of the HPV16 LCR increased with the severity of the cervical neoplasm (Hong et al., 2008; Ding et al., 2009). Nonetheless, it was also present in 71.4% of asymptomatic infection cases, and thus, the clinical implication of LCR methylation is not clear. Further studies have revealed that the level of hypermethylation of L1 gene of HPV16 and HPV18 also increases with the grade of the lesions (Turan et al., 2006, 2007; Kalantari et al., 2010), and moreover, L1 hypermethylation was more common than LCR hypermethylation (Turan et al., 2006) and may reflect the HPV genome integration into cellular DNA and could potentially be used as a clinical marker of cancer progression.

25.5.4.2 Methylation of Cellular Tumor Suppressor Genes

Hypermethylation and subsequent silencing of tumor suppressor genes (TSGs) is a typical feature of cancer progression. CpG island hypermethylation has been reported in CC (Szalmas and Konya, 2009) independently of the status of HPV infection. The TSGs involved participate in different pathways and some of them are related with SCC and others with adenocarcinoma (Dong et al., 2001; Kang et al., 2006, 2007).

It has been demonstrated that the identification of methylated TSGs in Pap smear could be an adjuvant test in CC screening for triage of women with HR-HPV, ASCUS, or LSIL. Promoter regions of genes coding for E-cadherin, FHIT, cyclin A1, p73, and DAPK are among the most frequently hypermethylated in cervical carcinogenesis, while the hypermethylation of *APC* and *RASSF1A* is more recurrently found in cervical adenocarcinoma (reviewed by Yang [2012]; Saavedra et al. [2012]).

25.5.4.3 miRNA Markers

MicroRNAs (miRNAs) are small noncoding short RNAs that regulate the stability and translational efficiency of target mRNA. Most of the miRNAs identified in cervical carcinoma or its precursor lesions for their diagnostic or prognostic value have been discovered by miRNA expression microarrays. Several such studies have highlighted the utility of individual miRNAs for its diagnostic or prognostic value, although none of them has been validated for the clinical practice. Among them, miR-100 and pri-miR-34a reduced expression has been associated with increasing grade of lesions from LSIL to CC (Li et al., 2010, 2011). Similarly, miR-218 was found underexpressed in HPV-positive cell lines, cervical lesions, and CC-containing HPV16 DNA (Martínez et al., 2008). The expression of other miRNAs, such as miR-21, has been found increased in cervical carcinogenesis (Defteros et al., 2011). Functional studies by Tang et al. (2013) and by Lee et al. (2008) have pointed out the upregulation of miR-182 and miR-199a, respectively, plays a role in CC development. Both studies demonstrated tumor growth regression in vitro using anti-miRNA oligonucleotides (Lee et al., 2008; Tang et al., 2013). Other miRNA patterns associated with CC development are the reduced expression of miR-143 as demonstrated by two independent groups (Lui et al., 2007; Wang et al., 2008) and the increased expression or miR-21 (Lui et al., 2007) and miR-146 (Wang et al., 2008).

A study on miRNA profiling has suggested that both miR-200a and miR-9 could play important regulatory roles in CC control, with miR-200a likely affecting the metastatic potential of CC cells by coordinating suppression of multiple genes controlling cell motility (Hu et al., 2010b).

Despite these evidences no robust studies have been published reporting the performance characteristic of miRNAs for cervical lesions diagnosis.

25.5.5 Cytological Protein Markers

25.5.5.1 p16

The molecular explanation of how p16 is involved in the cervical carcinogenic process has been commented earlier when dealing with histological protein markers. As shown in histological specimens, p16 expression in cytology is positively associated with the grade of dysplasia and HPV positivity in cytological specimen cervical squamous epithelium (Klaes et al., 1999; Longatto Filho et al., 2005; Tsoumpou et al., 2009). Nonetheless, absence of p16 in cytological smears can be found in some HPV-positive lesions (Nieh et al., 2005; Lambert et al., 2006; Samama et al., 2008), but it has a good negative predictive value (NPV) for ASCUS ending up in reactive changes after subsequent biopsies (Nieh et al., 2005). Conversely, positive p16 could also be observed in HPV-negative cervical specimens and in cell lines such as C33A, possibly due to mutation in the *Rb* gene (Milde-Landosch et al., 2001; Murphy et al., 2005). Of note, the alteration in p16 gene copy number by FISH has been recently studied in cervical cytologies, which reported that increase p16 copy number is associated with cytological abnormalities and has higher accuracy for predicting HSIL than cytology in HR-HPV-positive females (Zeng et al., 2011).

Tsoumpou et al. (2009) revised three studies in which the assessment of the accuracy of p16 staining was compared to HPV testing with the hybrid capture 2 (HC2) assay for an underlying CIN2 + in women with ASCUS (Nieh et al., 2005; Meyer et al., 2007) or LSIL (Guo et al., 2004; Meyer et al., 2007) and their performance characteristics are described in Table 25.5. Compared to the techniques for HPV

TABLE 25.5

Performance Characteristics of p16 versus HPV Detection by Hybrid Capture 2 (HC2) in Cytology

Study	Cutoff	Endpoint	Test	SN (%)	SP (%)	PPV (%)	NPV (%)
Guo et al. (2004)	LSIL	CIN 2	p16	92	49	33	96
			HC2	100	7	21	100
Nieh et al. (2005)	ASCUS	CIN 2	p16	95	56	50	96
			HC2	86	31	37	82
Meyer et al. (2007)	ASCUS	CIN 2	p16	0	93	0	93
			HC2	100	21	8	100
Meyer et al. (2007)	LSIL	CIN 2	p16	80	52	27	92
			HC2	100	17	21	100

Source: Tsoumpou, I. et al., *Cancer Treat. Rev.*, 35, 210, 2009.

Note: LSIL, low-grade squamous intraepithelial lesion; ASCUS, a typical squamous cell of undetermined significance; SN, sensitivity; SP, specificity; PPV, positive predictive value; NPV, negative predictive value.

detection in cytology, p16 has a equal or slightly lower sensitivity but quite higher specificity, and thus, it could be a perfect adjunct for HPV testing (Szarewski et al., 2008; Reuschenbach et al., 2010) appearing to be more effective than HR-HPV detection for the identification of reactive changes and LSIL from ASCUS-categorized Pap smears (Nieh et al., 2005).

25.5.5.2 Ki-67

As commented in the invasive marker section, Ki-67 is a nuclear protein expressed during the cell cycle that can be detected with the MIB-1 antibody. Similarly to the pattern observed in histological section, cytological Ki-67 is also useful in distinguishing nondiagnostic atypia from SIL (Wells et al., 2003), and its expression has been associated with ASCUS showing HPV positivity (Longatto Filho et al., 2005).

25.6 Omics-Based Molecular Biomarkers

Concerning microarrays analyzing genomic sequences, Ng et al. (2007) performed a comparative genomic hybridization (CGH) study and found that the gain of oncostatin M receptor gene occurs frequently in cervical SCC and is associated with adverse clinical outcome (Ng et al., 2007). Lee et al. (2010) compared hypermethylation patterns of SCC with adenocarcinoma by analyzing more that 10,000 promoter regions and identified that the hypermethylation of loci in PAK6 and NOGOR genes is strongly correlated with adenocarcinoma diagnosis and could be useful markers of the distinction of these two types of CCs. Integrated chromosomal and transcriptional profiling have identified chromosomal hotspots at 1q, 3q, 11q, and 20q with altered gene expression within large commonly altered chromosomal regions in CC (Wilting, 2008).

Experiments based on mRNA and miRNA expression microarrays might provide novel sensitive and specific markers. Some of these studies have revealed the importance of Wnt/β-catenin and TGF-β in CC progression (Kloth et al., 2005; Noordhuis et al., 2011). Kloth et al. (2005) reported that TGF-β excretion by tumor cells more likely contributes to paracrine stimulation of tumor development, whereas more recently Noordhuis et al. (2011), by comparing the expression profiles of CC with and without pelvic lymph node metastasis, observed that TGF-β- and p120-associated noncanonical β-catenin pathways were important in lymph metastasis in early-stage CC. In this line, other authors have proposed an 11-gene signature for predicting pelvic lymph node metastasis in cervical carcinoma (Huang et al., 2011).

A great body of studies analyzing the miRNA expression profile by microarrays has pointed out the important role of these molecules in cervical carcinogenesis. Huang et al. (2012) identified a signature of six miRNAs that were associated with advance stage, lymph node metastases, and poor prognosis in small cell CC. The study by Cheung et al. (2012) showed that the alteration of miRNA expression is already present in HSIL, and other investigators demonstrated that this expression pattern is different in CC specimens compared to that from normal adjacent tissue (Rao et al., 2012).

Despite the considerable amount of studies dealing with gene expression patterns in CC, not many novel biomarkers with clinical utility have been discovered. Recent transcriptional profiling studies have identified 2 cell cycle-related proteins, minichromosome maintenance protein-2 (MCM2) and topoisomerase IIα (TOP2A), whose genes are overexpressed in CC (Chen et al., 2003; Santin et al., 2005). Both proteins exert their function in early S phase, allowing recognition of replication origin and DNA unwinding (Romanowski et al., 1997). TOP2A is a nuclear enzyme that unknots and decatenates DNA through an adenosine triphosphate-dependent double-strand break followed by strand passing and relegation. In turn, MCM2 is a member of the MCM family of proteins, which, as we commented earlier, are required in an early stage of DNA replication to assemble replication origins and for replication progression as a replicative helicase (Chen et al., 2003; Santin et al., 2005).

25.7 Commercially Available Antibody Cocktails

25.7.1 MCM2/TOP2A (ProEx C)

ProEx C is a novel immunohistochemical marker for the detection of both MCM2 and TOP2A proteins, and its increased expression seems to be associated with HPV16 (Conesa-Zamora et al., 2009b) and HSIL (Shi et al., 2007; Badr et al., 2008; Pinto et al., 2008; Conesa-Zamora et al., 2009a). Studies dealing with cytological specimens have proven the ProEx C positivity in 100% of HSIL (Shroyer et al., 2006; Beccati et al., 2008) and 25% of LSIL biopsy-confirmed smears (Beccati et al., 2008) with higher sensitivity for the detection of HSIL than LBC (85.3% vs. 50%) when facing ASCUS (Kelly et al., 2006). ProEx C sensitivity and specificity for HSIL detection was also better than HR-HPV test (98.8% vs. 71.1% and 82.4% vs. 64.7%) on ASC-H (Siddiqui et al., 2008a) and on ASCUS cytology (98% vs. 82.4% and 74.5% vs. 73.2%, respectively) (Siddiqui et al., 2008b).

Recently, Depuydt et al. (2011) compared different combinations of cytological evaluation, HPV tests, and ProEx C stain demonstrating that primary HR-HPV DNA-based screening followed by ProEx C triage was the best screening strategy for the identification of HSIL in cytological specimens.

Several histological studies have reported that ProEx C is significantly associated with an increasing cell-layer level of expression and a higher grade of dysplasia (Shi et al., 2007; Conesa-Zamora et al., 2009a,b; Guo et al., 2011). These results indicate that cell cycle alteration continues beyond the restriction point G1-S to S phase where the proteins detected by ProEx C, TOP2A, and MCM2 exert their functions. Various evidences have detected ProEx C in the basal/parabasal layer of normal epithelia (Freeman et al., 1999; Badr et al., 2008; Beccati et al., 2008; Conesa-Zamora et al., 2009b). This constitutes an interesting staining internal control in contrast to p16 but, on the other hand, makes ProEx C only positive when considering the expression above the basal/parabasal layer. This fact should not have been a problem when handling cytology specimens although ProEx C staining was occasionally observed in normal-appearing endocervical cells, and thus, ProEx C should be evaluated paying attention to cell morphology (Shroyer et al., 2006). According to this evidence, ProEx C is positive in not necessarily neoplastic but proliferating lesions in a similar way of Ki-67. For these reasons, ProEx C does not have to be regarded as a strictly HPV-related marker. In fact, we reported both the ProEx C and Ki-67 expressions in neoplastic (SCC in situ of the skin) and also in nonneoplastic proliferating lesions (psoriasis and psoriasiform dermatitis) (Sánchez-Hernández et al., 2010). However, while ProEx C seems to be expressed as a diffuse discontinuous pattern in nonneoplastic lesions, the Ki-67 pattern is fully diffuse and continuous. These facts as well as the broader expression of ProEx C in neoplastic lesions compared to Ki-67 suggest that the former delineates neoplastic cells better than Ki-67 (Sánchez-Hernández et al., 2010) (Figure 25.5).

In fact, ProEx C expression was found to be significantly associated with infection by HR-HPV (Badr et al., 2008) and HPV16 (Conesa-Zamora et al., 2009b) being possible reasons for this finding that TOP2A expression is negatively regulated by Rb, and thus, HR-HPV E7-induced degradation of Rb may result in TOP2A overexpression (Santin et al., 2005). Along this line, ProEx C seems to be useful to distinguish dysplastic squamous and endocervical lesions from metaplasia (Badr et al., 2008; Sanati et al., 2010) and from menstruation-associated cytological changes (Ge et al., 2012). In addition, Aximu et al. observed a higher ProEx C expression in cervical adenocarcinoma in situ than in benign endocervical lesions (Aximu et al., 2009).

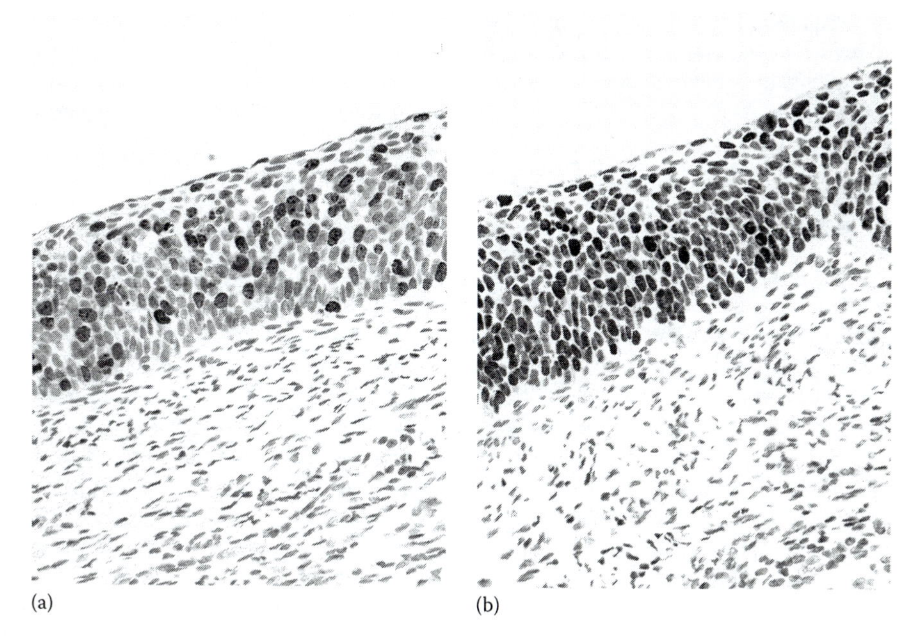

FIGURE 25.5 HSIL case showing Ki-67 (a) and ProEx C (b) positive staining (H&E counterstain, ×20).

25.7.2 p16/Ki-67 Dual

As explained earlier, Ki-67 and p16 correlate positively with cervical histological grade. However, Ki-67 is not specific enough for being used as a sole marker for SIL detection. On the other hand, it is the most widely used and robust marker of cell proliferation. The rationale for the development of the antibody cocktail to detect both p16 and Ki-67 (p16/Ki-67 dual) was that the lack of specificity of Ki-67 could be compensated with p16 staining, thus retaining the good sensitivity of both markers (Petry et al., 2011). This combination was useful in histology for distinguishing SIL from atrophic epithelium with atypia (Shidham et al., 2011). Besides, given the nuclear localization of Ki-67 staining and the predominantly cytoplasmic expression of p16, this antibody cocktail allows the evaluation of both proteins in a specific cell in only one slide since the design includes an anti-p16 antibody developed with a brown stain, whereas that of Ki-67 is red (Figure 25.6). There are not yet many studies with p16/Ki-67, but Petry et al. have

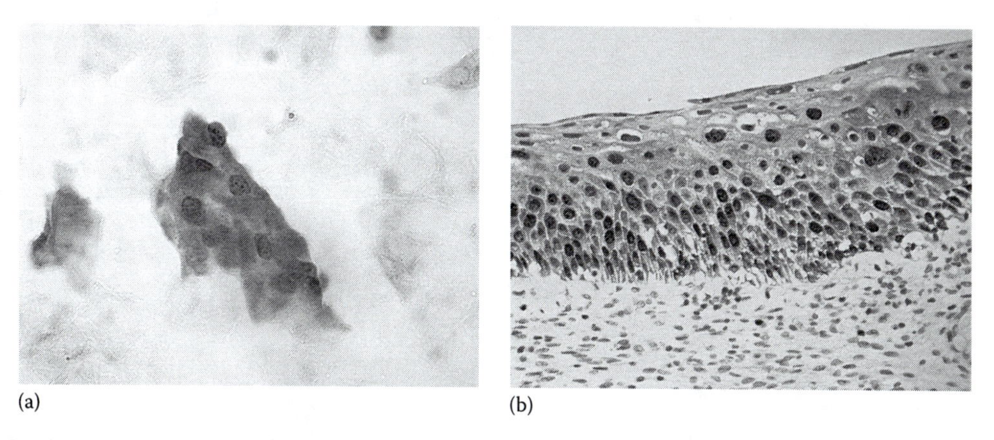

FIGURE 25.6 (See color insert.) p16/Ki-67 dual staining: (a) Cytological specimen showing a positive dysplastic cell (middle) with both Ki-67 nuclear red and p16 cytoplasmic brown stainings surrounded by negative squamous cells (H&E counterstain, ×40). (b) Histological specimen with dual positive staining in the lower two-thirds of the epithelium (H&E counterstain, ×20).

demonstrated its utility in cytology for triaging Pap-negative/HPV-positive women with high probability for underlying CIN 2+ (Petry et al., 2011). Very recently, an automated detection system for p16/Ki-67 dual clear detection in liquid cytology Pap tests has been developed for improving CC risk stratification with which a good correlation was obtained with readings by two cytopathologists (Gertych et al., 2012).

25.8 Cycle Marker Comparison

In order to determine the advantage and disadvantage of each of the revised markers compared to each other, Table 25.6 summarizes some studies reporting ProEx C, Ki-67, and p16 expressions according to the grade of dysplasia. Previous studies have demonstrated the correlation between ProEx C and the p16, Ki-67 (Badr et al., 2008; Conesa-Zamora et al., 2009a), and cyclin D1 (Conesa-Zamora et al., 2009a). Cytological studies with matched histology have revealed that ProEx C shows a direct correlation with Ki-67 expression although in LSIL the expression of ProEx was lower than that of Ki-67 (Beccati et al., 2008) that is in contrast with some other works in LSIL that report higher expression of ProEx C than Ki-67 (Badr et al., 2008; Pinto et al., 2008; Conesa-Zamora et al., 2009a). Besides, in NILM cases, this percentage was lower for ProEx C than for Ki-67 (12% vs. 23%) (Conesa-Zamora et al., 2009a). Table 25.7 revises the performance characteristics reported for these markers and their combinations in recent studies. In general, no great differences are observed in sensitivity and specificity among these markers. Some works have observed higher sensitivity for p16 than ProEx C in HSIL (Badr et al., 2008; Guo et al., 2011) and in SIL (Conesa-Zamora et al., 2012) followed by ProEx C and Ki-67, whereas Shi et al. (2007) observed better sensitivity of ProEx C for LSIL. In contrast, ProEx C showed higher specificity than p16 for CIN 3 + (Guo et al., 2011) and SIL detection (Conesa-Zamora et al., 2012). Concordantly, some authors have shown higher PPV and lower NPV for ProEx C compared to p16 (Halloush et al., 2008), whereas others revealed that p16 and ProEx C show higher expression in a group of LSIL that progressed to HSIL than in a group of stable or regressed LSIL (Ozaki et al., 2011). At this point it is important to point out that four independent studies (Shi et al., 2007; Badr et al., 2008; Pinto et al., 2008; Conesa-Zamora et al., 2012) concluded that the combination of p16/ProEx C shows the highest diagnostic value compared to other marker combinations (e.g., p16/Ki-67, ProEx C/Ki-67) for LSIL (Shi et al., 2007) and HSIL (Shi et al., 2007; Badr et al., 2008) and SIL compared to NILM (Pinto et al., 2008; Conesa-Zamora et al., 2012). Other authors support the use of p16/ProEx C initially followed by Ki-67 only when p16 and ProEx C yielded discordant

TABLE 25.6

Positivity for ProEx C, p16, and Ki-67 in Cervical Carcinoma and Its Precursor Lesions

Reference	n	Specimen	Marker	NILM (%)	LSIL (%)	HSIL (%)	CC (%)
Badr et al., 2008	73	Histology	ProEx C	1/38 (2.6)	11/23 (47.8)	34/37 (92.0)	
			p16		(26)	(93)	
			Ki-67		(32)	(91)	
Conesa-Zamora et al., 2009a	144	Histology	ProEx C	3/25 (12)	10/19 (53)	65/75 (87)	5/5 (100)
			p16	4/28 (14)	12/19 (63)	70/80 (88)	4/5 (80)
			Ki-67	6/26 (23)	10/21 (48)	72/81 (89)	4/4 (100)
Guo et al., 2011	136	Histology	ProEx C	0/20 (0)	7/27 (25.9)	33/60 (55.0)	27/29 (93.1)
			p16	0/20 (0)	7/27 (25.9)	44/60 (73.3)	26/29 (89.7)
			p16/ProEx C	0/20 (0)	0/27 (0)	27/60 (45.0)	24/29 (87.8)
Halloush et al., 2008	75	Cell blocks	ProEx C	2/29 (7)	2/27 (7)	16/19 (84)	
			p16	19/29 (66)	25/27 (92)	19/19 (100)	
			Ki-67	14/29 (48)	22/27 (82)	15/16 (94)	
Shi et al., 2007	62	Histology	ProEx C	0/14 (0)	32/34 (94.1)	11/14 (78.6)	
			p16	0/14 (0)	26/34 (76.5)	14/14 (100)	
			Ki-67	2/14 (14.3)	29/34 (85.3)	14/14 (100)	

Note: NILM, negative for intraepithelial lesion or malignancy; LSIL, low-grade squamous intraepithelial lesion; HSIL, high-grade squamous intraepithelial lesion; CC, cervical carcinoma.

TABLE 25.7

Revision of the Performance Characteristics of ProEx C, p16, and Ki-67 and Their Combinations for the Diagnosis of HPV-Induced Lesions

Reference	Evaluated Markers	Diagnostic Endpoint	SN (%)	SP (%)	Accuracy (%)
Badr et al., 2008	ProEx C	LSIL	48	53	
	p16		48	52	
	Ki-67		32	55	
	ProEx C	HSIL	92	80	
	p16		97	90	
	Ki-67		89	88	
	p16/ProEx C		89	93	
	p16/Ki-67		86	95	
	Ki-67/ProEx C		84	88	
	p16/Ki-67/ProEx C		81	95	
	ProEx C	SIL	75	97	
	p16		70	100	
	Ki-67		68	100	
Conesa-Zamora et al., 2012	ProEx C	SIL	80	87	81.2
	p16		80	84	81.2
	Ki-67		79	78	78.5
	p16/ProEx C		88	78	85.2
	p16/Ki-67		89	70	84.6
	Ki-67/ProEx C		88	76	85.5
	p16/Ki-67/ProEx C		93	70	87.2
Guo et al., 2011	ProEx C	HSIL	67	85	
	p16		79	85	
	p16/ProEx C		57	100	
Pinto et al., 2008	ProEx C	SIL	87	71	79
	p16		84	63	76
	Ki-67		94	52	73
	p16/ProEx C		92	61	76
	p16/Ki-67		94	43	69
	Ki-67/ProEx C		94	48	71

Note: SN, sensitivity; SP, specificity; SIL, squamous intraepithelial lesion; LSIL, low-grade SIL; HSIL, high-grade SIL.

results since this would provide similar diagnostic accuracy at reduced cost as only one-third of the cases will require the additional stain (Walts and Bose, 2009). Although we observed that a model composed by ProEx C plus p16 plus Ki-67 is a better SIL predictor than any combination of two markers, the integrated discrimination improvement (IDI) demonstrates no significant differences between ProEx C plus p16 and the combination of the three markers (Conesa-Zamora et al., 2012). In any case, an antibody cocktail containing p16/TOP2A/MCM2 could be very efficient for SIL detection. Besides, the combined evaluation could also be feasible because ProEx C has a nuclear location and p16 is cytoplasmic and no major technical problems have to be encountered when mixing two or more antibodies (Shi et al., 2007).

25.9 Patent Information of Molecular Markers

Table 25.8 summarizes a series of patents comprising different molecular tests for early detection of HPV infection and cervical lesions.

TABLE 25.8

Representative Patents for the Detection of HPV and Cervical Lesions

Patent Ref.	Applicants	Setting	Target Molecule/s	Molecule Type	Molecule Origin	Application
WO99/29890	Digene Corp	Cyto	E2, E6, E7, L1	mRNA	Viral	HPV detection
WO200208764	Medical Research Council, GB	Cyto and histo	Cell-cycle markers, E4, L1	Protein	Cellular and viral	HPV detection
WO2002/101075	Millennium Pharmaceuticals	Cyto and histo	Various	Nucleic acid and peptide	Cellular and viral	CC detection
WO2003/057914	NorChip	Cyto	E6, L1	mRNA	Viral	HPV detection
EP1510820	MTM lab	Cyto	Various	Nucleic acid and peptide	Cellular and viral	CC detection
WO2005/095964	Tripath	Cyto and histo	MCM2, TOP2A	Protein	Cellular	SIL detection
US2005/0037342	Mathur SP and RS	Cyto and serum	E6, E7, EGFR, IGF-II	Nucleic acid and protein	Cellular and viral	CC risk and response
WO2006/084155	Paterson, Bruce K	Cyto	E6, E7	mRNA	Viral	HPV detection
WO2006/116442	Tripath	Cyto and histo	MCM2	Protein	Cellular	SIL detection
US2009/0104597	Diamics, Inc.	Cyto	E1, E4, E5, E6, E7	Protein	Viral	HPV integration
US2009/0170087	Orion Genomics	Cyto and histo	Various	Methylated DNA	Cellular	CC detection
US2009/0186348	Asuragen, Inc.	Cyto and histo	Various	miRNA	Cellular	SIL and CC detection
US2010/0240049	Cepheid	Cyto and histo	Various	mRNA and miRNA	Cellular	CC risk and response
US2010/0234445	Stanford University	Cyto and histo	Various	miRNA	Cellular	CC detection

Note: Cyto, cytology; histo, histology; HPV, human papillomavirus; CC, cervical cancer; SIL, squamous intraepithelial lesion.

25.10 Future Perspectives

There is a need for a robust HPV marker that could identify not only the HPV genotype but also its integration status and its viral load. Forthcoming tests will probably be developed for detecting all these HPV features in order to improve the specificity of just HPV detection. The incidence of SCC of the cervix has been falling for some time, although that of adenocarcinoma of the cervix is now rising (Woodman et al., 2007). Therefore, future biomarkers must be useful to identify adenocarcinoma precursor lesions whose morphological identification is less evident. The introduction of the vaccine against main oncogenic HPV genotypes (HPV16, HPV18) either in its bivalent or tetravalent form will change the population of HPV genotypes that will be found in cytological specimens as well as the spectrum of lesions that cytopathologist will have to face. Recent clinical trials have revealed that both bivalent and tetravalent HPV vaccines show cross protection with other HPV genotypes not included in the vaccine (Einstein et al., 2011; Wheeler et al., 2012). Vaccination will cause the removal of not only HPV16 and HPV18 from cervical specimens but also other HR-HPV types, at least partially. As the incidence of SIL will decrease, biomarkers will have to be good enough to detect cell cycle abnormalities caused by less prevalent genotypes. Moreover, the percentage of nonmalignant lesions will certainly increase in cytological samples, and thus, markers will be very valuable for its ability to identify probable SIL to be referred to colposcopy from reactive or metaplastic lesions.

Besides, the biomarker usage will be probably influenced in the future by the genome-wide association studies (GWASs) that will help us to understand what is happening in the immune response of that small group of HPV-infected women who develop HSIL and which genetic profile is associated with this progression. Therefore, it would not be surprising that the use of information not only from HPV DNA but also from patient genome will be considered along with the expression of cell cycle marker in order to design an appropriate follow-up and management of HPV-infected patients. Although not yet developed, the demonstrated expression of some miRNAs in early stages of cervical carcinogenesis could be used for detecting LSIL. This identification would be especially useful if miRNA ISH could be performed in cytological specimens since both cell morphology and miRNA expression could be observed at the same glance.

25.11 Conclusions

Major advances in the reduction of CC mortality are due to the correct identification of its precursor lesions. Although Pap test is very specific for such identification, its sensitivity is poor. HPV testing could solve this problem but unfortunately HPV infection is too frequent and most HPV-induced lesions spontaneously regress. In this scenario, cell cycle markers are very useful for identifying cervical lesions with malignant potential and constitute important adjuncts of Pap test and HPV testing for an efficient identification of women referred to colposcopy. Although HSIL can easily be identified with p16, Ki-67, or ProEx C to date, no single marker is able to detect 100% of LSIL. Given the overlap between cell cycle activation in cervical carcinogenesis and other cervical lesions non-induced by HPV, the combinations of highly sensitive and highly specific markers are now providing the best efficiency for SIL diagnostic. Among them, the combination of p16, whose expression is characteristic of HR-HPV infection, with cell cycle proliferation markers such as Ki-67 and especially ProEx C, which can identify those SILs showing p16 negative stain, seems to be the best diagnostic strategy.

25.11.1 Conflict of Interest

The author disclosed no potential conflicts of interest.

Acknowledgments

We are grateful to "Fundación para la Formación e Investigación Sanitarias" from Healthcare Council of Murcia Region, Spain, for supporting our studies; to my coworkers Miguel Pérez-Guillermo, Alejandra Isaac, and Vicente Santaclara for providing the illustrations; and to Diego Arcas for reviewing the English version of the work.

References

American Cancer Society (ACS). Cervical cancer: Detailed guide. From http://www.cancer.org/Cancer/CervicalCancer/DetailedGuide/index; 2012, accessed on February 14, 2013.

Arbyn M, Bergeron C, Klinkhamer P, Martin-Hirsch P, Siebers AG, Bulten J. Liquid compared with conventional cervical cytology. A systematic review and meta-analysis. *Obstet Gynecol* 2008; 111:167–177.

Arias-Pulido H, Joste N, Chavez A et al. Absence of epidermal growth factor receptor mutations in cervical cancer. *Int J Gynecol Cancer* 2008; 18:749–754.

Arias-Pulido H, Peyton CL, Torrez-Martinez N, Anderson DN, Wheeler CM. Human papillomavirus type 18 variant lineages in United States populations characterized by sequence analysis of LCR-E6, E2, and L1 regions. *Virology* 2005; 338:22–34.

Avall-Lundqvist EH, Sjovall K, Nilsson BR, Eneroth PH. Prognostic significance of pretreatment serum levels of squamous cell carcinoma antigen and CA 125 in cervical carcinoma. *Eur J Cancer* 1992; 28A:1695–1702.

Aximu D, Azad A, Ni R, Colgan T, Nanji S. A pilot evaluation of a novel immunohistochemical assay for topoisomerase II-alpha and minichromosome maintenance protein 2 expression (ProEx C) in cervical adenocarcinoma in situ, adenocarcinoma, and benign glandular mimics. *Int J Gynecol Pathol* 2009; 28:114–119.

Baak JPA, Stoler MH, Bean SM, Anderson MC, Robboy SJ. Cervical precancer, including functional biomarkers and colposcopy. In: Robboy SL, Mutter GL, Prat J, Bently RC, Russell P, Anderson MC eds. *Pathology of the Female Reproductive Tract*. New York: Churchill Livingstone 2009; pp. 189–226.

Badr RE, Walts AE, Chung F et al. BD ProEx C: A sensitive and specific marker of HPV-associated squamous lesions of the cervix. *Am J Surg Pathol* 2008; 32:899–906.

Bae DS, Cho SB, Kim YJ et al. Aberrant expression of cyclin D1 is associated with poor prognosis in early stage cervical cancer of the uterus. *Gynecol Oncol* 2001; 81:341–347.

Bae SN, Namkoong SE, Jung JK, Kim CJ, Park JS, Kim JW et al. Prognostic significance of pretreatment squamous cell carcinoma antigen and carcinoembryonic antigen in squamous cell carcinoma of the uterine cervix. *Gynecol Oncol* 1997; 64:418–424.

Bahnassy AA, Zekri AR, Saleh M et al. The possible role of cell cycle regulators in multistep process of HPV-associated cervical carcinoma. *BMC Clin Pathol* 2007; 7:4.

Baldin V, Lukas J, Marcote MJ et al. Cyclin D1 is a nuclear protein required for cell cycle progression in G1. *Genes Dev* 1993; 7:812–821.

Beccati MD, Buriani C, Pedriali M, Rossi S, Nenci I. Quantitative detection of molecular markers ProEx C (minichromosome maintenance protein 2 and topoisomerase IIa) and MIB-1 in liquid-based cervical squamous cell cytology. *Cancer* 2008; 114:196–203.

Biedermann K, Dandachi N, Trattner M et al. Comparison of real-time PCR signal-amplified in situ hybridization and conventional PCR for detection and quantification of human papillomavirus in archival cervical cancer tissue. *J Clin Microbiol* 2004; 42:3758–3765.

Boronow RC. Death of the Papanicolaou smear? A tale of three reasons. *Am J Obstet Gynecol* 1998; 179:391–396.

Bosch FX, de Sanjosé S. Chapter 1: Human papillomavirus and cervical cancer—Burden and assessment of causality. *J Natl Cancer Inst Monogr* 2003; 31:3–13.

Branca M, Ciotti M, Giorgi C et al. Predicting high-risk human papillomavirus infection, progression of cervical intraepithelial neoplasia, and prognosis of cervical cancer with a panel of 13 biomarkers tested in multivariate modeling. *Int J Gynecol Pathol* 2008; 27:265–273.

Brinkman JA, Jones WE, Gaffga AM et al. Detection of human papillomavirus DNA in urine specimens from human immunodeficiency virus-positive women. *J Clin Microbiol* 2002; 40:3155–3161.

Busby-Earle RM, Steel CM, Williams AR, Cohen B, Bird CC. p53 mutations in cervical carcinogenesis—Low frequency and lack of correlation with human papillomavirus status. *Br J Cancer* 1994; 69:732–737.

Calleja-Macias IE, Kalantari M, Huh J et al. Genomic diversity of human papillomavirus-16, 18, 31, and 35 isolates in a Mexican population and relationship to European, African, and Native American variants. *Virology* 2004; 319:315–323.

Calleja-Macias IE, Villa LL, Prado JC et al. Worldwide genomic diversity of the high-risk human papillomavirus types 31, 35, 52, and 58, four close relatives of human papillomavirus type 16. *J Virol* 2005; 79:13630–13640.

Campitelli M, Jeannot E, Peter M et al. Human papillomavirus mutational insertion: Specific marker of circulating tumor DNA in cervical cancer patients. *PLoS One* 2012; 7:e43393.

Carreras R, Alameda F, Mancebo G et al. A study of Ki-67, c-erbB2 and cyclin D-1 expression in CIN-I, CIN-III and squamous cell carcinoma of the cervix. *Histol Histopathol* 2007; 22:587–592.

Chen Y, Miller C, Mosher R et al. Identification of cervical cancer markers by cDNA and tissue microarrays. *Cancer Res* 2003; 63:1927–1935.

Cheung TH, Lo KW, Yu MM et al. Aberrant expression of p21(WAF1/CIP1) and p27(KIP1) in cervical carcinoma. *Cancer Lett* 2001b; 172:93–98.

Cheung TH, Man KN, Yu MY et al. Dysregulated microRNAs in the pathogenesis and progression of cervical neoplasm. *Cell Cycle* 2012; 11:2876–2884.

Cheung TH, Yu MM, Lo KW et al. Alteration of cyclin D1 and CDK4 gene in carcinoma of uterine cervix. *Cancer Lett* 2001a; 166:199–206.

Chhabra S, Bhavani M, Mahajan N, Bawaskar R. Cervical cancer in Indian rural women: Trends over two decades. *J Obstet Gynaecol* 2010; 30:725–728.

Conesa-Zamora P, Doménech-Peris A, Orantes-Casado FJ et al. Effect of human papillomavirus on cell cycle-related proteins p16, Ki-67, Cyclin D1, p53, and ProEx C in precursor lesions of cervical carcinoma: A tissue microarray study. *Am J Clin Pathol* 2009a; 132:378–390.

Conesa-Zamora P, Doménech-Peris A, Ortiz-Reina S et al. Immunohistochemical evaluation of ProEx C in human papillomavirus-induced lesions of the cervix. *J Clin Pathol* 2009b; 62:159–162.

Conesa-Zamora P, Ortiz-Reina S, Moya-Biosca J et al. Genotype distribution of human papillomavirus (HPV) and co-infections in cervical cytologic specimens from two outpatient gynecological clinics in a region of southeast Spain. *BMC Infect Dis* 2009c; 9:124.

Conesa-Zamora P, Trujillo-Santos J, Orantes-Casado FJ, Ortiz-Reina S, Pérez-Guillermo M. Analysis of performance characteristics of five cell cycle-related immunohistochemical markers and human papillomavirus genotyping in the diagnosis of cervical squamous cell carcinoma precursor lesions. *Anal Quant Cytol Histol* 2012; 34:49–55.

Costa S, De Simone P, Venturoli S et al. Factors predicting human papillomavirus clearance in cervical intraepithelial neoplasia lesions treated by conization. *Gynecol Oncol* 2003; 90:358–365.

Cox JT, Schiffman M, Solomon D, ASCUS-LSIL Triage Study (ALTS) Group. Prospective follow-up suggests similar risk of subsequent cervical intraepithelial neoplasia grade 2 or 3 among women with cervical intraepithelial neoplasia grade 1 or negative colposcopy and directed biopsy. *Am J Obstet Gynecol* 2003; 188:1406–1412.

Crum CP, Egawa K, Fu YS et al. Atypical immature metaplasia (AIM). A subset of human papilloma virus infection of the cervix. *Cancer* 1983; 51:2214–2219.

Cui B, Zheng B, Zhang X, Stendahl U, Andersson S, Wallin KL. Mutation of PIK3CA: Possible risk factor for cervical carcinogenesis in older women. *Int J Oncol* 2009; 34:409–416.

Cuschieri KS, Whitley MJ, Cubie HA. Human papillomavirus type specific DNA and RNA persistence—Implications for cervical disease progression and monitoring. *J Med Virol* May 2004; 73(1):65–70.

De Marchi Triglia R, Metze K, Zeferino LC, Lucci De Angelo Andrade LA. HPV in situ hybridization signal patterns as a marker for cervical intraepithelial neoplasia progression. *Gynecol Oncol* 2009; 112:114–118.

Deftereos G, Corrie SR, Feng Q et al. Expression of mir-21 and mir-143 in cervical specimens ranging from histologically normal through to invasive cervical cancer. *PLoS One* 2011; 6:e28423.

DeMay RM. The Pap smear. In: DeMay RM ed. *The Art and Science of Cytopathology*. Chicago, IL: American Society of Clinical Pathologists Press 1996; pp. 61–205.

Denk C, Butz K, Schneider A, Dürst M, Hoppe-Seyler F. p53 mutations are rare events in recurrent cervical cancer. *J Mol Med (Berl)* 2001; 79:283–288.

Depuydt CE, Makar AP, Ruymbeke MJ, Benoy IH, Vereecken AJ, Bogers JJ. BD-ProExC as adjunct molecular marker for improved detection of CIN2 + after HPV primary screening. *Cancer Epidemiol Biomarkers Prev* 2011; 20:628–637.

Ding DC, Chiang MH, Lai HC et al. Methylation of the long control region of HPV16 is related to the severity of cervical neoplasia. *Eur J Obstet Gynecol Reprod Biol* 2009; 147:215–220.

Dong SM, Kim HS, Rha SH et al. Promoter hypermethylation of multiple genes in carcinoma of the uterine cervix. *Clin Cancer Res* 2001; 7:1982–1986.

Doorbar J. Molecular biology of human papillomavirus infection and cervical cancer. *Clin Sci (Lond)* 2006; 110:525–541.

Dueñas-Gonzalez A, Cetina L, Mariscal I, de la Garza J. Modern management of locally advanced cervical carcinoma. *Cancer Treat Rev* 2003; 29:389–399.

Duensing A, Duensing S. Centrosome-mediated chromosomal instability and steroid hormones as co factors in human papillomavirus-associated cervical carcinogenesis: Small viruses help to answer big questions. *Adv Exp Med Biol* 2008; 617:109–117.

Duggan MA. Cytologic and histologic diagnosis and significance of controversial squamous lesions of the uterine cervix. *Mod Pathol* 2000; 13:252–260.

Duggan MA, Akbari M, Magliocco AM. Atypical immature cervical metaplasia: Immunoprofiling and longitudinal outcome. *Hum Pathol* 2006; 37:1473–1481.

Duttagupta C, Romney SL, Palan PR, Slagle NS. Urinary cyclic nucleotides and the cytopathology of human uterine cervical dysplasias. *Cancer Res* 1982; 42:2938–2943.

Ebara T, Mitsuhashi N, Saito Y et al. Prognostic significance of immunohistochemically detected p53 protein expression in stage IIIB squamous cell carcinoma of the uterine cervix treated with radiation therapy alone. *Gynecol Oncol* 1996; 63:216–218.

Einstein MH, Baron M, Levin MJ et al. Comparison of the immunogenicity of the human papillomavirus (HPV)-16/18 vaccine and the HPV-6/11/16/18 vaccine for oncogenic non-vaccine types HPV-31 and HPV-45 in healthy women aged 18–45 years. *Hum Vaccin* 2011; 7:1359–1373.

Emig R, Magener A, Ehemann V et al. Aberrant cytoplasmic expression of the p16 protein in breast cancer is associated with accelerated tumour proliferation. *Br J Cancer* 1998; 78:1661–1668.

Esajas MD, Duk JM, de Bruijn HW et al. Clinical value of routine serum squamous cell carcinoma antigen in follow-up of patients with early-stage cervical cancer. *J Clin Oncol* 2001; 19:3960–3966.

Ferlay J, Shin HR, Bray F, Forman D, Mathers C, Parkin DM. GLOBOCAN 2008 v1.2, Cancer Incidence and Mortality Worldwide: IARC CancerBase No. 10 [Internet]. Lyon, France: International Agency for Research on Cancer; 2010. Available from: http://globocan.iarc.fr, accessed on February 14, 2013.

Freeman A, Morris LS, Mills AD et al. Minichromosome maintenance proteins as biological markers of dysplasia and malignancy. *Clin Cancer Res* 1999; 5:2121–2132.

Ge Y, Mody DR, Smith D, Anton R. p16(INK4a) and ProEx C immunostains facilitate differential diagnosis of hyperchromatic crowded groups in liquid-based Papanicolaou tests with menstrual contamination. *Acta Cytol* 2012; 56:55–61.

Geng L, Connolly DC, Isacson C et al. Atypical immature metaplasia (AIM) of the cervix: Is it related to high-grade squamous intraepithelial lesion (HSIL)? *Hum Pathol* 1999; 30:345–351.

Gerber D. Targeted therapies: A new generation of cancer treatments. *Am Fam Phys* 2008; 77:311–319.

Gertych A, Joseph AO, Walts AE, Bose S. Automated detection of dual p16/Ki67 nuclear immunoreactivity in liquid-based pap tests for improved cervical cancer risk stratification. *Ann Biomed Eng* January 4, 2012; 40:1192–1204.

Giannoudis A, Herrington CS. Differential expression of p53 and p21 in low grade cervical squamous intraepithelial lesions infected with low, intermediate, and high risk human papillomaviruses. *Cancer* 2000; 89:1300–1307.

Giarnieri E, Mancini R, Pisani T et al. Msh2, Mlh1, Fhit, p53, Bcl-2, and Bax expression in invasive and in situ squamous cell carcinoma of the uterine cervix. *Clin Cancer Res* 2000; 6:3600–3606.

Giuliano AR, Nielson CM, Flores R et al. The optimal anatomic sites for sampling heterosexual men for human papillomavirus (HPV) detection: The HPV detection in men study. *J Infect Dis* 2007; 196:1146–1152.

Goldhaber-Fiebert JD, Goldie SJ. Estimating the cost of cervical cancer screening in five developing countries. *Cost Eff Resour Alloc* 2006; 4:13.

Grace VM, Shalini JV, lekha TT, Devaraj SN, Devaraj H. Co-overexpression of p53 and bcl-2 proteins in HPV-induced squamous cell carcinoma of the uterine cervix. *Gynecol Oncol* 2003; 91:51–58.

Guo M, Baruch AC, Silva EG et al. Efficacy of p16 and ProExC immunostaining in the detection of high-grade cervical intraepithelial neoplasia and cervical carcinoma. *Am J Clin Pathol* 2011; 135:212–220.

Guo M, Hu L, Baliga M, He Z, Hughson MD. The predictive value of p16INK4a and hybrid capture 2 human papillomavirus testing for high-grade cervical intraepithelial neoplasia. *Am J Clin Pathol* 2004; 122:894–901.

Halloush RA, Akpolat I, Jim Zhai Q, Schwartz MR, Mody DR. Comparison of ProEx C with p16INK4a and Ki-67 immunohistochemical staining of cell blocks prepared from residual liquid-based cervicovaginal material: A pilot study. *Cancer* 2008; 114:474–480.

Heselmeyer-Haddad K, Sommerfeld K, White NM et al. Genomic amplification of the human telomerase gene (TERC) in pap smears predicts the development of cervical cancer. *Am J Pathol* 2005; 166:1229–1238.

Hiller T, Poppelreuther S, Stubenrauch F et al. Comparative analysis of 19 genital human papillomavirus types with regard to p53 degradation, immortalization, phylogeny, and epidemiologic risk classification. *Cancer Epidemiol Biomarkers Prev* 2006; 15:1262–1267.

Hong D, Ye F, Lu W et al. Methylation status of the long control region of HPV 16 in clinical cervical specimens. *Mol Med Rep* 2008; 1:555–560.

Hu X, Schwarz JK, Lewis JS Jr et al. A microRNA expression signature for cervical cancer prognosis. *Cancer Res* 2010a; 70:1441–1448.

Hu X, Zhang Z, Ma D et al. TP53, MDM2, NQO1, and susceptibility to cervical cancer. *Cancer Epidemiol Biomarkers Prev* 2010b; 19:755–761.

Huang EY, Huang YJ, Chanchien CC et al. Pretreatment carcinoembryonic antigen level is a risk factor for para-aortic lymph node recurrence in addition to squamous cell carcinoma antigen following definitive concurrent chemoradiotherapy for squamous cell carcinoma of the uterine cervix. *Radiat Oncol* 2012a; 7:13.

Huang L, Lin JX, Yu YH, Zhang MY, Wang HY, Zheng M. Downregulation of six microRNAs is associated with advanced stage, lymph node metastasis and poor prognosis in small cell carcinoma of the cervix. *PLoS One* 2012b; 7:e33762.

Huang L, Zheng M, Zhou QM et al. Identification of a gene-expression signature for predicting lymph node metastasis in patients with early stage cervical carcinoma. *Cancer* 2011; 117:3363–3373.

Huang LW, Chou YY, Chao SL, Chen TJ, Lee TT. p53 and p21 expression in precancerous lesions and carcinomas of the uterine cervix: Overexpression of p53 predicts poor disease outcome. *Gynecol Oncol* 2001; 83:348–354.

Huang LW, Lee CC. P16INK4A overexpression predicts lymph node metastasis in cervical carcinomas. *J Clin Pathol* 2012; 65:117–121.

Hunt CR, Hale RJ, Buckley CH, Hunt J. p53 expression in carcinoma of the cervix. *J Clin Pathol* 1996; 49:971–974.

Iaconis L, Hyjek E, Ellenson LH et al. p16 and Ki-67 immunostaining in a typical immature squamous metaplasia of the uterine cervix: Correlation with human papillomavirus detection. *Arch Pathol Lab Med* 2007; 131:1343–1349.

Jacob M, Broekhuizen FF, Castro W, Sellors J. Experience using cryotherapy for treatment of cervical precancerous lesions in low-resource settings. *Int J Gynaecol Obstet* 2005; 89:S13–S20.

Jain D, Srinivasan R, Patel FD, Kumari GS. Evaluation of p53 and Bcl-2 expression as prognostic markers in invasive cervical carcinoma stage IIb/III patients treated by radiotherapy. *Gynecol Oncol* January 2003; 88:22–28.

Kainz C, Kohlberger P, Gitsch G, Sliutz G, Breitenecker G, Reinthaller A. Mutant p53 in patients with invasive cervical cancer stages IB to IIB. *Gynecol Oncol* 1995; 57:212–214.

Kalantari M, Chase DM, Tewari KS et al. Recombination of human papillomavirus-16 and host DNA in exfoliated cervical cells: A pilot study of L1 gene methylation and chromosomal integration as biomarkers of carcinogenic progression. *J Med Virol* 2010; 82:311–320.

Kang S, Kim HS, Seo SS et al. Inverse correlation between RASSF1A hypermethylation, KRAS and BRAF mutations in cervical adenocarcinoma. *Gynecol Oncol* 2007; 105:662–666.

Kang S, Kim JW, Kang GH et al. Comparison of DNA hypermethylation patterns in different types of uterine cancer: Cervical squamous cell carcinoma, cervical adenocarcinoma and endometrial adenocarcinoma. *Int J Cancer* 2006; 118:2168–2171.

Kelly D, Kincaid E, Fansler Z, Rosenthal DL, Clark DP. Detection of cervical high-grade squamous intraepithelial lesions from cytologic samples using a novel immunocytochemical assay (ProEx C). *Cancer* 2006; 108:494–500.

Kim JW, Lee CG, Han SM et al. Loss of heterozygosity of the retinoblastoma and p53 genes in primary cervical carcinomas with human papillomavirus infection. *Gynecol Oncol* 1997; 67:215–221.

Kim K, Kang SB, Chung HH, Kim JW, Park NH, Song YS. XRCC1 Arginine194Tryptophan and GGH-401Cytosine/Thymine polymorphisms are associated with response to platinum-based neoadjuvant chemotherapy in cervical cancer. *Gynecol Oncol* 2008; 111:509–515.

Klaes R, Woerner SM, Ridder R et al. Detection of high-risk cervical intraepithelial neoplasia and cervical cancer by amplification of transcripts derived from integrated papillomavirus oncogenes. *Cancer Res* 1999; 59:6132–6136.

Kloth JN, Fleuren GJ, Oosting J et al. Substantial changes in gene expression of Wnt, MAPK and TNFalpha pathways induced by TGF-beta1 in cervical cancer cell lines. *Carcinogenesis* 2005; 26:1493–1502.

Korzeniewski N, Spardy N, Duensing A, Duensing S. Genomic instability and cancer: Lessons learned from human papillomaviruses. *Cancer Lett* 2011; 305:113–122.

Kulasingam SL, Hughes JP, Kiviat NB et al. Evaluation of human papillomavirus testing in primary screening for cervical abnormalities: Comparison of sensitivity, specificity, and frequency of referral. *JAMA* 2002; 288:1749–1757.

Kurvinen K, Syrjänen K, Syrjänen S. p53 and bcl-2 proteins as prognostic markers in human papillomavirus-associated cervical lesions. *J Clin Oncol* 1996; 14:2120–2130.

Lambert AP, Anschau F, Schmitt VM. p16INK4A expression in cervical premalignant and malignant lesions. *Exp Mol Pathol* 2006; 80:192–196.

Lee EJ, Mcclelland M, Wang Y, Long F, Choi SH, Lee JH. Distinct DNA methylation profiles between adenocarcinoma and squamous cell carcinoma of human uterine cervix. *Oncol Res* 2010; 18:401–408.

Lee JW, Choi CH, Choi JJ et al. Altered MicroRNA expression in cervical carcinomas. *Clin Cancer Res* 2008; 14:2535–2542.

Lee SH, Yang YJ, Kim KM, Chung BC. Altered urinary profiles of polyamines and endogenous steroids in patients with benign cervical disease and cervical cancer. *Cancer Lett* 2003; 201(2):121–131.

Li B, Hu Y, Ye F, Li Y, Lv W, Xie X. Reduced miR-34a expression in normal cervical tissues and cervical lesions with high-risk human papillomavirus infection. *Int J Gynecol Cancer* 2010; 20:597–604.

Li BH, Zhou JS, Ye F et al. Reduced miR-100 expression in cervical cancer and precursors and its carcinogenic effect through targeting PLK1 protein. *Eur J Cancer* 2011; 47:2166–2174.

Liang CW, Lin MC, Hsiao CH, Lin YT, Kuo KT. Papillary squamous intraepithelial lesions of the uterine cervix: Human papillomavirus-dependent changes in cell cycle expression and cytologic features. *Hum Pathol* 2010; 41:326–335.

Longatto Filho A, Utagawa ML, Shirata NK et al. Immunocytochemical expression of p16INK4A and Ki-67 in cytologically negative and equivocal pap smears positive for oncogenic human papillomavirus. *Int J Gynecol Pathol* 2005; 24:118–124.

Lui WO, Pourmand N, Patterson BK, Fire A. Patterns of known and novel small RNAs in human cervical cancer. *Cancer Res* 2007; 67:6031–6043.

Martinez I, Gardiner AS, Board KF, Monzon FA, Edwards RP, Khan SA. Human papillomavirus type 16 reduces the expression of microRNA-218 in cervical carcinoma cells. *Oncogene* 2008; 27:2575–2582.

Martín-Ezquerra G, Fuste P, Larrazabal F et al. Incidence of human papillomavirus infection in male sexual partners of women diagnosed with CIN II-III. *Eur J Dermatol* 2012; 22:200–204.

McWhinney SR, Goldberg RM, McLeod HL. Platinum neurotoxicity pharmacogenetics. *Mol Cancer Ther* 2009; 8:10–16.

Meyer JL, Hanlon DW, Andersen BT, Rasmussen OF, Bisgaard K. Evaluation of p16INK4a expression in ThinPrep cervical specimens with the CINtec p16INK4a assay. *Cancer* 2007; 111:83–92.

Milde-Langosch K, Riethdorf S, Kraus-Pöppinghaus A, Riethdorf L, Löning T. Expression of cyclin-dependent kinase inhibitors p16MTS1, p21WAF1, and p27KIP1 in HPV-positive and HPV-negative cervical adenocarcinomas. *Virchows Arch* 2001; 439:55–61.

Molina R, Filella X, Augé JM et al. CYFRA 21.1 in patients with cervical cancer: Comparison with SCC and CEA. *Anticancer Res* 2005; 25:1765–1771.

Monk BJ, Sill MW, Burger RA et al. Phase II trial of bevacizumab in the treatment of persistent or recurrent squamous cell carcinoma of the cervix: A Gynecologic Oncology Group Study. *J Clin Oncol* 2009; 27:1069–1074.

Mosher RE, Lee KR, Trivijitsilp P, Crum CP. Cytologic correlates of papillary immature metaplasia (immature condyloma) of the cervix. *Diagn Cytopathol* 1998; 18:416–421.

Mukherjea D, Rybak LP. Pharmacogenomics of cisplatin-induced ototoxicity. *Pharmacogenomics* 2011; 12:1039–1050.

Muñoz N, Bosch FX, de Sanjosé S et al., for the International Agency for Research on Cancer Multicenter Cervical Cancer Study Group. Epidemiologic classification of human papillomavirus types associated with cervical cancer. *N Engl J Med* 2003; 348:518–527.

Murphy N, Ring M, Heffron CC et al. p16INK4A, CDC6, and MCM5: Predictive biomarkers in cervical preinvasive neoplasia and cervical cancer. *J Clin Pathol* 2005; 58:525–534.

Mutirangura A. Serum/plasma viral DNA: Mechanisms and diagnostic applications to nasopharyngeal and cervical carcinoma. *Ann NY Acad Sci* 2001; 945:59–67.

Nam EJ, Kim JW, Kim SW et al. The expressions of the Rb pathway in cervical intraepithelial neoplasia: Predictive and prognostic significance. *Gynecol Oncol* 2007; 104:207–211.

Ng G, Winder D, Muralidhar B et al. Gain and overexpression of the oncostatin M receptor occur frequently in cervical squamous cell carcinoma and are associated with adverse clinical outcome. *J Pathol* 2007; 212:325–334.

Ngan HY, Cheng GT, Yeung WS, Wong LC, Ma HK. The prognostic value of TPA and SCC in squamous cell carcinoma of the cervix. *Gynecol Oncol* 1994; 52:63–68.

Ngan HY, Cheung AN, Lauder IJ, Cheng DK, Wong LC, Ma HK. Tumour markers and their prognostic value in adenocarcinoma of the cervix. *Tumour Biol* 1998; 19:439–444.

Ngan HY, Liu SS, Yu H, Liu KL, Cheung AN. Proto-oncogenes and p53 protein expression in normal cervical stratified squamous epithelium and cervical intra-epithelial neoplasia. *Eur J Cancer* 1999; 35:1546–1550.

Nichols GE, Williams ME, Gaffey MJ et al. Cyclin D1 gene expression in human cervical neoplasia. *Mod Pathol* 1996; 9:418–425.

Nieh S, Chen SF, Chu TY et al. Is p16(INK4A) expression more useful than human papillomavirus test to determine the outcome of atypical squamous cells of undetermined significance-categorized Pap smear? A comparative analysis using abnormal cervical smears with follow-up biopsies. *Gynecol Oncol* 2005; 97:35–40.

Noordhuis MG, Fehrmann RS, Wisman GB et al. Involvement of the TGF-beta and beta-catenin pathways in pelvic lymph node metastasis in early-stage cervical cancer. *Clin Cancer Res* 2011; 17:1317–1330.

Orbo A, Hanevik M, Jaeger R, Van Heusden S, Sager G. Urinary cyclic GMP after treatment of gynecological cancer. A prognostic marker of clinical outcome. *Anticancer Res* 2007; 27:2591–2596.

Orbo A, Jaeger R, Sager G. Urinary levels of cyclic guanosine monophosphate (cGMP) in patients with cancer of the uterine cervix: A valuable prognostic factor of clinical outcome? *Eur J Cancer* 1998; 34:1460–1462.

Ozaki S, Zen Y, Inoue M. Biomarker expression in cervical intraepithelial neoplasia: Potential progression predictive factors for low-grade lesions. *Hum Pathol* 2011; 42:1007–1012.

Park J, Sun D, Genest DR, Trivijitsilp P, Suh I, Crum CP. Coexistence of low and high grade squamous intraepithelial lesions of the cervix: Morphologic progression or multiple papillomaviruses? *Gynecol Oncol* 1998; 70:386–391.

Pecorelli S, Zigliani L, Odicino F. Revised FIGO staging for carcinoma of the cervix. *Int J Gynaecol Obstet* 2009; 105:107–108.

Pectasides D, Economides N, Bourazanis J et al. Squamous cell carcinoma antigen, tumor-associated trypsin inhibitor, and carcinoembryonic antigen for monitoring cervical cancer. *Am J Clin Oncol* 1994; 17:307–312.

Peto J, Gilham C, Fletcher O, Matthews FE. The cervical cancer epidemic that screening has prevented in the UK. *Lancet* 2004; 364:249–256.

Petry KU, Menton S, Menton M et al. Inclusion of HPV testing in routine cervical cancer screening for women above 29 years in Germany: Results for 8466 patients. *Br J Cancer* 2003; 88:1570–1577.

Petry KU, Schmidt D, Scherbring S et al. Triaging Pap cytology negative, HPV positive cervical cancer screening results with p16/Ki-67 Dual-stained cytology. *Gynecol Oncol* 2011; 121:505–509.

Pinto AP, Schlecht NF, Woo TY et al. Biomarker (ProEx C, p16(INK4A), and MiB-1) distinction of high-grade squamous intraepithelial lesion from its mimics. *Mod Pathol* 2008; 21:1067–1074.

Poljak M, Kocjan BJ. Commercially available assays for multiplex detection of alpha human papillomaviruses. *Expert Rev Anti Infect Ther* 2010; 8:1139–1162.

Pornthanakasem W, Shotelersuk K, Termrungruanglert W, Voravud N, Niruthisard S, Mutirangura A. Human papillomavirus DNA in plasma of patients with cervical cancer. *BMC Cancer* 2001; 1:2.

Prado JC, Calleja-Macias IE, Bernard HU et al. Worldwide genomic diversity of the human papillomaviruses-53, 56, and 66, a group of high-risk HPVs unrelated to HPV-16 and HPV-18. *Virology* 2005; 340:95–104.

Qiao X, Bhuiya TA, Spitzer M. Differentiating high-grade cervical intraepithelial lesion from atrophy in postmenopausal women using Ki-67, cyclin E, and p16 immunohistochemical analysis. *J Low Genit Tract Dis* 2005; 9:100–107.

Rao Q, Shen Q, Zhou H, Peng Y, Li J, Lin Z. Aberrant microRNA expression in human cervical carcinomas. *Med Oncol* 2012; 29:1242–1248.

Regauer S, Reich O. CK17 and p16 expression patterns distinguish (atypical) immature squamous metaplasia from high-grade cervical intraepithelial neoplasia (CIN 3). *Histopathology* 2007; 50:629–635.

Reuschenbach M, Clad A, von Knebel Doeberitz C et al. Performance of p16INK4a-cytology, HPV mRNA, and HPV DNA testing to identify high grade cervical dysplasia in women with abnormal screening results. *Gynecol Oncol* 2010; 119:98–105.

Reuschenbach M, Seiz M, von Knebel Doeberitz C et al. Evaluation of cervical cone biopsies for coexpression of p16INK4a and Ki-67 in epithelial cells. *Int J Cancer* 2012; 130:388–394.

Romanowski P, Madine MA. Mechanisms restricting DNA replication to once per cell cycle: The role of Cdc6p and ORC. *Trends Cell Biol* 1997; 7:9–10.

Ronco G, Cuzick J, Pierotti P et al. Accuracy of liquid based versus conventional cytology: Overall results of new technologies for cervical cancer screening: Randomised controlled trial. *BMJ* 2007; 335:28.

Saavedra KP, Brebi PM, Roa JC. Epigenetic alterations in preneoplastic and neoplastic lesions of the cervix. *Clin Epigenetics* 2012; 4:13.

Samama B, Schaeffer C, Boehm N. P16 expression in relation to human papillomavirus in liquid-based cervical smears. *Gynecol Oncol* 2008; 109:285–290.

Sanati S, Huettner P, Ylagan LR. Role of ProExC: A novel immunoperoxidase marker in the evaluation of dysplastic squamous and glandular lesions in cervical specimens. *Int J Gynecol Pathol* 2010; 29:79–87.

Sánchez-Hernández M, Conesa-Zamora P, García-Solano J, Corbalán-Vélez R, Martínez-Barba E, Pérez-Guillermo M. Expression profiles of ProEx C and Ki67 in squamous cell carcinoma in situ of the skin and their relationship with human papillomavirus genotypes. *J Cutan Pathol* 2010; 37:730–736.

Sano T, Oyama T, Kashiwabara K et al. Expression status of p16 protein is associated with human papillomavirus oncogenic potential in cervical and genital lesions. *Am J Pathol* 1998; 153:1741–1748.

Santin AD, Zhan F, Bignotti E et al. Gene expression profiles of primary HPV16- and HPV18-infected early stage cervical cancers and normal cervical epithelium: Identification of novel candidate molecular markers for cervical cancer diagnosis and therapy. *Virology* 2005; 331:269–291.

Santopietro R, Shabalova I, Petrovichev N et al. Cell cycle regulators p105, p107, Rb2/p130, E2F4, p21CIP1/WAF1, cyclin A in predicting cervical intraepithelial neoplasia, high-risk human papillomavirus infections and their outcome in women screened in three new independent states of the former Soviet Union. *Cancer Epidemiol Biomarkers Prev* 2006; 15:1250–1256.

Sarian LO, Derchain SF, Yoshida A, Vassallo J, Pignataro F, De Angelo Andrade LA. Expression of cyclooxygenase-2 (COX-2) and Ki67 as related to disease severity and HPV detection in squamous lesions of the cervix. *Gynecol Oncol* 2006; 102:537–541.

Schiffman M, Khan MJ, Solomon D et al. A study of the impact of adding HPV types to cervical cancer screening and triage tests. *J Natl Cancer Inst* 2005; 97:147–150.

Shi J, Liu H, Wilkerson M et al. Evaluation of p16INK4a, minichromosome maintenance protein 2, DNA topoisomerase IIalpha, ProEX C, and p16INK4a/ProEX C in cervical squamous intraepithelial lesions. *Hum Pathol* 2007; 38:1335–1344.

Shidham VB, Mehrotra R, Varsegi G, D'Amore KL, Hunt B, Narayan R. p16 immunocytochemistry on cell blocks as an adjunct to cervical cytology: Potential reflex testing on specially prepared cell blocks from residual liquid-based cytology specimens. *Cytojournal* 2011; 8:1.

Shinohara A, Yokoyama Y, Wan X et al. Cytoplasmic/nuclear expression without mutation of exon 3 of the beta-catenin gene is frequent in the development of the neoplasm of the uterine cervix. *Gynecol Oncol* 2001; 82:450–455.

Shroyer KR, Homer P, Heinz D, Singh M. Validation of a novel immunocytochemical assay for topoisomerase II-alpha and minichromosome maintenance protein 2 expression in cervical cytology. *Cancer* 2006; 108:324–330.

Siddiqui MT, Cohen C, Nassar A. Detecting high-grade cervical disease on ASC-H cytology: Role of BD ProEx C and digene hybrid capture II HPV DNA testing. *Am J Clin Pathol* 2008a; 130:765–770.

Siddiqui MT, Hornaman K, Cohen C, Nassar A. ProEx C immunocytochemistry and high-risk human papillomavirus DNA testing in papanicolaou tests with atypical squamous cell (ASC-US) cytology: Correlation study with histologic biopsy. *Arch Pathol Lab Med* 2008b; 132:1648–1652.

Siegel EM, Patel N, Lu B et al. Circulating biomarkers of iron storage and clearance of incident human papillomavirus infection. *Cancer Epidemiol Biomarkers Prev* 2012; 21:859–865.

Silva IH, Nogueira-Silva C, Figueiredo T et al. The impact of GGH -401C>T polymorphism on cisplatin-based chemoradiotherapy response and survival in cervical cancer. *Gene* 2013; 512:247–250.

Silva-Filho AL, Traiman P, Triginelli SA et al. Expression of p53, Ki-67, and CD31 in the vaginal margins of radical hysterectomy in patients with stage IB carcinoma of the cervix. *Gynecol Oncol* 2004; 95:646–654.

Solomon D, Davey D, Kurman R et al. The 2001 Bethesda System: Terminology for reporting results of cervical cytology. *JAMA* 2002; 287:2114–2119.

Sorbye SW, Arbyn M, Fismen S, Gutteberg TJ, Mortensen ES. HPV E6/E7 mRNA testing is more specific than cytology in post-colposcopy follow-up of women with negative cervical biopsy. *PLoS One* 2011; 6:e26022.

Southern SA, Herrington CS. Differential cell cycle regulation by low- and high-risk human papillomaviruses in low-grade squamous intraepithelial lesions of the cervix. *Cancer Res* 1998; 58:2941–2945.

Sproston AR, Roberts SA, Davidson SE, Hunter RD, West CM. Serum tumour markers in carcinoma of the uterine cervix and outcome following radiotherapy. *Br J Cancer* 1995; 72:1536–1540.

Storey A, Thomas M, Kalita A et al. Role of a p53 polymorphism in the development of human papillomavirus-associated cancer. *Nature* 1998; 393:229–234.

Sturgeon CM, Duffy MJ, Stenman UH et al. National Academy of Clinical Biochemistry laboratory medicine practice guidelines for use of tumor markers in testicular, prostate, colorectal, breast, and ovarian cancers. *Clin Chem.* 2008; 54:e11–e79.

Surendra S, Shastri SS, Ketayun Dinshaw K et al. Concurrent evaluation of visual, cytological and HPV testing as screening methods for the early detection of cervical neoplasia in Mumbai, India. *Bull World Health Organ* 2005; 83:186–194.

Szalmas A, Konya J. Epigenetic alterations in cervical carcinogenesis. *Semin Cancer Biol* 2009; 19:144–152.

Szarewski A, Ambroisine L, Cadman L et al. Comparison of predictors for high-grade cervical intraepithelial neoplasia in women with abnormal smears. *Cancer Epidemiol Biomarkers Prev* 2008; 17:3033–3042.

Szarewski A, Mesher D, Cadman L et al. Comparison of seven tests for high-grade cervical intraepithelial neoplasia in women with abnormal smears: The Predictors 2 study. *J Clin Microbiol* 2012; 50:1867–1873.

Tang T, Wong HK, Gu W et al. MicroRNA-182 plays an onco-miRNA role in cervical cancer. *Gynecol Oncol* 2013; 129:199–208.

Thrall MJ, Russell DK, Facik MS et al. High-risk HPV testing in women 30 years or older with negative Papanicolaou tests: Initial clinical experience with 18-month follow-up. *Am J Clin Pathol* 2010; 133:894–898.

Tindle RW. Immune evasion in human papillomavirus-associated cervical cancer. *Nat Rev Cancer* 2002; 2:59–65.

Trinh XB, Bogers JJ, Van Marck EA, Tjalma WA. Treatment policy of neuroendocrine small cell cancer of the cervix. *Eur J Gynaecol Oncol* 2004; 25:40–44.

Tseng CJ, Pao CC, Lin JD, Soong YK, Hong JH, Hsueh S. Detection of human papillomavirus types 16 and 18 mRNA in peripheral blood of advanced cervical cancer patients and its association with prognosis. *J Clin Oncol* 1999; 17:1391–1396.

Tsoumpou I, Arbyn M, Kyrgiou M et al. p16(INK4a) immunostaining in cytological and histological specimens from the uterine cervix: A systematic review and meta-analysis. *Cancer Treat Rev* 2009; 35:210–220.

Tsuda H, Hashiguchi Y, Nishimura S et al. Relationship between HPV typing and abnormality of G1 cell cycle regulators in cervical neoplasm. *Gynecol Oncol* 2003; 91:476–485.

Turan T, Kalantari M, Calleja-Macias IE et al. Methylation of the human papillomavirus-18 L1 gene: A biomarker of neoplastic progression? *Virology* 2006; 349:175–183.

Turan T, Kalantari M, Cuschieri K et al. High-throughput detection of human papillomavirus-18 L1 gene methylation, a candidate biomarker for the progression of cervical neoplasia. *Virology* 2007; 361:185–193.

Ueda M, Toji E, Nunobiki O et al. Germline polymorphisms of glutathione-S-transferase GSTM1, GSTT1 and p53 codon 72 in cervical carcinogenesis. *Hum Cell* 2010; 23:119–125.

Van de Putte G, Kristensen GB, Lie AK, Baekelandt M, Holm R. Cyclins and proliferation markers in early squamous cervical carcinoma. *Gynecol Oncol* 2004; 92:40–46.

Verheijen R, Kuijpers HJ, van Driel R et al. Ki-67 detects a nuclear matrix-associated proliferation-related antigen. II. Localization in mitotic cells and association with chromosomes. *J Cell Sci* 1989; 92:531–540.

Vijayalakshmi N, Selvaluxmi G, Majhi U et al. Alterations found in pl6/Rb/cyclin D1 pathway in the dysplastic and malignant cervical epithelium. *Oncol Res* 2007; 16:527–533.

Vogelstein B, Lane D, Levine AJ. Surfing the p53 network. *Nature* 2000; 408:307–310.

Walts AE, Bose S. p16, Ki-67, and BD ProExC immunostaining: A practical approach for diagnosis of cervical intraepithelial neoplasia. *Hum Pathol* 2009; 40:957–964.

Wang JL, Zheng BY, Li XD, Angström T, Lindström MS, Wallin KL. Predictive significance of the alterations of p16INK4A, p14ARF, p53, and proliferating cell nuclear antigen expression in the progression of cervical cancer. *Clin Cancer Res* 2004a; 10:2407–2414.

Wang SS, Sherman ME, Hildesheim A, Lacey JV Jr, Devesa S. Cervical adenocarcinoma and squamous cell carcinoma incidence trends among white women and black women in the United States for 1976–2000. *Cancer* 2004b; 100:1035–1044.

Wang X, Tang S, Le SY et al. Aberrant expression of oncogenic and tumor-suppressive microRNAs in cervical cancer is required for cancer cell growth. *PLoS One* 2008; 3:e2557.

Wells M, Östor AG, Crum CP et al. Tumors of the uterine cervix: Epithelial tumors. In: Tavassoli FA, Devilee P eds. *Pathology and Genetics of Tumours of the Breast and Female Genital Organs*. Lyon, France: IARC Press 2003; pp. 262–279.

Wheeler CM, Castellsagué X, Garland SM et al. Cross-protective efficacy of HPV-16/18 AS04-adjuvanted vaccine against cervical infection and precancer caused by non-vaccine oncogenic HPV types: 4-year end-of-study analysis of the randomised, double-blind PATRICIA trial. *Lancet Oncol* 2012; 13:100–110.

Wilting SM, de Wilde J, Meijer CJ et al. Integrated genomic and transcriptional profiling identifies chromosomal loci with altered gene expression in cervical cancer. *Genes Chromosomes Cancer* 2008; 47:890–905.

Wingo SN, Gallardo TD, Akbay EA et al. Somatic LKB1 mutations promote cervical cancer progression. *PLoS One* 2009; 4:e5137.

Woodman CB, Collins S, Winter H et al. Natural history of cervical human papillomavirus infection in young women: A longitudinal cohort study. *Lancet* 2001; 357:1831–1836.

Woodman CB, Collins SI, Young LS. The natural history of cervical HPV infection: Unresolved issues. *Nat Rev Cancer* 2007; 7:11–22.

Xi LF, Demers GW, Koutsky LA et al. Analysis of human papillomavirus type 16 variants indicates establishment of persistent infection. *J Infect Dis* 1995; 172:747–755.

Yang HJ. Aberrant DNA methylation in cervical carcinogenesis. *Chin J Cancer* 2012; doi: 10.5732/cjc.012.10033.

Yang HJ, Liu VW, Tsang PC et al. Quantification of human papillomavirus DNA in the plasma of patients with cervical cancer. *Int J Gynecol Cancer* 2004; 14:903–910.

Yin M, Zhao F, Lou G et al. The long-term efficacy of neoadjuvant chemotherapy followed by radical hysterectomy compared with radical surgery alone or concurrent chemoradiotherapy on locally advanced-stage cervical cancer. *Int J Gynecol Cancer* 2011; 21:92–99.

Yoon SM, Shin KH, Kim JY et al. Use of serum squamous cell carcinoma antigen for follow-up monitoring of cervical cancer patients who were treated by concurrent chemoradiotherapy. *Radiat Oncol* 2010; 5:78.

Zehbe I, Richard C, DeCarlo CA et al. Human papillomavirus 16 E6 variants differ in their dysregulation of human keratinocyte differentiation and apoptosis. *Virology* 2009; 383:69–77.

Zeng WJ, Li Y, Fei HL et al. The value of p16ink4a expression by fluorescence in situ hybridization in triage for high risk HPV positive in cervical cancer screening. *Gynecol Oncol* 2011; 120:84–88.

Zhao CY, Szekely L, Bao W, Selivanova G. Rescue of p53 function by small-molecule RITA in cervical carcinoma by blocking E6-mediated degradation. *Cancer Res* 2010; 70:3372–3381.

Zhao P, Mao X, Talbot IC. Aberrant cytological localization of p16 and CDK4 in colorectal epithelia in the normal adenoma carcinoma sequence. *World J Gastroenterol* 2006; 12:6391–6396.

zur Hausen H. Molecular pathogenesis of cancer of the cervix and its causation by specific human papillomavirus types. *Curr Top Microbiol Immunol* 1994; 186:131–156.

zur Hausen H. Papillomaviruses and cancer: From basic studies to clinical application. *Nat Rev Cancer* 2002; 2:342–350.

26

Biomarkers in Diagnosis of Papillary Thyroid Carcinoma

Marisa Cañadas-Garre, Nuria Muñoz Pérez, Jesús María Villar del Moral, José Antonio Ferrón Orihuela, and José Manuel Llamas-Elvira

CONTENTS

ABSTRACT Papillary thyroid carcinoma (PTC) is the most common among malignant thyroid neoplasms. Although incidence has been increasing in recent years, the prognosis remains excellent, with survival rates over 97%.

Fine-needle aspiration biopsy (FNAB) is the most valuable preoperative test to diagnose thyroid cancer. However, nondefinite results can rise up to 50% of the cases, making evident the need of molecular biomarkers that help improving its diagnostic accuracy.

The search of molecular biomarkers in thyroid cancer has been especially focused in gene mutations in components of the mitogen-activated protein kinase (MAPK) pathway, particularly mutations in BRAF, the most frequent gene alteration in PTC. The incorporation of this biomarker, and, in some cases, in combination with other gene mutations or rearrangements, to the routine FNAB has demonstrated a prominent improvement of the detection of PTC cases on FNAB. Many other gene markers have been explored in other to increase FNAB sensibility; among them, gene expression profiling, proteomic and immunohistochemical biomarkers, and epigenetic dysregulation are the best characterized. Some of these biomarkers have also showed prognostic and therapeutic values besides the diagnostic utility.

This thorough search for molecular biomarkers in PTC has led to the developing of different commercial platforms that are currently offered to the clinicians for the preoperative identification of PTC. It is still unknown if these available commercial tests will be soon entirely integrated in our health systems as an inseparable complement of FNAB.

26.1 Introduction

Thyroid cancers derived from follicular epithelial cells can be classified histologically into papillary, follicular, and anaplastic, corresponding to approximately 80%, 15%, and 2%–5%, respectively, of all thyroid malignancies (Hundahl et al., 1998). Benign tumors derived from thyroid follicular epithelial cells, including adenoma and hyperplasia, are more common than thyroid cancer.

World Health Organization (WHO) histological classification of thyroid carcinomas in its 2004 edition described as major subtypes of thyroid carcinoma (DeLellis et al., 2004):

1. Thyroid cancer derived from follicular cells
   a. Differentiated thyroid carcinoma (DTC)
      i. Papillary thyroid carcinoma (PTC)
      ii. Follicular thyroid carcinoma (FTC)

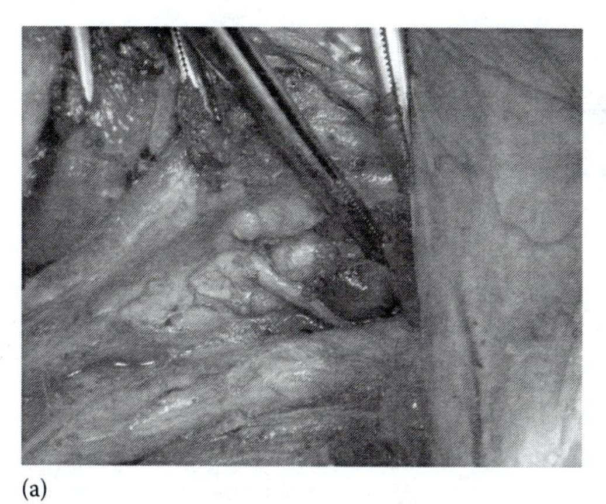
(a)

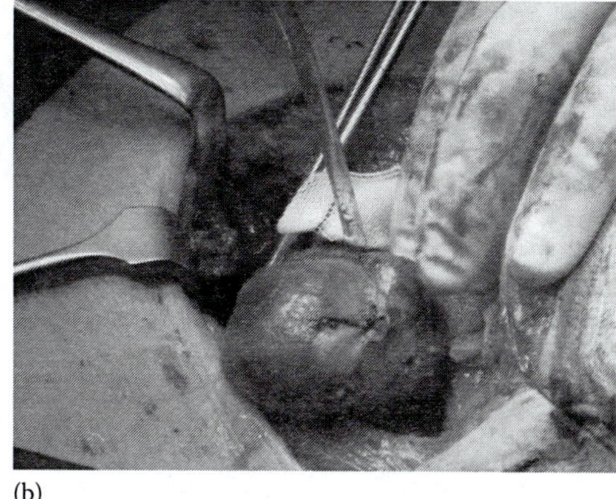
(b)

FIGURE 26.1 **(See color insert.)** Surgery images of PTC: (a) metastatic lymph nodes adjacent to right recurrent nerve in a case of PTC and (b) a case of PTC invading internal left jugular vein.

   b. Undifferentiated thyroid carcinoma (UTC)
      i. Poorly differentiated carcinoma (PDTC)
      ii. Anaplastic thyroid carcinoma (ATC)
2. Thyroid cancer derived from C cells
   a. Medullary thyroid carcinoma (MTC)

PTC constitutes approximately 80% of malignant thyroid neoplasms (Hundhal et al., 1998). It belongs to the subtype of well-differentiated carcinomas of follicular epithelial origin (PTC, FTC) and is defined as a malignant epithelial tumor showing evidence of follicular differentiation, which presents distinctive nuclear features (LiVolsi et al., 2004).

PTC tends to present intraglandular dissemination, lymph node metastasis, and local invasion (Figure 26.1). This tumor is often found located only in the thyroid gland in 68% of cases, in thyroid and lymph nodes in 13%, and only in lymph nodes in 20%. Distant metastases are rare and appear late (Carcangiu et al., 1985; Howlader et al., 2012).

Recurrence up to 30 years after initial treatment has been reported in long-term follow-up cases (Tubiana et al., 1985), although mortality is very low (6.5%) (McConahey et al., 1986).

26.1.1 Morphological Variants of Papillary Thyroid Carcinoma

Several histopathological variants have been described for PTC (LiVolsi, 1990; Kini, 2008). The 2004 classification of tumors of the WHO defines 16 variants, shown in Table 26.1 (LiVolsi et al., 2004).

Morphological variants of PTC are classified on the basis of the architectural pattern (growth) and cell type. Each variant must present more than 75% of the tumor composed of a specific pattern to be classified morphologically in that specific designation. The common denominator for all variants is the typical nuclear morphology, characterized by pale nuclei, nucleoli, nuclear grooves, and intranuclear cytoplasmic inclusions, except for the columnar cell variant. These features allow nuclear and cytological accurate histological diagnosis of PTC (Kini, 2008).

26.1.2 Epidemiology

26.1.2.1 Epidemiology of Thyroid Nodule

In geographic areas without iodine deficiency, about 4%–7% of the population will develop a palpable thyroid nodule throughout their lifetime, with a higher frequency in countries where goiter is endemic (Vander et al., 1968; Pacini et al., 2004). The prevalence of solitary or multiple thyroid nodules increases nearly

TABLE 26.1

Subtypes of PTC

Subtypes of PTC	Frequency
Classical or conventional	75%
Follicular variant	12%
Tall cell variant	10%
Diffuse sclerosing variant	2.3%
Macrofollicular variant	
Papillary microcarcinoma (occult sclerosing)	
Oncocytic cell variant (oxyphilic)	
Clear cell variant	
Columnar cell variant	
Solid-trabecular variant	
Cribriform-morular carcinoma	
PTC with fasciitis-like stroma	
PTC with focal insular component	
Mucoepidermoid papillary carcinoma or squamous cell carcinoma	
PTC with spindle and giant cell carcinoma	
Combined papillary and medullary carcinoma	

Source: LiVolsi, V.A. et al., *N. Engl. J. Med.*, 367(8),705, 2004.

70% when ultrasound is the screening method (Brander et al., 1992; Ezzat et al., 1994; Tan et al., 1995; Guth et al., 2009; Miller, 2010). Autopsy data also demonstrate the high frequency of this disease, reaching 50% in autopsies of patients without antecedents of thyroid disease (Mortensen et al., 1955). Published studies from different geographic areas indicate a prevalence of 2%–65% (Dean and Gharib, 2008).

Advanced age, female gender, iodine deficiency, and radiation exposure are considered risk factors for thyroid nodules; other factors include tobacco, alcohol, or pregnancy (Dean and Gharib, 2008). Even small changes in iodine diet intake significantly reduce the prevalence of goiter and the incidence of thyroid nodules and thyroid dysfunction (Knudsen et al., 2002). Irradiation, regardless accidental or therapeutically, induces the formation of nodules and increases the risk of cancer. The influence is higher on men and is more relevant when exposure occurs at an early age.

The evolution of the nodules during follow-up is variable: while approximately 30%–50% nodules decrease in volume, ≈30% are stable and 20%–89% increase their size (Quadbeck et al., 2002; Alexander et al., 2003; Imaizumi et al., 2006; Wémeau et al., 2011).

26.1.2.2 Epidemiology of Thyroid Cancer

Thyroid cancer is a low-incidence tumor but is the most common among those that affect the endocrine system. According to data from the International Agency for Research on Cancer (IARC), part of the WHO, thyroid cancer accounts for 1.7% of all malignancies (212,000 new cases in 2008) (Ferlay et al., 2010). The incidence is higher in women (163,000 vs. 49,000). The prognosis is good, with an estimated mortality of 0.5% of all cancer deaths, also higher in women (Ferlay et al., 2010; Howlader et al., 2012).

In the United States, approximately 1,638,910 new cancer cases and 577,190 deaths from this cause are estimated during 2012. Of these, 56,460 are expected to be thyroid cancer cases (13,250 men and 43,210 women), and 1,780 men and women will die of cancer of the thyroid (Howlader et al., 2012). The overall incidence (age-adjusted rate) is 11.6 per 100,000 inhabitants per year (data from 2005 to 2009), with a mean age at diagnosis of 50 years (Howlader et al., 2012). Since the 1990s, thyroid cancer is the malignancy that has experienced the fastest increase in incidence for both genders.

The overall age-adjusted mortality in the United States is 0.5 per 100,000 population per year (Howlader et al., 2012), and 1,780 deaths by thyroid cancer are estimated during 2012 (780 men). As the incidence, mortality has increased slightly from 2004 to 2008 (from 0.47 to 0.5 per 100,000 in men and from 0.47 to 0.52 in women) (Howlader et al., 2012).

TABLE 26.2

Stage Distribution and 5-Year Relative Survival by Stage at Diagnosis for 2002–2008, All Races, Both Sexes

Stage at Diagnosis	Stage Distribution (%)	5-Year Relative Survival (%)
Localized (confined to primary site)	68	99.9
Regional lymph nodes	25	97.1
Distant metastases	5	53.9
Unknown (unstaged)	2	87.4

Source: Data from Howlader, N. et al. (eds.), *SEER Cancer Statistics Review, 1975–2009 (Vintage 2009 Populations)*, National Cancer Institute, Bethesda, MD. http://seer.cancer.gov/csr/1975_2009_pops09/, based on November 2011 SEER data submission, posted to the SEER website, 2012.

In any case, the prognosis remains excellent, with an overall 5-year survival of 97% (Howlader et al., 2012). When the disease is localized (68% of the cases), the survival is ≈100%, ≈97% if there is regional node involvement and ≈54% if there is distant disease (Table 26.2). Prognosis is better if age is under 45 years, with 100% overall survival, and worsens with age (82% survival at age 75), with an average age of 73 years among deceased during 2005–2009 period (Howlader et al., 2012).

26.1.3 Current Methods for Early Diagnosis, Prognosis, and Therapy: Biochemical and Imaging Modalities Indicated for the Diagnosis of Thyroid Cancer

Newly diagnosed thyroid nodules must be evaluated mainly to rule out malignancy (Tan and Gharib, 1997; Hegedüs, 2004; Ross, 2005; Gharib and Papini, 2007). Clinical evaluation begins with a detailed history and thorough physical examination, focusing on the thyroid gland and adjacent cervical lymph nodes (Cooper et al., 2009).

Factors relevant to the prediction of malignancy in thyroid nodules are described in Table 26.3.

26.1.3.1 Determination of Serum Thyrotropin (TSH)

In the absence of specific clinical suspicion, initial thyroid evaluation requires only the determination of the serum TSH level, according to all Clinical practice guidelines for the diagnosis and management of thyroid nodules (American Association of Clinical Endocrinologists and Associazione Medici Endocrinologi [AACE/AME], American Thyroid Association [ATA], European Thyroid Association [ETA]).

Once a thyroid nodule >1–1.5 cm in any diameter is detected, after the determination of serum TSH, if its concentration is less than normal, a thyroid scan should be performed in order to document the functionality of the nodule. Since functioning nodules rarely carry malignancy, cytological evaluation is not necessary in those cases. In the case of evident or subclinical hyperthyroidism, the evaluation must continue with thyroid ultrasound (Cooper et al., 2009). The algorithm for evaluation of thyroid nodules is shown in Figure 26.2.

TABLE 26.3

High-Risk Factors Predictive of Malignancy in Thyroid Nodules

History of head/neck irradiation during childhood
Family history of papillary, MTC, or MEN2
Age below 20 years or over 70 years
Male sex
Growing nodule
Abnormal cervical lymphadenopathy
Nodule fixation
Vocal cord paralysis

Source: Gharib, H. and Papini, E., *Endocrinol. Metab. Clin. North Am.*, 36(3), 707, 2007.

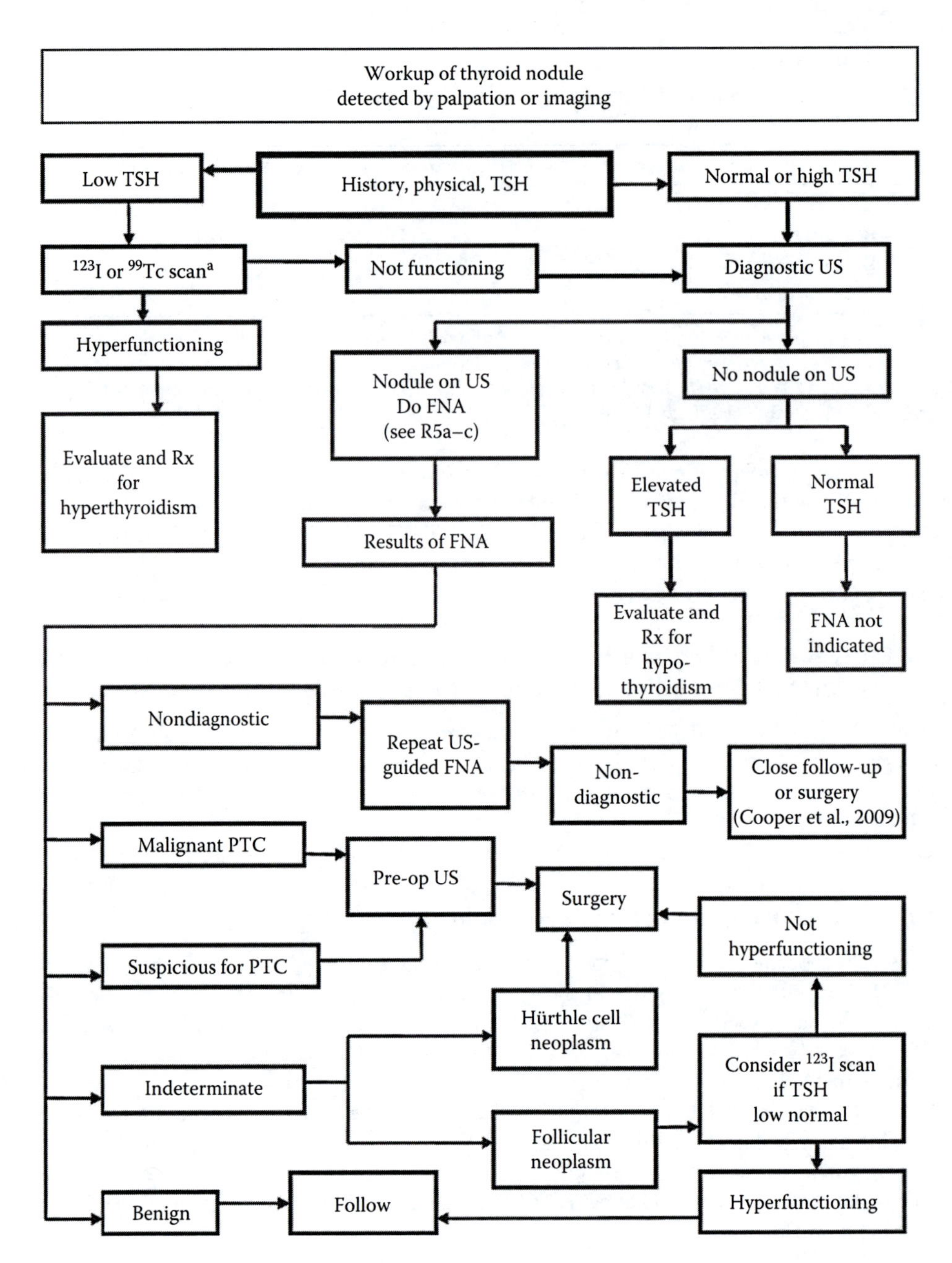

FIGURE 26.2 Algorithm for the evaluation of patients with one or more thyroid nodules. [a]If the scan does not show uniform distribution of tracer activity, ultrasound may be considered to assess for the presence of a cystic component. (From Cooper, D.S. et al., *Thyroid*, 19(11), 1167, 2009.)

26.1.3.2 Thyroid Ultrasound

Ultrasonography (US) is the most sensitive test for detecting lesions in the thyroid. It is recommended that all patients with nodular thyroid, with a palpable nodule or a multinodular goiter (MNG), are evaluated by US (Cooper et al., 2009), with the aim of

- Finding additional unsuspected nodules
- Measuring the number and size of nodules

- Locating the nodules (anterior/posterior)
- Registering the US characteristics (microcalcifications, irregular margins, vascular imaging, cystic or solid content, hypoechogenicity, shape), to evaluate the risk of malignancy
- Selecting lesions requiring US-guided FNAB (Tan and Gharib, 1997; Baskin, 2000)

26.1.3.3 Radionuclide Scan

Radionuclide thyroid scan is indicated by Clinical practice guidelines when TSH is suppressed and nodules present cytological diagnosis of follicular neoplasm (Gharib et al., 2008, 2010; Cooper et al., 2009).

This scan measures the ability of the nodule to uptake radiotracer compared to surrounding thyroid tissue. Thyroid scan is the only technique that allows the evaluation of nodular thyroid function and detects areas of functional autonomy within the thyroid gland. Based on the pattern of radioisotope uptake, nodules can be classified as (Cooper et al., 2009)

- Hyperfunctioning or "hot," if the nodule tracer uptake is greater than the parenchyma
- Nonfunctioning or "cold," when the nodule uptakes less tracer than the parenchyma
- Isofunctioning or "warm," if tracer uptake is homogeneous

Hot nodules are rarely malignant, while cold nodules present a risk of thyroid cancer varying among 5%–15%.

26.1.3.4 Fine-Needle Aspiration Biopsy

Fine-needle aspiration biopsy (FNAB), either palpation or ultrasound guided, is recognized as the diagnostic procedure of choice in the evaluation of thyroid nodules detected clinically or incidentally (recommendation rating: strongly recommended) (Gharib et al., 2008, 2010; Cooper et al., 2009).

US guidance for FNAB is recommended for those nodules that are nonpalpable, predominantly cystic, or located posteriorly in the thyroid lobe (recommendation rating: recommended) (Cooper et al., 2009).

FNAB is by far the most valuable preoperative method to identify patients with thyroid cancer, with a reported sensitivity (Se) of 97%, specificity (Sp) and diagnostic accuracy (Acc) values of 50.7% and 68.8%, respectively, and positive predictive value (PPV) of 55.9% and 96.3% for negative predictive value (NPV), according to a recent meta-analysis, comprising 25,445 FNAB results. Since its incorporation to the diagnostic routine, it has exerted a considerable impact on the management of patients with thyroid nodules, contributing to the reduction of surgery patients and obviously increasing the percentage of malignant nodules found at surgery (Hamberger et al., 1982; Suen, 1988; Galloway et al., 1991).

As a diagnostic test, FNAB can be used to diagnose PTC, PDTC, MTC, ATC, metastatic malignancy, thyroiditis, and most cysts and benign nodular goiters. However, follicular adenoma (FA), well-differentiated carcinoma, and some hypercellular goiters are indistinguishable in FNAB.

26.1.3.4.1 Guidelines for the Management of Patients with Thyroid Nodules, Based on Cytopathological Interpretation of FNAB Samples

Table 26.4 shows the frequency of results of FNAB and the percentage of malignancy associated with every FNAB category, plus the clinical management of the patient based on the FNAB diagnosis as recommended by several Clinical practice guidelines for the diagnosis and management of thyroid nodules.

26.1.3.4.2 Limitations of Fine-Needle Aspiration Biopsy

Current imaging and cytological techniques are not always capable to discriminate preoperatively between benign and malignant nodules. Palpation- or US-guided FNAB has been widely established as the most reliable diagnostic test in the initial clinical management of thyroid nodules, being the key diagnostic tool for preoperative selection of nodules at risk of malignancy (Gharib et al., 2008, 2010; Cooper et al., 2009). Nondefinite results (20%–50% of the cases) are the main limitation of FNAB, due to nondiagnostic results (4%–25%) or indeterminate cytological patterns (10%–30%) (Table 26.4).

TABLE 26.4

Frequency of Results for Thyroid FNAB with Their Respective Percentage of Malignancy and Clinical Management Recommendation

FNAB Category	Frequency	References	Malignancy	References	Recommendation	References
Nondiagnostic						
Nondiagnostic biopsies are those that fail to meet specified criteria for cytological adequacy.	4%–25%	Miller et al. (1985), Caruso and Mazzaferri (1991), Gharib and Goellner (1993), Hamburger (1994), Sangalli et al. (2006), Yang et al. (2007), Bongiovanni et al. (2012), Cañadas Garre et al. (2012)	2%–17%	McHenry et al. (1993), MacDonald and Yazdi (1996), Schmidt et al. (1997), Yang et al. (2007), Bongiovanni et al. (2012), Cañadas Garre et al. (2012)	Repetition by US-FNAB complemented with on-site cytological evaluation. Partially cystic nodules that repeatedly yield nondiagnostic aspirates need close observation or surgical excision. Surgery should be more strongly considered if the cytologically nondiagnostic nodule is solid.	Cooper et al. (2009)
Benign						
The sample shows no malignancy features (e.g., goiter, thyroiditis).	60%–70%	Yang et al. (2007), Baloch et al. (2008), Bongiovanni et al. (2012), Cañadas Garre et al. (2012)	1%–7%	Carmeci et al. (1998), Ylagan et al. (2004), Yang et al. (2007), Baloch et al. (2008), Bongiovanni et al. (2012)	The patient should be managed conservatively, so further immediate diagnostic studies or treatment is not routinely required.	Hegedüs (2004) Cooper et al. (2009)
Indeterminate						
Includes the following cytopathological patterns						
Follicular/Hürthle cell neoplasm						
Suitable cellularity, cytological features suggestive of malignancy, but no criteria for a definitive diagnosis (e.g., FA vs. differential diagnosis of FTC or follicular variant of PTC)	5%–30%	Caruso and Mazzaferri (1991), Gharib and Goellner (1993), Gharib et al. (1993), Gharib (2004), Hegedüs (2004), Sangalli et al. (2006), Yang et al. (2007), Cañadas Garre et al. (2012)	20%–32%	Caruso and Mazzaferri (1991), Raber et al. (2000), Baloch et al. (2002), Giorgadze et al. (2004), Yang et al. (2007), Bongiovanni et al. (2012), Cañadas Garre et al. (2012)	^{123}I thyroid scan may be considered, if not already done, especially if serum TSH is in the low-normal range. If a concordant autonomously functioning nodule is not detected, lobectomy or total thyroidectomy should be considered.	Cooper et al. (2009)

Atypia						
Suitable cellularity, with most, but not all, cytological features of PTC Inadequate cellularity, but cellular features strongly suggest malignancy	1%–3%	Yang et al. (2007), Baloch et al. (2008), Cañadas Garre et al. (2012)	19%–60%	Gharib (1994), Gharib and Goellner (1995), Castro and Gharib (2003), Yang et al. (2007)	Repeat FNAB	Baloch et al. (2008)
AUS/FLUS						
Bethesda System for Reporting Thyroid Cytopathology: ambiguous cytological findings that appear to be greater than what would be expected of a nonneoplastic process, yet the degree of cellular or architectural atypia is insufficient for an interpretation of "follicular neoplasm" or "suspicious for malignancy" (Cibas and Ali, 2009)	10%–16%	Yang et al. (2007), Bongiovanni et al. (2012), Chen et al. (2012)	5%–19%	Yang et al. (2007), Baloch et al. (2008), Bongiovanni et al. (2012), Chen et al. (2012)		
Suspicious for malignancy						
Suspicious for PTC, lymphoma, or other malignancies; metastatic/secondary thyroid tumor	≈3%	Yang et al. (2007), Bongiovanni et al. (2012)	50%–75%	Yang et al. (2007), Baloch et al. (2008), Bongiovanni et al. (2012)	Lobectomy or total thyroidectomy	Cooper et al. (2009)
Malignant						
PTC, Hürthle cell carcinoma, PDTC, FTC, MTC, anaplastic large cell lymphoma, and metastatic carcinoma	5%–8%	Filetti et al. (2006), Yang et al. (2007), Bongiovanni et al. (2012), Cañadas Garre et al. (2012)	97%–100%	Yang et al. (2007), Baloch et al. (2008), Bongiovanni et al. (2012), Cañadas Garre et al. (2012)	Surgery after US assessment	Cooper et al. (2009)

Note: AUS, atypia of uncertain significance; FLUS, follicular lesion of undetermined significance.

Surgical follow-up of these groups yields a percentage of malignancy of 2%–37% in the nondiagnostic category and 20%–60% in the indeterminate category, respectively (Chow et al., 2001; Table 26.4). These cases remain a diagnostic dilemma for patients and clinicians. Diagnostic thyroidectomy is still often required for definitive evaluation. In nonsurgical cases, misdiagnosing can delay therapy and result in poorer prognosis (Yeh et al., 2004; Tee et al., 2007). These intrinsic limitations of FNAB have prompted many efforts to improve its diagnostic Acc. Molecular testing of FNAB specimens for genetic alterations frequently associated with thyroid cancer has emerged as a valuable diagnostic tool.

26.2 Treatment Strategy

Treatment strategy is based on three resources.

26.2.1 Surgical Treatment

The treatment of choice for PTC is surgery: thyroidectomy with or without lymphadenectomy. The thyroid resection of choice is total or near-total thyroidectomy in most cases. In cases of incomplete thyroidectomy, thyroidectomy should be completed especially in cases of large tumors, multifocal, extrathyroidal extension, evidence of vascular invasion, local or distant metastases, history of exposure to radiation, or unfavorable histology. Completion surgery could be avoided for tumors <1 cm (microcarcinomas) in cases of unifocal neoplasms, with no history of radiation and no evidence of capsular or lymphatic involvement (Cooper et al., 2009).

The goal of nodal dissection can be therapeutic (always indicated if lymph nodes are clinically or US detected) or prophylactic in patients with T3 or T4 tumors (Cooper et al., 2009; Carling et al., 2012). The lateral compartment dissection (functional) is always therapeutic and is indicated when laterocervical nodes are proven to be metastatic on clinical and FNAB basis (Cooper et al., 2009; Stack et al., 2012).

26.2.2 Radioiodine Ablation Treatment

Thyroid ablation involves the application of postsurgical ^{131}I, whose aim is to destroy the thyroid remnants after surgery. Radioiodine ablation is always indicated in high-risk patients (T4, extrathyroidal extension, distant metastases) (Cooper et al., 2009). It is contraindicated in patients with very low risk (microcarcinoma without extrathyroidal extension and lymphatic metastases) (Paccini et al., 2006).

26.2.3 TSH Suppressive Treatment

The initial dose of FT4 should be enough to lower serum TSH values under 0.1 mU/L. TSH value is determined at least 3 months after beginning the treatment. TSH suppressive therapy (serum TSH <0.1 mU/L) is mandatory in patients with evidence of persistent disease. For high-risk patients who have reached an apparent remission after treatment, suppressive therapy for 3–5 years is suggested. In low-risk patients considered cured, FT4 dose can be decreased in order to maintain the level of TSH in the lower normal limit (0.5–1.0 mU/L) (Paccini et al., 2006; Cooper et al., 2009).

26.3 Invasive and Noninvasive Markers

For the purposes of this chapter, molecular markers used for the diagnosis of PTC will be classified in the basis of the invasive nature of the strategy required to obtain the sample to determine the marker:

- Invasive molecular biomarker: those that have been investigated in histological samples obtained by an invasive procedure for the individual, that is, FNAB or surgery
- Noninvasive molecular biomarkers: those that can be determined without performing an invasive procedure, that is, they can be determined in blood

26.3.1 Invasive Molecular Biomarkers Currently Used and under Development

26.3.1.1 Gene Mutations in Papillary Thyroid Carcinoma

PTCs often present mutations in genes encoding proteins that transduce signals through the mitogen-activated protein kinase (MAPK) signaling pathway (Figure 26.3). This ubiquitous intracellular cascade regulates important cellular processes as cell growth, proliferation, apoptosis, and survival in response to several ligands as growth factors, hormones, and cytokines that interact with transmembrane receptor tyrosine kinases located in the cell surface, transmitting signals to the cell nucleus (Robinson and Cobb, 1997).

Activating mutations of BRAF, RET, or RAS genes are found in approximately 70% of papillary carcinomas and rarely overlap each other in the same tumor, suggesting that signaling through the MAPK pathway is essential to tumor initiation and that the alteration of a single effector is sufficient for cell transformation (Kimura et al., 2003; Soares et al., 2003; Frattini et al., 2004) (Table 26.5). Despite their common ability to activate MAPK pathway, each of these mutations probably has unique and characteristic effects on cellular transformation, as they are associated with particular gene expression signatures and distinct phenotypical and biological properties of PTCs (Giordano et al., 2005; Adeniran et al., 2006).

Malignant cell transformation in PTCs can also be achieved by acquired gene silencing via aberrant methylation in CpG islands. Genetic and epigenetic alterations, affecting MAPK/ERK and PI3K/Akt signaling pathways, contribute and interact to cause altered patterns of gene expression and function (Xing et al., 2004a; Guan et al., 2008; Eze et al., 2011; Lee et al., 2011; Stephen et al., 2011).

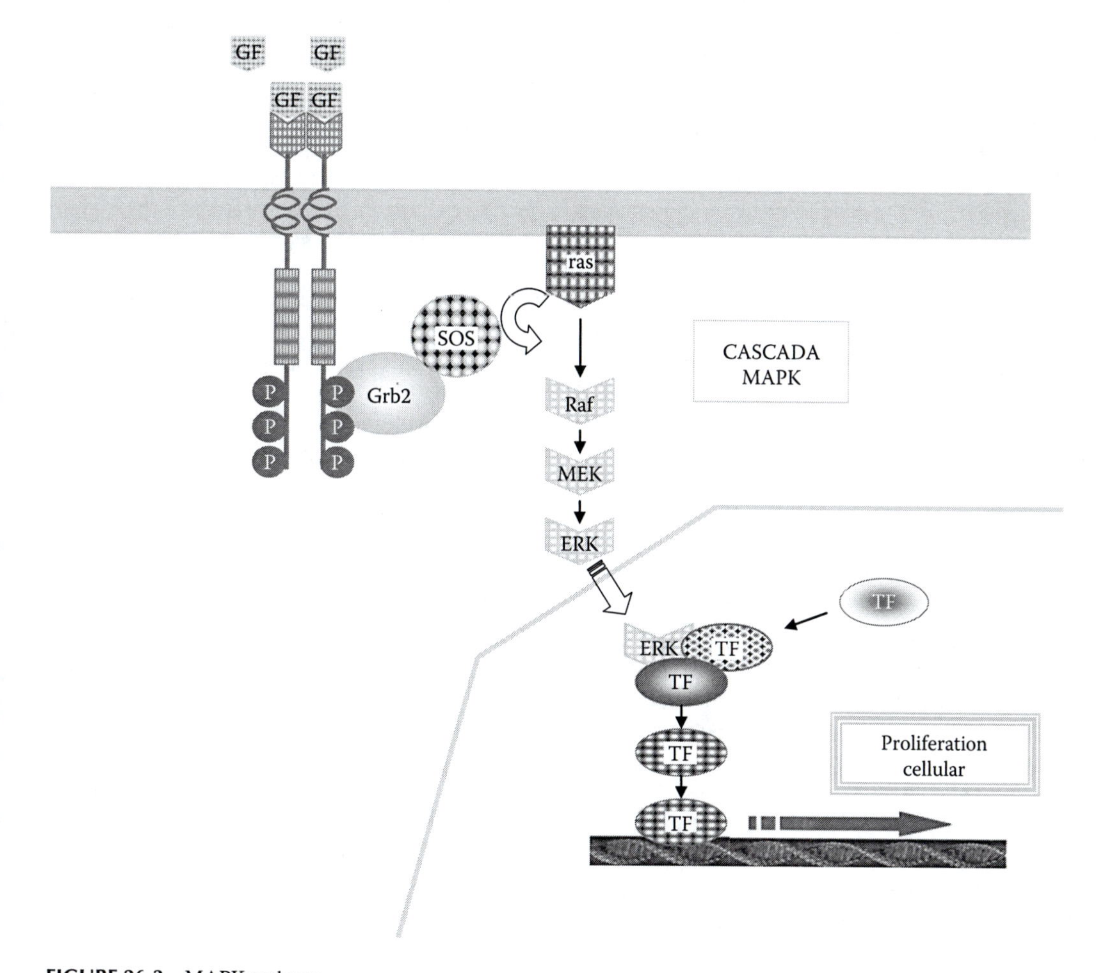

FIGURE 26.3 MAPK pathway.

TABLE 26.5

More Common Molecular Markers in PTC

Molecular Marker	Frequency (%)
BRAF	45
RAS	10–20
RET/PTC	20
PAX8/PPAR	37.5 (FV-PTC)
NTRK1	<10

Note: PTC, papillary thyroid carcinoma; FV-PTC, follicular variant of papillary thyroid carcinoma.

26.3.1.1.1 BRAF Mutations

BRAF is one of the three members of the conserved family of serine threonine kinases RAF (ARAF, BRAF, and CRAF), which are key effectors of the canonical MAPK pathway (RAF–MEK–ERK). This route is crucial in signal transduction by growth factors, hormones, and cytokines and is involved in regulating cell proliferation, differentiation, and apoptosis (Mercer and Pritchard, 2003; Tanoue and Nishida, 2003).

RAF genes have been described as oncogenes because RAF proteins are immediate effectors of RAS oncoproteins, and its initial description was the oncogenic viral form v-raf (Rapp et al., 1983). Activating mutations in the BRAF gene have been discovered in a large panel of human cancers, prominently in cutaneous melanoma (63%–66%) (Brose et al., 2002; Davies et al., 2002) but also in serous ovarian carcinoma (33%–40%) (Davies et al., 2002; Singer et al., 2003) and colorectal carcinoma (11%–20%) (Rajagopalan et al., 2002; Wang et al., 2003).

Point mutations on the BRAF serine–threonine kinase (located on chromosome 7q34) (Cohen et al., 2003; Xing et al., 2005) are mostly (≈90%) of a single type, involving transversion of the thymine at position 1799 of the gene sequence to an adenine (V600E), resulting in the substitution of the amino acid valine, located at position 600 of the protein, for a glutamate (V600E) (Smanik et al., 1995; Davies et al., 2002; Kimura et al., 2003). V600E mutation mimics phosphorylation at the activation segment of BRAF by inserting a negatively charged residue adjacent to an activating phosphorylation site at serine 599 (Davies et al., 2002), causing the conversion of BRAF to a catalytically active form by altering the association of this segment with the P-loop in the ATP binding domain, which normally maintains B-raf in an inactive conformation (Dhillon and Kolch, 2004; Hubbard, 2004; Wan et al., 2004). As a result, the MAPK pathway remains constitutively activated. This chronic stimulation of the MAPK pathway is tumorigenic for thyroid cells, as demonstrated by in vitro and in vivo transformation of thyroid cells (Knauf et al., 2005; Liu et al., 2007), thus confirming that $BRAF^{V600E}$ mutation is an oncogene for thyroid cancer. The role of $BRAF^{V600E}$ in thyroid cancer pathogenesis was explored by Knauf et al. (2005), by targeting its expression to thyroid cells of transgenic mice and demonstrating the origination of PTCs in those animals. The maintenance of proliferation, transformation, and tumorigenicity of BRAF-positive PTC cells was showed by Liu et al. (2007), using BRAF small interference RNA (siRNA) to stably transfect several BRAF-positive PTC cell lines in nude mice. PTC cell proliferation and transformation were only suppressed in specific BRAF siRNA clones, demonstrating the dependence of tumorigenicity and tumor growth on BRAF (Liu et al., 2007).

$BRAF^{V600E}$ mutation can be found in approximately 44% of PTCs (Xing, 2005; Cañadas Garre, 2010; Mathur et al., 2011), although the percentage varies depending on the series between 20% and 83% (Cohen et al., 2003; Kimura et al., 2003; Soares et al., 2003; Kim et al., 2004; Xing, 2005; Jung et al., 2012). $BRAF^{V600E}$ mutation is the main genetic alteration of PTC.

In addition to PTCs, BRAF mutations are found in ATCs and PDTCs, particularly in those tumors that also contain areas of well-differentiated PTC, suggesting that those PDTCs were probably derived from preexistent PTCs (Nikiforova et al., 2003a; Begum et al., 2004; Ciampi and Nikiforov, 2005; Xing, 2005).

Other much less common mechanisms of activation include BRAF K601E mutation, small insertions or deletions retaining the reading frame surrounding codon 600 (Trovisco et al., 2004; Carta et al., 2006;

Hou et al., 2007), and AKAP–BRAF rearrangement, which is more common in PTCs associated with radiation exposure (Ciampi et al., 2005). In the last years, new BRAF mutations have been described in different PTC subtypes (Table 26.6).

Many studies have compared the BRAF^{V600E} mutation distribution in different malignant (FTC, MTC, ATC) and benign thyroid pathologies (MNG, Graves' disease, FA) and in normal thyroid tissue, concluding that this mutation is specific for PTC and PDTCs derived from PTCs (Namba et al., 2003; Nikiforova et al., 2003a; Xu et al., 2003; Fugazzola et al., 2004; Hayashida et al., 2004; Puxeddu et al., 2004; Ciampi and Nikiforov, 2005; Kim et al., 2005b; Xing, 2005; Zhu et al., 2005; Castro et al., 2006; Erickson et al., 2007; Cañadas Garre, 2010; Chuang et al., 2010). Exceptionally, the presence of the BRAF^{V600E} mutation has been described in pathologies different from PTC: in 1 case of 73 patients with FTC (Kebebew et al., 2007), an FTC cell line (Xu et al., 2003), and in 2 cases of atypical nodular hyperplasia (Chung et al., 2006; Kim et al., 2011). BRAF^{K601E} and BRAF^{T599del} mutations have also been described in FTC and FA, respectively (Schulten et al., 2012).

According to previous observations, BRAF^{V600E} mutation is commonly associated with PTCs showing papillary architecture (conventional PTC, tall cell PTC, Warthin PTC, microPTC), with a frequency ranging between 26% and 83% (Fugazzola et al., 2004; Ciampi and Nikiforov, 2005; Trovisco et al., 2005a; Xing, 2005; Xing et al., 2005; Zhu et al., 2005; Riesco-Eizaguirre et al., 2006; Lupi et al., 2007; Costa et al., 2008; Frasca et al., 2008; Oler and Cerutti, 2009; Gao et al., 2012). BRAF^{V600E} mutation prevalence is particularly high (55%–100%) in a high aggressive variant of PTC, the tall cell subtype (Xing et al., 2005; Zhu et al., 2005; Lupi et al., 2007; Cañadas Garre, 2010; Cañadas Garre et al., 2011), whereas it is relatively low (7%–25%) in the follicular variant (Nikiforova et al., 2003a; Fugazzola et al., 2004, 2006; Salvatore et al., 2004; Trovisco et al., 2004, 2005a; Xing, 2005; Xing et al., 2005; Castro et al., 2006; Giannini et al., 2007; Riesco-Eizaguirre et al., 2006; Kebebew et al., 2007;

TABLE 26.6

BRAF Mutations in PTC

	BRAF Mutation		
Study	**Nucleotide Change**	**Amino Acid Change**	**PTC Subtype**
Davies et al. (2002)	V600E	V600E	Classic PTC
Soares et al. (2003) Trovisco et al. (2004)	A1801G	K601E	FV-PTC
Ciampi et al. (2005)		AKAP9–BRAF fusion	Nonspecified
Oler et al. (2005)	1799delTG	V600E + K601del	Conventional PTC
Trovisco et al. (2005b)	TGA 1799–1801	VK600–1E	Solid PTC
Xing et al. (2005)	T1799–1801del	V600E + K601del	Conventional PTC
Hou et al. (2007)	A1799–1816ins	V600D + FGLAT601–605ins	Nonspecified
Carta et al. (2006) Moretti et al. (2006)	1794–1795insGTT	V599Ins	Conventional PTC
Castro et al. (2006)		G474R	FV-PTC
Barzon et al. (2008)	1799–1814delinsATGT	V600–S605delinsDV	FV-PTC
Trovisco et al. (2008)	C1834T	Q612Stop	Conventional PTC
De Falco et al. (2008)	1796–1809delinsTC	T599I-VKSR(600–603)	FV-PTC
Chiosea et al. (2009)	C1796T; 1798_1799insCTT	T599I-V600delinsAL	Solid variant PTC
Santarpia et al. (2009)	C1793T	A598V	FV-PTC
Jung et al. (2012)	1795–1796insA; 1770–1795dup26	Ala598–Thr599insLys; Lys591–Ala598dup	MicroPTC
	1742–10T>C;1799T>A	Val600Glu	Conventional PTC
	1796C>G;1799T>A	Thr599–Val600>ArgGlu	MicroPTC
	1799_1800TG>AA	Val600Glu	MicroPTC
Schulten et al. (2012)	1794–1796delTAC	T599del	FA
	1796–1797insTAC	T599dup	Conventional PTC
Matsuse et al. (2013)	1798delinsTACA	V600delinsYM	Nonspecified

Lupi et al., 2007; Costa et al., 2008; Oler and Cerutti, 2009). The meta-analysis of Lee et al. (2007) confirmed that BRAF^{V600E} mutation is associated with PTC histological subtype, being more prevalent in the conventional (frequency: 59.1%, odds ratio [OR] = 3.521) and tall cell subtypes (frequency: 79.1%, OR = 4.319) than in the follicular variant (frequency: 16.9%, OR = 0.153), indicating that this mutation is associated with papillary growth pattern.

Many studies have investigated the association between the presence of BRAF^{V600E} mutation and more aggressive clinicopathological characteristics of PTC (Namba et al., 2003; Nikiforova et al., 2003a; Xu et al., 2003; Fugazzola et al., 2004; Kim et al., 2004, 2005a,b, 2006a,b; Puxeddu et al., 2004; Sedliarou et al., 2004; Liu et al., 2005; Powell et al., 2005; Trovisco et al., 2005a; Xing et al., 2005; Adeniran et al., 2006; Fugazzola et al., 2006; Jin et al., 2006; Jo et al., 2006; Lee et al., 2006; Park et al., 2006; Riesco-Eizaguirre et al., 2006; Sapio et al., 2006; Abrosimov et al., 2007; Durante et al., 2007; Kebebew et al., 2007; Lupi et al., 2007; Mitsiades et al., 2007; Rodolico et al., 2007; Frasca et al., 2008; Cañadas Garre, 2010; Cañadas Garre et al., 2011). Although the results are not entirely consistent, most studies of various ethnic and geographic demonstrate a significant association of the BRAF^{V600E} mutation with one or more high-risk clinicopathological features of PTC (Namba et al., 2003; Nikiforova et al., 2003a, Kim et al., 2004; Powell et al., 2005; Trovisco et al., 2005; Xing et al., 2005; Adeniran et al., 2006; Fugazzola et al., 2006; Jin et al., 2006; Jo et al., 2006; Kim et al., 2006a,b; Lee et al., 2006; Riesco-Eizaguirre et al., 2006; Durante et al., 2007; Kebebew et al., 2007; Lupi et al., 2007; Nakayama et al., 2007; Rodolico et al., 2007; Elisei et al., 2008; Frasca et al., 2008; Oler et al., 2008; Kwak et al., 2009; Lee et al., 2009; Xing, 2009; Xing et al., 2009; Cañadas Garre, 2010; Cañadas Garre et al., 2011). BRAF^{V600E} mutation has also been shown to be an independent predictor of tumor recurrence, even in patients with stages I–II disease (Xing et al., 2005; Kim et al., 2006b). This mutation has also been associated with decreased avidity to capture radioiodine and treatment failure of recurrent disease, which could be due to deregulation of the function of Na^+/I^- symporter (NIS) and other genes related to iodide metabolism in thyroid follicular cells (Xing et al., 2005; Kim et al., 2006b; Riesco-Eizaguirre et al., 2006). Lower functional NIS protein expression BRAF^{V600E} mutation has recently been observed in the conventional variant of PTC, what could reduce NIS-mediated ^{131}I uptake due to a lower functional NIS protein expression (Gao et al., 2012).

Among the various risk factors, extrathyroidal invasion, lymph node metastasis, and clinicopathological stage III/IV are the most reliable predictors of progression, recurrence, aggressiveness, and, ultimately, increased morbidity and mortality of PTC (DeGroot et al., 1990; Mazzaferri and Jhiang, 1994; Sherman et al., 1998, 2005; Mazzaferri and Kloos, 2001). Interestingly, among the various clinicopathological characteristics of PTC, many studies have shown that BRAF^{V600E} mutation is most frequently associated with these three risk predictors. In a recent review, gathering all studies with sufficient information to calculate the number of cases analyzed, there is a clear significant association of BRAF^{V600E} mutation with extrathyroidal invasion, lymph node metastasis, and advanced stages (III/IV), showing OR of 2.50 (95% CI: 2.11–2.97), 1.83 (95% CI: 1.58–2.13), and 2.14 (95% CI: 1.79–2, 56), respectively (Xing, 2007).

Four studies from the United States (Nikiforova et al., 2003a; Adeniran et al., 2006), Spain (Riesco-Eizaguirre et al., 2006), and Italy (Frasca et al., 2008) showed a significant association of BRAF^{V600E} mutation with extrathyroidal invasion and advanced stages (III–IV). The Italian study also revealed association with lymph node metastasis (Frasca et al., 2008). This association with nodal metastases, extrathyroidal invasion, and advanced stage has also been described in a large international multicenter study (Xing et al., 2005), a meta-analysis (Lee et al., 2007),and a recent study of 500 cases of PTC in a homogeneous Italian cohort from a single institution, which represents the largest study to date to determine the association between the BRAF^{V600E} mutation and clinicopathological features (Lupi et al., 2007). Interestingly, this study also found BRAF^{V600E} significantly associated with loss of the tumor capsule. It has been shown that PTC tumors that lose the capsule are associated with an increased risk of metastasis and recurrence (Ivanova et al., 2002; Kakudo et al., 2004; Lupi et al., 2007).

Another US study confirms the association of the presence of BRAF^{V600E} mutation with lymph node metastasis and advanced stages (III–IV) (Kebebew et al., 2007). In three Korean studies (Kim et al., 2004, 2006d; Lee et al., 2006) and one from the Mayo Clinic (Jin et al., 2006), a significant association of the BRAF^{V600E} mutation with lymph node metastases or extrathyroidal invasion is described; one of them also showed an independent association of the BRAF^{V600E} mutation with lymph node metastasis even when multivariate analysis adjusted for confounding factors was performed (Kim et al., 2006a).

In a recent study of PTC patients with lymph node metastases at diagnosis, the combined presence of BRAF and extranodal extension provided additive prognostic value for a lower disease-specific survival (79% at 10 years) than negativity for both or either variable (100% at 10 years) ($p = 0.004$) (Ricarte-Filho et al., 2012).

Despite this association between BRAF^{V600E} mutation and more aggressive tumor characteristics is not found in all studies (reviewed in Cañadas Garre [2010] and Lassalle et al. [2010]), BRAF^{V600E} is generally considered as a potential marker of aggressive PTC.

In summary, the association of the BRAF^{V600E} mutation with clinicopathological characteristics related to a more aggressive phenotype of PTC has been widely explored, with mixed results. Recently, two extensive reviews have addressed this controversial issue, showing that the most consistent associations observed for BRAF^{V600E} mutation are older age and more advanced tumor stage at diagnosis (Puxeddu and Moretti, 2007; Xing, 2007). The association between BRAF^{V600E} mutation and nodal metastasis appears to be less uniform, probably reflecting the fact that the neck dissection often varies among patients and studies.

The involvement of the mutant form of BRAF^{V600E} in tumor initiation and dedifferentiation and its correlation with more aggressive tumor characteristics has also been suggested in studies developed in transgenic mice with targeted thyroid expression of BRAF^{V600E} (Knauf et al., 2005). These animals developed PTCs with high penetrance and microscopic characteristics similar to those observed in human tumors. Furthermore, these tumors frequently appeared accompanied by invasion of blood vessels, thyroid capsule, and skeletal muscle, all characteristics of more aggressive behavior in humans, and also showed progression to PDTCs.

BRAF mutations are mutually exclusive with the relatively rare mutations of RAS genes, RET (RET/PTC), and NTRK1 rearrangements; all together account for approximately 70% of cases of gene alterations in PTCs (Kimura et al., 2003; Soares et al., 2003; Frattini et al., 2004; Puxeddu et al., 2004; Liu et al., 2005). This mutually exclusive oncogenic activation of RET/PTC, RAS, and BRAF in PTC supports the existence of a linear oncogenic signaling route that would involve RET/PTC–RAS–BRAF–MEK–ERK in these tumors, a concept also reinforced by in vitro functional experiments (Melillo et al., 2005; Mitsutake et al., 2006).

Post-Chernobyl childhood PTCs have shown a very low frequency of BRAF mutations (Kumagai et al., 2004; Lima et al., 2004; Nikiforova et al., 2004; Powell et al., 2005). On the contrary, these tumors present with a very high frequency of RET/PTC rearrangements (Kumagai et al., 2004; Lima et al., 2004). As in sporadic cases, BRAF gene alterations do not coexist with RET/PTC rearrangements. It has been suggested that ionizing radiation contributes to the incidence of PTC mainly by inducing breaks in double-stranded DNA and subsequent illegitimate recombination, leading thus to RET/PTC and NTRK1 rearrangements (Nikiforova et al., 2000, 2004).

26.3.1.1.2 RAS Mutations

The RAS genes (HRAS, KRAS, and NRAS) encode closely related G proteins that play a role in intracellular signal transduction originated from membrane receptors. They are frequently involved in human carcinogenesis; approximately 15% of all human cancers have mutations in these genes (Bos, 1989). Ras mutations found in tumors appear characteristically in codons 12, 13, and 61 of any of the three genes and lead to constitutive activation of RAS proteins. RAS proteins are key intracellular signal transducers that activate several routes, including RAF classical MEK–ERK pathway (Peyssonnaux and Eychène, 2001).

In its inactive state, RAS protein is bound to GDP. After activation, it releases GDP and binds GTP, thus activating the route and other MAPK signaling pathways, such as PI3K/Akt pathway. In normal conditions, the RAS–GTP-activated protein is rapidly inactivated due to its intrinsic GTPase activity and the action of cytoplasmic GTPase proteins. Point mutations in discrete domains of the RAS gene can increase its affinity for GTP (as is the case of mutations in codons 12 and 13) or inactivate its autocatalytic GTPase function (mutation in codon 61). As a result, the mutant protein remains in the active conformation.

Point mutations involving these specific sites (codons 12, 13, and 61) of HRAS, KRAS, and NRAS genes have been reported in approximately 10%–20% of PTCs (Namba et al., 1990; Ezzat et al., 1996; Vasko et al., 2004). PTCs positive for RAS mutations frequently show follicular variant histology, so this mutation also correlates with significantly less marked nuclear features of PTC, more frequent encapsulation, and low proportion of metastatic nodules (Zhu et al., 2003; Adeniran et al., 2006). Some studies have described the association between RAS mutations and a higher frequency of distant metastases (Hara et al., 1994). RAS gene mutations are not restricted to PTC but are found in other benign and malignant thyroid tumors and in tumors of other tissues.

RAS gene mutations are particularly prevalent in carcinomas and thyroid FAs and, less commonly, in PTC (Vasko et al., 2003). Its prevalence in PTC varies widely, depending on the series studied (0%–16%) (Lazzereschi et al., 1997; Sugg et al., 1999; Nikiforova et al., 2003b; Vasko et al., 2003). Mutations associated with PTC (and in general with thyroid lesions) predominantly involve codon 61 of NRAS and, to a lesser extent, of HRAS (Vasko et al., 2003; Zhu et al., 2003; Castro et al., 2006; Di Cristofaro et al., 2006).

26.3.1.1.3 RET/PTC Rearrangements

Growth factor receptors can also lead to cell transformation when its structure is modified by activating mutations. A relevant example to the pathogenesis of PTC is the RET/PTC oncogene (Grieco et al., 1990), a mutant form of the RET receptor tyrosine kinase. RET is the membrane receptor for the neurotrophic glial cell-derived growth factor (Sanicola et al., 1997) and is not normally expressed in thyroid follicular cells. A chromosomal rearrangement joins the promoters of genes related to C-terminal fragment of RET (which loses the transmembrane and extracellular domains), resulting in aberrant production of a truncated form of the receptor on thyroid cells. This chimeric protein contains the region involved in the transmission signal for growth but lacks the sites that allow the reception of the signal (ligand binding) and membrane anchor.

The normal expression of RET and its kinase activity are restricted to a subset of cells derived from embryo neural crest cells (Schuchardt et al., 1994). Consistent with this, the wild type of RET is expressed at high levels in parafollicular C cells, but its expression in thyroid follicular cells is debatable (Nikiforov, 2002).

Several types of Ret rearrangements have been found in human PTC, formed by the fusion of the 3′ intracellular tyrosine kinase domain gene with different 5′ gene fragments:

- *RET/PTC1*: Paracentric inversion formed by the long arm of chromosome 10, leading to fusion with a gene called H4/D10S170 (Grieco et al., 1990).
- *RET/PTC2*: Occurs by a reciprocal translocation between chromosomes 10 and 17, resulting in the juxtaposition of the tyrosine kinase domain of c-ret with a portion of the regulatory subunit of cAMP-dependent protein kinase A (PKA) (Bongarzone et al., 1993, 1994). Nine other types of interchromosome translocations have been identified recently (Nikiforova and Nikiforov, 2008).
- *RET/PTC3*: Paracentric inversion (both RET and ELE1 are on the long arm of chromosome 10) formed by the fusion with RFG/ELE1 (NCOA4) gene (Minoletti et al., 1994; Santoro et al., 1994; Fugazzola et al., 1996).

RET/PTC1, PTC2, and PTC3 are the most frequent RET gene alterations found in PTC, although at least 15 different types have been identified to date (Kondo et al., 2006).

Most unusual types of RET/PTC rearrangements have been identified in PTCs of patients with a history of exposure to ionizing radiation, either therapeutic or environmental (Bongarzone et al., 1993; Klugbauer et al., 1998a; Klugbauer and Rabes, 1999; Corvi et al., 2000; Klugbauer et al., 2000; Salassidis et al., 2000; Saenko et al., 2003), with the exception of ELKS–RET and HOOK3–RET fusions, described in PTCs without apparent history radiation exposure (Nakata et al., 1999; Ciampi et al., 2007). All fusions leave intact the tyrosine kinase domain of RET receptor and enable the RET/PTC oncoprotein bind SHC and activate the RAS–RAF–MAPK cascade (Knauf et al., 2003).

RET/PTC appears on about 20% of adult sporadic PTCs, although the reported frequency varies among different studies, both because of geographic variability as to the different detection Se (Nikiforov et al., 1997; Nikiforov, 2002). Somatic rearrangements of RET proto-oncogene have been detected in 3%–60% of sporadic PTCs (Nikiforov, 2002; Teng and Hempstead, 2004). The prevalence of RET/PTC in PTC varies significantly in different studies, probably reflecting the different methodologies, geographic sampling, and histological composition of the series. RET/PTC frequency is typically higher in patients with radiation exposure antecedents (50%–80%) and in children and younger patients (40%–70%) (Nikiforov et al., 1997; Soares et al., 1998; Fenton et al., 2000; Rabes et al., 2000). The homogeneity of the distribution of RET/PTC rearrangement within the tumor may be quite variable. RET/PTC rearrangements may be clonal (all tumor cells positive) or nonclonal (only a small percentage of tumor cells are positive) (Unger et al., 2004; Zhu et al., 2006). Clonal RET/PTC rearrangement is considered reasonably specific for PTCs (Nikiforova and Nikiforov, 2008) despite RET/PTC has been reported in adenomas and other benign thyroid (Ishizaka et al., 1991; Sheils et al., 2000; Elisei et al., 2001).

RET/PTC1 is the most common type, accounting for 60%–70% of the rearrangements in most series with sporadic PTC, whereas RET/PTC3 corresponds to 20%–30% (Soares et al., 1998; Sugg et al., 1998; Tallini et al., 1998; Nikiforov, 2002). In contrast to this, in thyroid cancers related to Chernobyl, RET/PTC3 rearrangements are the most common (Nikiforov et al., 1997; Motomura et al., 1998; Thomas et al., 1998; Nikiforov, 2002; Williams and Baverstock, 2006), at least for the "first wave" of cancers arising in this context, since RET/PTC1 seems to predominate in cases with a longer latency period (Williams, 2006). Other rarest types of RET/PTC rearrangements seem to be predominantly associated with exposure to radiation (Nikiforov, 2002).

Detection of RET/PTC rearrangements can be achieved on thyroid FNAB samples. Several studies have shown that the detection of RET/PTC on FNAB may improve the preoperative diagnosis of malignant disease in thyroid nodules, particularly in indeterminate or nondiagnostic samples (Cheung et al., 2001a; Salvatore et al., 2004; Domingues et al., 2005; Pizzolanti et al., 2007; Sapio et al., 2007b; Nikiforov et al., 2009; Yip et al., 2009; Cantara et al., 2010; Mathur et al., 2010; Moses et al., 2010; Musholt et al., 2010; Ohori et al., 2010; Nikiforov et al., 2011). Although these studies have demonstrated that RET/PTC rearrangements are capable to detect malignancy on FNAB, some results indicate that this marker is not completely specific of malignancy (Domingues et al., 2005; Nikiforov et al., 2009; Moses et al., 2010), therefore reducing its potential diagnostic utility in thyroid FNAB samples. Another limitation of this test is the need to isolate RNA with acceptable quality to perform the analysis, what can become an issue difficult to achieve in the clinical routine, even using preservative solutions, despite reported by some authors (Nikiforova et al., 2004b).

RET/PTC rearrangements, particularly RET/PTC1, are associated with earlier age, lower stage, higher proportion of lymph node metastases, and conventional papillary subtype (Adeniran et al., 2006). In PTCs with radiation exposure, RET/PTC1 has been found associated with the conventional papillary subtype, whereas RET/PTC3 is associated with the solid variant (Nikiforov et al., 1997).

26.3.1.1.4 NTRK1 (TRKA) Rearrangements

Chromosomal rearrangements detected in PTC also involve NTRK1 (also known as TRKA) (Tallini, 2002), which plays a role in regulating growth, differentiation, and programmed cell death neurons in the central and peripheral nervous system (Teng and Hempstead, 2004). The NTRK1 gene is located on chromosome 1, encoding the high-affinity receptor for nerve growth factor (NGF), whose activation allows the activation of the RAF–MEK–ERK pathway (Miller and Kaplan, 2001).

Rearrangements of NTRK1 involve their fusion to heterologous genes (Nikiforov, 2002) and give rise to chimeric proteins that have shown oncogenic properties derived from permanent abnormal activation of its tyrosine kinase domain (Tallini, 2002). Cell signaling through NTRK1 is modulated by the presence of p75 (NTR) (Miller and Kaplan, 2001). In contrast to NTRK1, p75 (NTR) is able to bind all neurotrophins but loses the intrinsic tyrosine kinase activity (Teng and Hempstead, 2004). Although initially described as a low-affinity receptor, p75 has the same affinity for NGF to NTRK1, and when it is coexpressed with NTRK1, it enhances the ability of the binding and response to neurotrophins. p75 also modulates and enhances the affinity for other receptor tyrosine kinases by their respective ligands (Teng and Hempstead, 2004).

NTRK1 rearrangements are rare, normally found in less than 10% of cases of sporadic PTC (Kuo et al., 2000; Musholt et al., 2000; Frattini et al., 2004; Liu et al., 2005).

The involvement of NTRK1 and p75 (NTR) in the etiopathogenesis of PTC is supported by the detection of NTRK1 rearrangements in PTC and the observation that thyroid-targeted expression of NTRK1 chimeric protein (TRKT1) leads to the development of PTC in transgenic mice (Russell et al., 2000; Rocha et al., 2006).

It has also been reported that the cellular localization of p75 seems to be related to the presence of the $BRAF^{V600E}$, although the biological relevance of this finding is yet unclear (Rocha et al., 2006).

Few studies investigated NTRK1 as a molecular marker on FNAB (Cantara et al., 2010; Mathur et al., 2010; Moses et al., 2010), but the results are unsatisfactory, with no positive results in more than 1100 cytologies analyzed.

26.3.1.1.5 PAX8/PPARγ Rearrangements

PAX8/PPARγ rearrangement is the result of t(2;3)(q13;p25) translocation. PAX8 gene, located in 2q13, encodes a transcription factor essential for the development of the follicular epithelial cell line (Mansouri et al., 1998), and PPARy gene, located on 3p25, encodes a ligand-dependent transcription factor nuclear, which is a member of the family of γ-peroxisome proliferator-activated receptor gamma, pparγ1 (Fajas et al., 1997). Kroll et al. showed that this translocation results in the fusion of the DNA binding domain of PAX8 thyroid transcription factor (2q13) with A–F domains of pparγ1 (3p25) (Kroll et al., 2000). The carcinogenic effect of this process seems to be due to loss of intrinsic transcriptional function of PAX8 and PPARγ1 in the pax8/pparγ rearranged form, as well as and PPARγ and PAX8 normal proteins, due to a PPARγ negative dominant effect on the function (Kroll et al., 2000; Au et al., 2006).

Initially, PAX8/PPARγ was only detected in FTC but not PTC or other thyroid benign neoplasms (FA and multinodular hyperplasia) and was presented as a marker for FTC (Kroll et al., 2000). However, this genetic alteration was subsequently described in several series of thyroid FAs (Marques et al., 2002; Nikiforova et al., 2002a; Cheung et al., 2003), which ruled out the possibility of considering PAX8/PPARγ rearrangements as molecular indicators of malignancy. Some authors even found PAX8/PPARγ fusion gene in a relatively large number of cases of follicular variant PTC (37.5%) (Castro et al., 2005, 2006).

PAX8/PPARγ appears in approximately 35% of classic FTCs and with a lower prevalence in oncocytic carcinomas or Hürthle cells (Dwight et al., 2003; French et al., 2003; Nikiforova et al., 2003b).

Several studies have included this marker to detect malignant nodules as an intent to improve diagnostic Acc on FNAB (French et al., 2008; Nikiforov et al., 2009; Cantara et al., 2010; Mathur et al., 2010; Moses et al., 2010; Ohori et al., 2010). However, its ability to enhance Se is not very high, only one group found 3 positive cases in more than 1000 indeterminate FNABs (Nikiforov et al., 2009, 2011).

26.3.1.1.6 Proteomic Markers in DTC

It is currently known that cancer not only starts at genome level but also achieves the proteomic level, although data obtained from genomic analysis and gene expression studies are limited (Krause et al., 2009).

The term proteomics refers to the global proteome analysis, comprising all the proteins expressed at any given time and in a specific physiological state of a particular biological entity (Wilkins et al., 1996; de Hoog and Mann, 2004). Transcriptome could also be defined as the complete set of RNA transcribed from the genome (Carpi et al., 2010a).

The human genome consists of about 30,000 genes that manifest at least 60,000 polymorphisms. Discrepancies between messenger RNA (mRNA) expression and proteins can be explained by posttranslational modifications (protein glycosylation, acetylation, and phosphorylation). Since these changes are essential for the functional properties of proteins, different modifications will lead to different tumor phenotypes. Proteomics offers the possibility of analyzing the impact of a genetic mutation in the activity of the transcribed protein (Krause et al., 2009).

Proteomic studies in human thyroid tissue are limited due to technical difficulties (Krause et al., 2009):

- There is a very wide range (more than 10 orders of magnitude) in the amount of measurable proteins in the thyroid proteome, which in some diseases will be below pmol/mL.
- Variations in the amount of thyroglobulin (Tg) in each sample of thyroid tissue (low in microfollicular structures and high in macrofollicular).

- The heterogeneity of the sample (follicles, stroma, vessels, erythrocytes, etc.) affects the proteome pattern.
- Tissue samples are not homogeneously classified.

Technical innovations in this field are aimed at that proteomics will become standard practice in the clinical laboratory by detecting tumor markers and even predicting the effect of a given treatment (Damante et al., 2009).

The techniques for the study of the proteome allow the analytical separation and identification of proteins. The most common separation methods include 1D or 2D gel electrophoresis or liquid chromatography, while the standard technique of characterization and identification is mass spectrometry (MS) (Damante et al., 2009). Some of these techniques have been developed to study phosphorylated proteins. The phosphorylation is a key mechanism for many cellular processes (metabolism, proliferation, apoptosis), and thus the phosphoproteomics provides specific cellular metabolic state. Over 1/3 proteins are phosphorylated, and many are protein kinases involved in cell signaling pathways associated with malignant transformation (Krause et al., 2009).

The combination of proteomic data together with gene expression profile provides a tool for deepening in the molecular biology of pathological processes, linking events in gene expression with functional pathways, revealing new targets for the diagnosis and treatment (Krause et al., 2009).

Current proteomic techniques require highly trained personnel and expensive instruments, which limits its use in clinical laboratories. In addition, the technique should be improved to enhance performing and reproducibility of the method, considering preanalytical variables, the variability in the analyses, and biological differences, including the heterogeneity of the tissue to be studied (Damante et al., 2009).

Table 26.7 summarizes the results of proteomic studies performed in thyroid tissue samples.

26.3.1.1.7 Epigenetic Dysregulation in Thyroid Oncogenesis

Epigenetic alterations are changes that occur in genes affecting their expression without altering the nucleotide sequence and play a role in human gene expression. Two epigenetic mechanisms are frequently used by cells to regulate gene expression: DNA methylation and histone modifications (Bird, 2002; Yoo and Jones, 2006). DNA methylation is an epigenetic process in which a methyl group is added to carbon in the fifth position of a cytosine residue in a CpG dinucleotide. Regions rich in CpG dinucleotides are called CpG islands and are located in regions typically flanking the 5′ promoters of the genes. Methylation of the promoter of a gene, particularly near the site of transcription initiation, occurs in close association with chromatin remodeling and is usually associated with gene silencing (Bird, 2002; Yoo and Jones, 2006). This induced gene silencing by methylation occurs by the recruitment of repressors of transcription of the DNA binding methyl groups or by blocking the binding of transcription factors to DNA.

26.3.1.1.8 Hypermethylation of Tumor Suppressor Genes in Thyroid Tumors

As in other human tumors, hypermethylation and therefore inadequate silencing of tumor suppressor genes are common in thyroid tumors. Epigenetic silencing of tumor suppressor genes or regulators of cell adhesion appears to play an important role in tumorigenesis. Detected aberrant DNA methylation (and therefore silencing) of some genes in thyroid cancer includes calcitonin (CALCA), E-cadherin (CDH1), tissue inhibitor of metalloproteinase 3 (TIMP3), death cell-associated protein kinase (DAPK), retinoic acid receptor β2 (RARβ2) (Hoque et al., 2005; Hu et al., 2006a,b), FGF receptor 2 (FGFR2), NIS, p16 (inhibitor of cyclin-dependent kinases: CDK4 and 6), PTEN (Alvarez-Nunez et al., 2006), Ras association domain family 1 (RASSF1A) signal protein (Schagdarsurengin et al., 2002, 2006; Xing et al., 2004a; Hoque et al., 2005; Santoro et al., 2013), RIZ1 nuclear methyltransferase, SLC5A8 and SLC26A4 iodine transporters, or TSH receptor (TSH-R) (Hoque et al., 2005; Russo et al., 2011). Epigenetic silencing of TTF-1 (no expression) through DNA methylation has also been described in more than half of undifferentiated thyroid tumors but not in normal thyroid or PTC (Kondo et al., 2009). These genes have tumor suppressor function that has been well established through several mechanisms. It is therefore conceivable that silencing by methylation of these genes has serious consequences and plays an important role in thyroid oncogenesis.

TABLE 26.7

Proteomic Studies Performed in Thyroid Cancer

Study	N	Comparison	Method	Results[a]
Agretti et al. (2012)	34	Normal tissue, benign pathological tissue, FTC, and PTC	2D-GE ESI-MS/MS	11 protein expression differences between neoplastic and nonneoplastic tissue The normal and nonneoplastic tissues have similar patterns of expression Cathepsin B protein is more distinctive between neoplastic and nonneoplastic tissues (upregulation in neoplasms: FA, FTC, and PTC) ATPQ and PHB are upregulated in PTC
Torres-Cabala et al. (2004)	94	Normal and pathological tissue	2-DE LC-MS	PTC: cytochrome C, S100C, galectin 1, cathepsin B, peroxide dismutase, cathepsin D FTC: polyubiquitin, thioredoxin peroxidase 2, glutathione S-transferase, cathepsin B, VDAC1
Brown et al. (2006)	8	Normal tissue and PTC	2D-DIGE MALDI-TOF-MS	Overexpression of galectin-3, CK-19, and cathepsin B. New proteins identified: S100A6, moesin, peroxiredoxin 2, protein phosphatase 2, 1 protein ligand selenium, vitamin binding protein 2, and mitochondrial functional proteins [HSP 70 (BiP)] IHC validation — Se[b]: ; Sp: ; PPV: ; NPV: S100A6 (>2+, ≥10% cells) — Se 85; Sp 69; PPV np; NPV np
Torres-Cabala et al. (2006)	33	Normal tissue, benign disease, FTC, and PTC. FNAB samples	2-DE LC-MS	PTC: S100C, galectin-1, galectin 1 and 3 cathepsin B, and cathepsin D precursor FTC (100%): VDAC1, cathepsin B IHC validation PTC: galectins especially 3 and S100C FTC: VDAC1
Braunschweig et al. (2007)	144	Normal tissue, FA, FTC, PTC, ATC, and MCT	Matrix of antibodies + IHC[b]	8 proteins detected (ErbB2, annexin IV, IL-11, caspase 9, RARα, FGF-7, STAT5A, c-myc) FA: elevated ErbB2 and secondly caspase 9 PTC: elevated RARα and IL-11. Second c-myc and FGF-7 FTC: elevation of c-myc and FGF-7 and after annexin IV and Stat5a MTC: increased annexin IV, STAT5A, c-myc, IL-11 ATC: low levels of all proteins studied IHC validation AF: ErbB2 PTC: ErbB2 and STAT5a FTC: Annexin IV MTC: All except ErbB2 ATC: ErbB2
Giusti et al. (2008)	13	Ex vivo FNAB. Normal tissue and PTC (classic and tall cell)	2-DE-MALDI-TOF-MS	Proteins overexpressed in PTC: annexin 5, annexin A1, moesin, galectin-3, TTR, β-actin, serum albumin, FLC, α-1 antitrypsin, Apo-A, 1 proteasome activator complex subunit 1 and 2, precursor of α-1 antitrypsin protein DJ-1, cofilin, lactate dehydrogenase-B, glyceraldehyde phosphate dehydrogenase PTC exclusive classic: villin, septin, annexin A1, S100A13, elongation factors 1 and 2, β chain of fibrinogen, glutathione peroxidase 3 precursor, intracellular channel protein chloro-3, carbonyl reductase, and macrophage limitation protein Exclusive of the tall cell variant: ferritin heavy chain, peroxiredoxin 1, and glucose-6-phosphate dehydrogenase

TABLE 26.7 (continued)

Proteomic Studies Performed in Thyroid Cancer

Study	N	Comparison	Method	Results[a]
Netea-Maier et al. (2008)	11	FTC vs. FA	2D-DIGE	FTC > AF: histone H2B, CK7 FTC < AF: CK8 78 kDA, glucose-regulated protein, calreticulin, annexin A3, β-actin IHC validation — Se / Sp / PPV / NPV HSP gp96 ≤+2 — 50 / 83 / 72 / 65 PDI A3 ≤+2 — 37 / 100 / 100 / 64 Calreticulin ≤+2 — 25 / 100 / 100 / 60 Three combinations — 12 / 100 / 100 / 56 HSP gp96 ≤+3 — 87 / 22 / 50 / 66 PDI A3 ≤+3 — 93 / 27 / 53 / 83 Calreticulin ≤+3 — 93 / 44 / 60 / 88
Sofiadis et al. (2010)	98	Normal tissue, PTC, PTC with antecedents of irradiation, FTC, and FA	SELDI-TOF-MS, LC-MS/MS	Overexpression of S100A6 in FTC vs. PTC, AF and normal tissue ($p < 0.001$) IHC validation • Cytoplasmic staining in PTC +3 vs. follicular tumors ($p = 0.004$), especially if a history of irradiation • % of nuclei stained higher in PTC vs. follicular tumors ($p = 0.01$), especially if irradiation antecedents
Krause et al. (2011)	27	Tejido normal, AF, FTC	RT-PCR 2-DE MALDI-TOF-MS/MS	FTC and FA: No mutation in RAS and PI3KCA. No PAX8-PPARγ rearrangement. Neither in normal tissue IHC validation[c]: n = 92 (46 AF and 46 CF) FTC: γ-H2AX (+4), Chk2 (+3). Negative or low in AF RT-PCR: Upregulation of cyclin-E ($p < 0.05$), E2F1 ($p < 0.001$), and Rb ($p < 0.006$) in FTC vs. AD Protein expression: ≥5 of the FTC and expressed ≥1–5 times more ($p < 0.05$): 6 FTC overexpressed in normal tissue vs. FA: SET protein, thioredoxin, β-amilode-A4,-A6 S100, precursor cathepsin B, nucleoside diphosphate kinase A
Sofiadis et al. (2012)	109	Tejido normal, PTC, PTC con antedentes de irradiación, FTC, and AF	2-DE MALDI-TOF-MS	Selection of 9 out of 25 proteins for predictive models: PLS-DA to FTC vs. AF and 19 of 27 for PLS-DA FTC vs. PTC Most significatives: 14-3-3 (isoforms β/α, ε, and ζ/δ), annexin 5, tubulin α chain 1B, peroxiredoxin 6, α1-antitrypsin precursor, selenium-binding protein 1, and disulfide precursor isomerase PLS-DA FTC vs. FA: PPV 100% PLS-DA FTC vs. PTC: PPV 94% IHC validation[c]: Annexin 5 (100% PTC and FA and 89% FTC) and 14-3-3 proteins (80% PTC, 67% FTC, and 33% FA)

Source: Modified from Krause, K. et al., *J. Clin. Endocrinol. Metab.*, 94(8), 2717, August 2009.

Note: np, not provided; PLS-DA, discriminant analysis partial least squares; RT-PCR, reverse-transcription polymerase chain reaction.

IL-11, interleukin 11; HSP gp96, heat shock protein glycoprotein 96; PDI A3 A3, protein disulfide isomerase; ATPQ, ATP synthase D chain; PHB, prohibitin; S100A6, S100 calcium binding, A6 isoform; TTR, transthyretin precursor; VDAC1, voltage protein anion channel 1; APOA1BP, apolipoprotein A-I binding precursor; FLC, serum-free light-chain measurement; γ-H2AX, histone H2AX phosphorylated; Chk2, serine/threonine protein kinase Chk2; SET = I2PP2A: protein inhibitor of tumor suppressor protein phosphatase 2A.

[a] Proteins expressed with differences ±2 times over control.

[b] Values of Se, Sp, PPV, and NPV given in percent.

[c] Validation in independent samples.

RARβ2 appears methylated in thyroid cancer with a frequency of 22%–32% (Hoque et al., 2005; Hu et al., 2006a,b).

Hypermethylation of some tumor suppressor genes has been observed both in thyroid cancer and in benign thyroid tumors, although it occurs more frequently and in greater amounts in malignancies, suggesting their early role in thyroid oncogenesis. PTEN and RASSF1A genes represent two such examples. PTEN encodes a phosphatase that dephosphorylates phosphatidylinositol-3,4,5-trisphosphate, ending the signaling through the PI3K/Akt route (Cantley and Neel, 1999). Inactivating germline mutations and deletions in this gene are the cause of Cowden syndrome, which is associated with the development of FTC and benign neoplasms of thyroid. Recently, hypermethylation of this gene was found in both thyroid benign neoplasms and thyroid cancer, including PTC and FTC (Alvarez-Nunez et al., 2006). Similarly, the RASSF1A gene, which encodes a signaling protein that could function through a route that would be involved Ras, is methylated in many human cancers and in benign thyroid tumors and thyroid cancer, including PTC, FTC, and ATC (Schagdarsurengin et al., 2002; Xing et al., 2004a). RASSF1A is found in PTC at frequencies ranging from 20% to 62% (Schagdarsurengin et al., 2002; Xing et al., 2004a; Nakamura et al., 2005; Xing, 2007). A small fraction of PTCs also exhibit RASSF1A methylation in a mutually exclusive manner with the BRAF mutation, suggesting that the loss of expression of RASSF1A in some PTCs and in follicular is an important process in oncogenesis, irrespective of BRAF/MEK/MAPK pathway (Xing et al., 2004a).

The p16 gene encodes an inhibitor of cyclin-dependent kinases and is recognized as a tumor suppressor gene found in many solid tumors and hematological malignancies (Esteller, 2002). In thyroid cancer, p16 frequency is detected around 25%–44% (Schagdarsurengin et al., 2002; Boltze et al., 2003; Ishida et al., 2007; Lam et al., 2007).

The association with more aggressive pathological features of PTC with methylation of several tumor suppressor genes (TIMP3, SLC5A8, and DAPK) suggests that silencing of these genes could play an important role in the oncogenesis of PTC (Hu et al., 2006b).

TIMP3 is a metalloproteinase tissue inhibitor, which has been shown to inhibit growth, angiogenesis, invasion, and metastasis of various cancers (Anand-Apte et al., 1996; Qi et al., 2003). This gene has been found hypermethylated in many human cancers (van der Velden et al., 2003; Feng et al., 2004; Brueckl et al., 2005; Darnton et al., 2005), including thyroid cancer (Hoque et al., 2005; Hu et al., 2006b). TIMP3 methylation has been associated with extrathyroidal invasion, lymph node metastasis, and multifocality in a large study of PTC cases (Hu et al., 2006b). This is consistent with the loss of function of TIMP3, promoting dissemination of cancer, and favoring angiogenesis, by lacking the ability to effectively block the binding of vascular endothelial growth factor (VEGF) to its receptor (Qi et al., 2003).

SLC5A8 is a member of the sodium symporter family (SLC5), which is expressed in many human tissues, including thyroid (Rodriguez et al., 2002; Lacroix et al., 2004; Porra et al., 2005). Its tumor suppressor function, promoting apoptosis, has been well documented and is frequently methylated in human cancers (Li et al., 2003; Ueno et al., 2004; Hong et al., 2005; Ganapathy et al., 2005), including thyroid cancer (Porra et al., 2005; Hu et al., 2006b). The methylation of this gene is associated with extrathyroidal invasion, multifocality, and PTC advanced stage (Hu et al., 2006b), which strongly supports the role of silencing in the progression of PTC.

DAPK is a calcium-/calmodulin-dependent serine–threonine kinase, which plays a role as a tumor suppressor through its proapoptotic function (Schildhaus et al., 2005). This gene is frequently hypermethylated and silenced in human cancers (Schildhaus et al., 2005), including thyroid cancer (Hoque et al., 2005; Hu et al., 2006b). The methylation of this gene is associated with multifocal PTC (Hu et al., 2006b).

26.3.1.1.9 Hypermethylation of Specific Genes in Thyroid Cancer

Epigenetic dysregulation of iodine metabolism in thyroid cancer is not fully known but seems to be related to the inhibition of genes involved in protein synthesis and loss of ability to concentrate iodine in the follicles (Kondo et al., 2008; Russo et al., 2011). A unique physiological function of the thyroid gland is its ability to capture, concentrate, and use iodine to synthesize thyroid hormones. This process involves several key proteins that are specifically expressed in follicular epithelial cells of the thyroid gland (Nilsson, 2001). The iodide is transported from the blood into the cell by NIS in the basal membrane, followed by transport, presumably by pendrin (also called SLC26A4) in the apical membrane of the cell to the follicular lumen where, by the action of thyroid peroxidase (TPO), iodide is oxidized and organified in Tg on tyrosine residues to form thyroid hormones. The entire process is coordinated by hormonal regulation, in which TSH, acting through binding to the TSH-R, plays a key role. The expression of these molecules responsible for thyroid iodide metabolism is often lost in thyroid cancer (Sheils and Sweeney, 1999; Venkataraman et al., 1999; Arturi et al., 2001; Ringel et al., 2001), and NIS dysfunction or mislocation often occurs, resulting in the loss of the ability of cancer cells to concentrate radioiodine. As a result, these thyroid cancer patients may fail radioiodine therapy, the main cause of mortality and morbidity associated with thyroid cancer (Ain, 2000; Sherman, 2003).

Although the molecular mechanisms underlying the silencing of thyroid-specific genes in thyroid cancer are not clear, hypermethylation is clearly an important mechanism. Many of these thyroid-specific genes are methylated in promoter regions in thyroid tumors, including NIS (Venkataraman et al., 1999; Neumann et al., 2004), TSH-R (Xing et al., 2003b), and the genes for the putative apical iodide transporters in thyroid follicular cells, SLC26A4 (Xing et al., 2003a) and SLC5A8 (Porra et al., 2005; Hu et al., 2006b).

The SLC5A8 tumor suppressor gene is also a putative iodide transporter located in the apical membrane of thyroid follicular cells. Methylation and silencing of this gene are closely associated with the mutation $BRAF^{V600E}$ PTC (Porra et al., 2005; Hu et al., 2006b).

As for the acetylation of histones, this seems to influence p53 and p27 overexpression and loss of expression of NIS, TPO, Tg, and RARβ. Currently, the remodeling of nucleosomes has not been associated with thyroid cancer (Hu et al., 2006a).

26.3.1.2 Gene Expression Profiling of Papillary Thyroid Carcinoma

Microarrays were described in the early 1990s, to analyze gene expression of tens of thousands of genes simultaneously in a single experiment, allowing identifying genes that are expressed in a particular cell at a particular time and under specific conditions. Thus, it has improved the understanding of different signaling pathways and carcinogenesis, described new targets, and new molecular markers for diagnostic and prognosis of cancer patients (Eszlinger et al., 2007).

Gene expression studies can be classified according to the nature of the platform used to analyze gene expression (Eszlinger et al., 2007):

- cDNA microarrays: Fragments of double-stranded DNA from 200 to 500 base pairs (bp), normally synthesized by polymerase chain reaction (PCR).
- Oligonucleotide microarrays: Single strands of 25–70 bp DNA.
- High-density oligonucleotide microarrays: GeneChips. These have permitted the miniaturization of assays. One array or matrix covers the human genome, with over 47,000 transcripts represented by more than 1 million different oligonucleotides.
- Serial analysis of gene expression (SAGE) (Velculescu et al., 1995): It is based on the fact that a short nucleotide sequence (9–10 bp) has enough information to uniquely identify a transcript. Thus, mRNA is obtained from cDNA, and the expression of multiple genes is analyzed quantitatively and simultaneously by multiple transcripts.

The first investigation of gene expression by microarray was performed by Huang et al. (2001). Since then, many studies have been developed, trying to find a marker or combination of markers, which would help distinguish benign from malignant tumors, also in FNAB samples.

Numerous articles have been published analyzing PTC (Huang et al., 2001; Wasenius et al., 2003; Finley et al., 2004a; Giordano et al., 2005; Hamada et al., 2005; Jarzab et al., 2005; Zhao et al., 2006; Delys et al., 2007; Fujarewicz et al., 2007; Murphy et al., 2008; Nikolova, et al., 2008; Kim et al., 2010a,b; Chung et al., 2012; Dom et al., 2012; Hebrant et al., 2012) and FTC gene profile (Barden et al., 2003; Cerutti et al., 2004; Chevillard et al., 2004; Weber et al., 2005; Zhao et al., 2008; Borup et al., 2010). Other studies compared gene profiles between benign and malignant lesions, leading in some cases to combinations of genes able to discriminate malignancy with high levels of Se and, to a lesser extent,

Sp (Aldred et al., 2004; Finley et al., 2004b; Mazzanti et al., 2004; Kebebew et al., 2005, 2006; Rosen et al., 2005; Lubitz et al., 2006; Yukinawa et al., 2006; Durand et al., 2008; Prasad et al., 2008, 2012; Kundel et al., 2010). Additionally to tissue obtained from surgical specimens, the search for markers has also been developed in samples obtained by FNAB in order to reach a preoperative prediction of benign or malignant lesions, irrespectively of demonstrating if the data are reproducible in other contexts (Hamada et al., 2005; Kebebew et al., 2005; Kebebew, 2006; Lubitz et al., 2006; Durand et al., 2008; Kundel et al., 2010; Li et al., 2011; Alexander et al., 2012).

All these studies have identified more than a thousand genes with differences in their expression profile in healthy tissue vs. benign vs. malignant disease. Many may correspond to false positives (FPs), and it is thought that only a small fraction of them will be diagnostically or prognostically useful (Eszlinger et al., 2006). The percentage of genes incorrectly identified by microarray analysis is supposed to be up to 30% (Kebebew et al., 2005). The sources of variability in gene expression in different studies might lay on immunity and immunoglobulin genes, most likely due to tumor infiltration by lymphocytes, a well-documented phenomenon in PTC. Finally, artifacts due to sample preparation or clinical or biological factors cannot be excluded (Jarzab et al., 2005). Given the differences in laboratory techniques or different studies, it is not considered that gene expression profiles can be compared at the level of individual genes but is best described in the terms of combinations of genes (Tamayo et al., 2007).

Validation of gene expression data has been performed using immunohistochemistry or by quantitative real-time reverse-transcription polymerase chain reaction (RT-PCR), which makes quantifiable the results of microarray and therefore more objective. This technique is easy and precise, with commercially available reagents; the results have good interobserver reproducibility, which requires only a small amount of RNA, such as obtained through FNAB (Hamada et al., 2005; Rosen et al., 2005; Weber et al., 2005; Kebebew, 2006; Zhao et al., 2006; Nikiforov et al., 2011).

The information published is so extensive that there have been two meta-analyses (Eszlinger et al., 2006; Griffith et al., 2006) providing external validity to the results. In the meta-analysis by Griffith et al. (2006), the authors determined a set of 12 genes over- or underexpressed in thyroid tumor tissue, relative to healthy controls or benign, with discriminative capacity (MET, TFF3, SERPINA1, TIMP1, FN1, TPO, TGFA, QPCT, CRABP1, FCGBP, EPS8, and PROS1). They started from 21 publications, and the choice of genes was based on the sample size, the magnitude of the differences in expression, and the number of publications that have documented this (Eszlinger et al., 2006). The second meta-analysis (Eszlinger et al., 2006) analyzed the validity of the methodology, that is, to assess whether, indeed, studies in different centers with high-density oligonucleotide microarrays (GeneChip) are comparable. To achieve this, they combined data from tissue samples (cold nodules and PTC), both paired (intraindividual comparison between pathological and healthy tissue) and unpaired (pathological and healthy tissue from different individuals). The aim, among others, was to assess whether it is feasible to compare data from different GeneChip generations. Microarray studies showed to be highly reproducible but only when the selected set of genes belonged to the same study. In addition, it showed that an intraindividual sample selection is necessary to detect subtle changes in the expression patterns of signaling pathways (Griffith et al., 2006).

Underexpression of genes associated with PTC is related to:

- Hormone synthesis (TPO deiodinases I and II or iodine symporter), reflecting the hypofunctionality of most thyroid tumors (Huang et al., 2001; Delys et al., 2007; Fujarewicz et al., 2007)
- Suppression of cell growth and regulation of transcription (Nikolova et al., 2008)

Overexpression of genes associated with PTC is related to:

- Cycle regulation and cell growth (Huang et al., 2001; Wasenius et al., 2003; Jarzab et al., 2005; Delys et al., 2007; Nikolova et al., 2008; Pita et al., 2009; Dom et al., 2012)
- Signal transduction (Chevillard et al., 2004; Jarzab et al., 2005; Griffith, 2006; Nikolova et al., 2008; Pita et al., 2009)
- Regulation of transcription (Wasenius et al., 2003; Griffith, 2006; Nikolova et al., 2008; Pita et al., 2009)

- Apoptosis (Wasenius et al., 2003; Jarzab et al., 2005; Nikolova et al., 2008)
- Proteolysis (Detours et al., 2005; Griffith, 2006; Delys et al., 2007; Nikolova et al., 2008; Banito et al., 2009; Pita et al., 2009)
- Adhesion molecules (Huang et al., 2001; Wasenius et al., 2003; Chevillard et al., 2004; Detours et al., 2005; Jarzab et al., 2005; Griffith et al., 2006; Delys et al., 2007; Nikolova et al., 2008; Pita et al., 2009; Dom et al., 2012)
- Immune response, immunoglobulins (Chevillard et al., 2004; Jarzab et al., 2005; Griffith et al., 2006; Delys et al., 2007; Nikolova et al., 2008)
- Cytoskeleton and cell matrix (Chevillard et al., 2004; Jarzab et al., 2005)

It has also been studied the association between gene expression profile and mutational status: RAS, BRAF, or RET/PTC (Giordano et al., 2005). They found a very strong correspondence between expressions, not only with gene and tumor morphology but also with the presence of RET/PTC rearrangements and the presence of mutations in RAS or BRAF. Interestingly, although the correlation between $BRAF^{V600E}$ mutation and aggressive form of PTC is controversial, underexpression of TPO in subjects with mutant $BRAF^{V600E}$ might be related to less iodine uptake and therefore less response to ablative therapy.

Other researchers have sought expression differences between PTC variants, showing that conventional PTC is distinguishable from tall cell and follicular variants (Chevillard et al., 2004; Wreesmann et al., 2004; Giordano et al., 2005).

PTC and ATC gene expressions have common points, so that the majority of all expressed genes in ATC are also expressed in some PTC and 43% of those expressed in all PTC are similarly expressed in all ATC. This fact supports the hypothesis that ATCs are especially derived from PTC (Hebrant et al., 2012). The function of genes differently expressed in ATC is related to inflammatory response, the transition from epithelial to mesenchymal tissue and invasion, a high rate of proliferation and dedifferentiation, the process of calcification and fibrosis, high glucose metabolism, lactate formation and chemoresistance. In the study by Hebrant et al. (2012), nine genes are capable of discriminating both types of tumor, underexpressed in ATC and overexpressed in PTC: Nell2, SPINT2, MARVELD2, DUOXA1, RPH3AL, TBX3, PCYOX1, c5orf41, and pKP4. This could be considered an aggressive profile associated with epithelial–mesenchymal transition, dedifferentiation, and glycolysis (Hebrant et al., 2012).

Table 26.8 shows the results of studies developed to investigate gene expression profile in PTC, providing details of Se, Sp, PPV, NPV, and Acc, if they are available. Since genes are expressed with their abbreviated nomenclature, a glossary is appended with complete identification.

26.3.1.3 Immunohistochemical Biomarkers

Immunohistochemistry studies protein expression and localization within the cell. Currently, a large number of tissue specific thyroid antigens have identified, allowing the characterization of certain diseases affecting the thyroid (Faggiano et al., 2007).

Thyroid-specific proteins useful in diagnosis for this technique are (Faggiano et al., 2007) as follows:

- Tg: It is present in all DTCs and confirms any thyroid tumor of follicular origin, including metastatic tumors of the thyroid.
- TPO: Staining negativity with MoAB47 monoclonal antibody is considered a marker of malignancy in follicular cell-derived tumors.
- TTF-1: It is expressed with great intensity in DTC. In PTC, its presence is associated with more aggressive tumors.
- NIS, SLC26A4 (pendrin), and SCL5A8 (AIT) are negative in most DTC. In some cases, NIS overexpression of PTC is positive staining at intracellular level.
- ATCs are negative for all thyroid-specific proteins and are positive for cytokeratins.

TABLE 26.8

Gene Expression Profile in PTC

Author	Sample	Method	Validation	Gen[a]	Results[b]
Takano et al. (2000)	Surgical thyroid samples 1 NT 4 thyroid tumors	SAGE	RT-PCR	600 tags in each tissue	CTSB: higher rate in PTC and FTC than NT or FA. SPARC, TBCA, GPX, GAPDHS, and Tg were expressed at different levels in differentiated and undifferentiated carcinomas.
Huang et al. (2001)	8 PTC 7 NT (paired)	Affymetrix HG-U95A oligonucleotide arrays	*RT-PCR*: 2 same PTC and 6 independent samples *IHC*: 42 PTC, 6 FTC, 1 CAT, 9 NT	*RT-PCR*: In PTC *U-R*: FN1, CITED1, CHI3L1, ODZ1, ADORA1, and SCEL *D-R*: GAS1, TFF3, FOSB, and ITPR1 *IHC*: CITED1, SFTPB	PTC is characterized by consistent and specific molecular changes.
Wasenius et al. (2003)	Surgical samples: 18 PTC 3 NT (not paired)	Atlas Human Cancer 1.2 cDNA array	*RT-PCR*: same sample *IHQ (TMA)*: same samples (16 PTC) + 107 (PTC) independent samples from Tissue Bank	*RT-PCR*: MET, FN, TIMP-1, and GADD153 *IHQ (TMA)*: FN, TIMP-1, MMP-11	MET and MMP-11 were only expressed in tumor tissues. PTC shows U-R: FN: 100%; IHQ 81% TIMP-1: 94%; IHQ 68% MET (94%) MMP-11: IHQ 87% PTC shows D-R: GADD153 (89%).
Aldred et al. (2004)	28 samples 6 PTC 9 FTC 13 NT (paired with PTC but not with FTC)	Affymetrix U95A_v2 GeneChips	RT-PCR Same samples + 10 FTC	CAV1 CAV2 CLDN10 IG-FBP	5 genes PTC vs. FTC *PTC*: U-R CITED1, CLDN10, IG-FBP6 *FTC*: no expression of CLDN10; D-R IGFBP6, CAV1, and CAV2.
Finley et al. (2004a)	Surgical samples 21 TBD 14 carcinomas (PTC, FV-PTC) Evaluation in 7 independent and unknown tumors	Affymetrix GeneChip Hu95 array	RT-PCR Immunoblot	*RT-PCR*: Adrenomedullin TROP-2, MET, NRP-2, trefoil *immunoblot*: NRP2	*Cancer vs. BTD*: S 93%; Sp 100% *FV-PTC vs. TBD*: S 91% Sp 100% *PTC vs. TBD*: S 100%, Sp 100%

TABLE 26.8 (continued)

Gene Expression Profile in PTC

Author	Sample	Method	Validation	Gen[a]	Results[b]
Chevillard et al. (2004)	Tissue Bank 6 NT/TBN (4 paired) 3 FTC 3 VF-PTC 2 PTC	Soares human infant brain 1NIB library (Genethon)	RT-PCR same samples	DUSP5, CYR61, and SDC4	Tumor vs. nontumor: gene expression differences Follicular neoplasm vs. FV-CPT: differentiated by set of 75 genes FA vs. FTC: similar gene expression (only 43 different genes) CPT vs. VF-CPT: differentiated by set of genes
Jarzab et al. (2005)	Surgical samples: 50 Training set: PTC 16 NT/ TBD (paired) 16 Validation set: PTC 7 NT/ TBD 11	Affymetrix GeneChip HG-U133A array	RT-PCR	DPP4, GJB3, ST14, SERPINA1, LRP4, MET, EVA1, SPUVE, LGALS3, HBB, MKRN2, MRC2, IGSF1, KIAA0830, RXRG, P4HA2, CDH3, IL13RA1, and MTMR4	*RFR-20 set*: Acc 94.4% (95% CI: 72.7–99.9 PTC diagnosis: S 85.7%, Sp 100%
Giordano et al. (2005)	Tissue Bank 51 PTC 4 NT (not paired)	Affymetrix GeneChip U133A array. Genotyping: RET/PTC1 y-3, HRAS, NRAS, KRAS, BRAF	IHC (TMA): 98 CPT, independent samples all but 6	IHQ: TPO	Mutational status determines gene expression variation. May predict success for therapies against the consequences of these mutations
Hamada et al. (2005)	18 PTC 18 NT (paired) 21 BTD 10 blood samples 38 FNAC in vivo	RT-PCR *U-R genes*: CITED1, CHI3L1, FN1, RIL, and SFTPB *D-R genes*: ITPR1, TFF3, and TPO	RT-PCR: 9 FNAC samples with final diagnosis 29 FNAC samples with only cytological diagnosis	*U-R genes*: CITED1, CHI3L1, FN1, RIL and SFTPB *D-R genes*: ITPR1, TFF3	9 FNAC samples: S 75%, Sp 100%, Acc 88.9% 29 FNAC samples: 24.1% shows a PTC gene expression pattern by RT-PCR without cytological signs of PTC. The remaining samples were classified correctly.
Zhao et al. (2006)	46 surgical samples 16 PTC (FV-PTC) 13 FTC	High-density cDNA filters (RZPD library 956, Human Unigene Set 2	RT-PCR in 12 random selected of the same samples	Tg PAX8 FN1 CNN3	CPT is similar to FV-CPT CFT minimally invasive vs. widely invasive: significant differences. VF-CPT vs. CFT: significant differences

(*continued*)

TABLE 26.8 (continued)

Gene Expression Profile in PTC

Author	Sample	Method	Validation	Gen[a]	Results[b]
Fujarewicz et al. (2007)	Tissue Bank (Huang et al., 2001; Eszlinger et al., 2004; Jarzab et al., 2005) 57 PTC 61 TBD 62 NT (paired or not)	Affymetrix 90 HG-U95A (Huang, Eszlinger) and Affymetrix 90 HG-U133A (Jarzab) oligonucleotide arrays	—	FN1, MET, DPP4, SERPINA1, KRT19, LGALS3, CITED1, DUSP6, SFTPB, TIMP1, MUC1, ADM, TROP2, NRP2, KIT, CDH1, LSM7, SYNGR2, FAM13A1, IMPACT	*20-gene classifier*: PTC diagnosis: Acc 98.5% (95% CI; 0.959–1) Benign vs. malignant: Acc 98.6% Lesions misclassified: 10.5%
Delys et al. (2007)	Tissue Bank: 12 Surgical samples: 14 26 PTC 26 NT (paired)	Agilent Human 1 cDNA microarray	RT-PCR (same samples). Combined with PTC microarray data sets from Jarzab et al. (2005), Huang et al. (2001)	*11 U-R*: ANXA1, CDH3, CLDN1, DUSP5, GPX1, HMGA2, NELL2, NRCAM, SLIT1, THBS2, TNC *4 D-R*: BCL2, EGR1, EGR2, FLRT2	44% of the transcriptome is regulated. Excellent agreement between 3 data sets
Durand et al. (2008)	Tissue Bank 6 FA 8 FTC 14 PTC (5 FV-PTC) 28 NT (paired)	Oligonucleotide-based low-density macroarray on nylon membrane	RT-PCR FNAC: 25 ex vivo samples	*RT-PTC*: ALDO A, GOT1, GAPD: increased in FTC. CDKN1A: increased in PTC and FTC. Lesser in FA SLC26A4 and TFF3: reduced expression in FTC and PTC	*Prediction models*: *PTC* (9/57 genes): S 86%, Sp 100% *PTC+FTC* (12/21 genes): S 91%, Sp 100% *FTC* (9/26 genes): S 100%, Sp 100% *Global* 19 common genes in 3 previous groups: median prediction strength = 0.92
Nikolova et al. (2008)	Surgical samples 18 PTC 18 NT (paired, adjacent). Human thyroid cancer cells: FTC-133	Affymetrix human genome U133 Plus 2.0 GeneChip arrays	Same samples RT-PCR northern blot	*RT-PCR*: CHI3L1 F AM20A KLHDC8A LRP4 NMU TM7SF4 RGS4 *Northern blot*: RGS4	Downregulation of RGS4 in thyroid cancer cells significantly attenuated its viability
Murphy et al. (2008)	Surgical samples PTC 9 NT 11	Affymetrix Human U133 GeneChip Set	IHQ of 88 independent Tissue Bank samples: TMA NT paired and adjacent 19 PTC 20 FV-PTC 9 FTC 14 HT 11 FA 15	U-R in PTC P-cadherin Bax Cytokeratin-19 Galectin-3	*CDH3* 0% NT 67% PTC *BAX* 0% NT 56% PTC *CK19* NT< CPT ($p < 0.0001$) FA< FV-PTC ($p = 0.0012$) *Galectin-3* NT< CPT ($p < 0.0001$) FV-PTC< PTC ($p = 0.0066$)

TABLE 26.8 (continued)

Gene Expression Profile in PTC

Author	Sample	Method	Validation	Gen[a]	Results[b]
Kim et al. (2010a)	Surgical paired samples PTC 5 samples NT 5 paired samples	Illumina HumanHT-12 v3 Expression BeadChip microarray	35 patients: RT-PCR IHC	*RT-PCR*: *U-R*: TM7SF4, SLC34A2, KCNJ2, COMP, KLK7 *D-R*: TFCP2L1, LYVE-1, FOXA2, SLC4A4 *IHC*: FOXA2, COMP, LYVE-1	—
Kim et al. (2010b)	80 CPT and mCPT 80 NT (paired)	Affymetrix Human Genome U133 Plus 2.0 arrays	—	—	mPTC and PTC show no difference in gene expression. mPTC should be considered an early stage of disease, which eventually evolves into PTC.
Hébrant et al. (2012)	Tissue Bank 11 ATC 48 PTC	Affymetrix HU 133 Plus 2.0 arrays	RT-PCR 5 ATC 5 PTC (independent samples)	NELL2, SPINT2, MARVELD2, DUOXA1, RPH3AL, TBX3, PCYOX1, c5 or f41, PKP4	43% of genes D-R in PTC were D-R in ATC. Signature of aggressiveness: 9 genes D-R in ATC and U-R in PTC
Dom et al. (2012)	Tissue Bank 50 thyroid cancer and paired NT: 22 radiation exposed 28 not exposed	Affymetrix Human Genome U133 Plus 2.0 arrays	RT-PCR External set (Jarzab)	SERPINE1, DUSP1, TRIB1, S100A10, ANXA1, GNAL, RDH12	793 probes gene set: Acc 69% Differentially expressed genes between exposed and nonexposed NT but not among tumors
Chung et al. (2012)		Illumina Human-8 Expression BeadChip microarray	RT-PCR (the same sample)	CDH3, NGEF, PROS1, TGFA, MET	90 probes gene set: Acc: 100%

Note: NT, normal tissue; PTC, papillary thyroid carcinoma; FV-PTC, follicular variant of CPT; mCPT, microCPT; FTC, follicular thyroid cancer; ATC, anaplastic thyroid carcinoma; BTD, benign thyroid disease; FA, follicular adenoma; HT, Hashimoto's thyroiditis; TMA, tissue microarray; U-R, upregulated; D-R, downregulated; IHC, immunohistochemical assay.

[a] Results from validated sample.

[b] Classification model tested; paired: NT obtained from contralateral lobe.

(*continued*)

Abbreviations: ACSL1, acyl-CoA synthetase long-chain family member 1; ADM, adrenomedullin; ADORA1, adenosine A1 receptor; ALDO A, aldolase A, fructose-bisphosphate; APOD, apolipoprotein D; ASCL1, achaete-scute complex homolog 1 (Drosophila); Bax, BCL2-associated X protein; BCL2, B-cell CLL/lymphoma 2; c5 or f41, novel junction protein; CAV1, CAVEOLIN 1; CAV2, CAVEOLIN 2; CCL21, chemokine (C-C motif) ligand 21; CCND1, cyclin D1; CD44, CD44 molecule (Indian blood group); CDH, cadherin 3, type 1, P-cadherin; CDH1, cadherin 1; CDH3, cadherin 3, type 1, P-cadherin (placental); CDK2AP1, cyclin-dependent kinase 2 associated protein 1; CDKN1A, cyclin-dependent kinase inhibitor 1A (p21, Cip1); CHI3L1, chitinase 3-like 1 (cartilage glycoprotein-39); CITED1, Cbp/p300-interacting transactivator; CITED2, Cbp/p300-interacting transactivator, with Glu/Asp-rich carboxy-terminal domain, 2; CLDN1, claudin 1; CLDN10, claudin 10; CNN3, calponin 3, acidic; COMP, cartilage oligomeric matrix protein; CTSB, cathepsin B; CYR61, cysteine-rich, angiogenic inducer, 61; DIO1, type I iodothyronine deiodinase; DIO2, type II iodothyronine deiodinase; DPP4, dipeptidyl peptidase 4; DPT, dermatopontin; DUOXA1, dual oxidase activator 1; DUSP1, dual specificity phosphatase 1; DUSP5, dual specificity phosphatase 5; DUSP6, dual specificity phosphatase 6; EBAG9, estrogen-responsive gene; EGR1, early growth response 1; EGR2, early growth response 2; EVA1, epithelial V-like antigen; FAM13A1, family with sequence similarity 13, member A1; FAM20A, family with sequence similarity 20, member A; FLRT2, fibronectin leucine-rich transmembrane protein 2; FN1, fibronectin 1; FOSB, FBJ murine osteosarcoma viral oncogene homolog B; FOXA2, forkhead box A2; GADD153, growth arrest and DNA damage-inducible; GAPDHS, glyceraldehyde-3-phosphate dehydrogenase; GAS1, growth arrest-specific 1; GJB3, gap junction protein, beta 3, 31 kDa; GNAL, guanine nucleotide-binding protein G(olf) subunit alpha; GOT1, glutamic–oxaloacetic transaminase 1, soluble (aspartate aminotransferase 1); GPX, glutathione peroxidase; GPX1, glutathione peroxidase 1; GRB2, growth factor receptor-bound protein 2; HBB, hemoglobin, beta; HMGA2, high mobility group AT-hook 2; Id4, inhibitor of DNA binding 4, dominant negative helix–loop–helix protein; IG- FBP, insulin-like growth factor binding; IGSF1, immunoglobulin superfamily, member 1; IL13RA1, interleukin 13 receptor, alpha 1; IMPACT, impact homolog; ITPR1, inositol 1,4,5-trisphosphate receptor, type 1; JUNB, jun B proto-oncogene; KCNJ2, potassium inwardly rectifying channel, subfamily J, member 2; KIT, v-kit Hardy-Zuckerman 4 feline sarcoma viral oncogene homolog; KLHDC8A, kelch domain containing 8A; KLK7, kallikrein-related peptidase; KRT19, keratin 19; LGALS3, galectin-3 (lectin, galactoside binding, soluble 3); LNK, SH2B adaptor protein 3; LRP4, low-density lipoprotein receptor-related protein gene; LSM7, LSM7 homolog, U6 small nuclear RNA associated; LYVE-1, lymphatic vessel endothelial hyaluronan receptor 1; MARVELD2, MARVEL domain containing 2; MATN2, matrilin 2; MET, hepatocyte grown factor receptor; MKRN2, makorin ring finger protein 2; MMP-11, matrix metallopeptidase 11 (stromelysin 3); MRC2, mannose receptor, C type 2; MSL3L1, male-specific lethal 3 homolog (Drosophila); MSN, binds to the osteopontin (OPN); MTMR4, myotubularin-related protein 4; MUC1, mucin 1, cell surface associated; NELL2, protein kinase C-binding protein NELL2; NGEF, neuronal guanine nucleotide exchange factor; NMU, neuromedin U; NRCAM, neuronal cell adhesion molecule; NRP2, neuropilin 2; NTRK2, neurotrophic tyrosine kinase, receptor, type 2; NTRK3, neurotrophic tyrosine kinase, receptor, type 3; ODZ1, tenascin M1, odz, odd Oz/ten-m homolog 1 (Drosophila); P4HA2, prolyl 4-hydroxylase, alpha polypeptide II; PAX8, paired box 8; PCYOX1, prenylcysteine oxidase 1; PKP4, plakophilin 4; PROS1, protein S; RDH12, retinol dehydrogenase 12; RGS4, regulator of G-protein signaling 4; RIL, PDZ and LIM domain 4; RPH3AL, rabphilin 3A-like (without C2 domains); RXRG, retinoid X receptor gene; S100A10, S100 calcium-binding protein A10; S100A6, calcyclin; SCEL, sciellin; SDC4, syndecan 4; SERPINA1, serpin peptidase inhibitor, clade A, member 1; a-1 antitrypsin; SERPINE1, serpin peptidase inhibitor, clade E (nexin, plasminogen activator inhibitor type 1), member 1; SFN, stratifin; SFTPB, surfactant, pulmonary-associated protein; SLC26A4, solute carrier family 26, member 4; SLC34A2, solute carrier family 34 (sodium phosphate), member 2; SLC4A4, solute carrier family 4, sodium bicarbonate cotransporter, member 4; SLC5A5, NIS, sodium iodide symporter; SLIT1, slit homolog 1 (Drosophila); SPARC, osteonectin, secreted protein, acidic, cysteine rich; SPINT2, serine peptidase inhibitor, Kunitz type, 2; SPUVE, protease, serine, 23; ST14, suppression of tumorigenicity 14 (colon carcinoma); SYNGR2, synaptogyrin 2; TBCA, a-tubulin; TBX3, T-box protein 3; TFCP2L1, transcription factor CP2-like 1; TFF, trefoil; TFF3, trefoil factor 3 (intestinal); Tg, thyroglobulin; TGFA, transforming growth factor alpha; THBS2, thrombospondin 2; TIMP1, metallopeptidase inhibitor 1; TM7SF4, transmembrane 7 superfamily member 4; TMPRSS4, transmembrane protease, serine 4; TNC, tenascin C; TNFRSF25, tumor necrosis factor, a proinflammatory cytokine; TPO, thyroid peroxidase; TRIB1, tribbles homologue 1; TROP2, tumor-associated calcium signal transducer.

TABLE 26.9

Immunohistochemical Markers in Thyroid Cancer

	Benign (%)	PTC (%)	FTC (%)	ATC (%)	MTC (%)
Galectin-3	4.5–11	72.6–98.9	21–66	100	0
HBME	2.3–31.5	85–94	50–88	0	0
CK19	0–16.9	72–96.7	21–50	0–25	20
HMWCK	59.7	59.7	0	—	—
Cyclin D1	66.9	66.9	40	—	—
p27 loss	83.4	83.4	60	—	—
CITED1	87	87	50	5.5	—
FN1	91	91	50	1.9	—

Sources: de Matos, P.S. et al., *Histopathology*, 47(4), 901, 2005; Prasad, M.L. et al., *Mod. Pathol.*, 18(1), 48, 2005; Park, Y.J. et al., *J. Korean Med. Sci.*, 22(4), 621, 2007.

Note: TB, benign; HBME1, Hector Battifora mesothelial antibody 1; CK19, cytokeratin 19; HMWCK, high molecular weight cytokeratin; p27, protein cyclin-dependent kinase inhibitor; CITED1, gene encoding the MSG1 protein (melanocyte-specific gene 1); FN1, fibronectin.

- Negativity for CEA and calcitonin excludes MTC.
- Negativity for common leukocyte antigen (CLA) excludes lymphoma.

In general, infra- or overexpression of proteins related to cell cycle or tumor invasion may help in differentiating benign from malignant tumors (Liang et al., 2009).

Table 26.9 shows a list of the markers most frequently detected by immunohistochemistry and with more capacity to discriminate between benign and malignant tumors.

26.3.1.4 MicroRNAs

MicroRNAs (miRNAs) are a new class of regulatory small molecules, not transcribed to proteins. They function as negative regulators of gene expression in all the processes involved in carcinogenesis: differentiation, proliferation, and cell survival. It is estimated that 1 miRNA can regulate over 200 genes and each gene has targets for multiple miRNAs. If miRNA binding to the mRNA molecule is perfect, protein synthesis continues. Otherwise, it produces the translational repression and thus inhibits protein synthesis (Figure 26.4). Imperfect binding is the feature that allows one miRNA to regulate multiple genes (Nikiforova et al., 2009).

There are at least 1600 (mirbase.org, release 19) of these 20–24 nt molecules already described in humans.

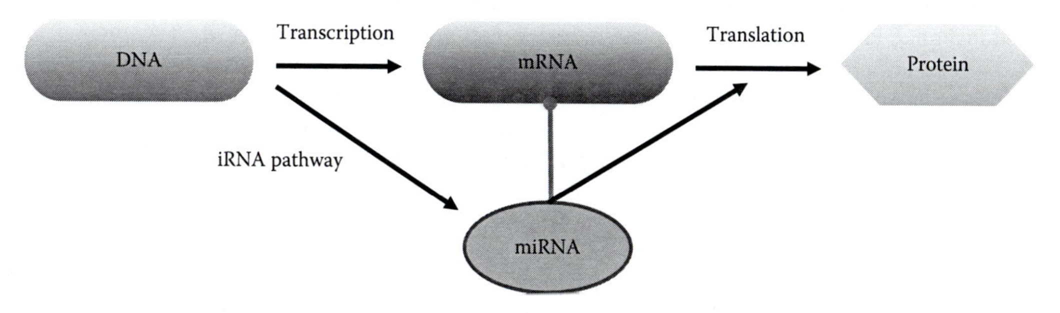

FIGURE 26.4 Regulation of miRNA-mediated gene expression. (Modified from Nikiforova, Y.E. et al., *J. Clin. Endocrinol. Metab.*, 94(6), 2092, 2009.)

Several miRNAs with specific gene targets have been identified:

- let-7 inhibits RAS in lung cancer, acting as a suppressor gene. It is also related to RET/PTC: RET/PTC3 oncogenic expression reduces let-7f expression in rat thyroid cell. Transfection of TCP-1 cells (with RET/PTC1) with let-7 inhibits the MAPK pathway activation, and consequently, cell growth is reduced. This fact is probably due to the reduction of the expression of cell cycle promoters (myc, CCND1) and stimulation of inhibitors as p21 (Ricarte-Filho et al., 2009).
- miR-221 and miR-222 expression can reduce p27 protein levels by direct action on their encoding genes, thus regulating the cell cycle (Visone et al., 2007). The overexpression of miR-221, miR-222, and miR-146, over 11–19-fold, determines a large decrease in KIT transcription and consequently in Kit protein synthesis.
- miR-16-1 and miR-15a both inhibit BCL2 (Nikiforova et al., 2009).
- Several target genes for miRNAs have been recently described as a potential diagnostic tool for thyroid cancer (Vriens et al., 2012). miR-100 acts on inhibitor of DNA binding 1 (ID1), fibroblast growth factor receptor 3 (FGFR3), early growth response 2 (EGR2), and matrix metallopeptidase 13 (MMP13). miR-125b affects Kruppel-like factor 13 (KLF13), chemokine (C-X-C motif) ligand 11 (CXCL11), and forkhead box A1 (FOXA1). miR-138 acts on telomerase reverse transcriptase (hTERT) and thyroid hormone receptor, beta (thrB). miR768-3p influences adaptor-related protein complex 1, gamma 1 subunit (AP1G1).

One well-established cause of thyroid cancer is ionizing radiation. Nikiforova et al. (2011) have studied its influence on the miRNA profile in cultured human thyroid cells, and, although they have found four different patterns of response during the first 4–24 h after radiation, these changes are not apparently linked to the processes of carcinogenesis, at least directly (Nikiforova et al., 2011).

miRNA overexpression results in inhibition of tumor suppressor genes, whereas miRNA downregulation will determine the stimulation of oncogenes, with the consequent effect on cell cycle regulation, proliferation, apoptosis, and other carcinogenic mechanisms (Vriens et al., 2012). Based on this, two different types of miRNA can be distinguished (Braun and Huttelmaier, 2011):

- OncomiRs: those that promote carcinogenesis
- Tumor suppressor miRNAs: those that antagonize cancer progression

miRNA expression profiles are specific for every tissue; therefore, those derived from C cell tumors (MTC) are significantly different from those arising from follicular cells (PTC, FTC, PDTC, ATC). Even among tumors derived from the same cells, profiles may vary greatly (Nikiforova et al., 2009).

In general, less aggressive tumors, like DTCs (PTC and FTC), often show oncomiRs (miR-221, miR-222, miR-146b) upregulated, stimulating cell proliferation and inhibiting apoptosis. Conversely, undifferentiated tumors (ATC, PDTC) are characterized by a significant suppression of the suppressor miRNAs, favoring dedifferentiation (Braun and Hüttelmaier, 2011). This dedifferentiation is merely the transformation of epithelial tissue into mesenchymal, promoted by downregulation of the -200 and -30 families of miRNAs. The expression of these miRNAs in mesenchymal ATC-derived cells causes a reduction in their invasive potential and induces the transformation of mesenchymal to epithelial tissue (Braun et al., 2010). In this sense, it seems that the epigenetic silencing of miRNAs suppressors could explain that miRNA transcription units are entirely downregulated in ATC (Braun and Hüttelmaier, 2011).

miRNAs not only have potential as a diagnostic tool but also provide therapeutic targets, based on the inhibition of oncomiR or increasing levels of suppressor miRNAs. However, the clinical utility as therapy is limited by their effects on nonneoplastic tissues (Braun and Hüttelmaier, 2011).

Table 26.10 summarizes the miRNA profile studies and potential tumor markers for PTC.

TABLE 26.10

miRNA Profile Studies in PTC

Study	N	Sample	miRNA	Validation	Methodology	S	E	PPV	NPV	Acc	Comments
He et al. (2005)	20	HT vs. PTC	miR-221 miR-222 miR-146 miR-21 miR-181a	miR-221 miR-222 miR-146b	N-blot RT-PCR	np	np	np	np	np	Discriminate HT from PTC. Relation with KIT
Pallante et al. (2006)	40	HT vs. PTC	miR-221 miR-222 miR-213 miR-220 miR-181b	miR-221 miR-222 miR-181b	N-blot RT-PCR 8 FNAB[a]	np	np	np	np	np	Discriminate HT from PTC
Nikiforova et al. (2008)	60	HT, BTD, cancer	148 mRNA: 47: over-e 57: down-r	miR-187 miR-221 miR-222 miR-146b miR-155 miR-224 miR-197	RT-PCR 62 FNAB[a] 1 miRNA ≥3 miRNA	100 88	94 100	np np	np np	95 98	Variation of the miRNA profile according to the mutational status: RAS ≠ BRAF, RET/PTC, and PAX/PPAR
Sheu et al. (2010)	113	Fixed tissue[b] PTC[c], FA, FTC, WDU, MNG	miR-146b miR-181b miR-21 miR-221 miR-222	— PTC-C vs. PTC-VF: miR-146b ($p = 0.043$) PTC-CA vs. PTC-VF: miR-146b, miR-21, miR-222 ($p < 0.028$) PTC (-C and -TC) vs. MNG: miR-146b ($p < 0.001$) PTC-VF vs. WDU and FTC: miR-146b ($p = 0.002$ and $p = 0.04$, respectively) PTC-VF vs. FA: miR-146b, miR-181b, miR-21, miR-221, miR-222 (significative p-value)	—	np	np	np	np	np	
Mazeh (2011)	47	FNAB[b] ex vivo BTD, PTC	miR-21 miR-31 miR-146b miR-187 miR-221 miR-222	No validation group miR-221 miR-222 miR-146b	95 90 80	100 100 100	100 100 100	96 93 87	98 96 91		
Keutgen et al. (2012)	29	FNAB[b] ex vivo Ind cyt	miR-328 miR-222 miR-197 miR-181a miR-146b miR-21	miR-328 miR-222 miR-197 miR-21	RT-PCR 72 FNAB[a] in vivo Global sin HC	100 100	84 95	np np	np np	90 97	5 out of 7 FN: oncocytic lesions. Improved test by not including FN in the calculations

(*continued*)

TABLE 26.10 (continued)

miRNA Profile Studies in PTC

Study	N	Sample	miRNA	Validation	Methodology	S	E	PPV	NPV	Acc	Comments
Shen et al. (2012)	60	Fixed FNAB[b] BTD (FA, HC), PTC, PTC-FV, FTC, ATC	miR-146b miR-221 miR-187 miR-197 miR-346 miR-30d miR-138 miR-302c	*Over-e*: miR-146b miR-221 miR-187 *Down-r*: miR-30d	RT-PCR 68 FNAB[a] 30 AUS The classifier predicts malignancy in 94.4% of PTC The classifier predicts malignancy in 62.5% of FTC	88.9 63.6	78.3 78.9	89 64	78 79	85,3 73,3	Improves PTC detection. If AUS: not useful for the diagnosis of follicular neoplasm and PTC-FV
	88	FNAB[b] in vivo BTD vs. PTC	miR-146b miR-155 miR-187 miR-197 miR-221 miR-222 miR-224	miR-146b miR-155 miR-221	RT-PCR 53 FNAB[a] in vivo Ind cyt	60	57.8	36	78.6	58.5	
Kitano et al. (2012)	95	FNAB[b] in vivo Ind cyt	miR-7	miR-7	RT-PCR 59 FNAB[a] in vivo Ind cyt	100	20	25	100	37	The benign outcome, based on the prediction model, would avoid diagnostic thyroidectomy
Vriens et al. (2012)	104	HT, BTD, cancer	*Down-r* miR-149 miR-100 miR-138 miR-125b miR-768-3p *Over-e* miR-628-3p miR-550 miR-564 miR-635 miR-584	miR-100, miR-138 miR-125b miR-768-3p	RT-PCR 125 FNAB[a] ex vivo *Tissue* BTD vs. cancer: miR-138 (79%) HC (benign vs. cancer): miR-138, miR-768-3p (98%) Follicular neoplasms: miR-125b *FNAB:* miR-138: Benign vs. malign: $p < 0.001$; Acc: 75% NPV (benign vs. malign): 81% NVP (follicular neoplasms): 100%	np	np	np	np	np	

Note: FNAB, fine-needle aspiration biopsy; HT, health tissue; BTD, benign thyroid disease; PTC, papillary thyroid carcinoma; FA, follicular adenoma; FTC, follicular thyroid carcinoma; WDU, well-differentiated tumor of undetermined malignant potential; HC, Hürthle or oncocytic cells; MNG, multinodular goiter; AUS, atypia of uncertain significance; over-e, overexpressed; down-r, downregulated; N-blot, northern blot; W-blot, western blot; RT-PCR, reverse-transcription polymerase chain reaction; Ind cyt, indeterminate cytology; FNs, false negatives.

Values of Se (sensitivity), Sp (specificity), PPV (positive predictive value), NPV (negative predictive value), and Acc (accuracy) given in %.

[a] Validation in independent samples.

[b] Determination of miRNA by RT-PCR.

[c] Conventional PTC (PTC-C), follicular variant (PTC-FV), and tall cells (PTC-TC).

26.3.1.5 Diagnostic Utility of Gene Alterations Associated with Papillary Thyroid Carcinoma

FNAB is the best tool for early diagnosis of thyroid lesions. When the risk of malignancy of a thyroid nodule is high, the patient is usually recommended for FNAB, which can be guided by ultrasound or by palpation.

The interpretation of thyroid FNAB by experienced cytopathologists is the gold standard for the detection of malignancy in thyroid nodules. Although the diagnostic Acc of FNAB interpreted as malignant or benign is high even in experienced hands, approximately 10%–30% of FNAB results are diagnosed as "indeterminate or follicular neoplasm" (Table 26.4), and about 20%–40% of them eventually become malignant after surgery (Caruso and Mazzaferri, 1991), which remains as a diagnostic dilemma for patients and clinicians. FNAB does not discriminate benign from malignant thyroid nodules in up to 30% of cases (Table 26.4; Yeh et al., 2004) and can appear as both false-negative (FN) and discordant cytology results. Therefore, it would be useful to have new diagnostic markers to increase the preoperative Acc of FNAB to distinguish benign from malignant thyroid neoplasms, improving patient outcome and reducing the cost of optimal care provided to patients with thyroid nodules.

Several genes have been proposed as diagnostic marker preoperative FNAB, both molecular (BRAF, RAS, RET/PTC, PAX8/PPARγ) and immunohistochemical (galectins, p27 [KIP1], DAP4, TPO). Unfortunately, data from several studies show the limitation of these markers, due to the lack of Sp, Se, or both (Henry et al., 1994; González-Cámpora et al., 1998; Troncone et al., 2000; Giannini et al., 2003; Salvatore et al., 2004; Sapio et al., 2007a,b; Bartolazzi et al., 2008; Shibru et al., 2008; Nikiforov et al., 2009).

Among all gene alterations in PTC, $BRAF^{V600E}$ mutation is the most promising and feasible biomarker with an actual potential to be implemented in the clinical routine. $BRAF^{V600E}$ mutation is the most common genetic alteration in thyroid cancer. It appears in 36%–65% of PTCs in Western countries (Table 26.15; Davies et al., 2002; Cohen et al., 2003; Fukushima et al., 2003; Kimura et al., 2003; Namba et al., 2003; Nikiforova et al., 2003a; Soares et al., 2003; Xu et al., 2003; Hayashida et al., 2004; Kroll, 2004; Salvatore et al., 2004; Trovisco et al., 2004; Xing et al., 2004b; Giordano et al., 2005; Xing, 2005; Xing et al., 2005; Cañadas Garre, 2010; Cañadas Garre et al., 2011). Its high frequency, combined with Sp for PTC, makes $BRAF^{V600E}$ mutation an attractive molecular marker for the diagnosis of PTC. Furthermore, the Sp (a single codon) and the nature of the mutation (single-nucleotide change) allow easy detection from a technical point of view. Furthermore, mutations in BRAF can be detected in genomic DNA from thyroid cytology (Cohen et al., 2003; Salvatore et al., 2004; Jin et al., 2006; Rowe et al., 2006; Sapio et al., 2007a,b; Cañadas Garre, 2010; Cañadas Garre et al., 2012).

As demonstrated by many authors, there is a very good correlation between the result of $BRAF^{V600E}$ in preoperative thyroid FNABs and histology tissue from thyroidectomy (Table 26.11; Nikiforov et al., 2009; Cañadas Garre, 2010; Cañadas Garre et al., 2012). Thus, the mutation $BRAF^{V600E}$ can be reliably detected in the material from thyroid smears obtained by FNAB, providing a representative result of $BRAF^{V600E}$ status in the thyroid nodule. This reliability and representativeness, together with the Sp of $BRAF^{V600E}$ for PTC/ATC, allows the detection of FN PTCs in thyroid smears obtained by FNAB with an Sp of 100% and a PPV for malignancy of 100%, as we have shown in 1031 FNAB specimens from 861 patients, the largest prospective cohort of occidental patients published to date (Cañadas Garre et al., 2012).

Many groups have investigated the capability of $BRAF^{V600E}$ mutation to diagnose PTC on FNAB (Table 26.11). Initially, those studies were small and conducted retrospectively or without the possibility of including $BRAF^{V600E}$ in the decision-making; however, in the last years, there has been developed a considerable amount of larger prospective studies aiming to improve PTC Se on FNAB (Table 26.11). Most of the studies only achieved good Se in the indeterminate category, concluding that $BRAF^{V600E}$ mutation was only or more helpful in this category. However, it is our opinion that the benefit of analyzing $BRAF^{V600E}$ mutation on thyroid FNAB also lies on the nonsurgical categories (inadequate/benign) in a significant way, and we proposed it for the routine analysis of the thyroid nodule, especially in clinical settings with moderate PTC detection on FNAB, procedure that we have implemented in the thyroid nodule diagnostic algorithm routine of our institution since January 2006 (Cañadas Garre et al., 2012). In our cohort of 966 FNABs, $BRAF^{V600E}$ mutation discriminated preoperatively 45.5%

TABLE 26.11

Recent Studies to Improve Diagnostic Accuracy of Cytopathology by Incorporating Genetic Markers

Study	Study Design	Cases		Gene Mutations	PTC Positive Cases by Cytological Categories				FP
		FNAB	Surgery		PTC	IND	NM	ND	
Cheung et al. (2001)	P	75	75	RET/PTC	6/12	9/23	0/16	2/22	
Elisei et al. (2001)	R	154	154	RET/PTC1 RET/PTC3	—	—	—	—	
Cohen et al. (2004)	R	91	91	BRAF	18/25	5/32	—	—	—
Hayashida et al. (2004)	PR	21	130	BRAF	29/47	1/8	0/3	—	
Salvatore et al. (2004)	R	96	96	BRAF RET/PTC1 RET/PTC3	22/54 5/33	4/11 0/11	—	0/4 1/4	
Xing et al. (2004b)	P	45	45	BRAF	6/10	2/25	0/5	—	
Domingues et al. (2005)	P	63	24	BRAF RET/PTC1 RET/PTC2 RET/PTC3	3/9 1/9 0/9 1/9	0/10 0/10 0/10 0/10	0/4 2/4 0/4 0/4	—	1 MNG (RET/PTC1)
Jin et al. (2006)	R	71	71	BRAF	??	??/12	??	??	
Rowe et al. (2006)	R	24	24	BRAF	—	3/19	—	—	
Chung et al. (2006)	R	137	137	BRAF	??	4/25	??	??	1 AHN
Kumagai et al. (2007)	P	237	208	BRAF	31/92	3/21	0/86	0/9	
Pizzolanti et al. (2007)	PRR	156	49	BRAF RET/PTC1 RET/PTC3	9/13 0/13 0/13	2/19 0/19 1/19	0/17 0/17 0/17	—	
Sapio et al. (2007b)	P	132	50	BRAF RET/PTC1 RET/PTC3 TRK	—	4/37 1/37	0/48 0/48 0/48	0/46 0/46 0/46	
Sapio et al. (2007a)	R	47	47	BRAF Galectine-3	—	9/47 23/47	—	—	
French et al. (2008)	P	24	17	PAX8/PPARγ		2/??			
Kim et al. (2008)	R	103	103	BRAF	50/60	13/27	0/16	—	
Bentz et al. (2009)	R	42	42	BRAF	14/19	3/17	0/6	—	
Jo et al. (2009)	P	101	101	BRAF	22/30	7/24	0/43	1/4	
Marchetti et al. (2009)	R	111	111	BRAF	41/55	18/52	0/1	—	
Moon et al. (2009)	R	91	91	BRAF	—	42/91	—	—	

TABLE 26.11 (continued)

Recent Studies to Improve Diagnostic Accuracy of Cytopathology by Incorporating Genetic Markers

Study	Study Design	Cases		Gene Mutations	PTC Positive Cases by Cytological Categories				FP
		FNAB	Surgery		PTC	IND	NM	ND	
Nikiforov et al. (2009)	P	470	141	BRAF	10/22	7/52	1/12	—	2 FA (RAS)
				RET/PTC	3/22	2/52	3/12		1 AHN (RET/PTC3)
				RAS	0/22	5/52	0/12		
				PAX8/PPARγ	0/22	1/52	0/12		
Yip et al. (2009)	R	332	332	BRAF	64/76	24/49	??	??	
				RAS					
				RET/PTC1					
				RET/PTC3					
Yip et al. (2009)	R	44	332	BRAF	29/??		??	2/??	
				RAS					
				RET/PTC1					
				RET/PTC3					
Zatelli et al. (2009)	P	469	166	BRAF	41/63	1/89	6/308	—	
Cantara et al. (2010)	R	235	174	BRAF	21/54	2/41	2/87	8/53	6 (RAS)
				RET/PTC	6/54	2/41	2/87	1/53	
				RAS	10/54	3/41	5/87	5/53	
				PAX8/PPARγ	0/54	0/41	0/87	0/53	
				TRK	0/54	0/41	0/87	0/53	
Kim et al. (2010b)	P	961	279	BRAF	162/180	50/80	2/688	7/111	5 (technique)
Mathur et al. (2010)	P	423	288	BRAF	/46	/84	/91	—	
				RET/PTC1,3					
				N,K-RAS					
				PAX8/PPARγ					
				TRK					
				ANGPT2					
				ECM1					
				EFNB2					
				EGFR					
				TMPRSS4					
				TIMP1					
Moses et al. (2010)	P	455		BRAF	10/57	13/137	0/257	0/2	1 (RET/PTC)
				RET/PTC	1/57	4/137	0/257	0/2	2 (NRAS)
				RAS	2/57	2/137	0/257	0/2	BTN
				PAX8/PPARγ	0/57	0/137	0/257	0/2	
				TRK	0/57	0/137	0/257	0/2	
Musholt et al. (2010)	P	290	93	BRAF	4/9	1/19	3/50	1/33	
				RET/PTC	0/9	1/19	1/50	0/33	
Ohori et al. (2010)	P	513	124	BRAF	—	?/513	—	—	
				RET/PTC					
				RAS					
				PAX8/PPARγ					
Troncone et al. (2010)	P	126	—	BRAF	3/5	1/5	0/116	—	
Adeniran et al. (2011)	P	83	46	BRAF	—	19/84	—	—	
Kim et al. (2011)	P	865	204	BRAF	175/194	46/151	0/504	0/16	1 AHN

(*continued*)

TABLE 26.11 (continued)

Recent Studies to Improve Diagnostic Accuracy of Cytopathology by Incorporating Genetic Markers

Study	Study Design	Cases		Gene Mutations	PTC Positive Cases by Cytological Categories				FP
		FNAB	Surgery		PTC	IND	NM	ND	
Nikiforov et al. (2011)	P	967	513	BRAF	10/52	7/461	—	—	9 (NRAS) FA
				RET/PTC	1/52	0/461			
				RAS	7/52	45/461			
				PAX8/PPARγ	1/52	3/461			
Pelizzo et al. (2011)	P	270	141	BRAF	93/138	2/119	1/4	2/9	
Yeo et al. (2011)	P	902	209	BRAF	97/184	2/15	0/10	—	
Cañadas Garre et al. (2012)	P	966	211	BRAF	6/7	5/57	5/664	1/233	
Marchetti et al. (2012)	R	95	85	BRAF	63/80	0/5	—	—	

Note: R, retrospective; P, prospective; FNAB, fine-needle aspiration biopsy; PTC, papillary thyroid carcinoma. Includes suspicious for malignancy; IND, indeterminate. Includes FLUS/AUS and follicular neoplasm; NM, negative for malignancy; ND, nondiagnostic; BTN, benign thyroid nodule; AHN, atypical hyperplastic nodule; FPs, false positives; —, cytological category not analyzed; MNG, multinodular goiter; ??, not specified.

of PTCs cytologically diagnosed as indeterminate and detected per se 33.3% (6/18) of FN PTCs misdiagnosed by cytopathological examination of the FNAB (Cañadas Garre et al., 2012). According to our results, the great advantage of the detection of $BRAF^{V600E}$ mutation on FNAB is the redefinition of FN PTCs in the nonsurgical FNAB categories (benign/inadequate), improving the Se of the preoperative FNAB test in 16.7% (Cañadas Garre et al., 2012). This improvement in the Se is achieved with a frequency of $BRAF^{V600E}$ mutation in PTC in the cohort of 47.2%, consequent with that reported for occidental countries (Table 26.15; Xing et al., 2005; Cañadas Garre, 2010; Cañadas Garre et al., 2011). This frequency was sufficient to promote an Se increment comparable to that reported for oriental countries (3.4%), where prevalence of $BRAF^{V600E}$ mutation is ≈80% (Kim et al., 2010c). These data also confirm the results of surgical series by Cantara et al. (2010), with similar rates for PTC detection on cytopathology FNs and Se for $BRAF^{V600E}$ mutation.

Therefore, the establishment of the mutation detection $BRAF^{V600E}$ as a complementary tool to determine the malignancy of the thyroid nodule in the diagnostic routine refines the preoperative diagnosis of thyroid nodules, not only in cases of indeterminate cytopathology diagnoses but also in cases in which the amount of cells is insufficient for histopathologic evaluation and in cases misdiagnosed as negative for malignancy (Cañadas Garre et al., 2012). The clinical impact of detection FNs of cytopathology can be quite important. The subjects whose tumors are not detected on the cytology may suffer a delay in their treatment, may have larger proportions of capsular and vascular invasion, and have a greater likelihood of persistent disease during follow-up (Yeh et al., 2004). $BRAF^{V600E}$ mutation can also partly clarify the diagnostic dilemma for indeterminate FNABs preoperatively, by direct confirmation of the positive cases as PTC (Marchetti et al., 2009; Zatelli et al., 2009; Cantara et al., 2010; Kim et al., 2010c), what allows a better surgical management of these patients and facilitates the possible choice of prophylactic lymphadenectomy or a more extensive primary resection. A second intervention for completion thyroidectomy could even be avoided in these cases if the routine determination of $BRAF^{V600E}$ mutation is implemented in the diagnosis of thyroid nodules by FNAB (Nikiforov et al., 2011; Cañadas Garre et al., 2012; McCoy et al., 2012).

Other authors have proposed the determination of a combination of the most frequent gene alterations in thyroid cancer (BRAF, RAS, RET/PTC, PAX8/PPARγ, TRK) on FNAB to achieve a higher Se for malignancy and improve the diagnostic Acc of the cytopathological analysis of thyroid FNAB (Table 26.11).

As the most frequent genetic alterations are mutually exclusive, presumably BRAF mutations, RET/PTC, NTRK, RAS, and PAX8-PPARy should be present in approximately 90% of all thyroid cancers of follicular origin. Therefore, the combined analysis of these genetic changes should result in higher proportions of improving the Acc of cytopathology. Some studies have tried to show the potential application of the combined mutation analysis on FNAB (Table 26.11). Although this approach could seem more powerful, it is noteworthy that most of the malignant lesions detected in those studies are cases detected by $BRAF^{V600E}$ mutation. Furthermore, among all genetic markers analyzed, only $BRAF^{V600E}$ and RET/PTC1 were specific for malignancy, whereas RAS and RET/PTC3 resulted in FP cases, corresponding to benign lesions: FA and hyperplastic nodule with atypia (Table 26.11; Nikiforov et al., 2009; Cantara et al., 2010; Moses et al., 2010). Therefore, the addition of RAS, equivalent to analyze two codons (12/13 and 61) in three genes (N, H, K), increases Se slightly and reduces Sp. Incorporating RET/PTC1, although does not alter Sp 100%, has the potential problem of the need to isolate RNA from an acceptable quality in cytological samples, while $BRAF^{V600E}$ determination is performed on genomic DNA, much more stable, with a very simple technique, easy to feasibly apply into the diagnostic routine. The predictive value of diagnostic tests for RAS and PAX8–PPARy is less clear, because these alterations can also occur in benign thyroid tumors.

Another possibility that has also been explored in the literature to increase the Se of FNAB has been the combination of genetic with immunohistochemical markers, as galectin-3, the immunohistochemical marker with higher potential in thyroid (Sapio et al., 2007a). In 2007, Sapio and colleagues conducted a retrospective study, incorporating $BRAF^{V600E}$ mutation analysis and expression of galectin-3 in indeterminate nodules, showing that the combination of both markers improves Se, Sp, PPV, and NPV of cytopathology. However, most of the PTC discovered corresponded to positive $BRAF^{V600E}$ (9/20, 45%), and the positivity for galectin-3 did not imply malignancy (6/23, 26.1% of patients with benign lesions were positive for galectin-3), that is, galectin-3 cannot be considered as a specific marker of malignancy.

In conclusion, among all gene alterations in PTC, $BRAF^{V600E}$ mutation, the most common of all the gene alterations in thyroid cancer, has been the only to demonstrate an evident clinical utility to guide the surgical management of thyroid nodules. It not only has proved diagnostic utility for the detection of FN PTCs on FNAB (Table 26.11) but also has been proposed as a prognostic marker for preoperative risk stratification of PTC on FNAB (Xing et al., 2009). Thus, the determination of the $BRAF^{V600E}$ mutation on preoperative FNABs could guide the need and extent of the surgical intervention in patients positive for this gene marker (Xing et al., 2009; Nikiforov et al., 2011; Cañadas Garre et al., 2012; McCoy et al., 2012).

26.3.2 Noninvasive Molecular Biomarkers Currently Used and under Development: Serum Biomarkers in PTC

The search for a serum marker for PTC in the recent years has finally rendered several markers that eventually have not entirely proven their usefulness (Hu et al., 2006a).

26.3.2.1 Circulating TSH

Measuring circulating TSH seems to be the most obvious and simple analysis. Boelaert et al. (2006, 2009) investigated its predictive value, concluding that the risk for DTC increases with increased TSH serum concentration, so that the incidence of cancer increases from 2.8%, when TSH is below the normal range, to 29.6%, when it is higher ($p < 0.001$). The risk is estimated to be 11.18 ($p < 0.001$, $CI_{95\%}$: 3.23–8.63). The rate of malignancy was also higher when TPO antibodies were detectable (11.9 vs. 6.7, $p = 0.02$) (Boelaert et al., 2006).

In this same line of work, Haymart et al. (2008) also tried to find an association between preoperative TSH and DTC. They found up to 46% of cancers with serum TSH levels above normal and, moreover, were able to correlate higher levels of TSH with tumor stage: TSH median rises to 4.9 ± 1 mIU/L in stages 7/IV vs. 2.1 ± 0.2 mIU/L in stages I/II ($p = 0.002$) (Haymart et al., 2008).

26.3.2.2 TSH-R mRNA

A further step has been to measure the mRNA of the TSH-R by RT-PCR using mononuclear cells of a blood sample (Milas et al., 2010). TSH-R mRNA is detected most frequently in PTC than FTC, in little or no differentiated tumors or MNG. Preoperative values of TSH-R mRNA > 1 ng/μg presented 61% Se, 83% Sp, 81% PPV, 64% NPV, and overall Acc of 71%. These authors found that most (55%) of FNs were incidental microcarcinomas of 1–2 mm, and when not considered, the test improved, 78% Se, 86% Sp, 81% PPV, 84% NPV, and 83% Acc, applied only to the PTC cohort of more than 1 cm, no FPs, and therefore the PPV was 100% with 78% Se.

Moreover, in detectable TSH-R mRNA, PPV for FNAB improved from 75% to 90% in patients with atypical or suspicious cytology. Only malignant tumors showed values above 5.5 ng/μg. Serum TSH-R mRNA levels became undetectable after total thyroidectomy in all patients with benign on the first postoperative day and in 85% of cancers. The remaining 15% were diagnosed with persistent or recurrent disease during the first year. The authors implemented this determination into clinical practice in patients with follicular neoplasm cytology: detectable levels of TSH-R mRNA together with ultrasound findings presented 97% Se, 84% Sp, 88% PPV, 95% NPV, and 91% Acc values (Milas et al., 2010).

26.3.2.3 Tg mRNA

The use of Tg as a marker of tumor progression is unquestioned, despite the antibody interference and variability in Se. Therefore, efforts have been made to measure Tg mRNA in serum by RT-PCR. However, its usefulness has been limited by the instability of the RNA molecule (conditioning a great variability in Se and Sp), the presence of mRNA-Tg from extrathyroid origin, and the loss of Tg expression in some recurrences (Ditkoff et al., 1996; Kaufmann et al., 2004; Ringel, 2004).

26.3.2.4 Proteomic Markers

Serum proteomic studies (peptidomic serum) are a special form of proteomics. It has been demonstrated that the activity of the exoproteases contributes to generate serum peptides specific for different tumor types, secreting various proteases that can generate a unique peptide profile through its catalytic action (Villanueva et al., 2006). The result is a low molecular weight protein set that shows, indirectly, the enzymatic activity of tumor cells and could serve as markers for both diagnosis and classification of disease (Moretz et al., 2008).

Following this line of investigation, Villanueva et al. developed a classifier (12-peptide signature thyroid cancer) using matrix-assisted laser desorption/ionization (MALDI)-TOF-MS, capable to differentiate between benign and malignant tumors, showing values of 95% Se and 95% Sp (Villanueva et al., 2006). The peptides involved were fibrinopeptide A, complement C3F, complement C4 precursor, H4 heavy chain of the inter-alpha-trypsin inhibitor, AI, A-IV, CI, E apolipoproteins, clusterin precursor, bradykinin, HMW kininogen, XIIIa factor, and transthyretin precursor (Villanueva et al., 2006).

Later, Moretz et al. (2008) analyzed serum samples in patients with PTC, using surface-enhanced laser desorption/ionization (SELDI)-TOF-MS (Moretz et al., 2008). They compared PTC with benign thyroid disease and tried to discriminate among them with 85.7% Se and 100% Sp, with the most remarkable difference in 11,101 Da protein of (downregulated in PTC). Although this was a pilot study with a small sample, it highlights the potential of serum proteomic studies.

A much larger study was developed by Wang et al. (2006), with 101 serum samples (mostly PTC, several other thyroid cancers, benign disease tissue, and normal thyroid). Their results were also promising, finding several protein expression profiles: a seven-protein profile capable to distinguish PTC from healthy individuals (80% Se, 88.9% Sp); other five-protein profile, which discriminates thyroid cancer from benign disease (80% Se, 80% Sp); a third profile consisting in three proteins that classify the patient as PTC or non-PTC; and the last profile, composed with four proteins that classify patients with stages I–II or more advanced. The last two patterns are not blind validated, but cross validation leaving one out yields values of 87% and 85% for Se and 74.1% and 91.4% for Sp, respectively (Wang et al., 2006). Biomarkers involved are listed in Table 26.12.

TABLE 26.12
Protein Expression Profiles

Expression Profile	*m/z* (Da)[a]
PTC vs. health tissue	Overexpressed in PTC: 2,672
	Overexpressed in health tissue: 6,651, 3,319, 5,597, 6,837, 6,855, 6,984
PTC vs. benign disease	Overexpressed in PTC: 8,762, 4,530, 14,115, 4,538
	Overexpressed in benign disease: 3,938, 2,799
Stages I–II vs. III–IV	Overexpressed in I–II: 228, 2,210, 2,085
	Overexpressed in III–IV: —
PTC vs. non-PTC	4,138, 5,842, 11,680, 13,953

Source: Wang, J.X. et al., *Proteomics*, 6, 5344, 2006.
[a] Protein by molecular weight in daltons in the mass spectrometer.

Advances in the study of protein profiling have allowed the developing of the xMAP technology, capable to simultaneously measure multiple markers in the serum of subjects. Using this technology, Linkov et al. (2008) studied serum concentrations of 32 factors belonging to 2 functional groups (cytokines/chemokines and growth factors) in 23 patients with thyroid cancer, 24 cases of benign disease, and 23 healthy controls. After an exhaustive statistical study, the panel of markers including IL-8 (IL-8), hepatocyte growth factor (HGF), induced monocyte interferon gamma (MIG), and interleukin 12p40 (IL-12p40) obtained an area under the curve of 80.3% for the empirical receiver operating characteristic (ROC) curve and 81.0% for the binormal, both with a $CI_{95}\% = 0.62–0.90$. These results conclude that this technology is a promising method that could help in the preoperative diagnosis of nodular thyroid disease patients and indeterminate results on FNAB.

Recently, great efforts have been done to find a protein serum pattern able to predict ^{131}I avidity in patients with PTC with pulmonary metastatic disease (Xu et al., 2011). Using SELDI-TOF-MS and seven proteins, these authors are able to distinguish between patients who will capture ^{131}I ($p < 0.05$), five proteins overexpressed in the avid group (*m/z* 13,578, 14,364.9, 14,792.4, 14,967.9, 15,512.8 Da) and two in the non-avid group (*m/z* 3,889.8, 4,193.8 Da). The ability to classify patients is high: 92.6% Se, 85.7 Sp, and Acc 90.2% (Xu et al., 2011).

26.3.2.5 Epigenetic Markers

Methylated DNA in circulating blood has been used by Hu et al. (2006a) as a marker for thyroid cancer diagnosis for several reasons: methylation commonly occurs in cancers, methylated DNA can be released by the tumor to the serum, DNA molecular stability and the possibility of quantitatively measuring by methylation specific PCR. With a set of five genes (CALCA, CDH1, TIMP3, DAPK, RARβ2), positive methylation was found in 70% of malignant tumors (including recurrences), whereas methylation levels were under cutoff in 95%–100% of benign cases, obtaining values of Se = 68% and Sp = 95% (Hu et al., 2006). It is noteworthy that 21% of recurrences detected by methylation, were not detected by any other means.

26.3.2.6 miRNA Markers

miRNA can be useful in discriminating between benign and malignant thyroid nodules, and circulating miRNA markers have been also described as minimally invasive potential in other tumors.

Yu et al. (2012) explored this potential usefulness in PTC, concluding that circulating miRNAs could be useful as markers of minimally invasive PTC. To achieve this, they compared the profile of circulating miRNA in PTC patients, healthy controls and benign nodules. Finally, from over 300 miRNA obtained in each group, 5 were selected based on 3 criteria: at least 30 copies in each group, difference in expression between PTC and the other groups of 5 or more times and overexpressed in the PTC group (Yu et al., 2012). Those selected for quantitative RT-PCR were circulating miR-100, miR-151-5p, miR-222, and miR-543, which met all the selection criteria and also included let-7e, with an expression of more than 3 times in PTC, and described in other tumors. Serum levels of let-7e, miR-151-5p, and miR-222 were significantly higher in PTC than in benign or healthy controls ($p < 0.001$). The three miRNA set is able to discriminate between benign pathology and PTC (area under the curve: 0.917, $CI_{95\%}$: 0.878–0.955), with 87.8% Se and 88.4% Sp, with a cutoff value of 0.41. This set also discriminates between PTC and healthy tissue (area under the curve: 0.897, 95% CI: 0.839–0.955), with 86.8% Se and 79.5% Sp, with a cutoff value of 0.58. The levels of miR-151-5p and mi-222 were well correlated with tissue levels (Pearson correlation coefficient $R = 0.33$, $p = 0.016$, and $R = 0.588$, $p < 0.001$, respectively) but not for let-7e. Clinicopathological association was also analyzed. miR-151-5p levels were higher in patients with positive nodes ($p = 0.012$) compared with those with no node affectation and were associated with tumor size ($p < 0.001$). miR-222 levels were also higher in patients with positive lymph nodes ($p = 0.001$) and with a more advanced stage ($p = 0.015$). Patients with multifocal tumors had also higher levels of let-7eo ($p < 0.001$).

26.3.2.7 Runx2 mRNA

There are other serum markers as Runx2 mRNA, a gene with an important role in the mesenchymal differentiation in osteogenic cells, relevant in PTC due to its expression in human PTC cell lines and its role in the development of other malignancies. Dalle Carbonare et al. (2012) proved that serum Runx2mRNA levels, measured by RT-PCR, are higher in 75% PTC rather than in benign nodular pathology ($p < 0.001$). They also observed a positive correlation with the expression of the same marker on FNAB ($p < 0.05$) and higher levels in patients with microcalcifications ($p > 0.05$).

26.3.2.8 Circulating DNA

In recent years, there has been much interest in the use of cell-free circulating DNA as diagnostic and prognostic marker in a variety of clinical situations. Although this DNA is present in the plasma of healthy subjects, it has been detected in much higher quantities in certain diseases and conditions such as cancer (Leon et al., 1977; Shapiro et al., 1983), autoimmune diseases (Steinman, 1984), and physical trauma (Lo et al., 2000). Free circulating DNA in plasma and serum has been shown to contain tumor markers such as oncogenic mutations, allelic loss, amplifications, microsatellite alterations, and hypermethylation of promoter regions in many cancers (Goessl, 2003). In the case of cancer, DNA level in plasma is associated with the severity of disease and poorer prognosis (Sozzi et al., 2003). It has been proposed that the mechanisms responsible for this release of plasma DNA include apoptotic and necrotic cell death and release of intact cells into the bloodstream with subsequent lysis (Gormally et al., 2007). Furthermore, larger amounts are found in plasma of patients with metastases, compared with patients with localized disease (Leon et al., 1977).

Few genes have been investigated in serum of patients with thyroid cancer. Among them, circulating mutant BRAF has been found specifically in patients with PTC, especially in patients with active disease and metastases (Cradic et al., 2009; Chuang et al., 2010).

Among methylation markers, RARβ2 has also shown great Sp (Hu et al., 2006a), making it an outstanding candidate for thyroid cancer, as it appeared not hypermethylated in any serum from patients with benign thyroid nodules, unlike p16 and RASSF1A, which are hypermethylated in FA (Boltze et al., 2003; Xing et al., 2004; Nakamura et al., 2005).

26.3.2.9 Galectin

Finally, Saussez et al. (2008) investigated whether, like in tissue expression, differences in serum levels of galectin can discriminate malign from benign lesions. This study prospectively determined concentrations of various galectins by ELISA. But while galectins 1 and 3 resulted higher in patients with malignant disease, there was a considerable overlap between the concentrations in both groups, so its discriminative ability is not specially good (73% Se, 74% Sp, 57% PPV, and 85% NPV, using a cutoff value of 3.2 ng/mL) (Saussez et al., 2008).

26.4 Integrative Omics-Based Molecular Markers for Early Diagnosis, Prognosis, and Therapy

26.4.1 BRAF

26.4.1.1 Diagnosis

Recent evidences have demonstrated that this biomarker can be used as an effective tool for PTC diagnosis (Cañadas Garre et al., 2012).

In thyroid, $BRAF^{V600E}$ mutation is restricted to malignant tumors, particularly PTC and PDTC/ATC originated from PTC (Namba et al., 2003; Nikiforova et al., 2003; Begum et al., 2004). Thus, detection of this mutation in thyroid FNAB samples or surgically removed lesions is virtually diagnostic of PTC (Cohen et al., 2004; Salvatore et al., 2004; Cañadas Garre, 2010; Cañadas Garre et al., 2012). BRAF mutation analysis may be particularly diagnostically useful in thyroid FNAB specimens diagnosed with atypical or indeterminate results, as it could help establish a diagnosis of PTC in a significant percentage of these samples (Cohen et al., 2004; Salvatore et al., 2004; Cañadas Garre et al., 2012). In addition, detection of the $BRAF^{V600E}$ mutation can be evaluated using several molecular techniques using DNA isolated from fresh or fixed FNAB samples. The comparison of four different methods (direct sequencing, colorimetric analysis, real-time PCR with FRET probes, and fluorescent allele-specific PCR) in the study of Jin et al. shows high Se and comparability of methods in archived thyroid cytologies (Jin et al., 2006).

26.4.1.2 Prognosis

BRAF has also shown an additional value as risk stratification biomarker and prognostication in the clinical practice, even on the preoperative FNAB (Xing et al., 2009; Zhou et al., 2012). The presence of the $BRAF^{V600E}$ mutation in the preoperative FNAB has been associated with the presence of occult contralateral microPTC, higher risk for extensive disease (extrathyroidal extension and lymph node metastases), and disease persistence/recurrence (Xing et al., 2009; Zhou et al., 2012). According to these results, total thyroidectomy, including the contralateral lobe, should be recommended for the treatment of patients with microPTC when preoperative $BRAF^{V600E}$ mutation is positive.

26.4.1.3 Therapy

$BRAF^{V600E}$ has demonstrated to be able to initiate PTC (Knauf et al., 2005) and also capable to maintain proliferation, transformation, and tumorigenicity of PTC cells (Liu et al., 2007). These results provide further support for potentially effective therapy targeted to PTCs positive for BRAF. Given that evidence aims to BRAF is also involved in the progression to ATC (Namba et al., 2003; Nikiforova et al., 2003; Begum et al., 2004), BRAF emerges as an attractive target in thyroid cancer, especially for the more aggressive subtypes, where there is an urgent need for treatment. Due to its high frequency and association with tumor dedifferentiation and resistance to conventional therapy with radioiodine, $BRAF^{V600E}$ mutation also represents an attractive therapeutic target for PTCs. Furthermore, as BRAF is lower than RET and RAS in the signaling cascade, BRAF inhibitors could potentially be effective in tumors with other mutations that affect this signaling pathway BRAF as previously mentioned.

In the last 5 years, a wide variety of multitargeted kinase inhibitors have been introduced in clinical trials for advanced or progressing metastatic thyroid cancers, yielding higher response rates than cytotoxic chemotherapy, even when responses were achieved in only few patients (Schlumberger et al., 2010). One of these promising agents is sorafenib (BAY 43-9006), a multikinase inhibitor with potent activity against RAF and other protein kinases (Wilhelm et al., 2004). Sorafenib effectively blocks the kinase activity of the wild-type $BRAF^{V600}$ and the mutant form, $BRAF^{600E}$ (Wan et al., 2004; Wilhelm et al., 2004).

The structural similarity between RET and VEGFR kinases results in the common ability to inhibit vascular endothelial growth factor receptors (VEGFRs) for most of these agents, which confers a potent antiangiogenetic effect; that is, sorafenib has RAF–RET and VEGFR-inhibiting activity; axitinib has

TABLE 26.13

Clinical Trials with Targeted Therapies in Patients with PTC

Study	Drug	Pathway Inhibited	Patients	Responses
Gupta-Abramson et al. (2008)	Sorafenib	RAF RET VEGFR	18 PTC	4 (22.2%) PR 11 (61.1%) SD
Kloos et al. (2009)	Sorafenib	RAF RET VEGFR	41 PTC	6 (14.6%) PR 23 (56.1%) SD
Hoftijzer et al. (2009)	Sorafenib	RAF RET VEGFR	9 PTC	2 (22.2%) PR 6 (66.7%) SD
Cohen et al. (2008a)	Sunitinib	E7080 VEGFR	37 DTC	4 (10.8%) PR 21 (56.8%) SD (DTC)
Carr et al. (2010)	Sunitinib	E7080 VEGFR	28 DTC	1 (3.6%) CR 7 (25.0%) PR 14 (50.0%) SD
Cohen et al. (2008b)	Axitinib	VEGFR KIT PDGFR	60 any histology	18 (30.0%) PR 23 (38.3%) SD
Pennel et al. (2008)	Gefitinib	EGFR	27 any histology	No response
Hayes et al. (2012)	Selumetinib	MEK1,2	32	1 (3.1%) PR 21 (65.6%) SD

Source: Modified from Antonelli, M., *Curr Genomics*, 12(8), 626, 2011.

Note: VEGFR, vascular endothelial growth factor receptor; PDGFR, platelet-derived growth factor receptors; EGFR, epidermal growth factor receptor; DTC, differentiated thyroid cancer; PTC, papillary thyroid carcinoma; PR, partial response; SD, stable disease; CR, complete response; RAF, raf protein kinases; RET, ret proto-oncogene; MEK, mitogen-activated protein kinase kinases.

VEGFR-, C-KIT-, and platelet-derived growth factor receptor (PDGFR)-inhibiting activity; pazopanib is an inhibitor of VEGFR and PDGFR; and sunitinib inhibits E7080 (a multikinase inhibitor) and VEGFR.

PTC patients seem to be more sensitive to the effects of these new drugs than FTC or PDTC patients, especially if they are positive for $BRAF^{V600E}$ or present lung rather than bone metastases (Schlumberger et al., 2010).

Table 26.13 shows several phase II trials conducted in PTC patients with different tyrosine kinase inhibitors. For PTC, the better responses have been achieved with sorafenib (Table 26.13), although the most encouraging results correspond to patients with the more aggressive thyroid cancer subtypes, that is, ATC and PDTC (Antonelli et al., 2011).

Vemurafenib (commercial name: Zelboraf) is a highly selective inhibitor of mutant B-Raf enzyme inhibitor (V600E mutated BRAF inhibition). In August 2011, the US Food and Drug Administration (FDA) approved Zelboraf (vemurafenib) for the treatment of patients with unresectable or metastatic melanoma positive for the $BRAF^{V600E}$ mutation as detected by an FDA-approved test (cobas 4800 BRAF V600 Mutation Test, Roche Molecular Systems, Inc.). Vemurafenib is the first molecularly targeted therapy to be licensed in the United States (since 2011) and Europe (since 2012) for the treatment of $BRAF^{V600E}$-positive advanced melanoma.

The discovery and approval of this new targeted drug, specific for $BRAF^{V600E}$ inhibition, open the field of action for patients with more aggressive PTCs, especially those with metastatic or unresectable PTC positive for the $^{BRAF\ V600}$ mutation and resistant to radioactive iodine therapy. Several clinical trials are currently being developed to investigate the influence, safety, and efficacy of vemurafenib in patients with PTC (Table 26.14).

TABLE 26.14

Ongoing Clinical Trials with Vemurafenib in Patients with Thyroid Cancer

Study	Condition	Status	Sponsor
Pharmacodynamic study of vemurafenib in the neoadjuvant setting in patients with locally advanced thyroid cancer	Thyroid cancer	Recruiting	MD Anderson Cancer Center
An open-label, multicenter phase II study of the BRAF inhibitor vemurafenib in patients with metastatic or unresectable papillary thyroid carcinoma (PTC) positive for the BRAF V600 mutation and resistant to radioactive iodine	Neoplasms	Recruiting	Hoffmann-La Roche

26.4.2 RET/PTC Arrangements

Targeted therapeutic inhibition by tyrosine kinase inhibitors has also been investigated in activated RET kinase.

Vandetanib (ZD6474) is an active low molecular weight molecule that inhibits receptor tyrosine kinases: it is a potent inhibitor of VEGFR-2,3 and RET tyrosine kinase (Herbst et al., 2007). This drug has been tested in phase II studies, demonstrating antitumor activity on advanced MTC, and has recently been approved for the treatment of unresectable locally advanced or metastatic MTCs (Brassard and Rondeau, 2012; Santarpia and Bottai, 2012).

The multikinase inhibitor sunitinib (SU12248) has been shown to inhibit efficient signaling from RET/PTC that has been tested in phase II clinical trials in unresectable differentiated thyroid cancer refractory to radioiodine, with promising results in response (Kim et al., 2006b; Cohen et al., 2008a; Carr et al., 2010; Antonelli et al., 2011).

26.4.3 MicroRNA Expression Profiling

Recently, differential expression analysis of miRNA has been proposed as a new tool to discriminate between benign and malignant thyroid neoplasms that are indeterminate on thyroid FNAB, based on the fact that certain miRNA expression differs for normal, benign, and malignant thyroid tissue. miR-100, miR-125b, miR-138, and miR-768-3p were overexpressed in malignant samples of follicular origin and in Hürthle cell carcinoma samples alone (Vriens et al., 2012). miR-125b was significantly overexpressed in FTC cases. The Acc for distinguishing benign from malignant thyroid neoplasms was 79% overall, 98% for Hürthle cell neoplasms, and 71% for follicular neoplasms. miR-138 was overexpressed in FNAB samples that were malignant on final pathology with an Acc of 75% (Vriens et al., 2012).

26.5 Ethnic Group Differences: BRAF Distribution Worldwide

BRAFV600E mutation represents the most frequent genetic alteration involved in the pathogenesis of sporadic PTC. There is a general agreement to its restriction to well-differentiated PTC and poorly differentiated or ATCs arising from preexisting PTCs (Ciampi and Nikiforov, 2005; Xing, 2005). However, there are discrepancies in the overall frequency of the mutant form of $BRAF^{V600E}$ in different ethnics (29%–83%: Table 26.15).

Table 26.15 summarizes the worldwide frequency of $BRAF^{V600E}$ in PTC. In these studies, a wide variation is observed for the frequency of $BRAF^{V600E}$ mutation, ranging from 26.7% to 82.9%, with an average of 52.1% (3741/7184). The breadth of this range is probably due to the heterogeneity of the histological variants conforming PTC, epidemiological factors, or age of the group analyzed. Gathering the cases from the same country, the prevalence of $BRAF^{V600E}$ mutation varies between 38.2% (Ireland) and 73.3% (Korea). Higher values have been reported in Asian countries such as China (62.8%) and Korea (73.3%) (Table 26.15). Indeed, excluding Korea from the calculus of the global frequency, the average drops to 44.9% (Table 26.15), rather similar to the prevalence calculated from a review of a series of 29 previous studies by Xing (2005), which was 44% (810/1856). The meta-analysis by Lee et al. (2007), which included 12 studies, showed a prevalence of 49% (570/1168). Although it has been proposed that variations in the prevalence of the $BRAF^{V600E}$ mutation in different ethnic could be due to genetic differences between races, in the few studies that addressed this issue, such as the meta-analysis by Lee et al. (2007) and the study by Sedliarou et al. (2004), no association between mutation $BRAF^{V600E}$ and ethnicity of patients (Caucasian/Asian) was found; therefore, the origin of these differences remains unclear. Probably, an important factor causing these differences is that many studies did not stratify by PTC subtype. On the other hand, evidence supporting the ethnical difference, at least in Korean population, is the study by Jung et al. (2012), compiling more than 1000 PTCs from different subtypes, showing higher $BRAF^{V600E}$ frequency in all PTC subtypes (Jung et al., 2012).

TABLE 26.15

Global Prevalence of $BRAF^{V600E}$ Mutation in PTC

				$BRAF^{V600E}$				
Study	**+**	**N**	**%**	**+**	**N**	**%**	**$IC_{95\%}$**	**Country**
Oler et al. (2005)	5	8	62.5	63	128	49.2	49.1–49.4	Brazil
Oler et al. (2009)	58	120	48.3					
Guan et al. (2009)	387	559	69.2	455	725	62.8	62.7–62.8	China
Zhou et al. (2012)	31	100	31					
Zhu et al. (2005)	37	66	56.1					
Porra et al. (2005)	38	61	62.3	38	61	62.3	—	France
Smyth et al. (2005)	13	34	38.2	13	34	38.2	—	Ireland
Barzon et al. (2008)	39	83	47	704	1810	38.9	38.9–38.9	Italy
Elisei et al. (2008)	38	102	37.3					
Frasca et al. (2008)	125	323	38.7					
Frattini et al. (2004)	19	60	31.7					
Fugazzola et al. (2004)	18	56	32.1					
Fugazzola et al. (2006)	99	260	38.1					
Lupi et al. (2007)	214	500	42.8					
Puxeddu et al. (2004)	24	60	40					
Romei et al. (2008)	28	78	35.9					
Salvatore et al. (2004)	26	69	37.7					
Sapio et al. (2006)	19	43	44.2					
Trovisco et al. (2005a)	55	176	31.3					
Fukushima et al. (2003)	40	76	52.6	398	1004	39.6	39.6–39.7	Japan
Hayashida et al. (2004)	37	72	51.4					
Ito et al. (2009)	242	631	38.4					
Nakayama et al. (2007)	26	40	65					
Namba et al. (2003)	49	170	28.8					
Sedliarou et al. (2004)	4	15	26.7					
Jo et al. (2006)	102	161	63.4	1331	1817	73.3	73.2–73.3	Korea
Jung et al. (2012)	835	1041	80.2					
Kim et al. (2004)	58	70	82.9					
Kim et al. (2005a)	64	79	81					
Kim et al. (2005b)	31	60	51.7					
Kim et al. (2006b)	149	203	73.4					
Kim et al. (2006a)	34	103	33					
Lee et al. (2006)	58	100	58					
Brzezianska et al. (2007)	12	25	48	17	38	44.7	44.4–45.1	Poland
Wojciechowska and Lewinski (2006)	5	13	38.5					
Domingues et al. (2005)	4	11	36.4	74	191	38.7	38.7–38.8	Portugal
Soares et al. (2003)	23	50	46					
Soares et al. (2004)	2	6	33.3					
Trovisco et al. (2004)	45	124	36.3					
Sedliarou et al. (2004)	9	31	29	64	122	52.5	52.1–52.8	Russia
Vasil'ev et al. (2004)	55	91	60.4					
Abubaker et al. (2008)	153	296	51.7	294	640	45.9	45.9–46.0	Saudi Arabia
Schulten et al. (2012)	91	238	38.2					
Cañadas Garre (2010)	50	106	47.2	105	222	47.3	47.2–47.4	Spain
Costa et al. (2008)	27	49	55.1					
Riesco-Eizaguirre et al. (2006)	28	67	41.8					
Perren et al. (2004)	7	15	46.7	7	15	46.7	—	Switzerland

TABLE 26.15 (continued)

Global Prevalence of BRAF^{V600E} Mutation in PTC

				BRAF^{V600E}				
Study	**+**	**N**	**%**	**+**	**N**	**%**	**IC$_{95\%}$**	**Country**
Kurt et al. (2012)	40	46	87	40	46	87	—	Turkey
Lima et al. (2004)	27	84	32.1	89	226	39.4	39.3–39.5	Ukraine-BR
Nikiforova et al. (2004)	30	82	36.6					
Powell et al. (2005)	18	32	56.3					
Xing et al. (2004c)	14	28	50					
Adeniran et al. (2006)	39	92	42.4	627	1371	45.7	45.7–45.7	United States
Cohen et al. (2003)	24	35	68.6					
Cohen et al. (2004)	36	95	37.9					
Kebebew et al. (2007)	133	274	48.5					
Kimura et al. (2003)	28	78	35.9					
Nikiforova et al. (2003a)	45	118	38.1					
Penko et al. (2005)	97	232	41.8					
Vasko et al. (2005)	21	33	63.6					
Xing (2005)	37	65	56.9					
Xing et al. (2004a)	18	30	60					
Xing et al. (2004b)	8	16	50					
Xing et al. (2004c)	14	28	50					
Xing et al. (2005)	106	219	48.4					
Xu et al. (2003)	21	56	37.5					
Total				3741	7184	52.1	52.1–52.1	Total
Total excluding Korea				2410	5367	44.9	44.9–44.9	

26.6 Commercially Available Molecular Diagnosis Tests for the Evaluation of Thyroid FNAB

Despite FNAB has been established as the best initial diagnostic test for clinical management of thyroid nodules, it presents the limitation of indeterminate and nondiagnostic results, up to 40% of the cases (Table 26.4). Current guidelines recommend total or partial thyroidectomy for most patients with indeterminate thyroid FNAB results in order to obtain a final diagnosis (Cooper et al., 2009; Gharib et al., 2010). Such surgery is invasive and expensive and can result in lifelong thyroid hormone therapy for the patient. In the last decade, numerous efforts have been made to develop genetic markers or marker panels that can be used as a complementary tool in the management of thyroid malignancy by identifying malignant nodular lesions.

As reviewed earlier, several genes have been investigated as diagnostic markers for preoperative FNAB. Among them, gene alterations (BRAF, RAS, RET/PTC, PAX8/PPARγ) and gene expression markers have overpassed the stage of research and have reached the commercial—ready to diagnose—point. These molecular tests are offered as an improvement of Se and Sp of the FNAB diagnosis. Here, we will review two commercially available tests that are used to complement FNAB: one based on gene expression (Veracyte Afirma® gene classifier) and the other based on gene alterations (Asuragen miRInform™ thyroid panel). We will also describe two tests based on unique molecular markers: Onc is based on the expression of TSH-R mRNA, and finally, as the most important gene marker for PTC, and the best molecular marker able to improve per se Se and Sp FNAB, we will also describe one commercial method to analyze BRAFT1799A mutation.

26.6.1 Veracyte Afirma® Gene Classifier

This method is intended to be a "rule out" test; the main goal is to identify benign lesions among those cytopathologically diagnosed as indeterminate in order to avoid unnecessary diagnostic thyroidectomies (Hodak and Rosenthal, 2013).

The procedure consists in a multigene expression classifier that assesses gene expression from mRNA isolated from needle washings during a standard FNAB.

The test includes 142 genes for general cases, identified through whole-genome analyses. An additional set of 25 supplemental genes is used to improve the classification of rare cancer subtypes.

This test has recently been validated in a multicenter study involving 3789 patients (Alexander et al., 2012). The analytical performance of the Afirma gene expression classifier for the classification of cytologically indeterminate thyroid nodule FNABs has also been verified, demonstrating that preserved samples are stable for up to 6 days at room temperature with no changes in RNA yield or quality, and storage and shipping temperatures were found to have no significant effect on results. The test has also demonstrated reproducibility, including variation across operators, runs, reagent lots, and laboratories (Walsh et al., 2012).

A cost-effectiveness analysis of the Veracyte Afirma® gene classifier method has been published by Li et al. (2011), concluding that its use for differential diagnosis of cytologically indeterminate thyroid nodules could potentially avoid almost 75% of currently diagnostic thyroidectomies, lowering overall costs and improving quality of life for patients with indeterminate thyroid nodules.

26.6.2 Asuragen miRInform™ Thyroid Panel

This method is intended to be a "rule in" test; the main goal is to identify malignant nodules with high Sp (Hodak and Rosenthal, 2013).

miRInform Thyroid is a panel of molecular markers that consists of seven RNA-based analytically validated molecular markers and utilizes FNAB specimens, collected in a nucleic acid preservation solution. These mutations include point mutations of BRAF (V600E) and RAS (N, H, K, 12/13/61 codons), as well as rearrangements of RET/PTC1,3 and PAX8/PPARγ.

The clinical validation of miRInform Thyroid is ongoing, but the test has been analytically validated, showing values of 95% and 99%, respectively. However, these gene alterations correspond to the most investigated molecular markers on FNAB and have been confirmed as good markers for PTC/FTC by many authors (Table 26.11). Establishing a parallelism with the study by Nikiforov et al. (2011), which analyzed the same markers and was performed in 1056 indeterminate FNAB samples with 513 histopathologic confirmations, the overall Se is 60%, and Sp varies between 96% and 99%, depending on the subclassification of indeterminate result (Nikiforov et al., 2011).

26.6.3 Cleveland Clinic TSH-R mRNA

This method detects thyroid-stimulating hormone receptor mRNA by quantitative reverse-transcription polymerase chain reaction (RT-PCR) to detect circulating thyroid cancer cells. Circulating thyroid cancer cells detected by peripheral blood TSH-R mRNA have demonstrated usefulness for thyroid cancer diagnosis and long-term surveillance (Milas et al., 2007, 2010).

This is a clinically useful blood test in the pre- and postoperative management of thyroid cancer, based on results from a prospective validation study in 1095 consecutive patients (Milas et al., 2010).

26.6.3.1 Preoperative Use

Preoperative TSH-R mRNA greater than 1 ng/mcg as a sole predictor of cancer had a PPV of 81% and Sp of 83% in 374 patients with surgically confirmed pathology (Table 26.16). Se and NPV were modest (61% and 64%, respectively), but PPV was rose to 100% in patients with PTCs larger than 1 cm.

TSH-R mRNA is particularly useful in detecting cancer in patients with follicular neoplasms on FNAB, increasing PPV (96%), Sp (96%), and Acc (85%). The Se of diagnosing cancer improved from

TABLE 26.16

Commercially Molecular Diagnosis Tests for the Evaluation of Thyroid FNAB

Test	Biomarkers	Se (%)	Sp (%)	PPV (%)	NPV (%)	Acc (%)
Veracyte Afirma® gene classifier		92	52		95 AUS 94 FN 85 SCF	
Asuragen miRInform™ thyroid panel		95[a]	99[a]			
Cleveland Clinic TSH-R mRNA						
All	TSH-R mRNA >1 ng/mcg	61	83	81[b]	64	
Patients with follicular neoplasms on FNAB		76		96	96	85

Note: Se, sensitivity; Sp, specificity; PPV, positive predictive value; NPV, negative predictive value; Acc, accuracy; AUS, atypia (or follicular lesion) of undetermined clinical significance; FN, follicular neoplasm or lesion suspicious for follicular neoplasm; SCF, suspicious cytological findings.

[a] Not clinically validated. Analytical Se and Sp.

[b] PPV was 100% in patients with PTCs greater than 1 cm.

76% to 97% when the blood test was combined with ultrasound. Ultrasound features such as irregular margins, hypervascularity, indistinct borders, and microcalcification are suggestive of cancer in follicular neoplasms, but none are independently diagnostic. The highest risk of an FP occurs with Hashimoto's disease (Milas et al., 2007, 2010).

26.6.3.2 Postoperative Use and Long-Term Surveillance

This test also presents an additional use as an early marker of adequate surgical clearance of disease or future recurrence after thyroidectomy and long-term follow-up of thyroid cancer, due to elevated TSH-R mRNA levels that became undetectable in all patients on postoperative day 1, except for those who had persistent or recurrent cancer within the year and unfavorable histological features (Milas et al., 2009). In patients with elevated Tg antibodies, detectable TSH-R mRNA was the only blood test to confirm cancer in four patients, and negative TSH-R mRNA reassured the absence of disease in patients whose imaging was also negative (Milas et al., 2010).

These data are based on the single institutional experience of the Cleveland Clinic and have not been reproduced by others to date. The test is available through direct arrangement with the Cleveland Clinic's clinical laboratory.

26.6.4 Galectin-3 ThyroTest Kit

The galectin-3 ThyroTest kit (Mabtech, Space Milan, Italy) is based on the expression analysis of galectin-3 on formalin-fixed and paraffin-embedded derived from FNAB cytological preparations, using purified galectin-3-specific monoclonal antibodies and a biotin-free immunohistocytochemical detection method. This test combines a morphological and a phenotypical evaluation of thyroid cells.

Galectin-3 is a β-galactosyl-binding molecule belonging to the lectin group, which is not normally expressed in the cytoplasm of thyroid cells, while it can be positive in well-differentiated carcinomas (Bartolazzi et al., 2001; Saggiorato et al., 2001).

Protocols for immunocytohistochemistry and the galectin-3-expression scoring system are described in the literature (Bartolazzi et al., 2001; Saggiorato et al., 2001; Papotti et al., 2005; Carpi et al., 2006; Bartolazzi et al., 2008; Carpi et al., 2010b).

This system has demonstrated an Acc of 88%, Se 78%, Sp 93%, PPV 82%, and NPV 91% in detecting thyroid malignancy in indeterminate FNAB, representing a good complementary tool for indeterminate nodules (Bartolazzi et al., 2008). The main limitations of this test are the rate of FPs (33/134; 24.6%) and the paucity of cells obtained from thyroid FNAB for cell-block preparation/galectin-3 immunostaining (Herrmann et al., 2002; Bartolazzi et al., 2008). The last issue can be minimized using preoperative US-guided large-needle aspiration biopsy (LNAB) instead of FNAB, which diminishes the frequency of inadequate and indeterminate nodules (Carpi et al., 2010b). The diagnostic performance of the galectin-3 ThyroTest associated with LNAB has also been investigated prospectively in 40 patients with a palpable thyroid nodule surgically excised, showing an Se of 100% and an Sp of 80%, demonstrating its utility in the preoperative evaluation of thyroid nodules, particularly in indeterminate cases, although the limitation of FPs remains (2/16; 12.5%) (Carpi et al., 2010b).

26.6.5 Cobas®4800 BRAF V600

There are numerous commercial tests for the detection of $BRAF^{V600E}$ mutation. As an example, we will describe the one developed by Roche Diagnostics, which is approved by the FDA.

The aim of this mutation test is the detection of DNA mutations in codon 600 of BRAF and was originally designed to detect $BRAF^{V600E}$ mutation in melanoma tissue extracted from formalin-fixed human paraffin samples in order to select vemurafenib as the therapeutic alternative for the treatment of patients with unresectable or metastatic melanoma positive for $BRAF^{V600E}$ mutation.

26.6.5.1 Principles of the Procedure

The BRAFV600 mutation test for cobas® 4800 is based on the amplification of the target DNA by real-time PCR, using a pair of complementary nucleotide probes with two different fluorescent markers, designed to detect nonmutated and mutated BRAF sequence.

26.6.5.2 Analytical Sensitivity and Specificity

This test is able to detect the $BRAF^{V600E}$ mutation with a mutation level of ≥5%, in samples containing at least 15% of tumor cells and a minimum of 2.3% mutation.

The overall concordance of BRAF V600 mutation test for cobas® 4800 was 98%, compared to 454 sequencing, with a 100% of concordance for positive and 95% for negative results and an Sp of 95%.

26.6.5.3 Reproducibility

Reproducibility is 98.8% (158/160) for every run, samples, replicates, operators and combined reagent lots.

26.7 Concluding Remarks and Future Perspectives

Currently, traditional cytopathological assessment of FNAB is the cornerstone for preoperative differentiation between benign and malignant thyroid nodules. However, limitations of FNAB, mainly due to inconclusive results (indeterminate and nondiagnostic), derivate in the need to find reliable and feasible molecular markers that help improving the diagnostic Acc of FNAB.

Given that the incidence of thyroid cancer is increasing, it would be helpful to complement existing risk stratification systems with reliable molecular markers, as has been suggested for $BRAF^{V600E}$ mutation, particularly for the surgical decision-making and clinical management (Xing, 2007).

It would be also very helpful to have an independent parameter of disease persistence/recurrence, as molecular markers, able to identify cases with increased risk of recurrence/persistence, to justify a more aggressive approach of the surgery, especially in patients whose tumor is located in thyroid without lymphatic involvement but that could be in risk of higher recurrence. Although $BRAF^{V600E}$ mutation has been associated with poor prognosis, disease recurrence and persistence in PTC remain unclear if the implementation of $BRAF^{V600E}$ mutation analysis on preoperative thyroid cytology must be really used as a risk factor to predict the aggressiveness of the disease at the time of deciding the extent of the surgery, the need of adjuvant therapy, and the follow-up interval.

New commercial tests developed to date have promising roles in the diagnosis and treatment of patients with nodular thyroid disease and thyroid cancer, although the actual knowledge regarding cost-effectiveness and clinical diagnostic improvement remains limited to their implementation in the routine.

New targeted therapies based on tyrosine kinase inhibitors for PTC are encouraging, especially for patients with more aggressive PTCs, metastatic or unresectable PTC positive for the $BRAF^{V600}$ mutation, and resistant to radioactive iodine therapy. However, the effects of resistance mechanisms related to $BRAF^{V600E}$ bypassing mechanisms via overamplification, upregulation, overexpression or activation of other components in the MAPK signaling cascade and therefore promoting alternative pathways with potential to enhance cell growth, proliferation, and survival are still unclear.

References

Abrosimov A, Saenko V, Rogounovitch T, Namba H, Lushnikov E, Mitsutake N, Yamashita S. Different structural components of conventional papillary thyroid carcinoma display mostly identical BRAF status. *Int J Cancer.* 2007;120(1):196–200.

Abubaker J, Jehan Z, Bavi P, Sultana M et al. Clinicopathological analysis of papillary thyroid cancer with PIK3CA alterations in a Middle Eastern population. *J Clin Endocrinol Metab.* Feb 2008;93(2):611–618.

Adeniran AJ, Hui P, Chhieng DC, Prasad ML, Schofield K, Theoharis C. BRAF mutation testing of thyroid fine-needle aspiration specimens enhances the predictability of malignancy in thyroid follicular lesions of undetermined significance. *Acta Cytol.* 2011;55(6):570–575.

Adeniran AJ, Zhu Z, Gandhi M, Steward DL, Fidler JP, Giordano TJ, Biddinger PW, Nikiforov YE. Correlation between genetic alterations and microscopic features, clinical manifestations, and prognostic characteristics of thyroid papillary carcinomas. *Am J Surg Pathol.* 2006;30(2):216–222.

Agretti P, Ferrarini E, Rago T, Candelieri A et al. MicroRNA expression profile helps to distinguish benign nodules from papillary thyroid carcinomas starting from cells of fine-needle aspiration. *Eur J Endocrinol.* Sep 2012;167(3):393–400.

Ain KB. Management of undifferentiated thyroid cancer. *Baillieres Best Pract Res Clin Endocrinol Metab.* Dec 2000;14(4):615–629.

Aldred MA, Huang Y, Liyanarachchi S, Pellegata NS, Gimm O, Jhiang S, Davuluri RV, de la Chapelle A, Eng C. Papillary and follicular thyroid carcinomas show distinctly different microarray expression profiles and can be distinguished by a minimum of five genes. *J Clin Oncol.* Sep 1, 2004;22(17):3531–3539.

Alexander EK, Hurwitz S, Heering JP, Benson CB, Frates MC, Doubilet PM, Cibas ES, Larsen PR, Marqusee E. Natural history of benign solid and cystic thyroid nodules. *Ann Intern Med.* 2003 Feb 18;138(4):315–318.

Alexander EK, Kennedy GC, Baloch ZW, Cibas ES et al. Preoperative diagnosis of benign thyroid nodules with indeterminate cytology. *N Engl J Med.* 2012 Aug 23;367(8):705–715.

Anand-Apte B, Bao L, Smith R, Iwata K, Olsen BR, Zetter B, Apte SS. A review of tissue inhibitor of metalloproteinases-3 (TIMP-3) and experimental analysis of its effect on primary tumor growth. *Biochem Cell Biol.* 1996;74(6):853–862.

Antonelli A, Fallahi P, Ferrari SM, Ruffilli I, Santini F, Minuto M, Galleri D, Miccoli P. New targeted therapies for thyroid cancer. *Curr Genomics.* 2011 Dec;12(8):626–631.

Arturi F, Russo D, Bidart JM, Scarpelli D, Schlumberger M, Filetti S. Expression pattern of the pendrin and sodium/iodide symporter genes in human thyroid carcinoma cell lines and human thyroid tumors. *Eur J Endocrinol.* 2001 Aug;145(2):129–135.

Baloch ZW, Fleisher S, LiVolsi VA, Gupta PK. Diagnosis of "follicular neoplasm": A gray zone in thyroid fine-needle aspiration cytology. *Diagn Cytopathol.* 2002 Jan;26(1):41–44.

Baloch ZW, LiVolsi VA, Asa SL, Rosai J et al. Diagnostic terminology and morphologic criteria for cytologic diagnosis of thyroid lesions: A synopsis of the National Cancer Institute Thyroid Fine-Needle Aspiration State of the Science Conference. *Diagn Cytopathol.* 2008 Jun;36(6):425–437.

Barden CB, Shister KW, Zhu B, Guiter G, Greenblatt DY, Zeiger MA, Fahey TJ 3rd. Classification of follicular thyroid tumors by molecular signature: Results of gene profiling. *Clin Cancer Res.* 2003 May;9(5):1792–1800.

Bartolazzi A, Gasbarri A, Papotti M, Bussolati G et al. Thyroid Cancer Study Group. Application of an immunodiagnostic method for improving preoperative diagnosis of nodular thyroid lesions. *Lancet*. 2001 May 26;357(9269):1644–1650.

Bartolazzi A, Orlandi F, Saggiorato E, Volante M et al. Galectin-3-expression analysis in the surgical selection of follicular thyroid nodules with indeterminate fine-needle aspiration cytology: A prospective multicentre study. *Lancet Oncol*. 2008;9(6):543–549.

Barzon L, Masi G, Boschin IM, Lavezzo E et al. Characterization of a novel complex BRAF mutation in a follicular variant papillary thyroid carcinoma. *Eur J Endocrinol*. 2008;159(1):77–80.

Baskin HJ. *Thyroid Ultrasound and Ultrasound-Guided FNA Biopsy*. Boston, MA: Kluwer Academic Publishers, 2000, pp. 71–86.

Begum S, Rosenbaum E, Henrique R, Cohen Y, Sidransky D, Westra WH. BRAF mutations in anaplastic thyroid carcinoma: Implications for tumor origin, diagnosis and treatment. *Mod Pathol*. 2004;17(11):1359–1363.

Bentz BG, Miller BT, Holden JA, Rowe LR, Bentz JS. B-RAF V600E mutational analysis of fine needle aspirates correlates with diagnosis of thyroid nodules. *Otolaryngol Head Neck Surg*. 2009 May;140(5):709–714.

Bird A. DNA methylation patterns and epigenetic memory. *Genes Dev*. 2002 Jan 1;16(1):6–21.

Boelaert K. The association between serum TSH concentration and thyroid cancer. *Endocr Relat Cancer*. 2009 Dec;16(4):1065–1072.

Boelaert K, Horacek J, Holder RL, Watkinson JC, Sheppard MC, Franklyn JA. Serum thyrotropin concentration as a novel predictor of malignancy in thyroid nodules investigated by fine-needle aspiration. *J Clin Endocrinol Metab*. 2006 Nov;91(11):4295–4301.

Boltze C, Zack S, Quednow C, Bettge S, Roessner A, Schneider-Stock R. Hypermethylation of the CDKN2/p16INK4A promotor in thyroid carcinogenesis. *Pathol Res Pract*. 2003;199(6):399–404.

Bongarzone I, Butti MG, Coronelli S, Borrello MG et al. Frequent activation of ret protooncogene by fusion with a new activating gene in papillary thyroid carcinomas. *Cancer Res*. 1994;54(11):2979–2985.

Bongarzone I, Monzini N, Borrello MG, Carcano C, Ferraresi G, Arighi E, Mondellini P, Della Porta G, Pierotti MA. Molecular characterization of a thyroid tumor-specific transforming sequence formed by the fusion of ret tyrosine kinase and the regulatory subunit RI alpha of cyclic AMP-dependent protein kinase A. *Mol Cell Biol*. 1993;13(1):358–366.

Bongiovanni M, Spitale A, Faquin WC, Mazzucchelli L, Baloch ZW. The Bethesda system for reporting thyroid cytopathology: A meta-analysis. *Acta Cytol*. 2012;56(4):333–339.

Borup R, Rossing M, Henao R, Yamamoto Y et al. Molecular signatures of thyroid follicular neoplasia. *Endocr Relat Cancer*. 2010 Jul 28;17(3):691–708.

Bos JL. ras oncogenes in human cancer: A review. *Cancer Res*. 1989;49(17):4682–4689. Erratum in: *Cancer Res*. 1990;50(4):1352.

Brander A, Viikinkoski P, Tuuhea J, Voutilainen L, Kivisaari L. Clinical versus ultrasound examination of the thyroid gland in common clinical practice. *J Clin Ultrasound*. 1992;20(1):37–42.

Brassard M, Rondeau G. Role of vandetanib in the management of medullary thyroid cancer. *Biologics*. 2012;6:59–66. doi: 10.2147/BTT.S24220. Epub March 8, 2012.

Braun J, Hoang-Vu C, Dralle H, Hüttelmaier S. Downregulation of microRNAs directs the EMT and invasive potential of anaplastic thyroid carcinomas. *Oncogene*. 2010 Jul 22;29(29):4237–4244. doi: 10.1038/onc.2010.169. Epub May 24, 2010.

Braun J, Hüttelmaier S. Pathogenic mechanisms of deregulated microRNA expression in thyroid carcinomas of follicular origin. *Thyroid Res*. 2011 Aug 3;4(Suppl 1):S1.

Braunschweig T, Kaserer K, Chung JY, Bilke S, Krizman D, Knezevic V, Hewitt SM. Proteomic expression profiling of thyroid neoplasms. *Proteomics Clin Appl*. 2007 Mar;1(3):264–271.

Brose MS, Volpe P, Feldman M, Kumar M et al. BRAF and RAS mutations in human lung cancer and melanoma. *Cancer Res*. 2002;62(23):6997–7000.

Brown LM, Helmke SM, Hunsucker SW, Netea-Maier RT, Chiang SA, Heinz DE, Shroyer KR, Duncan MW, Haugen BR. Quantitative and qualitative differences in protein expression between papillary thyroid carcinoma and normal thyroid tissue. *Mol Carcinog*. 2006 Aug;45(8):613–626.

Brueckl WM, Grombach J, Wein A, Ruckert S et al. Alterations in the tissue inhibitor of metalloproteinase-3 (TIMP-3) are found frequently in human colorectal tumours displaying either microsatellite stability (MSS) or instability (MSI). *Cancer Lett.* 2005 Jun 1;223(1):137–142.

Brzeziańska E, Pastuszak-Lewandoska D, Wojciechowska K, Migdalska-Sek M, Cyniak-Magierska A, Nawrot E, Lewiński A. Investigation of V600E BRAF mutation in papillary thyroid carcinoma in the Polish population. *Neuro Endocrinol Lett.* 2007;28(4):351–359.

Cañadas Garre M. Preoperative diagnosis of papillary thyroid carcinoma by the determination of the BRAFT1799A mutation on thyroid cytologies obtained by fine needle aspiration (FNA). PhD thesis, University of Granada, Granada, Spain, 2010.

Cañadas Garre M, Becerra-Massare P, de la Torre-Casares ML, Villar-Del Moral J et al. Reduction of false-negative papillary thyroid carcinomas by the routine analysis of BRAFT1799A mutation on fine-needle aspiration biopsy specimens: A prospective study of 814 thyroid FNAB patients. *Ann Surg.* 2012;255(5):986–992.

Cañadas Garre M, López de la Torre Casares M, Becerra Massare P, López Nevot MÁ, Villar Del Moral J, Muñoz Pérez N, Vílchez Joya R, Montes Ramírez R, Llamas Elvira JM. BRAF(T1799A) mutation in the primary tumor as a marker of risk, recurrence, or persistence of papillary thyroid carcinoma. *Endocrinol Nutr.* 2011 Apr;58(4):175–184.

Cantara S, Capezzone M, Marchisotta S, Capuano S et al. Impact of proto-oncogene mutation detection in cytological specimens from thyroid nodules improves the diagnostic accuracy of cytology. *J Clin Endocrinol Metab.* 2010 Mar;95(3):1365–1369.

Cantley LC, Neel BG. New insights into tumor suppression: PTEN suppresses tumor formation by restraining the phosphoinositide 3-kinase/AKT pathway. *Proc Natl Acad Sci USA.* 1999 Apr 13;96(8):4240–4245.

Carcangiu ML, Zampi G, Pupi A, Castagnoli A, Rosai J. Papillary carcinoma of the thyroid. A clinicopathologic study of 241 cases treated at the University of Florence, Italy. *Cancer.* 1985;55(4):805–828.

Carling T, Carty SE, Ciarleglio MM, Cooper DS et al. American Thyroid Association design and feasibility of a prospective randomized controlled trial of prophylactic lymph node dissection center for papillary thyroid carcinoma. *Thyroid.* 2012;22(3):237–244.

Carmeci C, Jeffrey RB, McDougall IR, Nowels KW, Weigel RJ. Ultrasound-guided fine-needle aspiration biopsy of thyroid masses. *Thyroid.* 1998 Apr;8(4):283–289.

Carpi A, Mechanick JI, Saussez S, Nicolini A. Thyroid tumor marker genomics and proteomics: Diagnostic and clinical implications. *J Cell Physiol.* 2010a Sep;224(3):612–619.

Carpi A, Naccarato AG, Iervasi G, Nicolini A et al. Large needle aspiration biopsy and galectin-3 determination in selected thyroid nodules with indeterminate FNA-cytology. *Br J Cancer.* 2006 Jul 17;95(2):204–209.

Carpi A, Rossi G, Coscio GD, Iervasi G, Nicolini A, Carpi F, Mechanick JI, Bartolazzi A. Galectin-3 detection on large-needle aspiration biopsy improves preoperative selection of thyroid nodules: A prospective cohort study. *Ann Med.* 2010b;42(1):70–78.

Carr LL, Mankoff DA, Goulart BH, Eaton KD, Capell PT, Kell EM, Bauman JE, Martins RG. Phase II study of daily sunitinib in FDG-PET-positive, iodine-refractory differentiated thyroid cancer and metastatic medullary carcinoma of the thyroid with functional imaging correlation. *Clin Cancer Res.* 2010 Nov 1;16(21):5260–5268.

Carta C, Moretti S, Passeri L, Barbi F et al. Genotyping of an Italian papillary thyroid carcinoma cohort revealed high prevalence of BRAF mutations, absence of RAS mutations and allowed the detection of a new mutation of BRAF oncoprotein (BRAF(V599lns)). *Clin Endocrinol (Oxf).* 2006;64(1):105–109.

Caruso D, Mazzaferri EL. Fine needle aspiration biopsy in the management of thyroid nodules. *Endocrinologist.* 1991;1:194–202.

Castro MR, Gharib H. Thyroid fine-needle aspiration biopsy: Progress, practice, and pitfalls. *Endocr Pract.* 2003;9(2):128–136.

Castro P, Rebocho AP, Soares RJ, Magalhães J, Roque L et al. PAX8-PPARgamma rearrangement is frequently detected in the follicular variant of papillary thyroid carcinoma. *J Clin Endocrinol Metab.* 2006 Jan;91(1):213–220.

Cerutti JM, Delcelo R, Amadei MJ, Nakabashi C, Maciel RM, Peterson B, Shoemaker J, Riggins GJ. A preoperative diagnostic test that distinguishes benign from malignant thyroid carcinoma based on gene expression. *J Clin Invest*. 2004 Apr;113(8):1234–1242.

Chen JC, Pace SC, Chen BA, Khiyami A, McHenry CR. Yield of repeat fine-needle aspiration biopsy and rate of malignancy in patients with atypia or follicular lesion of undetermined significance: The impact of the Bethesda System for Reporting Thyroid Cytopathology. *Surgery*. 2012 Dec;152(6):1037–1044.

Cheung CC, Carydis B, Ezzat S, Bedard YC, Asa SL. Analysis of ret/PTC gene rearrangements refines the fine needle aspiration diagnosis of thyroid cancer. *J Clin Endocrinol Metab*. 2001;86(5):2187–2190.

Cheung L, Messina M, Gill A, Clarkson A et al. Detection of the PAX8-PPAR gamma fusion oncogene in both follicular thyroid carcinomas and adenomas. *J Clin Endocrinol Metab*. 2003;88(1):354–357.

Chevillard S, Ugolin N, Vielh P, Ory K, Levalois C, Elliott D, Clayman GL, El-Naggar AK. Gene expression profiling of differentiated thyroid neoplasms: Diagnostic and clinical implications. *Clin Cancer Res*. 2004 Oct 1;10(19):6586–6897.

Chiosea S, Nikiforova M, Zuo H, Ogilvie J, Gandhi M, Seethala RR, Ohori NP, Nikiforov Y. A novel complex BRAF mutation detected in a solid variant of papillary thyroid carcinoma. *Endocr Pathol*. 2009;20(2):122–126.

Chow LS, Gharib H, Goellner JR, van Heerden JA. Nondiagnostic thyroid fine-needle aspiration cytology: Management dilemmas. *Thyroid*. 2001;11(12):1147–1151.

Chuang TC, Chuang AY, Poeta L, Koch WM, Califano JA, Tufano RP. Detectable BRAF mutation in serum DNA samples from patients with papillary thyroid carcinomas. *Head Neck*. 2010 Feb;32(2):229–234.

Chung KW, Kim SW, Kim SW. Gene expression profiling of papillary thyroid carcinomas in Korean patients by oligonucleotide microarrays. *J Korean Surg Soc*. 2012 May;82(5):271–280.

Chung KW, Yang SK, Lee GK, Kim EY et al. Detection of BRAFV600E mutation on fine needle aspiration specimens of thyroid nodule refines cyto-pathology diagnosis, especially in BRAF600E mutation-prevalent area. *Clin Endocrinol (Oxf)*. 2006 Nov;65(5):660–666.

Ciampi R, Giordano TJ, Wikenheiser-Brokamp K, Koenig RJ, Nikiforov YE. HOOK3-RET: A novel type of RET/PTC rearrangement in papillary thyroid carcinoma. *Endocr Relat Cancer*. 2007;14(2):445–452.

Ciampi R, Knauf JA, Kerler R, Gandhi M, Zhu Z, Nikiforova MN, Rabes HM, Fagin JA, Nikiforov YE. Oncogenic AKAP9-BRAF fusion is a novel mechanism of MAPK pathway activation in thyroid cancer. *J Clin Invest*. 2005;115(1):94–101.

Ciampi R, Nikiforov YE. Alterations of the BRAF gene in thyroid tumors. *Endocr Pathol*. 2005;16(3):163–172.

Cibas ES, Ali SZ. The Bethesda system for reporting thyroid cytopathology. *Thyroid*. 2009 Nov;19(11): 1159–1165.

Cohen EEW, Needles BM, Cullen KJ, Wong SJ et al. Phase 2 study of sunitinib in refractory thyroid cancer. In: *Proceedings of the 44 American Society of Clinical Oncology Meeting*, May 30–June 3, 2008a, Chicago, IL.

Cohen EE, Rosen LS, Vokes EE, Kies MS et al. Axitinib is an active treatment for all histologic subtypes of advanced thyroid cancer: Results from a phase II study. *J Clin Oncol*. 2008b Oct 10;26(29):4708–4713.

Cohen Y, Rosenbaum E, Clark DP, Zeiger MA, Umbricht CB, Tufano RP, Sidransky D, Westra WH. Mutational analysis of BRAF in fine needle aspiration biopsies of the thyroid: A potential application for the preoperative assessment of thyroid nodules. *Clin Cancer Res*. 2004;10(8):2761–2765.

Cohen Y, Xing M, Mambo E, Guo Z et al. BRAF mutation in papillary thyroid carcinoma. *J Natl Cancer Inst*. 2003;95(8):625–627.

Cooper DS, Doherty GM, Haugen BR, Kloos RT et al. Revised American Thyroid Association management guidelines for patients with thyroid nodules and differentiated thyroid cancer. *Thyroid*. 2009 Nov;19(11):1167–1214.

Corvi R, Berger N, Balczon R, Romeo G. RET/PCM-1: A novel fusion gene in papillary thyroid carcinoma. *Oncogene*. 2000;19(37):4236–4242.

Costa AM, Herrero A, Fresno MF, Heymann J, Alvarez JA, Cameselle-Teijeiro J, García-Rostán G. BRAF mutation associated with other genetic events identifies a subset of aggressive papillary thyroid carcinoma. *Clin Endocrinol (Oxf)*. 2008;68(4):618–634.

Cradic KW, Milosevic D, Rosenberg AM, Erickson LA, McIver B, Grebe SK. Mutant BRAF(T1799A) can be detected in the blood of papillary thyroid carcinoma patients and correlates with disease status. *J Clin Endocrinol Metab*. 2009 Dec;94(12):5001–5009.

Dalle Carbonare L, Frigo A, Francia G, Davì MV et al. Runx2 mRNA expression in the tissue, serum, and circulating non-hematopoietic cells of patients with thyroid cancer. *J Clin Endocrinol Metab.* 2012 Jul;97(7):E1249–E1256.

Damante G, Scaloni A, Tell G. Thyroid tumors: Novel insights from proteomic studies. *Expert Rev Proteomics.* 2009 Aug;6(4):363–376.

Darnton SJ, Hardie LJ, Muc RS, Wild CP, Casson AG. Tissue inhibitor of metalloproteinase-3 (TIMP-3) gene is methylated in the development of esophageal adenocarcinoma: Loss of expression correlates with poor prognosis. *Int J Cancer.* 2005 Jun 20;115(3):351–358.

Davies H, Bignell GR, Cox C, Stephens P et al. Mutations of the BRAF gene in human cancer. *Nature.* 2002;417(6892):949–954.

De Falco V, Giannini R, Tamburrino A, Ugolini C, Lupi C, Puxeddu E, Santoro M, Basolo F. Functional characterization of the novel T599I-VKSRdel BRAF mutation in a follicular variant papillary thyroid carcinoma. *J Clin Endocrinol Metab.* 2008;93(11):4398–4402.

de Hoog CL, Mann M. Proteomics. *Annu Rev Genomics Hum Genet.* 2004;5:267–293.

de Matos PS, Ferreira AP, de Oliveira Facuri F, Assumpção LV, Metze K, Ward LS. Usefulness of HBME-1, cytokeratin 19 and galectin-3 immunostaining in the diagnosis of thyroid malignancy. *Histopathology.* 2005 Oct;47(4):391–401.

Dean DS, Gharib H. Epidemiology of thyroid nodules. *Best Pract Res Clin Endocrinol Metab.* 2008 Dec;22(6):901–911.

DeGroot LJ, Kaplan EL, McCormick M, Straus FH. Natural history, treatment, and course of papillary thyroid carcinoma. *J Clin Endocrinol Metab.* 1990;71(2):414–424.

DeLellis RA, Lloyd RV, Heitz PU, Eng C. *Tumours of Endocrine Organs. Pathology and Genetics.* Lyon, France: World Health Organization IARC Press, 2004.

Delys L, Detours V, Franc B, Thomas G, Bogdanova T, Tronko M, Libert F, Dumont JE, Maenhaut C. Gene expression and the biological phenotype of papillary thyroid carcinomas. *Oncogene.* 2007 Dec 13;26(57):7894–7903.

Detours V, Wattel S, Venet D, Hutsebaut N et al. Absence of a specific radiation signature in post-Chernobyl thyroid cancers. *Br J Cancer.* 2005 Apr 25;92(8):1545–1552.

Dhillon AS, Kolch W. Oncogenic B-Raf mutations: Crystal clear at last. *Cancer Cell.* 2004;5(4):303–304.

Di Cristofaro J, Marcy M, Vasko V, Sebag F, Fakhry N, Wynford-Thomas D, De Micco C. Molecular genetic study comparing follicular variant versus classic papillary thyroid carcinomas: Association of N-ras mutation in codon 61 with follicular variant. *Hum Pathol.* 2006;37(7):824–830.

Ditkoff BA, Marvin MR, Yemul S, Shi YJ, Chabot J, Feind C, Lo Gerfo PL. Detection of circulating thyroid cells in peripheral blood. *Surgery.* 1996 Dec;120(6):959–964; discussion 964–995.

Dom G, Tarabichi M, Unger K, Thomas G, Oczko-Wojciechowska M, Bogdanova T, Jarzab B, Dumont JE, Detours V, Maenhaut C. A gene expression signature distinguishes normal tissues of sporadic and radiation-induced papillary thyroid carcinomas. *Br J Cancer.* 2012 Sep 4;107(6):994–1000.

Domingues R, Mendonça E, Sobrinho L, Bugalho MJ. Searching for RET/PTC rearrangements and BRAF V599E mutation in thyroid aspirates might contribute to establish a preoperative diagnosis of papillary thyroid carcinoma. *Cytopathology.* 2005 Feb;16(1):27–31.

Durand S, Ferraro-Peyret C, Selmi-Ruby S, Paulin C et al. Evaluation of gene expression profiles in thyroid nodule biopsy material to diagnose thyroid cancer. *J Clin Endocrinol Metab.* 2008 Apr;93(4):1195–1202.

Durante C, Puxeddu E, Ferretti E, Morisi R et al. BRAF mutations in papillary thyroid carcinomas inhibit genes involved in iodine metabolism. *J Clin Endocrinol Metab.* 2007;92(7):2840–2843.

Elisei R, Romei C, Vorontsova T, Cosci B et al. RET/PTC rearrangements in thyroid nodules: Studies in irradiated and not irradiated, malignant and benign thyroid lesions in children and adults. *J Clin Endocrinol Metab.* 2001 Jul;86(7):3211–3216.

Elisei R, Ugolini C, Viola D, Lupi C et al. BRAF(V600E) mutation and outcome of patients with papillary thyroid carcinoma: A 15-year median follow-up study. *J Clin Endocrinol Metab.* 2008 Oct;93(10):3943–3949.

Erickson LA, Jin L, Nakamura N, Bridges AG, Markovic SN, Lloyd RV. Clinicopathologic features and BRAF(V600E) mutation analysis in cutaneous metastases from well-differentiated thyroid carcinomas. *Cancer.* 2007;109(10):1965–1971.

Esteller M. CpG island hypermethylation and tumor suppressor genes: A booming present, a brighter future. *Oncogene.* 2002;21(35):5427–5440.

Eszlinger M, Krohn K, Kukulska A, Jarzab B, Paschke R. Perspectives and limitations of microarray-based gene expression profiling of thyroid tumors. *Endocr Rev*. 2007 May;28(3):322–338.

Eszlinger M, Wiench M, Jarzab B, Krohn K et al. Meta- and reanalysis of gene expression profiles of hot and cold thyroid nodules and papillary thyroid carcinoma for gene groups. *J Clin Endocrinol Metab*. 2006 May;91(5):1934–1942.

Eze OP, Starker LF, Carling T. The role of epigenetic alterations in papillary thyroid carcinogenesis. *J Thyroid Res*. 2011;2011:895470. doi: 10.4061/2011/895470.

Ezzat S, Sarti DA, Cain DR, Braunstein GD. Thyroid incidentalomas. Prevalence by palpation and ultrasonography. *Arch Intern Med*. 1994 Aug 22;154(16):1838–1840.

Ezzat S, Zheng L, Kolenda J, Safarian A, Freeman JL, Asa SL. Prevalence of activating ras mutations in morphologically characterized thyroid nodules. *Thyroid*. 1996;6(5):409–416.

Faggiano A, Caillou B, Lacroix L, Talbot M, Filetti S, Bidart JM, Schlumberger M. Functional characterization of human thyroid tissue with immunohistochemistry. *Thyroid*. 2007 Mar;17(3):203–211.

Fajas L, Auboeuf D, Raspé E, Schoonjans K et al. The organization, promoter analysis, and expression of the human PPARgamma gene. *J Biol Chem*. 1997;272(30):18779–18789.

Feng H, Cheung AN, Xue WC, Wang Y, Wang X, Fu S, Wang Q, Ngan HY, Tsao SW. Down-regulation and promoter methylation of tissue inhibitor of metalloproteinase 3 in choriocarcinoma. *Gynecol Oncol*. 2004 Aug;94(2):375–382.

Fenton CL, Lukes Y, Nicholson D, Dinauer CA, Francis GL, Tuttle RM. The ret/PTC mutations are common in sporadic papillary thyroid carcinoma of children and young adults. *J Clin Endocrinol Metab*. 2000;85(3):1170–1175.

Ferlay J, Shin HR, Bray F, Forman D, Mathers C, Parkin DM. Estimates of worldwide burden of cancer in 2008: GLOBOCAN 2008. *Int J Cancer*. 2010 Dec 15;127(12):2893–2917.

Filetti S, Durante C, Torlontano M. Nonsurgical approaches to the management of thyroid nodules. *Nat Clin Pract Endocrinol Metab*. 2006;2(7):384–394.

Finley DJ, Arora N, Zhu B, Gallagher L, Fahey TJ 3rd. Molecular profiling distinguishes papillary carcinoma from benign thyroid nodules. *J Clin Endocrinol Metab*. 2004a Jul;89(7):3214–3223.

Finley DJ, Zhu B, Barden CB, Fahey TJ 3rd. Discrimination of benign and malignant thyroid nodules by molecular profiling. *Ann Surg*. 2004b Sep;240(3):425–436; discussion 436–437.

Frasca F, Nucera C, Pellegriti G, Gangemi P et al. BRAF(V600E) mutation and the biology of papillary thyroid cancer. *Endocr Relat Cancer*. 2008;15(1):191–205.

Frattini M, Ferrario C, Bressan P, Balestra D et al. Alternative mutations of BRAF, RET and NTRK1 are associated with similar but distinct gene expression patterns in papillary thyroid cancer. *Oncogene*. 2004;23(44):7436–7440.

French CA, Fletcher JA, Cibas ES, Caulfield C, Allard P, Kroll TG. Molecular detection of PPAR gamma rearrangements and thyroid carcinoma in preoperative fine-needle aspiration biopsies. *Endocr Pathol*. 2008 Fall;19(3):166–174. Erratum in: *Endocr Pathol*. 2008 Winter;19(4):299.

Fugazzola L, Mannavola D, Cirello V, Vannucchi G, Muzza M, Vicentini L, Beck-Peccoz P. BRAF mutations in an Italian cohort of thyroid cancers. *Clin Endocrinol (Oxf)*. 2004;61(2):239–243.

Fugazzola L, Pierotti MA, Vigano E, Pacini F, Vorontsova TV, Bongarzone I. Molecular and biochemical analysis of RET/PTC4, a novel oncogenic rearrangement between RET and ELE1 genes, in a post-Chernobyl papillary thyroid cancer. *Oncogene*. 1996;13(5):1093–1097.

Fugazzola L, Puxeddu E, Avenia N, Romei C et al. Correlation between B-RAFV600E mutation and clinicopathologic parameters in papillary thyroid carcinoma: Data from a multicentric Italian study and review of the literature. *Endocr Relat Cancer*. 2006;13(2):455–464.

Fujarewicz K, Jarzab M, Eszlinger M, Krohn K et al. A multi-gene approach to differentiate papillary thyroid carcinoma from benign lesions: Gene selection using support vector machines with bootstrapping. *Endocr Relat Cancer*. 2007 Sep;14(3):809–826.

Fukushima T, Suzuki S, Mashiko M, Ohtake T, Endo Y, Takebayashi Y, Sekikawa K, Hagiwara K, Takenoshita S. BRAF mutations in papillary carcinomas of the thyroid. *Oncogene*. 2003; 22(41):6455–6457.

Galloway JW, Sardi A, DeConti RW, Mitchell WT Jr., Bolton JS. Changing trends in thyroid surgery. 38 Years' experience. *Am Surg*. 1991;57(1):18–20.

Ganapathy V, Gopal E, Miyauchi S, Prasad PD. Biological functions of SLC5A8, a candidate tumour suppressor. *Biochem Soc Trans*. 2005 Feb;33(Pt 1):237–240.

Gao WL, Wie LL, Chao YG, Wie L, Song TL. Prognostic prediction of BRAF(V600E) and its relationship with sodium iodide symporter in classic variant of papillary thyroid carcinomas. *Clin Lab.* 2012;58(9–10):919–926.

Gharib H. Changing trends in thyroid practice: Understanding nodular thyroid disease. *Endocr Pract.* 2004;10(1):31–39.

Gharib H. Fine-needle aspiration biopsy of thyroid nodules: Advantages, limitations, and effect. *Mayo Clin Proc.* 1994;69(1):44–49.

Gharib H, Goellner JR. Fine-needle aspiration biopsy of the thyroid: An appraisal. *Ann Intern Med.* 1993;118:282–289.

Gharib H, Goellner JR. Fine-needle aspiration biopsy of thyroid nodules. *Endocr Pract.* 1995;1(6): 410–417.

Gharib H, Goellner JR, Johnson DA. Fine-needle aspiration cytology of the thyroid. A 12-year experience with 11,000 biopsies. *Clin Lab Med.* 1993;13(3):699–709.

Gharib H, Papini E. Thyroid nodules: Clinical importance, assessment, and treatment. *Endocrinol Metab Clin North Am.* 2007;36(3):707–735, vi.

Gharib H, Papini E, Paschke R. Thyroid nodules: A review of current guidelines, practices, and prospects. *Eur J Endocrinol.* 2008;159(5):493–505.

Gharib H, Papini E, Paschke R, Duick DS, Valcavi R, Hegedüs L, Vitti P; AACE/AME/ETA Task Force on Thyroid Nodules. American Association of Clinical Endocrinologists, Associazione Medici Endocrinologi, and European Thyroid Association medical guidelines for clinical practice for the diagnosis and management of thyroid nodules. *Endocr Pract.* 2010 May–Jun;16(Suppl 1):1–43.

Giannini R, Faviana P, Cavinato T, Elisei R et al. Galectin-3 and oncofetal-fibronectin expression in thyroid neoplasia as assessed by reverse transcription-polymerase chain reaction and immunochemistry in cytologic and pathologic specimens. *Thyroid.* 2003;13(8):765–770.

Giannini R, Ugolini C, Lupi C, Proietti A et al. The heterogeneous distribution of BRAF mutation supports the independent clonal origin of distinct tumor foci in multifocal papillary thyroid carcinoma. *J Clin Endocrinol Metab.* 2007;92(9):3511–3516.

Giordano TJ, Kuick R, Thomas DG, Misek DE et al. Molecular classification of papillary thyroid carcinoma: Distinct BRAF, RAS, and RET/PTC mutation-specific gene expression profiles discovered by DNA microarray analysis. *Oncogene.* 2005;24(44):6646–6656.

Giorgadze T, Rossi ED, Fadda G, Gupta PK, Livolsi VA, Baloch Z. Does the fine-needle aspiration diagnosis of "Hürthle-cell neoplasm/follicular neoplasm with oncocytic features" denote increased risk of malignancy? *Diagn Cytopathol.* 2004 Nov;31(5):307–312.

Giusti L, Iacconi P, Ciregia F, Giannaccini G, Donatini GL, Basolo F, Miccoli P, Pinchera A, Lucacchini A. Fine-needle aspiration of thyroid nodules: Proteomic analysis to identify cancer biomarkers. *J Proteome Res.* 2008 Sep;7(9):4079–4088.

Goessl C. Diagnostic potential of circulating nucleic acids for oncology. *Expert Rev Mol Diagn.* 2003;3(4):431–442.

González-Cámpora R, Galera-Ruiz D, Armas-Padrón JR, Otal-Salaverri C, Galera-Davidson H. Dipeptidyl aminopeptidase IV in the cytologic diagnosis of thyroid carcinoma. *Diagn Cytopathol.* 1998;19(1):4–8.

Gormally E, Caboux E, Vineis P, Hainaut P. Circulating free DNA in plasma or serum as biomarker of carcinogenesis: Practical aspects and biological significance. *Mutat Res.* 2007;62:699–702.

Grieco M, Santoro M, Berlingieri MT, Melillo RM, Donghi R, Bongarzone I, Pierotti MA, Della Porta G, Fusco A, Vecchio G. PTC is a novel rearranged form of the ret proto-oncogene and is frequently detected in vivo in human thyroid papillary carcinomas. *Cell.* 1990;60(4):557–563.

Griffith OL, Melck A, Jones SJ, Wiseman SM. Meta-analysis and meta-review of thyroid cancer gene expression profiling studies identifies important diagnostic biomarkers. *J Clin Oncol.* 2006 Nov 1;24(31):5043–5051.

Guan H, Ji M, Bao R, Yu H, Wang Y, Hou P, Zhang Y, Shan Z, Teng W, Xing M. Association of high iodine intake with the T1799A BRAF mutation in papillary thyroid cancer. *J Clin Endocrinol Metab.* 2009;94(5):1612–1617.

Guan H, Ji M, Hou P, Liu Z, Wang C, Shan Z, Teng W, Xing M. Hypermethylation of the DNA mismatch repair gene hMLH1 and its association with lymph node metastasis and T1799A BRAF mutation in patients with papillary thyroid cancer. *Cancer.* 2008 Jul 15;113(2):247–255.

Gupta-Abramson V, Troxel AB, Nellore A, Puttaswamy K et al. Phase II trial of sorafenib in advanced thyroid cancer. *J Clin Oncol.* 2008 Oct 10;26(29):4714–4719.

Guth S, Theune U, Aberle J, Galach A, Bamberger CM. Very high prevalence of thyroid nodules detected by high frequency (13 MHz) ultrasound examination. *Eur J Clin Invest.* 2009 Aug;39(8):699–706.

Hamada A, Mankovskaya S, Saenko V, Rogounovitch T, Mine M, Namba H, Nakashima M, Demidchik Y, Demidchik E, Yamashita S. Diagnostic usefulness of PCR profiling of the differentially expressed marker genes in thyroid papillary carcinomas. *Cancer Lett.* 2005 Jun 28;224(2):289–301.

Hamberger B, Gharib H, Melton LJ 3rd, Goellner JR, Zinsmeister AR. Fine-needle aspiration biopsy of thyroid nodules. Impact on thyroid practice and cost of care. *Am J Med.* 1982;73:381–384.

Hamburger JI. Diagnosis of thyroid nodules by fine needle biopsy: Use and abuse. *J Clin Endocrinol Metab.* 1994;79(2):335–339.

Hayashida N, Namba H, Kumagai A, Hayashi T et al. A rapid and simple detection method for the BRAF(T1796A) mutation in fine-needle aspirated thyroid carcinoma cells. *Thyroid.* 2004;14(11):910–915.

Hayes DN, Lucas AS, Tanvetyanon T, Krzyzanowska MK et al. Phase II efficacy and pharmacogenomic study of Selumetinib (AZD6244; ARRY-142886) in iodine-131 refractory papillary thyroid carcinoma with or without follicular elements. *Clin Cancer Res.* 2012 Apr 1;18(7):2056–2065.

Haymart MR, Repplinger DJ, Leverson GE, Elson DF, Sippel RS, Jaume JC, Chen H. Higher serum thyroid stimulating hormone level in thyroid nodule patients is associated with greater risks of differentiated thyroid cancer and advanced tumor stage. *J Clin Endocrinol Metab.* 2008 Mar;93(3):809–814.

He H, Jazdzewski K, Li W, Liyanarachchi S et al. The role of microRNA genes in papillary thyroid carcinoma. *Proc Natl Acad Sci USA.* 2005 Dec 27;102(52):19075–19080.

Hébrant A, Dom G, Dewaele M, Andry G, Trésallet C, Leteurtre E, Dumont JE, Maenhaut C. mRNA expression in papillary and anaplastic thyroid carcinoma: Molecular anatomy of a killing switch. *PLoS One.* 2012;7(10):e37807.

Hegedüs L. Clinical practice. The thyroid nodule. *N Engl J Med.* 2004;351(17):1764–1771.

Henry JF, Denizot A, Porcelli A, Villafane M, Zoro P, Garcia S, De Micco C. Thyroperoxidase immunodetection for the diagnosis of malignancy on fine-needle aspiration of thyroid nodules. *World J Surg.* 1994;18(4):529–534.

Herbst RS, Heymach JV, O'Reilly MS, Onn A, Ryan AJ. Vandetanib (ZD6474): An orally available receptor tyrosine kinase inhibitor that selectively targets pathways critical for tumor growth and angiogenesis. *Expert Opin Investig Drugs.* 2007 Feb;16(2):239–249.

Herrmann ME, LiVolsi VA, Pasha TL, Roberts SA, Wojcik EM, Baloch ZW. Immunohistochemical expression of galectin-3 in benign and malignant thyroid lesions. *Arch Pathol Lab Med.* 2002 Jun;126(6):710–713.

Hodak SP, Rosenthal, DS. American Thyroid Association Clinical Affairs Committee. Information for clinicians: Commercially available molecular diagnosis testing in the evaluation of thyroid nodule fine-needle aspiration specimens. *Thyroid.* 2013 Feb;23(2);131–134. doi:10.1089/thy.2012.0320. Epub 2012 Nov 27.

Hoftijzer H, Heemstra KA, Morreau H, Stokkel MP et al. Beneficial effects of sorafenib on tumor progression, but not on radioiodine uptake, in patients with differentiated thyroid carcinoma. *Eur J Endocrinol.* 2009 Dec;161(6):923–931.

Hong C, Maunakea A, Jun P, Bollen AW, Hodgson JG, Goldenberg DD, Weiss WA, Costello JF. Shared epigenetic mechanisms in human and mouse gliomas inactivate expression of the growth suppressor SLC5A8. *Cancer Res.* 2005 May 1;65(9):3617–3623.

Hoque MO, Rosenbaum E, Westra WH, Xing M, Ladenson P, Zeiger MA, Sidransky D, Umbricht CB. Quantitative assessment of promoter methylation profiles in thyroid neoplasms. *J Clin Endocrinol Metab.* 2005;90(7):4011–4018. Erratum in: *J Clin Endocrinol Metab.* 2006 Sep;91(9):3278.

Hou P, Liu D, Xing M. Functional characterization of the T1799–1801del and A1799–1816ins BRAF mutations in papillary thyroid cancer. *Cell Cycle.* 2007;6(3):377–379.

Howlader N, Noone AM, Krapcho M, Neyman N et al. (eds). *SEER Cancer Statistics Review, 1975–2009 (Vintage 2009 Populations).* Bethesda, MD: National Cancer Institute. http://seer.cancer.gov/csr/1975_2009_pops09/, based on November 2011 SEER data submission, posted to the SEER website, 2012.

Hu S, Ewertz M, Tufano RP, Brait M et al. Detection of serum deoxyribonucleic acid methylation markers: A novel diagnostic tool for thyroid cancer. *J Clin Endocrinol Metab.* 2006a;91(1):98–104.

Hu S, Liu D, Tufano RP, Carson KA et al. Association of aberrant methylation of tumor suppressor genes with tumor aggressiveness and BRAF mutation in papillary thyroid cancer. *Int J Cancer*. 2006b;119(10):2322–2329.

Huang Y, Prasad M, Lemon WJ, Hampel H et al. Gene expression in papillary thyroid carcinoma reveals highly consistent profiles. *Proc Natl Acad Sci USA*. 2001 Dec 18;98(26):15044–15049.

Hundahl SA, Fleming ID, Fremgen AM, Menck HR. A National Cancer Data Base report on 53,856 cases of thyroid carcinoma treated in the U.S., 1985–1995. *Cancer*. 1998;83(12):2638–2648.

Hubbard SR. Oncogenic mutations in B-Raf: Some losses yield gains. *Cell*. 2004;116(6):764–766.

Imaizumi M, Usa T, Tominaga T, Neriishi K et al. Radiation dose-response relationships for thyroid nodules and autoimmune thyroid diseases in Hiroshima and Nagasaki atomic bomb survivors 55–58 years after radiation exposure. *JAMA*. 2006 Mar 1;295(9):1011–1022.

Ishida E, Nakamura M, Shimada K, Higuchi T, Takatsu K, Yane K, Konishi N. DNA hypermethylation status of multiple genes in papillary thyroid carcinomas. *Pathobiology*. 2007;74(6):344–352.

Ishizaka Y, Kobayashi S, Ushijima T, Hirohashi S, Sugimura T, Nagao M. Detection of retTPC/PTC transcripts in thyroid adenomas and adenomatous goiter by an RT-PCR method. *Oncogene*. 1991;6(9): 1667–1672.

Ito Y, Yoshida H, Maruo R, Morita S et al. BRAF mutation in papillary thyroid carcinoma in a Japanese population: Its lack of correlation with high-risk clinicopathological features and disease-free survival of patients. *Endocr J*. 2009;56(1):89–97.

Ivanova R, Soares P, Castro P, Sobrinho-Simões M. Diffuse (or multinodular) follicular variant of papillary thyroid carcinoma: A clinicopathologic and immunohistochemical analysis of ten cases of an aggressive form of differentiated thyroid carcinoma. *Virchows Arch*. 2002;440(4):418–424.

Jarzab B, Wiench M, Fujarewicz K, Simek K et al. Gene expression profile of papillary thyroid cancer: Sources of variability and diagnostic implications. *Cancer Res*. 2005 Feb 15; 65(4):1587–1597.

Jin L, Sebo TJ, Nakamura N, Qian X, Oliveira A, Majerus JA, Johnson MR, Lloyd RV. BRAF mutation analysis in fine needle aspiration (FNA) cytology of the thyroid. *Diagn Mol Pathol*. 2006;15(3):136–143.

Jo YS, Huang S, Kim YJ, Lee IS et al. Diagnostic value of pyrosequencing for the BRAF V600E mutation in ultrasound-guided fine-needle aspiration biopsy samples of thyroid incidentalomas. *Clin Endocrinol (Oxf)*. 2009 Jan;70(1):139–144.

Jo YS, Li S, Song JH, Kwon KH et al. Influence of the BRAF V600E mutation on expression of vascular endothelial growth factor in papillary thyroid cancer. *J Clin Endocrinol Metab*. 2006;91(9):3667–3670.

Jung CK, Im SY, Kang YJ, Lee H, Jung ES, Kang CS, Bae JS, Choi YJ. Mutational patterns and novel mutations of the BRAF gene in a large cohort of Korean patients with papillary thyroid carcinoma. *Thyroid*. 2012 Aug;22(8):791–797.

Kakudo K, Tang W, Ito Y, Mori I, Nakamura Y, Miyauchi A. Papillary carcinoma of the thyroid in Japan: Subclassification of common type and identification of low risk group. *J Clin Pathol*. 2004;57(10):1041–1046.

Kaufmann S, Schmutzler C, Schomburg L, Körber C, Luster M, Rendl J, Reiners C, Köhrle J. Real time RT-PCR analysis of thyroglobulin mRNA in peripheral blood in patients with congenital athyreosis and with differentiated thyroid carcinoma after stimulation with recombinant human thyrotropin. *Endocr Regul*. 2004 Jun;38(2):41–49.

Kebebew E, Peng M, Reiff E, Duh QY, Clark OH, McMillan A. ECM1 and TMPRSS4 are diagnostic markers of malignant thyroid neoplasms and improve the accuracy of fine needle aspiration biopsy. *Ann Surg*. 2005 Sep;242(3):353–361; discussion 361–363.

Kebebew E, Peng M, Reiff E, Duh QY, Clark OH, McMillan A. Diagnostic and prognostic value of cell-cycle regulatory genes in malignant thyroid neoplasms. *World J Surg*. 2006 May;30(5):767–774.

Kebebew E, Weng J, Bauer J, Ranvier G, Clark OH, Duh QY, Shibru D, Bastian B, Griffin A. The prevalence and prognostic value of BRAF mutation in thyroid cancer. *Ann Surg*. 2007;246(3):466–470; discussion 470–471.

Keutgen XM, Filicori F, Crowley MJ, Wang Y et al. A panel of four miRNAs accurately differentiates malignant from benign indeterminate thyroid lesions on fine needle aspiration. *Clin Cancer Res*. 2012 Apr 1; 18(7):2032 2038.

Kim HS, Kim do H, Kim JY, Jeoung NH, Lee IK, Bong JG, Jung ED. Microarray analysis of papillary thyroid cancers in Korean. *Korean J Intern Med*. 2010a Dec;25(4):399–407.

Kim J, Giuliano AE, Turner RR, Gaffney RE, Umetani N, Kitago M, Elashoff D, Hoon DS. Lymphatic mapping establishes the role of BRAF gene mutation in papillary thyroid carcinoma. *Ann Surg.* 2006a;244(5):799–804.

Kim KH, Kang DW, Kim SH, Seong IO, Kang DY. Mutations of the BRAF gene in papillary thyroid carcinoma in a Korean population. *Yonsei Med J.* 2004;45(5):818–821.

Kim KH, Suh KS, Kang DW, Kang DY. Mutations of the BRAF gene in papillary thyroid carcinoma and in Hashimoto's thyroiditis. *Pathol Int.* 2005a;55(9):540–545.

Kim SK, Hwang TS, Yoo YB, Han HS, Kim DL, Song KH, Lim SD, Kim WS, Paik NS. Surgical results of thyroid nodules according to a management guideline based on the BRAF(V600E) mutation status. *J Clin Endocrinol Metab.* 2011 Mar;96(3):658–664.

Kim SK, Kim DL, Han HS, Kim WS, Kim SJ, Moon WJ, Oh SY, Hwang TS. Pyrosequencing analysis for detection of a BRAFV600E mutation in an FNAB specimen of thyroid nodules. *Diagn Mol Pathol.* 2008 Jun;17(2):118–125.

Kim SW, Lee JI, Kim JW, Ki CS, Oh YL, Choi YL, Shin JH, Kim HK, Jang HW, Chung JH. BRAFV600E mutation analysis in fine-needle aspiration cytology specimens for evaluation of thyroid nodule: A large series in a BRAFV600E-prevalent population. *J Clin Endocrinol Metab.* 2010b;95(8):3693–3700.

Kim TY, Kim WB, Rhee YS, Song JY et al. The BRAF mutation is useful for prediction of clinical recurrence in low-risk patients with conventional papillary thyroid carcinoma. *Clin Endocrinol (Oxf).* 2006b;65(3):364–368.

Kim TY, Kim WB, Song JY, Rhee YS, Gong G, Cho YM, Kim SY, Kim SC, Hong SJ, Shong YK. The BRAF mutation is not associated with poor prognostic factors in Korean patients with conventional papillary thyroid microcarcinoma. *Clin Endocrinol (Oxf).* 2005b;63(5):588–593.

Kimura ET, Nikiforova MN, Zhu Z, Knauf JA, Nikiforov YE, Fagin JA. High prevalence of BRAF mutations in thyroid cancer: Genetic evidence for constitutive activation of the RET/PTC-RAS-BRAF signaling pathway in papillary thyroid carcinoma. *Cancer Res.* 2003;63(7):1454–1457.

Kini SR. *Thyroid Cytopathology. An Atlas and Text.* Philadelphia, PA: Lippincott Williams & Wilkins, 2008.

Kitano M, Rahbari R, Patterson EE, Steinberg SM, Prasad NB, Wang Y, Zeiger MA, Kebebew E. Evaluation of candidate diagnostic microRNAs in thyroid fine-needle aspiration biopsy samples. *Thyroid.* 2012 Mar;22(3):285–291.

Kloos RT, Ringel MD, Knopp MV, Hall NC et al. Phase II trial of sorafenib in metastatic thyroid cancer. *J Clin Oncol.* 2009 Apr 1;27(10):1675–1684. doi: 10.1200/JCO.2008.18.2717. Epub March 2, 2009.

Klugbauer S, Demidchik EP, Lengfelder E, Rabes HM. Detection of a novel type of RET rearrangement (PTC5) in thyroid carcinomas after Chernobyl and analysis of the involved RET-fused gene RFG5. *Cancer Res.* 1998a;58(2):198–203.

Klugbauer S, Jauch A, Lengfelder E, Demidchik E, Rabes HM. A novel type of RET rearrangement (PTC8) in childhood papillary thyroid carcinomas and characterization of the involved gene (RFG8). *Cancer Res.* 2000;60(24):7028–7032.

Klugbauer S, Rabes HM. The transcription coactivator HTIF1 and a related protein are fused to the RET receptor tyrosine kinase in childhood papillary thyroid carcinomas. *Oncogene.* 1999;18(30):4388–4393.

Knauf JA, Kuroda H, Basu S, Fagin JA. RET/PTC-induced dedifferentiation of thyroid cells is mediated through Y1062 signaling through SHC-RAS-MAP kinase. *Oncogene.* 2003;22(28):4406–4412.

Knauf JA, Ma X, Smith EP, Zhang L, Mitsutake N, Liao XH, Refetoff S, Nikiforov YE, Fagin JA. Targeted expression of BRAFV600E in thyroid cells of transgenic mice results in papillary thyroid cancers that undergo dedifferentiation. *Cancer Res.* 2005;65(10):4238–4245.

Knudsen N, Laurberg P, Perrild H, Bülow I, Ovesen L, Jørgensen T. Risk factors for goiter and thyroid nodules. *Thyroid.* 2002 Oct;12(10):879–888.

Kondo T, Asa SL, Ezzat S. Epigenetic dysregulation in thyroid neoplasia. *Endocrinol Metab Clin North Am.* 2008 Jun;37(2):389–400, ix.

Kondo T, Ezzat S, Asa SL. Pathogenetic mechanisms in thyroid follicular-cell neoplasia. *Nat Rev Cancer.* 2006;6(4):292–306.

Kondo T, Nakazawa T, Ma D, Niu D, Mochizuki K, Kawasaki T, Nakamura N, Yamane T, Kobayashi M, Katoh R. Epigenetic silencing of TTF-1/NKX2-1 through DNA hypermethylation and histone H3 modulation in thyroid carcinomas. *Lab Invest.* 2009 Jul;89(7):791–799. doi: 10.1038/labinvest.2009.50. Epub June 8, 2009.

Krause K, Jessnitzer B, Fuhrer D. Proteomics in thyroid tumor research. *J Clin Endocrinol Metab.* 2009 Aug;94(8):2717–2724.

Krause K, Prawitt S, Eszlinger M, Ihling C et al. Dissecting molecular events in thyroid neoplasia provides evidence for distinct evolution of follicular thyroid adenoma and carcinoma. *Am J Pathol.* 2011 Dec;179(6):3066–3074.

Kroll TG, Sarraf P, Pecciarini L, Chen CJ, Mueller E, Spiegelman BM, Fletcher JA. PAX8-PPARgamma1 fusion oncogene in human thyroid carcinoma [corrected]. *Science.* 2000;289(5483):1357–1360. Erratum in: *Science* 2000;289(5484):1474.

Kumagai A, Namba H, Akanov Z, Saenko VA et al. Clinical implications of pre-operative rapid BRAF analysis for papillary thyroid cancer. *Endocr J.* 2007 Jun;54(3):399–405.

Kumagai A, Namba H, Saenko VA, Ashizawa K et al. Low frequency of BRAFT1796A mutations in childhood thyroid carcinomas. *J Clin Endocrinol Metab.* 2004;89(9):4280–4284.

Kundel A, Zarnegar R, Kato M, Moo TA, Zhu B, Scognamiglio T, Fahey TJ 3rd. Comparison of microarray analysis of fine needle aspirates and tissue specimen in thyroid nodule diagnosis. *Diagn Mol Pathol.* 2010 Mar;19(1):9–14.

Kuo CS, Lin CY, Hsu CW, Lee CH, Lin HD. Low frequency of rearrangement of TRK protooncogene in Chinese thyroid tumors. *Endocrine.* 2000;13(3):341–344.

Kurt B, Yalçın S, Alagöz E, Karslıoğlu Y, Yigit N, Günal A, Deveci MS. The relationship of the BRAF(V600E) mutation and the established prognostic factors in papillary thyroid carcinomas. *Endocr Pathol.* 2012 Sep;23(3):135–140.

Kwak JY, Kim EK, Chung WY, Moon HJ, Kim MJ, Choi JR. Association of BRAFV600E mutation with poor clinical prognostic factors and US features in Korean patients with papillary thyroid microcarcinoma. *Radiology.* 2009;253(3):854–860.

Lacroix L, Pourcher T, Magnon C, Bellon N, Talbot M, Intaraphairot T, Caillou B, Schlumberger M, Bidart JM. Expression of the apical iodide transporter in human thyroid tissues: A comparison study with other iodide transporters. *J Clin Endocrinol Metab.* 2004 Mar;89(3):1423–1428.

Lam AK, Lo CY, Leung P, Lang BH, Chan WF, Luk JM. Clinicopathological roles of alterations of tumor suppressor gene p16 in papillary thyroid carcinoma. *Ann Surg Oncol.* 2007 May;14(5):1772–1779.

Lassalle S, Hofman V, Ilie M, Butori C, Bozec A, Santini J, Vielh P, Hofman P. Clinical impact of the detection of BRAF mutations in thyroid pathology: Potential usefulness as diagnostic, prognostic and theragnostic applications. *Curr Med Chem.* 2010;17(17):1839–1850.

Lazzereschi D, Mincione G, Coppa A, Ranieri A, Turco A, Baccheschi G, Pelicano S, Colletta G. Oncogenes and antioncogenes involved in human thyroid carcinogenesis. *J Exp Clin Cancer Res.* 1997;16(3):325–332.

Lee JH, Lee ES, Kim YS. Clinicopathologic significance of BRAF V600E mutation in papillary carcinomas of the thyroid: A meta-analysis. *Cancer.* 2007;110(1):38–46.

Lee JH, Lee ES, Kim YS, Won NH, Chae YS. BRAF mutation and AKAP9 expression in sporadic papillary thyroid carcinomas. *Pathology.* 2006;38(3):201–204.

Lee SJ, Lee MH, Kim DW, Lee S et al. Cross-regulation between oncogenic BRAF(V600E) kinase and the MST1 pathway in papillary thyroid carcinoma. *PLoS One.* 2011 Jan 13;6(1):e16180.

Lee X, Gao M, Ji Y, Yu Y, Feng Y, Li Y, Zhang Y, Cheng W, Zhao W. Analysis of differential BRAF(V600E) mutational status in high aggressive papillary thyroid microcarcinoma. *Ann Surg Oncol.* 2009;16(2):240–245.

Leon SA, Shapiro B, Sklaroff DM, Yaros MJ. Free DNA in the serum of cancer patients and the effect of therapy. *Cancer Res.* 1977;37:646–650.

Li H, Myeroff L, Smiraglia D, Romero MF et al. SLC5A8, a sodium transporter, is a tumor suppressor gene silenced by methylation in human colon aberrant crypt foci and cancers. *Proc Natl Acad Sci USA.* 2003 Jul 8;100(14):8412–8417.

Li H, Robinson KA, Anton B, Saldanha IJ, Ladenson PW. Cost-effectiveness of a novel molecular test for cytologically indeterminate thyroid nodules. *J Clin Endocrinol Metab.* 2011 Nov;96(11):E1719–E1726.

Liang HS, Zhong YH, Luo ZJ, Huang Y, Lin HD, Luo M, Zhan S, Su HX, Zhou SB, Xie KQ. Comparative analysis of protein expression in differentiated thyroid tumours: A multicentre study. *J Int Med Res.* 2009 May–Jun;37(3):927–938.

Lima J, Trovisco V, Soares P, Máximo V et al. BRAF mutations are not a major event in post-Chernobyl childhood thyroid carcinomas. *J Clin Endocrinol Metab.* 2004;89(9):4267–4271.

Linkov F, Ferris RL, Yurkovetsky Z, Marrangoni A et al. Multiplex analysis of cytokines as biomarkers that differentiate benign and malignant thyroid diseases. *Proteomics Clin Appl.* 2008 Oct 10;2(12):1575–1585.

Liu D, Liu Z, Condouris S, Xing M. BRAF V600E maintains proliferation, transformation, and tumorigenicity of BRAF-mutant papillary thyroid cancer cells. *J Clin Endocrinol Metab.* 2007 Jun;92(6):2264–2271. Epub March 20, 2007.

Liu RT, Chen YJ, Chou FF, Li CL, Wu WL, Tsai PC, Huang CC, Cheng JT. No correlation between BRAFV600E mutation and clinicopathological features of papillary thyroid carcinomas in Taiwan. *Clin Endocrinol (Oxf).* 2005;63(4):461–466.

LiVolsi VA. *Surgical Pathology of the Thyroid (Major Problems in Pathology).* Philadelphia, PA: Saunders, 1990.

LiVolsi VA, Albores-Saavedra J, Asa SL et al. Papillary carcinoma. In: DeLellis RA, Lloyd R, LiVolsi VA, Eng C, eds. *Pathology and Genetics of Tumours of the Endocrine Organs and Paraganglia.* Lyon, France: World Health Organization Classification of Tumours. IARC Press, 2004, pp. 57–66.

Lo YM, Rainer TH, Chan LY, Hjelm NM, Cocks RA. Plasma DNA as a prognostic marker in trauma patients. *Clin Chem.* 2000;46:319–323.

Lubitz CC, Ugras SK, Kazam JJ, Zhu B, Scognamiglio T, Chen YT, Fahey TJ 3rd. Microarray analysis of thyroid nodule fine-needle aspirates accurately classifies benign and malignant lesions. *J Mol Diagn.* 2006 Sep;8(4):490–498; quiz 528.

Lupi C, Giannini R, Ugolini C, Proietti A et al. Association of BRAF V600E mutation with poor clinicopathological outcomes in 500 consecutive cases of papillary thyroid carcinoma. *J Clin Endocrinol Metab.* 2007;92(11):4085–4090.

MacDonald L, Yazdi HM. Nondiagnostic fine needle aspiration biopsy of the thyroid gland: A diagnostic dilemma. *Acta Cytol.* 1996;40(3):423–428.

Mansouri A, Chowdhury K, Gruss P. Follicular cells of the thyroid gland require Pax8 gene function. *Nat Genet.* 1998;19(1):87–90.

Marchetti I, Iervasi G, Mazzanti CM, Lessi F et al. Detection of the BRAF(V600E) mutation in fine needle aspiration cytology of thyroid papillary microcarcinoma cells selected by manual macrodissection: An easy tool to improve the preoperative diagnosis. *Thyroid.* 2012 Mar;22(3):292–298.

Marchetti I, Lessi F, Mazzanti CM, Bertacca G, Elisei R, Coscio GD, Pinchera A, Bevilacqua G. A morpho-molecular diagnosis of papillary thyroid carcinoma: BRAF V600E detection as an important tool in preoperative evaluation of fine-needle aspirates. *Thyroid.* 2009 Aug;19(8):837–842.

Marques AR, Espadinha C, Catarino AL, Moniz S, Pereira T, Sobrinho LG, Leite V. Expression of PAX8-PPAR gamma 1 rearrangements in both follicular thyroid carcinomas and adenomas. *J Clin Endocrinol Metab.* 2002;87(8):3947–3952.

Mathur A, Moses W, Rahbari R, Khanafshar E, Duh QY, Clark O, Kebebew E. Higher rate of BRAF mutation in papillary thyroid cancer over time: A single-institution study. *Cancer.* 2011 Oct 1;117(19):4390–4395.

Mathur A, Weng J, Moses W, Steinberg SM et al. A prospective study evaluating the accuracy of using combined clinical factors and candidate diagnostic markers to refine the accuracy of thyroid fine needle aspiration biopsy. *Surgery.* 2010 Dec;148(6):1170–1176; discussion 1176–1177.

Matsuse M, Mitsutake N, Tanimura S, Ogi T et al. Functional characterization of the novel BRAF complex mutation, BRAF(V600delinsYM), identified in papillary thyroid carcinoma. *Int J Cancer.* 2013 Feb 1;132(3):738–743.

Mazeh H, Mizrahi I, Halle D, Ilyayev N et al. Development of a microRNA-based molecular assay for the detection of papillary thyroid carcinoma in aspiration biopsy samples. *Thyroid.* 2011 Feb;21(2):111–118.

Mazzaferri EL, Jhiang SM. Long-term impact of initial surgical and medical therapy on papillary and follicular thyroid cancer. *Am J Med.* 1994;97(5):418–428. Erratum in: *Am J Med.* 1995;98(2):215.

Mazzaferri EL, Kloos RT. Clinical review 128: Current approaches to primary therapy for papillary and follicular thyroid cancer. *J Clin Endocrinol Metab.* 2001;86(4):1447–1463.

Mazzanti C, Zeiger MA, Costouros NG, Umbricht C et al. Using gene expression profiling to differentiate benign versus malignant thyroid tumors. *Cancer Res.* 2004 Apr 15;64(8):2898–2903.

McConahey WM, Hay ID, Woolner LB, van Heerden JA, Taylor WF. Papillary thyroid cancer treated at the Mayo Clinic, 1946 through 1970: Initial manifestations, pathologic findings, therapy, and outcome. *Mayo Clin Proc*. 1986;61(12):978–996.

McCoy KL, Carty SE, Armstrong MJ, Seethala RR et al. Intraoperative pathologic examination in the era of molecular testing for differentiated thyroid cancer. *J Am Coll Surg*. 2012 Oct;215(4):546–554.

McHenry CR, Slusarczyk SJ, Askari AT, Lange RL, Smith CM, Nekl K, Murphy TA. Refined use of scintigraphy in the evaluation of nodular thyroid disease. *Surgery*. 1998;124(4):656–661; discussion 661–662.

McHenry CR, Walfish PG, Rosen IB. Non-diagnostic fine needle aspiration biopsy: A dilemma in management of nodular thyroid disease. *Am Surg*. 1993;59(7):415–419.

Melillo RM, Castellone MD, Guarino V, De Falco V et al. The RET/PTC-RAS-BRAF linear signaling cascade mediates the motile and mitogenic phenotype of thyroid cancer cells. *J Clin Invest*. 2005;115(4):1068–1081.

Mercer KE, Pritchard CA. Raf proteins and cancer: B-Raf is identified as a mutational target. *Biochim Biophys Acta*. 2003 Jun 5;1653(1):25–40.

Milas M, Barbosa GF, Mitchell J, Berber E, Siperstein A, Gupta M. Effectiveness of peripheral thyrotropin receptor mRNA in follow-up of differentiated thyroid cancer. *Ann Surg Oncol*. 2009 Feb;16(2):473–480.

Milas M, Mazzaglia P, Chia SY, Skugor M, Berber E, Reddy S, Gupta M, Siperstein A. The utility of peripheral thyrotropin mRNA in the diagnosis of follicular neoplasms and surveillance of thyroid cancers. *Surgery*. 2007 Feb;141(2):137–146; discussion 146.

Milas M, Shin J, Gupta M, Novosel T, Nasr C, Brainard J, Mitchell J, Berber E, Siperstein A. Circulating thyrotropin receptor mRNA as a novel marker of thyroid cancer: Clinical applications learned from 1758 samples. *Ann Surg*. 2010 Oct;252(4):643–651.

Miller FD, Kaplan DR. Neurotrophin signalling pathways regulating neuronal apoptosis. *Cell Mol Life Sci*. 2001;58(8):1045–1053.

Miller JM, Hamburger JI, Kini SR. Thyroid needle biopsy. *Arch Intern Med*. 1985 Apr;145(4):764–765.

Miller MC. The patient with a thyroid nodule. *Med Clin North Am*. 2010 Sep;94(5):1003–1015.

Minoletti F, Butti MG, Coronelli S, Miozzo M, Sozzi G, Pilotti S, Tunnacliffe A, Pierotti MA, Bongarzone I. The two genes generating RET/PTC3 are localized in chromosomal band 10q11.2. *Genes Chromosomes Cancer*. 1994;11(1):51–57.

miRBase. The microRNA database. http://www.mirbase.org/ (last accessed on December 12, 2012).

Mitsiades CS, Negri J, McMullan C, McMillin DW et al. Targeting BRAFV600E in thyroid carcinoma: Therapeutic implications. *Mol Cancer Ther*. 2007;6(3):1070–1078.

Mitsutake N, Miyagishi M, Mitsutake S, Akeno N, Mesa C Jr., Knauf JA, Zhang L, Taira K, Fagin JA. BRAF mediates RET/PTC-induced mitogen-activated protein kinase activation in thyroid cells: Functional support for requirement of the RET/PTC-RAS-BRAF pathway in papillary thyroid carcinogenesis. *Endocrinology*. 2006;147(2):1014–1019.

Moon HJ, Kwak JY, Kim EK, Choi JR, Hong SW, Kim MJ, Son EJ. The role of BRAFV600E mutation and ultrasonography for the surgical management of a thyroid nodule suspicious for papillary thyroid carcinoma on cytology. *Ann Surg Oncol*. 2009 Nov;16(11):3125–3131.

Moretti S, Macchiarulo A, De Falco V, Avenia N et al. Biochemical and molecular characterization of the novel BRAF(V599Ins) mutation detected in a classic papillary thyroid carcinoma. *Oncogene*. 2006 Jul 13;25(30):4235–4240.

Moretz WH 3rd, Gourin CG, Terris DJ, Xia ZS, Liu Z, Weinberger PM, Chin E, Adam BL. Detection of papillary thyroid carcinoma with serum protein profile analysis. *Arch Otolaryngol Head Neck Surg*. 2008 Feb;134(2):198–202.

Mortensen JD, Woolner LB, Bennett WA. Gross and microscopic findings in clinically normal thyroid glands. *J Clin Endocrinol Metab*. 1955;15(10):1270–1280.

Moses W, Weng J, Sansano I, Peng M, Khanafshar E, Ljung BM, Duh QY, Clark OH, Kebebew E. Molecular testing for somatic mutations improves the accuracy of thyroid fine-needle aspiration biopsy. *World J Surg*. 2010 Nov;34(11):2589–2594.

Motomura T, Nikiforov YE, Namba H, Ashizawa K, Nagataki S, Yamashita S, Fagin JA. ret rearrangements in Japanese pediatric and adult papillary thyroid cancers. *Thyroid*. 1998;8(6):485–489.

Murphy KM, Chen F, Clark DP. Identification of immunohistochemical biomarkers for papillary thyroid carcinoma using gene expression profiling. *Hum Pathol*. 2008 Mar;39(3):420–426.

Musholt TJ, Fottner C, Weber MM, Eichhorn W, Pohlenz J, Musholt PB, Springer E, Schad A. Detection of papillary thyroid carcinoma by analysis of BRAF and RET/PTC1 mutations in fine-needle aspiration biopsies of thyroid nodules. *World J Surg*. 2010 Nov;34(11):2595–2603.

Musholt TJ, Musholt PB, Khaladj N, Schulz D, Scheumann GF, Klempnauer J. Prognostic significance of RET and NTRK1 rearrangements in sporadic papillary thyroid carcinoma. *Surgery*. 2000;128(6):984–993.

Nakamura N, Carney JA, Jin L, Kajita S, Pallares J, Zhang H, Qian X, Sebo TJ, Erickson LA, Lloyd RV. RASSF1A and NORE1A methylation and BRAFV600E mutations in thyroid tumors. *Lab Invest*. 2005;85(9):1065–1075.

Nakata T, Kitamura Y, Shimizu K, Tanaka S, Fujimori M, Yokoyama S, Ito K, Emi M. Fusion of a novel gene, ELKS, to RET due to translocation t(10;12)(q11;p13) in a papillary thyroid carcinoma. *Genes Chromosomes Cancer*. 1999;25(2):97–103.

Nakayama H, Yoshida A, Nakamura Y, Hayashi H, Miyagi Y, Wada N, Rino Y, Masuda M, Imada T. Clinical significance of BRAF (V600E) mutation and Ki-67 labeling index in papillary thyroid carcinomas. *Anticancer Res*. 2007;27(5B):3645–3649.

Namba H, Nakashima M, Hayashi T, Hayashida N et al. Clinical implication of hot spot BRAF mutation, V599E, in papillary thyroid cancers. *J Clin Endocrinol Metab*. 2003;88(9):4393–4397.

Namba H, Rubin SA, Fagin JA. Point mutations of ras oncogenes are an early event in thyroid tumorigenesis. *Mol Endocrinol*. 1990;4(10):1474–1479.

Netea-Maier RT, Hunsucker SW, Hoevenaars BM, Helmke SM, Slootweg PJ, Hermus AR, Haugen BR, Duncan MW. Discovery and validation of protein abundance differences between follicular thyroid neoplasms. *Cancer Res*. 2008 Mar 1;68(5):1572–1580.

Neumann S, Schuchardt K, Reske A, Reske A, Emmrich P, Paschke R. Lack of correlation for sodium iodide symporter mRNA and protein expression and analysis of sodium iodide symporter promoter methylation in benign cold thyroid nodules. *Thyroid*. 2004 Feb;14(2):99–111.

Nikiforov YE, Ohori NP, Hodak SP, Carty SE et al. Impact of mutational testing on the diagnosis and management of patients with cytologically indeterminate thyroid nodules: A prospective analysis of 1056 FNA samples. *J Clin Endocrinol Metab*. 2011 Nov;96(11):3390–3397.

Nikiforov YE, Rowland JM, Bove KE, Monforte-Munoz H, Fagin JA. Distinct pattern of ret oncogene rearrangements in morphological variants of radiation-induced and sporadic thyroid papillary carcinomas in children. *Cancer Res*. 1997;57(9):1690–1694.

Nikiforov YE, Steward DL, Robinson-Smith TM, Haugen BR et al. Molecular testing for mutations in improving the fine-needle aspiration diagnosis of thyroid nodules. *J Clin Endocrinol Metab*. 2009;94(6):2092–2098.

Nikiforova MN, Biddinger PW, Caudill CM, Kroll TG, Nikiforov YE. PAX8-PPARgamma rearrangement in thyroid tumors: RT-PCR and immunohistochemical analyses. *Am J Surg Pathol*. 2002a;26(8):1016–1023.

Nikiforova MN, Chiosea SI, Nikiforov YE. MicroRNA expression profiles in thyroid tumors. *Endocr Pathol*. 2009 Summer;20(2):85–91.

Nikiforova MN, Ciampi R, Salvatore G, Santoro M et al. Low prevalence of BRAF mutations in radiation-induced thyroid tumors in contrast to sporadic papillary carcinomas. *Cancer Lett*. 2004;209(1):1–6.

Nikiforova MN, Gandhi M, Kelly L, Nikiforov YE. MicroRNA dysregulation in human thyroid cells following exposure to ionizing radiation. *Thyroid*. 2011 Mar;21(3):261–266.

Nikiforova MN, Kimura ET, Gandhi M, Biddinger PW et al. BRAF mutations in thyroid tumors are restricted to papillary carcinomas and anaplastic or poorly differentiated carcinomas arising from papillary carcinomas. *J Clin Endocrinol Metab*. 2003a;88(11):5399–5404.

Nikiforova MN, Lynch RA, Biddinger PW, Alexander EK, Dorn GW 2nd, Tallini G, Kroll TG, Nikiforov YE. RAS point mutations and PAX8-PPAR gamma rearrangement in thyroid tumors: Evidence for distinct molecular pathways in thyroid follicular carcinoma. *J Clin Endocrinol Metab*. 2003b;88(5):2318–2326.

Nikiforova MN, Stringer JR, Blough R, Medvedovic M, Fagin JA, Nikiforov YE. Proximity of chromosomal loci that participate in radiation-induced rearrangements in human cells. *Science*. 2000;290(5489): 138–141.

Nikiforova MN, Tseng GC, Steward D, Diorio D, Nikiforov YE. MicroRNA expression profiling of thyroid tumors: Biological significance and diagnostic utility. *J Clin Endocrinol Metab*. 2008 May;93(5):1600–1608.

Nikolova DN, Zembutsu H, Sechanov T, Vidinov K, Kee LS, Ivanova R, Becheva E, Kocova M, Toncheva D, Nakamura Y. Genome-wide gene expression profiles of thyroid carcinoma: Identification of molecular targets for treatment of thyroid carcinoma. *Oncol Rep*. 2008 Jul;20(1):105–121.

Nilsson M. Iodide handling by the thyroid epithelial cell. *Exp Clin Endocrinol Diabetes*. 2001;109(1):13–17.

Ohori NP, Nikiforova MN, Schoedel KE, LeBeau SO et al. Contribution of molecular testing to thyroid fine-needle aspiration cytology of "follicular lesion of undetermined significance/atypia of undetermined significance". *Cancer Cytopathol*. 2010 Feb 25;118(1):17–23.

Oler G, Camacho CP, Hojaij FC, Michaluart P Jr., Riggins GJ, Cerutti JM. Gene expression profiling of papillary thyroid carcinoma identifies transcripts correlated with BRAF mutational status and lymph node metastasis. *Clin Cancer Res*. 2008;14(15):4735–4742.

Oler G, Cerutti JM. High prevalence of BRAF mutation in a Brazilian cohort of patients with sporadic papillary thyroid carcinomas: Correlation with more aggressive phenotype and decreased expression of iodide-metabolizing genes. *Cancer*. 2009;115(5):972–980.

Oler G, Ebina KN, Michaluart P Jr., Kimura ET, Cerutti J. Investigation of BRAF mutation in a series of papillary thyroid carcinoma and matched-lymph node metastasis reveals a new mutation in metastasis. *Clin Endocrinol (Oxf)*. 2005;62(4):509–511.

Paccini F, Schlumberger M, Dralle H, Elisei R, Smit JW, Wiersinga F, and the European Thyroid Cancer Taskforce. European consensus for the management of patients with differentiated thyroid cancer of the epithelium. *Eur J Endocrinol*. 2006;154:787–803.

Pacini F, Burroni L, Ciuoli C, Di Cairano G, Guarino E. Management of thyroid nodules: A clinicopathological, evidence-based approach. *Eur J Nucl Med Mol Imaging*. 2004 Oct;31(10):1443–1449.

Pallante P, Visone R, Ferracin M, Ferraro A et al. MicroRNA deregulation in human thyroid papillary carcinomas. *Endocr Relat Cancer*. 2006 Jun;13(2):497–508.

Papotti M, Rodriguez J, De Pompa R, Bartolazzi A, Rosai J. Galectin-3 and HBME-1 expression in well-differentiated thyroid tumors with follicular architecture of uncertain malignant potential. *Mod Pathol*. 2005 Apr;18(4):541–546.

Park SY, Park YJ, Lee YJ, Lee HS et al. Analysis of differential BRAF(V600E) mutational status in multifocal papillary thyroid carcinoma: Evidence of independent clonal origin in distinct tumor foci. *Cancer*. 2006;107(8):1831–1818.

Park YJ, Kwak SH, Kim DC, Kim H et al. Diagnostic value of galectin-3, HBME-1, cytokeratin 19, high molecular weight cytokeratin, cyclin D1 and p27(kip1) in the differential diagnosis of thyroid nodules. *J Korean Med Sci*. 2007 Aug;22(4):621–628.

Patel A, Klubo-Gwiezdzinska J, Hoperia V, Larin A, Jensen K, Bauer A, Vasko V. BRAF(V600E) mutation analysis from May-Grünwald Giemsa-stained cytological samples as an adjunct in identification of high-risk papillary thyroid carcinoma. *Endocr Pathol*. 2011 Dec;22(4):195–199.

Pelizzo MR, Boschin IM, Barollo S, Pennelli G et al. BRAF analysis by fine needle aspiration biopsy of thyroid nodules improves preoperative identification of papillary thyroid carcinoma and represents a prognostic factor. A mono-institutional experience. *Clin Chem Lab Med*. 2011 Feb;49(2):325–329.

Penko K, Livezey J, Fenton C, Patel A, Nicholson D, Flora M, Oakley K, Tuttle RM, Francis G. BRAF mutations are uncommon in papillary thyroid cancer of young patients. *Thyroid*. 2005;15(4):320–325.

Pennell NA, Daniels GH, Haddad RI, Ross DS et al. A phase II study of gefitinib in patients with advanced thyroid cancer. *Thyroid*. 2008 Mar;18(3):317–323.

Perren A, Schmid S, Locher T, Saremaslani P, Bonvin C, Heitz PU, Komminoth P. BRAF and endocrine tumors: Mutations are frequent in papillary thyroid carcinomas, rare in endocrine tumors of the gastrointestinal tract and not detected in other endocrine tumors. *Endocr Relat Cancer*. 2004;11(4):855–860.

Peyssonnaux C, Eychène A. The Raf/MEK/ERK pathway: New concepts of activation. *Biol Cell*. 2001; 93(1–2):53–62.

Pita JM, Banito A, Cavaco BM, Leite V. Gene expression profiling associated with the progression to poorly differentiated thyroid carcinomas. *Br J Cancer*. 2009 Nov 17;101(10):1782–1791.

Pizzolanti G, Russo L, Richiusa P, Bronte V et al. Fine-needle aspiration molecular analysis for the diagnosis of papillary thyroid carcinoma through BRAF V600E mutation and RET/PTC rearrangement. *Thyroid*. 2007 Nov;17(11):1109–1115.

Porra V, Ferraro-Peyret C, Durand C, Selmi-Ruby S et al. Silencing of the tumor suppressor gene SLC5A8 is associated with BRAF mutations in classical papillary thyroid carcinomas. *J Clin Endocrinol Metab.* 2005;90(5):3028–3035.

Powell N, Jeremiah S, Morishita M, Dudley E, Bethel J, Bogdanova T, Tronko M, Thomas G. Frequency of BRAF T1796A mutation in papillary thyroid carcinoma relates to age of patient at diagnosis and not to radiation exposure. *J Pathol.* 2005;205(5):558–564.

Prasad ML, Pellegata NS, Huang Y, Nagaraja HN, de la Chapelle A, Kloos RT. Galectin-3, fibronectin-1, CITED-1, HBME1 and cytokeratin-19 immunohistochemistry is useful for the differential diagnosis of thyroid tumors. *Mod Pathol.* 2005 Jan;18(1):48–57.

Prasad NB, Kowalski J, Tsai HL, Talbot K et al. Three-gene molecular diagnostic model for thyroid cancer. *Thyroid.* 2012 Mar;22(3):275–284.

Prasad NB, Somervell H, Tufano RP, Dackiw AP et al. Identification of genes differentially expressed in benign versus malignant thyroid tumors. *Clin Cancer Res.* 2008 Jun 1;14(11):3327–3337.

Puxeddu E, Moretti S. Clinical prognosis in BRAF-mutated PTC. *Arq Bras Endocrinol Metabol.* 2007;51(5):736–747.

Puxeddu E, Moretti S, Elisei R, Romei C et al. BRAF(V599E) mutation is the leading genetic event in adult sporadic papillary thyroid carcinomas. *J Clin Endocrinol Metab.* 2004;89(5):2414–2420.

Qi JH, Ebrahem Q, Moore N, Murphy G, Claesson-Welsh L, Bond M, Baker A, Anand-Apte B. A novel function for tissue inhibitor of metalloproteinases-3 (TIMP3): Inhibition of angiogenesis by blockage of VEGF binding to VEGF receptor-2. *Nat Med.* 2003 Apr;9(4):407–415.

Quadbeck B, Pruellage J, Roggenbuck U, Hirche H, Janssen OE, Mann K, Hoermann R. Long-term follow-up of thyroid nodule growth. *Exp Clin Endocrinol Diabetes.* 2002 Oct;110(7):348–354.

Raber W, Kaserer K, Niederle B, Vierhapper H. Risk factors for malignancy of thyroid nodules initially identified as follicular neoplasia by fine-needle aspiration: Results of a prospective study of one hundred twenty patients. *Thyroid.* 2000 Aug;10(8):709–712.

Rabes HM, Demidchik EP, Sidorow JD, Lengfelder E, Beimfohr C, Hoelzel D, Klugbauer S. Pattern of radiation-induced RET and NTRK1 rearrangements in 191 post-chernobyl papillary thyroid carcinomas: Biological, phenotypic, and clinical implications. *Clin Cancer Res.* 2000;6(3):1093–1103.

Rajagopalan H, Bardelli A, Lengauer C, Kinzler KW, Vogelstein B, Velculescu VE. Tumorigenesis: RAF/RAS oncogenes and mismatch-repair status. *Nature.* 2002;418(6901):934.

Rapp UR, Goldsborough MD, Mark GE, Bonner TI, Groffen J, Reynolds FH Jr., Stephenson JR. Structure and biological activity of v-raf, a unique oncogene transduced by a retrovirus. *Proc Natl Acad Sci USA.* 1983;80(14):4218–4222.

Ricarte-Filho J, Ganly I, Rivera M, Katabi N, Fu W, Shaha A, Tuttle RM, Fagin JA, Ghossein R. Papillary thyroid carcinomas with cervical lymph node metastases can be stratified into clinically relevant prognostic categories using oncogenic BRAF, the number of nodal metastases, and extra-nodal extension. *Thyroid.* 2012 Jun;22(6):575–584.

Riesco-Eizaguirre G, Gutiérrez-Martínez P, García-Cabezas MA, Nistal M, Santisteban P. The oncogene BRAF V600E is associated with a high risk of recurrence and less differentiated papillary thyroid carcinoma due to the impairment of Na+/I- targeting to the membrane. *Endocr Relat Cancer.* 2006;13(1):257–269.

Ringel MD. Molecular detection of thyroid cancer: Differentiating "signal" and "noise" in clinical assays. *J Clin Endocrinol Metab.* 2004 Jan;89(1):29–32.

Ringel MD, Anderson J, Souza SL, Burch HB, Tambascia M, Shriver CD, Tuttle RM. Expression of the sodium iodide symporter and thyroglobulin genes are reduced in papillary thyroid cancer. *Mod Pathol.* 2001 Apr;14(4):289–296.

Robinson MJ, Cobb MH. Mitogen-activated protein kinase pathways. *Curr Opin Cell Biol.* 1997;9(2):180–186.

Rocha AS, Risberg B, Magalhães J, Trovisco V, de Castro IV, Lazarovici P, Soares P, Davidson B, Sobrinho-Simões M. The p75 neurotrophin receptor is widely expressed in conventional papillary thyroid carcinoma. *Hum Pathol.* 2006;37(5):562–568.

Rodolico V, Cabibi D, Pizzolanti G, Richiusa P et al. BRAF V600E mutation and p27 kip1 expression in papillary carcinomas of the thyroid < or = 1 cm and their paired lymph node metastases. *Cancer.* 2007;110(6):1218–1226.

Rodriguez AM, Perron B, Lacroix L, Caillou B, Leblanc G, Schlumberger M, Bidart JM, Pourcher T. Identification and characterization of a putative human iodide transporter located at the apical membrane of thyrocytes. *J Clin Endocrinol Metab.* 2002 Jul;87(7):3500–3503.

Romei C, Ciampi R, Faviana P, Agate L et al. BRAF V600E mutation, but not RET/PTC rearrangements, is correlated with a lower expression of both thyroperoxidase and sodium iodide symporter genes in papillary thyroid cancer. *Endocr Relat Cancer*. 2008 Jun;15(2):511–520.

Rosen J, He M, Umbricht C, Alexander HR, Dackiw AP, Zeiger MA, Libutti SK. A six-gene model for differentiating benign from malignant thyroid tumors on the basis of gene expression. *Surgery*. 2005 Dec;138(6):1050–1056; discussion 1056–1057.

Ross, DM. Diagnostic approach to and treatment of thyroid nodules. I. In: Rose BD, ed. Wellesley, MA: Uptodate, 2005. http://www.uptodate.com/contents/diagnostic-approach-to-and-treatment-of-thyroid-nodules.

Rowe LR, Bentz BG, Bentz JS. Utility of BRAF V600E mutation detection in cytologically indeterminate thyroid nodules. *CytoJournal*. 2006;3:10.

Russell JP, Powell DJ, Cunnane M, Greco A, Portella G, Santoro M, Fusco A, Rothstein JL. The TRK-T1 fusion protein induces neoplastic transformation of thyroid epithelium. *Oncogene*. 2000;19(50):5729–5735.

Russo D, Damante G, Puxeddu E, Durante C, Filetti S. Epigenetics of thyroid cancer and novel therapeutic targets. *J Mol Endocrinol*. 2011 Apr 28;46(3):R73–R81.

Saenko V, Rogounovitch T, Shimizu-Yoshida Y, Abrosimov A et al. Novel tumorigenic rearrangement, Delta rfp/ret, in a papillary thyroid carcinoma from externally irradiated patient. *Mutat Res*. 2003;527(1–2):81–90.

Saggiorato E, Cappia S, De Giuli P, Mussa A, Pancani G, Caraci P, Angeli A, Orlandi F. Galectin-3 as a presurgical immunocytodiagnostic marker of minimally invasive follicular thyroid carcinoma. *J Clin Endocrinol Metab*. 2001 Nov;86(11):5152–5258.

Salassidis K, Bruch J, Zitzelsberger H, Lengfelder E, Kellerer AM, Bauchinger M. Translocation t(10;14)(q11.2:q22.1) fusing the kinetin to the RET gene creates a novel rearranged form (PTC8) of the RET proto-oncogene in radiation-induced childhood papillary thyroid carcinoma. *Cancer Res*. 2000;60(11):2786–2789.

Salvatore G, Giannini R, Faviana P, Caleo A et al. Analysis of BRAF point mutation and RET/PTC rearrangement refines the fine-needle aspiration diagnosis of papillary thyroid carcinoma. *J Clin Endocrinol Metab*. 2004;89(10):5175–5180.

Sangalli G, Serio G, Zampatti C, Bellotti M, Lomuscio G. Fine needle aspiration cytology of the thyroid: A comparison of 5469 cytological and final histological diagnoses. *Cytopathology*. 2006 Oct;17(5):245–250.

Sanicola M, Hession C, Worley D, Carmillo P et al. Glial cell line-derived neurotrophic factor-dependent RET activation can be mediated by two different cell-surface accessory proteins. *Proc Natl Acad Sci USA*. 1997;94(12):6238–6243.

Santarpia L, Bottai G. Inhibition of RET activated pathways: Novel strategies for therapeutic intervention in human cancers. *Curr Pharm Des*. 2013;19(5):864–882.

Santarpia L, Sherman SI, Marabotti A, Clayman GL, El-Naggar AK. Detection and molecular characterization of a novel BRAF activated domain mutation in follicular variant of papillary thyroid carcinoma. *Hum Pathol*. 2009;40(6):827–833. Erratum in: *Hum Pathol*. 2009;40(8):1212.

Santoro A, Pannone G, Carosi MA, Francesconi A et al. BRAF mutation and RASSF1A expression in thyroid carcinoma of southern Italy. *J Cell Biochem*. 2012. May;114(5):1174–1182. doi: 10.1002/jcb.24460.

Santoro M, Dathan NA, Berlingieri MT, Bongarzone I, Paulin C, Grieco M, Pierotti MA, Vecchio G, Fusco A. Molecular characterization of RET/PTC3; a novel rearranged version of the RETproto-oncogene in a human thyroid papillary carcinoma. *Oncogene*. 1994;9(2):509–516.

Sapio MR, Guerra A, Posca D, Limone PP et al. Combined analysis of galectin-3 and BRAFV600E improves the accuracy of fine-needle aspiration biopsy with cytological findings suspicious for papillary thyroid carcinoma. *Endocr Relat Cancer*. 2007a;14(4):1089–1097.

Sapio MR, Posca D, Raggioli A, Guerra A et al. Detection of RET/PTC, TRK and BRAF mutations in preoperative diagnosis of thyroid nodules with indeterminate cytological findings. *Clin Endocrinol (Oxf)*. 2007b;66(5):678–683.

Sapio MR, Posca D, Troncone G, Pettinato G, Palombini L, Rossi G, Fenzi G, Vitale M. Detection of BRAF mutation in thyroid papillary carcinomas by mutant allele-specific PCR amplification (MASA). *Eur J Endocrinol*. 2006;154(2):341–348.

Saussez S, Glinoer D, Chayash antrain G, Pattou F, Carnaille B, André S, Gabius HJ, Laurent G. Serum galectin-1 and galectin-3 levels in benign and malignant nodular thyroid disease. *Thyroid*. 2008 Jul;18(7):705–712.

Schagdarsurengin U, Gimm O, Dralle H, Hoang-Vu C, Dammann R. CpG island methylation of tumor-related promoters occurs preferentially in undifferentiated carcinoma. *Thyroid.* 2006 Jul;16(7):633–642.

Schagdarsurengin U, Gimm O, Hoang-Vu C, Dralle H, Pfeifer GP, Dammann R. Frequent epigenetic silencing of the CpG island promoter of RASSF1A in thyroid carcinoma. *Cancer Res.* 2002 Jul 1;62(13):3698–3701.

Schildhaus HU, Kröckel I, Lippert H, Malfertheiner P, Roessner A, Schneider-Stock R. Promoter hypermethylation of p16INK4a, E-cadherin, O6-MGMT, DAPK and FHIT in adenocarcinomas of the esophagus, esophagogastric junction and proximal stomach. *Int J Oncol.* 2005 Jun;26(6):1493–1500.

Schlumberger M. Kinase inhibitors for refractory thyroid cancers. *Lancet Oncol.* 2010 Oct;11(10):912–913. doi: 10.1016/S1470-2045(10)70226-6. Epub Sep 17, 2010.

Schlumberger M. Kinase inhibitors for refractory thyroid cancers. *Lancet Oncol.* 2010 Oct;11(10):912–913.

Schmidt T, Riggs MW, Speights VO Jr. Significance of nondiagnostic fine-needle aspiration of the thyroid. *South Med J.* 1997;90(12):1183–1186.

Schuchardt A, D'Agati V, Larsson-Blomberg L, Costantini F, Pachnis V. Defects in the kidney and enteric nervous system of mice lacking the tyrosine kinase receptor Ret. *Nature.* 1994;367(6461):380–383.

Schulten HJ, Salama S, Al-Mansouri Z, Alotibi R et al. BRAF mutations in thyroid tumors from an ethnically diverse group. *Hered Cancer Clin Pract.* 2012 Aug 27;10(1):10.

Sedliarou I, Saenko V, Lantsov D, Rogounovitch T et al. The BRAFT1796A transversion is a prevalent mutational event in human thyroid microcarcinoma. *Int J Oncol.* 2004;25(6):1729–1735.

Shapiro B, Chakrabarty M, Cohn EM, Leon SA. Determination of circulating DNA levels in patients with benign or malignant gastrointestinal disease. *Cancer.* 1983;51:2116–2120.

Sheils OM, O'eary JJ, Uhlmann V, Lättich K, Sweeney EC. ret/PTC-1 Activation in hashimoto thyroiditis. *Int J Surg Pathol.* 2000;8(3):185–189.

Sheils OM, Sweeney EC. TSH receptor status of thyroid neoplasms—TaqMan RT-PCR analysis of archival material. *J Pathol.* 1999 May;188(1):87–92.

Shen R, Liyanarachchi S, Li W, Wakely PE Jr. et al. MicroRNA signature in thyroid fine needle aspiration cytology applied to "atypia of undetermined significance" cases. *Thyroid.* 2012 Jan;22(1):9–16.

Sherman SI. Thyroid carcinoma. *Lancet.* 2003 Feb 8;361(9356):501–511.

Sherman SI, Angelos P, Ball DW, Beenken SW et al. Thyroid carcinoma. *J Natl Compr Canc Netw.* 2005;3(3):404–457.

Sherman SI, Brierley JD, Sperling M, Ain KB et al. Prospective multicenter study of thyroid carcinoma treatment: Initial analysis of staging and outcome. National Thyroid Cancer Treatment Cooperative Study Registry Group. *Cancer.* 1998;83(5):1012–1021.

Sheu SY, Grabellus F, Schwertheim S, Worm K, Broecker-Preuss M, Schmid KW. Differential miRNA expression profiles in variants of papillary thyroid carcinoma and encapsulated follicular thyroid tumours. *Br J Cancer.* 2010 Jan 19;102(2):376–382.

Shibru D, Chung KW, Kebebew E. Recent developments in the clinical application of thyroid cancer biomarkers. *Curr Opin Oncol.* 2008;20(1):13–18.

Singer G, Oldt R 3rd, Cohen Y, Wang BG, Sidransky D, Kurman RJ, Shih IeM. Mutations in BRAF and KRAS characterize the development of low-grade ovarian serous carcinoma. *J Natl Cancer Inst.* 2003;95(6):484–486.

Smanik PA, Furminger TL, Mazzaferri EL, Jhiang SM. Breakpoint characterization of the ret/PTC oncogene in human papillary thyroid carcinoma. *Hum Mol Genet.* 1995;4(12):2313–2318.

Smyth P, Finn S, Cahill S, O'Regan E, Flavin R, O'Leary JJ, Sheils O. Ret/PTC and BRAF act as distinct molecular, time-dependant triggers in a sporadic Irish cohort of papillary thyroid carcinoma. *Int J Surg Pathol.* 2005;13(1):1–8.

Soares P, Fonseca E, Wynford-Thomas D, Sobrinho-Simões M. Sporadic ret-rearranged papillary carcinoma of the thyroid: A subset of slow growing, less aggressive thyroid neoplasms? *J Pathol.* 1998;185(1):71–78.

Soares P, Trovisco V, Rocha AS, Feijão T, Rebocho AP, Fonseca E, Vieira de Castro I, Cameselle-Teijeiro J, Cardoso-Oliveira M, Sobrinho-Simões M. BRAF mutations typical of papillary thyroid carcinoma are more frequently detected in undifferentiated than in insular and insular-like poorly differentiated carcinomas. *Virchows Arch.* 2004;444(6):572–576.

Soares P, Trovisco V, Rocha AS, Lima J et al. BRAF mutations and RET/PTC rearrangements are alternative events in the etiopathogenesis of PTC. *Oncogene.* 2003;22(29):4578–4580.

Sofiadis A, Becker S, Hellman U, Hultin-Rosenberg L et al. Proteomic profiling of follicular and papillary thyroid tumors. *Eur J Endocrinol.* 2012 Apr;166(4):657–667.

Sofiadis A, Dinets A, Orre LM, Branca RM et al. Proteomic study of thyroid tumors reveals frequent up-regulation of the Ca^{2+}-binding protein S100A6 in papillary thyroid carcinoma. *Thyroid.* 2010 Oct;20(10):1067–1076.

Sozzi G, Conte D, Leon M, Ciricione R et al. Quantification of free circulating DNA as a diagnostic marker in lung cancer. *J Clin Oncol.* 2003;21:3902–3908.

Stack BC, Ferris RL, Goldenberg D, Haymart M et al. American Thyroid Association review and consensus statement regarding the anatomy, terminology and rationale for lateral neck dissection in differentiated thyroid cancer. *Thyroid.* 2012;22(5):501–508.

Steinman CR. Circulating DNA in systemic lupus erythematosus. Isolation and characterization. *J Clin Investig.* 1984;73:832–841.

Stephen JK, Chitale D, Narra V, Chen KM, Sawhney R, Worsham MJ. DNA methylation in thyroid tumorigenesis. *Cancers (Basel).* 2011 Jun 1;3(2):1732–1743.

Suen KC. How does one separate cellular follicular lesions of the thyroid by fine-needle aspiration biopsy? *Diagn Cytopathol.* 1988;4(1):78–81.

Sugg SL, Ezzat S, Rosen IB, Freeman JL, Asa SL. Distinct multiple RET/PTC gene rearrangements in multifocal papillary thyroid neoplasia. *J Clin Endocrinol Metab.* 1998;83(11):4116–4122.

Sugg SL, Ezzat S, Zheng L, Freeman JL, Rosen IB, Asa SL. Oncogene profile of papillary thyroid carcinoma. *Surgery.* 1999;125(1):46–52.

Takano T, Hasegawa Y, Matsuzuka F, Miyauchi A, Yoshida H, Higashiyama T, Kuma K, Amino N. Gene expression profiles in thyroid carcinomas. *Br J Cancer.* 2000 Dec;83(11):1495–1502.

Tallini G. Molecular pathobiology of thyroid neoplasms. *Endocr Pathol.* 2002;13(4):271–288.

Tallini G, Santoro M, Helie M, Carlomagno F, Salvatore G, Chiappetta G, Carcangiu ML, Fusco A. RET/PTC oncogene activation defines a subset of papillary thyroid carcinomas lacking evidence of progression to poorly differentiated or undifferentiated tumor phenotypes. *Clin Cancer Res.* 1998;4(2):287–294.

Tamayo P, Scanfeld D, Ebert BL, Gillette MA, Roberts CW, Mesirov JP. Metagene projection for cross-platform, cross-species characterization of global transcriptional states. *Proc Natl Acad Sci USA.* 2007 Apr 3; 104(14):5959–5964.

Tan GH, Gharib H. Thyroid incidentalomas: Management approaches to nonpalpable nodules discovered incidentally on thyroid imaging. *Ann Intern Med.* 1997;126(3):226–231.

Tan GH, Gharib H, Reading CC. Solitary thyroid nodule. Comparison between palpation and ultrasonography. *Arch Intern Med.* 1995;155(22):2418–2423.

Tanoue T, Nishida E. Molecular recognitions in the MAP kinase cascades. *Cell Signal.* 2003;15(5):455–462.

Tee YY, Lowe AJ, Brand CA, Judson RT. Fine-needle aspiration may miss a third of all malignancy in palpable thyroid nodules: A comprehensive literature review. *Ann Surg.* 2007 Nov;246(5):714–720.

Teng KK, Hempstead BL. Neurotrophins and their receptors: Signaling trios in complex biological systems. *Cell Mol Life Sci.* 2004;61(1):35–48.

Thomas GA, Bunnell H, Cook HA, Williams ED, Nerovnya A, Cherstvoy ED, Tronko ND et al. High prevalence of RET/PTC rearrangements in Ukrainian and Belarussian post-Chernobyl thyroid papillary carcinomas: A strong correlation between RET/PTC3 and the solid-follicular variant. *J Clin Endocrinol Metab.* 1999;84(11):4232–4238.

Torres-Cabala C, Bibbo M, Panizo-Santos A, Barazi H, Krutzsch H, Roberts DD, Merino MJ. Proteomic identification of new biomarkers and application in thyroid cytology. *Acta Cytol.* 2006 Sep–Oct;50(5):518–528.

Torres-Cabala C, Panizo-Santos A, Krutzsch HC, Barazi H, Namba M, Sakaguchi M, Roberts DD, Merino MJ Differential expression of S100C in thyroid lesions. *Int J Surg Pathol.* 2004 Apr;12(2):107–115.

Troncone G, Cozzolino I, Fedele M, Malapelle U, Palombini L. Preparation of thyroid FNA material for routine cytology and BRAF testing: A validation study. *Diagn Cytopathol.* 2010 Mar;38(3):172–176.

Troncone G, Fulciniti F, Zeppa P, Vetrani A, Caleo A, Palombini L. Cyclin-dependent kinase inhibitor p27(Kip1) expression in thyroid cells obtained by fine-needle aspiration biopsy: A preliminary report. *Diagn Cytopathol.* 2000;23(2):77–81.

Trovisco V, Couto JP, Cameselle-Teijeiro J, de Castro IV, Fonseca E, Soares P, Sobrinho-Simões M. Acquisition of BRAF gene mutations is not a requirement for nodal metastasis of papillary thyroid carcinoma. *Clin Endocrinol (Oxf).* 2008;69(4):683–685.

Trovisco V, Soares P, Preto A, de Castro IV et al. Type and prevalence of BRAF mutations are closely associated with papillary thyroid carcinoma histotype and patients' age but not with tumour aggressiveness. *Virchows Arch*. 2005a;446(6):589–595.

Trovisco V, Soares P, Soares R, Magalhães J, Sá-Couto P, Sobrinho-Simões M. A new BRAF gene mutation detected in a case of a solid variant of papillary thyroid carcinoma. *Hum Pathol*. 2005b; 36(6):694–697.

Trovisco V, Vieira de Castro I, Soares P, Máximo V, Silva P, Magalhães J, Abrosimov A, Guiu XM, Sobrinho-Simões M. BRAF mutations are associated with some histological types of papillary thyroid carcinoma. *J Pathol*. 2004;202(2):247–251.

Tubiana M, Schlumberger M, Rougier P, Laplanche A, Benhamou E, Gardet P, Caillou B, Travagli JP, Parmentier C. Long-term results and prognostic factors in patients with differentiated thyroid carcinoma. *Cancer*. 1985;55(4):794–804.

Ueno M, Toyota M, Akino K, Suzuki H et al. Aberrant methylation and histone deacetylation associated with silencing of SLC5A8 in gastric cancer. *Tumour Biol*. 2004 May–Jun;25(3):134–140.

Unger K, Zitzelsberger H, Salvatore G, Santoro M et al. Heterogeneity in the distribution of RET/PTC rearrangements within individual post-Chernobyl papillary thyroid carcinomas. *J Clin Endocrinol Metab*. 2004;89(9):4272–4279.

van der Velden PA, Zuidervaart W, Hurks MH, Pavey S et al. Expression profiling reveals that methylation of TIMP3 is involved in uveal melanoma development. *Int J Cancer*. 2003 Sep 10;106(4):472–479.

Vander JB, Gaston EA, Dawber TR. The significance of nontoxic thyroid nodules. Final report of a 15-year study of the incidence of thyroid malignancy. *Ann Intern Med*. 1968;69(3):537–540.

Vasil'ev EV, Rumiantsev PO, Saenko VA, Il'in AA, Poliakova EI, Nemtsova MV, Zaletaev DV. Molecular analysis of structural abnormalities in papillary thyroid carcinoma gene. *Mol Biol (Mosk)*. 2004;38(4):642–653.

Vasko V, Ferrand M, Di Cristofaro J, Carayon P, Henry JF, de Micco C. Specific pattern of RAS oncogene mutations in follicular thyroid tumors. *J Clin Endocrinol Metab*. 2003;88(6):2745–2752.

Vasko V, Hu S, Wu G, Xing JC, Larin A, Savchenko V, Trink B, Xing M. High prevalence and possible de novo formation of BRAF mutation in metastasized papillary thyroid cancer in lymph nodes. *J Clin Endocrinol Metab*. 2005;90(9):5265–5269.

Vasko VV, Gaudart J, Allasia C, Savchenko V, Di Cristofaro J, Saji M, Ringel MD, De Micco C. Thyroid follicular adenomas may display features of follicular carcinoma and follicular variant of papillary carcinoma. *Eur J Endocrinol*. 2004;151(6):779–786.

Velculescu VE, Zhang L, Vogelstein B, Kinzler KW. Serial analysis of gene expression. *Science*. 1995 Oct 20;270(5235):484–487.

Venkataraman GM, Yatin M, Marcinek R, Ain KB. Restoration of iodide uptake in dedifferentiated thyroid carcinoma: Relationship to human Na+/I-symporter gene methylation status. *J Clin Endocrinol Metab*. 1999 Jul;84(7):2449–2457.

Villanueva J, Martorella AJ, Lawlor K, Philip J, Fleisher M, Robbins RJ, Tempst P. Serum peptidome patterns that distinguish metastatic thyroid carcinoma from cancer-free controls are unbiased by gender and age. *Mol Cell Proteomics*. 2006 Oct;5(10):1840–1852.

Visone R, Russo L, Pallante P, De Martino I et al. MicroRNAs (miR)-221 and miR-222, both overexpressed in human thyroid papillary carcinomas, regulate p27Kip1 protein levels and cell cycle. *Endocr Relat Cancer*. 2007 Sep;14(3):791–798.

Vriens MR, Weng J, Suh I, Huynh N, Guerrero MA, Shen WT, Duh QY, Clark OH, Kebebew E. MicroRNA expression profiling is a potential diagnostic tool for thyroid cancer. *Cancer*. 2012 Jul 1;118(13):3426–3432. doi: 10.1002/cncr.26587. Epub Oct 17, 2011.

Walsh PS, Wilde JI, Tom EY, Reynolds JD et al. Analytical performance verification of a molecular diagnostic for cytology-indeterminate thyroid nodules. *J Clin Endocrinol Metab*. 2012 Dec; 97(12):E2297–E2306.

Wan PT, Garnett MJ, Roe SM, Lee S et al. Cancer Genome Project. Mechanism of activation of the RAF-ERK signaling pathway by oncogenic mutations of B-RAF. *Cell*. 2004 Mar 19;116(6):855–867.

Wang JX, Yu JK, Wang L, Liu QL, Zhang J, Zheng S. Application of serum protein fingerprint in diagnosis of papillary thyroid carcinoma. *Proteomics*. 2006 Oct;6(19):5344–5349.

Wang L, Cunningham JM, Winters JL, Guenther JC et al. BRAF mutations in colon cancer are not likely attributable to defective DNA mismatch repair. *Cancer Res*. 2003;63(17):5209–5212.

Wasenius VM, Hemmer S, Kettunen E, Knuutila S, Franssila K, Joensuu H. Hepatocyte growth factor receptor, matrix metalloproteinase-11, tissue inhibitor of metalloproteinase-1, and fibronectin are up-regulated in papillary thyroid carcinoma: A cDNA and tissue microarray study. *Clin Cancer Res.* 2003 Jan;9(1):68–75.

Weber F, Shen L, Aldred MA, Morrison CD et al. Genetic classification of benign and malignant thyroid follicular neoplasia based on a three-gene combination. *J Clin Endocrinol Metab.* 2005 May;90(5):2512–2521.

Wémeau JL, Sadoul JL, d'Herbomez M, Monpeyssen H et al. Guidelines of the French society of endocrinology for the management of thyroid nodules. *Ann Endocrinol (Paris).* 2011 Sep;72(4):251–281.

Wilhelm SM, Carter C, Tang L, Wilkie D et al. BAY 43-9006 exhibits broad spectrum oral antitumor activity and targets the RAF/MEK/ERK pathway and receptor tyrosine kinases involved in tumor progression and angiogenesis. *Cancer Res.* 2004 Oct 1;64(19):7099–7109.

Wilkins MR, Pasquali C, Appel RD, Ou K et al. From proteins to proteomes: Large scale protein identification by two-dimensional electrophoresis and amino acid analysis. *Biotechnology (NY).* 1996 Jan;14(1):61–65.

Williams D, Baverstock K. Chernobyl and the future: Too soon for a final diagnosis. *Nature.* 2006; 440(7087):993–994.

Wojciechowska K, Lewinski A. BRAF mutations in papillary thyroid carcinoma. *Endocr Regul.* 2006 Dec;40(4):129–138.

Wreesmann VB, Sieczka EM, Socci ND, Hezel M et al. Genome-wide profiling of papillary thyroid cancer identifies MUC1 as an independent prognostic marker. *Cancer Res.* 2004 Jun 1; 64(11):3780–3789.

Xing M. BRAF mutation in thyroid cancer. *Endocr Relat Cancer.* 2005;12(2):245–262.

Xing M. BRAF mutation in papillary thyroid cancer: Pathogenic role, molecular bases, and clinical implications. *Endocr Rev.* 2007;28(7):742–762.

Xing M. Genetic-targeted therapy of thyroid cancer: A real promise. *Thyroid.* 2009;19(8):805–809.

Xing M. Prognostic utility of BRAF mutation in papillary thyroid cancer. *Mol Cell Endocrinol.* 2010;321(1):86–93.

Xing M, Clark D, Guan H, Ji M et al. BRAF mutation testing of thyroid fine-needle aspiration biopsy specimens for preoperative risk stratification in papillary thyroid cancer. *J Clin Oncol.* 2009;27(18):2977–2982.

Xing M, Cohen Y, Mambo E, Tallini G, Udelsman R, Ladenson PW, Sidransky D. Early occurrence of RASSF1A hypermethylation and its mutual exclusion with BRAF mutation in thyroid tumorigenesis. *Cancer Res.* 2004a Mar 1;64(5):1664–1668.

Xing M, Tokumaru Y, Wu G, Westra WB, Ladenson PW, Sidransky D. Hypermethylation of the Pendred syndrome gene SLC26A4 is an early event in thyroid tumorigenesis. *Cancer Res.* 2003a May 1;63(9):2312–2315.

Xing M, Tufano RP, Tufaro AP, Basaria S et al. Detection of BRAF mutation on fine needle aspiration biopsy specimens: A new diagnostic tool for papillary thyroid cancer. *J Clin Endocrinol Metab.* 2004b;89(6):2867–2872.

Xing M, Usadel H, Cohen Y, Tokumaru Y et al. Methylation of the thyroid-stimulating hormone receptor gene in epithelial thyroid tumors: A marker of malignancy and a cause of gene silencing. *Cancer Res.* 2003b May 1; 63(9):2316–2321.

Xing M, Vasko V, Tallini G, Larin A, Wu G, Udelsman R, Ringel MD, Ladenson PW, Sidransky D. BRAF T1796A transversion mutation in various thyroid neoplasms. *J Clin Endocrinol Metab.* 2004c;89(3):1365–1368.

Xing M, Westra WH, Tufano RP, Cohen Y et al. BRAF mutation predicts a poorer clinical prognosis for papillary thyroid cancer. *J Clin Endocrinol Metab.* 2005;90(12):6373–6379.

Xu X, Quiros RM, Gattuso P, Ain KB, Prinz RA. High prevalence of BRAF gene mutation in papillary thyroid carcinomas and thyroid tumor cell lines. *Cancer Res.* 2003;63(15):4561–4567.

Xu YH, Wang WJ, Song HJ, Qiu ZL, Luo QY. Serum differential proteomics analysis between papillary thyroid cancer patients with 131I-avid and those with non-131I-avid lung metastases. *Hell J Nucl Med.* 2011 Sep–Dec;14(3):228–233.

Yang J, Schnadig V, Logrono R, Wasserman PG. Fine-needle aspiration of thyroid nodules: A study of 4703 patients with histologic and clinical correlations. *Cancer.* 2007 Oct 25;111(5):306–315.

Yeh MW, Demircan O, Ituarte P, Clark OH. False-negative fine-needle aspiration cytology results delay treatment and adversely affect outcome in patients with thyroid carcinoma. *Thyroid.* 2004;14(3):207–215.

Yeo MK, Liang ZL, Oh T, Moon Y et al. Pyrosequencing cut-off value identifying BRAFV600E mutation in fine needle aspiration samples of thyroid nodules. *Clin Endocrinol (Oxf)*. 2011 Oct;75(4):555–560.

Yip L, Nikiforova MN, Carty SE, Yim JH et al. Optimizing surgical treatment of papillary thyroid carcinoma associated with BRAF mutation. *Surgery*. 2009 Dec;146(6):1215–1223.

Ylagan LR, Farkas T, Dehner LP. Fine needle aspiration of the thyroid: A cytohistologic correlation and study of discrepant cases. *Thyroid*. 2004 Jan;14(1):35–41.

Yoo CB, Jones PA. Epigenetic therapy of cancer: Past, present and future. *Nat Rev Drug Discov*. 2006 Jan;5(1):37–50. Erratum in: *Nat Rev Drug Discov*. 2006 Feb;5(2):121.

Yu S, Liu Y, Wang J, Guo Z et al. Circulating microRNA profiles as potential biomarkers for diagnosis of papillary thyroid carcinoma. *J Clin Endocrinol Metab*. 2012 Jun;97(6):2084–2092.

Yukinawa N, Oba S, Kato K, Taniguchi K, Iwao-Koizumi K, Tamaki Y, Noguchi S, Ishii S. A multi-class predictor based on a probabilistic model: Application to gene expression profiling-based diagnosis of thyroid tumors. *BMC Genomics*. 2006 Jul 27;7:190.

Zatelli MC, Trasforini G, Leoni S, Frigato G et al. BRAF V600E mutation analysis increases diagnostic accuracy for papillary thyroid carcinoma in fine-needle aspiration biopsies. *Eur J Endocrinol*. 2009 Sep;161(3):467–473.

Zhao J, Leonard C, Brunner E, Gemsenjäger E, Heitz PU, Odermatt B. Molecular characterization of well-differentiated human thyroid carcinomas by cDNA arrays. *Int J Oncol*. 2006 Nov;29(5):1041–1051.

Zhao J, Leonard C, Gemsenjäger E, Heitz PU, Moch H, Odermatt B. Differentiation of human follicular thyroid adenomas from carcinomas by gene expression profiling. *Oncol Rep*. 2008 Feb;19(2):329–337.

Zhou YL, Zhang W, Gao EL, Dai XX, Yang H, Zhang XH, Wang OC. Preoperative BRAF mutation is predictive of occult contralateral carcinoma in patients with unilateral papillary thyroid microcarcinoma. *Asian Pac J Cancer Prev*. 2012;13(4):1267–1272.

Zhu XL, Zhou XY, Zhu XZ. BRAFV599E mutation and RET/PTC rearrangements in papillary thyroid carcinoma. *Zhonghua Bing Li Xue Za Zhi*. 2005;34(5):270–274.

Zhu Z, Ciampi R, Nikiforova MN, Gandhi M, Nikiforov YE. Prevalence of RET/PTC rearrangements in thyroid papillary carcinomas: Effects of the detection methods and genetic heterogeneity. *J Clin Endocrinol Metab*. 2006;91(9):3603–3010.

27

Biomolecular Markers for Improving Management of Follicular and Medullary Thyroid Cancer

Umut Mousa, Cuneyd Anil, Serife Mehlika Isıldak, Alptekin Gursoy, and Angelo Carpi

CONTENTS

ABSTRACT Thyroid cancer usually presents as a thyroid nodule. According to different reports, more than 95% of thyroid nodules are benign. The gold standard for preoperative diagnosis of thyroid cancer is fine-needle aspiration cytology (FNAC). Especially in diagnosing medullary thyroid carcinoma (MTC) and some cases of well-differentiated thyroid carcinomas, biomolecular markers are proposed to increase the diagnostic value of FNAC. In this chapter, we mainly focused on classification, genetics, use of biomolecular and invasive markers, as well as treatment of follicular thyroid cancer

(FTC) and MTC. In the case of FTC, some molecular and immunohistochemical markers are proposed and are currently under investigation principally for improving preoperative diagnosis. Unlike MTC, there is no powerful biomarker such as calcitonin (Ct) for FTC diagnosis. In the follow-up, serum thyroglobulin (Tg) and whole-body iodine-131 scintigraphy are effective. MTC has relatively poor prognosis. Postsurgical therapy is scarcely effective. Blood Ct is the best studied and preferred marker in the diagnosis and follow-up of MTC. It can be measured in the basal state or after provocative stimuli such as pentagastrin and high-dose calcium. Carcinoembryonic antigen (CEA) and chromogranin A (CgA) are the other markers currently used for selected cases. Ct and CEA doubling times are gaining importance for the prognosis of MTC. The importance of rearranged during transfection (RET) proto-oncogene screening in MTC is also discussed in this chapter. RET has also become a therapeutic target. In conclusion, the management of FTC and MTC includes diagnostic and therapeutic problems. However, thanks to the development of translational medicine, the biomolecular marker studies are improving FTC and MTC diagnosis, prognosis, and therapy.

KEY WORDS: *medullary thyroid cancer, follicular thyroid cancer, calcitonin, RET proto-oncogene.*

Abbreviations

ATA	American Thyroid Association
ATC	anaplastic thyroid cancer
CCH	C cell hyperplasia
CEA	carcinoembryonic antigen
CGRP	calcitonin gene-related peptide
CMIA	chemiluminescent microparticle immunoassay
Ct	calcitonin
ELISA	enzyme-linked immunosorbent assay
ETA	European Thyroid Association
FDA	Food and Drug Administration
FDG PET/CT	fluorodeoxyglucose positron emission tomography/computed tomography
FMTC	familial medullary thyroid cancer
FNAC	fine-needle aspiration cytology
HCC	hurthle cell carcinoma
HMGA2	high-mobility group protein gene
ICMA	immunochemiluminescent assay
ILMA	immunoluminometric assay
IRMA	immunoradiometric assay
LNAB	large needle aspiration biopsy
LOH	loss of heterozygosity
MCM2	minichromosome maintenance protein 2
MEN	multiple endocrine neoplasia
MTC	medullary thyroid cancer
PA	plasminogen activator
RET	rearrangement during transfection
RIA	radioimmunoassay
TFF3	trefoil factor 3
Tg	thyroglobulin
TPO	thyroid peroxidase
TSH	thyroid-stimulating hormone
VEGFR	vascular endothelial growth factor receptor
VIP	vasoactive intestinal peptide

27.1 Introduction

27.1.1 General Aspects and Controversial Issues

The prevalence of thyroid cancer is increasing worldwide. This is most probably due to easier access to imaging techniques, most commonly ultrasonography (Carpi et al., 2012). The typical presentation pattern of thyroid cancer is a palpable thyroid nodule and/or a radiological image. The increasing use of thyroid ultrasonography by clinicians, especially endocrinologists and thyroidologists, has led to easier detection of micronodules (i.e., less than 10 mm diameter) that are normally nonpalpable on physical examination. The radiological characteristics of a thyroid nodule are beneficial but not specific in diagnosing thyroid cancer. Thus, tissue sampling remains the gold standard for preoperative diagnosis. Typically, more than 99% of thyroid cancers derive from thyroid follicular cells and parafollicular C cells. Most thyroid cancers (90%) are classified as differentiated, which means it has a close resemblance to the originating follicular epithelial cells and have two subtypes, papillary thyroid cancer (PTC) and follicular thyroid cancer (FTC).

Ultrasound-guided fine-needle aspiration cytology (FNAC) is the widely accepted method for tissue sampling today. Studies are continuing whether the large-needle biopsy method has any superiority, which is increasingly being proposed to be performed also for nondiagnostic FNAC results. Although the gold standard is FNAC, this method is not 100% specific and sensitive for thyroid cancer (Carpi et al., 2008), particularly medullary thyroid cancer (MTC) (Bugalho et al., 2005). In one study, FNAC had 63% sensitivity in detecting MTC, whereas basal calcitonin (Ct) measurement had 98% sensitivity (Bugalho et al., 2005). Such findings have led clinicians in search for alternative markers for aiding the diagnosis. Biomarkers are in use and under investigation to aid the clinicians both to decide whether to perform tissue sampling and in making diagnosis combined with the data obtained from the pathological characteristics. FTC is often reported as a follicular lesion by FNAC that complicates the differential diagnosis of follicular adenoma. PTC is discussed in a separate topic in this book; thus, this chapter will mainly include FTC and MTC.

27.2 Follicular Thyroid Cancer

27.2.1 Classification, Epidemiology, and Genetics

FTC is a malignant epithelial tumor with evidence of follicular cell differentiation and without the diagnostic features of PTC (Hedinger, 1988). This definition excludes the follicular variant of PTC (FVPTC), the poorly differentiated carcinoma, and the rare mixed medullary and follicular carcinoma (Carcangiu et al., 1984). The classification of tumors with predominant oncocytic features such as Hurthle cell carcinomas (HCC) is a matter of debate (Carcangiu et al., 1991). The World Health Organization (WHO) committee has acknowledged this tumor as an oxyphilic variant of FTC (Hedinger, 1988). However, the Armed Force Institute of Pathology (AFIF) monograph declared that tumors made up of this cell type have gross, microscopic, behavioral, cytogenetic, and possibly etiopathogenic features that separate from all others considering them in a distinct group (Rosai et al., 1992).

FTC is less frequent than PTC (5%–15% of thyroid malignancies) and occurs commonly in women with an F/M ratio about 2:1 (Schlumberger, 2007). FTC is likely to occur in older people; the mean age is about 10 years older than for typical PTC (i.e., greater than 50 years). In epidemiologic surveys, FTC made up 5%–50% of differentiated thyroid cancers with a tendency to be more common in areas with iodine deficiency (Grebe et al., 1996). Changes in diagnostic criteria and an increase in the incidence of PTC associated with dietary iodine supplementation, has led to a decrease in the frequency of FTC (Livolsi and Asa, 1994).

FTC usually presents as a solitary, painless nodule with an irregular border (Trovato et al., 2004). Clinically evident lymphadenopathy is exceptionally rare at presentation (Grebe et al., 1996).

FNAC of thyroid nodules has surpassed all other techniques for diagnosing thyroid cancer, with overall rates of sensitivity and specificity exceeding 90% in iodine-sufficient areas (Cooper et al., 2009,

Hegedus et al., 2003). The technique is easy to perform, safe, and well tolerated (Hales et al., 1990). Large series have revealed that around 70% (range, 53%–90%) of aspirates are benign; 4% (1%–10%) are malignant or suspicious for malignancy; 10% (5%–23%) are indeterminate, mainly represented by "follicular neoplasia"; and 17% (15%–20%) are inadequate for diagnosis (Carpi et al., 1996, Gharib and Goellner, 1993, Giuffrida and Gharib, 1995, Ridgway, 1992). The recent National Cancer Institute Thyroid Fine-Needle Aspiration State of the Science Conference proposed an expanded classification for FNA cytology (Baloch et al., 2008). Routine use of ultrasound-guided biopsy combined with on-site cytological examination improves the accuracy and decreases the risk of inadequacy of sampling (Baloch et al., 2000, Danese et al., 1998, Mikosch et al., 2000). Despite high sensitivity and specificity of FNAC approaching 100% for PTC, its performance for follicular neoplasms is lower. If a strict criterion for malignancy is used, sensitivity is as low as 8% in a series of 12 follicular carcinomas (Okamoto et al., 1994). In the case indeterminate cytology is considered malignant, sensitivity increases at the cost of seriously decreased specificity, ending up with a large number of false-positive results (Hamburger et al., 1994). In iodine-deficient regions, where FTC, follicular adenomas, and hyperplastic adenomatous nodules are prevalent, the usefulness of FNAC is limited (Mikosch et al., 2000). Results of FNAC should be combined with clinical and ultrasound characteristics to improve accuracy and to decrease the percentage of indeterminate cytology. However, compared to distinct sonographic features of PTC, follicular cancer is often isoechoic to hyperechoic and has a thick and irregular halo, with no microcalcifications; therefore, sonography in FTC has limited benefit (Moon et al., 2008, Reading et al., 2005).

Galectin 3 immunochemistry, alone or in combination with thyroid peroxidase (TPO), may be a valuable adjunct to the standard cytological techniques in cases of typical follicular lesions, either benign or malignant (Bartolazzi et al., 2008, Carpi et al., 2006). A combination of markers identified with microarray technology has also been advocated. However, independent confirmation of their usefulness is required (Barden et al., 2003, Cerutti et al., 2004, Chevillard et al., 2004, Weber et al., 2005).

The use of large-needle aspiration biopsy (LNAB), in addition to standard FNAC, has improved diagnostic accuracy of the nodules that are microfollicular at FNAC (Carpi and Nicolini, 2000).

In some centers, preoperative FNAC is combined with intraoperative frozen-section analysis. In the hands of experienced surgeon–pathologist teams, the rate of misdiagnosis with this approach is less than 5%, as evidenced by subsequent review of paraffin-embedded specimens. The approach avoids unnecessarily extensive surgery in patients with benign tumors, achieves resection of almost all malignant tumors, and rarely requires a second operation for completion of thyroidectomy (Furlan et al., 2004).

Imaging procedures other than ultrasonography and other tests may occasionally be helpful. Diagnostic thyroid scintiscanning, as traditionally practiced, is of little or no value and should be abandoned (Cooper et al., 2009, Hegedus et al., 2003, Pacini et al., 2006).

In areas where the prevalence of follicular tumors is higher, more patients require neck exploration because their FNAC is nonconclusive (Mikosch et al., 2000).

Usually cytology cannot differentiate malignant from a benign lesion in the case of follicular or Hurthle cell proliferation, and histological verification is required. Identification of FTC requires demonstration of invasion of the capsule, blood vessel, or adjacent thyroid tissue that cannot be seen on cytological smears (Grebe et al., 1996). Therefore, FTC diagnosis is assessed after surgery through the histological evaluation (Baloch et al., 2002, Deveci et al., 2006, Haugen et al., 2002).

The microscopic appearance of FTC varies from well-formed follicles to a predominantly solid growth pattern (Hedinger et al., 1988, Rosai et al., 1992). Poorly formed follicles and atypical patterns (e.g., cribriform) may occur, and combinations of multiple structural types may coexist. Details of the cellular morphology of FTC include a variant with dark nucleus and eosinophilic cytoplasm and a variant with dark nucleus and oncocytic cytoplasm that is less frequent but harbors a higher grade of malignancy (Trovato et al., 2004). FTC is divided into two categories on the basis of degree of invasion: minimally invasive with a more favorable prognosis and widely invasive. Differentiation of these also calls for histological examination. The outcome of FTC depends on patient's age, tumor size, histological type, extrathyroidal extension, and distant metastases at diagnosis (Hermanek et al., 2002, Schlumberger, 2007).

Minimally invasive FTC is an encapsulated tumor with a growth pattern similar to that of a trabecular, solid, microfollicular, or atypical adenoma, with virtually no potential of direct extrathyroidal extension.

Thus, the criteria for invasion of blood vessel and capsule should be absolute (Hedinger et al., 1988, Rosai et al., 1992). As the results may not be reproducible among pathologists and when the capsular and vascular invasion is minimal, the diagnosis may be challenging even at the final histological examination. Immunohistochemistry with markers such as TPO, galectin 3, or HMBE1 may help for this purpose. However, these techniques did not reliably improve the accuracy of pathology in case of suspicious findings (Bartolazzi et al., 2008). Global gene expression studies with the microarray technology demonstrated different profiles between papillary carcinoma and follicular tumors. Indeed, discriminating between follicular adenomas and minimally invasive follicular carcinoma depending on these studies of a limited number of genes needs verification (Barden et al., 2003, Cerutti et al., 2004, Chevillard et al., 2004, Weber et al., 2005).

The rare *widely invasive* form of FTC can be figured out easily from benign lesions. The tumor may be partially encapsulated; however, the margins are infiltrative even grossly, and vascular invasion is often widespread. A follicular element is always present among the heterogeneous structural features. Approximately 5%–20% of patients with FTC have distant metastases at presentation. These are most commonly to lungs or bones (Grebe et al., 1996, Rosai et al., 1992). In the case of poor or absent follicular differentiation or the existence of a trabecular, insular, or solid component, the tumor may be classified as a poorly differentiated carcinoma (Rosai et al., 1992, Volante et al., 2007). If a great majority of cells in a FTC display Hurthle cell (or oncocytic) features, the tumor is classified as a Hurthle cell or oncocytic carcinoma or as an oxyphilic variant FTC (Hedinger et al., 1988, Rosai et al., 1992, Watson et al., 1984).

Compared to PTC, FTC demonstrates a significant degree of aggressiveness. With a greater rate of recurrence, more frequent extraglandular extension, and distant metastases (leaning to spread through the bloodstream), FTC prognosis is less favorable than PTC (Grebe et al., 1996, Rosai et al., 1992). In a Mayo Clinic experience of longer than 50 years, local recurrences at 20 years were identified in 20% of FTCs and 30% of HCCs. Comparable distant metastasis rates were 23% and 28%, respectively (Grebe et al., 1996). In patients with invasive disease or distant metastases at the time of initial diagnosis, mortality over the 10–15 years following diagnosis has been reported to be 10%–50% (Grebe et al., 1996).

Though FVPTC is generally accepted to be related to PTC, its classification under PTC groups is still controversial. The prognosis of patients with FVPTC does not seem to be different from patients with the classical form. However, some studies have reported the behavior of FVPTC to be close to minimally invasive FTC having a low incidence of lymphatic and hematogenous spread. Thus, some have proposed a subclassification of FVPTC into nonencapsulated (infiltrative/diffuse) forms that are similar to PTC and encapsulated forms that are similar to FTC (Ghossein et al., 2009). Anyhow, FVPTC takes part in the differential diagnosis of pathological conditions demonstrating follicular structures, such as indeterminate cytology in FNAC (which include hyperplastic nodules, follicular adenomas, FTC, and follicular tumors with uncertain malignant potential). Molecular studies may potentially resolve this controversial issue (Carpi et al., 2011).

There is no established model for the pathogenesis of FTC. A multistep adenoma-to-carcinoma pathogenesis, similar to other adenocarcinomas, is not widely accepted because pathologists do not recognize follicular carcinoma in situ and documentation of the evolution of adenoma to carcinoma is not straightforward (Kondo et al., 2006, Pierotti et al., 1996, Vasko et al., 2003). Most follicular adenomas and all FTCs are probably of monoclonal origin. Point mutation of the *RAS* proto-oncogene, rendering oncogene activation, is common both in follicular adenomas (nearly 20%) and FTCs (nearly 40%), supporting a role in early tumorigenesis (Vasko et al., 2003). The rearranged during transfection (RET) oncogene does not appear to play a role in follicular tumors (Kondo et al., 2006, Pierotti et al., 1996). Also, cytogenetic abnormalities and genetic loss are more widespread in FTC than in PTC and also occur in follicular adenomas (Pierotti et al., 1996).

The most common cytogenetic abnormalities described in FTC are deletions, partial deletions, and deletion–rearrangements involving the short (p) arm of chromosome 3. A translocation, t (2; 3) (q13; p25), which ends in fusion of the DNA binding domains of the thyroid transcription factor PAX8 to domains of the peroxisome proliferator-activated receptor (PPARγ1), has been detected in 30% of FTCs (range, 11%–63%) and 10% of follicular adenomas but not in PTCs or multinodular hyperplasia (Kroll et al., 2000, Nikiforova et al., 2003, Powell et al., 2004). This chimeric protein may retard the growth inhibition and follicular differentiation normally induced by PPARγ1 (Powell et al., 2004). This mutation seems to be involved in progression of follicular adenoma to FTC (Schlumberger et al., 2011).

Loss of heterozygosity (LOH) on chromosomes 3p and 7q is frequently observed in the early steps of follicular tumoral transformation (Trovato et al., 2004, Zhang et al., 1998). The progression of follicular adenoma toward FTC is accentuated through the appearance of LOH on both 3p and 7q. LOH of chromosome 3 is more significantly found in FTC and follicular adenomas involving specific minimal common deleted regions corresponding to 3p25.3 and 3p21.2 loci, respectively (Trovato et al., 1999). Characteristically, LOH on 7q21.2 is specific for cell type. It increases along with neoplastic transformation reaching a 100% of expression in FTC correlating with the thyroid gland volume and the presence of multiple lesions (Trovato et al., 2004).

Mutations of RAS gene are encountered in FTC, FVPTC, and anaplastic thyroid cancer. This genetic abnormality seems more closely related with follicular cancers than PTC. It is virtually absent in tall-cell PTC and classical PTC. The incidence of RAS mutations is variable and is reported to be 14%–62% in FTC. RAS mutations occur also in benign follicular adenomas with a frequency ranging from 0% to 85% but are rarer than FTC (Ruggeri et al., 2008). These mutations may represent the earliest events in cancer progression along the malignant pathway leading to FTC and ATC (Namba et al., 1990). It has been suggested that activating mutations in RAS oncogenes could be related to chromosomal and genomic instability, thus rendering follicular cells amenable to the accumulation of additional molecular abnormalities. There are three types of RAS: H-RAS, K-RAS, and N-RAS. In thyroid tumors, *N-RAS* mutation is most common, and the other types of *RAS* mutations are relatively uncommon (Vasko et al., 2003). *RAS* mutations and *PAX8/PPARγ* translocations are rarely found in the same tumor, and these two mutations may represent two distinct tumor types (Nikiforova et al., 2003).

While the presence of RAS mutations in FVPTC favors its follicular origin, some specific *BRAF* mutations seem to confer the FVPTC phenotype, justifying the classification of this tumor under the PTC group (Kondo et al., 2006). This further complicates the issue of classification of FVPTC.

27.2.2 Noninvasive Serum and Tissue Biomarkers for Preoperative and Postoperative Evaluation

Many immunohistochemical and molecular biomarkers have been introduced to improve diagnostic accuracy of cytological and histopathological thyroid lesions; however, the clinical implications have been demonstrated only for some of them.

27.2.2.1 Immunohistochemical Biomarkers for Preoperative Evaluation

Immunohistochemistry recognizes specific proteins on cytological or histological specimens. As the expression of the currently studied biomarkers is variable in sensitivity and specificity, none of them have been routinely approved in cytological and/or histological diagnostic procedures, especially in FTC (Ruggeri et al., 2008).

27.2.2.1.1 Galectin 3

Galectin 3 is a member of the beta-galactoside binding family of lectins. It is strongly expressed in PTC. Immunostaining for galectin 3 has also been reported for preoperative diagnosis of FTC, and it may have some value in differentiating between benign and malignant follicular lesions (Gasbarri et al., 1999, Saggiorato et al., 2004). Immunocytochemistry with anti-galectin 3 antibodies has been introduced as a complementary procedure to conventional cytology in the diagnostic workup of thyroid nodules (Bartolazzi et al., 2001, Collet et al., 2005, Saggiorato et al., 2004). However, there had been reports exhibiting low sensitivity (Mehrotra et al., 2004, Oestreicher-Kedem et al., 2004) and low specificity (Mehrotra et al., 2004) before methodological aspects were defined (Bartolazzi et al., 2012). LNAB combined with galectin 3 immunodetection in cases of inadequate or indeterminate follicular FNAC can resolve the sensitivity and specificity issues (Bartolazzi et al., 2008, Carpi et al., 2006, 2010). Galectin 3 assay is commercially available (Galectin 3 Tireotest Mabtech, Space Import Export, Milan, Italy).

27.2.2.1.2 Other Immunohistochemical Markers

Minichromosome maintenance protein 2 (MCM2) is a cell proliferation marker such as Ki67. MCM2, but not Ki67, was helpful for differentiating minimally invasive follicular cancer from follicular adenoma in an immunohistochemical study (Cho Mar et al., 2006).

HBME-1, a strongly positive immunostaining marker for PTC, has also been extensively studied in tissue samples for FTC. Its predictivity to distinguish between follicular adenoma and FTC was not found to be sufficient (i.e., 60%) to propose its routine use (Ito et al., 2005b).

In a gene expression study, *QPRT*, a key enzyme in intracellular metabolic pathways, was expressed more profoundly in FTC than its adenoma counterpart. A successive confirmatory analysis using immunohistochemistry verified the result: 65% of follicular thyroid cancers and only 22% of follicular adenomas expressed the protein. QPRT was introduced as a potential new marker for the immunohistochemical screening of follicular thyroid nodules (Hinsch et al., 2009).

As compared with the use of single biomarker, the combination of two or three markers may represent a more accurate immunohistochemical approach in the preoperative differentiation of malignant tumors from their benign counterparts, especially in controversial categories (de Matos et al., 2005, Nasr et al., 2006).

27.2.2.2 Molecular Biomarkers for Preoperative Diagnosis

Different genes, genetic mutations, and signaling pathways involved in the development of thyroid cancer types have given way to the clinical use of thyroid molecular biomarkers recognizable by molecular biology techniques. The expression of each molecular marker may be studied on frozen specimens of the neoplastic tissue by using PCR techniques (Ruggeri et al., 2008).

27.2.2.2.1 PAX8/PPARγ

The expression of PAX8/PPARγ may be supposed as a marker of well-differentiated FTC, and its absence may represent tumor progression to undifferentiated forms of thyroid carcinomas. Some clinical trials have documented the effectiveness of this biomarker; however, they were not accurate enough for the routine use (Nakabashi et al., 2004, Puxeddu and Fagin, 2001). Nikiforov et al. performed a prospective study in which they proposed a set of molecular tests to 1056 consecutive FNAC samples with indeterminate cytology. The panel included PAX8/PPARγ translocation, and its positivity was associated with the presence of malignancy in almost 100% of cases (Nikiforov et al., 2011).

PAX8/PPARγ translocation within FTC may provide highly useful information regarding tumor behavior. Due to the fact that noncancerous tissues also harbor this genetic anomaly, detecting this mutation is not diagnostic (Shibru et al., 2008).

There is little information about the prognostic value of *PPAR-γ–PAX-8* rearrangements, although some authors have suggested a more aggressive phenotype. The *PPAR-γ–PAX-8* rearrangement has been detected rarely in poorly differentiated tumors (Kondo et al., 2006).

27.2.2.2.2 Loss of Heterozygosity

7q21.1 LOH has been suggested as a diagnostic key to assist pathologists for distinguishing FTC from benign thyroid lesions. It has been reported that suspected FTC lesions containing dark nucleus and eosinophilic cytoplasm cells may be included among benign lesions if they do not express LOH on 7q21.2. This may render it specific for cell type (Trovato et al., 1999, 2004). Unlike ongoing studies in the role of LOH in pathogenesis, diagnosis, and prognostication of some other cancer types such as colon, breast, and hematopoietic tissues, any clinical utility of LOH in thyroid cancer is currently unknown due to lack of novel data (Bertagnolli et al., 2011, Jerez et al., 2012, Schwarzenbach et al., 2012).

27.2.2.2.3 RAS Mutations

RAS mutation within FTC may provide useful information about tumor behavior. The presence of RAS mutations seems to be associated with a poor outcome, but they are also found in some adenomas as well as poorly differentiated thyroid tumors. Thus, they have not been determined to bear diagnostic significance to distinguish follicular adenoma from FTC (Kondo et al., 2006). In the aforementioned study by Nikiforov et al., RAS mutation was also included in the molecular panel applied on indeterminate FNAC cases, and about 85% of those positive for this mutation turned out to be malignant ultimately (Nikiforov et al., 2011).

27.2.2.2.4 Plasminogen Activator System

The plasminogen activator (PA) system, which consists of the urokinase PA (uPA) and the tissue-type PA (tPA), their two serpin inhibitors (PAI-1 and PAI-2), and the glycolipid-anchored receptor for the uPA (uPAR), is associated with cancer progression; it augments both distant metastasis and direct invasion (Ruggeri et al., 2008).

Most thyroid carcinomas (PTC, FTC, and ATC) overexpress uPA, uPAR, and PAI-1 (Chu et al., 2004, Kim et al., 2002, Ulisse et al., 2006). The highest levels of expression were found in anaplastic carcinomas (Horvatić Herceg et al., 2006), in well-differentiated carcinomas in which extrathyroidal invasion or distant metastases had been present (Horvatić Herceg et al., 2006, Ulisse et al., 2006), and in PTC whose size exceeded 1 cm in diameter (Horvatić Herceg et al., 2006, Ulisse et al., 2006). A clear correlation between PA system components and lymph node metastasis, distant metastasis, tumor stage, disease-free interval, and survival has been shown in thyroid cancer (Baldini et al., 2012). These data suggest that the PA system components have prognostic relevance in thyroid malignant tumors as shown in some other malignancies. When confirmed in large studies, they may represent candidate molecular biomarkers for prognostic evaluation both preoperative and postoperatively and also as potential therapeutic targets (Baldini et al., 2012, Ruggeri et al., 2008).

27.2.2.2.5 Other Molecular Markers

The expression of the *high mobility group protein gene (HMGA2)* and its protein has been studied in thyroid tissue samples as a possible marker detecting malignant growth of thyroid tumors. HMGA2 expression effectively distinguished between benign and malignant thyroid tissues and follicular adenoma and FTC. It was also reported that immunohistochemical examination would be possible with this marker (Belge et al., 2008).

Studies with other members of the HMG proteins have revealed that *HMGI(Y)* gene expression may also have a potential to differentiate between follicular adenoma and FTC (Czyz et al., 2004).

MicroRNAs (miRNAs or miRs) are a class of small endogenous noncoding RNAs of 19–23 nucleotides that negatively regulate gene expression (Bartel et al., 2004). Although most of the studies conducted so far on miR expression in thyroid cancer have focused on PTCs, some recent studies have also reported miR deregulation in FTCs (Table 27.1). The deregulated expression of these miRs together with their biological role suggests a correlation with diagnosis, prognosis, and therapeutic approaches. Very recently, different histopathological types of FTCs have been shown to have distinct miRNA expression profiles. A special miRNA profile has been demonstrated to be highly upregulated in oncocytic FTC, and together with it, a set of deregulated miRNAs have been reported to have a potential to discriminate between FTC and hyperplastic nodules in FNA samples (Dettmer et al., 2013). An assay for microRNAs is commercially available. (miRInform; chromosome point mutations and rearrangement panel, Asuragen, Texas, United States.)

Extensive studies are ongoing to discover novel candidate molecular markers that may distinguish follicular carcinomas from adenomas. Table 27.2 demonstrates a list of such markers. Among them, trefoil factor 3 (TFF3) mRNA expression, which is increased significantly in benign counterparts, seems to be more promising (Takano et al., 2009).

27.2.2.3 Molecular Biomarkers for Postoperative Evaluation

Unlike the case for BRAF mutation in PTC, none of the aforementioned molecular markers have been shown to have utility for postoperative diagnosis, surveillance, and prognosis. The PA system components seem to bear such a potential; however, they need validation in large studies (Baldini et al., 2012).

TABLE 27.1

Principal MicroRNA Profiles Associated with Follicular Thyroid Cancer

MicroRNA Type	Characteristics	Sensitivity (%)	Specificity (%)	Accuracy (%)	Tissue Studied and Purpose of Use	References
miR221	Upregulated in all TC	63–100	91–94	88–95	FNAC and surgical material; diagnostic (benign and malignant)	Nikiforova et al. (2008), Pai et al. (2012), Shen et al. (2012), Rossing et al. (2012)
miR222	Upregulated in all TC	81–100	91–94	84–95	FNAC and surgical material; diagnostic (benign and malignant)	Nikiforova et al. (2008), Pai et al. (2012), Rossing et al. (2012)
miR187	Upregulated in all TC	63–100	73–94	72–95	FNAC and surgical material; diagnostic (benign and malignant)	Nikiforova et al. (2008), Pai et al. (2012), Shen et al. (2012)
miR224	Upregulated in all TC	48–100	82–94	59–95	FNAC and surgical material; diagnostic (benign and malignant)	Nikiforova et al. (2008), Pai et al. (2012)
miR146b	Upregulated in all TC	63–100	94	95	FNAC and surgical material; diagnostic (benign and malignant)	Nikiforova et al. (2008), Shen et al. (2012)
miR155	Upregulated in all TC	100	94	95	FNAC and surgical material; diagnostic (benign and malignant)	Nikiforova et al. (2008)
miR197	Upregulated in all TC	86–100	89–94	87–95	FNAC and surgical material; diagnostic (benign and malignant)	Nikiforova et al. (2008), Rossing et al. (2012), Weber et al. (2006)
miR346	Upregulated in FTC	86	89	87	Surgical material; diagnostic	Weber et al. (2006)
miR30d	Downregulated in all TC	63–80	NA	NA	FNAC; diagnostic	Shen et al. (2012)
miR144	Downregulated in FTC	83–92	100	NA	Surgical material; diagnostic	Rossing et al. (2012)
miR199b	Downregulated in FTC	83–92	100	NA	Surgical material; diagnostic	Rossing et al. (2012)
miR191	Downregulated in FTC, FA	100	100	100	Surgical material; diagnostic	Colamaio et al. (2011)

TC, thyroid cancer; FNAC, fine-needle aspiration cytology; NA, not available; FTC, follicular thyroid cancer; FA, follicular adenoma.

27.2.2.4 Noninvasive Serum Biomarkers

For the detection of recurrent/residual thyroid cancer, serum thyroglobulin (Tg) remains the sole circulating marker but lacks high sensitivity and is unreliable in the presence of anti-thyroglobulin antibodies (TgAbs). New diagnostic and prognostic biomarkers are currently searched and tested (Table 27.3). However, up to date it is unclear if any of these biomarkers might be more accurate than the currently used methods (Ruggeri et al., 2008).

TABLE 27.2

Emerging Preoperative Molecular Markers to Distinguish Adenoma from Follicular Carcinoma

Gene/Reference	Sensitivity (%)	Specificity (%)	Accuracy (%)	Comments on Results
PAX8–PPARγ/Marques et al. (2002), Nikiforova et al. (2002)	63	100	89	Inconsistent 26%–63% positivity reported in FTC across studies
MET/Barden et al. (2003)	22	100	65	No further consistent data available
hTERT/Ito et al. (2005a), Liou et al. (2003)	100	71	85	Reported sensitivity 39%–100%, specificity 39%–90%
LGALS3/Mills et al. (2005), Niedziela et al. (2002), Takano et al. (2003)	100	98	99	No significant difference between FA and FTC in most studies
DDIT3/Cerutti et al. (2004)	85	91	88	No further consistent data available
ARG2/Cerutti et al. (2004)	85	91	88	No further consistent data available
ADM, BSG, ENPP/ Barden et al. (2003), Krause et al. (2008)	n.a.	n.a.	n.a.	No sensitivity data available
CCND2, PCSK2, PLAB/ Krause et al. (2008), Weber et al. (2005)	100	95	97	No further consistent data available
TFF3/Taniguchi et al. (2005), Foukakis et al. (2007), Durand et al. (2008)	72	83	80	Consistent; most similar studies report sensitivity 67%–77%, specificity 91%–98%, accuracy 83%–90%
HMGI (Y)/Czyz et al. (2004)	83	100	n.a.	No further consistent data available

n.a., not available.

TABLE 27.3

Potential Noninvasive Serum Biomarkers for Follicular Thyroid Cancer

Biomarker	Possible Clinical Use	Reference
Thyroglobulin	Preoperative diagnosis	Lee et al. (2012)
Thyroglobulin mRNA	Preoperative diagnosis Postoperative surveillance	Gupta and Chia (2007)
TSHR mRNA	Preoperative diagnosis Postoperative surveillance	Gupta and Chia (2007) Milas et al. (2010)
HMGIY	Preoperative diagnosis	Czyz et al. (2004)

mRNA, messenger ribonucleic acid; TSHR, thyroid-stimulating hormone receptor; HMGIY, high-mobility group protein gene IY.

27.2.2.5.1 Thyroglobulin

Tg is a glycoprotein produced only by normal or neoplastic thyroid follicular cells. Prediction of thyroid cancer outcome mostly depends on circulating Tg measurement in the complete absence of thyroid tissue. It is well established that Tg plays a reliable role in monitoring the course of well-differentiated carcinoma after total thyroidectomy. Tg assay allows detecting persistent or recurrent FTCs (Pacini et al., 2006).

Tg should not be detectable in patients who have had total thyroid ablation, which improves both the sensitivity and specificity for detection of persistent or recurrent disease (Eustatia-Rutten et al., 2004).

The trend in serum Tg level is probably more significant than the actual serum Tg level by itself. Modern Tg assays with a sensitivity of 0.1 ng/mL have an improved sensitivity for the detection of persistent disease during levothyroxine treatment, but this is accompanied by decreased specificity (Smallridge et al., 2007, Table 27.4). Schlumberger et al. evaluated 944 thyroid cancer patients after primary therapy (i.e., total thyroidectomy and RAI). Considering a cutoff for 7 Tg assays at 0.9 ng/mL under levothyroxine therapy, sensitivity ranged from 19% to 40% and specificity ranged from 92% to 97%. Using assays with a functional sensitivity at 0.2–0.3 ng/mL, sensitivity was 54%–63% and specificity was 89%. Using the two methods with a lowest functional sensitivity at 0.02 and 0.11 ng/mL resulted in a higher sensitivity for Tg (81% and 78%) but at the expense of a loss of specificity (42% and 63%). Using an optimized functional sensitivity according to receiver operating characteristic curves for these two methods at 0.22 and 0.27 ng/mL of Tg resulted in sensitivity at 65% and specificity at 85%–87% (Schlumberger et al., 2007).

Serum Tg should be measured every 6–12 months by an immunometric assay calibrated against the CRM-457 standard. Ideally, serum Tg should be assessed in the same laboratory and using the same assay, during follow-up of patients with DTC who have undergone total or near-total thyroidectomy (Cooper et al., 2009).

Besides specificity and sensitivity issues of Tg assays, hook effects, interference with TgAbs, and inability to reliably detect them are other factors that compromise the clinical utility of current Tg and TgAb methods. Tg assays employing radioimmunoassay (RIA) methods appear to be more resistant to TgAb interference than other immunometric assays (Baloch et al., 2003; Spencer et al., 2005).

Serum TgAbs may cause false negative results and should be determined with every measurement of serum Tg (Cooper et al., 2009, Pacini et al., 2006). Serum TgAbs in patients who are in complete remission after total thyroid ablation decline gradually to low or undetectable levels, with a median time of 3 years (Chiovato et al., 2003). Their persistence or reappearance during follow-up should be considered suspicious for persistent or recurrent disease.

In a retrospective study by Lee et al., preoperative serum Tg levels were found to have high value in predicting thyroid cancer in cytologically indeterminate nodules. They reported that Tg levels may be a useful marker for differentiating thyroid cancer from benign thyroid nodules in this group (Lee et al., 2012, Table 27.3). This issue should probably be reevaluated in prospective trials.

27.2.2.5.2 Circulating mRNAs of Thyroid-Specific Genes

Thyroid cancer cells in the circulation can be detected by measuring the mRNA of thyroid-specific genes. Among these, Tg mRNA and, more recently, thyroid-stimulating hormone receptor (TSHR) mRNAs have been reported to provide high diagnostic sensitivity and specificity for thyroid cancer detection. These markers may be used in synergy with current diagnostic modalities, that is, FNAC and ultrasound, for preoperative diagnosis and serum Tg measurement for monitoring (Gupta and Chia, 2007, Table 27.3).

Significant variability exists among various studies for Tg mRNA, questioning the strength of this marker. Recent studies have demonstrated high sensitivity and specificity (above 90%) of TSHR mRNA in detecting recurrent/residual disease even in the presence of TgAbs. TSHR mRNA measurement in patients with indeterminate FNAC may enhance cancer detection and save unnecessary surgery (Gupta and Chia, 2007). Besides guiding appropriate initial surgery for follicular neoplasms, TSHR mRNA has also been shown to represent a new blood test for the assessment of disease status in thyroid cancer follow-up (Milas et al., 2010, Table 27.3). TSH mRNA assay is commercially available (TSH mRNA Assay, Cleveland Clinic Laboratories, Ohio).

27.2.2.5.3 Other Potential Circulating Biomarkers

Gene products of some members of HMG proteins, that is, *HMGIY*, which were already mentioned, are currently being evaluated in FNAC samples and peripheral blood for their diagnostic role in thyroid cancer (Czyz et al., 2004, Table 27.3).

Measurement of the thyroid aspirate or peripheral blood levels of the product of the gene determined in tissues does not correlate with the activity or amount of tissue most of the time, and this seems to be a significant challenge to be resolved in this field.

TABLE 27.4

Some Commonly Employed Thyroglobulin Assays

Assay Name	Access Tg	Tg Plus	TgIRMA	Immulite 2000	Tg	TgRIA	Elecsys Tg	Tg
Manufacturer	Beckman Coulter, US	BRAHMS diagnostics, Germany	CISbio-Schering, Germany	Siemens, US	Genesis Diagnostics, UK	University of Southern California, US	Roche, Germany	Sanofi Pasteur, France
Assay type	Noncompetitive ICMA	Competitive IRMA	Competitive IRMA	Competitive ICMA	Noncompetitive ELISA	Competitive RIA	Competitive IECMA	Competitive IRMA
Reference range ng/mL (mcg/L)	3–32	2–34	2.1–43	1.6–60	2.0–50	3.0–40	1.4–78	1.5–50
Reference	Cooper et al. (2009), Smallridge et al. (2007), Spencer et al. (2005)	Spencer et al. (2005), Schlumberger et al. (2007)	Spencer et al. (2005)	Spencer et al. (2005), Schlumberger et al. (2007)	Spencer and Lopresti (2008)	Spencer et al. (2005)	Spencer and Lopresti (2008)	Spencer and Lopresti (2008)

27.2.3 Imaging for Postoperative Disease Detection

Nine to twelve months after total thyroidectomy is performed, an I-131 whole-body scan is advised for moderate- and high-risk patients (2 mCi imaging dose). The TSH level is advised to be >30 mU/L prior to this procedure to increase uptake by thyroid follicular cells. To accomplish this level, either thyroid hormone withdrawal (i.e., discontinuing levothyroxine replacement therapy at least 4 weeks before) or stimulation (i.e., with recombinant human TSH) is performed. A patient in remission is expected to have no iodine accumulation (references). Accumulation in the cervical area may represent a residual thyroid tissue or relapse. In such cases, other imaging techniques such as ultrasonography, computed tomography, and magnetic resonance imaging may help differentiate between residual thyroid tissue and relapse. The Tg level at the time of imaging is critical (stimulated Tg). A stimulated Tg level >2 ng/mL with a negative whole-body scan may indicate an early relapse; thus, the patient should be followed up more closely. 18-Fluorodeoxyglucose positron emission tomography/computed tomography (FDG PET/CT) can be used for localization of metastases of patients having elevated Tg levels (especially basal Tg levels >5–10 ng/mL) and negative whole-body scans (Cooper et al., 2009).

27.2.4 Treatment

The initial surgical procedure for FTC and HCC should be a near-total or total thyroidectomy unless there are contraindications to this surgery. As lymph node metastases are less frequent in FTC, lymph node dissection should be performed if involved lymph nodes are detected (Cooper et al., 2009, Pacini et al., 2006).

27.2.4.1 Radioactive Iodine Ablation and TSH Suppression

FTC and HCC are generally regarded as higher-risk tumors among differentiated thyroid cancers. Thus, the use of RAI in almost all of these cases is generally accepted. However, due to the favorable prognosis associated with surgical resection alone in minimally invasive follicular cancer, RAI ablation may not be required for all patients with this type (van Heerden et al., 1992).

Agents that may induce radioiodine uptake, such as histone deacetylase inhibitors and retinoids, represent another field in new drug development in thyroid cancer (Cras et al., 2007, Elisei et al., 2005).

As the inhibition of TSH secretion with levothyroxine is accepted to improve the recurrence and survival rates, levothyroxine treatment is recommended to all patients with FTC and HCC (Biondi et al., 2005). The initial effective dose is about 2 μg/kg body weight in adults. The basic aim is a serum TSH concentration of less than 0.1 mU/L for high-risk thyroid cancer patients; maintenance of the TSH at or slightly below the lower limit of normal (0.1–0.5 mU/L) is appropriate for low-risk patients (Cooper et al., 2009, Pacini et al., 2006).

Treatment with cytotoxic chemotherapy is generally limited to patients with symptomatic or rapidly progressive metastatic disease unresponsive to or unsuitable for surgery, RAI therapy, and external beam radiotherapy (Schlumberger et al., 2011).

27.2.4.2 Therapies Directed against Molecular Biomarkers

27.2.4.2.1 PA System Targeted Therapies

Therapeutic choices for aggressive and/or unresponsive thyroid cancers are limited. Therefore, developing new therapeutic strategies is a fundamental objective of research.

Experimental inhibitors of uPA and uPAR have opened a new field of therapeutic target for the development of antiangiogenic and antimetastatic therapeutic agents. It has been shown that inhibition of uPA catalytic activity or prevention of uPA binding to its receptor reduces tumor growth, angiogenesis, and metastasis (Duffy et al., 2004, Mazar et al., 1999). Hence, uPA and its receptor might become potential therapeutic biomarkers also for malignant thyroid neoplasms (Ruggeri et al., 2008).

27.2.4.2.2 MicroRNA-Targeted Therapies

Inhibition of upregulated miRs such as miR-221, miR-222, and miR-146 with “antagomirs” or “locked nucleic acid-modified anti-miRs” has been reported to have a potential attractive therapeutic option.

Similarly, restoration of downregulated miRs may be another possibility (Pallante et al., 2010, Weber et al., 2006). Interventions at the level of epigenetic silencing of tumor suppressive miRNAs have been proposed as another strategy in the treatment of thyroid cancer (Braun et al., 2011).

27.3 Medullary Thyroid Cancer

27.3.1 Classification, Epidemiology, and Genetics

MTC is a rare tumor that accounts for about 4% of all thyroid cancers (Hundahl et al., 1998). MTC arises from the parafollicular C cells of the thyroid gland. MTC is usually sporadic, whereas 25%–30% of MTC cases occur as inherited disorders (Kouvaraki et al., 2005).

MTC has unique histological properties. Macroscopically, MTC is a red to white firm tumor that is either well bordered or visibly invasive on cross section (Hedinger et al., 1988, LiVolsi et al., 1997). Histologically, MTC consists of sheets of spindle-shaped, round, or polygonal cells separated by fibrous stroma, arranged in a nested pattern that is typical for endocrine tumors. The cells have eosinophilic cytoplasms with a fine granular appearance and uniform nuclei. Amyloid deposits are seen between tumor cells in most of the cases (Figure 27.1). The diagnosis of MTC should be confirmed by positive immunohistochemical staining for Ct (Figure 27.2).

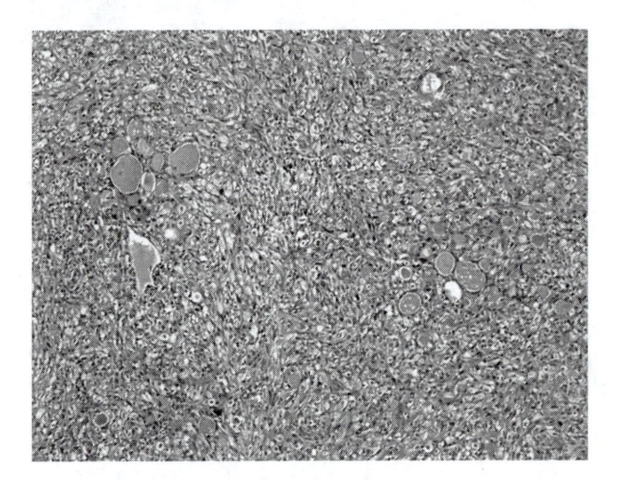

FIGURE 27.1 **(See color insert.)** Hematoxylin–eosin stain of a patient with MTC. Cancer cells destructing the normal thyroid follicular patterns are seen.

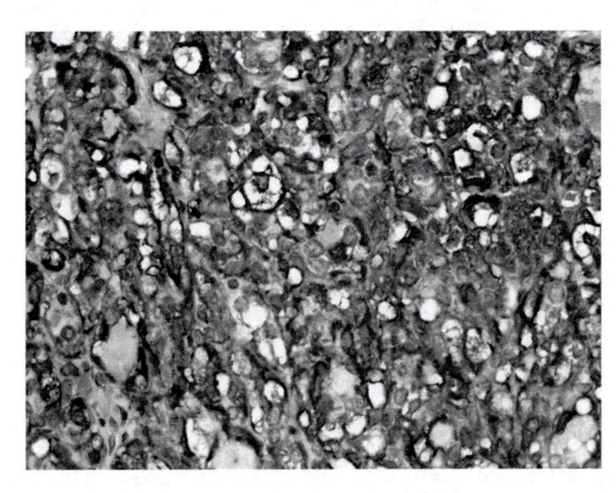

FIGURE 27.2 **(See color insert.)** Immunohistochemistry with Ct. Tumor cells stained positive. Diagnosis confirmed as MTC.

Lymph node metastases are common early in the course of the disease. This is mainly to lateral cervical or paratracheal lymph nodes. Lymph node metastases are present in 20%–30% of cases even with a tumor diameter of <1 cm (T1 tumor). This frequency rises to 50% and 90% in T2 and T3–T4 tumors, respectively (Moley et al., 1999, Scollo et al., 2003). Sites for distant metastases include primarily the liver followed by bones, brain, and skin. Distant metastases generally occur in multiple sites.

Hereditary MTC has specific histological features. C cell hyperplasia (CCH), defined as the presence of >40 C cells/cm^2 or as at least three x100 magnification fields containing >50 C cells, always points out hereditary MTC. CCH has only been reported in a few cases of sporadic MTC. Hereditary MTC is usually bilateral and multicentric, whereas sporadic MTC generally presents as a single tumor (Pacini et al., 1992).

Hereditary MTC can present as

1. A component of multiple endocrine neoplasia type 2A (MEN 2A)
2. A component of multiple endocrine neoplasia type 2B (MEN 2B)
3. As familial MTC being the only component

MEN 2 is a genetic syndrome that results from germ line mutations in the RET proto-oncogene (see later). It is transmitted in an autosomal dominant manner. Approximately 80%–90% of patients with hereditary MTC have MEN 2A and 100% of MEN 2A patients develop MTC. The other components of this syndrome, pheochromocytoma and hyperparathyroidism, are seen in approximately 50% and 20% of cases, respectively (Eng et al., 1996). Less common manifestations of MEN2A are cutaneous lichen amyloidosis and Hirschsprung's disease.

MEN 2B comprises 5%–10% of MEN cases and again MTC is a component of all MEN 2B patients. The second most prominent feature of the syndrome, pheochromocytoma, is present in 50% of cases. Other features of MEN 2B are enteric ganglioneuromas, a marfanoid body habitus and mucosal neuromas of the tongue, lips, and cornea.

The remaining 5%–15% of hereditary MTC cases is defined as familial medullary thyroid cancer (FMTC). This definition necessitates the presence of MTC in kindreds with four or more affected members without involvement of adrenal and parathyroid glands (Eng, 1999). FMTC can also occur as CCH (Phay et al., 2000).

The typical presentation of sporadic MTC is a single unilateral thyroid nodule or a palpable cervical lymph node, whereas hereditary MTC is usually bilateral and multicentric. Invasive hereditary MTC is considered to develop from a precursor multifocal CCH (Block et al., 1980). Rarely patients may present with systemic manifestations due to secretion of several peptides and substances, including Ct, chromogranin A (CgA), somatostatin, vasoactive intestinal peptide (VIP), carcinoembryonic antigen (CEA), calcitonin-gene-related peptide (CGRP), and even adrenocorticotropic hormone (ACTH) (Hoff et al., 2007). Ct is a 32 amino acid peptide coded by a gene located on chromosome 11 (Przepiorka et al., 1984). The importance of Ct in diagnosis and follow-up of MTC is discussed later in this chapter.

Association of MTC with one of the hereditary syndromes is important for the prognosis since the aggressiveness of MTC varies with the subtypes. Sporadic MTC cases often present between 50 and 60 years of age. FMTC presents between 20 and 40 years and is less aggressive when compared to other hereditary forms of MTC (Moley et al., 2007).

Hereditary MTC associated with MEN may present early in childhood with an aggressive course (Lemos et al., 2002). MEN 2B is the most aggressive hereditary form and has a high mortality. MTC with lymph node metastasis may be seen in patients as young as 3 years of age (Kaufman et al., 1982). Location of the RET mutation is strongly correlated with disease phenotype in MEN 2. Current literature recommends classifying the patients according to their RET mutation and suitable management such as prophylactic thyroidectomy before a certain age accordingly (Machens et al., 2007, Yip et al., 2003; de Groot et al., 2006). It should be noted that some mutations associated with disease aggressiveness and MTC-related deaths in some families were also reported in some FMTC families with no known cases of MTC-related deaths (Kouvaraki et al., 2005). Unknown genetic and environmental factors may be the other determinants of biological behavior of the tumor.

27.3.2 Noninvasive Serum Biomarkers

27.3.2.1 Calcitonin

Parafollicular C cells of the thyroid gland are neuroendocrine cells. They secrete a variety of peptides and hormones. Ct is the most commonly secreted substance from these cells. Ct is a very useful and highly sensitive tumor marker for both the diagnosis and the follow-up of MTC. Ct is a 32 amino acid peptide whose primary function is to inhibit osteoclastic bone resorption. Endogenous Ct seems to have no essential physiological role in humans since patients after thyroidectomy, with undetectable Ct levels, and MTC patients with extremely high Ct levels have no apparent alteration in their calcium and mineral homeostasis.

Although not widely accepted, routine measurement of serum Ct has been advocated for detection of MTC among patients with nodular thyroid diseases. In fact until the early 1990s, it was the only reliable tool for diagnosis of MTC. One crucial caveat of Ct measurement as a tumor marker is that it has a high sensitivity but low specificity for MTC. Ct can be elevated in cases of thyroid inflammation like Hashimoto's thyroiditis as well as nonthyroidal diseases like cirrhosis, kidney diseases, anemia, hypergastrinemia, and pregnancy. Other physiological and pathological states that can elevate serum Ct are seen in Table 27.5 (Toledo et al., 2009). Due to many non-MTC situations that can elevate serum Ct levels, close relatives of cases with multiple endocrine neoplasias should undergo prophylactic thyroidectomy based on carrying a mutation in the RET proto-oncogene rather than elevated serum Ct levels. Another debate is the cost-effectiveness of routine Ct evaluation in nodular thyroid diseases. A study performed in the United States reported that its measurement appeared to be cost-effective compared to TSH measurement (Cheung et al., 2008).

TABLE 27.5

Hypercalcitoninemia in Nonmedullary Thyroid Carcinoma Conditions

Physiological and lifestyle-related situations	Sex
	Men (<8.5 pg/mL) have higher basal values than women (<5 pg/mL)
	Age: Young show higher values than old people
	Obesity
	Cigarette smoking
	Physical activity
Drugs	Proton pump inhibitors (omeprazole, etc.)
	Glucocorticoids
	Beta blockers
	Glucagon
	Ct gene-related peptide
	Enteroglucagon
	Pancreozymin
Nonthyroid disease	Hypergastrinemias
	Hypercalcemias (hyperparathyroidism)
	Renal insufficiency
	Neuroendocrine tumors
	Pheochromocytoma
	Paraganglioma
	Enteropancreatic endocrine tumors
	VIPoma
	Insulinoma–carcinoids
	Small-cell pulmonary tumor
Thyroid disease	Follicular carcinoma
	Papillary carcinoma
	Chronic autoimmune thyroiditis

Source: Adapted from Toledo, S.P.A. et al., *Clinics (Sao Paolo)*, 64(7), 699, 2009. With permission.

TABLE 27.6

Some Commercially Available Ct Assays

Assay Name	Ct Immunoassay	Ct Assay	Liaison	IRMA-hCT	Advantage	Immulite 2000
Manufacturer	Biomerica, US	Scantibodies, US	DiaSorin, US	CisBio International, France	Nichols Institute, United Sates	DPC, France
Assay type	Two-site ELISA	IRMA	CLIA	Two-site IRMA	Chemiluminescent assay	Chemiluminescent assay
Reference range	<13 pg/mL female <30 pg/mL male	1–8 pg/mL female 3–21 pg/mL male	<10 pg/mL	<10 pg/mL	<5 pg/mL women <12 pg/mL men	<10 pg/mL

In 2006, the European Thyroid Association (ETA) recommended the measurement of basal Ct in the initial evaluation of thyroid nodules (Pacini et al., 2006). The American Thyroid Association (ATA) however does not advise for or against the routine measurement of Ct in nodular thyroid diseases (Kloos et al., 2009).

RIA and two-site immunoassay techniques such as immunoradiometric assay (IRMA), immunochemiluminescent assay (ICMA), and immunoluminometric assay (ILMA) are the main laboratory methods used for serum Ct evaluation today. IRMA, ICMA, and ILMA are the methods most widely used in tertiary centers today. They detect the monomeric form of Ct. It should be kept in mind that the normal values vary according to the commercial kit. Some commercially available Ct assays are shown in Table 27.6.

Rare cases of dedifferentiated MTC have been reported to have low serum Ct levels. Other tumor markers should be used to aid the diagnosis and follow-up in such cases.

27.3.2.1.1 Basal Ct

The upper limit of which Ct should be for suspicion of MTC is a matter of controversy. As previously stated in this chapter, FNAC of a thyroid nodule is the main tool in diagnosing differentiated thyroid cancers. However, diagnostic accuracy of this test is relatively low for MTC. With this caveat, many authorities suggest the use of routine Ct measurement as a screening method for MTC. Although markedly elevated Ct (i.e., >100 pg/mL) levels are compatible with the diagnosis of MTC, moderately elevated values of Ct are often nonconclusive. Ct levels higher than 100 pg/mL have an almost 100% probability for MTC, levels between 50 and 100 pg/mL have a moderate risk (25%), and levels between 20 and 50 pg/mL have a low risk (8.3%) (Constante et al., 2007). A study revealed that only 10%–40% of patients having thyroid nodules associated with hypercalcitoninemia had MTC (Borget et al., 2007). Other conditions that could elevate serum Ct levels should be evaluated especially in cases having basal serum Ct levels <100 pg/mL.

Many studies have been performed trying to estimate an exact cutoff level of Ct for MTC. ATA advises the further evaluation of subjects with nodular thyroid diseases having basal Ct levels >100 pg/mL. However, some researchers believe that this level should be lower. A recent study evaluated 2733 patients with thyroid nodules who underwent surgery. Ct levels were >10 pg/mL in 43 patients. Twelve of these were diagnosed as MTC, 31 had C cell hyperplasia, and 2 of the patients had MTC associated with C cell hyperplasia. Out of 2690 patients with normal Ct levels (<10 pg/mL), only 2 patients were diagnosed as micro-MTC. All patients with Ct levels >60 pg/mL had MTC diagnosis. In this study, the appropriate cutoff level of Ct for MTC diagnosis was 60 pg/mL. In patients with Ct levels between 10 and 59 pg/mL, only 11% of patients had MTC. The rest had C cell hyperplasia (Chambon et al., 2011).

As previously stated the ATA does not recommend for or against the routine use of serum Ct in the evaluation of thyroid nodules. On the other hand, further evaluation of subjects with nodular thyroid diseases having basal or stimulated Ct levels above 100 pg/mL is recommended (Kloos et al., 2009).

Basal Ct is also used in the postoperative setting in the follow-up of MTC. In the follow-up of MTC, Ct doubling time and stimulated Ct levels may be more informative for prognosis (see later).

27.3.2.1.2 Stimulated Serum Ct

Ct is stored in dense secretary granules and is released in the bloodstream through external stimulation of provocative agents such as calcium and pentagastrin.

27.3.2.1.2.1 Pentagastrin-Stimulated Ct Pentagastrin is a synthetic gastrin analog that stimulates Ct release from dense secretary granules of C cells via binding to the extracellular domain of the transmembrane cholecystokinin (CCK)-B/gastrin receptor (Machens et al., 2008).

A 6 h fasting period is necessary prior to the test. After an IV bolus of 0.5 μg/kg pentagastrin (Peptavlon® in 200 μg ampoules), serum Ct is measured at 0, 2, 5, and 15 min. Many different cutoff levels have been proposed, but generally a 3–20× increase of Ct relative to basal levels is considered as a positive response. Today pentagastrin is unavailable in many countries, so calcium stimulation is gaining more popularity.

A large prospective study involving patients with nodular thyroid diseases was performed in Italy. In this study, basal Ct levels and, in cases of moderate Ct elevation (i.e., between 20 and 100 pg/mL), a pentagastrin-stimulated Ct level were obtained in 5815 patients. The positive predictive value of basal Ct >100 pg/mL for MTC was 100%, whereas the pentagastrin-stimulated Ct >100 pg/mL was 40% (Constante et al., 2007).

In another study, 89 patients with untreated MTC were retrospectively analyzed. A pentagastrin-stimulated Ct to basal Ct ratio <10 was associated with a higher frequency and number of lymph node metastases. Thus, the authors argued that reduced stimulation to pentagastrin could reflect early dedifferentiation of the tumor that involves loss of the CCK-B/gastrin receptor (Machens et al., 2008).

Pentagastrin has some side effects such as retrosternal tightness, extremity paresthesia, dizziness, feeling of warmth, nausea, and metallic taste that can last 1–2 min after the injection (Doyle et al., 2009).

Today ATA recommends further evaluation of cases with nodular thyroid diseases having stimulated Ct levels above 100 pg/mL.

27.3.2.1.2.2 Calcium-Stimulated Ct Just like pentagastrin stimulation, a 6 h fasting period is advised prior to the test. After a 2.5 mg/kg calcium gluconate IV push over 4 min, serum Ct level is obtained at 0, 5, 10, and 20 min (Elisei, 2008).

A recent study analyzing 50 subjects with normal thyroid function and anatomy compared the potency and tolerance of Ct stimulation by high-dose calcium and compared this with pentagastrin. High-dose calcium was more potent and better tolerated than pentagastrin. Side effects associated with calcium infusion were temporary flushing, feeling of warmth, facial paresthesia, and altered gustatory sensation that lasted up to 15 min (Doyle et al., 2009).

A very recent study compared these two tests in the diagnosis and follow-up of MTC. The high-dose calcium stimulation test was found to be potent, well tolerated, and cost-effective. In this study, 16 cases were healthy controls, 13 cases had known RET mutation, 24 cases were treated for MTC and were present in remission, and 18 cases had persistent MTC disease. ROC analysis revealed that a calcium-stimulated Ct level >184 pg/mL in females and >1620 pg/mL in males differentiated MTC with normal/C cell hyperplasia subjects with high sensitivity and specificity. The highest accuracy level was 32.6 pg/mL for females and 192 pg/mL for males (Colombo et al., 2012).

These studies prove that high-dose calcium stimulation can be used as an alternative to pentagastrin stimulation in both the diagnosis and follow-up with advantages of better availability, cost-effectiveness, and higher tolerability.

27.3.2.1.3 Ct Doubling Time

Ct doubling time is a valuable prognostic factor for MTC cases. It can be used in the postoperative setting in the follow-up of MTC. Many studies have been performed proving Ct doubling time to have a higher prognostic value than preoperative Ct levels. A meta-analysis revealed that Ct and CEA doubling times less than 1 year were significant risk factors for recurrence and death due to MTC (Meijer et al., 2010). This meta-analysis involved data from 10 studies. In subjects where both data were available, CEA doubling time had a higher predictive value for survival and recurrence; thus, the authors advise the use of both tumor markers in the follow-up of subjects with MTC.

Another group performed a retrospective analysis of 70 patients with MTC. This study revealed that Ct and CEA doubling times of less than 2 years were negative prognostic factors for MTC disease-free and total survival (Gawlik et al., 2010).

27.3.2.2 Carcinoembryonic Antigen

This tumor marker has a low specificity for MTC so it should be used in the follow-up rather than diagnosis. In more than 50% of cases of MTC, CEA is elevated. In a study, Ct and CEA progression rates were found to be well correlated (Barbet et al., 2005). On the other hand, an increasing CEA level in the presence of stable Ct levels can be a sign of dedifferentiation of the tumor and is associated with worse prognosis. A preoperative CEA level of >30 ng/mL is associated to a surgically incurable disease (Sippel et al., 2008).

A multivariate analysis was designed aiming to correlate abnormal CEA levels and MTC progression. One hundred and fifty patients with MTC having preoperative CEA levels recorded were evaluated. Fifty four of these had elevated CEA levels prior to the initial surgery. CEA levels were significantly associated with the number of lymph node metastases and the frequency of distal metastases. Higher CEA levels were associated with more advanced disease. CEA levels >30 ng/mL were associated with central and ipsilateral lymph node metastases, whereas levels >100 ng/mL were associated with lateral lymph node and distant metastases. The authors also stated that CEA levels <30 ng/mL was associated with a local disease.

Postoperative CEA values are more valuable than the preoperative values especially with cases having lymph node metastases and distant metastases. Patients with preoperative CEA levels <30 mg/mL are considered surgically curable (Machens and Dralle, 2007, Sipple et al., 2008). Just as Ct doubling time, postoperative CEA doubling time is a fundamental parameter in the follow-up of MTC. A study performed emphasized the use of both Ct and CEA doubling times in the follow-up because CEA doubling time seemed to be more informative for prognosis of MTC (Meier et al., 2010). On the other hand, another study resulted in the opposite (Barbet et al., 2005).

As a result, preoperative and postoperative use of both markers in the follow-up of patients with MTC may be informative and necessary for risk stratification. However, in the latest guidelines, ATA recommends only the use of Ct in the detection, staging, postoperative management, and prognosis in patients with MTC (Kloos et al., 2009).

27.3.2.3 Chromogranin A

In 1992, a group measured serum CgA levels in 61 surgically confirmed MTC cases. CgA was elevated in only 14 of these cases, whereas Ct was elevated in 46 patients. Only one patient had elevated CgA levels despite normal Ct levels. CgA had also no response to pentagastrin. CgA was elevated mostly in cases with more advanced disease (Blind et al., 1992).

In a more recent study, a group reported their experience of CgA in MTC. CgA was increased in 12/45 cases of MTC with high Ct level and in 4/16 cases of undetectable Ct. During the follow-up, however, the CgA level reflected the tumor burden. The researchers advised possible usage of CgA in the follow-up of patients with MTC (Guignat et al., 2001).

Currently, the routine usage of CgA in the detection and follow-up of MTC is not advised. Its usage may be limited to rare cases of Ct negative MTC.

Other substances such as CGRP, ACTH, amyloid, somatostatin, serotonin, and VIP can be produced by MTC tumor cells. The use of these markers in the detection and follow-up of cases with MTC is currently not advised.

27.3.2.4 RET Proto-Oncogene

The tyrosine kinase encoded by RET has three domains:

1. The extracellular domain
2. The transmembrane domain
3. The intracellular tyrosine kinase domain

The extracellular domain contains four cadherin-like domains that interact with ligands and coreceptors (Takahashi et al., 1985, Airaksinen and Saarma, 2002, Anders et al., 2001). The two tyrosine kinase subdomains (TK1 and TK2) are located intracellularly and are involved in the activation of intracellular signal transduction pathways (Arighi et al., 2005).

In 1987, RET was defined as the predisposing gene for hereditary MTC that was followed by reports of its mutations in MEN2A, MEN2B, and FMTC (Hofstra et al., 1994, Mulligan et al., 1993, 1994).

In 1993 and 1994, it was demonstrated that MEN 2A, FMTC, and MEN 2B, respectively, were caused by germline RET mutations. Germline mutations in exons 5, 8, 10, 11, 13, 14, 15, or 16 of the RET gene have been identified in 98% of patients with MEN 2 (Eng et al., 1996).

Mutations leading to MEN 2A affect the cysteine-rich extracellular domain, each converting a cysteine to another amino acid—to arginine in half of the cases—in codons 609, 611, 618, and 620 of exon 10 and in codon 634 of exon 11 (Eng et al., 1996). Mutation of the extracellular cysteine in codon 634 of exon 11 causes ligand-independent activation of the receptor and constitutive cell transformation. Mutation of the intracellular tyrosine kinase (codon 918) causes activation of intracellular signaling pathways and also results in cellular transformation (Machens et al., 2003). The risk of progression from C cell hyperplasia to MTC increases with age. C cells are probably more susceptible to oncogenic RET activation because MTC usually develops prior to pheochromocytoma and parathyroid hyperplasia in patients with MEN2A. Other reported germ line mutations in MEN2A are in codons 630, 649, and 666 of exon 11; in codons 768, 776, 777, 790, and 791 of exon 13; in codon 804 of exon 14; in codons 866 and 891 of exon 15; in codon 912 of exon 16; in codons 515 and 533 of exon 8; in codon 912 of exon 16; and in codon 321 of exon 5.

Mutations defined in FMTC affect codons 609, 611, 618, and 620 of exon 10; codon 768 of exon 13; and codon 804 of exon 14. In several families, mutations affect codons 630, 631, 634, 649, and 666 in exon 11. Other mutations identified in FMTC kindreds are in codons 768, 776, 790, and 791 of exon 13; codons, 844, 833, and 819 of exon 14; and codons 866 and 891 of exon 15 in the intracellular domain of the gene (Eng et al., 1996). De novo mutations inherited through the paternal allele have been found in 4%–10% of index cases with MEN 2A and FMTC (Schuffenecker et al., 1997).

In MEN 2B, 95% of the patients have a single mutation converting methionine to threonine in codon 918 of exon 16 (Eng et al., 1996). It is frequently (>50%) a de novo mutation in the allele inherited through the paternal allele (Schuffenecker et al., 1997). Other rare mutations associated with MEN 2B involve codon 883 of exon 15 and double RET mutations.

Germ line mutations cause constitutive activation of the RET proto-oncogene. Mutations with strong activation of the RET proto-oncogene seem to lead to a more aggressive form of MTC, whereas mutations with weaker RET activation result in a less aggressive disease. These data have led to the development of genotype-based risk stratification by ATA (Kloos et al., 2009). ATA has classified the mutations into four levels, level D including the highest risk and level A the least risk. Level D mutations include codons 883 and 918 and are associated with the youngest age of onset, and highest risk of metastases and disease-specific mortality ATA level C mutations carry a high risk of aggressive MTC and include mutations in codon 634. ATA level B are mutations at RET codons 609, 611, 618, 620, and 630. ATA level A mutations carry the "least high" risk and are in codons 768, 790, 791, 804, and 891.

In 25%–33% of sporadic MTC, somatic mutations (occurring in the tumor alone) have been identified in codon 918 of the RET proto-oncogene and have been found to be associated with poor prognosis when compared to other sporadic tumors (Elisei et al., 2008; Romei et al., 1996, Schilling et al., 2001, Uchino et al., 1998). Other genetic abnormalities identified in a few cases of sporadic MTC include mutations in codons 618, 634, 768, 804, and 883 and partial deletion of the RET gene. Interestingly, somatic mutations of the RET proto-oncogene have been identified in 10%–20% of sporadic pheochromocytomas (codons 620, 630, 634, and 918).

ATA defines MTC as "an uncommon and challenging malignancy" (Kloos et al., 2009). ATA strongly recommends germ line RET testing for all patients with a personal medical history of primary C cell hyperplasia, MTC, or MEN 2. The guideline underlines the importance of early diagnosis in MTC and offers RET testing for all people with a family history consistent with MEN 2 or FMTC and at risk for autosomal dominant inheritance of the syndrome. This analysis should preferably be done before the age of recommended prophylactic thyroidectomy that is shortly after birth for MEN 2B and before 5 years of age for MEN 2A and FMTC. Analysis of the MEN 2–specific exons of RET is recommended as the method of initial testing. In patients with MEN 2B, M918T (exon 16) and A883F mutations of RET should be analyzed instead of sequencing the entire coding region of RET.

Prophylactic total thyroidectomy in a tertiary health-care setting is advised for children with ATA level C mutation (codon 634) before they are 5 years old. In cases with mutations of ATA level A and B risk, prophylactic thyroidectomy may be delayed beyond the first 5 years if serum Ct and annual cervical ultrasound are normal. If there is no clinical or radiological evidence of lymph node metastases, if the nodule is <5 mm in size (at any age), or if the serum basal Ct is <40 pg/mL in a child <6 months old, prophylactic level VI central compartment neck dissection may not be necessary in patients with MEN 2A/FMTC who undergo prophylactic thyroidectomy. However, children with MEN 2B are stratified as ATA level D risk and should have thyroidectomy within the first year of life preferably following a preoperative computed tomography assessment and cervical ultrasound. In RET mutation-positive patients, annual screening for pheochromocytoma begins by 8 years of age in carriers of the RET mutation associated with MEN 2B and codons 630 and 634 and by 20 years of age in carriers of other MEN 2A RET mutations. Patients with FMTC should be screened periodically from 20 years of age. For sporadic MTC, routine evaluation of somatic RET mutations is not advised currently.

A recent study carried out in 729 apparently sporadic MTC patients reported unsuspected germ line RET mutations in 6.5% of the cases (Romei et al., 2011). Another study suggests not to extend the mutation analysis in sporadic MTC beyond the hot spot regions of RET since it does not seem to be cost-effective (Lindsey et al., 2012).

27.3.3 Invasive Markers

27.3.3.1 Calcitonin Washout Evaluation

Ct can be evaluated from the washout fluid of thyroid nodules and suspicious lymph nodes (Ct washout). This method is recent and prospective studies are rare. After FNAC is performed, the same needle and syringe is washed with 1 mL of 0.9% sodium chloride solution and is sent to the laboratory for Ct evaluation.

The appropriate reference level of Ct from the washout fluid is understudied. In a very recent study, Ct washout evaluation was performed to 21 patients referred with either elevated serum Ct levels or suspicious MTC cytology. Out of these 21 patients, only 6 were diagnosed as MTC histologically. All of these six patients had basal serum Ct levels >100 pg/mL and similarly high washout Ct levels. Two patients had moderately elevated serum Ct levels, but their washout Ct levels were low and were eventually diagnosed as PTC in one patient and nodular hyperplasia in the other patient. The remaining patients had normal serum Ct levels and low washout levels. None of them were diagnosed as MTC histologically (Trimboli et al., 2012).

We previously reported a patient with Hashimoto's thyroiditis and an 8 mm nodule on the left thyroid lobe having a moderately elevated basal Ct level (49 pg/mL). Three FNACs were nonconclusive, whereas the Ct level from the washout fluid was 191,000 pg/mL. Eventually, total thyroidectomy was performed confirming the diagnosis of MTC (Mousa et al., 2013).

In a study in 2007, Ct washout was performed for five patients with MTC. The washout levels for Ct in these patients ranged from 17,000 to 560,000 pg/mL. A control group consisting of patients with PTC, normal thyroid gland, and Hashimoto's thyroiditis had Ct washout levels between 10 and 67 pg/mL. This study emphasized that Ct washout evaluation could be used as an alternative method for diagnosing MTC (Kudo et al., 2007). However, another study showed no correlation between serum Ct levels and Ct washout levels (Massaro et al., 2009). In a similar study in 2007, Ct washout was performed for thyroid nodules and lymph nodes. All patients with washout levels >36 pg/mL were diagnosed as MTC. Thus, this method had 100% sensitivity and specificity in this study (Boi et al., 2007).

Current knowledge from studies performed with Ct washout does not show a relevant advantage over cases with basal Ct levels >100 pg/mL. This method may have an advantage for cases with moderate serum Ct levels (i.e., <100 pg/mL), but larger prospective studies are needed.

A summary of sensitivity, specificity, and prognostic value of tumor markers in MTC is shown in Table 27.7.

TABLE 27.7
Sensitivity, Specificity, and Prognostic Importance of Tumor Markers in MTC

Marker and Cutoff	Diagnostic Sensitivity	Diagnostic Specificity	Prognostic Value in the Follow-Up
Basal Ct > 100 pg/mL	+++	++	++
Ct washout evaluation	+++	+++	
Stimulated Ct > 100 pg/mL	+++	+++	
Ct doubling time < 1 year			+++
CEA > 5 ng/mL	++	+	++
CEA doubling time < 1 year			+++
CgA > 18 ng/mL	+	+	+
RET proto-oncogene mutation			+++

Ct, calcitonin; CEA, carcinoembryonic antigen; CgA, chromogranin A; RET, rearrangement of transfection; +, low (<50%); ++, moderate (50%–90%); +++, high (>90%).

27.3.4 Treatment

MTC is a very chemoresistant and radioresistant cancer. Dacarbazine is the cytotoxic agent for metastatic MTC but does not seem to be of use regarding the survival (Hoff et al., 2007). External radiation beam therapy has a limited role in advanced MTC (Schwartz et al., 2008). Total thyroidectomy and lymph node dissection (central or lateral depending on the tumor characteristics) is the standard therapy of choice accepted today.

27.3.4.1 RET as a Therapeutic Target

In familial MTC, surgical resection before malignant transformation and/or metastases provides the highest chance of cure (Hoff et al., 2007).

Novel molecular treatment agents are under investigation for MTC. There are both preclinical studies targeting RET with various results in MTC treatment (Cakir and Grossman, 2009).

Trial of tyrosine kinase inhibitors on mice yielded promising results. Oral RET tyrosine kinase inhibitor RPI-1 administration to mice bearing subcutaneous xenograft tumors of the human MTC cell line MZ-CRC-1, harboring endogenous RET M918T mutation, resulted in a remarkable antitumor activity (Nicolini et al., 2011).

Vandetanib became the first agent approved by the Food and Drug Administration (FDA) in 2011 for the treatment of adults with symptomatic or progressive MTC. Vandetanib inhibits not only RET but also vascular endothelial growth factor receptor 2, 3 (VEGFR2, VEGFR3) and the epidermal growth factor receptor (EGFR). Vandetanib has shown to inhibit cell proliferation, as well as RET autophosphorylation, and to reduce RET expression especially in MEN 2B cells (Verbeek et al., 2011). In a phase II study, 30 patients with locally advanced or metastatic hereditary MTC received oral vandetanib. Six of 30 patients (20%) experienced a confirmed partial response and 53% of patients experienced stable disease for at least 24 weeks (Wells et al., 2011a). In another study investigating the efficacy of vandetanib in patients with advanced hereditary MTC, objective partial responses were observed in 16% and stable disease lasting 24 weeks or longer in 53% of the patients (Robinson et al., 2011). Similar therapeutic efficacy is observed in a phase III trial in patients with advanced MTC (Wells et al., 2011b).

Cabozantinib (XL184) is an inhibitor of VEGFR1, VEGFR2, hepatocyte growth factor receptor (MET), and RET. In preclinical studies, treatment with cabozantinib resulted in decreased tumor invasiveness (Sherman, 2011). Cabozantinib is studied in a group of patients with advanced solid tumors including 37 MTC patients. Ten out of 35 patients had a partial response (Kurzrock et al., 2011).

Sorafenib, which is an inhibitor of VEGFR2 and VEGFR3, RET, and BRAF, was evaluated in two phase II studies (Ahmed et al., 2011, Lam et al., 2011) and partial response was observed in 6%–15% of patients with MTC and stable disease lasting more than 6 months in 62%–74%.

Sunitinib and motesanib are other tyrosine kinase inhibitors targeting RET together with VEGFRs. Sunitinib has been mostly associated with stable disease in patients with MTC in a phase II trial (Carr et al., 2011). However, only 2% of patients with progressive MTC had confirmed partial response to motesanib (Schlumberger et al., 2009).

Another tyrosine kinase inhibitor affecting VEGFRs but not RET, axitinib, resulted in a low partial response (18%) in MTC patients in a phase II trial (Cohen et al., 2008).

Combination of tyrosine kinase inhibitors is under investigation for metastatic MTC. Hong et al. studied 13 patients (62% RET positive) with metastatic sporadic MTC treated with a combination of sorafenib and tipifarnib (inhibitor of RAS farnesylation) (Hong et al., 2011). MTC partial response rate was 38%. These findings suggest a potential role of RAS in the pathogenesis of MTC.

27.4 Conclusion

FTC and MTC are two malignancies with serious unresolved diagnostic and therapeutic issues. The principal problem concerns preoperative diagnosis of FTC or postsurgical treatment of MTC. Serum Ct remains to be the marker with the highest sensitivity and specificity for both the diagnosis and prognosis of MTC. Serum Tg is the sole marker used for the follow-up of patients with FTC undergone surgery. Today translational medicine is providing through biomolecular markers application the best tool for facing these clinical issues.

References

Ahmed M, Barbachano Y, Riddell A et al. Analysis of the efficacy and toxicity of sorafenib in thyroid cancer: A phase II study in a UK based population. *Eur J Endocrinol* 2011; 165: 315–322.

Airaksinen MS and Saarma M. The GDNF family: Signaling, biological functions and therapeutic value. *Nat Rev Neurosci* 2002; 3: 383–394.

Anders J, Kjar S, Ibanez CF et al. Molecular modeling of the extracellular domain of the RET receptor tyrosine kinase reveals multiple cadherin-like domains and a calcium-binding site. *J Biol Chem* 2001; 276: 35808–35817.

Arighi E, Borrello MG, and Sariola H. RET tyrosine kinase signaling in the development and cancer. *Cytokine Growth Factor Rev* 2005; 16: 441–467.

Baldini E, Sorrenti S, D'Armiento E et al. The urokinase plasminogen activating system in thyroid cancer: Clinical implications. *G Chir* October 2012; 33(10): 305–310.

Baloch Z, Carayon P, Conte-Devolx B et al. Laboratory medicine practice guidelines. Laboratory support for the diagnosis and monitoring of thyroid disease. *Thyroid* 2003; 13(1): 3–26.

Baloch ZW, Fleisher S, LiVolsi VA et al. Diagnosis of "follicular neoplasm": A gray zone in thyroid fine-needle aspiration cytology. *Diagn Cytopathol* 2002; 26: 41–44.

Baloch ZW, LiVolsi VA, Asa SL et al. Diagnostic terminology and morphologic criteria for cytologic diagnosis of thyroid lesions: A synopsis of the National Cancer Institute Thyroid Fine-Needle Aspiration State of the Science Conference. *Diagn Cytopathol* 2008; 36: 425–437.

Baloch ZW, Tam D, Langer J et al. Ultrasound-guided fine-needle aspiration biopsy of the thyroid: Role of on-site assessment and multiple cytologic preparations. *Diagn Cytopathol* 2000; 23: 425–429.

Barbet J, Campion L, Kraeber-Bodeber F et al. Prognostic impact of serum calcitonin and carcinoembryonic antigen doubling-times in patients with medullary thyroid carcinoma. *J Clin Endocrinol Metab* 2005; 90: 6077–6084.

Barden CB, Shister KW, Zhu B et al. Classification of follicular thyroid tumors by molecular signature: Results of gene profiling. *Clin Cancer Res* 2003; 9: 1792–1800.

Bartel DP. MicroRNAs: Genomics, biogenesis, mechanism, and function. *Cell* 2004; 116: 281–297.

Bartolazzi A, Bellotti C, and Sciacchitano S. Methodology and technical requirements of the galectin-3 test for the preoperative characterization of thyroid nodules. *Appl Immunohistochem Mol Morphol* January 2012; 20(1): 2–7.

Bartolazzi A, Gasbarri A, Papotti M et al. Application of an immunodiagnostic method for improving preoperative diagnosis of nodular thyroid lesions. *Lancet* 2001; 357: 1644–1650.

Bartolazzi A, Orlandi F, Saggiorato E et al. Galectin-3-expression analysis in the surgical selection of follicular thyroid nodules with indeterminate fine-needle aspiration cytology: A prospective multicentre study. *Lancet Oncol* 2008; 9: 543–549.

Belge G, Meyer A, Klemke M et al. Up regulation of HMGA2 in thyroid carcinomas: A novel molecular marker to distinguish between benign and malignant follicular neoplasias. *Genes Chromosomes Cancer* 2008; 47(1): 56–63.

Bertagnolli MM, Redston M, Compton CC et al. Microsatellite instability and loss of heterozygosity at chromosomal location 18q: Prospective evaluation of biomarkers for stages II and III colon cancer—A study of CALGB 9581 and 89803. *J Clin Oncol* August 10, 2011; 29(23): 3153–3162.

Biondi B, Filetti S, and Schlumberger M. Thyroid-hormone therapy and thyroid cancer: A reassessment. *Nat Clin Pract Endocrinol Metab* 2005; 1: 32–40.

Blind E, Schmidt-Gayk H, Sinn HP et al. Chromogranin A as a tumor marker in medullary thyroid carcinoma. *Thyroid* 1992; 2(1): 5–10.

Block MA, Jackson CE, Greenawald KA et al. Clinical characteristics distinguishing hereditary from sporadic medullary thyroid carcinoma. Treatment implications. *Arch Surg* 1980; 115: 142–148.

Boi F, Maurelli I, Pinna G et al. Calcitonin measurement in wash out fluid from fine needle aspiration of neck masses in patients with primary and metastatic medullary thyroid carcinoma. *J Clin Endocrinol Metab* 2007; 92: 2115–2118.

Borget I, De pouvourville G, and Schlumberger M. Editorial: Calcitonin determination in patients with nodular thyroid disease. *J Clin Endocrinol Metab* 2007; 92: 425–427.

Braun J and Hüttelmaier S. Pathogenic mechanisms of deregulated microRNA expression in thyroid carcinomas of follicular origin. *Thyroid Res* August 3, 2011; 4(Suppl 1): S1.

Bugalho MJM, Santos JR, and Sobrinho L. Preoperative diagnosis of medullary thyroid carcinoma: Fine needle aspiration cytology as compared with serum calcitonin measurement. *J Surg Oncol* 2005; 91: 56–60.

Cakir M and Grossman AB. Medullary thyroid cancer: Molecular biology and novel molecular therapies. *Neuroendocrinology* 2009; 90(4): 323–348.

Carcangiu MC, Zempi G, and Rosai J. Poorly differentiated ("insular") thyroid carcinoma: A reinterpretation of Langhans "wuchernde Struma". *Am J Surg Pathol* 1984; 8: 655–668.

Carcangiu ML, Bianchi S, Savino D et al. Follicular Hurthle cell neoplasm's of the thyroid gland: A study of 153 cases. *Cancer* 1991; 68: 1944–1953.

Carpi A, Di Concio G, Lervasi G et al. Thyroid fine needle aspiration: How to improve clinicians' confidence and performance with the technique. *Cancer Lett* 2008; 264(2): 163–171.

Carpi A, Ferrari E, Toni MG et al. Needle aspiration techniques in preoperative selection of patients with thyroid nodules: A long-term study. *J Clin Oncol* May 1996; 14(5): 1704–1712.

Carpi A, Mechanick JI, and Nicolini A. The Emerging role of percutaneous needle biopsy and molecular tumor marker analysis for the preoperative selection of thyroid nodules. In: *Thyroid Cancer from Emergent Biotechnologies to Clinical Practice Guidelines*, (eds.) A. Carpi and J.I. Mechanick, pp. 194–207. Taylor & Francis Group: Boca Raton, FL, 2011.

Carpi A, Naccarato AG, Iervasi G et al. Large needle aspiration biopsy and galectin-3 determination in selected thyroid nodules with indeterminate FNA-cytology. *Br J Cancer* July 17, 2006; 95(2): 204–209.

Carpi A and Nicolini A. The role of large-needle aspiration biopsy in the preoperative selection of palpable thyroid nodules: A summary of principal data. *Biomed Pharmacother* 2000; 54: 350–353.

Carpi A, Rossi G, Coscio GD et al. Galectin-3 detection on large-needle aspiration biopsy improves preoperative selection of thyroid nodules: A prospective cohort study. *Ann Med* 2010; 42(1): 70–78.

Carpi A, Rossi G, Romani R et al. Are risk factors common to thyroid cancer and nodule? A forty years observational time-trend study. *PLoS One* 2012; 7(10): e47758. doi: 10.1371/journal.pone.0047758. Epub October 31, 2012.

Carr LL, Mankoff DA, Goulart BH et al. Phase II study of daily sunitinib in FDG-PET-positive, iodine-refractory differentiated thyroid cancer and metastatic medullary carcinoma of the thyroid with functional imaging correlation. *Clin Cancer Res* 2011; 16: 5260–5268.

Cerutti JM, Delcelo R, Amadei MJ et al. A preoperative diagnostic test that distinguishes benign from malignant thyroid carcinoma based on gene expression. *J Clin Invest* 2004; 113: 1234–1242.

Chambon G, Alovisetti C, İdoux-Louche C et al. The use of preoperative measurement of basal serum thyrocalcitonin in candidates for thyroidectomy due to nodular thyroid disorders: Results from 2733 consecutive patients. *J Clin Endocrinol Metab* 2011; 96: 75–81.

Cheung K, Roman SA, Wang TS et al. Calcitonin measurement in the evaluation of thyroid nodules in the United States. *J Clin Endocrinol Metab* 2008; 93: 2173–2180.

Chevillard S, Ugolin N, Vielh P et al. Gene expression profiling of differentiated thyroid neoplasms: Diagnostic and clinical implications. *Clin Cancer Res* 2004; 10: 6586–6597.

Chiovato L, Latrofa F, Braverman LE et al. Disappearance of humoral thyroid autoimmunity after complete removal of thyroid antigens. *Ann Intern Med* 2003; 139: 346–351.

Cho Mar K, Eimoto T, Nagaya S et al. Cell proliferation marker MCM2, but not Ki67, is helpful for distinguishing between minimally invasive follicular carcinoma and follicular adenoma of the thyroid. *Histopathology* 2006; 48(7): 801–807.

Chu QD, Hurd TC, Harvey S et al. Overexpression of urinary plasminogen activator (uPA) protein and mRNA in thyroid carcinogenesis. *Diagn Mol Pathol* 2004; 13: 241–246.

Cohen EE, Rosen LS, Vokes EE et al. Axitinib is an active treatment for all histological subtypes of advanced thyroid cancer: Results from a phase II study. *J Clin Oncol* 2008; 26: 4708–4713.

Colamaio M, Borbone E, Russo L et al. miR-191 down-regulation plays a role in thyroid follicular tumors through CDK6 targeting. *J Clin Endocrinol Metab* December 2011; 96(12): E1915–E1924.

Collet JF, Hurbain I, Prengel C et al. Galectin-3 immunodetection in follicular thyroid neoplasm's: A prospective study on fine-needle aspiration samples. *Br J Cancer* 2005; 14: 1175–1181.

Colombo C, Verga U, Mian C et al. Comparison of calcium and pentagastrin tests for the diagnosis and follow up of medullary thyroid cancer. *J Clin Endocrinol Metab* 2012; 97(3): 905–913.

Constante G, Meringolo D, Durante C et al. Predictive value of serum calcitonin levels for preoperative diagnosis of medullary thyroid carcinoma in a cohort of 5817 consecutive patients with thyroid nodules. *J Clin Endocrinol Metab* 2007; 92: 450–455.

Cooper DS, Doherty GM, Haugen BR et al. Revised management guidelines for patients with thyroid nodules and differentiated thyroid cancer. *Thyroid* 2009; 19: 1167–1214.

Cras A, Darsin-Bettinger D, Balitrand N et al. Epigenetic patterns of the retinoic acid receptor beta2 promoter in retinoic acid-resistant thyroid cancer cells. *Oncogene* 2007; 26: 4018–4024.

Czyz W, Balcerczak E, Jakubiak M et al. HMGI(Y) gene expression as a potential marker of thyroid follicular carcinoma. *Arch Surg* 2004; 389(3): 193–197.

Danese D, Sciacchitano S, Farsetti A et al. Diagnostic accuracy of conventional versus sonography-guided fine-needle aspiration biopsy of thyroid nodules. *Thyroid* 1998; 8: 15–21.

de Groot JWB, Links TP, Plukker JTM et al. RET as a diagnostic and therapeutic target in sporadic and hereditary endocrine tumors. *Endocr Rev* 2006; 27: 535–560.

de Matos PS, Ferreira AP, de Oliveira Facuri F et al. Usefulness of HBME-1, cytokeratin 19 and galectin-3 immunostaining in the diagnosis of thyroid malignancy. *Histopathology* 2005; 47: 391–401.

Dettmer M, Vogetseder A, Durso MB et al. MicroRNA expression array identifies novel diagnostic markers for conventional and oncocytic follicular thyroid carcinomas. *J Clin Endocrinol Metab* January 2013; 98(1): E1–E7.

Deveci MS, Deveci G, LiVolsi VA et al. Fine-needle aspiration of follicular lesions of the thyroid. Diagnosis and follow-up. *Cytojournal* 2006; 7: 3–9.

Doyle P, Düren C, Nerlich K et al. Potency and tolerance of calcitonin stimulation with high-dose calcium versus pentagastrin in normal adults. *J Clin Endocrinol Metab* 2009; 94(8): 2970–2974.

Duffy MJ and Duggan C. The urokinase plasminogen activator system: A rich source of tumour markers for the individualised management of patients with cancer. *Clin Biochem* 2004; 37: 541–548.

Durand S, Ferraro-Peyret C, Selmi-Ruby S et al. Evaluation of gene expression profiles in thyroid nodule biopsy material to diagnose thyroid cancer. *J Clin Endocrinol Metab* April 2008; 93(4): 1195–1202.

Elisei R. Routine serum calcitonin measurement in the evaluation of thyroid nodules. *Best Pract Res Clin Endocrinol Metab* 2008; 22(6): 941–953.

Elisei R, Cosci B, Romei C et al. Prognostic significance of somatic RET oncogene mutations in sporadic medullary thyroid cancer: A 10-year follow-up study. *J Clin Endocrinol Metab* 2008; 93: 682–687.

Elisei R, Vivaldi A, Agate L et al. All-trans-retinoic acid treatment inhibits the growth of retinoic acid receptor beta messenger ribonucleic acid expressing thyroid cancer cell lines but does not reinduce the expression of thyroid-specific c genes. *J Clin Endocrinol Metab* 2005; 90: 2403–2411.

Eng C. RET proto-oncogene in the development of human cancer. *J Clin Oncol* 1999; 17: 380–393.

Eng C, Clayton D, Schuffenecker I et al. The relationship between specific RET proto-oncogene mutations and disease phenotype in multiple endocrine neoplasia type 2. International RET mutation consortium analysis. *JAMA* 1996; 276: 1575–1579.

Eustatia-Rutten CFA, Smit JWA, Romijn JA et al. Diagnostic value of serum thyroglobulin measurements in the follow-up of differentiated thyroid carcinoma: A structured meta-analysis. *Clin Endocrinol (Oxford)* 2004; 61: 61–74.

Foukakis T, Gusnanto A, Au AY et al. A PCR-based expression signature of malignancy in follicular thyroid tumors. *Endocr Relat Cancer* 2007; 14(2): 381–391.

Furlan JC, Bedard YC, and Rosen IB. Role of fine-needle aspiration biopsy and frozen section in the management of papillary thyroid carcinoma subtypes. *World J Surg* 2004; 28: 880–885.

Gasbarri A, Martegani MP, Del Prete F et al. Galectin-3 and CD44v6 isoforms in the preoperative evaluation of thyroid nodules. *J Clin Oncol* 1999; 17: 3494–3502.

Gawlik T, d'amico A, Szpak-Ulczok S et al. The prognostic value of tumor markers doubling times in medullary thyroid carcinoma-preliminary report. *Thyroid Res* 2010; 3: 10.

Gharib H and Goellner JR. Fine-needle aspiration of the thyroid: An appraisal. *Ann Intern Med* 1993; 118: 282–289.

Ghossein R. Problems and controversies in the histopathology of thyroid carcinomas of follicular cell origin. *Arch Pathol Lab Med* 2009; 133: 683–691.

Giuffrida D and Gharib H. Controversies in the management of cold, hot, and occult thyroid nodules. *Am J Med* 1995; 99: 642–650.

Grebe SKG and Hay ID. Follicular thyroid cancer. *Endocrinol Metab Clin North Am* 1996; 24: 761–801.

Guignat L, Bidart JM, Nocera M et al. Chromogranin A and the α-subunit of glycoprotein hormones in medullary thyroid carcinoma and pheochromocytoma. *Br J Cancer* 2001; 84(6): 808–812.

Gupta M and Chia SY. Circulating thyroid cancer markers. *Curr Opin Endocrinol Diabetes Obes* 2007; 14(5): 383–388.

Hales MS and Hsu FS. Needle tract implantation of papillary carcinoma of the thyroid following aspiration biopsy. *Acta Cytol* 1990; 34: 801–804.

Hamburger JI. Diagnosis of thyroid nodules by fine needle biopsy: Use and abuse. *J Clin Endocrinol Metab* 1994; 79: 335–339.

Haugen BR, Woodmansee WW, and McDermott MT. Towards improving the utility of fine needle aspiration biopsy for the diagnosis of thyroid tumors. *Clin Endocrinol* 2002; 56: 281–290.

Hedinger C, Williams ED, and Sobin LH. Histological typing of thyroid tumors. In: *International Classification of Tumors*, (eds.) C. Hedinger, ED. Williams, and L.H. Sobin, 2nd edn. Springer-Verlag: Berlin, Germany, 1988, pp. 3–4.

Hegedus L, Bonnema SJ, and Bennedbaek FN. Management of simple nodular goiter: Current status and future perspectives. *Endocr Rev* 2003; 24:102–132.

Hermanek P and Sobin LH. Thyroid gland (ICD-OC73). *TNM Classification of Malignant Tumors,* 6th edn. International Union against Cancer, Springer-Verlag: New York, 2002.

Hinsch N, Frank M, Döring C et al. QPRT: A potential marker for follicular thyroid carcinoma including minimal invasive variant; a gene expression, RNA and immunohistochemical study. *BMC Cancer* 2009; 9: 93.

Hoff AO and Hoff PM. Medullary thyroid carcinoma. *Hematol Oncol Clin North Am* 2007; 21: 475–488.

Hofstra RM, Landsvater RM, Ceccherini I. A mutation in RET proto-oncogene associated with multiple neoplasia type 2B and sporadic medullary thyroid carcinoma. *Nature*, 1994; 367: 375–376.

Hong DS, Cabanillas ME, Wheler J et al. Inhibition of the Ras/Raf/MEK/ERK and RET kinase pathways with the combination of the multikinase inhibitor sorafenib and the farnesyltransferase inhibitor tipifarnib in medullary and differentiated thyroid malignancies. *J Clin Endocrinol Metab* 2011; 96: 997–1005.

Horvatić Herceg G, Herceg D, Kralik M et al. Urokinase-type plasminogen activator and its inhibitor in thyroid neoplasms: A cytosol study. *Wien Klin Wochenschr* 2006; 118: 601–609.

Hundahl SA, Fleming ID, Fremgen AM et al. A National Cancer Data Base report on 53,856 cases of thyroid carcinoma treated in the US, 1985–1995. *Cancer* 1998; 83: 2638–2648.

Ito Y, Yoshida H, Tomoda C et al. Telomerase activity in thyroid neoplasms evaluated by the expression of human telomerase reverse transcriptase (hTERT). *Anticancer Res* January–February 2005a; 25(1B): 509–514.

Ito Y, Yoshida H, Tomoda C et al. HBME-1 expression in follicular tumor of the thyroid: An investigation of whether it can be used as a marker to diagnose follicular carcinoma. *Anticancer Res* 2005b; 25(1A): 179–182.

Jerez A, Sugimoto Y, Makishima H et al. Loss of heterozygosity in 7q myeloid disorders: Clinical associations and genomic pathogenesis. *Blood* June 21, 2012; 119(25): 6109–6117.

Kaufman FR, Roe TF, Isaacs H Jr et al. Metastatic medullary thyroid carcinoma in young children with mucosal neuroma syndrome. *Pediatrics* 1982; 70: 263–267.

Kim SJ, Shiba E, Taguchi T et al. uPA receptor expression in benign and malignant thyroid tumors. *Anticancer Res* 2002; 22: 387–393.

Kloos RT, Eng C, and Evans DB. Medullary thyroid cancer: Management guidelines of the American Thyroid Association. *Thyroid* 2009; 19(6): 565–612.

Kondo T, Ezzat S, and Asa SL. Pathogenetic mechanisms in thyroid follicular-cell neoplasia. *Nat Rev Cancer* 2006; 6: 292–303.

Kouvaraki MA, Shapiro SE, Perrier ND et al. RET proto-oncogene: A review and update of genotype-phenotype correlations in hereditary medullary thyroid cancer and associated endocrine tumors. *Thyroid* 2005; 15: 531–544.

Krause K, Eszlinger M, Gimm O et al. TFF3-based candidate gene discrimination of benign and malignant thyroid tumors in a region with borderline iodine deficiency. *J Clin Endocrinol Metab* April 2008; 93(4): 1390–1393.

Kroll TG, Sarraf P, Pecciarini L et al. PAX8-PPARγ1 fusion oncogene in human thyroid carcinoma. *Science* 2000; 289: 1357–1360.

Kudo T, Miyauchi A, Ito Y et al. Diagnosis of medullary thyroid carcinoma by calcitonin measurement in fine needle aspiration biopsy specimens. *Thyroid* 2007; 17(7): 635–638.

Kurzrock R, Sherman SI, Ball DW et al. Activity of XL184 (Cabozantinib), an oral tyrosine kinase inhibitor, in patients with medullary thyroid cancer. *J Clin Oncol* 2011; 29: 2660–2666.

Lam ET, Ringel MD, Kloos RT et al. Phase II clinical trial of sorafenib in metastatic medullary thyroid cancer. *J Clin Oncol* 2011; 28: 2323–2330.

Lee EK, Chung KW, Min HS et al. Preoperative serum thyroglobulin as a useful predictive marker to differentiate follicular thyroid cancer from benign nodules in indeterminate nodules. *J Korean Med Sci* 2012; 27(9): 1014–1018.

Lemos MC, Carrilho F, and Rodrigues FJ. Early onset of medullary thyroid carcinoma in kindred with multiple endocrine neoplasia type IIA associated with Cutaneous lichen amyloidosis. *Endocr Pract* 2002; 8: 19–22.

Lindsey SC, Kunii IS, Germano-Neto F et al. Extended RET gene analysis in patients with apparently sporadic medullary thyroid cancer: Clinical benefits and cost. *Horm Cancer* 2012; 3(4): 181–186.

Liou MJ, Chan EC, Lin JD et al. Human telomerase reverse transcriptase (hTERT) gene expression in FNA samples from thyroid neoplasms. *Cancer Lett* March 10, 2003; 191(2): 223–227.

LiVolsi VA. C cell hyperplasia/neoplasia. *J Clin Endocrinol Metab* 1997; 82: 39–41.

LiVolsi VA and Asa SL. The demise of follicular carcinoma of the thyroid gland. *Thyroid* 1994; 4: 233–236.

Machens A and Dralle H. Genotype-phenotype based surgical concept of hereditary medullary thyroid carcinoma. *World J Surg* 2007; 31: 957–968.

Machens A, Hauptmann S, and Dralle H. Medullary thyroid cancer responsiveness to pentagastrin stimulation: An early surrogate parameter of tumor dissemination? *J Clin Endocrinol Metab* 2008; 93(6): 2234–2238.

Machens A, Niccoli-Sire P, Hoegel J et al. European Multiple Endocrine Neoplasia (EUROMEN) Study Group. Early malignant progression of hereditary medullary thyroid cancer. *N Engl J Med* 2003; 349(16): 1517–1525.

Machens A, Ukkat J, and Hauptmann S. Abnormal carcinoembryonic antigen levels and medullary thyroid cancer progression. *Arch Surg* 2007; 142: 289–293.

Marques AR, Espadinha C, Catarino AL et al. Expression of PAX8-PPAR gamma 1 rearrangements in both follicular thyroid carcinomas and adenomas. *J Clin Endocrinol Metab* August 2002; 87(8): 3947–3952.

Massaro F, Dolcino M, Degrandi R et al. Calcitonin assay in wash-out fluid after fine needle aspiration biopsy in patients with a thyroid nodule and borderline value of the hormone. *J Endocrinol Invest* 2009; 32(4): 308–312.

Mazar AP, Henkin J, and Goldfarb RH. The urokinase plasminogen activator system in cancer: Implications for tumor angiogenesis and metastasis. *Angiogenesis* 1999; 3: 15–32.

Mehrotra P, Okpokam A, Bouhaidar R et al. Galectin-3 does not reliably distinguish benign from malignant thyroid neoplasm's. *Histopathology* 2004; 45: 493–500.

Meijer JA, Cessie S, van den Hout WB et al. Calcitonin and carcinoembryonic antigen doubling times as prognostic factors in medullary thyroid carcinoma: A structured meta-analysis. *Clin Endocrinol (Oxford)* 2010; 72: 534–542.

Mikosch P, Gallowitsch HJ, Kresnik E et al. Value of ultrasound-guided fine-needle aspiration biopsy of thyroid nodules in an endemic goiter area. *Eur J Nucl Med* 2000; 27: 62–69.

Milas M, Shin J, Gupta M et al. Circulating thyrotropin receptor mRNA as a novel marker of thyroid cancer: Clinical applications learned from 1758 samples. *Ann Surg* 2010; 252(4): 643–651.

Mills LJ, Poller DN, and Yiangou C. Galectin-3 is not useful in thyroid FNA. *Cytopathology* June 2005; 16(3): 132–138.

Moley JF and DeBenedetti MK. Patterns of nodal metastases in palpable medullary thyroid carcinoma: Recommendations for extent of node dissection. *Ann Surg* 1999; 229: 880–887.

Moley JF and Fialkowski EA. Evidence-based approach to the management of sporadic medullary thyroid carcinoma. *World J Surg* 2007; 31: 946–956.

Moon WJ, Jung SL, Lee JH et al. Benign and malignant thyroid nodules: US differentiation-multicenter retrospective study. *Radiology* 2008; 247: 762–770.

Mousa U, Gursoy A, Ozdemir H et al. Medullary thyroid carcinoma in a patient with Hashimoto's thyroiditis diagnosed by calcitonin washout from a thyroid nodule. *Diagn Cytopath* 2013; 41(7): 644–646.

Mulligan LM, Eng C, Healey CS et al. Specific mutations of the RET proto-oncogene are related to disease phenotype in MEN2A and FMTC. *Nat Genet* 1994; 6: 70–74.

Mulligan LM, Kwok JB, and Healey CS. Germ-line mutations of the RET proto-oncogene in multiple endocrine Neoplasia type 2A. *Nature* 1993; 363: 458–460.

Nakabashi CC, Guimarães GS, Michaluart P et al. The expression of PAX8-PPARgamma rearrangements is not specific to follicular thyroid carcinoma. *Clin Endocrinol (Oxford)* 2004; 61: 280–282.

Namba H, Rubin SA, and Fagin JA. Point mutations of ras oncogenes are an early event in thyroid tumorigenesis. *Mol Endocrinol* 1990; 4: 1474–1479.

Nasr MR, Mukhopadhyay S, Zhang S et al. An immunohistochemical panel consisting of GAL3, FN.1 and HBME1 may be useful in the diagnosis of follicular cell-derived thyroid tumors. *Mol Pathol* 2006; 19: 1631–1637.

Nicolini V, Cassinelli G, Cuccuru G et al. Interplay between Ret and Fap-1 regulates CD95-mediated apoptosis in medullary thyroid cancer cells. *Biochem Pharmacol* 2011; 82: 778–788.

Niedziela M, Maceluch J, and Korman E. Galectin-3 is not a universal marker of malignancy in thyroid nodular disease in children and adolescents. *J Clin Endocrinol Metab* September 2002; 87(9): 4411–4415.

Nikiforov YE, Ohori NP, Hodak SP et al. Impact of mutational testing on the diagnosis and management of patients with cytologically indeterminate thyroid nodules: A prospective analysis of 1056 FNA samples. *J Clin Endocrinol Metab* 2011; 96(11): 3390–3397.

Nikiforova MN, Biddinger PW, Caudill CM et al. PAX8-PPARgamma rearrangement in thyroid tumors: RT-PCR and immunohistochemical analyses. *Am J Surg Pathol* August 2002; 26(8): 1016–1023.

Nikiforova MN, Lynch RA, Biddinger PW et al. RAS point mutations and PAX8-PPAR gamma rearrangement in thyroid tumors: Evidence for distinct molecular pathways in thyroid follicular carcinoma. *J Clin Endocrinol Metab* 2003; 88: 2318–2326.

Nikiforova MN, Tseng GC, Steward D et al. MicroRNA expression profiling of thyroid tumors: Biological significance and diagnostic utility. *J Clin Endocrinol Metab* 2008; 93: 1600–1608.

Oestreicher-Kedem Y, Halpern M, Roizman P et al. Diagnostic value of galectin-3 as a marker for malignancy in follicular patterned thyroid lesions. *Head Neck* 2004; 26: 960–966.

Okamoto T, Yamashita T, Harasawa A et al. Test performances of three diagnostic procedures in evaluating thyroid nodules: Physical examination, ultrasonography and fine needle aspiration cytology. *Endocr J* 1994; 41: 243–247.

Pacini F, Fugazzola L, Basolo F et al. Expression of calcitonin gene-related peptide in medullary thyroid cancer. *J Endocrinol Invest* 1992; 15: 539–542.

Pacini F, Schlumberger M, Dralle H et al. The European Thyroid Cancer Taskforce. Consensus for the management of patients with differentiated carcinoma of the follicular epithelium. *Eur J Endocrinol* 2006; 154: 787–803.

Pai R, Nehru GA, Samuel P et al. Discriminating thyroid cancers from benign lesions based on differential expression of a limited set of miRNA using paraffin embedded tissues. *Indian J Pathol Microbiol* April–June 2012; 55(2): 158–162.

Pallante P, Visone R, Croce CM et al. Deregulation of microRNA expression in follicular-cell-derived human thyroid carcinomas. *Endocr Relat Cancer* 2010; 17(1): F91–F104.

Phay JE, Moley JF, and Lairmore TC. Multiple endocrine neoplasias. *Semin Surg Oncol* 2000; 18: 324–332.

Pierotti MA, Bongarzone I, Borrello MG et al. Cytogenetics and molecular genetics of carcinomas arising from thyroid epithelial follicular cells. *Genes Chromosomes Cancer* 1996; 16: 1–14.

Powell GJ, Wang X, Allard BL et al. The PAX8/PPAR gamma fusion oncoprotein transforms immortalized human thyrocytes through a mechanism probably involving wild-type PPAR gamma inhibition. *Oncogene* 2004; 23: 3634–3641.

Przepiorka D, Baylin SB, McBride OW et al. The human CT gene is located on the short arm of chromosome 11. *Biochem Biophys Res Commun* 1984; 120: 493–499.

Puxeddu E and Fagin JA. Genetic markers in thyroid neoplasia. *Endocrin Metab Clin North Am* 2001; 30: 493–513.

Reading CC, Charboneau JW, Hay ID et al. Sonography of thyroid nodules: A "classic pattern" diagnostic approach. *Ultrasound Q* 2005; 21: 157–165.

Ridgway EC. Clinician's evaluation of a solitary thyroid nodule. *J Clin Endocrinol Metab* 1992; 74: 231–235.

Robinson BG, Paz-Ares L, Krebs A et al. Vandetanib (100 mg) in patients with locally advanced or metastatic hereditary medullary thyroid cancer. *J Clin Endocrinol Metab* 2011; 95: 2664–2671.

Romei C, Cosci B, Renzini G et al. RET genetic screening of sporadic medullary thyroid cancer (MTC) allows the preclinical diagnosis of unsuspected gene carriers and the identification of a relevant percentage of hidden familial MTC (FMTC). *Clin Endocrinol (Oxford)* 2011; 74(2): 241–247.

Romei C, Elisei R, Pinchera A et al. Somatic mutations of the RET proto-oncogene in sporadic medullary thyroid carcinoma are not restricted to exon 16 and are associated with tumor recurrence. *J Clin Endocrinol Metab* 1996; 81: 1619–1622.

Rosai J, Carganio ML, and Delellis RA. *Tumors of the Thyroid Gland*. Armed Force Institute of Pathology: Washington, DC, 1992.

Rossing M, Borup R, Henao R et al. Down-regulation of microRNAs controlling tumourigenic factors in follicular thyroid carcinoma. *J Mol Endocrinol* January 25, 2012; 48(1): 11–23.

Ruggeri RM, Campennì A, Baldari S et al. What is new on thyroid cancer biomarkers. *Biomark Insights* 2008; 3: 237–252.

Saggiorato E, Aversa S, Deandreis D et al. Galectin-3: Presurgical marker of thyroid follicular epithelial cell-derived carcinomas. *J Endocrinol Invest* 2004; 27: 311–317.

Schilling T, Bürck J, Sinn HP et al. Prognostic value of codon 918 (ATGe>ACG) RET proto-oncogene mutations in sporadic medullary thyroid carcinoma. *Int J Cancer* 2001; 95: 62–66.

Schlumberger M. Papillary and follicular thyroid carcinoma. *Ann Endocrinol (Paris)* 2007, 68: 120–128.

Schlumberger M, Hitzel A, Toubert ME et al. Comparison of seven serum thyroglobulin assays in the follow-up of papillary and follicular thyroid cancer patients. *J Clin Endocrinol Metab* July 2007; 92(7): 2487–2495.

Schlumberger MJ, Elisei R, Bastholt L et al. Phase II study of safety and efficacy of motesanib in patients with progressive or symptomatic, advanced or metastatic medullary thyroid cancer. *J Clin Oncol* 2009; 27: 3794–3801.

Schlumberger MJ, Filetti S, and Hay ID. Nontoxic diffuse and nodular goiter and thyroid neoplasia. In: *Williams Textbook of Endocrinology*, (eds.) S. Melmed, K.S. Polonsky, R.R. Larsen, and H.M. Kronenberg, 12th edn. Elsevier/Saunders: Philadelphia, PA, 2011, pp. 446–481.

Schuffenecker I, Ginet N, Goldgar D et al. Prevalence and parental origin of de novo RET mutations in multiple endocrine neoplasia type 2A and familial medullary thyroid carcinoma. Le Groupe d'Etude des Tumeurs a Calcitonine. *Am J Hum Genet* 1997; 60: 233–237.

Schwartz DL, Rana V, Shaw S et al. Postoperative radiotherapy for advanced medullary thyroid cancer: Local disease control in the modern era. *Head Neck* 2008; 30: 883–888.

Schwarzenbach H, Eichelser C, Kropidlowski J et al. Loss of heterozygosity at tumor suppressor genes detectable on fractionated circulating cell-free tumor DNA as indicator of breast cancer progression. *Clin Cancer Res* October 15, 2012; 18(20): 5719–5730.

Scollo C, Baudin E, Travagli JP et al. Rationale for central and bilateral lymph node dissection in sporadic and hereditary medullary thyroid cancer. *J Clin Endocrinol Metab* 2003; 88: 2070–2075.

Shen R, Liyanarachchi S, Li W et al. MicroRNA signature in thyroid fine needle aspiration cytology applied to "atypia of undetermined significance" cases. *Thyroid* January 2012; 22(1): 9–16.

Sherman SI. Targeted therapies for thyroid tumors. *Mod Pathol* 2011; 24(Suppl 2): 44–52.

Shibru D, Chung KW, and Kebebew E. Recent developments in the clinical application of thyroid cancer biomarkers. *Curr Opin Oncol* January 2008; 20(1): 13–18.

Sippel RS, Kunnimalaiyaan M, and Chen H. Current management of medullary thyroid cancer. *The Oncologist* 2008; 13: 539–547.

Smallridge RC, Meek SE, Morgan MA et al. Monitoring thyroglobulin in a sensitive immunoassay has comparable sensitivity to recombinant human TSH-stimulated thyroglobulin in follow-up of thyroid cancer patients. *J Clin Endocrinol Metab* 2007; 92: 82–87.

Spencer CA, Bergoglio LM, Kazarosyan M et al. Clinical impact of thyroglobulin (Tg) and Tg autoantibody method differences on the management of patients with differentiated thyroid carcinomas. *J Clin Endocrinol Metab* October 2005; 90(10): 5566–5575.

Spencer CA and Lopresti JS. Measuring thyroglobulin and thyroglobulin autoantibody in patients with differentiated thyroid cancer. *Nat Clin Pract Endocrinol Metab* 2008; 4: 223–233.

Takahashi M, Ritz J, and Cooper GM. Activation of a novel human transforming gene, ret, by DNA rearrangement. *Cell* 1985; 42: 581–588.

Takano T, Miyauchi A, Matsuzuka F et al. Ubiquitous expression of galectin-3 mRNA in benign and malignant thyroid tumors. *Cancer Lett* September 10, 2003; 199(1): 69–73.

Takano T and Yamada H. Trefoil factor 3 (TFF3): A promising indicator for diagnosing thyroid follicular carcinoma. *Endocr J* 2009; 56(1): 9–16.

Taniguchi K, Takano T, Miyauchi A et al. Differentiation of follicular thyroid adenoma from carcinoma by means of gene expression profiling with adapter-tagged competitive polymerase chain reaction. *Oncology* 2005; 69(5): 428–435.

Toledo SPA, Lourenço Jr DM, Santos MA et al. Hypercalcitoninemia is not pathognomonic of medullary thyroid carcinoma. *Clinics (Sao Paolo)* 2009; 64(7): 699–706.

Trimboli P, Rossi F, Baldelli R et al. Measuring calcitonin in washout of the needle in patients undergoing fine needle aspiration with suspicious medullary thyroid cancer. *Diagn Cytopathol* 2012; 40(5): 394–398.

Trovato M, Fraggetta F, Villari D et al. Loss of heterozygosity of the long arm of chromosome 7 in follicular and anaplastic thyroid cancer, but not in papillary thyroid cancer. *J Clin Endocrinol Metab* 1999; 84: 3235–3240.

Trovato M, Ulivieri A, Dominici R et al. Clinico-pathological significance of cell-type-specific loss of heterozygosity on chromosome 7q21: Analysis of 318 microdissected thyroid lesions. *Endocr Relat Cancer* 2004; 11: 365–376.

Uchino S, Noguchi S, Adachi M et al. Novel point mutations and allele loss at the RET locus in sporadic medullary thyroid carcinomas. *Jpn J Cancer Res* 1998; 89: 411–418.

Ulisse S, Baldini E, Toller M et al. Differential expression of the components of the plasminogen activating system in human thyroid tumour derived cell lines and papillary carcinomas. *Eur J Cancer* 2006; 42: 2631–2638.

van Heerden JA, Hay ID, Goellner JR et al. Follicular thyroid carcinoma with capsular invasion alone: A nonthreatening malignancy. *Surgery* 1992; 112: 1130–1136.

Vasko V, Ferrand M, Di Cristofaro J et al. Specific pattern of RAS oncogene mutations in follicular thyroid tumors. *J Clin Endocrinol Metab* 2003; 88: 2745–2752.

Verbeek HH, Alves MM, de Groot JW et al. The effects of four different tyrosine kinase inhibitors on medullary and papillary thyroid cancer cells. *J Clin Endocrinol Metab* 2011; 96: 991–995.

Volante M, Collini P, Nikiforov YE et al. Poorly differentiated thyroid carcinoma: The turin proposal for the use of uniform diagnostic criteria and an algorithmic diagnostic approach. *Am J Surg Pathol* 2007; 31: 1256–1264.

Watson RG, Brennan MD, Goellner JR et al. Invasive Hurthle cell carcinoma of the thyroid: Natural history and management. *Mayo Clin Proc* 1984; 59: 851–855.

Weber F, Shen L, Aldred MA et al. Genetic classification of benign and malignant thyroid follicular neoplasia based on a three-gene combination. *J Clin Endocrinol Metab* 2005; 90: 2512–2521.

Weber F, Teresi RE, Broelsch CE et al. A limited set of human microRNA is deregulated in follicular thyroid carcinoma. *J Clin Endocrinol Metab* September 2006; 91(9): 3584–3591.

Wells SA, Jr, Gosnell JE, Gagel RF et al. Vandetanib for the treatment of patients with locally advanced or metastatic hereditary medullary thyroid cancer. *J Clin Oncol* 2011a; 28: 767–772.

Wells SA, Jr, Robinson BG, Gagel RF et al. Vandetanib in patients with locally advanced or metastatic medullary thyroid cancer: A randomized, double-blind phase III trial. *J Clin Oncol* 2011b; 30: 134–141.

Yip L, Cote GJ, Shapiro SE et al. Multiple endocrine neoplasia type 2: Evaluation of the genotype-phenotype relationship. *Arch Surg* 2003; 138: 409–416.

Zhang JS, Nelson M, McIver B et al. Differential loss of heterozygosity at 7q31.2 in follicular and papillary thyroid tumors. *Oncogene* 1998; 17(6): 789–793.

Part VII

Hematological Cancers

28

Biomarkers in Myelodysplastic Syndrome

Néstor L. López Corrales and Vasco Ariston de Carvalho Azevedo

CONTENTS

ABSTRACT This chapter focuses on the review and characterization of the most common biological markers in the diagnosis, prognosis, and treatment of myelodysplastic syndrome (MDS). First, the basic concepts about definition, categories, diagnosis, as well as systems to classify the syndrome are explained, and then the chapter proceeds with the description of the biological markers recognized and accepted by international standards. Finally, the main features of markers currently under testing and developments with potential usefulness in MDS treatment are described. Special emphasis is given to the use of noninvasive markers.

28.1 Introduction

The use of biological markers (biomarkers) in oncology is growing fast and currently covers virtually every aspect from diagnosis to outcomes, including classification, prognosis, and treatment. Although the standards used for diagnosis and evaluation of the status and progression of myelodysplastic syndrome (MDS) highlight the importance of cytogenetic subgroups, marrow blast percentages and cytopenias, there are innovative technological tools with the potential to complement and expand findings obtained by conventional means. Considering the wide heterogeneity of MDS, the simultaneous use of biological indicators (markers) of different nature is fully justified. Presently, there are markers for diagnosis, prognosis, and stratification as well as for treatment responses and follow-up, but the bibliography reflects a constant identification of new markers, especially at the molecular level. A major drawback of standard techniques is that the main MDS markers are obtained by invasive methodologies like bone marrow (BM) sampling. This inconvenience has led to a major effort aimed at finding valuable markers through the use of noninvasive methodologies, such as the analysis of plasma profiles.

Although their potential is indisputable, the incorporation of new markers into clinical practice requires a deep understanding of the basic biological changes behind each pathologic process, the assays used to measure the resulting phenotypes and genotypes, and the regulatory processes that new biomarkers must face to be accepted for clinical use. The main hurdles faced by new markers are the use of a common terminology, the definition of their prognostic and predictive use, and companion diagnostic markers, as well as analytic and clinical validity and utility. In this context, the objective of this chapter is, first, to describe the current markers considered and accepted by international standards and, second, to give an overview of the principal markers under testing and development, with a special emphasis on noninvasive indicators.

28.2 Definition of MDS

By definition, MDS represents a heterogeneous group of myeloid neoplasms. MDS is characterized by BM failure with peripheral cytopenia and morphologic dysplasia in one or more of the following hematopoietic cell lineages: (1) erythroid cells (also ringed sideroblasts >15% considered diagnostic), (2) neutrophils and their precursors, and (3) megakaryocytes.

According to Steensma (2012), the defining characteristic of MDS as currently understood by the international medical community is the failure of injured and diseased bone marrow (BM) to successfully execute its primary physiologic task of sustained hematopoiesis. This catastrophic hematopoietic failure results in cytopenias (i.e., peripheral blood cell counts lower than the expected range for the healthy, unaffected population), especially anemia. Another important characteristic of MDS is the tendency for the disease to worsen over time, unpredictably but inexorably, eventually killing the afflicted individual if he or she does not first die from an unrelated cause.

28.3 Classification of MDS

An interesting review about the classification of MDS can be found in the work of Bennett (2005). MDS can be classified according to its etiology (primary = de novo or following a known mutagenic, event = secondary), cytologic features of BM and peripheral blood cells (PBCs), and specific karyotypes.

28.3.1 Primary MDS

1. *MDS in elderly patients.* MDS can be considered a disease of the elderly, with a median age of 60–75 years and being much less frequent in patients under 50, but the distribution varies greatly between categories and subtypes of MDS.
2. *The childhood MDS.* It is an uncommon disease characterized by an aggressive progression to acute leukemia. In some cases it can be similar to adult MDS or have a more myeloproliferative presentation in others. *Familial cases of MDS* are rare, and one of the best characterized is that of familial platelet disorder with propensity to myeloid malignancy, caused by heterozygous germ line *RUNX1* mutations.

28.3.2 Secondary MDS

These are cases of MDS mainly related in fact to specific treatments like chemotherapy, radiotherapy and previous contact with toxic substances. Secondary MDS (sMDS) have been described as a complication in cancer therapies. The majority of sMDS/acute myeloid leukemia (AML) are morphologically characterized by multilineage myeloid dysplasia: the great majority having chromosome abnormalities. sMDS has a rapid course and a short survival rate.

In the new update, 4th edition, the World Health Organization (WHO) incorporates new scientific and clinical information to refine the diagnostic criteria for previously described neoplasms and to introduce newly recognized disease entities (Vardiman et al., 2009).

28.3.3 Categories of MDS according to WHO

The WHO (2009) has determined the following seven categories for MDS: (1) refractory cytopenia with unilineage dysplasia (RCUD) involving refractory anemia (RA), refractory neutropenia (RN), and refractory thrombocytopenia (RT); (2) RA with ring sideroblasts (RARS); (3) refractory cytopenia with multilineage dysplasia (RCMD); (4) RA with excess blasts (RAEB1 and RAEB2); (5) MDS with isolated del(5q); (6) MDS, unclassifiable; and (7) childhood MDS and provisional entity: refractory cytopenia of childhood (Vardiman et al., 2009; Vardiman, 2012).

Table 28.1 describes the main categories and blood findings on each.

28.4 Diagnosis of MDS

The diagnosis of MDS is essentially based on morphological evidence of dysplasia through the analysis of BM aspirates and biopsy. Usually, additional studies such as karyotype, flow cytometry, or molecular genetics are also conducted, giving complementary information and in many cases defining the type of pathology.

BM sampling followed by biopsy remains the routine process to determine cellular morphology, evaluate of percent of blasts, and determine BM cellularity and architecture as well.

Diagnosis is confirmed by the presence of dysplasia. A number of morphological classifications are in place to classify patients with MDS (see WHO's classification). So far, diagnosis still depends on cytomorphology of PB and BM smears.

28.4.1 Minimal Diagnostic Criteria

In most of the patients, the diagnosis of MDS can be straightforward just following the WHO standards, but there are cases where signs and main indicators are not clear. In 2007, a standard minimum criterion for the diagnosis of MDS was proposed mainly due to the difficulties to determine or exclude the diagnosis of MDS in cases where cytopenias and cytogenetic markers are not conclusive. For a complete explanation of this consensus statement, it is recommended to see the original work of Valent et al. (2007).

TABLE 28.1

Categories of MDS and Findings in Blood and BM

Category of MDS	PB	BM
RCUD: RA, RN, RT	Unicytopenia or bicytopenia[a] No or rare blasts (<1%)	Unilineage dysplasia: >10% of the cells in one myeloid lineage; <5% blasts; <15% of erythroid precursors are ring sideroblasts
RARS	Anemia no blast	≥15% of erythroid precursors are ring sideroblasts. Erythroid dysplasia only <5% blast
RCMD	Cytopenia(s) No or rare blasts (<1%)[b] No Auer rods <1 × 10^9/L monocytes	Dysplasia in ≥10% of the cells in >2 myeloid lineages (neutrophil and/or erythroid precursors and/or megakaryocytes) <5% blasts in marrow No Auer rods 15% ring sideroblasts
RAEB1	Cytopenia(s) <5% blasts[b] No Auer rods <1 × 10^9/L monocytes	Unilineage or multilineage dysplasia 5%–9% blasts[b] No Auer rods
RAEB2	cytopenia(s) 5%–19% blasts[c] Auer rods[c] <1 × 10^9/L monocytes	Unilineage or multilineage dysplasia 10%–19% blasts[c] Auer rods[c]
MDS—unclassified (MDS-U)	Cytopenias <1% blasts[b]	Unequivocal dysplasia in <10% of cells in one or more myeloid lineages when accompanied by a cytogenetic abnormality considered as presumptive evidence for a diagnosis of MDS <5% blasts
MDS associated with isolated del(5q)	Anemia Usually normal or increased platelet count No or rare blasts (<1%)	Normal to increased megakaryocytes with hypolobated nuclei <5% blasts Isolated del(5q) cytogenetic abnormality No Auer rods

Source: The 2008 revision of the World Health Organization (WHO) classification of myeloid neoplasms and acute leukemia: rationale and important changes, Vardiman, J.W. et al., *Blood*, 114(5), 937, 2009.

[a] Bicytopenia may occasionally be observed. Cases with pancytopenia should be classified as MDS-U.

[b] If the marrow myeloblast percentage is <5% but there are 2%–4% myeloblasts in the blood, the diagnostic classification is RAEB-1. Cases of RCUD and RCMD with 1% myeloblasts in the blood should be classified as MDS-U.

[c] Cases with Auer rods and <5% myeloblasts in the blood and less than 10% in the marrow should be classified as RAEB-2. Although the finding of 5%–19% blasts in the blood is, in itself, diagnostic of RAEB-2, cases of RAEB-2 may have <5% blasts in the blood if they have Auer rods or 10%–19% blasts in the marrow or both. Similarly, cases of RAEB-2 may have <10% blasts in the marrow but may be diagnosed by the other 2 findings, Auer rod+ and/or 5%–19% blasts in the blood.

In case of inconclusive morphological features, the WHO indicates that a presumptive diagnosis of MDS can be made if a specific clonal chromosomal abnormality is present (Table 28.2).

28.5 Prognosis of MDS: Main Standards

There are several sources/standards that can be used in order to estimate diagnosis and prognosis of MDS.

28.5.1 IPSS

Published in 1997 (Greenberg et al., 1997), the International Prognostic Scoring System (IPSS) combined cytogenetic, morphological, and clinical data, determining number of cytopenias, percentage of BM myeloblasts, and cytogenetic abnormalities as features for the syndrome in the outcome of AML.

TABLE 28.2

Chromosomal Abnormalities Admitted by the WHO as Presumptive Evidence of MDS

Balanced	Unbalanced
7 or del(7q)	t(11;16)(q23;p13.3)
5 or del(5q)	t(3;21)(q26.2;q22.1)
i(17q) or t(17p)	t(1;3)(p36.3;q21.1)
13 or del(13q)	t(2;11)(p21;q23)
del(11q)	inv(3)(q21;q26.2)
del(12p) or t(12p)	t(6;9)(p23;q34)
del(9q)	
idic(X)(q13)	
Complex karyotype (three or more chromosomal abnormalities) may involve one or more of the previously mentioned abnormalities.	

Source: Adapted from Vardiman, J.W. et al., *Blood*, 114(5), 937, 2009.

In addition to those variables, age and gender were considered to have an impact on the survival as well. Owing to several difficulties with the original (see Hasle et al., 2004), the IPSS was revised recently (Greenberg et al., 2012). For specific and detailed information, the reader should consult the original papers of Greenberg et al. (2012) and Haasle et al. (2004).

28.5.2 WHO Classification-Based Prognostic Scoring System

Based on the WHO classification, karyotype, and transfusion requirement, survival is shorter in patients who require regular blood transfusions versus those who do not. Early observations signaled that the transfusion dependency would be not only associated with worse overall survival (OS) but also with increased risk of transformation to AML (Sanz et al., 2008).

Recently the WHO Classification-Based Prognostic Scoring System (WPSS) has been modified to include hemoglobin levels instead of transfusion needs.

28.5.3 MDACC Risk Stratification

It was developed to obtain a more precise model to evaluate IPSS in low-risk patients (Garcia Manero, 2010, 2012; Bejar et al., 2012). It adds the feature of comorbidities and their effect on the prognosis. For a detailed explanation and better understanding of the implications of comorbidities in the prognosis and outcome of MDS, the studies of Stauder et al. (2008), Della Porta et al. (2011), Wang et al. (2009), Naqvi et al. (2011), and Pfeilstocker et al. (2012) are recommended to the reader.

28.6 Markers in MDS

Since MDS is a BM pathology, biopsy of BM and cytogenetic analysis of PB and BM, as well as serum parameters, are implicated in the diagnosis, prognosis, and treatment of the disease. Consequently, most of the main biological markers currently used in this syndrome are necessarily included in the group of invasive biological markers.

28.6.1 Chromosomal Instabilities as Markers in MDS

In MDS the presence of chromosomal abnormalities is a common feature and a key to achieve diagnosis, estimate prognosis, and evaluate treatments. The chromosomal instabilities can be detected in about 50% of patients with MDS and about 30%–40% of those with MDS/myeloproliferative neoplasia (MPN) using standard metaphase karyotyping. There is an important proportion of patients showing either normal or non-informative cytogenetics, which represents a bottleneck in managing the disease. Consequently, the routine cytogenetic analysis is still an important tool in MDS.

As indicated earlier, the WHO has a list of chromosomal abnormalities accepted as the cytogenetic markers to be used in the diagnostic of MDS (Table 28.2), but there are other abnormalities taken into account to establish the prognosis of MDS. At present, using the cytogenetic component of the IPSS-R, more than 85% of all cytogenetic findings can be classified according to their prognostic impact. The problem is the remaining proportion of cases where the cytogenetic abnormalities cannot determine a prognosis: in other words, cases presenting chromosome instabilities with unknown prognostic meaning. This has been recently reevaluated and a modified version of the score has been published (see references).

28.6.2 IPSS Cytogenetic Risk Group and Comprehensive Cytogenetic Scoring System

Recently, a new comprehensive system based up on cytogenetic features has been proposed by Schanz et al. (2012). This system was developed using the information provided by the German-Austrian MDS Study Group (n = 1193), the International MDS Risk Analysis Workshop (IMRAW) (n = 816), the Spanish Hematological Cytogenetics Working Group (n = 849), and the International Working Group on MDS Cytogenetics (n = 44) databases and considering only patients with primary MDS (pMDS) and oligoblastic AML after MDS treated with supportive care, cases being evaluated for OS and AML evolution. Five different risk subgroups are proposed considering OS and hazard ratio (HR): very good (median OS, 61 months; HR, 0.5; n = 81); good (49 months; HR, 1.0; n = 1,809); intermediate (26 months; HR, 1.6; n = 529); poor (16 months; HR, 2.6; n = 148); very poor (6 months; HR, 4.2; n = 187).

The IPSS-R has included these five cytogenetic prognostic subgroups with specific classification of a number of less common cytogenetic subsets and alteration of others. The classification added data extracted from MDS databases of primary untreated MDS patients from multiple international institutions, 11 countries, including data from the Spanish, French, Piemonte (Italy), and Brazilian MDS registries and that from the IMRAW. Table 28.3 shows the main details of this comprehensive system.

In addition to these categories of cytogenetic prognosis, it is possible to identify different subgroups between those cases with complex karyotypes (mix of abnormalities). The presence of subsets with complex karyotypes, categorized according to the number of abnormalities, indicates that the prognosis in those cases would deteriorate with increasing numbers of alterations, giving an idea about the clonal evolution and genetic instability.

Originally, the IPSS scoring systems assigned rare abnormalities, often found in complex karyotypes, to the intermediate cytogenetic risk group.

Some of the most common chromosomal abnormalities associated to MDS suggest a role in prognosis and diagnosis as well as in treatment responses. Examples of common chromosome alterations in MDS are depicted in Table 28.4.

TABLE 28.3

Cytogenetics Risk Subgroups according to IPSS-R Score System

Prognostic Subgroup	Cytogenetic Abnormality	Survival Years, Median
Very good (4%[a]/3%[b])	-Y, del(11q)	5.4
Good (72%[a]/66%[b])	Normal, del(5q), del(12p), del(20q); double including del(5q)	4.8
Intermediate (13%[a]/19%[b])	del(7q), +8, +19, i(17q), any other single or double independent clones	2.7
Poor (4%[a]/5%[b])	-7, inv(3)/t(3q)/del(3q); double including -7/del(7q); complex: 3 abnormalities	1.5
Very poor (7%[a]/7%[b])	Complex: >3 abnormalities	0.7

Source: Adapted from Greenberg, P.L. et al., *Blood*, 120(12), 2454, 2012.

[a] Data from patients in this IWG-PM database, multivariate analysis (n = 7012).

[b] Data from Schanz et al. 2012 (n = 2754).

TABLE 28.4

Some Chromosome Alterations in MDS

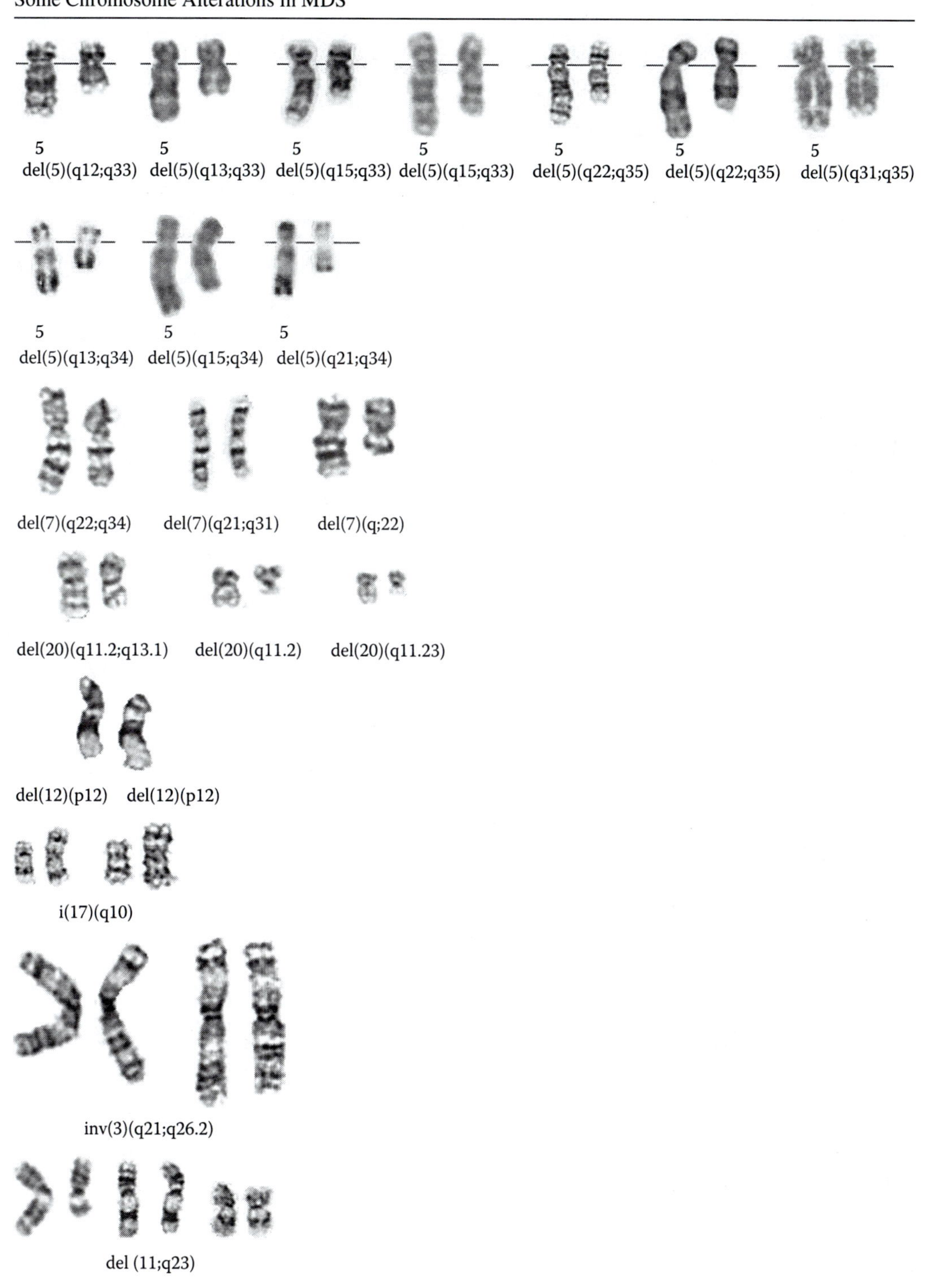

(continued)

TABLE 28.4 (continued)

Some Chromosome Alterations in MDS

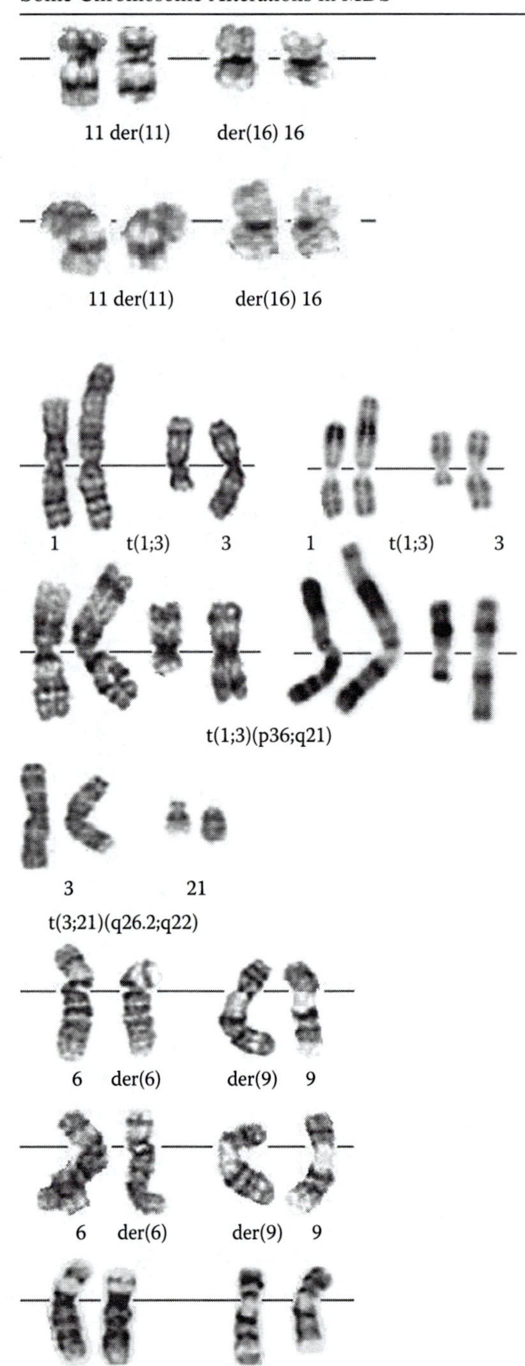

TABLE 28.4 (continued)

Some Chromosome Alterations in MDS

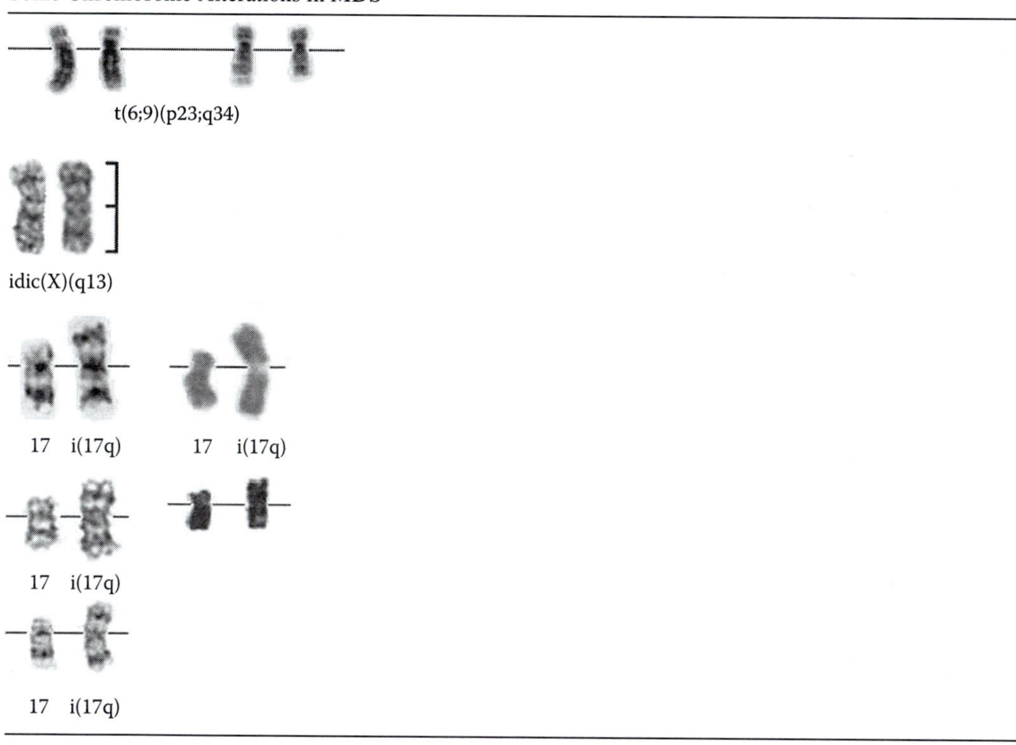

Source: Pictures obtained from Wisconsin University, http://www.slh.wisc.edu/cytogenetics/cancer/bmdeletion_tabl.dot.

It is almost impossible to provide a detailed explanation for each chromosome abnormality found in MDS. For a detailed description of the implications and incidence of cytogenetic rearrangements in MDS, the websites http://www.slh.wisc.edu/cytogenetics/cancer/mds.dot and http://AtlasGeneticsOncology.org are recommended to the reader. Of particular interest is the paper published by Haase et al. (2007), which links specific chromosomal abnormalities to survival curves. The authors pointed some rare chromosomal abnormalities associated with good prognosis in MDS as well. The most interesting feature is that the work was based upon cytogenetic results from more than 2000 patients of MDS.

28.6.2.1 Description of Some Common Chromosomal Instabilities in MDS

28.6.2.1.1 del(5q) Syndrome

Described as deletions in the long arm of chromosome 5 (del(5q)), it is one of the most common structural abnormalities in MDS, detected in up to 10% cases either as an isolated instability or with additional rearrangements. In sMDS/AML, this alteration has been frequently associated with abnormalities on chromosome 7.

The WHO defined del(5q) as a specific type of MDS presenting isolated interstitial deletion of long arm on chromosome 5, del(5q), and a percentage of blasts below 5% in BM samples. Breakpoints and size of deletions are highly variable (see figure in Table 28.4), with a most critical area in between bands q31and q33. The region is extremely rich in genes encoding growth factors and del(5q) has been also detected in other pathologies distinct from the del(5q) syndrome associated to MDS. When reexamined by FISH, some cases of del(5q) are found to be more complex than expected (e.g., with cryptic t(5;7)).

This "5q-" syndrome is characterized by a high prevalence in elderly females with a relatively good prognosis. Currently, there is a new category called therapy-related MDS/AML, excluding cases with previous chemotherapy from 5q- syndrome.

28.6.2.1.2 Monosomy 7 and Partial Deletion of the Long Arm of Chromosome 7

(Partial) monosomies of chromosome 7 are typical rearrangements in sMDS but rare in pMDS. In principle, the monosomy 7 and del(7q) losing a segment at 7q22.1 (deletions are variable in size and are always interstitial with two main zones at 7q22 and 7q32–34; see figure in Table 28.4) have different implications. Monosomy 7 is associated to bad/poor prognosis and del(7q) is related to intermediate prognosis with better OS. In fact, monosomy 7 in pMDS is often found in children "childhood monosomy 7" with juvenile chronic myelomonocytic leukemia (JCML) and in familial -7 MDS (although nonspecific, monosomy 7 is the most common cytogenetic abnormality in childhood MDS). According to the reference, RAS, gene mutations, or loss of the NF1 gene would be critical in the pathogenesis of MDS with -7. Additionally monosomy 7 is often associated with other chromosome changes. In sMDS, 40%–60% of cases have simultaneous del(7q)/-7 and del(5q)/-5. Patients with del(7)q and -7 have a severe outcome with sensitivity to infections and therapy resistance. According to the Atlas of Genetics and Cytogenetics in Oncology and Haematology, the balanced translocation t(1;7)(q10;p10) and several unbalanced translocations resulting in a partial monosomy 7 of the 7q22–7q34 bands can be considered as variants of this alteration.

28.6.2.1.3 Chromosome 20 Deletion

A chromosome 20q deletion is associated with about 5% of pMDS. The majority of cases with an interstitial deletion between 20q11.2 and q13.3. Del(20q) can be associated with all subtypes of MDS ([refractory anemia (RA) to refractory anemia with excess of blasts (RAEB) and chronic myelomonocytic leukemia (CMML)]) and myeloproliferative syndromes (MPS). Del(20q) is frequently associated with del(7q)/-7 and/or 3 del(13q). As a single anomaly, the del(20)(q) has a favorable prognosis.

28.6.2.1.4 Deletion of 12p (Del(12p))

Deletions of the short arm of chromosome 12 are usually present together with multiple karyotypic changes in sMDS. This is synonymous of poor prognosis. The deletions involve loss of material between band p11 and p13. The genomic analysis of this region indicates that ETV6 and CDKN1B genes are deleted in all malignancies harboring this type of abnormality. Inversion inv(3)(q21q26).

28.6.2.1.5 Translocation t(3;5)(q25.1;q34)

A balanced translocation of chromosome 3q25.1 and 5q34 is associated with MDS and AML and described in subsets of patients with multilineage dysplasia. Originally, the rearrangement was described joining part of the nucleophosmin (NPM) gene on chromosome 5 with sequences from a novel gene on chromosome 3, but recently the NPM/MLF1 gene fusion was also identified suggesting that an NPM/MLF1 fusion could be the primary molecular abnormality in t(3;5) MDS and AML with multilineage dysplasia. The histological spectrum of the cases is variable (Yoneda-Kato et al., 1996; Arber et al., 2003).

28.6.2.1.6 Translocation t(5;12)(q33;p13)

A balanced translocation of chromosome 5q33 and 12p13 is considered as a recurrent chromosomal abnormality in a subgroup of myeloid malignancies with features of both myeloproliferative disorders and MDS. The molecular consequence of t(5;12) is a fusion between the platelet-derived growth factor receptor-B gene on chromosome 5 and a novel ETS-like gene, TEL, on chromosome 12 (Wlodarska et al., 1995). The variant translocations involving TEL/ETV6 and chromosomes 3, 6, or 10 have been identified and can define a molecular subgroup of MDS with ETV6 rearrangement.

28.6.2.1.7 Trisomy of Chromosome 8 (+8)

Trisomy 8 is a quite common instability observed in 15%–20% of MDS cases. Many of them are found in treatment-related cases of MDS (sMDS). This abnormality has been detected in MDS with RA, RARS, and RAEB and it is often observed with other alterations like -5/del(5q), t(1;7), or del(20q) but in separate clones.

28.6.2.1.8 Translocation t(11;16)(q23;p13.3)

Translocation t(11;16)(q23;p13.3) is a common rearrangement originally observed in leukemia. This translocation is widely considered a common therapy-related (secondary) AML (Glassman and Hayes,

2003). Specifically, the involvement of 11q23-balanced translocations in acute leukemia after treatment with inhibitors of DNA topoisomerases has been recognized frequently (sMDS). Rowley et al. (1997) cloned the region showing the involvement of two genes, MLL (mixed-lineage leukemia) and CBP (CREB binding protein). As result of the recurring translocation t(11;16)(q23;p13.3), MLL is fused in frame to CBP, MLL on 11q23 and CBP at 16p13 (CREB binding protein) (Lavau et al., 2000).

28.6.2.1.9 Translocation t(3;21)(q26.2;q22)

The translocation t(3;21)(q26.2;q22) is rare in cases of MDS and AML but commonly related to previous therapy and with poor outcome. This abnormality is reported in approximately 1% of all cases. A feature of this instability is the disruption of chromosome locus 3q26, a rare but recurrent cytogenetic aberration that occurs in AML or MDS. A recent comparative study between this translocation and inv(3)(q21;q26.2)/t(3;3)(q21;q26.2) (both sharing 3q26 locus abnormalities) has shown that multilineage dysplasia and frequent association with -7/7q are similar in both groups, but MDS/AML cases associated with t(3;21) have a higher frequency of therapy-related disease and shorter survival times, suggesting that they are distinct from MDS/AML cases associated with inv(3)/t(3;3) (Li et al., 2012).

28.6.2.1.10 Translocation t(2;11)(p21;q23)

The translocation t(2;11)(p21;q23) has been cloned in several cases of MDS and AML. The alteration is associated with a strong upregulation of miR-125b (from 6- to 90-fold). In principle, the effect of miR-125b is greatly dependent on the stage and the pathway of differentiation of targeted cells. In those cases with t(2;11) translocation, there is an upregulation of miR-125b, which is directly linked to the chromosomal changes. In addition, miR-125b acts in an opposite direction by blocking the process of differentiation (Bousquet et al., 2008). From experiments using mouse models, it was suggested that miR-125b confers a proliferative advantage to the leukemic cells. The overexpression of miR-125b could be sufficient for both to shorten the latency of BCR-/ABL-induced leukemia and to independently induce leukemia in this animal model (Bousquet et al., 2010).

28.6.2.1.11 Translocation t(6;9)(p23;q34)

The translocation t(6;9)(p23;q34) is a rare recurring cytogenetic aberration resulting in the formation of a chimeric DEK/NUP214 fusion gene on the der(6) chromosome. This alteration has been reported in de novo AML, AML preceded by MDS, and in sAML. Because of the low percentage of cases harboring these alterations, most of the observations have been made in just a few patients. Nevertheless, it has been proposed to add AML with t(6;9)(p23;q34), DEK/NUP214 as a separate disease entity to the WHO Classification of Hematological Malignancies, which in turn would cover the potential MDS associated to the AML (Slovak et al., 2006). The t(6;9)-positive AML cases would have distinctive morphologic features, an immunophenotype suggesting an origin from an early hematopoietic progenitor cell, and a high frequency of flt3 gene mutation (Oyarzo et al., 2004). DEK is a proto-oncogene and there are evidences that chromosomal aberrations involving this region increase its level of expression. In addition, the presence of antibodies against this protein is associated with various diseases.

28.6.2.1.12 Deletion in Long Arm of Chromosome 13 (Del(13q))

Del(13q) is occasionally seen in cases with BM failure without signs of myelodysplasia and described as MDS unclassified syndromes. It was originally classified as a marker for intermediate risk by the WHO, but recently del(13q) has been associated with a positive prognosis and good response to therapy (immunosuppressive therapy [IST]) (Hosokawa et al., 2012). At a molecular level, cases with del(13q) show high prevalence of increased glycosylphosphatidylinositol-anchored protein (GPI-AP)-deficient cells. There are indications that the presence of small populations of GPI-AP-deficient blood cells would be a significant factor predicting a good response to IST in patients with AML and low-risk MDS.

28.6.2.1.13 i(17q) or t(17p)

Originally related to the deletion of the p53 gene, 17p deletion was described as having a variable extent but with a pathogenetic role for inactivation of tumor suppressor gene(s) located in the region, especially the p53 gene (Soenen et al., 1998). The formation of isodicentric 17q (i(17q)) has been reported in connection with loss of p arm and duplication of q arm. Most of the time, this instability is found with other alterations as part of complex karyotypes including t(17p).

The inv(3)(q21q26.2) or t(3;3)(q21;q26.2) is present in approximately 1% of cases of MDS. This alteration has been observed associated to other abnormalities such as -7/7q and -5/5q and more complex cytogenetic aberrations. The cases presenting this inversion are prone to develop AML in comparison with those not harboring the instability. In fact, AML with inv(3)(q21q26.2) or t(3;3)(q21;q26.2) is a distinct subtype in the WHO classification (Cui et al., 2011). At the molecular level, proto-oncogene *EVI1* at 3q26.2.2 or its longer form *MDS1-EVI1* (also known as *MECOM*) and *RPN1* at 3q21 involve overexpression of EVI1, or MECOM, and/or an *RPN1/EVI1* fusion transcript.

28.7 Molecular Markers

Until just a few years ago the genetics of MDS was largely defined by cytogenetic abnormalities. However, the last decade has seen a growing interest in finding new markers at the molecular level to improve the diagnosis, prognosis, and treatment of MDS. As stated by Graubert and Walter (2011), *"technology development has been a major driver of recent discoveries in MDS genetics as the field has moved from 'low-resolution genome scans' using conventional cytogenetics and candidate gene resequencing to array-based karyotyping, genome-wide mRNA/miRNA expression profiling, and now genome- wide sequence analysis."* This has also been highlighted by Davids and Steensma (2010), who stressed that thanks to the advent of new techniques such as array comparative genomic hybridization (aCGH) and single-nucleotide polymorphic array (SNPa), clonal chromosomal deletions and segments of copy-neutral loss of heterozygosity (CN-LOH) can be considered common findings in cases of MDS showing no cytogenetic alterations (i.e., with normal karyotype). These findings would also suggest sites of recurrently mutant genes located all across the genome in MDS.

A logical consequence of these technical achievements is the identification of recurrent mutations in MDS, which will give new insights into the pathophysiology of the disorder. An example is the notion that multiple mutations would be required for MDS initiation and progression to AML. In MDS a wide variety of genomic instabilities like gene point mutations, copy number alterations, break points, microdeletions, and uniparental disomies (UPDs) have been constantly reported within the last few years. This underscores the need to complement the classical karyotype studies with molecular analysis to provide independent prognostic value for MDS patients while digging deeper into the molecular basis of the syndrome.

28.7.1 Role of Genetic Point Mutation in MDS

Molecular abnormalities such as somatic point mutations can be identified in most MDS cases. Taking into account that recurrent mutations could alter different cellular process, including gene expression, response to DNA damage, signaling, or just the splicing machinery, it is understandable that, in some cases, those mutations could be linked to specific features of the disease.

There are several databases describing specific mutations in cancer. Two of these are the Cancer Genome Anatomy Project, at http://cgap.nci.nih.gov, and Catalog of Somatic Mutations in Cancer (COSMIC), at the Sanger Institute, http://www.sanger.ac.uk/genetics/CGP/cosmic/, which is one of the most complete sources of information about gene mutations in tumors (for specific information about COSMIC, see Forbes et al., 2008). Both provide useful information about genomic abnormalities and mutations affecting MDS.

The data retrieved from COSMIC indicate the presence of mutations in 222 genes in the context of the following types of MDS:

1. Myelodysplastic/myeloproliferative neoplasm—unclassifiable
2. Myelodysplastic/myeloproliferative disease—unclassifiable
3. MDS
4. MDS—therapy related

The list of the mutated genes is not static but updated regularly based on new published data. Just to have an idea, according to the Cancer Gene Census (http://www.sanger.ac.uk/genetics/CGP/Census/), more than 1% of human genes are implicated in cancer and 90% of those would have somatic mutations; 20% bear germ line mutations that predispose to cancer and 10% show both somatic and germ line mutations.

Figure 28.1 describes the top 20 genes mutated in MDS and Table 28.5 describes some of the main features of this group of genes found in the COSMIC database.

Several points can be highlighted in the analysis of this table. First, and as mentioned before, the number of mutated genes is not static and it is expected to have variations in the proportion of genes mutated, number and location of those mutations, and the number of analyzed samples (increases). Second, in order to obtain accurate estimations of the proportions of mutations and their possible effects, it is critical to consider the number of samples analyzed for each gene. For example, ATRX1 presents the highest ratio of mutations but obtained from a small number of cases. In contrast, SF3B, the following gene in the list, shows 21% of mutations but calculated from more than 1000 samples. Only six genes of this group (top 20) show data obtained from more than 1000 samples. This indicates that, in most cases, a larger number of samples would be necessary to obtain proper statistics. Similar conclusions can be reached regarding the impact of the type of mutations in the prognosis, diagnosis, or treatment of MDS. With a few exceptions such as U2AF1, NRAS, or IDH1 (where missense mutations are the only type reported), most genes harbor a wide variety of alterations such as frameshift insertion and deletions; nonsense, missense, and undefined mutations; or gene fusions. In the vast majority, there is no specific location for the mutation, which gives us an idea about the potential heterogeneity in their impact/effect, if any, on the phenotype of the disease. Another important issue is the estimation of the possible implications of each gene in the context of their biological function and pathways involved. The bibliography shows recurrent somatic mutations affecting genes involved in RNA splicing in up to 85% of MDS cases (Lindsley and Ebert, 2012). Reports about splicing mutations in diseases with

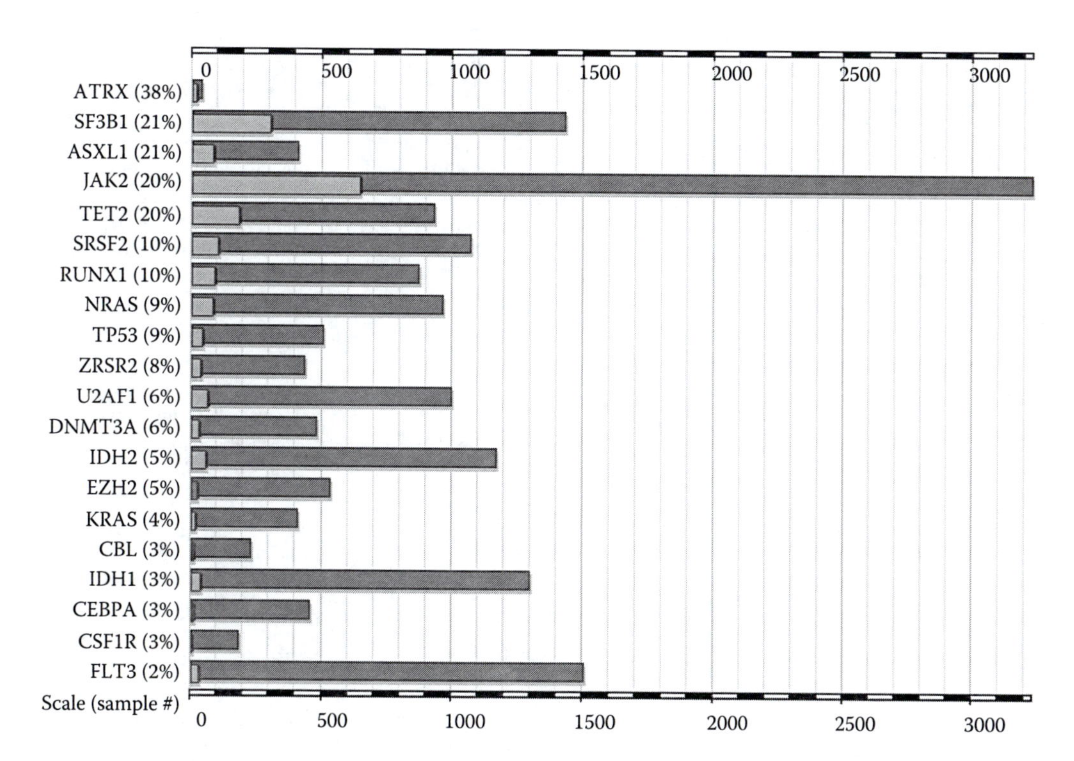

FIGURE 28.1 The most significantly mutated genes (cancer gene census) in myelodysplastic syndromes considering myelodysplastic/myeloproliferative neoplasm—unclassifiable; myelodysplastic/myeloproliferative disease—unclassifiable; myelodysplastic syndrome; and myelodysplastic syndrome—therapy related. (From COSMIC, data from October 2012.) Dark gray bars: Total number of samples in the database. Light gray bars: Proportion of the samples harboring mutations.

TABLE 28.5

Features of the Top 20 Genes Mutated in MDS

Gene	Type of Mutations	Location	Frequency	Features and Implications
ATRX	Substitution missense in nine locations (64%), insertions, and deletions	Xq21.1	34% in MDS (n = 37) (COSMIC), mutated in alpha-thalassemia MDS (ATMDS), 100% in MMNU	Under investigation for its predictive role for response to hypomethylating agents
SFB3B1	Substitutions missense (99%) in 11 different positions. Main mutation located at p.kE700. Cases of deletion and complex mutations in different locations	2q33.1	Up to 21% in MDS (n = 1434) (COSMIC). Prevalent in low-risk MDS and associated with ring sideroblasts	Favorable prognosis
ASXL1	15% missense substitution in three different locations, 39% insertions, and 15% deletions. Involved in complex rearrangements	20q11.1	21% (n = 408) but can be up to 43% in MDS/MPN patients. More frequent in the MDS high-risk group	Epigenetic regulator. May play a role in driving proliferation. Possible independent predictor of unfavorable prognostic and associated with a median survival of 1.33 months
JAK2	Substitutions missense in three locations. Most on position 617. Deletions at 543. Fusions with BCR, ETV6 PAX5, PCM1, SSBP2 SEC31A	9p24	9% and 2% in MDS and therapy-related MDS (sMDS), respectively. (COSMIC) (n = 3226)	Tyrosine kinase. Valid to differentiate diagnosis (RARS-T) from others. High frequency in RARS and thrombocytosis associated to SF3B1 mutations 51% in MMNU
TET2	Nonsense and missense substitution, 33% and 36% resp; deletions, 16%; insertions, 10%. Complex and other mutations, 18%. No signs of relationships between specific mutation and pathological features of MDS	4q24	Up to 20%. (n = 935); frequent in low-risk patients; higher in myelodysplastic/ myeloproliferative neoplasm—unclassifiable	Control of cytosine hydroxymethylation. Potential utility as a predictive biomarker for response to 5-azacitidine but overall clinical significance of TET2 remains unclear. TET2 and EZH2 mutations together could be a new category/class mol. alterations.
SRSF2	79% missense substitutions in three positions (most at AA95) and 13.5% deletions. Mutations often associated to RUNX1 and IDH1	17q25.1	10%–12% most in pMDS.(n = 1072)	Splicing factor. Possible negative prognostic impact. In univariate analysis, mutated SRSF2 predicted shorter OS and more frequent acute myeloid leukemia progression compared with wild-type SRSF.
RUNX-1 (AML 1)	36% missense substitutions; 17% deletions; 15%, insertions; 12%, other mutations. Bi-allelic and heterozygous mutations	21q22, Involved in t(3;21) (q26;q22), rearranging with MDS1/ EVI1	More frequent in sMDS (22%). 8% in pMDS	Transcription factor. Its loss affect multilineage hematopoiesis, maturation of progenitors, and inefficient platelet production (mice models). Rearrangement of RUNX-1/MDS1 helps on diagnosis. Independent unfavorable predictor
NRAS	100% missense substitutions. Most substitutions located on positions (AA) 12, 13, and 61	1p32	9% (n = 965) N-Ras mutations at codon 12 were more strongly associated with hematopoietic tumors	Role in signal transduction. Possible poor prognosis: Increased risk of leukemic transformation but not conclusive data

TABLE 28.5 (continued)

Features of the Top 20 Genes Mutated in MDS

Gene	Type of Mutations	Location	Frequency	Features and Implications
TP53	54.3% missense substitution (20 locations, mainly AA 248). Few deletions and insertions. LOH worst prognosis	i(17q) or t(17p). Complex karyotypes	Up to 9% (n = 506); common in sMDS	Ubiquitous tumor suppressor gene in human cancers. Transcription factor. Strong independent predictor factor of poor prognosis. Decreased response to hypomethylating agents. Strongly associated with thrombocytopenia and elevated blast proportion
ZRSR2	31% nonsense substitutions and 25% missense substitutions (16 positions); 11.4% deletions; 31.4% other mutations	Xp22.1	8% (n = 451)	No impact on prognostic of MDS till present
U2AF1	96.7% missense substitution (four positions)	21q22.3	6% in MDS (n = 999)	Splicing factor. No impact on prognosis of MDS till present
DNMT3A	76.7% missense substitutions, nonsense substitutions, insertions, and deletions. Most substitutions on position 882	2p23	6% in MDS (n = 473) (COSMIC)	Epigenetic regulation. Function in de novo methylation DNMT3A mutations would have a worse OS than the wild-type gene. Faster development to AML. DNMT3A R882 mutations are recurrent molecular aberrations in AML and MDS and may be an adverse prognostic event in MDS
IDH2	R140 and R172 in IDH2. Mutations are always heterozygous and tend to occur in a mutually exclusive manner with *TET2* mutations.	15q26.1	5% (n = 1123)	Cell metabolism, epigenetic regulation. Gain of function. Induces global DNA hypermethylation leading to impaired hematopoietic differentiation and increased stem cell and progenitor cell marker expression. Higher median platelet counts in patients with mutations. No impact on OS were observed.
EZH2	54% missense substitutions, 29% deletions, 8% complex and others. Different positions. Mono- and bi-allelic mutations	7q35–q36 frequently associated with UPD7q or 7q36.1 but not with deletions of 7q in MDS	2%–6% in MDS but more frequent in MDS/MPN (n = 415)	Epigenetic regulation. Possible dual effect as tumor suppressor and oncogene, according to the context. Mutations would produce loss of gene function. Independent negative prognostic factor especially in MDS/MPN patients. Mutations together with TET2 as possible new class of molecular lesions conveying a clonal epigenetic instability. Mutations together with ASXL1 could confer better OS

(continued)

TABLE 28.5 (continued)

Features of the Top 20 Genes Mutated in MDS

Gene	Type of Mutations	Location	Frequency	Features and Implications
KRAS	100% missense substitutions (AA 12 and 13). Fusions with UBE2L3	12p12	3% in pMDS (n = 271) Up to 5% in sMDS (n = 102)	Signal transduction. Possible coexistence of RAS activation and monosomy 7 in MDS cooperating in the multistep process of leukemogenesis
CBL	90% missense substitution (nine positions)	11q23.3	4% in MDS (n = 211) Frequently seen in MDS/MPN cases association with 11q-CN-LOH	Signal transduction. CBL mutation may lead to MPN by driving cellular proliferation. Nonsignificant on the OS. C-CBL mutations play a role at least in part in a subset of MDS patients during sAML transformation. C-CBL mutation is very rare in MDS, but acquisition and/or expansion of C-CBL mutant clones occurs in 11.8% of patients during sAML transformation
IDH1	97% missense substitution in AA 132	2q33.3	3% (n = 1240)	IDH1 mutations associated with unfavorable prognostic but pendent of validation. Metabolic changes induced by an IDH1 mutation may influence chemoresistance in a manner that is context dependent
CEBP alpha	In frame and frameshift insertions and deletions. Missense and nonsense substitutions. Possible loss of function	19q13.1	3% in pMDS and 25% in MDS, therapy related (n = 455). Dif. sources	Myeloid-specific transcription factor required for normal myeloid differentiation. The loss of function of CEBP alpha has leukemogenic potential
CSF1R	Missense and nonsense substitutions	5q32	3% (n = 181)	Codify for cytokine that controls the production, differentiation, and function of macrophages. Mutations can be linked to a predisposition to myeloid malignancy
FLT3	Insertions and missense substitutions	13q12	2% (n = 1506)	FLT3 occurs in MDS and CMML at a lower frequency than AML. It does not predict poor outcomes

Source: Data extracted from COSMIC.

morphologic dysplasia like MDS suggest the presence of aberrant splicing in the pathophysiology of some types of MDS, especially involving multiple components like *U2AF35*, *ZRSR2*, *SRSF2*, and *SF3B1* (Yoshida et al., 2011).

Two genes that are part of the splicing machinery are in the list of top 20 mutated genes: *SF3B1*, associated with the presence of ring sideroblasts but without additional prognostic value (thus far), and *U2AF1*, associated with an increased rate of progression to AML but only present in a reduced percentage of MDS cases (6% in COSMIC). Several genes implicated in epigenetics regulation would be the second group of coding sequences most commonly mutated in MDS. These code for epigenetic regulators, specifically proteins involved in DNA methylation and histone modification. The review by Graubert and

Walter (2011) is an important source about the mutations in regulators of methylation and their effect on MDS. As pointed out, abnormalities in these genes would have an effect on transcription, which is in itself maintained trough cell division. In fact, MDS and secondary AML have already been linked to alterations in DNA methylation in hematopoietic progenitors, suggesting an important role of DNA methylation abnormalities in the pathophysiology of MDS (Figueroa et al., 2009; Jiang et al., 2009). It has also been suggested that the effects on methylation could be helpful to analyze the impact of DNA methyltransferase (DNMT) inhibitors in MDS therapy.

In this set of epigenetic regulators is *EZH2*. It belongs to the polycomb group, composed of transcription repressor genes. The literature suggests a possible dual function: tumor suppressor and oncogene, depending on the context. In MDS, it presents several types of mutations linked to a loss of enzymatic function. In principle, these mutations are more prevalent in lower-risk MDS but are paradoxically associated with reduced OS, which is somewhat controversial.

Within the same group, mutations in *DMNT3* are observed in up to 6% of MDS and are associated with short survival and fast transformation to leukemia. The gene presents a variety of mutations conducive to loss of function and there are indications that it may play a role in the balance between hematopoietic self-renewal and differentiation.

TET2, another member of the previously mentioned group, presents a high percentage of mutations, up to 20%. TET family proteins (Tet1, Tet2, and Tet3) catalyze the conversion of 5-methyl-cytosine to 5-hydroxymethyl-cytosine (5HOmC). In embryonal stem cells, TET1 plays a functional role in maintaining the pluripotent state (Sanada and Ogawa, 2012). In principle, there is no specific significance of TET2 mutations in the prognosis of MDS, but Kosmider et al. (2009) reported TET2 as a favorable prognostic factor (independent from IPSS-R) in MDS. Data obtained from mouse models indicated that its deficiency could be linked to initial myeloid transformation in humans, and there are also indications that *TET2* mutations also occur frequently during progression of MPN or MDS to secondary AML. However, Smith et al. (2010), in a study covering more than 300 MDS and CMML patients, did not find any significant association between mutations occurring on TET2 and the prognostic scoring system, cytogenetic status, or the probability to transform to AML. Recently mutations in this gene have been associated to the response to azacitidine treatments (Itzykson R et al. in Garcia Manero, 2012). It does make sense considering that TET2 is a protein involved in the conversion of 5mC to 5OHmC and could therefore result in passive induction of DNA methylation. In general, it is possible to assume that more specific studies in a bigger cohort of patients will be necessary for a better knowledge of the relationship, if any, of TET2 mutations with the phenotype of MDS.

IDH1 and IDH2 are two isocitrate dehydrogenase genes that belong to the group of epigenetic regulators and present low incidence of mutations in MDS. IDH1 and IDH2 are components of TCA enzymes that catalyze isocitrate to alpha-ketoglutarate conversion in the cytoplasm and mitochondria, respectively. Cancer-associated IDH1 and IDH2 mutations confer a neomorphic enzymatic activity producing oncometabolites capable to interfere with global DNA methylation. As a result, the mutated enzymes show severely compromised activity of the intrinsic isocitrate to alpha-ketoglutarate conversion but in turn acquire a de novo activity to catalyze alpha-ketoglutarate to 2 hydroxyglutarate (2HG) conversion. The mutations detected would produce a gain more than a loss of function (Sanada and Ogawa, 2012). Interestingly, mutations in IDH have been hypothetically implicated in a model explaining the development of either secondary AML or AML without preleukemic phase, starting in human stem cells. The model arose from the analysis of 12 genes, including some of the very well-known mutated genes in AML and MDS like TET2, RUNX1 ASXL1, or CBL (Rocquain et al., 2010).

The last gene in this group, *ASXL1*, has been associated with the regulation of homeotic gene expression during embryogenesis (repressing/activating depending on the context). It is located on chromosome 20q but outside of the common deleted region (CDR) in MDS. This gene presents high frequency of mutations in MDS, up to 21%, more frequent in high-risk MDS group and associated with signs of aggressiveness and poor clinical outcome (Gelsi-Boyer et al., 2012). Multivariate analysis indicated an association with high risk and shorter time to develop leukemia. Animal models with disrupted gene function have shown defective hematopoiesis with progenitor defects. Mutations in ASXL1 have been associated with TET2 and RUNX anomalies in MDS as well as in AML. These genes would be part of the hypothetical model to develop the disease described in the research of Rocquain et al. (2010).

Another interesting group of mutated genes is that of transcription factors. The importance of this group of genes is based on the fact the hematopoietic function is coordinated by transcription factors and that some of them are usually mutated in myeloid malignancies (Lam and Zhang, 2012). MDS is not an exception and we find that *RUNX1* presents a high ratio of mutations, up to 21% in sMDS and 8% in pMDS. Mutations in this gene have been associated with activation of *RTK–RAS pathway*, through mutations in several other genes (Mangan and Speck, 2011). Different types of mutation according to the origin of MDS (sMDS or pMDS), with diverse phenotypic implications, have been observed in mouse models. Specifically, N-terminal missense and C-terminal frameshift mutations would be related to leukemic transformation. In addition, and an interesting factor to take into account, is that mutations in RUNX1 located in germ lines produce familial platelet disorders with tendency to myeloid malignancies. *ETV6* is another member of the transcription factor group found mutated in MDS and considered an independent prognostic factor. However, its frequency of mutation is low (around 2%) and it has been involved in translocations with other genes (several partners). Its main function is the maintenance of hematopoiesis and several mechanisms are hypothesized to explain its implication in the MDS pathogenesis. The group of genes belonging to signaling pathways is represented in this list of top mutated genes in MDS by *NRAS* (approximately 10% of MDS cases) and *KRAS* (1%–2%, up to 5% in sMDS). These are involved in signal cascades critical for cell growth and survival. NRAS is associated with poor outcome but without independent prognostic value yet. *CBL* is implicated in the negative regulation of the RTK pathway. In principle, it has a low frequency of mutations in MDS (3%–4%), but this gene would have a tumor suppressor function. *JAK2* is mutated at low frequency in MDS, and there are differences between sMDS and pMDS. Its association with SF3B1 mutations can be considered as part of the composite MDS/MPN phenotype of RARS-T.

28.7.1.1 Gene Mutations as Independent Risk Factors

It is evident that somatic gene mutations are quite common in MDS and many of them would be associated with specific clinical features. The value of somatic mutations as independent prognostic factors for a set of specific genes is supported by several lines of research. The works of Bejar et al. (2011) and Torsten (2012) presented strong evidence that a group of five genes, *TP53*, *EZH2*, *ETV6*, *RUNX1*, and *ASXL1*, would have a specific value as independent prognostic factors and is associated to poor survival from multivariate studies. Their findings indicate that mutations in specific genes help explain the clinical heterogeneity of MDS and that the identification of these abnormalities would improve the prediction of prognosis in MDS. In all patients except those at highest risk, the presence of these mutations was associated with an OS similar to that of patients in the next-highest IPSS risk group. Thus far, these are the only genes recognized as independent prognostic factors regardless of the IPSS classification.

Considering that somatic point mutations can be identified in more than 70% of MDS, including most cases with a normal karyotype, and the fact that some of the mutations can be powerful predictors of clinical phenotype (predicting prognosis independently of existing clinical variables) (Lindsley and Ebert, 2012), the logical next approach would be to integrate mutational analysis results into the IPSS-R.

However, authors such as Tiu et al. (2011) still contend that the clinical outcomes and clinicomorphologic associations for cases with some of the mutated and wild-type genes are, at least, conflictive, if not downright negative in many studies. Again, a more comprehensive clinical analysis involving a large number of patients is a must to test the clinical impact of these abnormalities.

28.8 Implication of Noncoding Sequences in the Pathogenesis of MDS: MicroRNA

As with other molecular markers (i.e., gene point mutations), recent research has established the aberrant expression and function of microRNAs (miRNAs) in MDS. The unique expression of miRNA patterns has been identified and modeled in mice in an attempt to reproduce features of MDS.

28.8.1 MicroRNA and Its Relationship with MDS

miRNAs are 18–25 nucleotide noncoding RNAs highly conserved from invertebrates to vertebrates. Once the status of mature miRNA is reached, it is incorporated into the RNA interfering silencing complex to repress protein translation as well as RNA decay. miRNAs play important roles in the regulation of DNA methylation and histone modification and can function as oncogenes, tumor suppressor genes, or both.

Recently, miRNAs have been specifically implicated in the development of solid and hematopoietic malignancies (Rhyasen and Starczynowski, 2012). Regarding MDS, this syndrome is thought to arise from a CD34+ HSC (CD34+ human stem cells where CD34 represents a marker for primitive blood- and BM-derived progenitor cells, especially for hematopoietic and endothelial stem cells) that has acquired genetic and/or epigenetic abnormalities. Studies conducted on human CD34+ cells described relative miRNA abundance using microarray and RT-PCR techniques. In normal conditions, human stem and progenitor cells obtained from BM (CD34+ cells) differentially express a set of specific miRNAs (see Georgantas et al., 2007; Liao et al., 2008; Rhyasen and Starczynowski, 2012). This is a good starting point to study the expression of those miRNA families in MDS.

Recent communications have pointed out the differences and aberrations in the expression of these sequences in MDS patients. An extensive review of the most relevant analyses of the possible effects of miRNA on MDS can be found in the works of Rhyasen and Starczynowski (2012) and Fang et al. (2012).

Other examples can be found in Sokol et al. (2011). These authors present evidence that the overexpression of miRNAs such as miR-181a, b, c, d, miR-121, miR-376, miR 125b, miR-155, and miR-130a and underexpression of miR486-5p would be associated with high-risk MDS. Studies on CD34+ cells have yielded even more specific results that point at 22 miRNAs differentially expressed across all types of MDS, 13 upregulated and 9 downregulated. In principle, these can be grouped into five distinct clusters distinguishing normal from MDS patients and MDS subtypes (Dostalova Merkerova et al., 2011).

Looking at the published results, the primary observation is the tendency of aberrant expression (over and under) of miRNAs, mainly in del(5q) syndrome, and, second, it is difficult to separate between different MDS subtypes according to miRNA expression. The interpretation of the data is additionally complicated by observations such as the reduced expression of miRNA 146 in isolated CD34+ cells from del(5q), which, at same time, is upregulated in the PB granulocytes of these patients (Starczynowski et al., 2010).

miRNAs located in the region of del(5q) have been repeatedly analyzed. According to Sokol et al. (2011), there is a subset of 13 miRNAs with altered expression when compared with normal samples, mostly significant underexpression of miR 146 and miR 145 in CD34+ cells isolated from BM, which suggests a direct implication in the phenotype of del(5q) syndrome (see Starczynowski et al., 2010). This hypothesis makes sense in view of the findings of Oliva et al. (2010) regarding the increased expression of these two miRNAs in patients treated with lenalidomide (a derivative of thalidomide initially intended as a treatment for multiple myeloma and currently used in MDS). In clinical trials, these two miRNAs have shown low expression in del(5q) but are elevated following lenalidomide treatment. This increase in the expression is also associated with erythroid responses and cytogenetic remission. The mechanism by which lenalidomide increases the expression of both miRNAs is not clear. Lenalidomide may induce miR-145 and 146 in CD34+ cells in MDS but not in CD34-, which suggests that these two miRNAs could be used as markers for drug response in this context.

Erdogan et al. (in Fang et al., 2012) described 13 miRNAs differentially expressed between MDS and normal samples, of which 8 (miR103, miR-140, miR-150, miR-342, miR-378, miR-483, miR-632, and miR-636) were statistically significant and with the highest discriminatory power between low-risk MDS patients and control samples.

Focusing on diagnosis and prognosis of MDS, it has been shown that miR-422a and miR-617 are correlated with disease progression: low expression in normal and low-risk samples and high in advanced MDS and AML. Similarly, overexpression of miR-181 has been related to high-risk cohort with progress to AML, but more studies are necessary to convincingly correlate miRNA expression profiles to outcome, prognosis, and treatment response in MDS. Table 28.6 shows the analysis of expression of specific miRNAs related to MDS. Data were obtained from different sources.

TABLE 28.6

Expression Analysis of Specific miRNAs and Its Contribution to MDS

MiRNA	Expression	MDS/Cell Type	Functions Implicated
miRNA 145	Down	del(5q) CD34+ HSC/progenitor cells	Self-renewal
		Mature cells	Self-renewal Thrombocytosis
miRNA 146a	Down	Mature	Dysplasia and neutropenia
miR/150	Down	HSC/progenitor	Marrow failure
	Down	Mature cells	
miR 378	Down	MDS del(5q) and with good cytogenetic risk profiles del(5q)	Thrombocytopenia
miR-125b	Up	MDS with t(2;11)/CD34+ HSC/progenitor	Self-renewal
mir 155	Down	Mature cells	Self-renewal
miR 135a	Up	Mature cells	Neutropenia
miR 222	Up	Mature cells	Neutropenia
miR 148	Up	Mature cells	Neutropenia
miR 342	Up	Mature cells	Neutropenia
miR 181	Up	Mature cells	Effect on progenitors
miR 10a	Down	Mature cells	Thrombocytopenia
miR 206	Down		Thrombocytopenia

Source: Data coincident from several sources.

As it was mentioned, it is important to have into account the miR-125b (see Translocation t(2;11)(p21;q23). In those cases with t(2;11) translocation, there is an upregulation of miR-125b, which is directly linked to the chromosomal changes.

Of note, it is important to consider that diagnosis and prognosis of MDS are most challenging in those cases grouped as low and intermediate-1 risk, where the majority of patients would show normal cytogenetic parameters. Therefore, miRNA biomarkers of MDS are expected to be beneficial in this particular group of patients. For Fang et al. (2012), the promise of miRNAs in the clinic has been realized in part by miRNA expression profile studies that successfully distinguish different cancer types and the fact that unique miRNA expression profiles have been identified and can be used to discriminate between different MDS subtypes. Another important feature of miRNAs in the context of their potential use as diagnostic and prognostic markers is their stability.

Perhaps the most interesting aspect to explore in the relationship of miRNA and the pathophysiology of MDS relates to their therapeutic possibilities. In contrast to the targeted inhibition/activation of single genes, miRNAs regulate multiple gene groups. Thus, the prospective use of miRNA mimics or antagomiRs as therapeutic agents for hematological malignancies is potentially important.

28.9 Copy Number Changes UPD/CN-LOH in MDS

UPD arises when an individual inherits two copies of a particular chromosome from the same parent, either maternal or paternal, and no copies of this chromosome from the other parent. The origin of UPD can be meiotic but this event also occur in a portion of somatic cells through mitotic cell division. To have a proper idea about the impact of UPD, we could consider a constitutional genotype as heterozygous and its conversion to homozygous or hemizygous in a tumor or other somatic cell is called LOH. In fact, somatic recombination in mitosis leading to UPD is an important mechanism leading to LOH.

UPD has recently awakened considerable interest in the cancer field mainly because it would be a common but previously unrecognized mechanism in tumor development.

An extensive review and description of mechanisms of UPD/CN-LOH in developmental disorders as well as in cancer can be found in Tuna et al. (2009) and O'Keefe et al. (2010).

Emerging data demonstrate that some hematological malignancies such as chronic lymphocytic leukemia (CLL), MPN, MDS, and AML are all associated with significant increased incidence with age and exhibit abundant CN-LOH. The genesis of the acquired CN-LOH in these diseases is not very well known. A main cause is likely to be the effect of extrinsic factors such as treatment with DNA damaging agents leading to genomic DNA alterations upstream of sites of mitotic. Other potential mechanisms that have been postulated are time acquired or inherited weakness of components of DNA repair machinery, mitotic spindle checkpoints, telomere shortening, and a possible supersaturating overwhelming of some DNA repair components. For a complete description of the possible mechanisms behind this phenomenon, the reader should consult O'Keefe et al. (2010).

28.9.1 Analysis of UPD/CN-LOH in MDS and Myeloid Malignancies

SNP microarrays allow the simultaneous analysis of large numbers of polymorphic loci across the genome, which provides information on copy number change and/or LOH.

In MDS, particularly in del(5q) patients, this methodology has allowed to detect not only gene deletions but also regions of UPD that can be used to pinpoint particular regions for mutation analysis. The early study of Wang et al. (2008), focused on the 5q-syndrome group, revealed several regions of UPD in most of samples, the largest one being 7.6 Mb. The authors concluded that all the cases studied with del(5q) MDS had UPD, with a total of 32 regions identified in the patients. In summary, UPD was observed in the 95% of del(5q) MDS cases used in the study.

Similarly, Gondek et al. (2008) detected both chromosomal aberrations and UPD using SNPa in MDS, MDS/MPD, and secondary AML patients (n = 174), with evident somatic origin. According to the authors, acquired segmental UPD (produced by mitotic recombination) would be a common event in MDS (20% of MDS and 23% of sAML patients) as either the sole abnormality or a concurrent defect. More interesting is the possible diagnostic implications of UPD in this syndrome. For example, cryptic lesions found in patients with normal metaphase cytogenetics (across all sub-entities studied) were associated with reduced OS as demonstrated for sAML and MDS/MPD, whereas selected subtypes of MDS and those patients free of genomic imbalances detected by SNPa and metaphase cytogenetics had a more favorable prognosis.

Another good example of SNPa in MDS is provided by Heinrichs et al. (2009). This group detected clonal acquired abnormalities in up to 41% of patients harboring chromosomal abnormalities and in 15% of cases without cytogenetic alterations. Particularly interesting is the fact that in malignancies like MDS/AML and pAML, the distribution of acquired CN-LOH is not at random. Chromosome pairs 4, 7, 11, 13, and 21 show frequently recurrent UPD (hot spots) and they are mainly located in telomeric regions.

28.9.2 Clinical Significance in MDS

As indicated by O'Keefe et al. (2010), there is strong evidence that the addition of SNPa karyotyping to standard metaphase cytogenetics would increase the ability to identify clonal markers in different myeloid pathologies. Focusing on MDS, it can be particularly helpful in those cases with normal cytogenetics but with a wide range of clinical outcomes. For example, UPDs affecting chromosome 7q were identified in patients who had a rapidly deteriorating clinical course despite a low-risk IPSS score (see Heinrichs et al., 2009). This was one of the first report that applied genome-wide SNPa analysis to paired BM and normal DNA specimens from a large cohort of patients with MDS, unveiling the need to differentiate acquired from inherited abnormalities.

From a technical point of view, since SNPa technology does not require cell culture, the number of evaluable samples is increased. This is particularly true of hematologic malignancies associated with BM fibrosis, through the use of PBCs in selected situations.

From a clinical standpoint, however, only a few recurrent areas of CN-LOH have been acknowledged to be of use (ex homozygous JAK2 mutations; UPD13q linked to FLT-3, ITD, or UPD17p and homozygous TP53 mutation; as well as UPD11q and C-CBL), all related to unfavorable outcomes.

It is quite clear that the assignment of prognostic significance will require systematic application of SNPa as a routine diagnostic tool complementing metaphase cytogenetics, particularly on patients with normal cytogenetics or lesions associated with favorable prognosis. The detection of UPD may effectively upstage the prognosis and allow for better prognostic resolution explaining heterogeneity of outcomes in patients with otherwise comparable clinical features.

In addition, and looking for the initial diagnosis of MDS, the possibility to detect clonal genomic aberrations in cases of normal karyotype by SNPa analysis would help distinguish MDS from other causes of BM cell dysplasia and pancytopenia due to the effects of drugs, environmental toxins, or aberrant immune responses.

It is important to have into account that additional research is still needed to determine the exact effect of UPDs on prognostic information considering the number of specific genomic regions. This can be achieved by evaluating significant cohorts of patients with MDS in clinical trials and developing prospective studies.

28.10 Noninvasive Biomarkers in MDS

Despite the discovery of chromosomal abnormalities, gene mutations, aberrant hypermethylation, and the potential implication of noncoding sequences, the pathophysiology of MDS has remained elusive.

Until now, the diagnosis and prognosis of MDS syndromes have been performed by cytogenetic and BM analyses coupled to clinical parameters from PB. As previously mentioned in this chapter, the IPSS-R is the internationally recognized tool to assess the risk of patients with MDS transforming to AML. However, there is a general agreement that the current system may still be improved by tracking the disease through molecular markers.

There is a special concern for those patients with low-grade FAB/WHO subtypes but high-risk cytogenetic findings (according to IPSS-R), in whom a frequent cytogenetic monitoring during therapy is desirable for an adequate clinical management. In these cases the BM morphology alone is not helpful to assess response to therapy, because blast counts are not informative and dysplastic changes may persist because of the therapy itself. There is no way to monitor these patients under treatment except by cytogenetic analyses of BM in informative cases.

Consequently, an important remaining challenge in MDS is to obtain useful molecular markers in a noninvasive way. A significant effort is being made to use circulating markers, which are more attractive because they can be measured from a simple blood drawn rather than a BM biopsy. In the following are some circulating markers currently under use as well under study and development.

28.10.1 Circulating miRNA in the Diagnosis of MDS

There is a general consensus that circulating miRNAs are potential biomarkers for cancer (Mitchell et al., 2008). As previously described, there is strong evidence that noncoding sequences such as miRNA play a role in the pathogenesis of MDS. There are reports that plasmatic levels of two different miRNAs, let-7a and miR-16, can be possible predictors of progression for MDS (Zuo et al., 2011). This team reported significantly low levels of these two miRNAs in MDS patients in a study that analyzed 126 subjects. The authors found that miRNA levels predicted OS and progression-free survival (PFS). This is just a first line of evidence on the potential use of miRNA as markers.

Moreover, miRNA levels could be used to further stratify patients in each IPSS-R category into different survival groups, especially considering that let-7a and miR-16 both play important roles in myeloid leukemogenesis by regulating cell cycle and apoptosis (functions affected in MDS syndrome). Let-7a would act as tumor suppressor that regulates oncogenes such as RAS and HMGA2, and miR-16 targets multiple oncogenes, including BCL2, MCL1, CCND1, and WNT3A. Both of these miRNAs are downregulated in CLL, pituitary adenomas, and prostate carcinoma. These preliminary findings thus suggest that the detection of specific miRNAs in plasma is an appealing, noninvasive possible biomarker for diagnosis or prognosis of MDS patients.

28.10.2 Serum Proteome Profiling in MDS

Obtaining protein profiles from serum is another possible methodology to use in the routine analysis of MDS. In the study of Aivado et al. (2007), proteome profiles obtained from serum could be used to distinguish MDS from non-MDS cytopenias. This report was developed studying 218 patients, and it helped identify two different members of the CXC chemokine family, namely CXC chemokine ligands 4 (CXCL4) and 7 (CXCL7), whose serum levels were significantly decreased in MDS patients. The analysis performed in subtypes of MDS also confirms low levels of the two proteins in advanced MDS. At present, however, there are no indications of an impending introduction of this type of analysis in the current international standards for prognosis and diagnosis. In a similar context, the utility of measuring pretreatment proteasome chymotrypsin-like, caspase-like, and trypsin-like activities in plasma to predict response and survival of patients with AML or advanced-stage MDS has also been tested (Ma et al., 2009). The enzymatic activity of these three proteins would be increased significantly in patients of MDS compared to healthy subjects, but only chymotrypsin-like activity was an independent predictor of response to treatment from age grouping (<70 vs. ≥ 70 years), cytogenetics, and blood urea nitrogen (results from multivariate analysis).

28.10.3 Prognostic Significance of Serum Ferritin Level in MDS

This is a prognostic predictor already included in the last revised version of IPSS. Elevated levels of serum ferritin (SF) due to ineffective erythropoiesis and increased iron absorption from the gut are often observed in non-transfused MDS patients, suggesting involvement of iron overload in its pathogenesis. Iron overload results from high transfusion requirements and retrospective studies have shown an association with relatively poor survival in a subset of the low-risk patients in MDS (Mahesh et al., 2008). A retrospective study in Japan has shown higher mortality in heavily iron-overloaded patients, with liver and cardiac dysfunction being the primary cause (Takatoku et al., 2007).

The literature shows SF levels in MDS patients with chromosomal abnormality to be significantly higher than in subjects with a normal karyotype, and considering its negative effects, body iron accumulation could arguably aggravate the prognosis of MDS (Kikuchi et al., 2012).

Interestingly, a relationship between iron accumulation and genomic instability has been pointed out already. Excess iron would increase the levels of reactive oxygen species (ROS), mainly superoxide and hydroxyl radical. These are inductors of lipid peroxidation, oxidative DNA damage, and subsequent mutation of genes and DNA breaks, all of which could potentially lead to leukemic transformation in MDS.

There is growing evidence to assume that SF levels at diagnosis are a valuable tool, and as such it has been internationally recognized. SF at diagnosis can be an independent prognostic factor for the OS in MDS patients, it can be related to chromosomal abnormality, and, finally, high levels of SF have been associated with poor leukemia-free survival (LFS) on those transfusion-dependent MDS patients.

28.10.4 Significance of Levels of Beta-2-Microglobulin (B2M) in MDS

Beta-2 microglobulin (B2M) is a subunit of human leukocyte antigen class I (HLA-I), and it has been well established as a prognostic marker in various solid tumors and hematologic malignancies. This sHLA-I has been reported to be an immunomodulator inhibiting the cytotoxic effects of T lymphocytes, which may offset its predictive value for disease aggressiveness in patients with MDS (Albitar et al., 2007).

The level of beta-2 microglobulin (B2M) is also considered in the reviewed IPSS standard to have an important role on prognosis of MDS. This marker has been associated to the risk of AML evolution. Accordingly, the risk is higher in patients with B2M> or = 2 mg/dL. B2M level at diagnosis can be an independent prognostic parameter for survival and for the risk of developing AML in high-risk MDS patients (Neumann et al., 2009).

The hypothesis about the implications of B2M in prognosis is based on its role in the immunological response of the host to the malignancy. Since most circulating B2M is derived from the cellular surface, increased levels may relate to increased cell turnover, increased tumor mass, or both (Gatto et al., 2003).

28.10.5 Prognostic Significance of Lactate Dehydrogenase

Lactate dehydrogenase (LDH) is another marker considered by the IPSS-R. Early studies have shown that an elevated serum LDH is associated with a poor prognosis in MDS (Aul et al., 1992). In 2005, the IPSS was refined by including the serum level of LDH as a variable to improve risk assessment in pMDS (Germing et al., 2005). At that time, elevated LDH at diagnosis was associated with a reduced probability of survival and an increased probability of AML evolution. Recently, the value of developing serial test of LDH has been suggested as a predictor of disease progression (Wimazal et al., 2008). An increase in LDH over time is associated with disease progression and an increase in LDH in the follow-up is associated with a significantly reduced survival. One of the problems is our lack of knowledge to explain the biochemical reason for an increased LDH in these patients, as well as the lack of information about other parameters that could be associated to LDH levels (cytogenetic evolution, association with molecular markers, potential concomitance of elevated LDH with other signs of disease progression, etc). In any case, LDH levels are important not just at diagnosis of MDS but also as a potentially useful follow-up parameter, especially when disease progression is an important decision point for treatment.

28.10.6 Chromosomal Markers in Peripheral Blood: FISH and Conventional Cytogenetic Analysis

Cytomorphology and cytogenetic analysis of BM cells are the two workhorses of diagnosis and prognosis of MDS. Cytogenetic analysis of BM is also a methodology widely used in the routine monitoring of the progress of the disease as well as in clinical trials and to evaluate treatments. Considering the invasive nature of BM biopsy, there is an interest to replace it by more patient-friendly means to periodically monitor the status/progression of the disease.

It is clear that for all MDS patients harboring chromosomal aberrations, a technique allowing a frequent cytogenetic monitoring performed from PB would be much less invasive than BM biopsy and would help to more efficiently guide treatment based on molecular–cytogenetic response. While the analysis of PB should not be substituted for BM at diagnosis, this is a viable alternative for monitoring patients using the appropriate FISH probe(s) (Cherry et al., 2012).

Consequently, significant efforts have been made over the past few years to analyze cytogenetic markers for diagnosis and prognosis of MDS directly from PB. In 2001, research on the colony-forming capacity of PB stem/progenitor cells (PBSC) indicated that in cases of RA with unfavorable chromosomal aberrations, RARS, and in advanced stages of MDS such as RAEB and RA in transformation (RAEB-t), the number of myeloid progenitor cells increased up to 100-fold. The most important conclusions of these study were (1) the possibility that the marked increase of circulating colony-forming cells (CFC) could be associated with disease progression, and, as logical consequence, (2) the evaluation of PBSC could be an important parameter in the diagnosis of MDS (Vehmeyer et al., 2001).

Based on these preliminary results, the analysis of cytogenetic abnormalities directly in those CD34+ cells from PB was considered as an alternative to BM studies to monitor progression and response to treatments. First, the clone sizes of enriched circulating CD34+ cells analyzed by FISH (specific probes) were very close to the results of classical cytogenetic analyses of BM metaphases. Second, the comparison of FISH analyses of enriched and non-enriched PB and BM cells with conventional chromosome banding analyses of metaphases confirms that the analysis of circulating CD34+ cells by FISH is a sensitive, reliable method to measure the abnormal cell clones in PB. According to the authors of the study, the method was practical, noninvasive, representative for the clonal situation in the BM and had a predictive value (Braulke et al., 2010). At that time the main problem was its feasibility. It was proven in a small cohort of cases, and a test in a more large set of patients as well as diversity in MDS status and treatments was necessary to prove its usefulness.

The same group (Dr. Haase, personal communication) is currently testing FISH and conventional cytogenetic analysis in peripheral CD34+ cells in a bigger cohort of patients. Using results from a database of 14,000 FISH analysis performed, they detected abnormalities in 50% of MDS patients (a similar proportion to that observed with BM cytogenetics analysis). In this study, the combination of banding analysis and FISH with a specific set of probes in CD34+ PBCs allowed to detect almost any cytogenetic abnormality related to MDS. In addition, they got successful results in therapy trials (azacitidine). There is a multicenter nationwide German long-term study (CD34 FISH study) under development, and the preliminary results indicate the feasibility and high rate of success of applying FISH and cytogenetic studies in PB. For example, most abnormalities detected by conventional banding analysis (CBA) can also be identified by FISH and SNPa, which can be performed on CD34+ PBCs. Furthermore, the presence of SNPa-detected abnormalities could contribute to poorer prognosis. FISH and SNPa of PBC of MDS patients allow a comprehensive genetic analysis even if BM is not available. Supporting the use of SNPa, there are also data about aCGH directly applied to circulating granulocytes to detect gross karyotypic alterations in patients with MDS, especially when marrow examination has failed or not been done (Vercauteren et al., 2010).

Similarly, another group examining the safety of lenalidomide monotherapy and markers for disease progression in MDS patients with <5% blasts and isolated del(5q) coupled the BM analysis with FISH on enriched CD34+ stem cells from PB, carried out every 2–3 months to monitor cytogenetic response and detect possible cytogenetic progressions. They reported the treatment response based on the reduction of the clone size, from the data obtained in CD34+ PBC.

Additional data about a strategy for FISH testing in PB and BM have been provided by Coleman et al. (2011) using a specific set of FISH probes, MDS FISH panel. The overall results show that PB FISH testing would provide a useful noninvasive technique for the detection of cytogenetic abnormalities in patients with suspected disease, although a normal PB FISH result clearly does not exclude the possibility of disease. The objective of this work was to serially monitor an abnormal clone in the PB, allowing for less frequent follow-up BM evaluations.

Additionally, there are indications about the role of circulating CD34+ cells in the prognostic value of MDS by itself. It has been reported that specific counts (>10/microl) were associated with worse LFS. In principle, separating newly diagnosed patients on the basis of 10/microl cutoff of circulating CD34+ cells may have prognostic utility, especially in intermediate-risk MDS (Cesana et al., 2008).

28.11 Concluding Remarks and Future Perspectives

Till present the major features present in the IPSS-R system (cytogenetic subgroups, marrow blast%, and cytopenias) are retaining a major prognostic impact in this syndrome. At same time, there is a growing interest to find markers covering several aspects in MDS like (1) markers for accurate prognosis in low- and intermediate-risk cases, (2) markers where cytogenetics abnormalities can't determine a prognostic or cases presenting chromosome instabilities with unknown prognostic meaning, (3) markers for routine evaluation of the progress of the disease, and (4) markers for treatment responses, and quite important, to increase the use of noninvasive markers for routine analysis.

At molecular level there are evidences about the usefulness of specific point gene mutations as independent prognosis factors. Unfortunately, and considering the wide spectrum of clinical outcomes and clinicomorphologic associations in MDS, they cannot predict prognosis independently of existing clinical variables in all subtypes of MDS. Consequently a deep effort is necessary to find a bigger number of markers as well as amplifying the cohort of analyzed cases. In addition it seems that not only a single gene but a group of genes/sequences will be necessary to obtain useful information to define molecular profiles in MDS.

Into this group of potential molecular markers, noncoding sequences as miRNA seem to be very promising. In principle cytogenetic alterations are likely to be the main contributor of altered miRNA expression. In fact the majority of miRNAs maps to copy number alterations and data suggest that subsets of these are altered miRNA and likely relevant to the syndrome. Second, and because a single miRNA can affect different mRNA targets, the information about its implications in MDS as well as manipulation of few miRNAs can have an important impact not just in the diagnosis and prognostic but in therapeutic possibilities. Third and more relevant is the possibility to use miRNAs from PB as markers, having in mind that overexpressed miRNA could be the best candidates to pursue further investigations. As counterpart and till present, there are no enough studies implicating a large patient cohort to provide a consistent sample source to uncover deregulated miRNA expression signatures in MDS. Again, as in gene point mutations, the miRNA expression needs to be carefully analyzed according to MDS subtypes, risk groups, and cell populations before estimating its validity as markers in the syndrome.

The other interesting group of potential markers are those sequences involved in UPD regions. This arises by the fact that key genes involved in tumorigenesis have been identified in these regions and that UPD might be a far more common, nonrandom contributing factor to the development of cancer previously unrecognized. This can be very interesting in MDS patients with normal chromosomal complement because UPD karyotype and genotype appear normal when examined by conventional cytogenetic analysis, FISH, or aCGH. The main limitation in using SNPa to identify UDP is the need of a minimum level of cells/DNA harboring abnormalities to be properly detected (>20% app. considering a first-line screening), and the use of SNPa analysis requires to differentiate acquired CN-LOH from germ line-encoded CN-LOH (up to 15% of control persons).

Regarding to the noninvasive markers, some are being used to complement the diagnosis and prognosis already (plasmatic levels of LDH, SF, beta-2 microglobulin), but the need to increase the use of noninvasive markers facing the routine monitoring of patients is clear. The impossibility to replace an initial BM biopsy (complete cytomorphological examination and conventional chromosome analysis) just by the analysis of PB is clear, but it is possible to assume it, PB study, as a viable alternative for monitoring patients using the appropriate FISH probe(s). In fact it looks like the combination of FISH CBA and SNPa on peripheral CD34+ cells would reproduce the results obtained in the BM study. In addition to the mentioned, peripheral circulant miRNA looks for other promising door in the search of noninvasive markers for MDS.

References

Aivado M, Spentzos D, Germing U, Alterovitz G, Meng XY, Grall F, Giagounidis AA et al. 2007. Serum proteome profiling detects myelodysplastic syndromes and identifies CXC chemokine ligands 4 and 7 as markers for advanced disease. *Proc Natl Acad Sci USA*. January 23, 2007;104(4):1307–1312. Epub January 12, 2007.

Albitar M, Johnson M, Do KA, Day A, Jilani I, Pierce S, Estey E et al. 2007. Levels of soluble HLA-I and beta2M in patients with acute myeloid leukemia and advanced myelodysplastic syndrome: Association with clinical behavior and outcome of induction therapy. *Leukemia*. March;21(3):480–488. Epub January 11, 2007.

Arber DA, Chang KL, Lyda MH, Bedell V, Spielberger R, and Slovak ML. 2003. Detection of NPM/MLF1 fusion in t(3;5)-positive acute myeloid leukemia and myelodysplasia. *Hum Pathol*. August 2003;34(8):809–813.

Aul C, Gattermann N, Heyll A, Germing U, Derigs G, and Schneider W. 1992. Primary myelodysplastic syndromes: Analysis of prognostic factors in 235 patients and proposals for an improved scoring system. *Leukemia*. January;6(1):52–59.

Bejar R, Stevenson K, Abdel-Wahab O, Galili N, Björn NB, Garcia-Manero G, Hagop KH et al. 2011. Clinical effect of point mutations in myelodysplastic syndromes. *Engl J Med*. June 30;364(26):2496–2506. doi: 10.1056/NEJMoa1013343.

Bejar R, Stevenson KE, Caughey BA, Abdel-Wahab O, Steensma DP, Galili N, Raza A et al. 2012. Validation of a prognostic model and the impact of mutations in patients with lower-risk myelodysplastic syndromes. *J Clin Oncol*. September 20, 2012;30:3376–3382.

Bennett JM. 2005. A comparative review of classification systems in myelodysplastic syndromes (MDS). *Semin Oncol*. August;32(4 Suppl 5):S3–S10. Review.

Bousquet M, Harris MH, Zhou B, and Lodish HF. 2010. MicroRNA miR-125b causes leukemia. *Proc Natl Acad Sci USA*. December 14, 2010;107(50):21558–21563. Epub November 30, 2010.

Bousquet M, Quelen C, Rosati R, Mansat-DeMas V, LaStarza R, Bastard C, Lippert E et al. 2008. Myeloid cell differentiation arrest by miR-125b-1 in myelodysplastic syndrome and acute myeloid leukemia with the t(2;11)(p21;q23) translocation. *Exp Med*. October 7, 2008;205(11):2499–2506. Epub October 20, 2008.

Braulke F, Schanz J, Jung K, Shirneshan K, Schulte K, Schuetze C, Steffens R, Trümper L, and Haase D. 2010. FISH analysis of circulating CD34+ cells as a new tool for genetic monitoring in MDS: Verification of the method and application to 27 MDS patients. *Leuk Res*. October;34(10):1296–1301. Epub March 11, 2010.

Cesana C, Klersy C, Brando B, Nosari A, Scarpati B, Scampini L, Molteni A et al. 2008. Prognostic value of circulating CD34+ cells in myelodysplastic syndromes. *Leuk Res*. November;32(11):1715–1723. Epub May 5, 2008.

Cherry AM, Slovak ML, Campbell LJ, Chun K, Eclache V, Haase D, Haferlach C et al. 2012. Will a peripheral blood (PB) sample yield the same diagnostic and prognostic cytogenetic data as the concomitant bone marrow (BM) in myelodysplasia? *Leuk Res*. July;36(7):832–840. Epub April 25, 2012.

Coleman JF, Theil KS, Tubbs RR, and Cook JR. 2011. Diagnostic yield of bone marrow and peripheral blood fish panel testing in clinically suspected myelodysplastic syndromes and/or acute myeloid leukemia a prospective analysis of 433 cases. *Am J Clin Pathol*. 135:915–920. doi: 10.1309/AJCPW10YBRMWSWYE.

Cui W, Sun J, Cotta CV, Medeiros LJ, and Lin P. 2011. Myelodysplastic syndrome with inv(3)(q21q26.2) or t(3;3)(q21;q26.2) has a high risk for progression to acute myeloid leukemia. *Am J Clin Pathol*. August 2011;136(2):282–288.

Davids MS and Steensma DP. 2010. The molecular pathogenesis of myelodysplastic syndromes. *Cancer Biol Ther*. August 15, 2010;10(4):309–319.

DellaPorta MG, Malcovati L, Strupp C, Ambaglio I, Kuendgen A, Zipperer E, Travaglino E et al. 2011. Risk stratification based on both disease status and extra-hematologic comorbidities in patients with myelodysplastic syndrome. *Haematologica*. March;96(3):441–449. Epub December 6, 2010.

Dostalova Merkerova M, Krejcik Z, Votavova H, Belickova M, Alzbeta Vasikova A, and Cermak J. 2011. Distinctive microRNA expression profile in CD34+ bone marrow cells from patients with myelodysplastic syndrome. *Eur J Hum Genet*. 2011;19:313–319.

Fang J, Varney M, and Starczynowski DT. 2012. Implication of microRNAs in the pathogenesis of MDS. *Curr Pharm Des*. 18:3170–3179.

Figueroa ME, Skrabanek L, Li Y, Jiemjit A, Fandy TE, Paietta E, Fernandez H et al. 2009. MDS and secondary AML display unique patterns and abundance of aberrant DNA methylation. *Blood*. October 15;114(16):3448–3458. Epub August 3.

Forbes SA, Bhamra G, Bamford S, Dawson E et al. 2008. The catalogue of somatic mutations in cancer (COSMIC). *Curr Protoc Hum Genet*. April;10(11). doi:10.1002/0471142905.hg1011s57.

Garcia-Manero G. 2010. Prognosis of myelodysplastic syndromes. *Hematol Am Soc Hematol Educ Program*. 2010;2010:330–337.

Garcia-Manero G. 2012. Myelodysplastic syndromes: Update on diagnosis, risk-stratification, and management. *Am J Hematol*. July;87(7):692–701. doi: 10.1002/ajh.23264. Review.

Gatto S, Ball G, Onida F, Kantarjian HM, Estey EH, and Beran M. 2003. Contribution of beta-2 microglobulin levels to the prognostic stratification of survival in patients with myelodysplastic syndrome (MDS). *Blood*. 102(5):1622–1625.

Gelsi-Boyer V, Brecqueville M, Devillier R, Murati A, Mozziconacci M-J, and Birnbaum D. 2012. Mutations in ASXL1 are associated with poor prognosis across the spectrum of malignant myeloid. *J Hematol Oncol*. March 21;5:12. doi: 10.1186/1756-8722-5-12.

Georgantas RW, Hildreth R, Morisot S, Alder J, Liu CG, Heimfeld S, Calin GA, Croce CM, Civin CI. 2007. CD34+ hematopoietic stem-progenitor cell microRNA expression and function: A circuit diagram of differentiation control. *Proc Natl Acad Sci USA*. February 20;104(8):2750–2755. Epub February 9, 2007.

Germing U, Hildebrandt B, Pfeilstöcker M, Nösslinger T, Valent P, Fonatsch C, Lübbert M et al. 2005. Refinement of the international prognostic scoring system (IPSS) by including LDH as an additional prognostic variable to improve risk assessment in patients with primary myelodysplastic syndromes (MDS). *Leukemia*. 19:2223–2231.

Glassman AB and Hayes KJ. 2003. Translocation (11;16)(q23;p13) acute myelogenous leukemia and myelodysplastic syndrome. *Ann Clin Lab Sci*. 33(3):285–288.

Gondek LP, Tiu R, O'Keefe CL, Sekeres MA, Thei KS, and Maciejewski JP. 2008. Chromosomal lesions and uniparental disomy detected by SNP arrays in MDS, MDS/MPD, and MDS-derivedAML. *Blood*. February 1;111(3):1434–1442.

Graubert T and Walter MJ. 2011. Genetics of myelodysplastic syndromes: New insights. *Hematol Am Soc Hematol Educ Program*. 2011;2011:543–549. Review.

Greenberg P, Cox C, LeBeau MM, Fenaux P, Morel P, Sanz G, Sanz M et al. 1997 International scoring system for evaluating prognosis in myelodysplastic syndromes. *Blood*. March 15;89(6):2079–2088. Erratum in: *Blood*. February 1, 1998;91(3):1100.

Greenberg PL, Tuechler H, Schanz J, Sanz G, Garcia-Manero G, Solé F, Bennett JM et al. 2012. Revised international prognostic scoring system for myelodysplastic syndromes. *Blood*. September 20, 2012;120(12):2454–2465. Epub June 27, 2012.

Haase D, Germing U, Schanz J, Pfeilstöcker M, Nösslinger T, Hildebrandt B, Kundgen A et al. 2007. New insights into the prognostic impact of the karyotype in MDS and correlation with subtypes: Evidence from a core dataset of 2124 patients. *Blood*. December 15;110(13):4385–4395. Epub August 28, 2007.

Hasle H, Baumann I, Bergsträsser E, Fenu S, Fischer A, Kardos G, Kerndrup G et al. 2004. The International Prognostic Scoring System (IPSS) for childhood myelodysplastic syndrome (MDS) and juvenile myelomonocytic leukemia (JMML). *Leukemia*. December 2004;18(12):2008–2014.

Heinrichs S, Kulkarni RV, Bueso-Ramos CE, Levine RL, Loh ML, Cheng Li, Neuberg D et al. 2009. Accurate detection of uniparental disomy and microdeletions by SNP array analysis in myelodysplastic syndromes with normal cytogenetics. *Leukemia*. September; 23(9):1605–1613. doi: 10.1038/leu.2009.82.

Hosokawa K, Katagiri T, Sugimori N, Ishiyama K et al. 2012. Favorable outcome of patients who have 13q deletion: A suggestion for revision of the WHO "MDS-U" designation. *Haematologica*. June 11, 2012;97(12):1845–1849. [Epub ahead of print]

Jiang Y, Dunbar A, Gondek LP, Mohan S, Rataul M, O'Keefe C, Sekeres M, Saunthararajah Y, and Maciejewski JP. 2009. Aberrant DNA methylation is a dominant mechanism in MDS progression to AML. *Blood*. February 5, 2009;113(6):1315–1325.

Kikuchi S, Kobune M, Iyama S, Sato T, Murase K, Kawano Y, Takada K et al. 2012. Prognostic significance of serum ferritin level at diagnosis in myelodysplastic syndrome. *Int J Hematol*. May;95(5):527–534. Epub March 11, 2012.

Kosmider O, Gelsi-Boyer V, Cheok M, Grabar S, Della-Valle V, Picard F, Viguié F et al. 2009. *TET2* mutation is an independent favorable prognostic factor in myelodysplastic syndromes (MDSs). *Blood*. October 8;114(15):3285–3291. Epub August 7, 2009.

Lam K and Zhang DE. 2012. RUNX1 and RUNX1-ETO: Roles in hematopoiesis and leukemogenesis. *Front Biosci*. September;17:1120–1139.

Lavau C, Du C, Thirman M, and Zeleznik-Le N. 2000. Chromatin-related properties of CBP fused to MLL generate a myelodysplastic-like syndrome that evolves into myeloid leukemia. *EMBO J*. September 1;19(17):4655–4664.

Li S, Yin CC, Medeiros LJ, Bueso-Ramos C, Lu G, Lin P. 2012. Myelodysplastic syndrome/acute myeloid leukemia with t(3;21)(q26.2;q22) is commonly a therapy-related disease associated with poor outcome. *Am J Clin Pathol*. July 2012;138(1):146–152.

Liao R, Sun J, Zhang L, Lou G, Chen M, Zhou D, Chen Z, and Zhang S. 2008. Micro RNAs play a role in the development of human hematopoietic stem cells. *J Cell Biochem*. 104:805–817.

Lindsley RC and Ebert BL. 2012. Molecular pathophysiology of myelodysplastic syndromes. *Annu Rev Pathol*. August 28. [Epub ahead of print]

Ma W, Kantarjian H, Bekele B, Donahue AC, Zhang X, Zhang ZJ, O'Brien S et al. 2009. Proteasome enzymatic activities in plasma as risk stratification of patients with acute myeloid leukemia and advanced-stage myelodysplastic syndrome. *Clin Cancer Res*. June 1, 2009;15(11):3820–3826. Epub May 19.

Mahesh S, Ginzburg Y, and Verma A. 2008. Iron over load in myelodysplastic syndromes. *Leuk Lymphoma*. March;49(3):427–438.

Mangan JK and Speck NA. 2011. *RUNX1* mutations in clonal myeloid disorders: From conventional cytogenetics to next generation sequencing, a story 40 years in the making. *Crit Rev Oncog*. 16(1–2):77–91.

Mitchell PS, Parkin RK, Kroh EM, Fritz BR, Wyman SK, Pogosova-Agadjanyan EL, Peterson A et al. 2008. Circulating microRNAs as stable blood-based markers for cancer detection. *Proc Natl Acad Sci USA*. July 29, 2008;105(30):10513–10518. Epub July 28, 2008.

Naqvi K, Garcia-Manero G, Sardesai S, Oh J et al. 2011. Association of comorbidities with overall survival in myelodysplastic syndrome: Development of a prognostic model. *J Clin Oncol*. June 1;29(16):2240–2246. Epub May 2, 2011.

Neumann F, Gattermann N, Barthelmes HU, Haas R, and Germing U. 2009. Levels of beta 2 microglobulin have a prognostic relevance for patients with myelodysplastic syndrome with regard to survival and the risk of transformation into acute myelogenous leukemia. *Leuk Res*. 2009;33(2):232–236.

O'Keefe C, McDevitt MA, and Maciejewski JP. 2010. Copy neutral loss of heterozygosity: A novel chromosomal lesion in myeloid malignancies. *Blood*. April 8; 115(14):2731–2739.
Oliva EN, Nobile F, and Iacopino P. 2010. Increases in miRNA-145 and miRNA-146a expression in patients with IPSS lower-risk myelodysplastic syndromes and del(5q) treated with lenalidomide. ASH Annual Meeting 2010 116: Abstracts 3631.
Oyarzo MP, Lin P, Glassman A, Bueso-Ramos CE, Luthra R, and Medeiros LJ. 2004. Acute myeloid leukemia with t(6;9)(p23;q34) is associated with dysplasia and a high frequency of flt3 gene mutations. *Am J Clin Pathol*. September 2004;122(3):348–358.
Pfeilstöcker M, Tüchler H, Schönmetzler A, Nösslinger T, Pittermann E. 2012. Time changes in predictive power of established and recently proposed clinical, cytogenetical and comorbidity scores for myelodysplastic syndromes. *Leuk Res*. February;36(2):132–139.
Rhyasen GW and Starczynowski DT. 2012. Deregulation of microRNAs in myelodysplastic syndrome. *Leukemia*. January;26(1):13–22. doi: 10.1038/leu.2011.221.
Rocquain J, Nadine C, Virginie T, Stéphane R, Anne M, Meyer N, Zoulika T et al. 2010. Combined mutations of ASXL1, CBL, FLT3, IDH1, IDH2, JAK2, KRAS, NPM1, NRAS, RUNX1, TET2 and WT1 genes in myelodysplastic syndromes and acute myeloid leukemias. *BMC Cancer*. 10:401.
Rowley JD, Reshmi S, Sobulo O, Musvee T, Anastasi J, Raimondi S, Schneider NR et al. 1997. All patients with the t(11;16)(q23;p13.3) that involves MLL and CBP have treatment-related hematologic disorders. *Blood*. July 15, 1997;90(2):535–541.
Sanada M and Ogawa S. 2012. Genome-wide analysis of myelodysplastic syndromes. *Curr Pharm Des*. 18(22):3163–3169.
Sanz G, Nomdedeu B, Such E, Bernal T, Belkaid M, Ardanaz MT, Marco V et al. 2008. Independent impact of iron overload and transfusion dependency on survival and leukemic evolution in patients with myelodysplastic syndrome. *Blood* (ASH Annual Meeting Abstracts). November 2008;112:640.
Schanz J, Tüchler H, Solé F, Mallo M, Luño E, Cervera J, Granada I et al. 2012. New comprehensive cytogenetic scoring system for primary myelodysplastic syndromes (MDS) and oligoblastic acute myeloid leukemia after MDS derived from an international database merge. *J Clin Oncol*. March 10;30(8):820–829. Epub February 13, 2012.
Slovak ML, Gundacker H, Bloomfield CD, Dewald G, Appelbaum FR, Larson RA, Tallman MS et al. 2006. A retrospective study of 69 patients with t(6;9)(p23;q34) AML emphasizes the need for a prospective, multicenter initiative for rare "poor prognosis" myeloid malignancies. *Leukemia*. 2006;20:1295–1297. doi: 10.1038/sj.leu.2404233. Published online April 20, 2006.
Smith AE, Mohamedali AM, Kulasekararaj A, Lim Z, Gäken J, Lea NC, Przychodzen B et al. 2010. Next-generation sequencing of the TET2 gene in 355MDS and CMML patients reveal slow-abundance mutant clones with early origins, but indicates node finite prognostic value. *Blood*. November 11;116(19):3923–3932. Epub August 6, 2010.
Soenen V, Preudhomme C, Roumier C, Daudignon A, Laï JL, Fenaux P. 1998. 17p Deletion in acute myeloid leukemia and myelodysplastic syndrome. Analysis of breakpoints and deleted segments by fluorescence in situ. *Blood*. February 1, 1998;91(3):1008–1015.
Sokol L, Caceres G, Volinia S, Alder H, Nuovo GJ, Liu CG, McGraw K et al. 2011. Identification of a risk dependent microRNA expression signature in myelodysplastic syndromes. *Br J Haematol*. April;153(1):24–32. doi: 10.1111/j.1365-2141.2011.08581.x. Epub February 21, 2011.
Starczynowski DT, Kuchenbauer F, Argiropoulos B, Sung S, Morin R, Muranyi A, Hirst M et al. 2010. Identification of miR 145 NS Mir 146 as mediators of the 5q syndrome phenotype. *Nat Med*. 2010;16:49–58.
Stauder R, Nösslinger T, Pfeilstöcker M, Sperr WR, Wimazal F, Krieger O, and Valent P. 2008. Impact of age and comorbidity in myelodysplastic syndromes. *J Natl Compr Canc Netw*. October;6(9):927–934.
Steensma DP. 2012. Historical perspectives on myelodysplastic syndromes. *Leuk Res*. August 23, 2012. pii: S0145–2126(12)00340–2. doi: 10.1016/j.leukres.2012.08.007.
Takatoku M, Uchiyama T, Okamoto S, Kanakura Y, Sawada K, Tomonaga M, Nakao S et al. 2007. Japanese National Research Group on Idiopathic Bone Marrow Failure Syndromes. Retrospective nationwide survey of Japanese patients with transfusion-dependent MDS and aplastic anemia highlights the negative impact of iron overload on morbidity/mortality. *Eur J Haematol*. June;78(6):487–494. Epub March 28, 2007.
Tiu RV, Visconte V, Traina F, Schwandt A, and Maciejewski JP. 2011. Updates in cytogenetics and molecular markers in MDS. *Curr Hematol Malig Rep*. 6:126–135.

Torsten H. 2012. Molecular genetics in myelodysplastic syndromes. *Leuk Res*. 36(2012):1459–1462.

Tuna M, Knuutila S, and Mill GB. 2009. Uniparental disomy in cancer. *Trends Mol Med*. March 2009;15(3):120–128. Epub February 25, 2009.

Valent P, Horny HP, Bennett JM, Fonatsch C, Germing U, Greenberg P, Haferlach T et al. 2007. Definitions and standards in the diagnosis and treatment of the myelodysplastic syndromes: Consensus statements and report from a working conference. *Leuk Res*. June;31(6):727–736. Epub January 25, 2007.

Vardiman J. 2012. The classification of MDS: From FAB to WHO and beyond. *Leuk Res*. December 2012;36(12):1453–1458. doi: 10.1016/j.leukres.2012.08.008. Epub August 30, 2012.

Vardiman JW, Thiele J, Arber DA, Brunning RD, Borowitz MJ, Porwit A, Harris NL et al. 2009. The 2008 revision of the World Health Organization (WHO) classification of myeloid neoplasms and acute leukemia: Rationale and important changes. *Blood*. July 30;114(5):937–951. doi: 10.1182/blood-2009-03-209262. Epub April 8, 2009. Review.

Vehmeyer K, Haase D, and Alves F. 2011. Increased peripheral stem cell pool in MDS: An indication of disease progression? *Leuk Res*. November;25(11):955–959.

Vercauteren SM, Sung S, Starczynowski DT, Lam WL, Bruyere H, Horsman DE, Tsang P, Leitch H, and Karsan A. 2010. Array comparative genomic hybridization of peripheral blood granulocytes of patients with myelodysplastic syndrome detects karyotypic abnormalities. *Am J Clin Pathol*. July;134(1):119–126.

Wang L, Fidler C, Nadig N, Giagounidis A, Della Porta MG, Malcovati L, Killick S et al. 2008. Genome-wide analysis of copy number changes and loss of heterozygosity in myelodysplastic syndrome with del(5q) using high-density single nucleotide polymorphism arrays. *Haematologica*. July;93(7):994–1000. Epub May 2, 2008.

Wang R, Gross CP, Halene S, and Ma X. 2009. Comorbidities and survival in a large cohort of patients with newly diagnosed myelodysplastic syndromes. *Leuk Res*. December 2009;33(12):1594–1598. Epub March 25, 2009.

Wimazal F, Sperr WR, Kundi M, Vales A, Fonatsch C, Thalhammer-Scherrer R, Schwarzinger I, and Valent P. 2008. Prognostic significance of serial determinations of lactate dehydrogenase (LDH) in the follow-up of patients with myelodysplastic syndromes. *Ann Oncol*. 2008;19:970–976. doi: 10.1093/annonc/mdm595.

Wlodarska I, Mecucci C, Marynen P, Guo C et al. 1995. TEL gene is involved in myelodysplastic syndromes with either the typical t(5;12)(q33;p13) translocation or its variant t(10;12)(q24;p13,). *Blood*. May 15, 1995;85(10):2848–2852.

Yoneda-Kato N, Look AT, Kirstein MN, Valentine MB, Raimondi SC, Cohen KJ, Carroll AJ, and Morris SW. 1996. The t(3;5)(q25.1;q34) of myelodysplastic syndrome and acute myeloid leukemia produces a novel fusion gene, NPM-MLF1. *Oncogene*. January 18, 1996;12(2):265–275.

Yoshida K, Sanada M, Shiraishi Y, Nowak D, Nagata Y, Yamamoto R, Sato Y et al. 2011. Frequent pathway mutations of splicing machinery in myelodysplasia. *Nature*. September 11;478(7367):64–69. doi: 10.1038/nature10496.

Zuo Z, Calin GA, dePaula HM, Medeiros LJ, Fernandez MH, Shimizu M, Garcia-Manero G, and Bueso-Ramos CE. 2011. Circulating microRNAs let-7a and miR-16 predict progression-free survival and overall survival in patients with myelodysplastic syndrome. *Blood*. 118:413–415.

29

Markers for Diagnosis, Prognosis, and Therapy of Acute Myeloid Leukemia

Ota Fuchs

CONTENTS

ABSTRACT Acute myeloid leukemia (AML) is a broad range of disorders that are all characterized by a block in the differentiation and by uncontrolled proliferation of hematopoietic progenitor cells. AML is the most frequent hematological malignancy in adults, with an annual incidence of three to four cases per 100,000 individuals. In approximately 20% of AML patients, the leukemia is secondary, arising from prior myelodysplastic syndrome or other hematological disorders, or is therapy-related (t-AML) following chemotherapy and radiotherapy. Complex karyotype and a high prevalence of tumor suppressor *TP53* mutation are typical for t-AML. Specific recurrent chromosomal abnormalities can be identified in approximately 55% of cases by cytogenetic analysis. These detected chromosomal aberrations are the most important tools to classify patients at their initial diagnosis and to divide them into favorable, intermediate, and unfavorable subgroups. Core-binding-factor AML characterized by translocation t(8;21)(q22;q22) and fusion gene *RUNX1-RUNX1T1* and inv(16)(p13.1;q22) or t(16;16)(p13.1;q22) and fusion gene *CBFB-MYH11* belongs to the genetic favorable-risk category. High-risk cytogenetics includes complex karyotypes, monosomy 7, monosomy 5, del(5q), or abnormalities of 3q. The age of the patient is also an important prognostic factor. Older patients have higher comorbidities and they tolerate the complications of chemotherapy poorly with a significant risk of death. However, approximately 45% of adult patients with AML have normal karyotype (cytogenetically normal AML; CN-AML patients) and are usually classified as an intermediate-risk group. These patients have a 5-year overall survival rate between 24% and 42%, but clinical outcome may vary greatly. The prognosis of AML with normal cytogenetics may be further subdivided based on genetic lesions. In recent years, a number of gene mutations as well as deregulated expression of genes have been reported. Additional molecular markers (gene expression profiles and microRNA (miR) expression signatures, single-nucleotide polymorphism arrays, and DNA methylation signatures) are studied and incorporated into clinical practice. Proteomic profiling helped also in identification of the new targets for specific therapies. Blood-based noninvasive methods and bone-marrow-based invasive methods are used for collection of starting material for analysis. Cytogenetic and molecular characterization has become not only a part of the standard diagnostic approach but also the basis for molecularly targeted therapies, such as all-trans-retinoic acid and arsenic trioxide in PML-RARA positive acute promyelocytic leukemia or FLT3 inhibitors in AML with FLT3 mutation.

KEY WORDS: *acute myeloid leukemia, prognosis, cytogenetics, mutations, expression, microRNA, proteomics.*

29.1 Introduction

Acute myeloid leukemia (AML) is a relatively rare cancer with a median age of presentation over 60 years but is the most common type of acute leukemia in adults. AML is a neoplasm of myeloid blasts resulting in rapid mortality if untreated. In younger patients, the incidence is two to three per 100,000, which rises to 13–15 per 100,000 in the seventh and eighth decades of age (Burnett et al., 2011). AML is characterized by uncontrolled proliferation of hematopoietic progenitor cells, an arrest of maturation due to blocked normal differentiation pathways, and activation of antiapoptotic pathways. AML is a highly heterogeneous disease in terms of morphology, cytochemistry of the leukemic population, immunophenotype, cytogenetics, and molecular abnormalities including, which may either be mutations, gene overexpression. To assist with patient diagnosis and management, classifications, such as the French–American–British (FAB) (Bennett et al., 1976, 1985) and the World Health Organization (WHO) classification (Vardiman et al., 2009; Döhner et al., 2010) (Table 29.1), were developed to define clinically relevant disease subtypes. FAB classification is still widely used in clinical setting that groups AML into eight subgroups (M0–M7) based on its degree of differentiation and morphology. Treatment for all subtypes of AML, except the M3 subtype, acute promyelocytic leukemia (APL), involves combination chemotherapy and a possible hematopoietic stem cell transplantation (SCT) as a part of consolidation therapy (Burnett, 2012; Paun and Lazarus, 2012). In APL, the balanced t(15;17) translocation rearranges the promyelocytic leukemia gene PML on chromosome 15 with retinoic acid receptor-α (RARA) located on chromosome 17. APL with fusion gene PML-RARA is treated with molecularly targeted therapy such as the differentiation-inducing agent all-trans-retinoic acid (ATRA) and arsenic trioxide (ATO), especially in cases where ATRA plus anthracycline-based chemotherapy cannot be used (Lo-Coco et al., 2008; Baljevic et al., 2011).

TABLE 29.1

WHO Classification (2008) of AML and Related Neoplasms

AML with recurrent genetic abnormalities
AML with t(8;21)(q22;q22); *RUNX1-RUNX1T1*
AML with inv(16)(p13.1q22) or t(16;16)(p13;q22); *CBFB-MYH11*
APL with t(15;17)(q22;q12); *PML-RARA*
AML with t(9;11)(p22;q23); *MLLT3-MLL*
AML with t(6;9)(p23;q34); *DEK-NUP214*
AML with inv(3)(q21q26.2) or t(3;3)(q21;q26.2); *RPN1-EVI1*
AML (megakaryoblastic) with t(1;22)(p13;q13); *RBM15-MKL1*
Provisional entity: AML with mutated *NPM1*
Provisional entity: AML with mutated *CEBPA*
AML with myelodysplasia-related changes
Therapy-related myeloid neoplasma
AML, not otherwise specified
AML with minimal differentiation
AML without maturation
AML with maturation
Acute myelomonocytic leukemia
Acute monoblastic/monocytic leukemia
Acute erythroid leukemia
Pure erythroid leukemia
Erythroleukemia, erythroid/myeloid
Acute megakaryoblastic leukemia
Acute basophilic leukemia
Acute panmyelosis with myelofibrosis
Myeloid sarcoma
Myeloid proliferations related to Down's syndrome
Transient abnormal myelopoiesis
Myeloid leukemia associated with Down's syndrome
Blastic plasmacytoid dendritic cell neoplasm

29.2 Diagnosis of AML

The diagnosis of APL must be confirmed by demonstration of t(15;17) translocation using fluorescent in situ hybridization (FISH) or reverse transcription polymerase chain reaction (Miller et al., 1992; Sanz et al., 2009).

The diagnosis of non-APL AML requires >20% blasts of myeloid lineage in marrow or blood (Vardiman et al., 2009). Weinkauff et al. (1999) found no differences in morphological features, cytochemistry, or immunophenotype between the blasts in peripheral blood (PB) and bone marrow (BM) samples in any of 30 cases studied. However, in 10 (23%) of 44 cases in which cytogenetic analysis was performed, PB but not BM samples were insufficient for analysis. The converse never occurred. PB and BM were collected after written informed consent was obtained from all patients in accordance with the Declaration of Helsinki. In cases with adequate metaphases, there was strong correlation between the cytogenetic results for PB and BM samples. Some PB samples with blast counts of 30% or more are adequate for diagnosis of AML, especially when therapy can be delayed until it is known that an adequate number of analyzable metaphases are recovered from the PB samples. Multicolor flow cytometry (MFC) has largely replaced histochemical staining for establishment of blast lineage (Kern et al., 2010; Hoffmann et al., 2012). Myeloid lineage antigens include CD33, CD13, CD117 (CKIT), CD14, CD64, CD41, and glycophorin A. Immunophenotyping is one of the independent prognostic factors in AML. Relevance of immunophenotypes to prognostic subgroups of age, white blood cells (WBCs), platelet count, and cytogenetics in de novo AML was studied (Li et al., 2011b). Human leukocyte antigen (HLA)-DR and CD14 expression associated with the elderly, highest WBC count, and unfavorable-risk cytogenetics. CD4, CD7, and CD11b expression correlated with highest WBC count and unfavorable-risk cytogenetics. CD64 expression was associated with higher WBC count, while that of CD13 was associated with lower platelet count. CD22, CD34, CD123, and terminal deoxynucleotidyl transferase (TdT) expression correlated with unfavorable-risk cytogenetics. CD5 expression was associated with normal platelet count, while that of CD19 was associated with children-favorable-risk cytogenetics. CD117 expression was associated with low WBC and lower platelet count. MPO and glycophorin A expression was associated with lower WBC count and favorable-risk cytogenetics. The results of the relevance analysis revealed the distribution characteristics of antigen expression in different AML prognostic subgroups.

The European Group for the Immunological Classification of Leukemias (EGIL) has proposed that AML could be defined immunologically by the expression of two or more of the following myeloid markers: MPO, CD13, CD33, CDw65, and CD117. With regard to classification, the prognostic significance of 21 antigens taken separately and with immunophenotype subgroups was evaluated and compared with other clinical and biological variables in 177 adult AML patients (Legrand et al., 2000). None of the antigens tested were associated with treatment outcome. However, patients with blasts disclosing a full expression of panmyeloid phenotype (defined by the expression of all five myeloid markers) had a higher complete remission (CR) rate and differed significantly in disease-free survival (DFS) and overall survival (OS) than patients whose cells expressed fewer than five of these markers. In multivariate analysis, only age, panmyeloid phenotype, performance status, and permeability glycophorin activity influenced treatment outcome. Three risk groups were defined based on CD34 and CD33 antigen expression (Plesa et al., 2008). The poor-risk group included patients with CD34-positive/CD33-positive or CD34-negative/CD33-negative disease. The intermediate-risk group included patients with CD34-positive/CD33-negative disease, and the favorable-risk group included patients with CD34-negative/CD33-positive disease.

Expression patterns of CD33 and CD15 also predicted outcome in AML patients (Derolf et al., 2008). CD33+/CD15– group had the highest frequency of unfavorable cytogenetic aberrations, the highest relapse rate and shortest median OS. CD33–/CD15+ group had high remission rate and did not have unfavorable cytogenetics.

Differences between childhood and adult AML, recommendations that are specific to children, and new diagnostic and prognostic molecular markers in pediatric AML have been recently presented by Creutzig et al. (2012).

29.3 Age and Performance Status of AML Patients

Biological age is an important prognostic variable adversely affecting both attainment of remission and relapse risk (Smith et al., 2011). Both response to therapy and OS worsen with increasing age of AML patients (Appelbaum et al., 2006; Juliusson et al., 2009, 2012; Szotkowski et al., 2010). This reflects concurrent comorbidities and higher frequencies of adverse cytogenetics. Older patients tolerate the intensive chemotherapy poorly with a significant risk of death during induction, mainly related to sepsis. The proportion of AML patients with unfavorable-risk cytogenetics increased markedly from 35% in patients' age younger than 56% to 51% in patients older than age 75 (Appelbaum et al., 2006). Much of the increase in unfavorable cytogenetics was due to a marked increase in the proportion of patients with loss of part or all of chromosomes 5 or 7, a finding seen in 12% of AML patients younger than age 56 but in 34% of patients older than age 75. Multidrug resistance was found in 33% of AML patients younger than 56, but in between 57% and 62% of cases in the higher age categories.

Poor performance status at diagnosis affects adversely prognosis. The presence of hepatosplenomegaly, a raised serum lactate dehydrogenase (LDH), and high PB white cell count (WBC) is associated with a worse prognosis (Ferrara and Mirto, 1996; Dalley et al., 2001; Greenwood et al., 2006).

Presence of secondary AML that arose from myelodysplastic syndrome (MDS), chronic myeloproliferative disorder, or was therapy-related AML (t-AML) does not per se convey unfavorable prognosis, and patients with secondary AML should be offered the chance benefiting from treatment according to the current frontline AML protocols (Larson, 2007; Ostgärd et al., 2010).

29.4 Cytogenetics

Cytogenetics remains the most important disease-related prognostic factor and powerful independent prognostic indicator in AML (Ferrara et al., 2008; Foran, 2010; Grimwade and Mrózek, 2011; Röllig et al., 2011). Till now, more than 100 balanced chromosomal rearrangements (translocations, insertions, and inversions) have been identified and cloned.

These chromosomal rearrangements are critical initiating events in the pathogenesis of AML. Karyotype analysis identifies biologically distinct subsets of AML that differ in their response to therapy and treatment outcome (Mrózek et al., 2004; Smith et al., 2011).

The latest revision (2008) of the WHO classification (Vardiman et al., 2009) is shown in Table 29.2.

Approximately 10% of adult AML and 20% of children AML are classified as having core-binding factor (CBF) leukemia with balanced chromosomal rearrangements that disrupt gene *RUNX1* (also known as *CBFA2* or *AML1*), which plays a critical role in hematopoiesis and leukemogenesis (Yamagata et al., 2005;

TABLE 29.2

Cytogenetic Abnormalities Used in the WHO Classification (2008) of AML

Cytogenetic abnormalities used to define entities within the WHO category of AML with recurrent genetic abnormalities
t(8;21)(q22;q22); *RUNX1-RUNX1T1*
inv(16)(p13.1q22) or t(16;16)(p13;q22); *CBFB-MYH11*
t(15;17)(q22;q12–21); *PML-RARA*
t(9;11)(p22;q23); *MLLT3-MLL*
t(6;9)(p23;q34); *DEK-NUP214*
inv(3)(q21q26.2) or t(3;3)(q21;q26.2); *RPN1-EVI1*
t(1;22)(p13;q13); *RBM15-MKL1*
Cytogenetic abnormalities sufficient to diagnose the WHO category of AML with myelodysplasia-related changes
Complex karyotype
(Defined as three or more unrelated abnormalities, none of which can be a translocation or
inversion associated with AML with recurrent genetic abnormalities)
Unbalanced abnormalities
−7 or del(7q)
−5 or del(5q)
i(17q), an isochromosome for long arm of chromosome 17 or t(17p)
−13 or del(13q)
del(11q)
del(12p) or t(12p)
del(9q)
idic(X)(q13), isodicentic X-chromosome
Balanced abnormalities
t(11;16)(q23;p13.3)
t(3;21)(q26.2;q22.1)
t(1;3)(p36.3;q21.1)
t(2;11)(p21;q23)
t(5;12)(q33;p12)
t(5;7)(q33;q11.2)
t(5;17)(q33;p13)
t(5;10)(q33;q21)
t(3;5)(q25;q34)

TABLE 29.3

Variation in Cytogenetic Risk Group—The UK Medical Research Council Cytogenetic Group Assignment 2010

Risk Group Assignment	Cytogenetic Abnormality	Comments
Favorable	t(15;17)(q22;q12–21) cytogenetic abnormalities	Irrespective of additional
		t(8;21)(q22;q22)
		inv(16)(p13.1q22) or t(16;16)(p13.1q22)
Intermediate		Other noncomplex entities, not classified as favorable or adverse
		Normal karyotype
Adverse		abn(3q) [excluding t(3;5)(q21–25;q31–35)], inv(3)(q21q26) or t(16;16)(p13;q22), add(5q), del(5q), −5, −7, add(7q), del(7q), t(6;11)(q27;q23), t(10;11)(p11–13;q23), other t(11;q23) [excluding t(9;11)(p21–22;q23) and t(11;19)(q23;p13)], t(9;22)(q34;q11), −17, abn(17p)
		Complex (>4 unrelated abnormalities)

Source: Grimwade, D. et al., *Blood*, 116, 354, 2010.
The table is based on multivariable analysis conducted in 5876 adults (16–59 years) treated in the UK Medical Research Council AML10, 12, and 15 trials.

Marcucci, 2006; Mrózek et al., 2008; Sangle and Perkins, 2011; Lam and Zhang, 2012). Patients with two specific, clonal, recurring cytogenetic abnormalities t(8;21)(q22;q22), inv(16)(p13.1q22) and t(16;16)(p13.1q22) are called CBF AML. Compared to other cytogenetic AML subgroups, CBF AML is considered a more favorable subset of AML (Table 29.3). CBF AML results in the formation of hybrid fusion genes called *RUNX1-RUNX1T1* (also known as *AML1-ETO*) and *CBFB-MYH11*, which can be quantified in patients before, during, and after the therapy, including SCT (Yin et al., 2012). Favorable karyotype patients have a good prognosis with CR rates exceeding 90%, a 5-year survival of at least 65%, and relapse rates too low and salvage rates too high to benefit from routine use of allograft in first complex remission (Smith et al., 2011). Patients with CBF AML and mutations in the *KIT* gene (exon 17) have a higher relapse risk (Paschka et al., 2006; Shimada et al., 2006). The mechanism underlying *KIT* gene mutations that adversely affects the prognosis involves phosphorylation of the KIT receptor after physiologic binding of KIT ligand, which activates downstream pathways supporting cell proliferation and survival (Lennartsson et al., 2005).

About 10%–20% of AML patients have adverse cytogenetics, which includes monosomal karyotype (monosomies of chromosomes 5 and/or 7 [−5/−7]) (Perrot et al., 2011; Kayser et al., 2012), abnormalities of 3q [abn(3q)] (Lugthart et al., 2010), or a complex karyotype often associated with TP53 alterations (Rücker et al., 2012). These patients are usually older (>60 years) and had MDS or were treated by chemotherapy or radiation. CR rates are around 60% and a 5-year survival about 10%. Due to this very poor prognosis with current therapies, an allograft in first CR or an experimental treatment approach may be justified (Fang et al., 2011; Paun and Lazarus, 2012).

The mixed-lineage leukemia (*MLL*) gene (also known as *ALL1* or *HRX*), located on chromosome 11q23, encodes a histone methyltransferase and is frequently rearranged in AML. Recurrent translocations of *MLL* are generally considered to confer a poor prognosis (Meyer et al., 2009). Fusion proteins with more than 60 partners were characterized, and these partners have also a significant effect on disease outcome (Coenen et al., 2011). Other entities that have been associated with poor prognosis are t(6;9)(p23;q34), t(9;22)(q34;q11), and 17p deletions (Smith et al., 2011).

Since cytogenetics provides the framework for current risk stratification schemes in AML with a major role in determining whether patients are candidates for allogenic transplant in first remission, it is important to have clearly defined risk groups not only for direction of patient management but also for of the comparison of data between different clinical results (Smith et al., 2011).

29.5 Mutations in the Molecular Markers

Approximately 45% of adult patients with AML have normal karyotype (cytogenetically normal AML [CN-AML] patients) and are usually classified as an intermediate-risk group.

Cytogenetic analysis is uninformative for these patients because they have vastly different clinical outcomes within this intermediate-risk group. Analysis of specific genetic abnormalities, not detectable by cytogenetics, and quantification of expression of specific genes with prognostic significance are valuable tools for more accurate risk stratification and clinical outcome prediction of these CN-AML patients (Ley et al., 2003, 2008; Schlenk et al., 2008; Foran, 2010; Abdel-Wahab et al., 2011; Burnett et al., 2011; Dombret, 2011; Rockova et al., 2011; Shen et al., 2011; Smith et al., 2011; Walker and Marcucci, 2011; Estey, 2012).

29.5.1 Mutations in the NPM1 Gene

Nucleophosmin 1 (NPM1) (also called nucleolar protein B23, numatrin, or NO38) is a multifunctional phosphoprotein that contains 294 amino acids (Okuwaki, 2008). NPM1 is one of the three nucleophosmin isoforms that are generated through alternative splicing. NPM1 resides predominantly in the nucleoli, but also continuously shuttles between nucleus and cytoplasm (Frehlick et al., 2007; Falini et al., 2009). The *NPM1* gene is located on chromosome 5q35 and is composed of 12 exons (Chan et al., 1989). NPM1 is essential for processing and transportation of ribosomal RNA and proteins, molecular chaperoning, and regulation of the stability of tumor suppressors, such as p53 and ARF (Borer et al., 1989; Herrera et al., 1995; Savkur and Olson, 1998; Colombo et al., 2002, 2005; Enomoto et al., 2006; Grisendi et al., 2006; Mariano et al., 2006; Yu et al., 2006; Maggi et al., 2008; Li and Hann, 2009). The ARF tumor suppressor is a protein that is transcribed from an alternate reading frame of the inhibitor of cyclin-dependent kinase CDK4. NPM1 can affect DNA replication, repair, and transcription by interacting with the components of chromatin such as histones and chromatin-remodeling proteins (Angelov et al., 2006; Amin et al., 2008a,b; Koike et al., 2010). NPM1 plays important roles in cell cycle (Ugrinova et al., 2007; Xiao et al., 2009). In addition, NPM1 may preferentially promote ribosome biogenesis in G1 and facilitate DNA replication during S-phase while supporting chromosome segregation in mitosis (Hisaoka et al., 2010).

Almost 40% of CN-AML patients have mutations in exon 12 of the *NPM1* gene that result in loss of tryptophan residues normally required for NPM1 binding to the nucleoli and in the generation of an additional nuclear export signal motif at the C-terminus of NPM1 that causes its abnormal cytoplasmic localization (Falini et al., 2005, 2006a, 2009, 2010a; Bolli et al., 2007; Liso et al., 2008; Falini, 2010b; Oelschlaegel et al., 2010). These mutations are the most common genetic alterations in adult CN-AML patients and are associated with female sex, higher WBC, increased blast percentage, and low or absent CD34 expression. Cytoplasmic nucleophosmin leukemic mutant is also rarely generated by an exon-11 NPM1 mutation (Albiero et al., 2007). AMLs with mutated NPM1 (NPM1c+) have distinct characteristics, including a significant association with a normal karyotype, involvement of different hematopoietic lineages, a specific gene expression profile, and, clinically, a better response to induction therapy and a favorable prognosis (Meani and Alcalay, 2009; Rau and Brown, 2009; Falini et al., 2010a). NPM1c+ maintains the capacity of wild-type NPM to interact with a variety of cellular proteins and impairs their activity by delocalizing them to the cytoplasm. NPM1c+ specifically inhibits the activities of the cell-death proteases, caspase-6 and caspase-8, through direct interaction with their cleaved, active forms, but not the immature procaspases. NPM1c+ not only affords protection from death ligand-induced cell death but also suppresses caspase-6/caspase-8-mediated myeloid differentiation (Leong et al., 2010).

After the discovery of NPM1-mutated AML in 2005 and its subsequent inclusion as a provisional entity in the 2008 WHO classification of myeloid neoplasms, several controversial issues remained to be clarified (Falini et al., 2011). It was unclear whether the NPM1 mutation was a primary genetic lesion and whether additional chromosomal aberrations and multilineage dysplasia (MLD) had any impact on the biologic and prognostic features of NPM1-mutated AML. Moreover, it was uncertain how to classify AML patients who were double-mutated for NPM1 and CCAAT/enhancer-binding protein alpha (CEBPA). Recent studies have shown that (1) the NPM1 mutant perturbs hematopoiesis in experimental models, (2) leukemic stem cells from NPM1-mutated AML patients carry the mutation, and (3) the NPM1 mutation is usually mutually exclusive of biallelic CEBPA mutations. Moreover, the biologic and clinical features of NPM1-mutated AML do not seem to be significantly influenced by concomitant chromosomal aberrations or MLD. NPM1-mutated AML with and without MLD showed overlapping immunophenotype (CD34 negativity) and gene expression profile (CD34 downregulation, homeobox (*HOX*) genes upregulation) suggesting NPM1-mutated AML as a founder genetic event that defines a distinct leukemia entity accounting for approximately one-third of all AML. Distinctive gene expression and microRNA (miR) signatures were found associated with AML bearing cytoplasmic mutated NPM1 (Verhaak et al., 2005; Garzon et al., 2008; Becker et al., 2010).

Approximately 40% of patients with *NPM1* mutations also carry *FLT3* internal tandem duplication (*FLT3-ITD*). Patients with *NPM1* mutations, who did not also have *FLT3* mutation, have generally more favorable prognosis (Gale et al., 2008; Scholl et al., 2008; Luo et al., 2009). The favorable prognosis of NPM1-mutated/FLT3-ITD negative patients might be explained by a higher bax/bcl-2 ratio (Del Poeta et al., 2010). These patients respond to induction therapy and stay in remission more likely. These patients may be exempted from allogenic hematopoietic SCT during the first CR because their outcome after conventional consolidation chemotherapy is the same as after allogenic transplantation. However, patients with *NPM1* mutations who also carry *FLT3* mutation have bad prognosis.

Moreover, *NPM1* mutations due to their frequency and stability may be used for minimal residual disease (MRD) monitoring in AML patients with a normal karyotype (Jaeger and Kainz, 2003; Bacher et al., 2009; Schnittger et al., 2009; Shook et al., 2009; Dvorakova et al., 2010).

29.5.2 FLT3 Mutations

The feline c-fms proto-oncogene product is a 170 kd glycoprotein with associated tyrosine kinase activity. Fms-like tyrosine kinase 3 (FLT3) and its ligand (FL) are important in hematopoietic progenitor cell proliferation and differentiation (Gilliland and Griffin, 2002). As a result of ligand binding, FLT3 receptor on the cell surface of hematopoietic progenitors dimerizes, resulting in activation of its tyrosine kinase domain (TKD), receptor autophosphorylation, and recruitment of downstream signaling molecules such as signal transducer and activator of transcription 5a (STAT5a) and the mitogen-activated protein kinase (MAPK) pathways leading to proliferative and pro-survival effects.

Internal tandem duplication (ITD) of base pairs within the juxtamembrane coding portion or point mutations in the second kinase domain occur in approximately 30% of patients with newly diagnosed AML and result in constitutive activation of the *FLT3* gene on chromosome 13q12 (Nakao et al., 1996; Yamamoto et al., 2001; Naoe and Kiyoi, 2004). *FLT3* mutations in the case of ITDs are associated with chemoresistance in the leukemic stem cells, shorter DFS and OS, and higher rate of relapse (Fröhling et al., 2002; Ravandi et al., 2010; Whitman et al., 2010; Patel et al., 2012). Specific gene expression signature associated with *FLT3*-ITD was described (Bullinger et al., 2008; Whitman et al., 2010). Overexpression of *FLT3*, HOX genes, and immunotherapeutic targets and decreased expression of erythropoiesis-associated genes are connected with *FLT3*-ITD. The prognostic significance of *FLT3* point mutations is less clear with conflicting results (Mead et al., 2008).

In clinical practice, a frequent approach to patients with poor prognostic AML is to offer allogenic SCT. Gale et al. (2005) found no benefit from any form of transplantation consolidation for patients with *FLT3-ITD*. Several inhibitors of FLT3 have entered clinical trials and are studied alone or mainly in combination with chemotherapy (Small, 2008; Weisberg et al., 2009; Kindler et al., 2010; Wiernik, 2010).

29.5.3 CCAAT/Enhancer-Binding Protein Alpha Mutations

The C/EBPα is the founding member of a family of related leucine zipper transcription factors that play important roles in myeloid differentiation (Tenen et al. 1997; Keeshan et al., 2003; Suh et al., 2006; Friedman, 2007; Pabst and Mueller, 2007). Members of this family consist of N-terminal transactivation domains, a DNA-binding basic domain, and a C-terminal leucine-rich dimerization region (Figure 29.1). The dimerization domain, known as "leucine zipper," contains leucine repeats that intercalate with leucine repeats of the dimer partner forming a coiled coil of α-helices in parallel orientation. C/EBPα

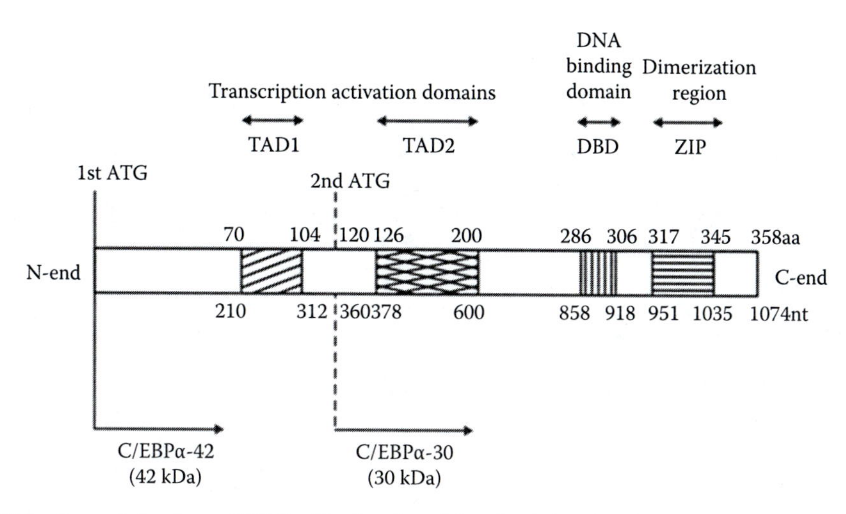

FIGURE 29.1 Transcription factor C/EBPα: The location of functional domain within the C/EBPα protein. Numbers directly above the schema indicate the amino acids of the human C/EBPα. Numbers directly under the schema indicate nucleotides (GenBank Accession No. NM_004364.2). The full-length 42 kDa form of C/EBPα protein and the shorter, dominant negative 30 kDa form of this protein are also shown.

mRNA is translated into two major proteins, C/EBPα p42 (42 kDa) and C/EBPα p30 (30 kDa), by ribosomal scanning mechanism in which a fraction of ribosomes ignore the first two AUG codons and initiate translation at the third AUG codon located 357 nucleotides downstream of the first one (Figure 29.1). The 30 kDa protein lacks the transactivating domain TAD1 (Figure 29.1) and was shown to inhibit DNA binding and transactivation by C/EBPα p42 (Pabst et al., 2001). C/EBPα p30 fails to induce myeloid differentiation (D'Alo' et al., 2003; Friedman, 2007). Targeted inactivation of C/EBPα in mice demonstrates its importance in the proper development and function of liver, adipose tissue, lung, and hematopoietic tissues (Wang et al., 1995; Flodby et al., 1996; Zhang et al., 1997). C/EBPα is highly expressed in these differentiated tissues where it controls differentiation-dependent gene expression and inhibits cell proliferation (Fuchs, 2007). Learning more about the precise molecular functions of the C/EBPα protein and how these are affected by leukemogenic mutations should lead to an improved understanding of the cellular functions that are disrupted in patients with AML.

CEBPA mutations were found in 10%–19% of CN-AML patients (Pabst et al., 2001; Gombart et al., 2002; Preudhomme et al., 2002; Fröhling et al., 2004; Lin et al., 2005; Fuchs et al., 2008, 2009). Two kinds of mutations were mainly described: (1) truncating, frameshift mutations occurring near the N-terminus in one of the two transcription activation domains (TAD1 and TAD2) on one allele and (2) in-frame insertions or deletions clustering within the C-terminal basic domain-leucine zipper (DBD and ZIP) on the other allele. Often, CN-AML patients with *CEBPA* mutations belong to FAB subtypes M1 or M2 and have one mutation toward N-end and one toward C-end, but other cases of mutations were also detected. Kato et al. (2011) showed that a mutation of *CEBPA* in one allele was observed in AML after MDS, while the two alleles are mutated in de novo AML. Favorable impact of *CEBPA* mutations was mainly observed in patients with biallelic mutation and with lack of *FLT3*-ITD (Radomska et al. 2006; Hou et al., 2009; Pabst et al., 2009; Wouters et al., 2009b; Dufour et al., 2010; Taskesen et al., 2011).

29.5.4 Partial Tandem Duplications of the *MLL* Gene

The *MLL* gene (also known as *ALL1* or *HRX*), located on chromosome 11q23, encodes a histone methyltransferase and is frequently rearranged in AML. Wild-type *MLL* is schematically presented in Figure 29.2. To date, *MLL* has been found in more than 60 different translocations with different fusion partners (De Braekeleer et al., 2005; Basecke et al., 2006). Partial tandem duplications of the *MLL* gene were first observed in CN-AML by Caligiuri et al. (1994). These duplications consist of an in-frame repetition of *MLL* exons in a 5′–3′ direction and lead to the change of the resulting transcript and protein. *MLL*-PTD is named according to the fused exons (mainly e9/e3, e10/e3, e11/e3).

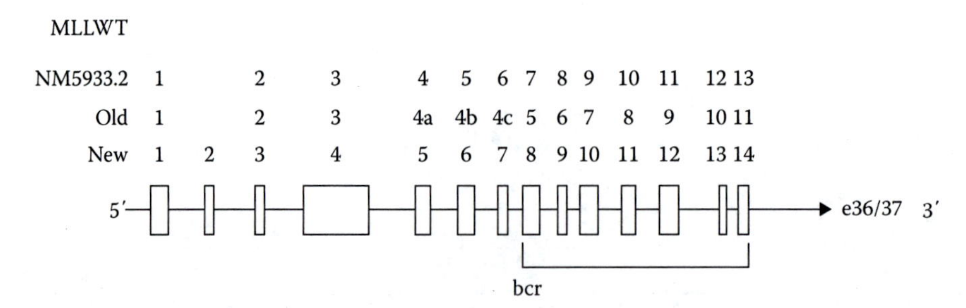

FIGURE 29.2 Exon–intron structure of the wild-type *MLL* gene involved in tandem and nontandem duplications. The nomenclature is different in various studies. (From Nilson, I. et al., *Br. J. Haematol.*, 93, 966, 1996; Strout, M.P. et al., *Proc. Natl. Acad. Sci. USA*, 95, 2390, 1998; Šárová, I. et al., *Cancer Genet. Cytogenet.*, 195, 150, 2009.) The *MLL* gene as a whole contains 36 or 37 exons according to the different nomenclatures, and the resulting product of its expression contains 3969 amino acids. In the case of *MLL*-PTD, e9/e3 are exons and introns between exons 3 and 9 inserted between exons 9 and 10 of the wild-type *MLL* and are duplicated by this way (the fusion of introns 2 and 9).

MLL-PTD is detectable in 5%–11% of patients with CN-AML (Schnittger et al., 2000; Döhner et al., 2002; Steudel et al., 2003; Döhner and Döhner 2008). *MLL*-PTD has been found also in PB and BM samples of healthy adults. However, in exon–intron structure of the wild-type *MLL* gene involved in tandem and nontandem duplications. The nomenclature is different in various studies (Nilson et al., 1996; Strout et al., 1998; Šárová et al., 2009). The *MLL* gene as a whole contains 36 or 37 exons according to the different nomenclatures, and the resulting product of its expression contains 3969 amino acids. In the case of *MLL*-PTD, e9/e3 are exons and introns between exons 3 and 9 inserted between exons 9 and 10 of the wild-type *MLL* and are duplicated by this way (the fusion of introns 2 and 9).

In contrast to the *MLL*-PTD in AML, *MLL*-PTD in healthy adults had often unusual exon fusions and showed a ladder on gel electrophoresis after the nested RT-PCR (Marcucci et al., 1998; Schnittger et al., 1998; Basecke et al., 2006). *MLL*-PTDs cooperate with silencing of the *MLL* wild-type allele by epigenetic mechanisms (Whitman et al., 2008a). *MLL*-PTDs contribute to leukemogenesis through hypermethylation of DNA and epigenetic silencing of tumor suppressor genes (Dorrance et al., 2006; Whitman et al., 2008a). Inhibitors of DNA methyltransferase and histone acetylase inhibitors and their combination can reactivate the wild-type allele in *MLL*-PTD-positive blasts (Whitman et al., 2005).

MLL-PTDs are associated with shorter duration of the CR and shorter relapse-free survival and event-free survival, but *MLL*-PTDs have no effect on OS (Döhner and Döhner 2008).

29.5.5 WT1 Mutations

The Wilms' tumor 1 (*WT1*) gene is located on chromosome 11p13 and encodes a zinc-finger transcriptional regulator that can function as tumor suppressor in patients with the WAGR (Wilms' tumor predisposition, aniridia, genitourinary abnormalities, and mental retardation) tumor predisposition syndrome (Haber et al., 1990) and as an oncogene in various leukemias, as well as other cancers (Miwa et al., 1992; King-Underwood et al., 1996; Ariyaratana and Loeb, 2007; Yang et al., 2007). Mutations in *WT1* gene were found in approximately 10% of AML patients (Paschka et al., 2008; Virappane et al., 2008; Gaidzik et al., 2009; Hou et al., 2010; Owen et al., 2010). Mutations are mainly localized in zinc-finger domains in exons 7 and 9 but can be also found in exons 1, 2, 3, and 8. The truncated WT1 protein is the result of frameshift mutations in exon 7. Truncated WT1 is without nuclear localization signal and does not bind to other interacting proteins as p53 and its homologue p73. Frameshift mutations in exon 9 are less frequent but there are also missense mutations. *WT1* mutations have been reported as an adverse prognostic factor in adult CN-AML and independently predict for poor outcome (Paschka et al., 2008; Virappane et al., 2008; Gaidzik et al., 2009; Renneville et al., 2009; Hou et al., 2010; Owen et al., 2010). *WT1* mutations lead to inferior rate of CR, higher incidence of relapse, and shorter relapse-free survival and OS. A recent study demonstrated that a single-nucleotide polymorphism (SNP) rs16754 in the WT1 mutational hot spot predicted favorable outcome in CN-AML (Damm et al., 2010a).

29.5.6 Isocitrate Dehydrogenase 1 and 2 Gene Mutations

Mardis et al. (2009) found recurring mutations in codon 132 of the isocitrate dehydrogenase 1 (*IDH1*) gene by sequencing a whole AML genome by next-generation sequencing (Mardis, 2011). The protein encoded by this gene is the enzyme that catalyzes the oxidative carboxylation of isocitrate to α-ketoglutarate leading to nicotinamide adenine dinucleotide phosphate production in Krebs cycle and was found in the cytoplasm and peroxisomes (Geisbrecht and Gould, 1999). Three classes of IDH isoenzymes exist in mammalian cells (two forms of mitochondrial IDH and cytosolic IDH). *IDH1* gene is localized to chromosome band 2q33.3 and *IDH2* gene to chromosome band 15q26.1 (Narahara et al., 1985; Oh et al., 1996). *IDH2* encodes the mitochondrial isoform that uses nicotinamide adenine dinucleotide phosphate as a cofactor. The same cofactor is also used by IDH1.

Most cancer-associated enzyme mutations result in constitutive activation or inactivation of the mutated enzyme. *IDH1* and *IDH2* mutations result in the new enzyme activity, production of 2-hydroxyglutarate, not shared by wild-type enzymes (Ward et al., 2010). This accumulation of 2-hydroxyglutarate induces global DNA hypermethylation, disrupts TET2 function because this enzyme is α-ketoglutarate-dependent, and impairs hematopoietic differentiation (Figueroa et al., 2010a). *TET2* is a homolog of the gene originally discovered at the chromosome ten–eleven translocation (TET) site in a subset of patients with AML. TET2 catalyzes the conversion of methylcytosine to 5-hydroxymethylcytosine, suggesting a potential role for TET proteins in epigenetic regulation (Gaidzik et al., 2012). Blocking the accumulation of 2-hydroxyglutarate through the inhibition of mutant IDH enzymes could represent a therapeutic target (Cazzola, 2010; Dang et al., 2010).

IDH1 mutations at codon R132 occur in CN-AML patients with a frequency of 5.5%–11% (Boissel et al., 2010; Gross et al., 2010; Schnittger et al., 2010; Wagner et al., 2010; Patel et al., 2011). A strong association between *IDH1* mutations and the *NPM1* mutation and M1 FAB subtype was observed. On the other hand, *IDH1* mutations are inversely associated with the M4 FAB subtype and expression of HLA-DR, CD13, and CD14 antigens. The prognostic impact of *IDH1* mutations in CN-AML is associated with a higher risk of relapse and a shorter OS (Abbas et al., 2010; Boissel et al., 2010; Marcucci et al., 2010; Paschka et al., 2010; Schnittger et al., 2010). Others (Chou et al., 2010a; Wagner et al., 2010; Patel et al., 2011), however, found no significant impact of *IDH1* mutations on CN-AML patients outcome. *IDH2* mutations in exon 4, including mainly codon R140 and in rare cases codon R172, had no prognostic impact (Thol et al., 2010). Both *IDH1* mutations and *IDH2* mutations can be also identified using high-resolution melting curve analysis (Noordermeer et al., 2011). Recent studies of Chou et al. (2011) and of Patel et al. (2012) showed high stability of *IDH2* mutations during disease evolution and their connection with favorable prognosis and with improved OS. Contrary to this observation, Boissel et al. (2010) found *IDH2* mutations independently associated with a higher risk of relapse and shorter OS. The prognostic impact of *IDH1* mutations and *IDH2* mutations needs further study as very controversial results were obtained. Green et al. (2010) observed no difference in outcome between *IDH1*-mutated and nonmutated patients when the results were stratified by an *NPM1* mutation status but an adverse outcome for *IDH1*-mutated patients when the results were correlated with *FLT3*-ITD mutation.

29.5.7 Mutations in Gene for DNA Methyltransferase 3A

About 22% of CN-AML patients have DNA methyltransferase 3A (*DNMT3A*) mutations. The most common *DNMT3A* mutation affects amino acid R882, but other parts of *DNMT3A* gene are also affected by mutations in CN-AML patients (Ley et al., 2010). *DNMT3A* mutations were mostly found in patients with acute myelomonocytic leukemia and acute monoblastic/monocytic leukemia and were significantly associated with increased white cell counts at diagnosis (Thiede, 2012).

Aberrant DNA methylation contributes to the pathogenesis of cancer (Watanabe and Maekawa, 2010; Rodríguez-Paredes and Esteller 2011; Taberlay and Jones, 2011). Clusters of CpG dinucleotides in promoters of tumor-suppressor genes are hypermethylated in cancer (HIC) genomes, and this hypermethylation results in reduced expression of the downstream gene. However, inhibition of DNA methyltransferases is only one potential mechanism of function of demethylating agents (5-azacytidine and decitabine). *DNMT3A* mutations do not change 5-methylcytosine content in AML genomes but are associated with poor survival (Markova et al., 2012; Ribeiro Tibúrcio et al., 2012). *DNMT3A* mutations are in many cases found together with *FLT3* mutations, *NPM1* mutations, and *IDH1* mutations. All these combinations of mutations have a significantly worse outcome.

29.5.8 *RAS* Mutations in CN-AML

Ras-signaling cascade contributes to the molecular pathogenesis of myeloproliferative disorders (Chan et al., 2004). Ras oncogenes (small GTPases) regulate mechanism of proliferation, differentiation, and apoptosis. *NRAS* (neuroblastoma RAS) mutations were detected in 9% of adult CN-AML patients and 14% of CN-AML patients younger than 56 or 60 years (Bowen et al., 2005; Bacher et al., 2006). There was no prognostic impact of these mutations in most studies (Ritter et al., 2004; Gaidzik and Döhner, 2008; Schlenk and Döhner, 2009). Mutations in other members of *Ras* family are rare in CN-AML and there was also no consistent effect on prognosis, but the presence of *Ras* mutations appears to sensitize AML blasts to high-dose cytarabine in vivo (Motyckova and Stone, 2010).

29.5.9 *BCOR* and *BCORL1* Mutations in CN-AML

Both *BCOR* and *BCORL1* genes are located on the X-chromosome and encode for large nuclear proteins that are ubiquitously expressed in human tissues. The BCOR protein acts as corepressor of BCL6; it can bind to other transcriptional factors and appears to play a key role in the regulation of hematopoiesis. BCORL1 is also a transcriptional corepressor and functional studies have shown that it can bind to class II histone deacetylases (HDAC4, HDAC5, and HDAC7) to interact with the CTBP1 corepressor and to affect the repression of E-cadherin (Tiacci et al., 2012). In AML, the *BCOR* gene is targeted by both translocations and mutations. *BCOR* mutations were detected in about 4% (10 of 262) of an unselected cohort of de novo CN-AML (Tiacci et al., 2012). *BCORL1* somatic mutations were found in about 6% of a series of 173 AML patients. Similarly to mutations of *BCOR* gene, most of the alterations affecting *BCORL1* gene were nonsense mutations. Analysis of a large series of CN-AML patients suggests that *BCOR* mutations may confer a poorer prognosis (Grossmann et al., 2011). Till now, no prognostic information is available for *BCORL1* mutations (Li et al., 2011a).

29.5.10 Other Gene Mutations in CN-AML

Mutations in *RUNX1* have been shown in approximately 10%–13% of CN-AML (Döhner and Döhner, 2008; Harada and Harada, 2009; Tang et al., 2009). These mutations were positively associated with *MLL*-PTD and negatively associated with *NPM1* and *CEBPA* mutations. They predicted a lower CR rate and shorter DFS and OS.

TET2, first described in 2008, includes frameshift, nonsense, and missense mutations lying across several of its 12 exons located on chromosome 4q24 (Abdel-Wahab et al., 2009; Bacher et al., 2010; Nibourel et al., 2010; Mohr et al., 2011). The direct influence of mutations in *TET2* on patient survival in CN-AML remains a disputable issue. *TET2* mutations were revealed in 10%–25% of CN-AML patients. Abdel-Wahab et al. (2009) showed a decreased survival rate in mutated *TET2* in comparison with wild-type *TET2* group of CN-AML. However, Nibourel et al. (2010) did not find significant impact of *TET2* mutation on clinical outcome of CN-AML patients, but they observed mutated *TET2* strongly associated with mutated *NPM1.* Recently, Metzeler et al. (2011) have found *TET2* mutations in 23% of CN-AML patients, and these mutations were associated with older age. In favorable-risk group of CN-AML patients with *CEBPA* mutation and/or mutated *NPM1* without *FLT3*-ITD, *TET2*-mutated patients had shorter event-free survival, lower CR rate, and shorter DFS and OS. In CN-AML patients with intermediate risk with wild-type *CEBPA* and wild-type *NPM1* without *FLT3*-ITD, *TET2* mutations were not associated with outcomes.

Casitas B-cell lymphoma (*CBL*) mutations were identified in rare cases of CN-AML (Makishima et al., 2009; Reindl et al., 2009; Bacher et al., 2010). Cbl is E3 ubiquitin ligase involved in degradation of activated receptor tyrosine kinases, including Src kinases (Makishima et al., 2009). Presence of these mutations was suggested to be involved in aberrant *FLT3* expression. FLT3 ligand-dependent hyperproliferation of *CBL* mutant cells could be abrogated by treatment with the specific inhibitor, midostaurin (PKC412).

Mutations in the additional sex comblike 1 (*ASXL1*) gene were analyzed in exon 12 in CN-AML patients, and 8.9% mutations were detected (Chou et al., 2010b). This mutation was closely associated with older age, male sex, *RUNX1* mutation, and expression of HLA-DR and CD34 (Chou et al., 2010b; Rocquain et al., 2010). Association with *FLT3*-ITD, *NPM1* mutation, *WT1* mutation, and expression of CD33 and CD15 were not detected. *ASXL1*-mutated patients had a shorter OS than patients without this mutation (Schnittger et al., 2013), but the mutation was not an independent adverse prognostic factor in multivariate analysis.

Phosphoinositide phospholipase Cβ1 (*PI-PLCβ1*) gene mutations are very rare in CN-AML (Damm et al., 2010b). Follo et al. (2009) described greater representation of these mutations (monoallelic deletions) in AML and their association with a worse clinical outcome.

Loss of function mutations and deletions encompassing the plant homeodomain finger 6 (*PHF6*) gene are present in 10/353 adult AMLs (Van Vlierberghe et al., 2011) and are associated with reduced OS (Patel et al., 2012).

29.5.11 European LeukemiaNet Standardized Reporting System for Correlation of Cytogenetics and Molecular Genetic Data in AML with Clinical Data

The karyotype is so far the most important prognostic parameter in AML. Molecular mutations have been analyzed to subdivide AML with normal karyotype into prognostic subsets. Grossmann et al. (2012) tried to develop a prognostic model for the entire AML cohort solely based on molecular markers. They studied 1000 patients with cytogenetic data for the following molecular alterations: *PML-RARA*, *RUNX1-RUNX1T1*, *CBFB-MYH11*, *FLT3*-ITD, and *MLL*-PTD, as well as mutations in *NPM1*, *CEBPA*, *RUNX1*, *ASXL1*, and *TP53*. *PML-RARA* rearrangement or *CEBPA* double mutations were very favorable. *RUNX1-RUNX1T1*, *CBFB-MYH11*, or *NPM1* without FLT3-ITD were favorable. *MLL*-PTD and/or *RUNX1* mutation and/or *ASXL1* mutation was unfavorable, and *TP53* mutations very unfavorable (Grossmann et al., 2012; Patel et al., 2012; Sebaa et al., 2012). This comprehensive molecular characterization provides a more powerful model for prognostication than cytogenetics.

29.6 Overexpression of Marker Genes with Prognostic Relevance

Alterations in the expression of genes belonging to signal transduction pathways as well as transcription factors are known to play a functional role in the pathogenesis of AML (Baldus and Bullinger, 2008). Therefore, these marker genes are implicated in the process of leukemogenesis, and their overexpression may be useful to predict outcome in CN-AML patients.

29.6.1 WT1 Gene Expression

The *WT1* gene overexpression was found in several leukemias, including AML (Cilloni et al., 2009). WT1 mRNA levels in the PB can predict relapse after achieving CR, and its levels after consolidation therapy are closely correlated with DFS and OS and with early relapse (Cilloni et al., 2009; Gianfaldoni et al., 2010; Miyawaki et al., 2010). Monitoring of *WT1* expression is significant predictor of relapse in AML patients after hematopoietic cell transplantation (Lange et al., 2011). At least 36 isoforms of WT1 protein are produced from the same DNA template as a result of alternative transcription initiation, alternative pre-mRNA splicing and mRNA editing, and alternative translation initiation (Kramarzova et al., 2012; Lopotová et al., 2012). Isoform profiles were independent of total *WT1* expression. There was a trend toward higher risk of relapse associated with the overexpression of isoform B in adult AML (Kramarzova et al., 2012).

29.6.2 Brain and Acute Leukemia, Cytoplasmic Expression

The *BAALC* gene, located on chromosome 8q22.3, is primarily expressed in neuroectoderm-derived tissues and in hematopoietic precursors and encodes a protein with unknown function (Baldus et al., 2003, 2006; Langer et al., 2008; Santamaria et al., 2010). High level of *BAALC* expression showed a higher refractoriness to induction treatment, lower CR rate after salvage therapy, and lower OS and relapse-free survival in intermediate-risk AML (Santamaria et al., 2010). The *BAALC* expression is considered an independent prognostic factor in CN-AML. High *BAALC* expression was associated with *FLT3*-ITD and high *ETS*-related gene (*ERG*) expression in multivariable analysis (Baldus et al., 2006). High *BAALC* expression is also connected with overexpression of genes involved in drug resistance (*MDR1*) and stem cell markers (*CD133, CD34, KIT*). In low *BAALC* expressers, genes associated with undifferentiated hematopoietic precursors and unfavorable outcome predictors were downregulated, while *HOX* genes and *HOX* gene-embedded miR were upregulated (Schwind et al., 2010). Insulin-like growth factor-binding protein 7 (IGFBP7) has been identified as a tumor suppressor in solid tumors. IGFBP7 is BAALC associated protein and is abberantly overexpressed in majority of AML at diagnosis (Heesch et al., 2010). Furthermore, high IGFBP7 was associated with the regulation of the proliferation of leukemic cells and might be involved in chemotherapy resistance. Global *miR* expression analysis did not reveal significant differences between different rate *BAALC* expression groups (Langer et al., 2008). Inverse association between the expression of *miR-148a* and *BAALC* was revealed (Schwind et al., 2010).

29.6.3 *ERG* (V-ETS Erythroblastosis Virus E26 Oncogene Homolog) Expression

ERG, located at chromosome band 21q22, is downstream effector of signaling transduction pathways involved in the regulation of cell proliferation, differentiation, and apoptosis (Marcucci et al., 2005, 2007; Mrózek et al., 2007; Metzeler et al. 2009; Schwind et al., 2010). CN-AML patients with overexpression of *ERG* have been reported to have a poor clinical outcome. When combined with other known prognostic markers, *ERG* expression can improve the molecular risk-based stratification of patients with CN-AML. Low *ERG* expression is associated with downregulation of genes involved in the DNA methylation machinery and upregulation of *miR-148a*, which targets DNA methyltransferase 3B (*DNMT3B*) and with better outcome (Schwind et al., 2010).

29.6.4 Meningioma 1 Expression

Meningioma 1 (*MN1*) is located at 22q11 and its overexpression is associated with lower response rate after first course of induction therapy and poor clinical outcome for CN-AML patients. Moreover, high *MN1* expression was connected with a higher relapse rate and worse relapse-free survival and OS (Heuser et al., 2006; Grosveld, 2007; Langer et al., 2009). *MN1* expression levels were directly correlated with *BAALC* expression levels and with the expression of genes reported as associated with a *BAALC* expression signature, specifically with expression of *CD34* and *ABCB1* (*MDR1*) and several other genes (Langer et al., 2008, 2009). *MN1* expression levels were negatively connected with expression of *HOX* genes and with *NPM1*-mutated CN-AML (Langer et al., 2009). *MN1*-associated miR expression signature comprises 15 miRs, and expression of 8 miRs (*hsa-miR-126* family) was positively correlated and expression of 7 miRs (*hsa-miR-16, hsa-miR-19a,* and *hsa-miR-20a*, all members of *miR-17–92* polycistron) negatively correlated with *MN1* expression (Langer et al., 2009). *MN1* overexpression conferred resistance to the differentiation activity of all-trans-retinoic acid (ATRA) in AML (Heuser et al., 2007).

29.6.5 Ecotropic Viral Integration Site 1 Expression

Human ecotropic viral integration site 1 (EVI1) is localized to chromosome 3 band q26, spans 60kb, and contains 16 exons (Goyama and Kurokawa, 2010). High *EVI1* expression occurs in approximately 8% of patients with de novo AML (Barjesteh van Waalwijk van Doom-Khosrovani et al., 2003). High *EVI1* expression was observed not only in AML carrying the chromosome 3 abnormalities but also in CN-AML (Lugthart et al., 2008; Santamaria et al., 2009; Gröschel et al., 2010) and in both groups connected with poor treatment response. *EVI1* overexpression defines a poor prognostic subset of *MLL*-rearranged AML (Gröschel et al., 2013).

29.6.6 Other Molecular Marker Gene Expressions

The preferentially expressed antigen of melanoma (*PRAME*) gene was shown to be expressed in high levels in AML. PRAME mRNA was observed in about one-third of AML cases, and there was a good correlation between PRAME mRNA level and hematological remission and relapse. It may be also a useful marker to detect MRD after allogenic transplantation (Paydas et al., 2005; Qin et al., 2009). Epping et al. (2005) showed that PRAME is a repressor of retinoic acid signaling, but Steinbach et al. (2007) did not confirm this mechanism in the pathogenesis of AML. Specific immunotherapies for patients with AML using leukemia-associated antigens (LAAs) as target structures might be a therapeutic option. Expression of genes for these antigens has prognostic importance (Greiner et al., 2008).

ALL1-fused gene from chromosome 1q (*AF1q*) gene overexpression in CN-AML patients is associated with a significantly greater incidence of concurrent *FLT3*-ITD and with a poor outcome (Strunk et al., 2009). NC-AML patients with low *AF1q* expression had better OS and CR rate than patients with high AF1q mRNA level.

High *MLL5* expression is associated with a favorable outcome of CN-AML patients and enables identification of a significant proportion of patients with favorable prognosis that is not identified by other markers' analyses (Damm et al., 2011b).

Increased expression of the phosphoinositide phospholipase Cβ1 (*PI-PLC β1*) gene is an independent prognostic factor in CN-AML and is associated with a significantly shorter OS but with no difference for relapse-free survival (Damm et al., 2010b).

The Rho family of small GTPases, including Rho, Rac, and Cdc42, functions as critical mediators of signaling pathways from plasma membrane regulating actin assembly, migration, proliferation, and survival in hematopoietic cells. *RhoH* gene, also known as translocation three four (*TTF*), encodes a 191-amino acid protein belonging to the Rho family (Gu et al., 2005; Iwasaki et al., 2008). Rho H functions as a negative regulator for interleukin 3 (IL3)-induced signals through modulation of the JAK-STAT (Janus kinase signal transducer and activator of transcription)-signaling pathway (Gündogdu et al., 2010). Low RhoH levels are connected with an upregulation of IL3-dependent cell growth, STAT5 activity, and an increase of CD123 surface expression that has been described in AML patients (Gündogdu et al., 2010). Multivariate analysis demonstrated that low expression of *RhoH* was an independent unfavorable prognostic factor for both OS and DFS of AML in the intermediate-risk group (Iwasaki et al., 2008).

Activation of notch signal pathway (expression of *Notch1*, *Jagged1*, and *Delta1* as members of this pathway) is associated with a poorer prognosis for AML patients with intermediate risk (Xu et al., 2011).

The forkhead transcription factors (FOXOs) are direct target of the PI3/AKT (protein kinase B) signaling, and they integrate the signals of several other transduction pathways at the transcriptional level. The PI3/AKT/FOXO signaling pathway is upregulated in AML. High *FOXO3a* expression is associated with a poorer prognosis in CN-AML (Santamaria et al., 2009), and the increased levels of both total and highly phosphorylated FOXO3a correlate with higher proliferation and blood blasts, and these high levels of FOXO3a are an adverse prognostic factor in AML (Kornblau et al., 2010).

BM neoangiogenesis plays an important pathogenetic and possible prognostic role in AML (Loges et al., 2005; Lee et al., 2007; Hou et al., 2008; Mourah et al. 2009). Multivariable analysis showed that the levels of vascular endothelial growth factor (VEGF) transcript isoform 121 (VEGF121) remained an independent prognostic factor for either event-free survival or OS (Mourah et al., 2009). High levels of VEGF121 were significantly related to a worse prognosis. Angiopoietin-2 (*Ang2*) gene expression represents also an independent prognostic factor in AML with intermediate risk, and high *Ang2* expression is associated with an unfavorable prognosis (Loges et al., 2005; Lee et al., 2007; Hou et al., 2008). High vascular endothelial growth factor C (*VEGFC*) expression appeared strongly associated with reduced CR rate and reduced OS and event-free survival in adult AML independent of cytogenetic risk and WBC count (de Jonge et al., 2010). High *VEGFC* expression was related to enhanced chemoresistance and predicted adverse long-term prognosis.

Transforming growth factor beta (TGFβ) superfamily receptors activin receptor-like kinase (ALK)-1 and ALK-5 have an important role in endothelial cells behavior and might be involved in the pathogenesis of AML. *ALK-1* and *ALK-5* are both expressed by the majority of AML patients. *ALK-5* expression has a significant negative impact on CR achievement and OS of AML patients (Otten et al., 2011).

Dysregulation of the Wnt/β-catenin pathway has been observed in various malignancies, including AML (Gandillet et al., 2011). Overexpression of β-catenin is an independent adverse prognostic factor in AML (Ysebaert et al., 2006; Chen et al., 2009).

Chemokine (C-X-C motif) receptor 4 (CXCR4) retains hematopoietic progenitors and leukemia cells within the marrow microenvironment. Multivariate analysis revealed *CXCR4* expression as an independent prognostic factor for disease relapse and survival (Konoplev et al., 2007; Spoo et al., 2007; Tavernier-Tardy et al., 2009). Low *CXCR4* expression correlated with a better prognosis, resulting in a longer relapse-free survival and OS.

Many studies of AML have linked the overexpression of ABCB1 (also named permeability glycoprotein, Pgp), a member of ATP-binding proteins coded by the multidrug resistance gene (*MDR1*), to poor prognosis (Leith et al., 1999; Steinbach and Legrand, 2007; Trnkova et al., 2007). Other drug resistance proteins BCRP (breast cancer resistance protein) (also named ABCG2) and LRP (lung resistance protein) have also an adverse impact (Huh et al., 2006; Damiani et al., 2010).

29.7 Gene Expression Profiling in CN-AML

Gene expression profiling (GEP) was described 12 years ago by Golub et al. (1999). GEP analyses on the basis of microarrays allow the simultaneous characterization of thousands of genes. GEP is useful for the classification of leukemias. In CN-AML, microarray GEP has been applied to identify expression signatures in order to predict clinical outcome within this very heterogeneous group of patients (Kohlmann et al., 2010).

Bullinger et al. (2004, 2006), Bullinger and Valk (2005) and Radmacher et al. (2006) defined by GEP two novel molecular subclasses of CN-AML with significant differences in survival times with respect to the presence or absence of *FLT3* mutations and the FAB subtypes.

NPM1 gene mutations are connected with specific gene expression pattern in CN-AML (Alcalay et al., 2005; Verhaak et al., 2005; Wilson et al., 2006; Garzon et al., 2008; Becker et al., 2010). This specific gene expression signature was characterized by the activation of *HOX* genes including a particular subset of HOX *TALE* (three amino acid loop extension); genes distinguish themselves from typical homeodomains containing genes. Downregulated in the *NPM1* mutation group were genes whose low expression is associated with better prognosis in CN-AML as *BAALC, MN1, ERG*, and multidrug resistance genes.

Comparison of gene expression between biallelic *CEBPA* mutation and monoallelic *CEBPA* mutation AML was described by Dufour et al. (2010). Expression of multiple members of the HOX gene family (*HOXA5, HOXA9, HOXA10, HOXB2,* and *HOXB6*), *CD34*, and lymphoid markers *CD6, CD52,* and *TSPO* (gene for translocator protein, benzodiazepine receptor) is downregulated in CN-AML patients with biallelic *CEBPA* mutation.

Specific gene expression signatures associated with *FLT3*-ITD and *FLT3*-TKD (mutations in the TKD) were described (Neben et al., 2005; Bullinger et al., 2008; Whitman et al., 2008b, 2010). Overexpression of *FLT3*, HOX genes (*HOXB3, HOXB5, PBX3, MEIS1*), and immunotherapeutic targets (*WT1, CD33*) and underexpression of leukemia-associated (*MLLT3, TAL1*) and erythropoiesis-associated genes (*GATA3, EPOR, ANK1, HEMGN*) is typical for *FLT3*-ITD, whereas overexpression of gene for transcription factor FOXA1 containing forkhead box was observed in *FLT3*-TKD (Neben et al., 2005; Whitman et al., 2010). Whereas the predictive value for *FLT3*-ITD was relatively high (77%), the high number of false predictions eliminates GEP as an investigational tool for research studies waiting on an entrance to clinical practice and decision making (Verhaak et al., 2009; Wouters et al., 2009a; Marcucci et al., 2011a). GEP technique seems not to be in future a primary diagnostic tool but will be used in many cases as a confirmative method.

29.8 MicroRNA Expression Profiling

miRs are small noncoding RNAs of 19–25 nucleotides that function as negative regulators of gene expression by causing target mRNA cleavage or by interfering with target mRNA translation. Dysregulation of miRs plays an important role in the pathogenesis of many cancers based on their involvement in basic cellular functions (Nana-Sinkam and Croce, 2010; Zhu et al., 2012). In addition, miRs have the capacity to target tens to hundreds of genes simultaneously. Thus, they are attractive candidates as prognostic and diagnostic biomarkers and therapeutic targets in cancer.

miR expression signatures have been correlated with recurrent molecular aberrations in AML. *NPM1* mutations associate with upregulation of *miR-10a, miR-10b, and miR-196a*, all lying in the genomic cluster of *HOX* genes that are overexpressed (Garzon et al., 2008; Becker et al., 2010). Upregulation of *miR-181a* and *miR-181b* expression is associated with *CEBPA* mutations in CN-AML (Marcucci et al., 2008, 2009, 2011b). Another miR significantly associated with a prolonged OS is *miR-212* (Sun et al., 2013). *miR-212* is also associated with prolonged event-free and relapse-free survival. High *miR-212* expression levels are associated with a gene expression profile that is significantly enriched for genes involved in the immune response. However, the prognostic significance of *miR-212* did not correlate with specific AML subtype (Sun et al., 2013). *FLT3*-ITD was observed to be associated with *miR-155* upregulation and *miR-144* and *miR-451* downregulation (Whitman et al., 2010). Genome-wide profiling identified aberrantly expressed miR associated with R172 *IDH2*-mutated CN-AML patients (Marcucci et al., 2010). The most upregulated *miR* genes were genes of *miR-125* family (*miR-125a* and *miR-125b*), *miR-1,* and *miR-133.* The most downregulated *miR* genes were *miR-194-1*, *miR-526*, *miR-520a-3p,* and *miR-548b*. Recently, *miR-3151* was discovered in intron 1 of *BAALC*. AML patients exhibiting high *miR-3151* expression had worse outcome than patients expressing low levels. High expression of *miR-3151* is an independent prognosticator for poor outcome in CN-AML (Eisfeld et al., 2012).

Recent studies have also shown that clinical outcome in CN-AML is affected by changes in miR expression (Ramsingh et al., 2010). Overexpression of *miR-20a, miR-25, miR-191, miR-199a,* and *miR-199b* adversely affected OS (Garzon et al., 2008; Fatica, 2012).

29.9 DNA Methylation Arrays

DNA cytosine methylation in CpG islands regulates gene expression. Aberrant methylation of specific genes was observed in cancer including leukemia, although little is known about the mechanisms of this specific gene set methylation (Saied et al., 2012). Genome-wide promoter DNA methylation profiling revealed unique AML subgroups and methylation patterns that are associated with clinical outcome (Bullinger and Armstrong, 2010; Figueroa et al., 2010b). DNA methylation profiles segregate patients with *CEBPA* mutations from other subtypes of leukemia and defined four epigenetically distinct forms of AML with *NPM1* mutations. Epigenetic modification of the *CEBPA* promoter regions was also described, and *CEBPA* hypermethylation appeared to be favorable prognostic marker in addition to *NPM1* mutation with lack of *FLT3*-ITD and *CEBPA* biallelic, double mutations (Hackanson et al., 2008; Lin et al., 2011; Szankasi et al., 2011). Lugthart et al. (2011) found that the promoter DNA methylation signature of *EVI1* AML blast cells differed from normal BM cells and other AMLs and contained many hypermethylated genes. EVI1 was observed to physically interact with *DNMT3A* and *DNMT3B* and colocalize with them in nuclei, and complex is involved in EVI1-mediated transcriptional repression. Cases with the significantly higher levels of EVI1 are associated with many more methylated genes (Lugthart et al., 2011). In high-risk MDS and in AML after MDS, methylation of *CDKN2b* (p15/INK4b/, inhibits CDK4), *CDH* (E-cadherin) and *HIC1* was associated with failure to achieve CR after induction chemotherapy (Grovdal et al., 2007). Low global luminometric methylation assay (LUMA) levels correlated with an increased CR rate and methylation of *CDKN2b* correlated with better DFS and OS in uni- and multivariate analysis (Deneberg et al., 2010). In order to fully understand the role of DNA methylation in AML, a global view of the AML methylome is required (Saied et al., 2012). Integration of genetic and epigenetic information is an important predictor of outcome and treatment response in AML, including response to allogeneic hematopoietic SCT. Many of the identified genetic alterations not only represent independent prognostic factors but also may constitute targets for specific therapeutic intervention (Marcucci et al., 2011a).

29.10 Conclusion and Future Directions

Cytogenetic analysis was the major tool for predicting outcome and guiding therapy. Improved molecular knowledge and more reliable information concerning rarer recurring cytogenetic aberrations have led to reclassification of a significant proportion of patients as adverse risk, which includes those with *FLT3*-ITD, *RUNX1* mutation, *MLL*-PTD, or *EVI1* overexpression and who lack a favorable cytogenetic abnormality.

CN-AML is very heterogeneous on the molecular level and harbors many genetic alterations that define new molecular subgroups. This molecular heterogeneity of CN-AML is not fully reflected in current classification systems (Vardiman et al., 2008; Döhner et al., 2010). Molecular markers with prognostic significance are very important for future therapies. Decision over whether to allograft a patient in first CR depends on the evaluation in a risk/benefit analysis in prognostic scoring system (Smith et al., 2011). The favorable cytogenetic risk group is now supplemented by CN-AML with mutant *NPM1* or biallelic *CEBPA* mutations in the absence of *FLT3*-ITD (Döhner et al., 2010). These CN-AML patients may not need to be referred for allogenic SCT in first CR (Table 29.4) (Burnett et al., 2011).

TABLE 29.4

The Ability of the Four European LeukemiaNet (ELN) Groups to Predict Treatment Outcome

Risk Genetic Group	Subsets
Favorable	t(8;21)(q22;q22); *RUNX1-RUNX1T1*
	inv(16)(p13.1q22) or t(16;16)(p13.1q22); *CBFB-MYH11*
	Mutated *NPM1* without FLT3-ITD (normal karyotype)
	Mutated *CEBPA* (normal karyotype)
Intermediate-I	Mutated *NPM1* and *FLT3*-ITD (normal karyotype)
	Wild-type *NPM1* and *FLT3*-ITD (normal karyotype)
	Wild-type *NPM1* without *FLT3*-ITD (normal karyotype)
Intermediate-II	t(9;11)(p22;q23); *MLLT3-MLL*
	Cytogenetic abnormalities not classified as favorable or adverse
Adverse	inv(3)(q21q26.2) or t(3;3)(q21q26.2), *RPN1-EVI1*
	t(6;9)(p23;q34); *DEK-NUP214*
	t(v;11)(v;q23); *MLL* rearranged
	−5 or del(5q)
	−7
	abn(17p)
	Complex karyotype
	t(10;11)(p11–13;q23),
	other t(11;q23) [excluding t(9;11)(p21–22;q23)
	and t(11;19)(q23;p13)],
	t(9;22)(q34;q11),
	−17, abn(17p)
	Complex karyotype (three or more chromosome abnormalities in the absence of abnormalities described earlier in this table)

Source: Mrózek, K. et al., *J. Clin. Oncol.*, 30, 4515, 2012.

The table is based on analysis conducted in a relatively large cohort of 1550 adult patients with primary AML similarly treated. The patients did not undergo allogenic SCT in the first CR.

Low expression of *BAALC* is also associated with favorable outcome in CN-AML (Santamaria et al., 2010), but not in association with *FLT3, NPM1,* and *CEBPA* mutations, and may not be prognostic in older patients (Langer et al., 2008). Low *BAALC* expression is an important factor for CR achievement and longer DFS. Even better OS is reached in CN-AML patients who had low *ERG* expression in addition to low *BAALC* expression (Burnett et al., 2011). The similarity of *BAALC* and *ERG* expression signatures between younger and older CN-AML patients and the fact that these molecular markers affect similarly outcomes in the group of younger and older than 60-year CN-AML patients suggest that older patients with favorable molecular risk factors, such as low *BAALC* and *ERG* expression, if treated more intensively, might have outcomes comparable with those of younger CN-AML patients with the same molecular markers (Schwind et al., 2010). Patients with low *ERG,* low *EVI1,* and high *PRAME* expression levels were also shown to have a good prognosis (Santamaria et al., 2009). Recently, Damm et al. (2011a) proposed an integrative prognostic risk score (IPRS) for CN-AML patients based on clinical and molecular markers. Nine clinical, hematological, and molecular factors including age; WBC count; mutation status of *NPM1, FLT3*-ITD, *CEBPA, and WT1* SNP rs16754; and expression levels of *BAALC, ERG, MN1,* and *WT1* (Damm et al., 2011a). Other molecular markers like *NRAS, MLL-PTD, WT1, IDH1,* or *IDH2* mutations were not significant and thus not included in the IPRS. Dolnik et al. (2012) used microarray-based comparative genomic hybridization and SNP profiling data of 391 AML cases to further study genomic regions of interest, and they resequenced 1000 genes located in the critical regions in a representative cohort of 50 AML samples comprising all major cytogenetic subgroups. They identified 120 missense/nonsense mutations as well as 60 insertions/deletions affecting 73 different genes, about 3.6 tumor-specific aberrations/AML. Not only recurrent mutations in well-known genes implicated in AML (described in paragraph 5) but mostly nonrecurrent single-nucleotide variations, insertions, or deletions (indels) in other transcription factors including *E2F1, RUNX1, SPI1/PU.1,* and *IKZF1* were found. Recurrent mutation refers to the same mutation reappearing many times. Furthermore, mutations in the splicing factor *SFPQ* and in the nonclassic regulators of mRNA processing *CTCF* and *RAD21* were also detected. These splicing-related mutations affected 10% of AML patients. Screening of AMLs derived from MDS revealed mutations of splicing-associated genes in about 26% of the cases, whereas only in 7% of de novo AML (Yoshida et al., 2011).

Awaiting efficient targeted therapies, the open question is how gene mutation patterns may help physicians to guide the management of AML patients in the daily practice. Given the large number of mutations already described and their partial overlap, the definition of a standardized and well-accepted prognostic algorithm based on mutation patterns will not be an easy task. The delineation of all mutations that lead to deregulated splicing or epigenetic silencing will provide the basis for a better understanding of the complex nature of common leukemia phenotypes, which then could be directly targeted in the future (Dolnik et al., 2012). SNP arrays in CN-AML show that approximately one-third of patients have a uniparental disomy (i.e., the copy neutral loss of heterozygosity undetectable by standard cytogenetics) (Tiu et al., 2009). Uniparental disomy appears to be a previously unappreciated but common genetic lesion in AML (Bullinger et al., 2010). Other tools, such as GEP and MRD monitoring, might also be useful for integrating all the important knowledge from known information in a single signature or measure. Genome-wide search and new technologies will help to subcategorize CN-AML. Array-based cytogenetic approaches, gene and miR signatures, and DNA methylation signatures may detect potential targets for new therapies and have been shown to have prognostic significance in patients with CN-AML (Bullinger and Fröhling, 2012).

Acknowledgments

This work was supported by the research grant NT/13836–4/2012 from the Ministry of Health of the Czech Republic and by the project (Ministry of Health, Czech Republic) for conceptual development of research organization (Institute of Hematology and Blood Transfusion, Prague).

References

Abbas, S., Lugthart, S., Kavelaars, F.G., Schelen, A., Koenders, J.E., Zeilemaker, A., van Putten, W.J. et al. 2010. Acquired mutations in the genes encoding IDH1 and IDH2 both are recurrent aberrations in acute myeloid leukemia: Prevalence and prognostic value. *Blood* 116: 2122–2126.

Abdel-Wahab, O., Mullally, A., Hedvat, C., Garcia-Manero, G., Patel, J., Wadleigh, M., Malinge, S. et al. 2009. Genetic characterization of TET1, TET2, and TET3 alterations in myeloid malignancies. *Blood* 114: 144–147.

Abdel-Wahab, O., Patel, J., and R.L. Levine. 2011. Clinical implications of novel mutations in epigenetic modifiers in AML. *Hematology/Oncology Clinics of North America* 25: 1119–1133.

Albiero, E., Madeo, D., Bolli, N., Giaretta, I., Bona, E.D., Martelli, M.F., Nicoletti, I. et al. 2007. Identification and functional characterization of a cytoplasmic nucleophosmin leukaemic mutant generated by a novel exon-11 NPM1 mutation. *Leukemia* 21: 1099–1103.

Amin, M.A., Matsunaga, S., Uchiyama, S., and K. Fukui. 2008a. Depletion of nucleophosmin leads to distortion of nucleolar and nuclear structures in HeLa cells. *Biochemical Journal* 415: 345–351.

Amin, M.A., Matsunaga, S., Uchiyama, S., and K. Fukui. 2008b. Nucleophosmin is required for chromosome congression, proper mitotic spindle formation, and kinetochore-microtubule attachment in HeLa cells. *FEBS Letters* 582: 3839–3844.

Angelov, D., Bondarenko, V.A., Almagro, S., Menoni, H., Mongélard, F., Hans, F., Mietton, F. et al. 2006. Nucleolin is a histone chaperone with FACT-like activity and assists remodeling of nucleosomes. *EMBO Journal* 25: 1669–1679.

Appelbaum, F.R., Gundacker, H., Head, D.R., Slovak, M.L., Willman, C.L., Goodwin, J.E., Anderson, J.E., and S.H. Petersdorf. 2006. Age and acute myeloid leukemia. *Blood* 107: 3481–3485.

Ariyaratana, S. and D.M. Loeb. 2007. The role of the Wilms tumour gene (WT1) in normal and malignant haematopoiesis. *Expert Reviews in Molecular Medicine* 9: 1–17.

Bacher, U., Badbaran, A., Fehse, B., Zabelina, T., Zander, A.R., and N. Kröger. 2009. Quantitative monitoring of NPM1 mutations provides a valid minimal residual disease parameter following allogeneic stem cell transplantation. *Experimental Hematology* 37: 135–142.

Bacher, U., Haferlach, C., Schnittger, S., Kohlmann, A., Kern, W., and T. Haferlach. 2010. Mutations of the TET2 and CBL genes: Novel molecular markers in myeloid malignancies. *Annals of Hematology* 89: 643–652.

Bacher, U., Haferlach, T., Schoch, C., Kern, W., and S. Schnittger. 2006. Implications of NRAS mutations in AML: A study of 2502 patients. *Blood* 107: 3847–3853.

Bacher, U., Kohlmann, A., Haferlach, C., and T. Haferlach, T. 2009. Gene expression profiling in acute myeloid leukaemia (AML). *Best Practice & Research Clinical Haematology* 22: 169–180.

Baldus, C.D. and L. Bullinger. 2008. Gene expression with prognostic implications in cytogenetically normal acute myeloid leukemia. *Seminars in Oncology* 35: 356–364.

Baldus, C.D., Tanner, S.M., Ruppert, A.S., Whitman, S.P., Archer, K.J., Marcucci, G., Caligiuri, M.A. et al. 2003. BAALC expression predicts clinical outcome of de novo acute myeloid leukemia patients with normal cytogenetics: A Cancer and Leukemia Group B Study. *Blood* 102: 1613–1618.

Baldus, C.D., Thiede, C., Soucek, S., Bloomfield, C.D., Thiel, E., and G. Ehninger. 2006. BAALC expression and FLT3 internal tandem duplication mutations in acute myeloid leukemia patients with normal cytogenetics: Prognostic implications. *Journal of Clinical Oncology* 24: 790–797.

Baljevic, M., Park, J.H., Stein, E., Douer, D., Altman, J.K., and M.S. Tallman. 2011. Curing all patients with acute promyelocytic leukemia: Are we there yet? *Hematology/Oncology Clinics of North America* 25: 1215–1233.

Barjesteh van Waalwijk van Doorn-Khosrovani, S., Erpelinck, C., van Putten, W.L., Valk, P.J., van der Poel-van de Luytgaarde, S., Hack, R., Slater, R. et al. 2003. High EVI1 expression predicts poor survival in acute myeloid leukemia: A study of 319 de novo AML patients. *Blood* 101: 837–845.

Basecke, J., Whelan, J.T., Griesinger, F., and F.E. Bertrand. 2006. The MLL partial tandem duplication in acute myeloid leukaemia. *British Journal of Haematology* 135: 438–449.

Becker, H., Marcucci, G., Maharry, K., Radmacher, M.D., Mrózek, K., Margeson, D., Whitman, S.P. et al. 2010. Favorable prognostic impact of NPM1 mutations in older patients with cytogenetically normal de novo acute myeloid leukemia and associated gene- and microRNA-expression signatures: A Cancer and Leukemia Group B Study. *Journal of Clinical Oncology* 28: 596–604.

Bennett, J.M., Catovsky, D., Daniel, M.T., Flandrin, G., Galton, D.A., Gralnick, H.R., and C. Sultan. 1976. Proposals for the classification of the acute leukemias. French-American-British (FAB) co-operative group. *British Journal of Haematology* 33: 451–458.

Bennett, J.M., Catovsky, D., Daniel, M.T., Flandrin, G., Galton, D.A., Gralnick, H.R., and C. Sultan. 1985. Proposed revised criteria for the classification of acute myeloid leukemia. A report of the French-American-British cooperative group. *Annals of Internal Medicine* 10: 620–625.

Boissel, N., Nibourel, O., Renneville, A., Gardin, C., Reman, O., Contentin, N., Bordessoule, D. et al. 2010. Prognostic impact of isocitrate dehydrogenase enzyme isoforms 1 and 2 mutations in acute myeloid leukemia: A Study by the Acute Leukemia French Association Group. *Journal of Clinical Oncology* 28: 3717–3723.

Bolli, N., Nicoletti, I., De Marco, M.F., Bigerna, B., Pucciarini, A., Mannucci, R., Martelli, M.P. et al. 2007. Born to be exported: COOH-terminal nuclear export signals of different strengthen sure cytoplasmic accumulation of nucleophosmin leukemic mutants. *Cancer Research* 67: 6230–6237.

Borer, R.A., Lehner, C.F., Eppenberger, H.M., and E.A. Nigg. 1989. Major nucleolar proteins shuttle between nucleus and cytoplasm. *Cell* 56: 379–390.

Bowen, D.T., Frew, M.E., Hills, R., Gale, R.E., Wheatley, K., Groves, M.J., Langabeer, S.E. et al. 2005. RAS mutation in acute myeloid leukemia is associated with distinct cytogenetic subgroups but does not influence outcome in patients younger than 60 years. *Blood* 106: 2113–2119.

Bullinger, L. 2006. Gene expression profiling in acute myeloid leukemia. *Haematologica* 91: 733–738.

Bullinger, L. and S.A. Armstrong. 2010. HELP for AML: Methylation profiling opens new avenues. *Cancer Cell* 17: 1–3.

Bullinger, L., Döhner, K., Bair, E., Fröhling, S., Schlenk, R.F., Tibshirani, R., Döhner, H., and J.R. Pollack. 2004. Use of gene-expression profiling to identify prognostic subclasses in adult acute myeloid leukemia. *New England Journal of Medicine* 350: 1605–1616.

Bullinger, L., Döhner, K., Kranz, R., Stirner, C., Fröhling, S., Scholl, C., Kim, Y.H. et al. 2008. An FLT3 gene-expression signature predicts clinical outcome in normal karyotype AML. *Blood* 111: 4490–4495.

Bullinger, L. and S. Fröhling. 2012. Array-based cytogenetic approaches in acute myeloid leukemia: Clinical impact and biological insights. *Seminars in Oncology* 39: 37–46.

Bullinger, L., Krönke, J., Schön, C., Radtke, I., Urlbauer, K., Botzenhardt, U., Gaidzik, V. et al. 2010. Identification of acquired copy number alterations and uniparental disomies in cytogenetically normal acute myeloid leukemia using high-resolution single-nucleotide polymorphism analysis. *Leukemia* 24: 438–449.

Bullinger, L. and P.J. Valk. 2005. Gene expression profiling in acute myeloid leukemia. *Journal of Clinical Oncology* 23: 6296–6305.

Burnett, A., Wetzler, M., and B. Löwenberg. 2011. Therapeutic advances in acute myeloid leukemia. *Journal of Clinical Oncology* 29: 487–494.

Burnett, A.K. 2012. New induction and postinduction strategies in acute myeloid leukemia. *Current Opinion in Hematology* 19: 76–81.

Caligiuri, M.A., Schichman, S.A., Strout, M.P., Mrózek, K. et al. 1994. Molecular rearrangement of the ALL-1 gene in acute myeloid leukemia without cytogenetic evidence of 11q23 chromosomal translocations. *Cancer Research* 54: 370–373.

Cazzola, M. 2010. IDH1 and IDH2 mutations in myeloid neoplasms-Novel paradigms and clinical implications. *Haematologica* 95: 1623–1627.

Chan, I.T., Kutok, J.L., Williams, I.R., Cohen, S., Kelly, L., Shigematsu, H., Johnson, L. et al. 2004. Conditional expression of oncogenic K-ras from its endogenous promoter induces a myeloproliferative disease. *Journal of Clinical Investigation* 113: 528–538.

Chan, W.Y., Liu, Q.R., Borjigin, J., Busch, H., Rennert, O.M., Tease, L.A., and P.K. Chan. 1989. Characterization of the cDNA encoding human nucleophosmin and studies of its role in normal and abnormal growth. *Biochemistry* 28: 1033–1039.

Chen, C.C., Gau, J.P., You, J.Y., Lee, K.D., Yu, Y.B., Lu, C.H., Lin, J.T. et al. 2009. Prognostic significance of beta-catenin and topoisomerase II alpha in de novo acute myeloid leukemia. *American Journal of Hematology* 84: 87–92.

Chou, W.C., Hou, H.A., Chen, C.Y., Tang, J.L., Yao, M., Tsay, W., Ko, B.S. et al. 2010a. Distinct clinical and biologic characteristics in adult acute myeloid leukemia bearing the isocitrate dehydrogenase 1 mutation. *Blood* 115: 2749–2754.

Chou, W.C., Huang, H.H., Hou, H.A., Chen, C.Y., Tang, J.L., Yao, M., Tsay, W. et al. 2010b. Distinct clinical and biological features of de novo acute myeloid leukemia with additional sex comb-like 1(ASXL1) mutations. *Blood* 116: 4086–4094.

Chou, W.C., Lei, W.C., Ko, B.S., Hou, H.A., Chen, C.Y., Tang, J.L., Yao, M. et al. 2011. The prognostic impact and stability of Isocitrate dehydrogenase 2 mutation in adult patients with acute myeloid leukemia. *Leukemia* 25: 246–253.

Cilloni, D., Renneville, A., Hermitte, F., Hills, R.K., Daly, S., Jovanovic, J.V., Gottardi, E. et al. 2009. Real-time quantitative polymerase chain reaction detection of minimal residual disease by standardized WT1 assay to enhance risk stratification in acute myeloid leukemia: A European Leukemia Net Study. *Journal of Clinical Oncology* 27: 5195–5201.

Coenen, E.A., Zwaan, C.M., Meyer, C., Marschalek, R., Pieters, R., van der Veken, L.T., Beverloo, H.B., and M.M. van den Heuvel-Eibrink. 2011. KIAA1524: A novel MLL translocation partner in acute myeloid leukemia. *Leukemia Research* 35: 133–135.

Colombo, E., Bonetti, P., Lazzerini Denchi, E., Martinelli, P., Zamponi, R., Marine, J.C., Helin, K., Falini, B., and P.G. Pelicci. 2005. Nucleophosmin is required for DNA integrity and p19Arf protein stability. *Molecular and Cellular Biology* 25: 8874–8886.

Colombo, E., Marine, J.C., Danovi, D., Falini, B., and P.G. Pelicci. 2002. Nucleophosmin regulates the stability and transcriptional activity of p53. *Nature Cell Biology* 4: 529–533.

Creutzig, U., van den Heuvel-Elbrink, M.M., Gibson, B., Dworzak, M.N., Adachi, S., de Bont, E., Harbott, J. et al. 2012. Diagnosis and management of acute myeloid leukemia in children and adolescents: Recommendations from an international expert panel. *Blood* 120: 3187–3205.

Dalley, C.D., Lister, T.A., Cavenagh, J.D., and A.Z.S. Rohatiner. 2001. ICRF Medical Oncology Unit. 2001. Serum LDH, a prognostic factor in elderly patients with acute myeloid leukaemia. *British Journal of Cancer* 84: 147.

D'Alo', F., Johansen, L.M., Nelson, E.A., Radomska, H.S., Evans, E.K., Zhang, P., Nerlov, C., and D.G. Tenen. 2003. The amino terminal and E2F interaction domains are critical for C/EBP alpha-mediated induction of granulopoietic development of hematopoietic cells. *Blood* 102: 3163–3171.

Damiani, D., Tiribelli, M., Michelutti, A., Geromin, A., Cavallin, M., Fabbro, D., Pianta, A. et al. 2010. Fludarabine-based induction therapy does not overcome the negative effect of ABCG2 (BCRP) over-expression in adult acute myeloid leukemia patients. *Leukemia Research* 34: 942–945.

Damm, F., Heuser, M., Morgan, M., Wagner, K., Görlich, K., Grosshennig, A., Hamwi, I. et al. 2011a. Integrative prognostic risks core in acute myeloid leukemia with normal karyotype. *Blood* 117: 4561–4568.

Damm, F., Heuser, M., Morgan, M., Yun, H., Grosshennig, A., Göhring, G., Schlegelberger, B. et al. 2010a. Single nucleotide polymorphism in the mutational hotspot of WT1 predicts a favorable outcome in patients with cytogenetically normal acute myeloid leukemia. *Journal of Clinical Oncology* 28: 578–585.

Damm, F., Lange, K., Heuser, M., Oberacker, T., Morgan, M., Wagner, K., Krauter, J. et al. 2010b. Phosphoinositide phospholipase C beta 1(PI-PLC beta 1) gene in myelodys plastic syndromes and cytogenetically normal acute myeloid leukemia: Not a deletion, but increased PI-PLC beta 1 expression is an independent prognostic factor. *Journal of Clinical Oncology* 28: e384–e387.

Damm, F., Oberacker, T., Thol, F., Surdziel, E., Wagner, K., Chaturvedi, A., Morgan, M. et al. 2011b. Prognostic importance of histone methyl transferase MLL5 expression in acute myeloid leukemia. *Journal of Clinical Oncology* 29: 682–689.

Dang, L., Jin, S., and S.M. Su. 2010. IDH mutations in glioma and acute myeloid leukemia. *Trends in Molecular Medicine* 16: 387–397.

De Braekeleer, M., Morel, F., LeBris, M.J., Herry, A., and N. Douet-Guilbert. 2005. The MLL gene and translocations involving chromosomal band 11q23 in acute leukemia. *Anticancer Research* 25: 1931–1944.

de Jonge, H.J.M., Valk, P.J., Veeger, N.J., ter Elst, A., den Boer, M.L., Cloos, J., de Haas, V. et al. 2010. High VEGFC expression is associated with unique gene expression profiles and predicts adverse prognosis in pediatric and adult acute myeloid leukemia. *Blood* 116: 1747–1754.

Del Poeta, G., Ammatuna, E., Lavorgna, S., Capelli, G., Zaza, S., Luciano, F., Ottone, T. et al. 2010. The genotype nucleophosmin mutated and FLT3-ITD negative is characterized by high bax/bcl-2 ratio and favourable outcome in acute myeloid leukaemia. *British Journal of Haematology* 149: 383–387.

Deneberg, S., Grövdal, M., Karimi, M., Jansson, M., Nahi, H., Corbacioglu, A., Gaidzok, V. et al. 2010. Gene-specific and global methylation patterns predict outcome in patients with acute myeloid leukemia. *Leukemia* 24: 932–941.

Derolf, A.R., Björklund, E., Mazur, J., Björkholm, M., and A. Porwit. 2008. Expression patterns of CD33 and CD15 predict outcome in patients with acute myeloid leukemia. *Leukemia and Lymphoma* 49: 1279–1291.

Döhner, H., Estey, E.H., Amadori, S., Appelbaum, F.R., Büchner, T., Burnett, A.K., Dombret, H. et al. 2010. Diagnosis and management of acute myeloid leukemia in adults: Recommendations from an international expert panel, on behalf of the European Leukemia Net. *Blood* 115: 453–474.

Döhner, K. and H. Döhner. 2008. Molecular characterization of acute myeloid leukemia. *Haematologica* 93: 976–982.

Döhner, K., Tobis, K., Ulrich, R., Fröhling, S., Benner, A., Schlenk, R.F., and H. Döhner. 2002. Prognostic significance of partial tandem duplications of the MLL gene in adult patients 16 to 60 years old with acute myeloid leukemia and normal cytogenetics: A study of the Acute Myeloid Leukemia Study Group Ulm. *Journal of Clinical Oncology* 20: 3254–3261.

Dolnik, A., Engelmann, J.C., Scharfenberger-Schmeer, M., Mauch, J., Kelkenberg-Schade, S., Haldemann, B., Fries, T. et al. 2012. Commonly altered genomic regions in acute myeloid leukemia are enriched for somatic mutations involved in chromatin remodeling and splicing. *Blood* 120: e83–e92.

Dombret, H. 2011. Gene mutation and AML pathogenesis. *Blood* 118: 5366–5367.

Dorrance, A.M., Liu, S., Yuan, W., Becknell, B., Arnoczky, K.J., Guimond, M., Strout, M.P. et al. 2006. MLL partial tandem duplication induces aberrant Hox expression in vivo via specific epigenetic alterations. *Journal of Clinical Investigation* 116: 2707–2716.

Dufour, A., Schneider, F., Metzeler, K.H., Hoster, E., Schneider, S., Zellmeier, E., Benthaus, T. et al. 2010. Acute myeloid leukemia with biallelic CEBPA gene mutations and normal karyotype represents a distinct genetic entity associated with a favorable clinical outcome. *Journal of Clinical Oncology* 28: 570–577.

Dvorakova, D., Racil, Z., Jeziskova, I., Palasek, I., Protivankova, M., Lengerova, M., Razga, F., and J. Mayer. 2010. Monitoring of minimal residual disease in acute myeloid leukemia with frequent and rare patient-specific NPM1 mutations. *American Journal of Hematology* 85: 926–929.

Eisfeld, A.K., Marcucci, G., Maharry, K., Schwind, S., Radmacher, M.D., Nicolet, D., Becker, H. et al. 2012. *miR-3151* interplays with its host gene *BAALC* and independently affects outcome of patients with cytogenetically normal acute myeloid leukemia. *Blood* 120: 249–258.

Enomoto, T., Lindström, M.S., Jin, A., Ke, H., and Y. Zhang. 2006. Essential role of the B23/NPM core domain in regulating ARF binding and B23 stability. *Journal of Biological Chemistry* 281: 18463–18472.

Epping, M.T., Wang, L., Edel, M.J., Carlée, L., Hernandez, M., and R. Bernards. 2005. The human tumor antigen PRAME is a dominant repressor of retinoic acid receptor signaling. *Cell* 122: 835–847.

Estey, E.H. 2012. Acute myeloid leukemia: 2012 Update on diagnosis, risk stratification, and management. *American Journal of Hematology* 87: 90–99.

Falini, B. 2010b. Acute myeloid leukemia with mutated nucleophosmin (NPM1): Molecular, pathological, and clinical features. *Cancer Treatment and Research* 145: 149–168.

Falini, B., Bolli, N., Liso, A., Martelli, M.P., Mannucci, R., Pileri, S., and I. Nicoletti. 2009. Altered nucleophosmin transport in acute myeloid leukaemia with mutated NPM1: Molecular basis and clinical implications. *Leukemia* 23: 1731–1743.

Falini, B., Bolli, N., Shan, J., Martelli, M.P., Liso, A., Pucciarini, A., Bigerna, B. et al. 2006b. Both carboxy-terminus NES motif and mutated tryptophan(s) are crucial for aberrant nuclear export of nucleophosmin leukemic mutants in NPMc+AML. *Blood* 107: 4514–4523.

Falini, B., Martelli, M.P., Bolli, N.,, Bonasso, R., Ghia, E., Pallotta, M.T., Diverio, D. et al. 2006a. Immunohistochemistry predicts nucleophosmin (NPM) mutations in acute myeloid leukemia. *Blood* 108: 1999–2005.

Falini, B., Martelli, M.P., Bolli, N., Sportoletti, P., Liso, A., Tiacci, E., and T. Haferlach. 2011. Acute myeloid leukemia with mutated nucleophosmin (NPM1): Is it a distinct entity? *Blood* 117: 1109–1120.

Falini, B., Martelli, M.P., Pileri, S.A., and C. Mecucci. 2010a. Molecular and alternative methods for diagnosis of acute myeloid leukemia with mutated NPM1: Flexibility may help. *Haematologica* 95: 529–534.

Falini, B., Mecucci, C., Tiacci, E., Alcalay, M., Rosati, R., Pasqualucci, L., LaStarza, R. et al. 2005. Cytoplasmic nucleophosmin in acute myelogenous leukemia with a normal karyotype. *The New England Journal of Medicine* 352: 254–266.

Fang, M., Storer, B., Estey, E., Othus, M., Zhang, L., Sandmaier, B.M., and F.R. Appelbaum. 2011. Outcome of patients with acute myeloid leukemia with monosomal karyotype who undergo haematopoietic cell transplantation. *Blood* 118: 1490–1494.

Fatica, A. 2012. Noncoding RNAs in acute myeloid leukemia: From key regulators to clinical players. *Scientifica* 2012: 1–10, Article ID 925758.

Ferrara, F. and S. Mirto. 1996. Serum LDH value as a predictor of clinical outcome in acute myelogenous leukemia of the elderly. *British Journal of Haematology* 92:627–631.

Ferrara, F., Palmieri, S., and F. Leoni. 2008. Clinically useful prognostic factors in acute myeloid leukemia. *Critical Reviews in Oncology/Hematology* 66: 181–193.

Figueroa, M.E., Abdel-Wahab, O., Lu, C., Ward, P.S., Patel, J., Shih, A., Li, Y. et al. 2010a. Leukemic IDH1 and IDH2 mutations result in a hypermethylation phenotype, disrupt TET2 function, and impair hematopoietic differentiation. *Cancer Cell* 18: 553–567.

Figueroa, M.E., Lugthart, S., Li, Y., Erpelinck-Verschueren, C., Deng, X., Christos, P.J., Schifano, E. et al. 2010b. DNA methylation signatures identify biologically distinct subtypes in acute myeloid leukemia. *Cancer Cell* 17: 13–17.

Flodby, P., Barlow, C., Kylefjord, H., Ahrlund-Richter, L., and K.G. Xanthopoulos. 1996. Increased hepatic cell proliferation and lung abnormalities in mice deficient in CCAAT/enhancer binding protein alpha. *Journal of Biological Chemistry* 271: 24753–24760.

Follo, M.Y., Finelli, C., Clissa, C., Mongiorgi, S., Bosi, C., Martinelli, G., Baccarani, M. et al. 2009. Phosphoinositide-phospholipase C beta1 mono-allelic deletion is associated with myelodysplastic syndromes evolution into acute myeloid leukemia. *Journal of Clinical Oncology* 27: 782–790.

Foran, J.M. 2010. New prognostic markers in acute myeloid leukemia: Perspective from the clinic. *Hematology ASH Education Program Book* 2010: 47–55.

Frehlick, L.J., Eirín-López, J.M., and J. Ausió. 2007. New insights into the nucleophosmin/nucleoplasmin family of nuclear chaperones. *BioEssays* 29: 49–59.

Friedman, A.D. 2007. C/EBP alpha induces PU.1 and interacts with AP-1 and NF-kappa B to regulate myeloid development. *Blood Cells, Molecules and Diseases* 39: 340–343.

Fröhling, S., Schlenk, R.F., Breitruck, J., Benner, A., Kreitmeier, S., Tobis, K., Döhner, H., and K. Döhner. 2002. AML Study Group Ulm. Acute myeloid leukemia. Prognostic significance of activating FLT3 mutations in younger adults (16 to 60 years) with acute myeloid leukemia and normal cytogenetics: A study of the AML Study Group Ulm. *Blood* 100: 4372–4380.

Fröhling, S., Schlenk, R.F., Stolze, I., Bihlmayr, J., Benner, A., Kreitmeier, S., Tobis, K., Döhner, H., and K. Döhner. 2004. CEBPA mutations in younger adults with acute myeloid leukemia and normal cytogenetics: Prognostic relevance and analysis of cooperating mutations. *Journal of Clinical Oncology* 22: 624–633.

Fuchs, O. 2007. Growth-inhibiting activity of transcription factor C/EBP alpha, its role in haematopoiesis and its tumour suppressor or oncogenic properties in leukaemias. *Folia Biologica* (Praha) 53: 97–108.

Fuchs, O., Kostecka, A., Provaznikova, D., Krasna, B., Brezinova, J., Filkukova, J., Kotlin, R. et al. 2009. Nature of frequent deletions in CEBPA. *Blood Cells, Molecules and Diseases* 43: 260–263.

Fuchs, O., Provaznikova, D., Kocova, M., Kostecka, A., Cvekova, P., Neuwirtova, R., Kobylka, P. et al. 2008. CEBPA polymorphisms and mutations in patients with acute myeloid leukemia, myelodysplastic syndrome, multiple myeloma and non-Hodgkin's lymphoma. *Blood Cells, Molecules and Diseases* 40: 401–405.

Gaidzik, V. and K. Döhner. 2008. Prognostic implications of gene mutations in acute myeloid leukemia with normal cytogenetics. *Seminars in Oncology* 35: 346–355.

Gaidzik, V.I., Paschka, P., Späth, D., Habdank, M., Köhne, C.-H., Germing, U., von Lilienfeld-Toal M. et al. 2012. TET2 mutations in acute myeloid leukemia (AML): Results from a comprehensive genetic and clinical analysis of the AML Study Group. *Journal of Clinical Oncology* 30: 1350–1357.

Gaidzik, V.I., Schlenk, R.F., Moschny, S., Becker, A., Bullinger, L., Corbacioglu, A., Krauter, J. et al. 2009. Prognostic impact of WT1 mutations in cytogenetically normal acute myeloid leukemia: A study of the German-Austrian AML Study Group. *Blood* 113: 4505–4511.

Gale, R.E., Green, C., Allen, C., Mead, A.J., Burnett, A.K., Hills, R.K., Linch, D.C., and Medical Research Council Adult Leukaemia Working Party. 2008. The impact of FLT3 internal tandem duplication mutant level, number, size, and interaction with NPM1 mutations in a large cohort of young adult patients with acute myeloid leukemia. *Blood* 111: 2776–2784.

Gale, R.E., Hills, R., Kottaridis, P.D., Srirangan, S., Wheatley, K., Burnett, A.K., and D.C. Linch. 2005. No evidence that FLT3 status should be considered as an indicator for transplantation in acute myeloid leukemia (AML): An analysis of 1135 patients, excluding acute promyelocytic leukemia, from the UK MRC AML10 and 12 trials. *Blood* 106: 3658–3665.

Gandillet, A., Park, S., Lassailly, F., Griessinger, E., Vargafting, J., Filby, A., Lister, T.A., and Bonnet, D. 2011. Heterogeneous sensitivity of human acute myeloid leukemia to β- catenin down-modulation. *Leukemia* 25: 770–780.

Garzon, R., Garofalo, M., Martelli, M.P., Briesewitz, R., Wang, L., Fernandez-Cymering, C., Volinia, S. et al. 2008. Distinctive microRNA signature of acute myeloid leukemia bearing cytoplasmic mutated nucleophosmin. *The Proceedings of the National Academy of Sciences of the USA* 105: 3945–3950.

Geisbrecht, B.V. and S.J. Gould. 1999. The human PICD gene encode sacytoplasmic andperoxisomal NADP(+)-dependent isocitrate dehydrogenase. *Journal of Biological Chemistry* 274: 30527–30533.

Gianfaldoni, G., Mannelli, F., Ponziani, V., Longo, G., Bencini, S., Bosi, A., and A.M. Vannucchi. 2010. Early reduction of WT1 transcripts during induction chemotherapy predicts for longer disease free and overall survival in acutemyeloid leukemia. *Haematologica* 95: 833–836.

Gilliland, D.G. and J.D. Griffin. 2002. The roles of FLT3 in hematopoiesis and leukemia. *Blood* 100: 1532–1542.

Golub, T., Slonim, D.K., Tamayo, P., Huard, C., Gaasenbeek, M., Mesirov, J.P., Coller, H. et al. 1999. Molecular classification of cancer: Class discovery and class prediction by gene expression monitoring. *Science* 286: 531–537.

Gombart, A.F., Hofmann, W.K., Kawano, S., Takeuchi, S., Krug, U., Kwok, S.H., Larsen, R.J. et al. 2002. Mutations in the gene encoding the transcription factor CCAAT/enhancer binding protein alpha in myelodysplastic syndromes and acute myeloid leukemias. *Blood* 99: 1332–1340.

Goyama, S., and Kurokawa, M. 2010. Evi-1 as a critical regulator of leukemic cells. *International Journal of Hematology* 91: 753–757.

Green, C.L., Evans, C.M., Hills, R.K., Burnett, A.K., Linch, D.C., and R.E. Gale. 2010. The prognostic significance of IDH1 mutations in younger adult patients with acute myeloid leukemia is dependent on FLT3/ITD status. *Blood* 116: 2779–2782.

Greenwood, M.J., Seftel, M.D., Richardson, C., Barbaric, D., Barnett, M.J., Bruyere, H., Forrest, D.L. et al. 2006. Leukocyte count as a predictor of death during remission induction in acute myeloid leukemia. *Leukemia and Lymphoma* 47: 1245–1252.

Greiner, J., Bullinger, L., Guinn, B.A., Döhner, H., and M. Schmitt. 2008. Leukemia-associated antigens are critical for the proliferation of acute myeloid leukemia cells. *Clinical Cancer Research* 14: 7161–7166.

Grimwade, D., Hills, R.K., Moorman, A.V., Walker, H., Chatters, S., Goldstone, A.H., Wheatley, K., Harrison, C.J., and A.K. Burnett. 2010. Refinement of cytogenetic classification in acute myeloid leukemia: Determination of prognostic significance of rare recurring chromosomal abnormalities among 5876 younger adult patients treated in the United Kingdom Medical Research Council trials. *Blood* 116: 354–365.

Grimwade, D. and K. Mrózek. 2011. Diagnostic and prognostic value of cytogenetics in acute myeloid leukemia. *Hematology/Oncology Clinics of North America* 25: 1135–1161.

Grisendi, S., Mecucci, C., Falini, B., and P.P. Pandolfi. 2006. Nucleophosmin and cancer. *Nature Reviews Cancer* 6: 493–505.

Gröschel, S., Lugthart, S., Schlenk, R.F., Valk, P.J., Eiwen, K., Goudswaard, C., van Putten, W.J. et al. 2010. High EVI1 expression predicts outcome in younger adult patients with acute myeloid leukemia and is associated with distinct cytogenetic abnormalities. *Journal of Clinical Oncology* 28: 2101–2107.

Gröschel, S., Schlenk, R.F., Engelmann, J., Rockova, V., Teleanu, V., Kühn M.W.M., Eiwen, K. et al. 2013. Deregulated expression of EVI1 defines a poor půrognostic subset of MLL-rearranged acute myeloid leukemias: A study of the German-Austrian Acute Myeloid Leukemia Study Group and the Dutch-Belgian-Swiss HOVON/SAKK Cooperative Group. *Journal of Clinical Oncology* 31: 95–103.

Gross, S., Cairns, R.A., Minden, M.D., Driggers, E.M., Bittinger, M.A., Jang, H.G., Sasaki, M. et al. 2010. Cancer-associated metabolite 2-hydroxyglutarate accumulates in acute myelogenous leukemia with isocitrate dehydrogenase 1 and 2 mutations. *Journal of Experimental Medicine* 207: 339–344.

Grossmann, V., Schnittger, S., Kohlmann, A., Eder, C., Roller, A., Dicker, F., Schmid, C. et al. 2012. A novel hierarchical prognostic model of AML solely based on molecular mutations. *Blood* 120: 2963–2972.

Grossmann, V., Tiacci, E., Holmes, A.B., Kohlmann, A., Martelli, M.P., Kern, W., Spanhol-Rosseto, A. et al. 2011. Whole-exome sequencing identifies mutations of BCOR in acute myeloid leukemia with normal karyotype. *Blood* 118: 6153–6163.

Grosveld, G.C. 2007. MN1, a novel player in human AML. *Blood Cells Molecules and Diseases* 39: 336–339.

Grövdal, M., Khan, R., Aggerholm, A., Abtunovic, P., Astermak, J., Bernell, P., Engström, L.M. et al. 2007. Negative effect of DNA hypermethylation on the outcome of intensive chemotherapy in older patients with high-risk myelodysplastic syndromes and acute myeloid leukemia following myelodysplastic syndrome. *Clinical Cancer Research* 13: 7107–7112.

Gu, Y., Jasti, A.C., Jansen, M., and J.E. Siefring. 2005. RhoH, a hematopoietic-specific RhoGTPase, regulates proliferation, survival, migration, and engraftment of hematopoietic progenitor cells. *Blood* 105: 1467–1475.

Gündogdu, M.S., Liu, H., Metzdorf, D., Hildebrand, D., Aigner, M., Aktories, K., Heeg, K., and K.F. Kubatzky. 2010. The haematopoietic GTPase RhoH modulates IL3 signalling through regulation of STAT activity and IL3 receptor expression. *Molecular Cancer* 25: 225.

Haber, D.A., Buckler, A.J., Glaser, T., Call, K.M., Pelletier, J., Sohn, R.L., Douglass, E.C., and D.E. Housman. 1990. An internal deletion within an 11p13 zinc finger gene contributes to the development of Wilms' tumor. *Cell* 61: 1257–1269.

Hackanson, B., Bennett, K.L., Brena, R.M., Jiang, J., Claus, R., Chen, S.S., Blagitko-Dorfs, N. et al. 2008. Epigenetic modification of CCAAT/enhancer binding protein alpha expression in acute myeloid leukemia. *Cancer Research* 68: 3142–3151.

Harada, Y. and H. Harada. 2009. Molecular pathways mediating MDS/AML with focus on AML1/RUNX1 point mutations. *Journal of Cellular Physiology* 220: 16–20.

Heesch, S., Schlee, C., Neumann, M., Stroux, A., Kühnl, A., Schwartz, S., Haferlach, T. et al. 2010. BAALC-associated gene expression profiles define IGFBP7 as a novel molecular marker in acute leukemia. *Leukemia* 24: 1429–1436.

Herrera, J.E., Savkur, R., and M.O. Olson. 1995. The ribonuclease activity of nucleolar protein B23. *Nucleic Acids Research* 23: 3974–3979.

Heuser, M., Argiropoulos, B., Kuchenbauer, F., Yung, E., Piper, J., Fung, S., Schlenk, R.F. et al. 2007. MN1 overexpression induces acute myeloid leukemia in mice and predicts ATRA resistance in patients with AML. *Blood* 110: 1639–1647.

Heuser, M., Beutel, G., Krauter, J., Döhner, K., von Neuhoff, N., Schlegelberger, B., and A. Ganser. 2006. High meningioma 1(MN1) expression as a predictor for poor outcome in acute myeloid leukemia with normal cytogenetics. *Blood* 108: 3898–3905.

Hisaoka, M., Ueshima, S., Murano, K., Nagata, K., and M. Okuwaki. 2010. Regulation of nucleolar chromatin by B23/nucleophosmin jointly depends upon its RNA binding activity and transcription factor UBF. *Molecular and Cellular Biology* 30: 4952–4964.

Hoffmann, M.H., Klausen, T.H., Boegsted, M., Larsen, S.F., Schmitz, A., Leinoe, E.B., Schmiegelow, K. et al. 2012. Clinical impact of leukemic blast heterogeneity at diagnosis in cytogenetic intermediate-risk acute myeloid leukemia. *Cytometry Part B: Clinical Cytometry* 82: 123–131.

Hou, H.A., Chou, W.C., Lin, L.I., Tang, J.L., Tseng, M.H., Huang, C.F., Yao, M. et al. 2008. Expression of angiopoietins and vascular endothelial growth factors and their clinical significance in acute myeloid leukemia. *Leukemia Research* 32: 904–912.

Hou, H.A., Huang, T.C., Lin, L.I., Liu, C.Y., Chen, C.Y., Chou, W.C., Tang, J.L. et al. 2010. WT1 mutation in 470 adult patients with acute myeloid leukemia: Stability during disease evolution and implication of its incorporation into a survival scoring system. *Blood* 115: 5222–5231.

Hou, H.A., Lin, L.I., Chen, C.Y., and H.F. Tien. 2009. Reply to heterogeneity within AML with CEBPA mutations, only CEBPA double mutations, but not single CEBPA mutations are associated with favorable prognosis. *British Journal of Cancer* 101: 738–740.

Huh, H.J., Park, C.J., Jang, S., Seo, E.J., Chi, H.S., Lee, J.H., Lee, K.H. et al. 2006. Prognostic significance of multidrug resistance gene 1 (MDR1), multidrug resistance-related protein (MRP) and lung resistance protein (LRP) mRNA expression in acute leukemia. *Journal of Korean Medical Science* 21: 253–258.

Iwasaki, T., Katsumi, A., Kiyoi, H., Tanizaki, R., Ishikawa, Y., Ozeki, K., Kobayashi, M. et al. 2008. Prognostic implication and biological roles of RhoH in acute myeloid leukaemia. *European Journal of Haematology* 81: 454–460.

Jaeger, U. and B. Kainz. 2003. Monitoring minimal residual disease in AML: The right time for real time. *Annals of Hematology* 82: 139–147.

Juliusson, G., Antunovic, P., Derolf, A., Lehmann, S., Möllgård, L., Stockelberg, D., Tidefelt, U., Wahlin, A., and M. Höglund. 2009. Age and acute myeloid leukemia: Real world data on decision to treat and outcomes from the Swedish Acute Leukemia Registry. *Blood* 113: 4179–4187.

Juliusson, G., Lazarevic, V., Hörstedt, A.-S., Hagberg, O., and M. Höglund. 2012. Acute myeloid leukemia in the real world: Why population–based registries are needed. *Blood* 119: 3890–3899.

Kato, N., Kitaura, J., Doki, N., Komeno, Y., Watanabe-Okochi, N., Togami, K., Nakahara, F. et al. 2011. Two types of C/EBPα mutations play distinct but collaborative roles in leukemogenesis: Lessons from clinical data and BMT models. *Blood* 117: 221–233.

Kayser, S., Zucknick, M., Döhner, K., Krauter, J., Köhne, C.-H., Horst, H.A., Held, G. et al. 2012. Monosomal karyotype in adult acute myeloid leukemia: Prognostic impact and outcome after different treatment strategies. *Blood* 118: 551–558.

Keeshan, K., Santilli, G., Corradini, F., Perrotti, D., and B. Calabretta. 2003. Transcription activation function of C/EBPα is required for induction of granulocyte differentiation. *Blood* 102: 1267–1275.

Kern, W., Bacher, U., Haferlach, C., Schnittger, S., and T. Haferlach. 2010. The role of multiparameter flow cytometry for disease monitoring in AML. *Best Practice & Research Clinical Haematology* 23: 379–390.

Kindler, T., Lipka, D.B., and T. Fischer. 2010. FLT3 as a therapeutic target in AML: Still challenging after all these years. *Blood* 116: 5089–5102.

King-Underwood, L., Renshaw, J., and K. Pritchard-Jones. 1996. Mutations in the Wilms' tumor gene WT1 in leukemias. *Blood* 87: 2171–2179.

Kohlmann, A., Bullinger, L., Thiede, C., Schaich, M., Schnittger, S., Döhner, K., Dugas, M. et al. 2010. Gene expression profiling in AML with normal karyotype can predict mutations for molecular marker sand allows novel insights into perturbed biological pathways. *Leukemia* 24: 1216–1220.

Koike, A., Nishikawa, H., Wu, W., Okada, Y., Venkitaraman, A.R., and T. Ohta. 2010. Recruitment of phosphorylated NPM1 to sites of DNA damage through RNF8-dependent ubiquitin conjugates. *Cancer Research* 70: 6746–6756.

Konoplev, S., Rassidakis, G.Z., Estey, E., Kantarjian, H. et al. 2007. Over expression of CXCR4 predicts adverse overall and event-free survival in patients with unmutated FLT3 acute myeloid leukemia with normal karyotype. *Cancer* 109: 1152–1156.

Kornblau, S.M., Singh, N., Qiu, Y., Chen, W., Zhang, N., and K.R. Coombes. 2010. Highly phosphorylated FOXO3A is an adverse prognostic factor in acute myeloid leukemia. *Clinical Cancer Research* 16: 1865–1874.

Kramarzova, K., Stuchly, J., Willasch, A., Gruhn, B., Schwarz, J., Cermak, J., Machova-Polakova, K. et al. 2012. Real-time PCR quantification of major Wilms' tumor gene 1 (WT1) isoforms in acute myeloid leukemia, their characteristic expression patterns and possible functional consequences. *Leukemia* 26: 2086–2095.

Lam, K. and D.E. Zhang. 2012. RUNX1 and RUNX1-ETO: Roles in hematopoiesis and leukemogenesis. *Frontiers in Bioscience* 17: 1120–1139.

Lange, T., Hubmann, M., Burkhardt, R., Franke, G.N., Cross, M., Scholz, M., Leiblein, S. et al. 2011. Monitoring of WT1 expression in PB and CD34(+) donor chimerism of BM predicts early relapse in AML and MDS patients after hematopoietic cell transplantation with reduced-intensity conditioning. *Leukemia* 25: 498–505.

Langer, C., Marcucci, G., Holland, K.B., Radmacher, M.D., Maharry, K., Paschka, P., Whitman, S.P. et al. 2009. Prognostic importance of MN1 transcript levels, and biologic insights from MN1-associated gene and microRNA expression signatures in cytogenetically normal acute myeloid leukemia: A Cancer and Leukemia Group B Study. *Journal of Clinical Oncology* 27: 3198–3204.

Langer, C., Radmacher, M.D., Ruppert, A.S., Whitman, S.P., Paschka, P., Mrózek, K., Baldus, C.D. et al. 2008. High BAALC expression associates with other molecular prognostic markers, poor outcome, and a distinct gene-expression signature in cytogenetically normal patients younger than 60 years with acute myeloid leukemia: A Cancer and Leukemia Group B (CALGB) Study. *Blood* 111: 5371–5379.

Larson, R.A. 2007. Is secondary leukemia an independent poor prognostic factor in acute myeloid leukemia? *Best Practice and Research Clinical Haematology* 20: 29–37.

Lee, C.Y., Tien, H.F., Hu, C.Y., Chou, W.C., and L.I. Lin. 2007. Marrow angiogenesis-associated factors as prognostic biomarkers in patients with acute myelogenous leukaemia. *British Journal of Cancer* 97: 877–882.

Legrand, O., Perrot, J.Y., Baudard, M., Cordier, A., Lautier, R., Simonin, G., Zittoun, R., Casadevall, N., and J.P. Marie. 2000. The immunophenotype of 177 adults with acute myeloid leukemia: Proposal of a prognostic score. *Blood* 96: 870–877.

Leith, C.P., Kopecky, K.J., Chen, I.M., Eijdems, L., Slovak, M.L., McConnell, T.S., Head, D.R. et al. 1999. Frequency and clinical significance of the expression of the multi drug resistance proteins MDR1/P-glycoprotein, MRP1, and LRP in acute myeloid leukemia: A Southwest Oncology Group Study. *Blood* 94: 1086–1099.

Lennartsson, J., Jelacic, T., Linnekin, D., and R. Shivakrupa. 2005. Normal and oncogenic forms of the receptor tyrosine kinase kit. *Stem Cells* 23: 16–43.

Leong, S.M., Tan, B.X., Bte Ahmad, B., Yan, T., Chee, L.Y., Ang, S.T., Tay, K.G. et al. 2010. Mutant nucleophosmin deregulates cell death and myeloid differentiation through excessive caspase-6 and -8 inhibition. *Blood* 116: 3286–3296.

Ley, T.J., Ding, L., Walter, M.J., McLellan, M.D., Lamprecht, T., Larson, D.E., Kandoth, C. et al. 2010. DNMT3A mutations in acute myeloid leukemia. *The New England Journal of Medicine* 363: 2424–2433.

Ley, T.J., Mardis, E.R., Ding, L., Fulton, B., McLellan, M.D., Chen, K., Dooling, D. et al. 2008. DNA sequencing of acytogenetically normal acute myeloid leukaemia genome. *Nature* 456: 66–72.

Ley, T.J., Minx, P.J., Walter, M.J., Ries, R.E., Sun, H., McLellan, M., DiPersio, J.F. et al. 2003. A pilot study of high-throughput, sequence-based mutational profiling of primary human acute myeloid leukemia cell genomes. *The Proceedings of the National Academy of Sciences of the USA* 100: 14275–14280.

Li, M., Collins, R., Jiao, Y., Ouiellette, P., Bixby, D., Erba, H.,Vogelstein, B. et al. 2011a. Somatic mutations in the transcriptional corepressor gene BCORL1 in adult acute myelogenous leukemia. *Blood* 118: 5914–5917.

Li, X., Li, J., Du, W., Zhang, J., Liu, W., Chen, X., Li, H., Huang, S., and X. Li. 2011b. Relevance of immunophenotypes to prognostic subgroups of age, WBC, platelet count, and cytogenetics in de novo acute myeloid leukemia. *APMIS* 119: 76–84.

Li, Z. and S.R. Hann. 2009. The Myc-nucleophosmin-ARF network: A complex web unveiled. *Cell Cycle* 8: 2703–2707.

Lin, L.I., Chen, C.Y., Lin, D.T., Tsay, W., Tang, J.L., Yeh, Y.C., Shen, H.L. et al. 2005. Characterization of CEBPA mutations in acute myeloid leukemia: Most patients with CEBPA mutations have biallelic mutations and show a distinct immunophenotype of the leukemic cells. *Clinical Cancer Research* 11: 1372–1379.

Lin, T.C., Hou, H.A., Chou, W.C., Ou, D.L., Yu, S.L., Tien, H.F., and L.I. Lin. 2011. CEBPA methylation as a prognostic biomarker in patients with de novo acute myeloid leukemia. *Leukemia* 25: 32–40.

Liso, A., Bogliolo, A., Freschi, V., Martelli, M.P., Pileri, S.A., Santodirocco, M., Bolli, N., Martelli, M.F., and B. Falini. 2008. In human genome, generation of a nuclear export signal through duplication appears unique to nucleophosmin (NPM1) mutations and is restricted to AML. *Leukemia* 22: 1285–1289.

Lo-Coco, F., Ammatuna, E., Montesinos, P., and M.A. Sanz. 2008. Acute promyelocytic leukemia: Recent advances in diagnosis and management. *Seminars in Oncology* 35: 401–409.

Loges, S., Heil, G., Bruweleit, M., Schoder, V., Butzal, M., Fischer, U., Gehling, U.M. et al. 2005. Analysis of concerted expression of angiogenic growth factors in acute myeloid leukemia: Expression of angiopoietin-2 represents an independent prognostic factor for overall survival. *Journal of Clinical Oncology* 23: 1109–1117.

Lopotová, T., Nádvorníková, S., Žáčková, M., Polák, J., Schwarz, J., Klamová, H., and J. Moravcová. 2012. N-terminally truncated WT1 variant (SWT1) is expressed at very low levels in acute myeloid leukemia and advanced phases of chronic myeloid leukemia. *Leukemia Research* 36: e81–e83.

Lugthart, S., Figueroa, M.E., Bindels, E., Skrabanek, L. et al. 2011. Aberrant DNA hypermethylation signature in acute myeloid leukemia directed by EVI1. *Blood* 117: 234–241.

Lugthart, S., Gröschel, S., Baverloo, H.B., Kayser, S., Valk, P.J., van Zelderen-Bhola S.L., Ossenkoppele, G.J. et al. 2010. Clinical, molecular, and prognostic significance of WHO type inv(3)(q21q26.2)/t(3,3)(q21,q26.2) and various other 3q abnormalities in acute myeloid leukemia. *Journal of Clinical Oncology* 28: 3890–3898.

Lugthart, S., van Drunen, E., van Norden, Y., van Hoven, A., Erpelinck, C.A., Valk, P.J., Beverloo, H.B. et al. 2008. High EVI1 levels predict adverse outcome in acute myeloid leukemia: Prevalence of EVI1 overexpression and chromosome 3q26 abnormalities underestimated. *Blood* 111: 4329–4337.

Luo, J., Qi, C., Xu, W., Kamel-Reid, S., Brandwein, J., and H. Chang. 2010. Cytoplasmic expression of nucleophosmin accurately predicts mutation in the nucleophosmin gene in patients with acute myeloid leukemia and normal karyotype. *American Journal of Clinical Pathology* 133: 34–40.

Maggi, L.B. Jr., Kuchenruether, M., Dadey, D.Y., Schwope, R.M., Grisendi, S., Townsend, R.R., Pandolfi, P.P., and J.D. Weber. 2008. Nucleophosmin serves as a rate-limiting nuclear export chaperone for the mammalian ribosome. *Molecular and Cellular Biology* 28: 7050–7065.

Makishima, H., Cazzolli, H., Szpurka, H., Dunbar, A., Tiu, R., Huh, J., Muramatsu, H. et al. 2009. Mutations of e3 ubiquitin ligase cbl family members constitute a novel common pathogenic lesion in myeloid malignancies. *Journal of Clinical Oncology* 27: 6109–6116.

Marcucci, G. 2006. Core binding factor acute myeloid leukemia. *Clinical Advances in Hematology and Oncology* 4: 339–341.

Marcucci, G., Baldus, C.D., Ruppert, A.S., Radmacher, M.D., Mrózek, K., Whitman, S.P., Kolitz, J.E. et al. 2005. Overexpression of the ETS-relatedgene, ERG, predicts a worse outcome in acute myeloid leukemia with normal karyotype: A Cancer and Leukemia Group B Study. *Journal of Clinical Oncology* 23: 9234–9242.

Marcucci, G., Haferlach, T., and H. Döhner. 2011a. Molecular genetics of adult acute myeloid leukemia: Prognostic and therapeutic implications. *Journal of Clinical Oncology* 29: 475–486.

Marcucci, G., Maharry, K., Radmacher, M.D., Mrózek, K., Vukosavljevic, T., Paschka, P., Whitman, S.P. et al. 2008. Prognostic significance of, and gene and microRNA expression signatures associated with, CEBPA mutations in cytogenetically normal acute myeloid leukemia with high-risk molecular features: A Cancer and Leukemia Group B Study. *Journal of Clinical Oncology* 26: 5078–5087.

Marcucci, G., Maharry, K., Whitman, S.P., Vukosavljevic, T., Paschka, P., Langer, C., Mrózek, K. et al. 2007. High expression levels of the ETS-relatedgene, ERG, predict adverse outcome and improve molecular risk-based classification of cytogenetically normal acute myeloid leukemia: A Cancer and Leukemia Group B Study. *Journal of Clinical Oncology* 25: 3337–3343.

Marcucci, G., Maharry, K., Wu, Y.Z., Radmacher, M.D., Mrózek, K., Margeson, D., Holland, K.B. et al. 2010. IDH1 and IDH2 gene mutations identify novel molecular subsets within de novo cytogenetically normal acute myeloid leukemia: A Cancer and Leukemia Group B Study. *Journal of Clinical Oncology* 28: 2348–2355.

Marcucci, G., Mrózek, K., Radmacher, M.D., Bloomfield, C.D., and C.M. Croce. 2009. MicroRNA expression profiling in acute myeloid and chronic lymphocytic leukaemias. *Best Practice and Research Clinical Haematology* 22: 239–248.

Marcucci, G., Mrózek, K., Radmacher, M.D., Garzon, R., and C.D. Bloomfield. 2011b. The prognostic and functional role of microRNAs in acute myeloid leukemia. *Blood* 117: 1121–1129.

Marcucci, G., Strout, M.P., Bloomfield, C.D., and M.A. Caligiuri. 1998. Detection of unique ALL1 (MLL) fusion transcripts in normal human bone marrow and blood: Distinct origin of normal versus leukemic ALL1 fusion transcripts. *Cancer Research* 58: 790–793.

Mardis, E.R. 2011. Adecade's perspective on DNA sequencing technology. *Nature* 470: 198–203.

Mardis, E.R., Ding, L., Dooling, D.J., Larson, D.E., McLellan M.D., Chen, K., Koboldt, D.C. et al. 2009. Recurring mutations found by sequencing an acute myeloid leukemia genome. *The New England Journal of Medicine* 361: 1058–1066.

Mariano, A.R., Colombo, E., Luzi, L., Martinelli, P., Volorio, S., Bernard, L., Meani, N. et al. 2006. Cytoplasmic localization of NPM in myeloid leukemias is dictated by gain-of-function mutations that create a functional nuclear export signal. *Oncogene* 25: 4376–4380.

Marková, J., Michková, P., Burčková, K., Březinová, J., Michalová, K., Dohnalová, A., Maaloufová, J.S. et al. 2012. Prognostic impact of DNMT3A mutations in patients with intermediate cytogenetic risk profile acute myeloid leukemia. *European Journal of Haematology* 88: 128–135.

Mead, A.J., Gale, R.E., Hills, R.K., Gupta, M., Young, B.D., Burnett, A.K., and D.C. Linch. 2008. Conflicting data on the prognostic significance of FLT3/TKD mutations in acute myeloid leukemia might berelated to the incidence of biallelic disease. *Blood* 112: 444–445.

Meani, N. and M. Alcalay. 2009. Role of nucleophosmin in acute myeloid leukemia. *Expert Review of Anticancer Therapy* 9: 1283–1294.

Metzeler, K.H., Dufour, A., Benthaus, T., Hummel, M., Sauerland, M.C., Heinecke, A., Berdel, W.E. et al. 2009. ERG expression is an independent prognostic factor and allows refined risk stratification in cytogenetically normal acute myeloid leukemia: A comprehensive analysis of ERG, MN1, and BAALC transcript levels using oligo nucleotide microarrays. *Journal of Clinical Oncology* 27: 5031–5038.

Metzeler, K.H., Maharry, K., Radmacher, M.D., Mrózek, K., Margeson, D., Becker, H., Curfman, J. et al. 2011. TET2 mutations improve the New European leukemia net risk classification of acute myeloid leukemia: A Cancer and Leukemia Group B Study. *Journal of Clinical Oncology* 29: 1373–1381.

Meyer, C., Kowarz, E., Hofmann, J., Renneville, A., Zuna, J., Trka, J., Ben Abdelali, R. et al. 2009. New insights to the *MLL* recombinome of acute leukemias. *Leukemia* 23: 1490–1499.

Miller, W.H. Jr., Kakizuka, A., Frankel, S.R., Warrell, R.P. Jr., DeBlasio, A., Levine, K., Evans, R.M., and E. Dmitrovsky. 1992. Reverse transcription polymerase chain reaction for the rearranged retinoic acid receptor alpha clarifies diagnosis and detects minimal residual disease in acute promyelocytic leukemia. *The Proceedings of the National Academy of Sciences of the USA* 89: 2694–2698.

Miwa, H., Beran, M., and G.F. Saunders. 1992. Expression of the Wilms' tumor gene (WT1) in human leukemias. *Leukemia* 6: 405–409.

Miyawaki, S., Hatsumi, N., Tamaki, T., Naoe, T., Ozawa, K., Kitamura, K., Karasuno, T. et al. 2010. Prognostic potential of detection of WT1 mRNA level in peripheral blood in adult acute myeloid leukemia. *Leukemia and Lymphoma* 51: 1855–1861.

Mohr, F., Döhner, K., Buske, C., and V.P. Rawat. 2011. TET genes: New players in DNA demethylation and important determinants for stemness. *Experimental Hematology* 39: 272–281.

Motyckova, G. and R.M. Stone. 2010. The role of molecular tests in acute myeloid leukemia treatment decisions. *Current Hematology Malignancies Report* 5: 109–117.

Mourah, S., Porcher, R., Lescaille, G., Rousselot, P., Podgorniak, M.P., Labarchède, G., Naimi, B. et al. 2009. Quantification of VEGF isoforms and VEGFR transcripts by qRT-PCR and their significance in acute myeloid leukemia. *The International Journal of Biological Markers* 24: 22–31.

Mrózek, K., Döhner, H., and C.D. Bloomfield. 2007. Influence of new molecular prognostic markers in patients with karyotypically normal acute myeloid leukemia: Recent advances. *Current Opinion in Hematology* 14: 106–114.

Mrózek, K., Heerema, N.A., and C.D. Bloomfield. 2004. Cytogenetics in acute leukemia. *Blood Reviews* 18: 115–136.

Mrózek, K., Marcucci, G., Nicolet, D., Maharry, K.S., Becker, H., Whitman, S.P., Metzeler, K.H. et al. 2012. Prognostic significance of the European LeukemiaNet standardized system for reporting cytogenetic and molecular alterations in adults with acute myeloid leukemia. *Journal of Clinical Oncology* 30: 4515–4523.

Mrózek, K., Marcucci, G., Paschka, P., and C.D. Bloomfield. 2008. Advances in molecular genetics and treatment of core-binding factor acute myeloid leukemia. *Current Opinion in Oncology* 20: 711–718.

Nakao, M., Yokota, S., Iwai, T., Kaneko, H., Horiike, S., Kashima, K., Sonoda, Y., Fujimoto, T., and S. Misawa. 1996. Internal tandem duplication of the flt3 gene found in acute myeloid leukemia. *Leukemia* 10: 1911–1918.

Nana-Sinkam, P. and C.M. Croce. 2010. MicroRNAs in diagnosis and prognosis in cancer: What does the future hold? *Pharmacogenomics* 11: 667–669.

Naoe, T. and H. Kiyoi. 2004. Normal and oncogenic FLT3. *Cellular and Molecular Life Sciences* 61: 2932–2938.

Narahara, K., Kimura, S., Kikkawa, K., Takahashi, Y., Wakita, Y., Kasai, R., Nagai, S., Nishibayashi, Y., and H. Kimoto. 1985. Probable assignment of soluble isocitrate dehydrogenase (IDH1) to 2q33.3. *Human Genetics* 71: 37–40.

Neben, K., Schnittger, S., Brors, B., Tews, B., Kokocinski, F., Haferlach, T., Müller, J. et al. 2005. Distinct gene expression patterns associated with FLT3- and NRAS-activating mutations in acute myeloid leukemia with normal karyotype. *Oncogene* 24: 1580–1588.

Nibourel, O., Kosmider, O., Cheok, M., Boissel, N., Renneville, A., Philippe, N., Dombret, H. et al. 2010. Incidence and prognostic value of TET2 alterations in de novo acute myeloid leukemia achieving complete remission. *Blood* 116: 1132–1135.

Nilson, I., Löchner, K., Siegler, G., Greil, J., Beck, J.D., Fey, G.H., and P. Marschalek. 1996. Exon/intron structure of the human ALL-1 (MLL) gene involved in translocations to chromosomal region 11q23 and acute leukaemias. *British Journal of Haematology* 93: 966–972.

Noordermeer, S.M., Tönnissen, E., Vissers, I., van der Heijden, A., van de Locht, L.T., Deutz-Terlouw, P.P., Marijt, E.W., Jansen, J.H., and B.A. van der Reijden. 2011. Rapid identification of IDH1 and IDH2 mutations in acute myeloid leukaemia using high resolution melting curve analysis. *British Journal of Haematology* 152: 493–496.

Oelschlaegel, U., Koch, S., Mohr, B., Schaich, M., Falini, B., Ehninger, G., and C. Thiede. 2010. Rapid flow cytometric detection of a berrant cytoplasmic localization of nucleophosmin (NPMc) indicating mutant NPM1 gene in acute myeloid leukemia. *Leukemia* 24: 1813–1816.

Oh, I.U., Inazawa, J., Kim, Y.O., Song, B.J., and T.L. Huh. 1996. Assignment of the human mitochondrial NADP(+)-specific isocitrate dehydrogenase (IDH2) gene to 15q26.1 by in situ hybridization. *Genomics* 38: 104–106.

Okuwaki, M. 2008. The structure and functions of NPM1/Nucleophosmin/B23, a multifunctional nuclear acidic protein. *The Journal of Biochemistry* 143: 441–448.

Ostgärd, L.S., Kjeldsen, E., Holm, M.S., Brown Pde, N., Pedersen, B.B., Bendix, K., Johansen, P., Kristensen, J.S., and J.M. Nørgaard. 2010. Reasons for treating secondary AML as de novo AML. *European Journal of Haematology* 85: 217–226.

Otten, J., Schmitz, L., Vettorazzi, E., Schultze, A., Marx, A.H., Simon, R., Krauter, J. et al. 2011. Expression of TGF-β receptor ALK-5 has a negative impact on outcome of patients with acute myeloid leukemia. *Leukemia* 25: 375–379.

Owen, C., Fitzgibbon, J., and P. Paschka. 2010. The clinical relevance of *Wilms Tumor I* (WT1) gene mutations in acute leukaemia. *Hematological Oncology* 28: 13–19.

Pabst, T., Eyholzer, M., Fos, J., and B.U. Mueller. 2009. Heterogeneity within AML with CEBPA mutations, only CEBPA double mutations, but not single CEBPA mutations are associated with favourable prognosis. *British Journal of Cancer* 100: 1343–1346.

Pabst, T. and B.U. Mueller. 2007. Transcriptional dysregulation during myeloid transformation in AML. *Oncogene* 26: 6829–6837.

Pabst, T., Mueller, B.U., Zhang, P., Radomska, H.S., Narravula, S., Schnittger, S., Behre, G., Hiddemann, W., and D.G. Tenen. 2001. Dominant-negative mutations of CEBPA, encoding CCAAT/enhancer binding protein-alpha (C/EBP alpha), in acute myeloid leukemia. *Nature Genetics* 27: 263–270.

Paschka, P., Marcucci, G., Ruppert, A.S., Mrózek, K., Chen, H., Kittles, R.A., Vukosavljevic, T. et al. 2006. Adverse prognostic significance of KIT mutations in adult acute myeloid leukemia with inv(16) and t(8;21): A Cancer and Leukemia Group B Study. *Journal of Clinical Oncology* 24: 3904–3911.

Paschka, P., Marcucci, G., Ruppert, A.S., Whitman, S.P., Mrózek, K., Maharry, K., Langer, C. et al. 2008. Wilms' tumor 1 gene mutations independently predict poor outcome in adults with cytogenetically normal acute myeloid leukemia: A Cancer and Leukemia Group B Study. *Journal of Clinical Oncology* 26: 4595–4602.

Paschka, P., Schlenk, R.F., Gaidzik, V.I., Habdank, M., Krönke, J., Bullinger, L., Späth, D. et al. 2010. IDH1 and IDH2 mutations are frequent genetic alterations in acute myeloid leukemia and confer adverse prognosis in cytogenetically normal acute myeloid leukemia with NPM1 mutation without FLT3 internal tandem duplication. *Journal of Clinical Oncology* 28: 3636–3643.

Patel, J.P., Gönen, M., Figueroa, M.E., Fernandez, H., Sun, Z., Racevskis, J., Van Vlierberghe, P. et al. 2012. Prognostic relevance of integrated genetic profiling in acute myeloid leukemia. *The New England Journal of Medicine* 366: 1079–1089.

Patel, K.P., Ravandi, F., Ma, D., Paladugu, A., Barkoh, B.A., Medeiros, L.J., and R. Luthra. 2011. Acute myeloid leukemia with IDH1 or IDH2 mutation: Frequency and clinicopathologic features. *American Journal of Clinical Pathology* 135: 35–45.

Paun, O. and H.M. Lazarus. 2012. Allogeneic hematopoietic cell transplation for acute myeloid leukemia in first complete remission: Have the indications changed? *Current Opinion in Hematology* 19: 95–101.

Paydas, S., Tanriverdi, K., Yavuz, S., Disel, U., Baslamisli, F., and R. Burgut. 2005. PRAME mRNA levels in cases with acute leukemia: Clinical importance and future prospects. *American Journal of Hematology* 79: 257–261.

Perrot, A., Luquet, I., Pigneux, A., Mugneret, F., Delaunay, J., Harousseau, J.-L., Barin, C. et al. 2011. Dismal prognostic value of monosomal karyotype in elderly patients with acute myeloid leukemia: A GOELAMS Study of 186 patients with unfavorable cytogenetic cytogenetic abnormalities. *Blood* 118: 679–685.

Plesa, C., Chelghoum, Y., Plesa, A., Elhamri, M., Tigand, I., Michallet, M., Dumontet, C., and X. Thomas. 2008. Prognostic value of immunophenotyping in elderly patients with acute myeloid leukemia: A single-institution experience. *Cancer* 112: 572–580.

Preudhomme, C., Sagot, C., Boissel, N., Cayuela, J.M., Tigaud, I., de Botton, S., Thomas, X. et al. 2002. Favorable prognostic significance of CEBPA mutations in patients with de novo acute myeloid leukemia: A study from the Acute Leukemia French Association (ALFA). *Blood* 100: 2717–2723.

Qin, Y., Zhu, H., Jiang, B., Li, J., Lu, X., Li, L., Ruan, G. et al. 2009. Expression patterns of WT1 and PRAME in acute myeloid leukemia patients and their usefulness for monitoring minimal residual disease. *Leukemia Research* 33: 384–390.

Radmacher, M.D., Marcucci, G., Ruppert, A.S., Mrózek, K., Whitman, S.P., Vardiman, J.W., Paschka, P. et al. 2006. Independent confirmation of aprognostic gene-expression signature in adult acute myeloid leukemia with a normal karyotype: A Cancer and Leukemia Group B Study. *Blood* 108: 1677–1683.

Radomska, H.S., Bassères, D.S., Zheng, R., Zhang, P., Dayaram, T., Yamamoto, Y., Sternberg, D.W. et al. 2006. Block of C/EBP alpha function by phosphorylation in acute myeloid leukemia with FLT3 activating mutations. *The Journal of Experimental Medicine* 203: 371–381.

Ramsingh, G., Koboldt, D.C., Trissal, M., Chiappinelli, K.B., Wylie, T., Koul, S., Chang, L.W. et al. 2010. Complete characterization of the micro RNAome in a patient with acute myeloid leukemia. *Blood* 116: 5316–5326.

Rau, R. and P. Brown. 2009. Nucleophosmin (NPM1) mutations in adult and childhood acute myeloid leukaemia: Towards definition of a new leukaemia entity. *Hematological Oncology* 27: 171–181.

Ravandi, F., Kantarjian, H., Faderl, S., Garcia-Manero, G., O'Brien, S., Koller, C., Pierce, S. et al. 2010. Outcome of patients with FLT3-mutated acute myeloid leukemia in first relapse. *Leukemia Research* 34: 752–756.

Reindl, C., Quentmeier, H., Petropoulos, K., Greif, P.A., Benthaus, T., Argiropoulos, B., Mellert, G. et al. 2009. CBL exon 8/9 mutants activate the FLT3 pathway and cluster in core binding factor/11q deletion acute myeloid leukemia/myelodysplastic syndrome subtypes. *Clinical Cancer Research* 15: 2238–2247.

Renneville, A., Boissel, N., Zurawski, V., Llopis, L., Biggio, V., Nibourel, O., Philippe, N. et al. 2009. Wilms tumor 1 gene mutations are associated with a higher risk of recurrence in young adults with acute myeloid leukemia: A study from the Acute Leukemia French Association. *Cancer* 115: 3719–3727.

Ribeiro Tibúrcio, A.F., Pratcorona, M., Erpelinck-Verschueren, C., Rockova, V., Sanders, M., Abbas, S., Figueroa, M.E. et al. 2012. Mutant *DNMT3A*: A new marker of poor prognosis in acute myeloid leukemia. *Blood* 119: 5824–5831.

Ritter, M., Kim, T.D., Lisske, P., Thiede, C., Schaich, M., and A. Neubauer. 2004. Prognostic significance of N-RAS and K-RAS mutations in 232 patients with acute myeloid leukemia. *Haematologica* 89: 1397–1399.

Rockova, V., Abbas, S., Wouters, B.J., Erpelinck, C.A.J., Beverloo, H.B., Delwel, R., van Putten, W.L.J., Löwenberg, B., and P.J.M. Valk. 2011. Risk-stratification of intermediate-risk acute myeloid leukemia: Integrative analysis of a multitude of gene mutation and expression markers. *Blood* 118: 1069–1076.

Rocquain, J., Carbuccia, N., Trouplin, V., Raynaud, S., Murati, A., Nezri, M., Tadrist, Z. et al. 2010. Combined mutations of ASXL1, CBL, FLT3, IDH1, IDH2, JAK2, KRAS, NPM1, NRAS, RUNX1, TET2 and WT1 genes in myelodysplastic syndromes and acute myeloid leukemias. *BMC Cancer* 10: 401.

Rodríguez-Paredes, M. and M. Esteller. 2011. Cancer epigenetics reaches mainstream oncology. *Nature Medicine* 17: 330–339.

Röllig, C., Bornhäuser, M., Thiede, C., Taube, F., Kramer, M., Mohr, B., AYulitzky, W. et al. 2011. Long-term prognosis of acute myeloid leukemia according to the new genetic risk classification of the European LeukemiaNet recommendations: Evaluation of the proposed reporting system. *Journal of Clinical Oncology* 29: 2758–2765.

Rücker, F.G., Schlenk, R.F., Bullinger, L., Kayser, S., Teleanu, V., Kett, H., Habdank, M. et al. 2012. TP53 alterations in acute myeloid leukemia with complex karyotype correlate with specific copy number alterations, monosomal karyotype, and dismal outcome. *Blood* 119: 2114–2121.

Saied, M.H., Marzec, J., Khalid, S., Smith, P., Down, T.A., Rakyan, V.K., Molloy, G. et al. 2012. Genome wide analysis of acute myeloid leukemia reveal leukemia specific methylome and subtype specific hypomethylation of repeats. *PLOS One* 7: e33213.

Sangle, N.A. and S.L. Perkins. 2011. Core-binding factor acute myeloid leukemia. *Archives of Pathology and Laboratory Medicine* 135: 1504–1509.

Santamaría, C., Chillón, M.C., García-Sanz, R., Pérez, C., Caballero, M.D., Mateos, M.V., Ramos, F. et al. 2010. BAALC is an important predictor of refractoriness to chemotherapy and poor survival in intermediate-risk acute myeloid leukemia (AML). *Annals of Hematology* 89: 453–458.

Santamaría, C.M., Chillón, M.C., García-Sanz, R., Pérez, C., Caballero, M.D., Ramos, F., de Coca, A.G. et al. 2009. Molecular stratification model for prognosis in cytogenetically normal acute myeloid leukemia. *Blood* 114: 148–152.

Sanz, M.A., Grimwade, D., Tallman, M.S., Lowenberg, B., Fenaux, P., Estey, E.H., Naoe, T. et al. 2009. Management of acute promyelocytic leukemia: recommendations from an expert panel on behalf of the European LeukemiaNet. *Blood* 113: 1875–1891.

Sárová, I., Brezinová, J., Zemanová, Z., Lizcová, L., Berková, A., Izáková, S., Malinová, E. et al. 2009. A partial nontandem duplication of the MLL gene in four patients with acute myeloid leukemia. *Cancer Genetics and Cytogenetics* 195: 150–156.

Savkur, R.S. and M.O. Olson. 1998. Preferential cleavage inpre-ribosomal RNA by protein B23 endoribonuclease. *Nucleic Acids Research* 26: 4508–4515.

Schlenk, R.F. and K. Döhner. 2009. Impact of new prognostic markers in treatment decisions in acute myeloid leukemia. *Current Opinion in Hematology* 16: 98–104.

Schlenk, R.F., Döhner, K., Krauter, J., Fröhling, S., Corbacioglu, A., Bullinger, L., Habdank, M. et al. 2008. Mutations and treatment outcome in cytogenetically normal acute myeloid leukemia. *The New England Journal of Medicine* 358: 1909–1918.

Schnittger, S., Eder, C., Jeromin, S., Alpermann, T., Fasan, A., Grossmann, V., Kohlmann, A. et al. 2013. *ASXL1* exon 12 mutations are frequent in AML with intermediate risk karyotype and are independently associated with an adverse outcome. *Leukemia* 27: 82–91.

Schnittger, S., Haferlach, C., Ulke, M., Alpermann, T., Kern, W., and T. Haferlach. 2010. IDH1 mutations are detected in 6.6% of 1414 AML patients and are associated with intermediate risk karyotype and unfavorable prognosis in adults younger than 60 years and unmutated NPM1 status. *Blood* 116: 5486–5496.

Schnittger, S., Kern, W., Tschulik, C., Weiss, T., Dicker, F., Falini, B., Haferlach, C., and T. Haferlach. 2009. Minimal residual disease levels assessed by NPM1 mutation-specific RQ-PCR provide important prognostic in formation in AML. *Blood* 114: 2220–2231.

Schnittger, S., Kinkelin, U., Schoch, C., Heinecke, A., Haase, D., Haferlach, T., Büchner, T. et al. 2000. Screening for MLL tandem duplication in 387 unselected patients with AML identify a prognostically unfavorable subset of AML. *Leukemia* 14: 796–804.

Schnittger, S., Wörmann, B., Hiddemann, W., and F. Griesinger. 1998. Partial tandem duplications of the MLL gene are detectable in peripheral blood and bone marrow of nearly all healthy donors. *Blood* 92: 1728–1734.

Scholl, S., Theuer, C., Scheble, V., Kunert, C., Heller, A., Mügge, L.O., Fricke, H.J., Höffken, K., and U. Wedding. 2008. Clinical impact of nucleophosmin mutations and Flt3 internal tandem duplications in patients older than 60 year with acute myeloid leukaemia. *European Journal of Haematology* 80: 208–215.

Schwind, S., Marcucci, G., Maharry, K., Radmacher, M.D., Mrózek, K., Holland, K.B., Margeson, D. et al. 2010. BAALC and ERG expression levels are associated without come and distinct gene and microRNA expression profiles in older patients with de novo cytogenetically normal acute myeloid leukemia: A Cancer and Leukemia Group B Study. *Blood* 116: 5660–5669.

Sebaa, A., Ades, L., Baran-Marzack, F., Mozziconacci, M.-J., Penther, J., Dobbelstein, S., Stamatoullas, A. et al. 2012. Incidence of 17p deletions and *TP53* mutation in myelodysplastic syndrome and acute myeloid leukemia with 5q deletion. *Genes, Chromosomes and Cancer* 51: 1086–1092.

Shen, Y., Zhu, Y.M., Fan, X., Shi, J.Y., Wang, Q.R., Yan, X.J., Gu, Z.H. et al. 2011. Gene mutation patterns and their prognostic impact in a cohort of 1185 patients with acute myeloid leukemia. *Blood* 118: 5593–5603.

Shimada, A., Taki, T., Tabuchi, K., Tawa, A, Horibe, K., Tsuchida, M., Hanada, R., Tsukimoto, I., and Y. Hayashi. 2006. KIT mutations, and not FLT3 internal tandem duplication, are strongly associated with a poor prognosis in pediatric acute myeloid leukemia with t(8,21): A study of the Japanese Childhood AML Cooperative Study Group. *Blood* 107: 1806–1809.

Shook, D., Coustan-Smith, E., Ribeiro, R.C., Rubnitz, J.E., and D. Campana. 2009. Minimal residual disease quantitation in acute myeloid leukemia. *Clinical Lymphoma and Myeloma* 9(Suppl 3): S281–S285.

Small, D. 2008. Targeting FLT3 for the treatment of leukemia. *Seminars in Hematology* 45: S17–S21.

Smith, M.L., Hills, R.K., and D. Grimwade. 2011. Independent prognostic variables in acute myeloid leukaemia. *Blood Reviews* 25: 39–51.

Spoo, A.C., Lübbert, M., Wierda, W.G., and J.A. Burger. 2007. CXCR4 is a prognostic marker in acute myelogenous leukemia. *Blood* 109: 786–791.

Steinbach, D. and O. Legrand. 2007. ABC transporters and drug resistance in leukemia: Was P-gp nothing but the first head of the Hydra? *Leukemia* 21: 1172–1176.

Steinbach, D., Pfaffendorf, N., Wittig, S., and B. Gruhn. 2007. PRAME expression is not associated with down-regulation of retinoic acid signaling in primary acute myeloid leukemia. *Cancer Genetics and Cytogenetics* 177: 51–54.

Steudel, C., Wermke, M., Schaich, M., Schäkel, U., Illmer, T., Ehninger, G., and C. Thiede. 2003. Comparative analysis of MLL partial tandem duplication and FLT3 internal tandem duplication mutations in 956 adult patients with acute myeloid leukemia. *Genes Chromosomes Cancer* 37: 237–251.

Strout, M.P., Marcucci, G., Bloomfield, C.D., and M.A. Caligiuri. 1998. The partial tandem duplication of ALL1 (MLL) is consistently generated by Alu-mediated homologous recombination in acute myeloid leukemia. *The Proceedings of the National Academy of Sciences of the USA* 95: 2390–2395.

Strunk, C.J., Platzbecker, U., Thiede, C., Schaich, M., Illmer, T., Kang, Z., Leahy, P. et al. 2009. Elevated AF1q expression is a poor prognostic marker for adult acute myeloid leukemia patients with normal cytogenetics. *American Journal of Hematology* 84: 308–309.

Suh, H.C., Gooya, J., Renn, K., Friedman, A.D., Johnson, P.F., and J.R. Keller. 2006. C/EBP alpha determines hematopoietic cell fate in multipotential progenitor cells by inhibiting erythroid differentiation and inducing myeloid differentiation. *Blood* 107: 4308–4316.

Sun, S.M., Rockova, V., Bullinger, L., Dijkstra, M.K., Döhner, H., Löwenberg, B., and Jongen-Lavrencic, M. 2013. The prognostic relevance of miR-212 expression with survival in cytogenetically and molecularly heterogeneous AML. *Leukemia* 27: 100–106.

Szankasi, P., Ho, A.K., Bahler, D.W., Efimova, O., and T.W. Kelley. 2011. Combined testing for CCAAT/enhancer-binding protein alpha (CEBPA) mutations and promoter methylation in acute myeloid leukemia demonstrates shared phenotypic features. *Leukemia Research* 35: 200–207.

Szotkowski, T., Muzik, J., Voglova, J., Koza, V., Maaloufova, J., Kozak, T., Jarosova, M. et al. 2010. Prognostic factors and treatment outcome in 1,516 adult patients with de novo and secondary acute myeloid leukemia in 1999–2009 in 5 hematology intensive care centers in the Czech Republic. *Neoplasma* 57: 578–589.

Taberlay, P.C. and P.A. Jones. 2011. DNA methylation and cancer. *Progress in Drug Research*. 67: 1–23.

Tang, J.L., Hou, H.A., Chen, C.Y., Liu, C.Y., Chou, W.C., Tseng, M.H., Huang, C.F. et al. 2009. AML1/RUNX1 mutations in 470 adult patients with de novo acute myeloid leukemia: Prognostic implication and interaction with other gene alterations. *Blood* 114: 5352–5361.

Taskesen, E., Bullinger, L., Corbacioglu, A., Sanders, M.A., Erpelinck, C.A., Wouters, B.J., van der Poel-van de Luytgaarde, S.C. et al. 2011. Prognostic impact, concurrent genetic mutations, and gene expression features of AML with CEBPA mutations in a cohort of 1182 cytogenetically normal AML patients: Further evidence for CEBPA double mutant AML as a distinctive disease entity. *Blood* 17: 2469–2475.

Tavernier-Tardy, E., Cornillon, J., Campos, L., Flandrin, P., Duval, A., Nadal, N., and D. Guyotat. 2009. Prognostic value of CXCR4 and FAK expression in acute myelogenous leukemia. *Leukemia Research* 33: 764–768.

Tenen, D.G., Hromas, R., Licht, J.D., and D.E. Zhang. 1997. Transcription factors, normal myeloid development, and leukaemia. *Blood* 90: 489–519.

Thiede, C. 2012. Mutant *DNMT3A*: Teaming up to transform. *Blood* 119: 5615–5617.

Thol, F., Damm, F., Wagner, K., Göhring, G., Schlegelberger, B., Hoelzer, D., Lübbert, M. et al. 2010 Prognostic impact of IDH2 mutations in cytogenetically normal acute myeloid leukemia. *Blood* 116: 614–616.

Tiacci, E., Grossmann, V., Martelli, M.P., Kohlmann, A., Haferlach, T., and B. Falini. 2012. The corepressors BCOR and BCORL1: Two novel players in acute myeloid leukemia. *Haematologica* 97: 3–5.

Tiu, R.V., Gondek, L.P., O'Keefe, C.L., Huh, J., Sekeres, M.A., Elson, P., Mc Devitt, M.A. et al. 2009. New lesions detected by single nucleotide polymorphism array-based chromosomal analysis have important clinical impact in acute myeloid leukemia. *Journal of Clinical Oncology* 27: 5219–5226.

Trnková, Z., Bedrlíková, R., Marková, J., Michalová, K., Stöckbauer, P., and J. Schwarz. 2007. Semiquantitative RT-PCR evaluation of the MDR1 gene expression in patients with acute myeloid leukemia. *Neoplasma* 54: 387–390.

Ugrinova, I., K. Monier, K., Ivaldi, C., Thiry, M., Storck, S., Mongelard, F., and P. Bouvet. 2007. Inactivation of nucleolin leads to nucleolar disruption, cell cycle arrest and defects in centrosome duplication. *BMC Molecular Biology* 8: 66.

Van Vlierberghe, P., Patel, J., Abdel-Wahab, O., Lobry, C., Hedvat, C.V., Balbin, M., Nicolas, C. et al. 2011. PHF6 mutations in adult acute myeloid leukemia. *Leukemia* 25: 130–134.

Vardiman, J.W., Thiele, J., Arber, D.A., Brunning, R.D., Borowitz, M.J., Porwit, A., Harris, N.L. et al. 2009. The 2008 revision of the World Health Organization (WHO) classification of myeloid neoplasms and acute leukemia: Rationale and important changes. *Blood* 114: 937–951.

Verhaak, R.G., Goudswaard, C.S., van Putten, W., Bijl, M.A., Sanders, M.A., Hugens, W., Uitterlinden, A.G. et al. 2005. Mutations in nucleophosmin (NPM1) in acute myeloid leukemia (AML): Association with other gene abnormalities and previously established gene expression signatures and their favorable prognostic significance. *Blood* 106: 3747–3754.

Verhaak, R.G., Wouters, B.J., Erpelinck, C.A., Abbas, S., Beverloo, H.B., Lugthart, S., Löwenberg, B., Delwel, R., and P.J. Valk. 2009. Prediction of molecular subtypes in acute myeloid leukemia based on gene expression profiling. *Haematologica* 94: 131–134.

Virappane, P., Gale, R., Hills, R., Kakkas, I., Summers, K., Stevens, J., Allen, C. et al. 2008. Mutation of the Wilms' tumor 1 gene is a poor prognostic factor associated with chemotherapy resistance in normal karyotype acute myeloid leukemia: The United Kingdom Medical Research Council Adult Leukaemia Working Party. Mutation of the Wilms' tumor 1 gene is a poor prognostic factor associated with chemotherapy resistance in normal karyotype acute myeloid leukemia: The United Kingdom Medical Research Council Adult Leukaemia Working Party. *Journal of Clinical Oncology* 26: 5429–5435.

Wagner, K., Damm, F., Göhring, G., Görlich, K., Heuser, M., Schäfer, I., Ottmann, O. et al. 2010. Impact of IDH1 R132 mutations and an IDH1 single nucleotide polymorphism in cytogenetically normal acute myeloid leukemia: SNP rs11554137 is an adverse prognostic factor. *Journal of Clinical Oncology* 28: 5078–5087.

Walker, A. and G. Marcucci. 2011. Impact of molecular prognostic factors in cytogenetically normal acute myeloid leukemia at diagnosis and relapse. *Haematologica* 96: 640–643.

Wang, N.D., Finegold, M.J., Bradley, A., Ou, C.N., Abdelsayed, S.V., Wilde, M.D., Taylor, L.R., Wilson, D.R., and G. Darlington. 1995. Impaired energy homeostasis in C/EBP alpha knockout mice. *Science* 269: 1108–1112.

Ward, P.S., Patel, J., Wise, D.R., Abdel-Wahab, O., Bennett, B.D., Coller, H.A., Cross, J.R. et al. 2010. The common feature of leukemia-associated IDH1 and IDH2 mutations is a neomorphic enzyme activity converting alpha-ketoglutarate to 2-hydroxyglutarate. *Cancer Cell* 17: 225–234.

Watanabe, Y. and M. Maekawa. 2010. Methylation of DNA in cancer. *Advances in Clinical Chemistry* 52: 145–167.

Weinkauff, R., Estey, E.H., Starostik, P., Hayes, K., Huh, Y.O., Hirsch-Ginsberg, A., Andreeff, M. et al. 1999. Use of peripheral blood blasts for diagnosis of acute myeloid leukemia. *American Journal of Clinical Pathology* 111: 733–740.

Weisberg, E., Barrett, R., Liu, Q., Stone, R., Gray, N., and J.D. Griffin. 2009. FLT3 inhibition and mechanisms of drug resistance in mutant FLT3-positive AML. *Drug Resistance Updates* 12: 81–89.

Whitman, S.P., Hackanson, B., Liyanarachchi, S., Liu, S., Rush, L.J., Maharry, K., Margeson, D. et al. 2008a. DNA hypermethylation and epigenetic silencing of the tumor suppressor gene, SLC5A8, in acute myeloid leukemia with the MLL partial tandem duplication. *Blood* 112: 2013–2016.

Whitman, S.P., Liu, S., Vukosavljevic, T., Rush, L.J., Yu, L., Liu, C., Klisovic, M.I. et al. 2005. The MLL partial tandem duplication: Evidence for recessive gain-of-function in acute myeloid leukemia identifies a novel patient subgroup for molecular-targeted therapy. *Blood* 106: 345–352.

Whitman, S.P., Maharry, K., Radmacher, M.D., Becker, H., Mrózek, K., Margeson, D., Holland, K.B. et al. 2010. FLT3 internal tandem duplication associates with adverse outcome and gene- and microRNA-expression signatures in patients 60 years of age or older with primary cytogenetically normal acute myeloid leukemia: A Cancer and Leukemia Group B Study. *Blood* 116: 3622–3626.

Whitman, S.P., Ruppert, A.S., Radmacher, M.D., Mrózek, K., Paschka, P., Langer, C., Baldus, C.D. et al. 2008b. FLT3D835/I836 mutations are associated with poor disease-free survival and a distinct gene-expression signature among younger adults with de novo cytogenetically normal acute myeloid leukemia lacking FLT3 internal tandem duplications. *Blood* 111: 1529–1559.

Wiernik, P.H. 2010. FLT3 inhibitors for the treatment of acute myeloid leukemia. *Clinical Advances in Hematology and Oncology* 8: 429–444.

Wilson, C.S., Davidson, G.S., Martin, S.B., Andries, E., Potter, J., Harvey, R., Ar, K. et al. 2006. Gene expression profiling of adult acute myeloid leukemia identifies novel biologic clusters for risk classification and outcome prediction. *Blood* 108: 685–696.

Wouters, B.J., Löwenberg, B., and R. Delwel. 2009a. A decade of genome-wide gene expression profiling in acute myeloid leukemia: Flashback and prospects. *Blood* 113: 291–298.

Wouters, B.J., Löwenberg, B., Erpelinck-Verschueren, C.A., van Putten, W.L., Valk, P.J., and R. Delwel. 2009b. Double CEBPA mutations, but not single CEBPA mutations, define a subgroup of acute myeloid leukemia with a distinctive gene expression profile that is uniquely associated with a favorable outcome. *Blood* 113: 3088–3091.

Xiao, J., Zhang, Z., Chen, G.G., Zhang, M., Ding, Y., Fu, J., Li, M., and J.P. Yun. 2009. Nucleophosmin/B23 interacts with p21WAF1/CIP1 and contributes to its stability. *Cell Cycle* 8: 889–895.

Xu, X., Zhao, Y., Xu, M., Dai, Q., Meng, W., Yang, J., and R. Qin. 2011. Activation of Notch signal pathway is associated with a poorer prognosis in acute myeloid leukemia. *Medical Oncology* 28(Suppl 1): S483–S489.

Yamagata, T., Maki, K., and K. Mitani. 2005. RUNX1/AML1 in normal and abnormal hematopoiesis. *International Journal of Hematology* 82: 1–8.

Yamamoto, Y., Kiyoi, H., Nakano, Y., Suzuki, R., Kodera, Y., Miyawaki, S., Asou, N. et al. 2001. Activating mutation of D835 within the activation loop of FLT3 in human hematologic malignancies. *Blood* 97: 2434–2439.

Yang, L., Han, Y., Suarez Saiz, F., and M.D. Minden. 2007. A tumor suppressor and oncogene: The WT1 story. *Leukemia* 21: 868–876.

Yin, J.A.L., O'Brien, M.A., Hills, R.K., Daly, S.B., Wheatley, K., and A.K. Burnett. 2012. Minimal residual disease monitoring by quantitative RT-PCR in core binding factor AML allows risk stratification and predicts relapse: Results of the United Kingdom MRC AML-15 trial. *Blood* 120: 2826–2835.

Yoshida, K., Sanada, M., Shiraishi, Y., Nowak, D., Nagata, Y., Yamamoto, R., Sato, Y. et al. 2011. Frequent pathway mutations of splicing machinery in myelodysplasia. *Nature* 478: 64–69.

Ysebaert, L., Chicanne, G., Demur, C., De Toni, F., Prade-Houdellier, N, Ruidavets, J.B., Mansat-De Mas, V. et al. 2006. Expression of beta-catenin by acute myeloid leukemia cells predicts enhanced clonogenic capacities and poor prognosis. *Leukemia* 20: 1211–1216.

Yu, Y., Maggi, Jr., L.B., Brady, S.N., Apicelli, A.J., Dai, M.S., Lu, H., and J.D. Weber. 2006. Nucleophosmin is essential for ribosomal protein L5 nuclear export. *Molecular and Cellular Biology* 26: 3798–3809.

Zhang, D.E., Zhang, P., Wang, N.D., Hetherington, C.J., Darlington, G.J., and D.G. Tenen. 1997. Absence of granulocytecolony-stimulating factor signaling and neutrophil development in CCAAT enhancer binding protein alpha-deficient mice. *The Proceedings of the National Academy of Siences of the USA* 94: 569–574.

Zhu, Y.D., Wang, L., Sun, C., Fan, L., Zhu, D.X., Fang, C., Wang, Y.H. et al. 2012. Distinctive microRNA signature is associated with the diagnosis and prognosis of acute leukemia. *Medical Oncology* 29: 2323–2331.

30

Biomarkers in Hodgkin's Lymphoma

Esin Demir, Burak Yılmaz, Mehmet Gunduz, and Esra Gunduz

CONTENTS

ABSTRACT Lymphoma is a type of hematological cancer which occurs in the immune system, and specifically starts in lymphocytes. Lymphoma is basically of two types: Hodgkin's and non-Hodgkin's lymphoma (NHL). This chapter will specifically focus on Hodgkin's lymphoma (HL), whose subtypes are nodular lymphocyte-predominant Hodgkin's lymphoma (NLPHL) and classical Hodgkin's lymphoma (cHL). The characteristic cell types involved in these subtypes are different from each other. Biomarkers are another critical factor in making the correct identification of each subtype. Biomarkers can be categorized into different groups such as origin-related, chromosomal, cytokine, chemokine, and some important pathways-related markers. These biomarkers are not only important to distinguish subtypes but also critical to determine further treatment strategies for disease. Due to the importance of biomarker knowledge, we have reviewed significant HL biomarkers in this chapter.

KEY WORDS: *Hodgkin's lymphoma, biomarker, NLPHL, cHL, pathway, treatment.*

30.1 Introduction

30.1.1 Why Is It Important?

Hodgkin's lymphoma (HL) accounts for approximately 11% of all lymphoma diagnoses. In 2012, 9060 people were diagnosed with HL and 1190 of those died (SEER Stat Fact Sheets: Hodgkin Lymphoma, 2012). HL incidences worldwide are still on the rise. On the other hand, HL is a curable cancer type. However, treatment strategies change according to specific subtypes of the disease.

Biomarkers have critical importance in the diagnosis of HL. Clinicians might be confused about HL subclass identification and sometimes other lymphoma types can be mistaken for HL. With the help of biomarkers, such confusions will eventually disappear. Once the HL subclass is specifically identified, treatment can be determined together with other criteria such as stage of disease and patient-specific determinants. Biomarker identification is not only important for determining treatment strategy but also critical for early diagnosis and prevention of disease. Most early diagnosed cancer patients go on with their normal life with some routine control tests. Therefore, biomarker knowledge in HL will be beneficial in saving most HL patients' lives. Furthermore, biomarkers identified under different titles (chromosomal, cytokine, etc.) can be used together. This will increase the sensitivity and specificity of the biomarkers.

30.1.2 Epidemiology

There is a changing epidemiological pattern in HL with time, ethnic origin, gender, and age across the world. As HL is a complex disease, there are other critical factors in the occurrence of the disease such as infectious diseases, immune deficits, and genetic susceptibilities (Cartwright and Watkins et al., 2004). Disorder generally strikes about 5 in every 100,000 people (Sathiya and Muthuchelian et al., 2009). Between 2000 and 2007, 16,710 HL cases were diagnosed and reported in the United States Surveillance, Epidemiology, and End Results (SEER) database. In terms of sex and race, males had significantly higher incidence compared to females and HL was predominantly seen in whites than in other races (Shenoy et al., 2011). HL diagnosis and mortality distribution in the United States between 2005 and 2009 according to different age intervals have been demonstrated in two charts (Figure 30.1).

Furthermore, in 2010, approximately 8490 new cases were diagnosed and HL was the cause of 1320 deaths in the United States (American Cancer Society, 2010). There are also epidemiological studies for the UK population. Age-dependent incidence of HL for males in the United Kingdom is 20–34 and 75–79 years of age; and for females, it is 20–24 and 70–74 years of age (Office for National Statistics, 2011). Furthermore, there is wide international variation of HL across the world according to the 2008 dataset. Southern Europe and Northern America have the highest incidence rates of HL (Ferlay et al., 2010). General HL distribution can be visualized in Figure 30.2. The figure may indicate that geographical factors are also effective in the variety of HL incidence.

30.1.3 Lymphoma Classification

Lymphoma is the most commonly seen hematological cancer type, which occurs in the lymphatic system. Lymphatic vessels and lymph nodes are the basic components of the lymphatic system. This system aids the human immune system by removing and destroying toxins, pathogens, and wastes. The malignancy is derived from lymphocytes, which are classified into B, T, and NK (natural killer) cells.

Lymphoma classification is important in terms of understanding disease biology and developing treatment options. There are many classification systems. These systems can be biologically rational or clinically useful classifications. The World Health Organization (WHO) classifies lymphoma and updates its

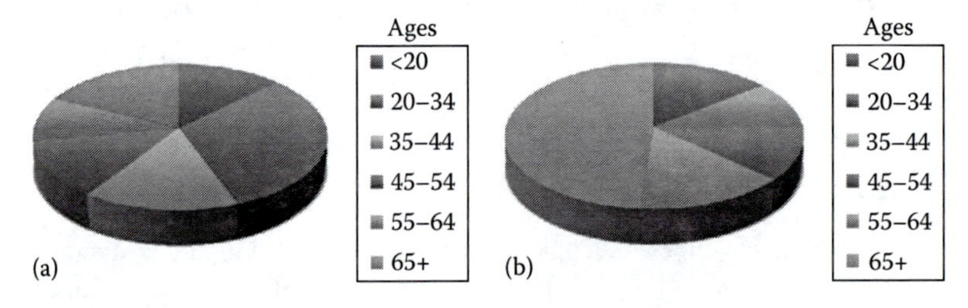

FIGURE 30.1 Hodgkin's lymphoma (a) diagnosis and (b) mortality distribution with respect to different age intervals between 2005 and 2009 in the United States. Median age for diagnosis is 35 and median age for mortality is 64. (From SEER stat fact sheet, Hodgkin's lymphoma, Surveillance epidemiology and end results, 2012, Available from http://seer.cancer.gov/statfacts/html/hodg.html, 2012.)

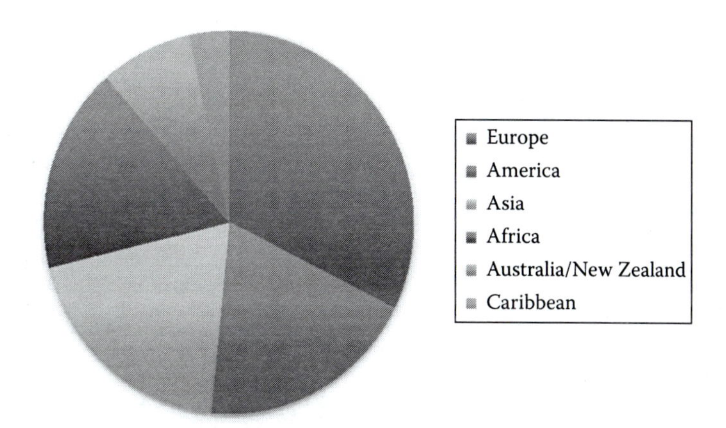

FIGURE 30.2 Hodgkin's lymphoma worldwide distribution.

classification in definite times. The last classification was made in 2008 and is adopted by most pathologists, clinicians, and biologists. This is the latest form of lymphoma classification (Jaffe, 2009).

30.1.3.1 Hodgkin's Lymphoma

1. *Nodular lymphocyte-predominant Hodgkin's lymphoma*
2. *Classical Hodgkin's lymphoma*
   a. Nodular sclerosis classical Hodgkin's lymphoma
   b. Lymphocyte-rich classical Hodgkin's lymphoma
   c. Mixed-cellularity classical Hodgkin's lymphoma
   d. Lymphocyte-depleted classical Hodgkin's lymphoma

30.1.3.2 Non-Hodgkin's Lymphoma

1. *Mature T-cell neoplasms*
2. *Mature B-cell neoplasms*
   a. Mature T-cell and B-cell neoplasms also have some subtypes

30.1.4 Current Methods for Early Diagnosis, Prognosis, and Therapy

Early diagnosis might be possible with the detection of some HL symptoms: painless, swollen lymph nodes in the neck (or underarm and groin), fever for no known reason, drenching night sweats, weight loss for no known reason, itchy skin, and feeling of extreme tiredness. Even though these symptoms give some cue about HL, it is not possible to diagnose only with these symptoms. Therefore, physical exam and patient's medical history are necessary. Then, a complete blood count (CBC), blood chemistry, and sedimentation rate analysis might be requested (National Cancer Institute, 2012). However, a more accurate and specific diagnostic tool is to do a biopsy. This invasive test enables the pathologist to analyze the tissue sample under microscope morphologically. Reed–Sternberg cells, which are characteristic cell types of classical Hodgkin's lymphoma (cHL), can be easily distinguished morphologically. However, further tests (the most commonly used test is immunohistochemistry) are required to determine subtypes of cHL or nodular lymphocyte-predominant Hodgkin's lymphoma (NLPHL). Currently, CD30 and CD15 are the most common biomarkers that are used to identify Reed–Sternberg cells. Although there are markers commonly used for cHL, it is not easy to identify subtypes of cHL. There are no commonly used biomarkers to distinguish subtypes of cHL and also NLPHL from cHL.

Prognosis and treatment options of HL can change according to the stage of the disease (basically four stages), the patient's specific symptoms and health, the subtype of the disease, and the blood test results. To be able to determine the stage and metastatic status of HL, computerized tomography (CT) scan, magnetic resonance imaging (MRI), and positron emission tomography (PET) can be used as noninvasive imaging tools. Invasive tests are bone marrow aspiration and biopsy. The disadvantage of invasive tools from the aspect of the patient is pain and psychological inconvenience due to the instruments used during invasive processes such as needles. However, they give the histological appearance of cells and most biomarker expressions. Therefore, biopsy samples are specific and sensitive diagnostic tools that are used to determine disease stage and appropriate treatments for patients. In the following sections, most of the presented biomarker candidates are determined from patient biopsy samples, which may exemplify the importance of invasive methods.

Treatment of early-stage HL is successful because 90% of patients survive at least 5 years after diagnosis. Chemotherapeutic agents (bleomycin, doxorubicin, prednisone, procarbazine, and vincristine) and radiotherapy (20–40 Gy) are used for the treatment of HL. Doxorubicin and bleomycin include the ABVD (adriamycin, bleomycin, vinblastine, dacarbazine) regimen, which is associated with treatment-related complications such as congestive heart failure and pulmonary fibrosis. Other chemotherapeutic drugs (prednisone, procarbazine, and vincristine) have an MOPP (mustargen, oncovin, procarbazine, prednisone) regimen, which increases the risk of myelodysplasia and acute myeloid leukemia (Armitage et al., 2010). Researchers have been carrying out studies to decrease the side effects of treatment. Long-term complications increase with the use of radiotherapy compared to the ABVD-alone group, especially for low-risk patients (van Leeuwen et al., 2003). These types of studies will eventually reveal the effectiveness of combined (radio- and chemotherapy) versus only ABVD, and patients will most likely survive to lead a better life. In addition, general statistics show that with the effectiveness of today's therapy, 90% of patients diagnosed with stage I HL have a chance of living 10 years or more, while 50% of stage IV HL patients may live 10 years or more (Seth et al., 2006).

From a different point of view, biomarker identification in subtypes of HL can be useful in targeted therapies, and in the future, it might be possible to use biomarkers for pharmacogenomic approaches. Currently, there is no targeted therapy or pharmacogenomic approach in the treatment of HL. There is a large gap in the identified HL biomarkers. This chapter will hopefully fill this gap and also contribute to easier and cheaper diagnosis of HL by clinicians. Despite the high costs of diagnostic imaging tools (PET, MRI), newly identified biomarkers with their special diagnostic capabilities can replace these as cheaper tools. However, further studies need to be performed in this area. Furthermore, these newly identified biomarkers will most likely help in developing more effective, less toxic therapies for early- and advanced-stage HL patients.

30.2 Noninvasive Biomarkers in Hodgkin's Lymphoma

Serum samples from 101 chemotherapy-treated patients were analyzed via capture enzyme-linked immunoassay specific for Interleukin 10 (IL-10) (Sarris et al., 1999; Table 30.1). Of these, 74 were nodular sclerosis cHL (NS-cHL), 12 were mixed-cellularity cHL (MC-cHL), 6 were lymphocyte-predominant, and others were unclassified HL cases. ABVD (chemotherapeutic regimen)-treated patients had an elevated level of IL-10, a symptom that is found to be associated with inferior failure-free survival (FFS). Bohlen's group also studied IL-10 with a similar experimental setup (Bohlen et al., 2000). Serum levels of 64 HL patients were investigated for IL-10 via sensitive enzyme-linked immunosorbent assay (ELISA). Of these, 14.1% demonstrated an elevated IL-10 level compared to the control group whose IL-10 level is undetectable. Multivariate analysis shows a correlation between higher age (>45) and elevation in IL-10 level. Furthermore, Viviani's group has proved that IL-10 is a poor prognostic marker (Viviani et al., 2000). In this study, they argue that altered (mostly elevated) cytokine secretion may play a role in HL-related immunosuppression. For this purpose, they specifically analyzed IL-10 serum levels in 73 chemotherapy-naive HL patients. IL-10 secretion is significantly higher (patient: 56% versus control: 32% with $p < 0.03$) in patients with advanced HL. Therefore, IL-10 is associated with poor prognosis.

Nadali's group has demonstrated prognostic significance of soluble CD30 (sCD30) with 303 patients' serum samples (Nadali et al., 1998). Of these, 210 patients were NS subtype of cHL, 53 were MC-cHL, 21 were lymphocyte-predominant (LP), 6 were lymphocyte-depleted (LD)-cHL, and others were unclassified. The methodology they used to analyze sCD30 was the sandwich ELISA. They concluded that high level of sCD30 and advanced stage of HL are independently associated with an unfavorable prognosis of the disease.

TABLE 30.1

Noninvasive Biomarkers in Hodgkin's Lymphoma

Noninvasive Biomarkers	Sample Source	Detection Method	Importance	References
IL-10	101 HL patients' serum samples 64 HL patients' serum samples 73 HL patients' serum samples	Capture enzyme-linked immunoassay ELISA ELISA	Elevated level of IL-10 is associated with inferior FFS 14% of patients have elevated IL-10 level and higher age relation IL-10 is significantly associated with poor prognosis	Sarris et al. (1999) Bohlen et al. (2000) Viviani et al. (2000)
sCD30	303 patients' serum samples	Sandwich ELISA	High level of sCD30 and advanced stage of HL are associated with an unfavorable prognosis of the disease	Nadali et al. (1998)
Peripheral blood absolute lymphocyte count (ALC)/absolute monocyte count (AMC) ratio	476 cHL patients' blood samples	Statistical survival analysis of patients according to absolute lymphocyte count/absolute monocyte count ratio	If patients' ALC/AMC-DX ratio is bigger than 1.1, they have better survival This study is specific to cHL patients	Porrata et al. (2012)
sCD163, sTARC	41 cHL patients' blood samples at different time points of treatment	Serum ELISA (markers are also investigated IHC, flow cytometry, RT-PCR)	At different points of treatment, these biomarker levels are also different, so these markers can be used to determine treatment response of patients (further studies are necessary)	Jones et al. (2013)
TARC	322 HL patients' blood samples (patients at different stages of the disease are examined in separate groups)	Sandwich ELISA	High level of TARC is associated with poor response to HL treatment	Sauer et al. (2013) Ma et al. (2008)
YKL-40, IL-6	470 HL patients' blood samples (patients at different stages of the disease are examined in separate groups)	Sandwich ELISA	Untreated and advanced-stage HL patients have higher level of these biomarkers	Biggar et al. (2008)
ALCAM, cathepsin S, CD26, CD44, IL1R2, MIF	*4 cell lines: L1236, KMH2 (MC-cHL) L428 (NS-cHL-derived) and DEV (NLPHL-derived) cell lines *28 cHL patients' plasma samples	ELISA (also IHC, some proteomic studies have been performed)	These proteins are most likely important in the cross talk between HRS and infiltrating cells	Ma et al. (2008)
Alpha-1-Antitrypsin	22 pediatric HL patients' serum samples (different disease stages exist)	SELDI-TOF MS Western blotting	Its expression correlates with severity of disease	Qi et al. (2008)
DLC1 (Epigenetic marker)	14 HL patients' serum samples	RT-PCR Bisulfite treatment and promoter methylation analysis	It is possible to use it as a noninvasive, tumor-specific epigenetic biomarker of HL	Ying et al. (2007)

Note: HL, Hodgkin's lymphoma; ELISA, enzyme-linked immunosorbent assay; FFS, failure-free survival; HRS, Hodgkin and Reed–Sternberg cells; SELDI-TOF MS, type of mass spectrophotometer; RT-PCR, real-time polymerase chain reaction; cHL, classical Hodgkin's lymphoma.

Although cHL disease treatment has high cure rates, there are still patients for whom treatment has been ineffective. For this purpose, it is important to find prognostic cHL biomarkers to obtain fully effective treatment results in all patients. Porrata's group followed up 476 cHL patients between 1974 and 2010 at the Mayo Clinic (Porrata et al., 2012). Of these, 84% of patients were NS-cHL, 76% MC, 13% LD, and 0.6% both LD and lymphocyte-rich (LR) subclasses of cHL. Patients' peripheral blood absolute lymphocyte count/absolute monocyte count ratio (ALC/AMC-DX) was determined at diagnosis and then their survival analysis was made. The results demonstrated that peripheral blood ratio of absolute lymphocyte count to absolute monocyte count can be a single predictive biomarker for the prognosis of cHL patients. Patients whose AMC-DX count was smaller than 900 cells (total 80 events) had better survival compared to other group of patients whose AMC-DX count was bigger than 900 cells. Several analytic groups were also examined in this study. Importantly, the overall survival analysis of cHL patients reveals that patients have better prognosis if their ALC/AMC-DX ratio is bigger than 1.1 compared to the patient group whose ratios are smaller than 1.1.

Serum CD163 (sCD163) and serum thymus and activation-regulated chemokine (sTARC) proteins were examined by taking blood samples from 41 cHL patients to see whether they were informative biomarkers for the treatment response of patients (Jones et al., 2013). Blood samples of patients were taken at different time points such as prior to, during, and after therapy. Before therapy, patient results showed that they all had elevated levels of sCD163 and sTARC. During therapy, sCD163 had a significant value compared to the control, which indicates tumor burden. After therapy, serum ELISA results showed that sTARC had greater value. Thus, it would be more informative to use a combination of biomarkers to obtain estimation about disease prognosis throughout the entire treatment process. Furthermore, Sauer's group were also interested in sTARC protein levels in HL patients (Sauer et al., 2013). TARC/CCL17 is highly expressed by malignant Hodgkin Reed–Sternberg cells and is secreted into the serum. Thus, they specifically examined sTARC levels of 322 patients, whose samples were characterized according to their treatment status (before, during, or after). The results of the study showed that all HL patients, who were not yet treated, had high levels of TARC in their serum compared to healthy patients. Moreover, sTARC protein levels of early-stage patients were lower than those of advanced-stage HL patients. This along with other results of the study shows that a high level of sTARC is related with poor response to HL treatment. There is more information about TARC in the "Chemokine Markers" section.

Biggar's group initially hypothesized that YKL-40 (chitinase 3-like-1 protein) and its possible regulator, interleukin 6 (IL-6), can be possible biomarkers of HL because their serum levels have been found elevated in many cancers but they are not examined in HL (Biggar et al., 2008). Blood samples from 470 HL patients were taken and then their serum YKL-40 and IL-6 protein levels were analyzed via ELISA. According to ELISA results, untreated and advanced-stage HL patients had higher levels of YKL-40 and IL-6 compared to the control group. Therefore, serum YKL-40 and IL-6 can be HL biomarkers.

Elevated levels of seven proteins (ALCAM, cathepsin S, CD26, CD44, IL1R2, MIF, and TARC) were detected in patient plasma samples via ELISA (Ma et al., 2008). In fact, in addition to these seven, other proteins were initially analyzed in the secretome of HRS cells via LC-MS/MS. As many as 37 proteins were found related with immune response. Hodgkin lymphoma cell lines were used for the validation of 16 of 37 proteins and 15 of those 37 proteins were also validated in HL tissues. However, the seven proteins mentioned earlier revealed the most significant results, so they can be used as HL noninvasive biomarkers if further studies correlate with this one.

Analysis of serum samples from 22 children with HL at different stages (13 with stage II, and 9 with stage III or IV) reveals a potential marker protein, alpha-1-antitrypsin (Qi et al., 2008). Its corresponding peak has been differentially identified via SELDI-TOF MS. Alpha-1-antitrypsin's differential expression was validated via Western blotting and it was shown that the protein expression increased when the stage of HL became more severe. Thus, it is possible to use this protein as a prognostic marker for pediatric HL patients.

Deleted in liver cancer 1 (DLC1) gene was epigenetically regulated, specifically methylated, and silenced in a series of 4 of 6 HL cell lines It was also detected not only in tumor biopsies but also in patient serum samples (Ying et al., 2007). DLC1 gene was aberrantly methylated in most HL primary tumors (44%) and its expression was also detected in 29% of HL patient serum samples via bisulfite treatment and promoter methylation analysis.

A summary of noninvasive markers is shown in Table 30.1.

30.3 Invasive Biomarkers in Hodgkin's Lymphoma

30.3.1 Based on Hodgkin's Lymphoma Subtype

30.3.1.1 Nodular Lymphocyte-Predominant Hodgkin's Lymphoma Biomarkers

HL has two subtypes: NLPHL and cHL is a rare subtype (approximately 5% of HL cases) and has distinct clinical and pathological features (Tsai and Mauch, 2007; Table 30.2). This lymphoma subtype is characterized by atypical variants of Reed–Sternberg cells, which are sometimes called "popcorn cells" or "lymphocytic and histiocytic cells" (L&H cells) (Nogová et al., 2006; Tsai and Mauch, 2007).

NLPHL cells (L&H cells) express CD20 (B-cell marker) and B-cell-associated antigens CD19, CD22, CD45, CD79a and epithelial membrane antigen (EMA) but does not express CD30 and CD15, which are typical markers of cHL (Nogová et al., 2006; Smith, 2010). Although transcription factors B-cell Oct-binding protein 1 (BOB1) and B-cell-associated transcription factor PU.1 are not expressed in cHL cells (or Reed–Sternberg cells), NLPHL cells are positive for both of them (Lee and Ann, 2009; Smith, 2010).

In addition, NLPHL cells express some particular signaling molecules such as Fyn, Syk (spleen tyrosine kinase), BLNK, and phospholipase C-gamma 2. Especially Syk, BLNK, and phospholipase C-gamma2 have been found to be negative in cHL cells, whereas positively stained in immunohistochemical studies of L&H cells (Lee and Ann, 2009). It is possible to relate the known features of HL with the functions of these proteins. For example, BLNK is responsible for phospholipase C-gamma2 activation, which is involved in intracellular Ca^{2+} metabolism and NF-κB activation (Marafioti et al., 2004). Previously, cHL cells were shown to have constitutively active NF-κB (Bargou et al., 1997; Petro and Khan, 2001). This will be explained in the "Classical Hodgkin's Lymphoma" section in detail.

Other cell signaling related to the marker Syk plays a critical role in the proper activity of immunoreceptors (B-cell, T-cell and Fc receptors). Syk activity is mostly related with Fc receptors (Izban et al., 2001). Thus, the differential existence of Syk in NLPHL (not in cHL) makes this tyrosine kinase a possible marker of NLPHL. Generally, these mentioned markers are demonstrated in L&H cells via immunohistochemical assays at the protein level. Gene-profiling assays of these markers have not been performed.

Furthermore, single-cell polymerase chain reactions using L&H cells isolated from tumor tissue reveal rearranged immunoglobulin V genes (Ig V genes). Mutation detection in these genes enables us to interpret the tumor cells' origin. For example, Ig V gene somatic mutations suggest that the origin of L&H cells is most likely from the germinal center (GC) of B cells as this type of somatic mutation of Ig V gene specifically occurs in this region (Braeuninger et al., 1997; Marafioti et al., 1997; Bonnerot et al., 1998). In addition, comparative genomic hybridization assays introduce a large number of chromosomal abnormalities detected in L&H cells. The abnormalities found in approximately two-thirds of analyzed cases are gain of chromosome 1, 2q, 3, 4q, 5q, 6, 8q, 11q, 12q, x and loss of chromosome 17. Some of these genomic imbalances have also been observed in non-HL but gain of 2q, 4q, 5q, 6, and 11q is rarely detected in non-HL (Marafioti et al., 2000). Thus, these rearrangements could be possible markers of NLPHL in the future if there is more supporting information in the literature.

Another possible genetic marker is the BCL6 gene. This gene located at 3q27 and its protein is a DNA-binding transcription repressor, which is responsible for the expression of at least 14 genes (Franke et al., 2001). Chromosomal translocations related with BCL6 frequently make the gene active. BCL6 translocations in NLPHL—t(3;22) (q27;q11), t(3;7) (q27;p12), t(3;9) (q27;q11), and t(3;14) (q27;q32)—which involve immunoglobulin heavy chain locus (Smith, 2010), are mostly found in diffuse large B-cell lymphoma (DLBCL), but aberrations found in DLBCL are similar to those in NLPHL (Staudt et al., 1999). This might imply that BCL6 genetic arrangements need to be further investigated to qualify as a distinct marker of NLPHL, but still these findings imply that there can be a relationship of origin between these two lymphoma types (Staudt et al., 1999; Wlodarska et al., 2004).

A summary of NLPHL markers is given in Table 30.2.

TABLE 30.2
NLPHL Markers

NLPHL Markers	Sample Source and Detection Method	Expression l Level	Importance	References
Octamer transcription factor Oct2 (+)	Tissue samples of 35 NLPHL cases and 32 cHL cases Method: IHC, in situ hybridization	Highly overexpressed in all NLPHL cases (100%)	Oct2 is absent in 87.5% of cHL cases and partially present in 9.4% of cHL cases *Useful for cHL/NLPHL distinction	Re et al. (2001)
Cluster of differentiation antigens CD20 (+) and CD79a (+)	Primary tumor samples of NLPHL Method: IHC	100% (large nodule appearance)	B-cell marker *Possible evidence for B-cell origin of NLPHL *CD20 is useful for NLPHL/THRLBCL distinction	Marafioti et al. (2003) Nogová et al. (2006) Smith (2010)
Cluster of differentiation antigens CD19 (+), CD22 (+)	Primary tumor samples of NLPHL Method: IHC	100% expression in NLPHL (simply positive for these antigens)	B-cell-associated antigens *Possible evidence for B-cell origin of NLPHL	Lee and Ann (2009)
B-cell Oct-binding protein 1 BOB1 (+)	Primary tumor samples of cHL and NLPHL Method: IHC	100% in NLPHL tumors (rarely expressed in cHL)	BOB1 (−/+) in cHL *Stronger expression in NLPHL, possible marker for cHL/NLPHL distinction	Marafioti et al. (2003) Smith (2010)
B-cell-associated transcription factor PU.1 (+)	Primary tumor samples of CHL, NLPHL, and THRLBCL Method: H&E staining and IHC	All expressed in NLPHL tumors (no expression in cHL and THRLBCL)	PU.1 is (−) in cHL and in T-cell/histiocyte-rich large B-cell lymphoma (THRLBCL) *Useful marker for cHL/NLHL distinction	Marafioti et al. (2003) Smith (2010)
Signal molecules BLNK (+) Phospholipase C- gamma2 (+)	Paraffin-embedded biopsy samples of NLPHL, cHL Method: IHC, IF	Expressed in great majority of tested NLPHL cases	BLNK activates phospholipase C-gamma2 *Important for intracellular Ca^{2+} metabolism and NF-κB activation *Useful in NLPHL/cHL distinction *Gene expression levels are down-regulated in cHL	Marafioti et al. (2003) Lee and Ann (2009)
Spleen tyrosine kinase (SYK) (+)	Paraffin-embedded biopsies of NLPHL, cHL Method: IHC, IF	Expressed in great majority of tested NLPHL cases	Syk (−) in cHL *Important for immunoreceptor (Fc) activity *Gene expression is down-regulated in cHL	Marafioti et al. (2003) Lee and Ann (2009)
Chromosomal abnormalities Gain of 2q, 4q, 5q, 6, 11q	19 NLPHL patient samples Method: cytogenetic analysis, FISH, CGH	2q (36.8%), 4q (47.4%), 5q (52.6%), 6p (36.8%), 6q (47.4%), 11q (36.8%)	Rare detection in non-Hodgkin lymphoma (NHL) *Possible marker for NLPHL/cHL and NHL distinction	Franke et al. (2001) Lee and Ann (2009)
Immunoglobulin V gene mutations (rearranged V_H gene)	11 NLPHL patient samples: primarily their isolated L&H cells Method: single-cell isolation, PCR and sequence analysis	7.5%–27.2% somatic mutation frequency	Useful to demonstrate GC B-cell origin	Marafioti et al. (1997)

Note: NLPHL, nodular lymphocyte-predominant Hodgkin's lymphoma; cHL, classical Hodgkin's lymphoma; THRLBCL, T-cell histiocyte-rich large B-cell lymphoma; GC, germinal center; Ref, reference; (+), gene expression; (−), non-expression of gene; L&H cells, lymphocytic and histiocytic cells; (−/+), usually non-expression and rarely expression; FISH, fluorescence in situ hybridization; CGH, comparative genomic hybridization; IHC, immunohistochemistry; IF, immunofluorescence; (*), important.

30.3.1.2 Classical Hodgkin's Lymphoma Biomarkers

cHL is another important subtype of HL. It is more common than NLPHL, approximately 95% of HL cases. cHL is characterized by malignant cells called Hodgkin and Reed–Sternberg cells (HRS cells). Hodgkin cells are mononucleated and Reed–Sternberg cells are multinucleated structures.

In 2008, WHO classified four subtypes of cHL: NS-cHL, LR-cHL, MC-cHL, LD-cHL. NS-cHL is the most abundant type and accounts for approximately 60% of cases. Its characterization is based on fibrotic bands that function in the separation of nodules consisting of HRS cells, but this kind of bands does not exist in MC-cHL (approximately 30% of cases) (Renné et al., 2005).

Similar to NLPHL cells (L&H cells), cHL cells (HRS cells) are also most likely derived from germinal B-cells. The difference is that L&H cells are probably derived from antigen-selected GC B-cells but HRS cells are mutated GC B-cells, which have undergone disadvantageous mutation in their Ig variable chains (Renné et al., 2005). As both L&H cells and HRS cells are rarely found in tumor tissue, approximately 1% of tissue, detection of certain markers in the tissue is critical for diagnosis and later for treatment. An understanding of the origin and microenvironment of HRS cells is an important basis for obtaining cHL markers.

30.3.1.2.1 Based on Type of Marker

30.3.1.2.1.1 cHL Markers Related with HRS Cell Origin

As HRS cells are mostly known to derive from GC B-cells, they are expected to have B-cell-associated features (Table 30.3). CD40 (or TNFRS5) and CD80 expression of HRS cells are two of these features. However, in general, HRS cells lose their B-cell-related phenotype more commonly than L&H cells, which means that B-cell-characteristic gene expressions are mostly down-regulated in HRS cells (Kuppers, 2009). Detection of low-level Oct2 transcript (no protein) and no Bob-1 transcript (B-cell-specific cofactor of Oct2) is related with loss of B-cell phenotype mechanisms in HRS cells (Re et al., 2001). No protein detection of transcriptional activators Oct2 and Bobl is an important characteristic of HRS cells and potential markers because Oct2 is overexpressed in NLPHL cells or L&H cells (Stein et al., 2001). The difference in Oct2 expression is likely to have a relation with Ig V gene expression. Oct2 presence and Ig expression have been detected in L&H cells but not in HRS cells. Therefore, Oct2 is a possible marker for cHL.

HRS cells do not retain some of the B-cell-specific gene expressions. EBF1 (early B-cell factor 1) is involved in the B-cell differentiation program and it is an activator of B-cell-specific genes in mouse. HRS cells have a low level of EBF1 expression (Stein et al., 2001; Pongubala et al., 2008). Furthermore, other down-regulated B-cell lineage-related genes are the targets of Pax5, which is a critical transcription factor through B-cell maturation. Despite Pax5 expression in HRS cells, most Pax5 targets are not expressed in HRS cells (Kuppers, 2009). Pax5 expression is an important sign showing B-cell origin of HRS cells but absence of Pax5 target gene expression is probably related with impairment of Pax5 function because Notch1 binding to Pax5 causes nonfunctional Pax5 (Pongubala et al., 2008). Notch1 (T-cell transcription factor) is highly expressed in HRS cells and it is one of the negative regulators involved in losing the B-cell phenotype (Jundt et al. 2008). However, Notch1 is expressed not only in cHL cells at a high level but also in anaplastic large cell lymphoma (ALCL), and therefore Notch1 may not be a good marker to distinguish cHL and ALCL (Jundt et al., 2002). In addition, B-cell-specific activator protein (BSAP) is another protein expressed in HRS cells. BSAP plays an important role in B-cell antigen expression (Foss et al., 1999). These two protein expressions can be evidences of B-cell lineage of HRS cells and these genes might be used as supportive markers together with other normally used cHL markers (e.g., CD20 (−), CD45 (−), and CD30 (+)). As an example, Pax5 nuclear staining helped to reclassify two cases as cHL which were initially diagnosed as ALCL. ALCL and cHL are both CD30 (+) lymphoproliferative disorders but Pax5 staining in immunohistochemical assays caused a change in initial diagnosis, which will be critical for subsequent treatment strategy. Thus, Pax5 can be used as a distinctive marker in some cases (Desouki et al., 2010).

GATA (1–3) are important transcription factors in hematopoietic cells, especially GATA-2 normally expressed in early erythroid cells, mast cells, and megakaryocytes (Orkin, 1992; Weiss and Orkin et al., 1995). Overexpression of GATA-2 inhibits terminal differentiation of some hematopoietic stem cells

TABLE 30.3

HRS Cells' Origin-Related cHL Markers

Origin-Related Markers	Sample Source and Detection Method	Expression Level	Importance	References
Octamer transcription factor Oct2 low transcript, Oct2 protein (–) B-cell Oct-binding protein 1 BOB1 (–)	-35 NLPHL, 32 cHL patients' paraffin-embedded tissue samples IHC, in situ hybridization, Western and Northern blotting	88% cHL (–) for Oct2 and 75% cHL (–) for BOB1 mRNA Oct2 protein strong (+) in cHL	Oct2 (+) in NLPHL *Oct2 (+) and Ig V mutation (+) → two related issues especially in NLPHL	Stein et al. (2001) Re et al. (2001)
Paired box protein, Pax5 (+) Pax5 target genes (–) Notch1 (+)	Paraffin-embedded tissue samples of 41 cHL and 71 other lymphoma types Tissue microarray and IHC	Pax5 88% (+) in HL cases but (–) in ALCL	Pax5 is transcription factor in B-cell maturation *Pax5 is important to distinguish cHL and ALCL	Jundt et al. (2002) Hertel et al. (2002) Kuppers (2009) Desouki et al. (2010)
GATA-2 (+) PU.1 (–)	50 cHL, 10 NLPHL, 30 DLBCL,10 BL biopsy samples, and cHL cell lines IHC and IF	50% GATA-2 expression in cHL	GATA-2: Deregulator of HSC differentiation PU.1: Suppressor of GATA- 2 *GATA-2 (–) in other lymphomas	Schneider et al. (2004) Hertel et al. (2002)
HSC regulators PcG genes BMI-1 (+), EZH2 (+), HPC1 (+)	HL-derived cell lines and 54 primary biopsy samples of NLPHL patients IHC and IF	Strong and unique expression pattern in HRS cells	BMI-1 (+), EZH2 (+) in GC B cells so show origin of HRS cells *HPC1 (–) in other B-cell-originated malignant lymphomas, important marker	Vlag and Otte (1999), Sewalt et al. (2002) Dukers et al. (2004)
Multiple mMyeloma-1; MUM-1 (+)	75 cHL and 13 NLPHL patient samples IHC	100% in cHL but 69% expression in NLPHL	*It can be used to distinguish NLHL and cHL	Carbone et al. (2002)

Note: NLPHL, nodular lymphocyte-predominant Hodgkin's lymphoma; cHL, classical Hodgkin's lymphoma; DLBCL, diffuse large B-cell lymphomas; BL, Burkitt lymphoma; GC, germinal center; (+), gene expression; (–), non-expression of gene; FISH, fluorescence in situ hybridization; CGH, comparative genomic hybridization; IHC, immunohistochemistry; IF, immunofluorescence; (*), important.

(HSC) such as differentiation of erythroid progenitors to erythroids (Kitajima et al., 2002). This type of deregulators of HSC differentiation may also be involved in HRS cells' reprogramming (Kuppers, 2009). Another reason for GATA-2 examination in HRS cells is that B-cell-associated transcription factor PU.1 is not expressed in HRS cells and early transcription factor GATA-2 is normally repressed by PU.1. Thus, GATA-2 is analyzed in cHL and GATA-2 expression is detected in HRS cells. GATA-2 was also examined and no expression was detected in NLPHL, Burkitt lymphoma, and DLBCL. Specific expression of GATA-2 (at the level of mRNA, protein, and 50% of patient biopsy samples) in HRS cells makes it a suitable marker of cHL (Schneider et al., 2004).

Some HSC regulators can have unique expression patterns in HRS cells due to their roles in HRS cells' reprogramming from GC B-cell origin through malignant cells in cHL. Polycomb group (PcG) proteins have functions in the HSC self-renewal progress, cell cycle regulation, and repression of gene expression by modifying histones (Vlag and Otte, 1999; Sewalt et al., 2002). HRS cells express both BMI-1 and EZH2 PcG genes, and these PcG complexes are separately expressed during normal B-cell development in the GC. Therefore, co-expression of PcG complexes in HRS cells is related with B-cell origin of HRS cells. Two PcG complexes are known and they have different core proteins, such as BMI-1, MEL-18, RING1, HPH1, HPC1, and -2, EED, EZH2, YY1, and the HPC2 binding partner, CtBP. HRS cells express all these core proteins of PcG complexes. Especially HPC1 is not expressed in other B-cell-originated malignant lymphomas. This PcG gene expression profile of HRS cells is unique and can be used as a marker in further studies (Dukers et al., 2004).

Bcl-6 translocations are mainly involved in B-cell differentiation and they are almost not seen in HRS cells compared to L&H cells. In one study including 23 NLPHL cases and 40 cHL cases, Bcl-6 status was explored and none of the cHL patients showed Bcl-6 translocations although 48% of NLPHL patients did (Wlodarska et al., 2003). However, in another study, Bcl-6 breakpoints were detected in 4 out of 70 cHL patients and Bcl-6 translocations were demonstrated to exist in cHL patients (Martin-Subero, 2006). Therefore, Bcl-6 translocations seem not to be appropriate as a marker.

Multiple myeloma-1/interferon regulatory factor-4 (MUM1/IRF4) is a member of the interferon regulatory factor (IRF) family and is expressed by post GC B-cells. MUM1 expression has been found to be present in all cHL cases, but not in all NLPHL cases (69%). Its different expression in cHL versus NLPHL cases is most likely due to the differentiation stages from GC B-cell origin (Carbone et al., 2002). MUM1 can be useful as a marker in combination with other cHL markers.

30.3.1.2.1.2 Chromosomal Markers

Most researchers do not prefer to analyze the subtypes of cHL separately. Even when the subtypes of cHL are analyzed, the results (markers found in research) are not specific to cHL subgroups, but are rather generalized as cHL markers (Table 30.4). Comparative genomic hybridization analysis of 1 NLPHL and 11 cHL patients (1 case of LR-cHL, 4 cases of MC-cHL, 5 cases of NS-cHL, and 1 case of LD-cHL) revealed that one MC-cHL (4p16) and one NS-cHL (4q23-q24) patient had subregional high-level amplification of chromosome 4, whereas an NLPHL patient had chromosome 9 subregional amplification (9p23-p24). Tyrosine kinase gene JAK2 also amplifies via (9p23-p24) amplification in NLPHL and HRS

TABLE 30.4

Chromosomal cHL Markers

Chromosomal Markers	Sample Source and Detection Method	Importance	References
Amplification of 4p16	1 NLPHL and 11 cHL patients' biopsy materials Method: CHG and FISH	*Associated with specifically MC-cHL subtype, so it can be used as a marker of MC-cHL	Joos et al. (2000)
Amplification of 4q23-24	1 NLPHL and 11 cHL patients' biopsy materials Method: CHG and FISH	*Associated with specifically NS-cHL subtype	Joos et al. (2000)
2p chromosomal gains 2p (54% in cHL) and (88% in NS-cHL)	41 cHL patient biopsy samples Method: CHG and FISH	2p15-16 includes REL oncogene *Associated with specifically NS-cHL	Joos et al. (2002)
Other possible chromosomal gains with these frequencies: 2q (37%), 17p (27%), 9p (24%) 16p (24%), 20q (20%), 17q (20%)	41 cHL patient biopsy samples Method: CHG and FISH	*These frequencies can change according to different studies	Joos et al. (2002)
Chromosomal gains with this frequencies: 2p (40%), 17p (40%), 9p (30%), 14q (30%), 16p (30%), 22q (35%), 17q (70%)	20 cHL patients' primary tumor samples and 4 cHL-derived cell lines Method: CHG	The most significant change in 17q chromosomal gain frequency *17q abnormalities are not frequent in NLPHL and other lymphomas, so possible marker for cHL.	Chui et al. (2003)

Note: NLPHL, nodular lymphocyte-predominant Hodgkin's lymphoma; cHL, classical Hodgkin's lymphoma; MC-cHL, mixed cellularity classical Hodgkin's lymphoma; NS-cHL, nodular sclerosis classical Hodgkin's lymphoma; FISH, fluorescence in situ hybridization; CGH, comparative genomic hybridization; (*), important.

cells (Joos et al., 2000; Kuppers, 2009). This genetic change is similar to those in primary mediastinal B-cell lymphoma, so this most likely demonstrates B-cell origin (Joos et al., 2000).

Another study investigating 41 cHL patients (8 LR-cHL, 16 NS-cHL, 15 MC-cHL, and 2 LD-cHL) via comparative genomic hybridization revealed chromosomal imbalances. These are mostly in the form of chromosomal gains and have the following frequencies: chromosome 2p (54%), 12q (37%), 17p (27%), 9p and 16p (24% each), and 17q and 20q (20% each). Other than these chromosomal gains, 22% of cHL cases show loss of chromosome 13q. The most frequent chromosomal gain 2p includes REL oncogene amplification, which is a member of the NF-κB transcription factor family. REL amplification via 2p chromosomal gain is mostly seen in NS-cHL with 88% frequency. The investigated cHL cases have demonstrated an imbalance in genetic changes between subtypes (Joos et al., 2002). Molecular and cytogenetic markers will most probably be identified for each subtype in further studies.

Samples of 20 cHL patients were subjected to comparative genomic hybridization analysis and the results of chromosomal gains were 17q with 70% frequency, 2p (40%), 12q (40%), 17p (40%), 22q (35%), 9p (30%), 14q (30%), and 16p (30%). Chromosomal loss results were 13q with 35% frequency, 6q (30%), 11q (25%), and 4q (25%). The 17q abnormalities especially are the most likely cHL markers, which are not frequent in NLPHL or other lymphomas (Chui et al., 2003).

30.3.1.2.1.3 Cytokine Markers

Cytokines are involved in immune and inflammatory responses, hematopoiesis, intracellular communication, and many other biologic processes (Table 30.5). T-cell helper-2 (Th2) cytokines IL-5 and IL-13 are expressed in approximately 95% of primary cHL tumors (Samoszuk and Nansen,

TABLE 30.5

Cytokine cHL Markers

Cytokine Markers	Sample Source and Detection Method	Expression Level	Importance	References
T-cell helper-2 cytokines IL-5 (+), IL-13 (+), IL-13 specific receptor chain (IL-13R alpha1) (+)	36 cHL, 5 NLPHL, and 23 NHL primary tumors and cell lines Methods: in situ hybridization, single-cell RT-PCR	IL-13R alpha1 (+) in 89% of cHL cases IL5 and IL13 (+) in 95% of primary tumors	*Especially IL-13 and IL-13R alpha1 high expression are not seen in NLPHL and low-level expression exists in non-Hodgkin's lymphoma	Samoszuk and Nansen (1990) Skinnider and Mak (2002) Skinnider et al. (2001)
T-cell helper-2 cytokines IL-6 (+), IL-9 (+)	Primary tumors and cell lines are used (numbers change in different studies)	IL-6 (+) in 75% and IL-9 (+) in 58% of cHL cases	*IL-9 is not useful for distinction of cHL-ALCL	Merz et al. (1991) Herbst et al. (1997)
T-cell differentiation related marker IL-12 (+)	Methods: IHC, in situ hybridization	IL-12 (+) in 85% of cHL cases	*IL-6 (+) and IL-12 (+) more found in (EBV)$^+$ cases of cHL	Schwaller et al. (1995) Skinnider et al. (2002)
Transforming growth factor beta1; TGF-β1 (+)	43 primary cHL and NHL samples Method: in situ hybridization	TGF-β1 (+) in 61% of primary cHL tumors and 100% (+) in NS-cHL	*Associated with specifically NS-cHL subtype	Newcom and Gu (1995)
Macrophage colony-stimulating factor; M-CSF (+)	Cell lines are used Method: IHC	M-CSF (+) in 75% of cHL cases and M-CSF (+) in 18% of NHL cases	*M-CSF (+) in NHL but less than cHL	Zheng et al. (1999) Skinnider et al. (2002)

Note: NLPHL, nodular lymphocyte-predominant Hodgkin's lymphoma; cHL, classical Hodgkin's lymphoma; NHL, non-Hodgkin lymphoma; NS-cHL, nodular sclerosis classical Hodgkin's lymphoma; ALCL, anaplastic large cell lymphoma; RT-PCR, reverse transcriptase polymerase chain reaction; IHC, immunohistochemistry; (+), gene expression; (*), important.

1990; Skinnider and Mak, 2002). IL-5 is essential for eosinophil growth and differentiation. IL-13 is involved in the growth and differentiation of B-cells. Especially IL-13 and IL-13-specific receptor chain (IL-13R alpha1) are expressed not only in cHL primary tumors but also in cHL-derived cell lines. They function as autocrine growth factors in HRS cells (Skinnider et al., 2001). Analysis of 36 cHL, 5 NLPHL, and 23 NHL patient samples revealed positivity in 86% of cHL patients (irrespective of subtypes) and IL-13 expression in 17% of NHL but no IL-13 expression for NLPHL. In addition, IL-13R alpha1 is expressed in 89% of cHL cases (Skinnider et al., 2001). As IL-13 and IL-13R alpha1 expressions are uncommon in non-Hodgkin's lymphoma (NHL) and are not seen in NLPHL, IL-13 and IL-13R alpha1 can be used as markers of cHL.

Other Th2 cytokines are expressed in primary cHL tumors with the following frequencies: IL-6 (75%) and IL-9 (58%). IL-9 expression is also shown in two of six cases of ALCL and therefore does not seem appropriate in distinguishing cHL and ALCL (Merz et al., 1991). IL-6 is expressed not only in primary tumors but also in five of seven cHL cell lines. Although IL-6 has been considered an autocrine growth factor, treatment strategies neutralizing IL-6 did not affect HRS cells proliferation. Also, IL-12 involved in Th1 differentiation is expressed in primary cHL tumors with 85% frequency (Skinnider and Mak, 2002). Both IL-6 and IL-12 expressions are significantly higher in Epstein–Barr virus $(EBV)^+$ cases of cHL compared to $(EBV)^-$ cases (Schwaller et al., 1995; Herbst et al., 1997).

Transforming growth factor beta-1 (TGF-β1) is an immunosuppressive cytokine, which is expressed in 61% of primary cHL tumors. Its expression is predominantly associated with NS-cHL (Newcom and Gu, 1995). Therefore TGF-β1 can be used as a marker to distinguish the NS-cHL subtype from other cHL subtypes.

The membrane-bound form of the macrophage colony-stimulating factor (M-CSF) is one of the hematopoietic growth factors, which is expressed at 75% frequency in primary cHL samples. It is also expressed in NHL but the frequency is lower than in cHL samples (18%). Membrane-bound M-CSF expression is also associated with other hematologic malignancies such as myeloid leukemia and myelodysplastic syndromes (MDS) (Zheng et al., 1999). Still the expression of M-CSF in all primary cHL cases is significantly higher, so it is possible to use membrane-bound M-CSF as a marker. However, only membrane-bound M-CSF as cHL marker may not be convenient to distinguish cHL from other malignancies, so other cHL markers could be used together with membrane-bound M-CSF.

30.3.1.2.1.4 Chemokine Markers

Chemokines are a specific group of cytokines which have important abilities in the selective migration of cells such as leukocytes (Table 30.6). TARC is expressed in 88% of cHL primary tumors (Skinnider and Mak, 2002). TARC is mostly expressed in NS-cHL and MC-cHL but not in NLPHL and most NHL cases, except for a small number of ALCL and T-cell–rich B-cell lymphoma (TCRBCL) cases (Van den Berg et al., 1999; Peh et al., 2001). The differential expression of TARC makes it useful as a marker.

Macrophage-derived chemokine (MDC) expression is detected via immunohistochemistry in 87% of cHL cases and it is has been found to be specific to cHL cases. A high level of MDC distinguishes cHL from NLPHL (Hedvat et al., 2001). It can also be used as a marker among cHL subtypes because it has a higher expression level in NS-cHL than in MC-cHL (52). Eotaxin is another chemokine and its expression type is similar to MDC. It is highly expressed in cHL, and especially higher in subtype NS-cHL compared to MC-cHL (Skinnider and Mak, 2002).

Th1-associated chemokines interferon gamma-inducible protein-10 (IP-10), monokine induced by interferon gamma (Mig-1), and MIP-1alpha are highly expressed in cHL, especially in the MC-cHL subtype. Their expression was detected in all primary cHL tumors (Skinnider and Mak, 2002), so they seem to be potential biomarkers to distinguish cHL.

Chemokine receptors CCR7 and CXCR4 are up-regulated in cHL, whereas CCR7 is not expressed in NLPHL. CXCR4 also has strong expression in NLPHL. CCR7 expression is NF-κB pathway-related when constitutive NF-κB activity is down-modulated via specific suppressors. CCR7 expression is significantly reduced whereas CXCR4 expression is not reduced. Thus, CCR7 can be used as an NF-κB-dependent chemokine marker, which can distinguish cHL from NLPHL but CXCR4 is not a marker of cHL (Höpken et al., 2002).

TABLE 30.6
Chemokine cHL Markers

Chemokine Markers	Sample Source and Detection Method	Expression Level	Importance	References
Thymus- and activation-regulated chemokine; TARC (+)	99 cHL and 20 NLPHL patients' samples Method: IHC	88% in cHL cases	*Associated specifically with NS-cHL and MC-cHL *Useful marker to distinguish cHL from ALCL and TCRBCL	Van den Berg et al. (1999) Peh et al. (2001)
Macrophage-derived chemokine; MDC (+)	39 cHL, 18 NLPHL, and 102 NHL patients' samples Method: IHC	MDC (+) in 87% of cHL cases	*Associated specifically with NS-cHL and MC-cHL	Teruya-Feldstein et al. (1999) Hedvat et al. (2001)
Eotaxin T-cell helper-1-associated chemokines: IP-10 (+), Mig-1 (+), MIP-1alpha (+)	Further investigation is necessary	All of them are expressed in all cHL cases, especially higher expressed in NS-cHL and MC-cHL	*Eotaxin is associated specifically with NS-cHL *Others are associated specifically with MC-cHL subtype	Skinnider et al. (2002)
NF-κB pathway-related chemokine receptor CCR7 (+)	HL-derived cell lines Method: Northern blot, flow cytometry, IHC, in situ hybridization	Highly expressed in cHL, not in NLPHL	*NF-κB pathway suppression causes down-regulation of CCR7	Höpken et al. (2002)

Note: HL, Hodgkin's lymphoma; NLPHL, nodular lymphocyte-predominant Hodgkin's lymphoma; cHL, classical Hodgkin's lymphoma; NS-cHL, nodular sclerosis classical Hodgkin's lymphoma; MC-cHL, mixed cellularity classical Hodgkin's lymphoma; ALCL, anaplastic large cell lymphoma; TCRBCL, T-cell-rich B-cell lymphoma; RT-PCR, reverse transcriptase polymerase chain reaction; IHC, immunohistochemistry; (+), gene expression; (*), important.

30.3.1.2.1.5 Tumor Necrosis Factor (TNF) Family-Related cHL Markers

TNF family is critical in the pathogenesis of cHL, so some TNF family ligands and receptors have high expression levels in cHL primary tumors (Table 30.7). In cHL tumor tissue, $CD4^+$ T-cells express CD40L on their surface. Approximately 2–5 $CD4^+$ T-cells expressing CD40L are found in the environment of single HRS cells. CD40L expression frequency in cHL primary tumors is 100% (Skinnider and Mak, 2002). CD40L positivity may imply high CD40 expression of adjacent HRS cells, which is approximately 94% (Kim et al., 2003). However, only CD40 positivity may not be an appropriate biomarker because 76% of diffuse large B-cell NHL cases also showed positivity for CD40 (Linderoth et al., 2003).

CD30 (tumor necrosis factor receptor super-family member 8-or TNFRSF8) is a well-known cHL marker that is expressed in HRS cells. The expression of its ligand CD30L is also found in primary cHL tumors with 100% frequency. It is mostly expressed by eosinophils, mast cells, which are adjacent to HRS cells in a tumor. However, CD30 is expressed not only on the surface of HRS cells but also in ALCL (Deutsch et al., 2011). Therefore, using CD30 together with other cHL markers may be more appropriate than using only CD30. In another study, CD30 positivity was investigated in subgroups of cHL (Tzankov et al., 2003). LD-cHL and MC-cHL subclasses of cHL have 100% expression of CD30 and NS-cHL has 97% expression frequency of CD30, whereas CD30 expression frequency is relatively lower in LR-cHL. Similar to CD30 expression analysis in the subtypes of cHL, CD15, CD20, CD79a, and latent membrane protein-1 (LMP1) expression levels were also investigated in each subtype. In this study, 330 cHL case tissue samples were collected and separated according to the WHO classification. Immunohistochemistry and tissue microarray were used to analyze the cases. CD15 expression level was 80% in LD-cHL, 70% in NS-cHL, 58% in MC-cHL, and 40% in LR-cHL. CD20 expression level was 42% in MC-cHL, 30% in LR-cHL, 28% in NS-cHL, and 20% in

TABLE 30.7

TNF Family-Related cHL Markers

TNF Family-Related Markers	Sample Source and Detection Method	Expression Level	Importance	References
Cluster of differentiation antigens CD40 (+), CD ligand CD40L (+) and CD95 (+)	66 cHL patients' frozen tissue samples Method: IHC	CD40 (+) in 94%, CD95 (+) in 91% of cHL cases	*CD40 (+) in non-Hodgkin's lymphoma, so may not be a good marker	Kim et al. (2003) Linderoth et al. (2003) Georgakis et al. (2006)
Cluster of differentiation antigen CD30 (+)	66 cHL patients' frozen tissue samples Method: IHC There are many studies related with cHL and CD30	100%	*Well-known marker but also high expression in ALCL	Kim et al. (2003) Deutsch et al. (2011) Georgakis et al. (2006)
Other CD antigens CD15, CD20, CD79a	330 cHL cases	CD30 > CD15 > CD20 > CD79a (expression is generally in this pattern: details in text)	Different subtypes have varying expression frequencies. These markers can be used in combination with others	Tzankov et al. (2003)
Receptor activator of NFκ-B; RANK (+) RANK ligand; RANKL (+)	cHL cell lines Method: flow cytometry, Western blotting, IHC, ELISA	Co-expressed RANK and RANKL in cHL	*Associated specifically with NS-cHL and MC-cHL	Bosshart (2002) Georgakis et al. (2006)

Note: HL, Hodgkin's lymphoma; NLPHL, nodular lymphocyte-predominant Hodgkin's lymphoma; cHL, classical Hodgkin's lymphoma; NS-cHL, nodular sclerosis classical Hodgkin's lymphoma; MC-cHL, mixed-cellularity classical Hodgkin's lymphoma; ALCL, anaplastic large cell lymphoma; IHC, immunohistochemistry; ELISA, enzyme-linked immunosorbent assay; (+), gene expression; (*), important; (>), more expression in cHL.

LD-cHL. CD79a expression level was lower than CD15 and CD20. The maximum expression level of CD79a was 17% in MC-cHL. Other frequencies were 10% in LR-cHL and 8% in NS-cHL. LMP1 was highly expressed in LD-cHL (60%) and it had low expression frequencies in other subtypes (33% in MC-cHL, 18% in NS-cHL, 10% in LR-cHL). In future studies, it will be possible to use these markers (such as CD15 and CD20) in combination with others.

RANKL is a ligand that belongs to the TNF family and its expression frequency is 100% in all RANK$^+$ cHL cases. RANK is a receptor activator of NFκ-B (Bosshart, 2002). RANK is expressed especially in NS-cHL and MC-cHL subtypes of cHL.

30.3.1.2.1.6 NFκ-B Pathway-Related cHL Markers

TNFα-induced protein 3 (TNFAIP3) is a TNF family protein but is mostly associated with the NFκ-B pathway and negatively regulates NFκ-B signaling (Table 30.8). Generally, point mutations and deletions are detected in this gene and these alterations are observed in 40% of HRS cells, which increases up to 60% when the case is EBV$^-$ (Kuppers, 2009).

The cHL tumor includes HRS cells as well as background non-neoplastic inflammatory cells. Constitutive activation of nuclear NFκ-B is an important characteristic feature of HRS cells. This high-level NFκ-B distinguishes HRS cells from background cells, which have low NFκ-B (Jungnickel et al., 2000). NFκ-B deregulated signaling is not only important in HL but also in NHL types such as DLBCL, mucosa-associated lymphoid tissue (MALT) lymphoma, primary effusion lymphoma (PEL), and adult T-cell lymphoma/leukemia (ATL) (Jost and Ruland, 2007). Thus, any NFκ-B-related biomarker might have aberrant expressions in one of these NHL types but their expression level is most likely different from each other.

NFKBIA gene encoding IκBα, which is an inhibitor of NFκ-B, has point mutations or deletions in approximately 20% of cHL cases (Emmerich et al., 2003; Kuppers, 2009). For example, one frameshift

TABLE 30.8

NFκ-B Pathway-Related cHL Markers

NFκ-B-Related Markers	Sample Source and Detection Method	Expression Level	Importance	References
TNFα-induced protein 3; TNFAIP3 (+)	Point mutations and deletions are detected	40% of cHL tumor cells	*Higher expressed in EBV⁻ cHL	Kuppers (2009)
NFκ-B pathway constitutive activation	cHL cell lines and 1 primary case sample Method: IF, Northern blotting	Constitutively active p50, p65, and c-Rel	*NFκ-B (+) in non-Hodgkin lymphoma	Bargou et al. (1996) Jost and Ruland (2007)
Point mutations and deletions in inhibitor of NFκ-B; IκBα (+)	cHL cell lines and primary samples (3 NLPHL, 2 cHL) Method: PCR and sequencing	Point mutations and deletions are detected in IκBα	*Important role in deregulated NFκ-B activity	Jungnickel et al. (2000) Emmerich et al. (2003)
Jun proteins c-Jun (+) and JunB (+)	HL and NHL cell lines and cHL patient samples Method: IHC, IF, Metabolic labeling and IP	High level of c-Jun and JunB expression is detected	*c-Jun (+) and JunB (+) also in ALCL but lesser than cHL	Mathas et al. (2002)
Cell cycle regulator cyclin D2 (+)	103 cHL patients' samples Method: IHC	Cyclin D2 (+) in 72% of cHL cases	*Its expression is induced by NFκ-B	Bai et al. (2004)

Note: HL, Hodgkin's lymphoma; NLPHL, nodular lymphocyte-predominant Hodgkin's lymphoma; cHL, classical Hodgkin's lymphoma; ALCL, anaplastic large cell lymphoma; IHC, immunohistochemistry; IF, immunofluorescence; IP, immunoprecipitation; (+), gene expression; (*), important.

mutation in the NFKBIA gene causes the generation of a truncated inhibitor protein of NFκ-B, so this can be one of the mechanisms explaining the constitutive activity of the NFκ-B pathway in the pathogenesis of cHL (Emmerich et al., 2003).

Jun proteins c-Jun and JunB are aberrantly expressed in cHL primary tumors. c-Jun up-regulated expression is autoregulatory in HRS cells but JunB is controlled by the NFκ-B pathway. c-Jun and JunB are sometimes called complex activator protein 1 (AP-1). This type of c-Jun and JunB up-regulated expression is also seen in ALCL but not in other lymphoma types. Furthermore, AP-1 together with NFκ-B induces the expression of cell cycle regulator cyclin D2, proto-oncogene c-met, and lymphocyte homing receptor CCR7 in HRS cells (Mathas et al., 2002). Cyclin D2, c-met, and CCR7 have been studied previously in cHL samples. Cyclin D2 is overexpressed in 72% of cHL cases (Bai et al., 2004). c-met and its ligand hepatocyte growth factor were analyzed in two independent groups of cHL patients and c-met expression was found to be associated with a favorable prognosis of cHL patients despite the oncogenic role of c-met (Xu et al., 2012). This striking finding can be used as a marker, but before that, controversy between the known oncogenic role of c-met and its favorable prognostic effect on cHL patients should be illuminated. For CCR7, the "Chemokine Markers" section includes related information.

30.3.1.2.1.7 Jak-Stat Pathway-Related cHL Markers

The genomic region of Janus kinase 2 (JAK2) can amplify in HRS cells with 40% frequency (JAK2 is also explained in the "Chromosomal Markers" section) (Table 30.9). The negative regulator of the Jak-Stat pathway, SOCS1, can also have genomic changes such as point mutations with 45% frequency in cHL. The frequency of SOCS1 expression in NLPHL is slightly more than in cHL, which is 50%. Thus, SOCS1 may not be a good marker to distinguish cHL from NLPHL (Kuppers, 2009).

Jak-Stat pathway changes in cHL pathogenesis are not only due to changes at the genomic level. Autocrine/paracrine signaling events also affect cHL pathology. Signal transducer and activator of transcription (STAT) family plays an important role in this signaling. STAT3 and STAT6 were examined in different lymphoma types. STAT6 was constitutively phosphorilated in 78% of cHL cases. STAT3 was active in 87% of cases. The phosphorilated STAT6 level in NHL was approximately 17%.

TABLE 30.9
Jak-Stat Pathway-Related cHL Markers

Jak-Stat-Related Markers	Sample Source and Detection Method	Expression Level	Importance	References
Negative regulator of Jak-Stat pathway; SOCS1 (+)	SOCS1 point mutations are detected in cHL	SOCS1 (+) in 45% of cHL and SOCS1 (+) 50% of NLPHL cases	*SOCS1 (+) in NLPHL *cHL has slightly lower expression than NLPHL	Kuppers (2009)
Signal transducer and activator of transcription (STAT) family protein; STAT3 (+), STAT6 (+)	32 cHL and 4 NLPHL patients' samples and cHL cell lines Method: immunoblotting, IHC, in situ hybridization	STAT6 (+) in 87% of cHL and STAT3 (+) in 78% of cHL Also, STAT3 (+) in 73% of T-cell NHL cases	*STAT3 (+), STAT6 (+) in non-Hodgkin's lymphoma *STAT6 as cHL marker more appropriate than STAT3	Skinnider and et al. (2002)

Note: NHL, non-Hodgkin's lymphoma; NLPHL, nodular lymphocyte-predominant Hodgkin's lymphoma; cHL, classical Hodgkin's lymphoma; IHC, immunohistochemistry; (+), gene expression; (*), important.

However, STAT3 has been found in 73% of T-cell NHL cases, which is not so far from 87%. Thus, STAT6 can be used as a marker, whereas STAT3 may not be an appropriate marker (Skinnider et al., 2002). Furthermore, up-regulated IL-13 expression is a characteristic feature of cHL, and IL-13 (detailed information is available in the "Cytokine Markers" section)-mediated signaling affects STAT6 expression so that their high expression levels in cHL are not surprising and they are potential markers that can be used together.

30.3.1.2.1.8 PI3K-Akt Pathway-Related Markers

CD30L, CD40L, and activator of NFκ-B ligand (RANKL) induce Akt phosphorilation in HRS cells (Table 30.10). These ligands are expressed in all cHL primary cases (detailed information is provided in the "TNF Family-Related cHL Markers" section) and they induce Akt activity. Phoshorilated Akt exists in 64% of primary cHL tumors (Georgakis et al., 2006). As Akt activity is not associated with loss of PTEN expression, Akt can be used with CD30L, CD40L, and RANKL as a marker. Using only Akt as a marker does not seem appropriate because the Akt pathway is active in almost all tumors and primarily causes tumor growth and resistance to therapy. In addition, the activity of Akt via phosphorilation induces phosphorilation of its downstream targets glycogen synthase kinase 3 (GSK-3) and mTOR substrates 4E-BP1, p70 S6 kinases in HRS cells. However, these downstream targets should be further investigated in order to qualify as a marker of cHL (Dutton et al., 2005).

TABLE 30.10
PI3K-Akt Pathway-Related cHL Markers

PI3K-Akt-Related Markers	Sample Source and Detection Method	Expression Level	Importance	References
Phosphorilated Akt (+)	cHL cell lines Method: Western blotting, IHC, tissue microarray	Phosphorilated Akt (+) in 65% of cHL	*Associated with CD30L, CD40L, and activator of NFκ-B ligand (RANKL)	Georgakis et al. (2006)
Akt downstream targets; glycogen synthase kinase 3;GSK-3(+) and mTOR substrates 4E-BP1, p70 S6 kinases (+)	Further investigation is necessary	Further investigation is necessary	*Their further investigation is necessary to be able to use these as markers	Dutton et al. (2005)

Note: NHL, non-Hodgkin's lymphoma; NLPHL, nodular lymphocyte-predominant Hodgkin's lymphoma; cHL, classical Hodgkin's lymphoma; IHC, immunohistochemistry; (+), gene expression; (*), important.

30.4 Patent Information

The US patent number US006372441B has been ascribed to the inventors Karl-Heinz Heider, Kurt Zatloukal, and Christine Beham-Schmid (Heider et al., 2002) for the diagnosis and treatment of Hodgkin's lymphoma. Basically, it describes the correlation between the variant exon v4 of the CD44 gene expression level and the disease prognosis. One more recent patent number US008211649B2, also about the same subject (Hodgkin's lymphoma diagnosis and treatment), is ascribed to its inventors Thi-Sau Migone, Jerry Klein, Yasuhiro Oki, and Anas Younes (Migone et al., 2012). This patent is related to the nucleotide sequences and antibodies of neutrokine-alpha and/or neutrokone-alphaSV. Diagnostic and therapeutic methods using parts of the invention are also provided in the patent document for immune system-related disorders. Furthermore, another patent number US008067472B2 is about methods of treating non-Hodgkin and Hodgkin's lymphoma (Richon et al., 2011). Its inventors are Victoria Richon, Judy Chiao, William Kelly, and Thomas Miller. This patent provides a method for the apoptosis of neoplastic cells using histon deacetylase (HDAC) inhibitors. This invention is important especially from the pharmaceutical perspective of Hodgkin's and non-Hodgkin's lymphoma.

30.5 Concluding Remarks and Future Perspectives

As NLPHL is a rare type of Hodgkin's disease (5%) compared to cHL (95%), research on NLPHL is less than cHL studies. For this reason, NLPHL biomarkers are all presented in one section but cHL biomarkers are analyzed in many different sections. Understanding cHL molecular biology helps identifying more biomarkers than NLPHL. Some of these biomarkers need more investigation to be used as markers because other lymphoma types might demonstrate similar expression patterns. If one or more lymphoma types express the same biomarker at a similar frequency, then it is possible to use additional biomarkers in the research or clinical diagnosis to be able to get certain results. In addition, there are less noninvasive biomarkers than invasive biomarkers due to the fact that new biomarkers are mostly defined from patients' biopsy samples.

Biomarker knowledge in Hodgkin's lymphoma is important for the proper diagnosis and treatment of the disease. Current diagnostic tools are relatively expensive and the discovered biomarkers will definitely help in improving the specific diagnosis of Hodgkin's lymphoma (e.g., MC-cHL distinction from NS-cHL) and new targeted therapies can be developed according to novel markers. Future studies will most likely validate the markers discussed in this chapter and most validated markers could be used in clinics. Further studies are necessary to be able to transfer these markers from research to clinics.

References

American Cancer Society, Cancer facts & figures. 2010, http://www.cancer.org/acs/groups/content/@nho/documents/document/acspc-024113.pdf

Armitage J., Early stage Hodgkin's lymphoma. *N Engl J Med.* 2010; 363:653–662.

Bai M., Tsanou E., Agnantis NJ. et al., Proliferation profile of classical Hodgkin's lymphomas. Increased expression of the protein cyclin D2 in Hodgkin's and Reed-Sternberg cells. *Mod Pathol.* November 2004; 17(11):1338–1345.

Bargou R., Emmerich F., Krappmann D. et al., Constitutive nuclear factor-kB-RelA activation is required for proliferation and survival of Hodgkin's disease tumor cells. *J Clin Invest.* December 15, 1997; 100(12):2961–2969.

Bargou RC., Leng C., Krappmann D. et al., High-level nuclear NF-kappa B and Oct-2 is a common feature of cultured Hodgkin/Reed-Sternberg cells. *Blood.* May 15, 1996; 87(10):4340–4347.

Biggar R., Johansen J., Smed K. et al., Serum YKL-40 and IL-6 levels in Hodgkin lymphoma. *Clin Cancer Res.* November 1, 2008; 14(21):6974–6978.

Bohlen H., Kessler M., Sextro M. et al., Poor clinical outcome of patients with Hodgkin's disease and elevated interleukin-10 serum levels. Clinical significance of interleukin-10 serum levels for Hodgkin's disease. *Ann Hematol.* March 2000; 79(3):110–113.

Bonnerot C., Briken V., Brachet V. et al., Syk protein tyrosine kinase regulates Fc receptor -chain-mediated transport to lysosomes. *EMBO J.* 1998; 17(16):4606–4616.

Bosshart H., Expression of survival receptors in Hodgkin's disease cell lines. *Blood.* May 2002; 99(9):3484–3485.

Braeuninger A., Kuppers R., Strickler JG. et al., Hodgkin's and Reed–Sternberg cells in lymphocyte predominant Hodgkin's disease represent clonal populations of germinal center-derived tumor B cells. *Proc Natl Acad Sci USA.* 1997; 94:9337–9342.

Carbone A., Gloghini A., Aldinucci D. et al., Expression pattern of MUM1/IRF4 in the spectrum of pathology of Hodgkin's disease. *Br J Haematol.* May 2002; 117(2):366–372.

Cartwright RA. and Watkins G., Epidemiology of Hogkin's disease: A review. *Hematol Oncol.* 2004; 22:11–26.

Chui DT., Hammond D., Baird M. et al., Classical Hodgkin's lymphoma is associated with frequent gains of 17q. *Genes Chromosomes Cancer.* 2003; 38(2):126–136.

Desouki MM., Post GR., Cherry D., and Lazarchick J., PAX-5: A valuable immunohistochemical marker in the differential diagnosis of lymphoid neoplasms. *Clin Med Res.* July 2010; 8(2):84–88.

Deutsch YE., Tadmor T., Podack ER. et al., CD30: An important new target in hematologic malignancies. *Leuk Lymphoma.* September 2011; 52(9):1641–1654. Epub May 27, 2011.

Dukers DF., vanGalen JC., Giroth C. et al., Unique polycomb gene expression pattern in Hodgkin's lymphoma and Hodgkin's lymphoma-derived cell lines. *Am J Pathol.* 2004; 164:873–881.

Dutton A., Reynolds GM., Dawson CW. et al., Constitutive activation of phosphatidyl-inositide 3 kinase contributes to the survival of Hodgkin's lymphoma cells through a mechanism involving Akt kinase and mTOR. *J Pathol.* 2005; 205:498–506.

Emmerich F., Theurich S., Hummel M. et al., Inactivating I kappa B epsilon mutations in Hodgkin/Reed–Sternberg cells. *J Pathol.* 2003; 201:413–420.

Ferlay J., Shin HR., Bray F., Forman D., Mathers C., and Parkin DM., *GLOBOCAN 2008 v1.2, Cancer Incidence and Mortality Worldwide: IARC CancerBase No. 10 [Internet].* Lyon, France: International Agency for Research on Cancer, 2010. Available from: http://globocan.iarc.fr

Foss HD., Reusch R., Demel G. et al., Frequent expression of the B-cell-specific activator protein in Reed-Sternberg cells of classical Hodgkin's disease provides further evidence for its B-cell origin. *Blood.* November 1, 1999; 94(9):3108–3113.

Franke S., Wlodarska I., and Maes B., Lymphocyte predominance Hodgkin's disease is characterized by recurrent genomic imbalances. *Blood.* 2001; 97:1845–1853.

Georgakis GV., Li Y., Rassidakis GZ. et al., Inhibition of the phosphatidylinositol-3 kinase/Akt promotes G1 cell cycle arrest and apoptosis in Hodgkin's lymphoma. *Br J Haematol.* 2006; 132:503–511.

Hedvat CV., Jaffe ES., Qin J. et al., Macrophage derived chemokine expression in classical Hodgkin's lymphoma: Application of tissue microarrays. *Mod Pathol.* 2001; 14:1270–1276.

Heider K., Zatloukal K., Schmid C. et al., Method for diagnosis and therapy of Hodgkin's lymphoma. 2002, United States patent information: http://www.google.com//patents//US6372441

Herbst H., Samol J., Foss HD. et al., Modulation of interleukin-6 expression in Hodgkin'sand Reed-Sternberg cells by Epstein- Barr virus. *J Pathol.* 1997; 182:299–306.

Hertel CB., Zhou XG., Hamilton-Dutoit SJ. et al., Loss of B cell identity correlates with loss of B cell-specific transcription factors in Hodgkin/Reed-Sternberg cells of classical Hodgkin's lymphoma. *Oncogene.* 2002; 21:4908–4920.

Höpken UE., Foss HD., Meyer D. et al., Up-regulation of the chemokine receptor CCR7 in classical but not in lymphocyte-predominant Hodgkin disease correlates with distinct dissemination of neoplastic cells in lymphoid organs. *Blood.* February 15, 2002; 99(4):1109–1116.

Izban K., Ergin M., Huang Q. et al., Characterization of NF-kB expression in Hodgkin's disease: Inhibition of constitutively expressed NF-kB results in spontaneous caspase-independent apoptosis in Hodgkin's and Reed-Sternberg cells. *Mod Pathol.* 2001; 14(4):297–310.

Jaffe E. The 2008 WHO classification of lymphomas: Implications for clinical practice and translational research. *Hematology.* 2009; 523–531.

Jones K., Vari F., Keane C. et al., Serum CD163 and TARC as disease response biomarkers in classical Hodgkin lymphoma. *Clin Cancer Res.* February 1, 2013; 19(3):731–742. doi: 10.1158/1078-0432.CCR-12-2693. Epub 2012 Dec 5.

Joos S., Küpper M., Ohl S. et al., Genomic imbalances including amplification of the tyrosine kinase gene JAK2 in CD30+ Hodgkin's cells. *Cancer Res.* 2000; 60:549–552.

Joos S., Menz CK., Wrobel G. et al., Classical Hodgkin's lymphoma is characterized by recurrent copy number gains of the short arm of chromosome 2. *Blood.* 2002; 99:1381–1387.

Jost PJ. and Ruland J., Aberrant NF-kappaB signaling in lymphoma: Mechanisms, consequences, and therapeutic implications. *Blood.* April 1, 2007; 109(7):2700–2707.

Jundt F., Acikgöz O., Kwon SH. et al., Aberrant expression of Notch1 interferes with the B-lymphoid phenotype of neoplastic B cells in classical Hodgkin's lymphoma. *Leukemia.* 2008; 22:1587–1594.

Jundt F., Anagnostopoulos I., Förster R. et al., Activated Notch 1 signaling promotes tumor cell proliferation and survival in Hodgkin's and anaplastic large cell lymphoma. *Blood.* May 1, 2002; 99(9):3398–3403.

Jungnickel B., Staratschek-Jox A., Bräuninger A. et al., Clonal deleterious mutations in the IκBα gene in the malignant cells in Hodgkin's disease. *J Exp Med.* 2000; 191:395–401.

Kim LH., Eow GI., Peh SC. et al., The role of CD30, CD40 and CD95 in the regulation of proliferation and apoptosis in classical Hodgkin's lymphoma. *Pathology.* October 2003; 35(5):428–435.

Kitajima K., Masuhara M., Era T. et al., GATA-2 and GATA-2/ER display opposing activities in the development and differentiation of blood progenitors. *EMBO J.* 2002; 21:3060–3069.

Kuppers R., The biology of Hodgkin's lymphoma. *Nat Rev Cancer.* 2009; 9:15–27.

Lee A. and Ann L., Nodular lymphocyte predominant Hodgkin's lymphoma. *Oncologist.* 2009; 14:739–751.

Linderoth J., Jerkeman M., Cavallin-Ståhl E. et al., Immunohistochemical expression of CD23 and CD40 may identify prognostically favorable subgroups of diffuse large B-cell lymphoma: A Nordic Lymphoma Group Study. *Clin Cancer Res.* February 2003; 9(2):722–728.

Ma Y., Visser L., Roelofsen H. et al., Proteomics analysis of Hodgkin lymphoma: Identification of new players involved in the cross-talk between HRS cells and infiltrating lymphocytes. *Blood.* 2008; 111:2339–2346.

Marafioti T., Hummel M., Anagnostopoulos I. et al., Origin of nodular lymphocyte predominant Hodgkin's disease from a clonal expansion of highly mutated germinal-center B cells. *N Engl J Med.* 1997; 337:453–458.

Marafioti T., Hummel M., Foss HD. et al., Hodgkin's and Reed-Sternberg cells represent an expansion of a single clone originating from a germinal center B-cell with functional immunoglobulin gene rearrangements but defective immunoglobulin transcription. *Blood.* 2000; 95:1443–1450.

Marafioti T., Jabri L., Pulford K. et al., Leucocyte-specific protein (LSP1) in malignant lymphoma and Hodgkin's disease. *Br J Haematol.* February 2003; 120(4):671–678.

Marafioti T., Pozzobon M., Hansmann M. et al., Expression of intracellular signaling molecules in classical and lymphocyte predominance Hodgkin's disease. *Blood.* January 1, 2004; 103(1):188–193. Epub July 24, 2003.

Martin-Subero JI., Chromosomal breakpoints affecting immunoglobulin loci are recurrent in Hodgkin's and Reed-Sternberg cells of classical Hodgkin's lymphoma. *Cancer Res.* 2006; 66:10332–10338.

Mathas S., Hinz M., Anagnostopoulos I. et al., Aberrantly expressed c-Jun and JunB are a hallmark of Hodgkin lymphoma cells, stimulate proliferation and synergize with NF-kappa B. *EMBO J.* August 1, 2002; 21(15):4104–4113.

Merz H., Houssiau FA., Orscheschek K. et al., Interleukin-9 expression in human malignant lymphomas: Unique association with Hodgkin's disease and large cell anaplastic lymphoma. *Blood.* 1991; 78:1311–1317.

Migone T., Klein J., Oki Y. et al., Methods of diagnosing and prognosing Hodgkin's lymphoma. 2012, Patent information: http://www.google.com/patents/US8211649

Nadali G., Tavecchia L., Zanolin E. et al., Serum level of the soluble form of the CD30 molecule identifies patients with Hodgkin's disease at high risk of unfavorable outcome. *Blood.* 1998; 91:3011–3016.

National Cancer Institute, 2012. http://www.cancer.gov/cancertopics/pdq/treatment/adulthodgkins/Patient/page1

Newcom SR. and Gu L., Transforming growth factor beta 1 messenger RNA in Reed-Sternberg cells in nodular sclerosing Hodgkin's disease. *J Clin Pathol.* 1995; 48:160–163.

Nogová L., Rudiger T., and Engert A., Biology, clinical course and management of nodular lymphocyte predominant Hodgkin's lymphoma. *Curr Hematol Malig Rep.* March 2006; 1(1):60–65. doi: 10.1007/s11899-006-0019-2.

Office for National Statistics, Cancer Statistics registrations: Registrations of cancer diagnosed in 2008, England. 2011, Series MB1 no.39.2011.

Orkin SH., GATA-binding transcription factors in hematopoietic cells. *Blood.* 1992; 80:575–581.

Peh SC., Kim LH., and Poppema S., TARC, a CC chemokine, is frequently expressed in classic Hodgkin's lymphoma but not in NLP Hodgkin's lymphoma, T-cell-rich B-cell lymphoma, and most cases of anaplastic large cell lymphoma. *Am J Surg Pathol.* 2001; 25:925–929.

Petro J. and Khan W., Phospholipase C-gamma2 couples Bruton's tyrosine kinase to the NF-kB signaling pathway in B lymphocytes. *J Biol Chem*. January 19, 2001; 276(3):1715–1719. Epub October 19, 2000.

Pongubala JM., Northrup DL., Lancki DW. et al., Transcription factor EBF restricts alternative lineage options and promotes B cell fate commitment independently of Pax5. *Nat Immunol*. February 2008; 9(2):203–215. Epub January 6, 2008.

Porrata L., Ristow K., Colgan J. et al., Peripheral blood lymphocyte/monocyte ratio at diagnosis and survival in classical Hodgkin's lymphoma. *Haematologica*. 2012; 97(2):262–269.

Qi L., Cazares L., Johnson C. et al., Serum protein expression profiling in pediatric Hodgkin lymphoma: A report from the Children's Oncology Group. *Pediatr Blood Cancer*. 2008; 51:216–221.

Re D., Muschen M., Tahamtan A. et al., Oct-2 and Bob-1 deficiency in Hodgkin's and Reed Sternberg cells. *Cancer Res*. 2001; 61:2080–2084.

Renné C., Martín-Subero JI., Hansmann ML. et al., Molecular cytogenetic analyses of immunoglobulin loci in nodular lymphocyte predominant Hodgkin's lymphoma reveal a recurrent IGH-BCL6 juxtaposition. *J Mol Diagn*. 2005; 7:352–356.

Richon V., Chiao J., Kelly W. et al., Methods of treating Hodgkin and Non-Hodgkin's lymphoma. 2011, Patent information: http://www.google.com/patents/US8067472

Samoszuk M. and Nansen L., Detection of interleukin-5 messenger RNA in Reed-Sternberg cells of Hodgkin's disease with eosinophilia. *Blood*. 1990; 75:13–16.

Sarris AH., Kliche KO., Pethambaram P. et al., Interleukin-10 levels are often elevated in serum of adults with Hodgkin's disease and are associated with inferior failure-free survival. *Ann Oncol*. April 1999; 10(4):433–440.

Sathiya M. and Muthuchelian K., Significance of immunologic markers in the diagnosis of lymphoma. *Acad J Cancer Res*. 2009; 2(1):40–50.

Sauer M., Plütschow A., Jachimowicz RD. et al., Baseline serum TARC levels predict therapy outcome in patients with Hodgkin lymphoma. *Am J Hematol*. February 2013; 88(2):113–115. doi: 10.1002/ajh.23361. Epub 2012 Dec 8.

Schneider EM., Torlakovic E., Stühler A. et al., The early transcription factor GATA-2 is expressed in classical Hodgkin's lymphoma. *J. Pathol*. 2004; 204:538–545.

Schwaller J., Tobler A., Niklaus G. et al., Interleukin-12 expression in human lymphomas and nonneoplastic lymphoid disorders. *Blood*. 1995; 85:2182–2188.

SEER stat fact sheet: Hodgkin's lymphoma, Surveillance epidemiology and end results, 2012. Available from http://seer.cancer.gov/statfacts/html/hodg.html 2012

Seth ET., *Etiology of Hodgkin's Lymphoma, in New Development in Lymphoma and Hodgkin's Disease Record*. Nova Publishers, New York, NY, 2006.

Sewalt RG., Lachner M., Vargas M. et al., Selective interactions between vertebrate polycomb homologs and the SUV39H1 histone lysine methyltransferase suggest that histone H3–K9 methylation contributes to chromosomal targeting of polycomb group proteins. *Mol Cell Biol*. 2002; 22:5539–5553.

Shenoy P., Maggioncalda, A., Malik, N. et al., Incidence patterns and outcomes for Hodgkin lymphoma patients in the United States. *Adv Hematol*. 2011; 2011:1–11. doi:10.1155/2011/725219.

Skinnider BF., Elia AJ., Gascoyne RD. et al., Interleukin 13 and interleukin 13 receptor are frequently expressed by Hodgkin's and Reed-Sternberg cells of Hodgkin's lymphoma. *Blood*. January 1, 2001a; 97(1):250–255.

Skinnider BF., Elia AJ., Gascoyne RD. et al., Signal transducer and activator of transcription 6 is frequently activated in Hodgkin's and Reed-Sternberg cells of Hodgkin's lymphoma. *Blood*. January 15, 2002; 99(2):618–626.

Skinnider BF., Kapp U., and Mak TW., Interleukin 13: A growth factor in Hodgkin's lymphoma. *Int Arch Allergy Immunol*. December 2001b; 126(4):267–276.

Skinnider BF. and Mak TW., The role of cytokines in classical Hodgkin's lymphoma. *Blood*. June 15, 2002; 99(12):4283–4297.

Smith L., Nodular lymphocyte predominant Hodgkin lymphoma; diagnostic pearls and pitfalls. *Arch Pathol Lab Med*. 2010; 134:1434–1439.

Staudt LM., Dent AL., Shaffer AL. et al., Regulation of lymphocyte cell fate decisions and lymphomagenesis by BCL-6. *Int Rev Immunol*. 1999; 18:381–403.

Stein H., Marafioti T., Foss HD. et al., Down-regulation of BOB.1/OBF.1 and Oct2 in classical Hodgkin's disease but not in lymphocyte predominant Hodgkin's disease correlates with immunoglobulin transcription. *Blood*. January 15, 2001; 97(2):496–501.

Teruya-Feldstein J., Jaffe ES., Burd PR. et al., Differential chemokine expression in tissues involved by Hodgkin's disease: Direct correlation of eotaxin expression and tissue eosinophilia. *Blood.* 1999; 93:2463–2470.

Tsai H. and Mauch P., Nodular lymphocyte-predominant Hodgkin's lymphoma. *Semin Radiat Oncol.* 2007; 17:184–189.

Tzankov A., Zimpfer A., Pehrs A. et al., Expression of B-Cell markers in classical Hodgkin lymphoma: A tissue microarray analysis of 330 cases. *Mod Pathol.* 2003; 16(11):1141–1147.

Van den Berg A., Visser L., Poppema S. et al., High expression of the CC chemokine TARC in Reed-Sternberg cells. A possible explanation for the characteristic T-cell infiltrate in Hodgkin's lymphoma. *Am J Pathol.* 1999; 154:1685–1691.

van Leeuwen FE., Klokman WJ., Stovall M., et al. Roles of radiation dose, chemotherapy, and hormonal factors in breast cancer following Hodgkin's disease. *J Natl Cancer Inst.* 2003; 95:971–980.

Viviani S., Notti P.; Bonfante V. et al., Elevated pretreatment serum levels of Il-10 are associated with a poor prognosis in Hodgkin's disease, the milan cancer institute experience. *Med Oncol.* February 2000; 17(1):59–63.

Vlag J. and Otte AP., Transcriptional repression mediated by the human polycomb-group protein EED involves histone deacetylation. *Nat Genet.* 1999; 23:474–478.

Weiss MJ. and Orkin SH., Transcription factor GATA-1 permits survival and maturation of erythroid precursors by preventing apoptosis. *Proc Natl Acad Sci USA.* 1995; 92:9623–9627.

Wlodarska I. et al., Frequent occurrence of BCL6 rearrangements in nodular lymphocyte predominance Hodgkin's lymphoma but not in classical Hodgkin's lymphoma. *Blood.* 2003; 101:706–710.

Wlodarska I., Stul M., De Wolf-Peeters C. et al., Heterogeneity of BCL6 rearrangements in nodular lymphocyte predominant Hodgkin's lymphoma. *Haematologica.* 2004; 89:965–972.

Xu C., Plattel W., vanden Berg A. et al., Expression of the c-Met oncogene by tumor cells predicts a favorable outcome in classical Hodgkin's lymphoma. *Haematologica.* April 2012; 97(4):572–578. Epub December 16, 2011.

Ying J., Li H., Murray P. et al., Tumor-specific methylation of the 8p22 tumor suppressor gene *DLC1* is an epigenetic biomarker for Hodgkin, Nasal NK/T-Cell and other types of lymphomas. *Epigenetics.* 2007; 2:15–21.

Zheng GG., Wu KF., Geng YQ. et al., Expression of membrane-associated macrophage colony stimulating factor (M-CSF) in Hodgkin's disease and other hematologic malignancies. *Leuk Lymphoma.* 1999; 32:339–344.

31

Multiple Myeloma and Evolution of Novel Biomarkers and Therapies

Michael Byrne, Joseph Katz, and Jan S. Moreb

CONTENTS

ABSTRACT Multiple myeloma (MM) is a malignant plasma cell (PC) dyscrasia of the bone marrow (BM) that could be preceded by monoclonal gammopathy of undetermined significance (MGUS) or smoldering MM (SMM), and it can evolve into extramedullary disease with more aggressive disease in the form of primary or secondary PC leukemia. The recent advances in molecular cytogenetic and genomic profiling studies have provided better understanding of the pathogenesis and mechanisms of the multistep model of disease progression. Few biomarkers, invasive and noninvasive, have been identified, which could be divided into multiple categories related to the diagnosis, prognosis, and treatment of myeloma. Due to the nature of cancer, many of these biomarkers overlap in their potential clinical applications, and many are still awaiting clinical validation. The use of bioinformatics to integrate the massive complexity of the data sets generated by the whole genome profiling techniques should help improve the management of MM and may hasten the arrival of a new era of personalized therapies guided by specific biomarkers.

31.1 Introduction

The need to personalize medicine has had its advocates for a long time. The Canadian scientist William Osler (1849–1919) said: "Variability is the law of life, and as no two faces are the same, so no two bodies are alike, and no two individuals react alike and behave alike under the abnormal conditions which we know as disease." Indeed, we have inched closer to targeted and personalized medicine since then, and the popularity of the biomarkers field is one of the main manifestations in this drive. Over the last decade, the number of physicians and scientists exploring biomarkers, their role in treatment, and their implications on prognosis and long-term survival has increased dramatically. Many have suggested that biomarkers are an important step toward individualized therapy and the reduction of treatment-related adverse effects. Others have speculated that biomarkers will enable clinicians to provide individualized treatments to their patients avoiding ineffective therapy and reducing healthcare costs. Thus, new technologies such as gene expression profiling (GEP) and proteomics are being utilized to understand the pathophysiology of cancer and provide clues that can be used to design better targeted therapies.

Multiple myeloma (MM) is a malignant plasma cell (PC) disorder that accounts for 15% of all PC dyscrasias and 10% of all hematologic malignancies. It is more frequent in developed countries. The American Cancer Society (ACS) estimates that in 2012, about 21,700 new MM cases will be diagnosed in the United States, while 10,710 deaths are expected to occur (www.cancer.org/multiple-myeloma). MM is characterized by a wide heterogeneity in clinical presentation and course. Recent advances have led to better understanding of the makeup of the disease and its microenvironment, leading to new and novel therapies that have resulted in significant improvement in overall survival of patients with MM. The 2012 ACS's statistics estimates that the 5-year relative overall survival rate for MM patients is around 40%.

In this chapter, we will review the achievements so far and discuss new discoveries of biomarkers as it relates to MM diagnosis, prognosis, treatments, and treatment toxicities. We will focus on noninvasive biomarkers, their classification, and their development into useful clinical assets in the overall treatment for MM patients.

31.2 Background

31.2.1 General

PC dyscrasias is a group of multiple malignant and premalignant disorders originating from abnormal monoclonal PCs in the bone marrow (BM) with a wide spectrum of manifestations that may overlap and clinically may provide diagnostic and therapeutic challenges. Differentiating early stages of active myeloma from monoclonal gammopathy of undetermined significance (MGUS) or smoldering myeloma is in the center of this challenge. Moreover, the ability to predict which patients with MGUS or smoldering myeloma are likely to progress to active MM may have therapeutic implications especially in the era of novel targeted therapies. Few clinical and laboratory features have been shown to help in such quandary (Hervé et al., 2011; Sawyer, 2011). Available novel drugs that can induce long-term remission may be appropriate for early treatment of such disease categories prior to their full transformation into active MM. Thus, biomarkers that can predict such progression may be of clinical importance in this arena (Fonseca et al., 2009).

MM is a disease of terminally differentiated PCs whose principal manifestations are bone lytic lesions, renal failure, anemia, and hypercalcemia, with the production of measurable serum and/or urine paraprotein. MM is unique by the fact that the malignant cells produce measurable markers that usually correspond with the disease activity and make it easy to determine the diagnosis and response to treatment. However, at the cellular level, MM has a high degree of genetic and biologic heterogeneity that results in variable responses to chemotherapy, clinical course, and ultimately outcomes (Hervé et al., 2011; Sawyer, 2011). This is illustrated by survival in MM ranging from 6 months to greater than 10 years. Unfortunately, despite recent advances, MM is a disease that is uniformly fatal with most patients relapsing more than once in their lifetimes. Numerous prognostic factors ranging from BM cytogenetics and fluorescence in situ hybridization (FISH) to peripheral blood markers have been identified and are used to guide the treatment of these patients (Hervé et al., 2011; Sawyer, 2011). However, most of the diagnostic and prognostic criteria for MM require an invasive procedure to obtain BM aspirate and biopsy.

Current MM markers and prognostic criteria cannot predict the constantly changing nature of MM. The natural history of MM is one of recurrent resistant relapse, and only recent studies have provided a long suspected explanation for such natural history of clonal evolution (Egan et al., 2012; Keats et al., 2012). Thus, the initial markers at diagnosis may not predict these changing characters and response to therapies of these emerging resistant clones.

Significant advances in understanding the cellular interactions and signaling mechanisms that are integral to establishing an environment conducive to cell survival and tumor growth—the so-called microenvironment—have revolutionized the field of MM therapeutics. Within the microenvironment, a variety of proinflammatory cytokines are responsible for PC survival and the pathogenesis of the disease in general and the destructive bone lesions specifically. The study of this microenvironment has provided us with many important clues with regard to cellular growth, adhesion, and even resistance to chemotherapy. With further study, these cell-signaling pathways may become important targets for drug therapy. The quantification of these peptides/genes may provide important clues with regard to prognosis and disease response.

31.2.2 Significance of Biomarkers for MM

The field of biomarkers in oncology is rapidly advancing, and many are already in the stages of analytical and clinical validation. Although tumor markers have been used for decades, such as prostate-specific antigen and carcinoembryonic antigen, however, with the technological advances and discoveries, it is realized that the genetics of cancer is more complex involving multiple genes; thus, the development of actionable molecular assays is still needed to guide the treatment of the most common and deadly malignancies (NCCN task force) (Engstrom et al., 2011). There are several categories of cancer biomarker types: diagnostic, prognostic, predictive, and companion diagnostic markers (Engstrom et al., 2011). Validation of these biomarkers for clinical use could be complex and expensive.

For MM, biomarkers that do not depend on performing BM biopsy (noninvasive biomarkers) will be clinically welcome and will have to cover the following diagnostic and prognostic aspects of MM: (1) Which MGUS or smoldering MM (SMM) patient is at high risk for transformation to active MM; (2) which MM patient will live long or even be cured; (3) who will respond better to one drug more than others and who will need tandem autologous stem cell transplantation (ASCT) upfront to get the survival benefit; (4) which patients will have the serious complications of DVT/PE, peripheral neuropathy, osteonecrosis of the jaw (ONJ), second malignancies, etc.; (5) which prognostic biomarkers to use at relapse versus at initial diagnosis; and (6) how to identify biomarker strategies for therapeutic purposes.

The challenges for the biomarker field have been discussed widely in the last decade (De Gruttola et al., 2001; Lesko and Atkinson, 2001; Rolan et al., 2003), and the main obstacle remains the amount of validation needed that will meet multiple regulatory determinations and guidelines put forward by medical societies and governmental agencies such as the US Food and Drug Administration (FDA) (Food and Drug Administration Modernization Act, 1997). Especially challenging is the development of diagnostic and prognostic markers for use in diseases with asymptomatic phase that can take a long time for validation necessary to obtain long-term clinical outcomes (Frank and Hargreaves, 2003). Such conditions certainly exist within PC dyscrasias such as MGUS and SMM. On the other hand, such biomarkers might be very useful in assessing new medicines that can prevent costly chronic progressive diseases.

31.2.3 Current Treatment for MM

Going forward, it will be important to outline in broad strokes the current therapeutic approach to MM treatment. The current algorithm for the treatment of active MM in our institution is outlined in Figure 31.1. This is somewhat similar to what many medical centers do for patients not enrolled on clinical trials, although some others may provide different approach to high- versus low-risk MM patients, such as the Mayo Stratification of Myeloma and Risk-Adapted Therapy (mSMART) consensus guidelines (www.msmart.org), and others offer extensive prolonged treatment plan that includes tandem ASCT

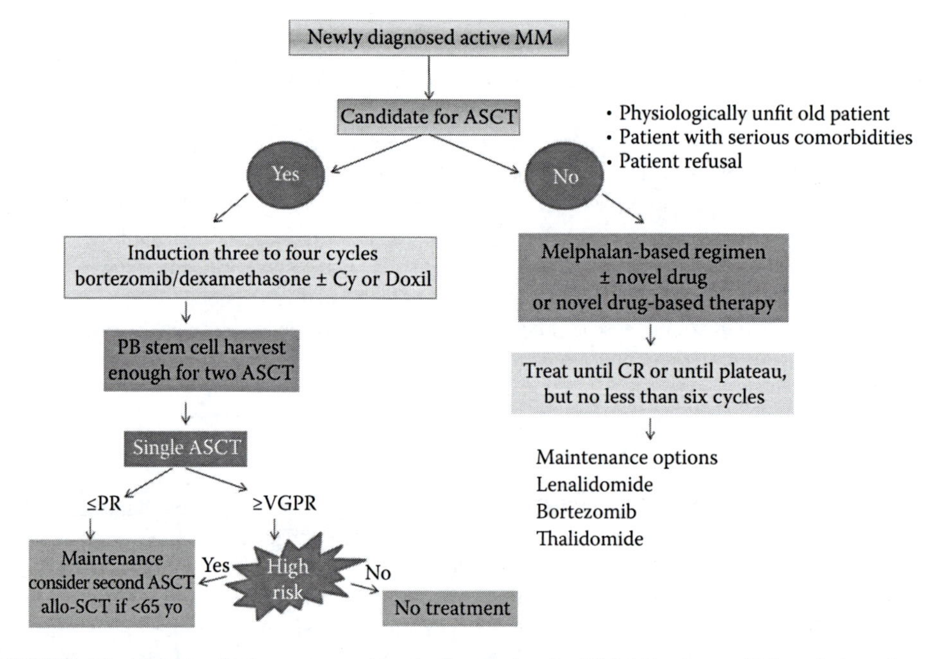

FIGURE 31.1 Our algorithm for the treatment of newly diagnosed active MM. All patients with bone lesions also receive treatment with BP. Cy, cyclophosphamide; allo-SCT, allogeneic stem cell transplantation; ASCT, autologous stem cell transplantation; CR, complete remission; PR, partial remission; VGPR, very good partial remission.

with the intention of inducing complete remissions and possibly cure (van Rhee et al., 2010). Because bortezomib has been shown to be effective in the presence of many of adverse prognostic chromosomal abnormalities (Chang et al., 2007), our induction regimen is always bortezomib based, and therefore all patients are treated with the same induction therapy. There have been several novel drugs approved for treatment of newly diagnosed and relapsed MM that include thalidomide, bortezomib, Doxil, lenalidomide, carfilzomib, and pomalidomide. Lenalidomide has been recently shown to be an effective drug in maintenance with improved overall survival (McCarthy et al., 2012). Relapsed/refractory MM patients should be considered for clinical trials, salvage ASCT or allogeneic SCT, or combination chemotherapies including novel agents or just known combination chemotherapy.

31.3 Current Invasive and Noninvasive Markers

The majority of testing performed in MM patients is noninvasive. While blood/serum samples account for the bulk of tests ordered in MM patients, there is a role in testing the urine for secretion of paraprotein (discussed later). The advantages of such noninvasive testing are significant. Only rarely do patients object to phlebotomy or provide their health-care providers with a urine sample. Furthermore, such unobtrusive means allow for testing at regular intervals in order to determine response to therapy or relapse of MM.

BM biopsy represents the sole invasive test routinely offered to MM patients at diagnosis. BM biopsy is the only way of obtaining important information about BM cellularity and architecture, percentage of abnormal PC involvement, and cytogenetics. While the test is generally well tolerated, its invasiveness precludes its use at regular intervals.

Finally, a small percentage of patients will present with solitary bone or extramedullary tissue mass, called plasmacytoma, for which biopsy will be recommended. Biopsies of presumed plasmacytomas, if conclusive, are generally only done to confirm the diagnosis and are not repeated.

31.3.1 Invasive Biomarkers

31.3.1.1 Marrow Morphology and Flow Cytometry

BM biopsy is recommended at the time of diagnosis and during regular intervals during the treatment of patients with MM. Slides should be reviewed by an experienced pathologist or hematopathologist and provide important information about PC involvement and response to therapy. Review of the core biopsy provides information about the cellularity of the BM and the extent of PC involvement (Figure 31.2a and b). The percentage of PC involvement is critical for discerning patients with MGUS from those with asymptomatic myeloma. Treatment-related changes in these percentages are important in assessing response to antimyeloma therapy. Flow cytometry is often undertaken and reveals a population of abnormal PCs that are CD38, CD138, and CD56 positive; CD19 and CD45 negative or variable; and CD117 positive (Figure 31.2b).

31.3.1.2 Plasma Cell Labeling Index (PCLI)

PCLI is a staining procedure done usually on the BM sample to estimate the percentage of myeloma cells in S phase. This percentage can be measured using a slide-based immunofluorescence method using an antibody against 5-bromo-2′-deoxyuridine (BU-1), which is actively incorporated by DNA of the dividing PCs. S-phase cells are detected using the BU-1 antibody and a rhodamine-conjugated antimouse Ig reagent. This procedure allowed the determination of the PCLI within 4 h of receipt of the sample (Greipp et al., 1993). The technique, which can be performed using BM or peripheral blood specimens (Kumar et al., 2004), also utilizes concurrent cytoplasmic staining against immunoglobulin as well as κ and λ light chains (LCs). Employment of cytoplasmic immunoglobulin staining allows more specific identification of PCs as well as confirmation of the monoclonal nature of the PC population. The staining procedure can be done manually or using an automated stainer (Greipp et al., 1993). The normal average is 1%, and only about 5% of MM patients will have elevated PCLI in excess of 5%. PCLI is an

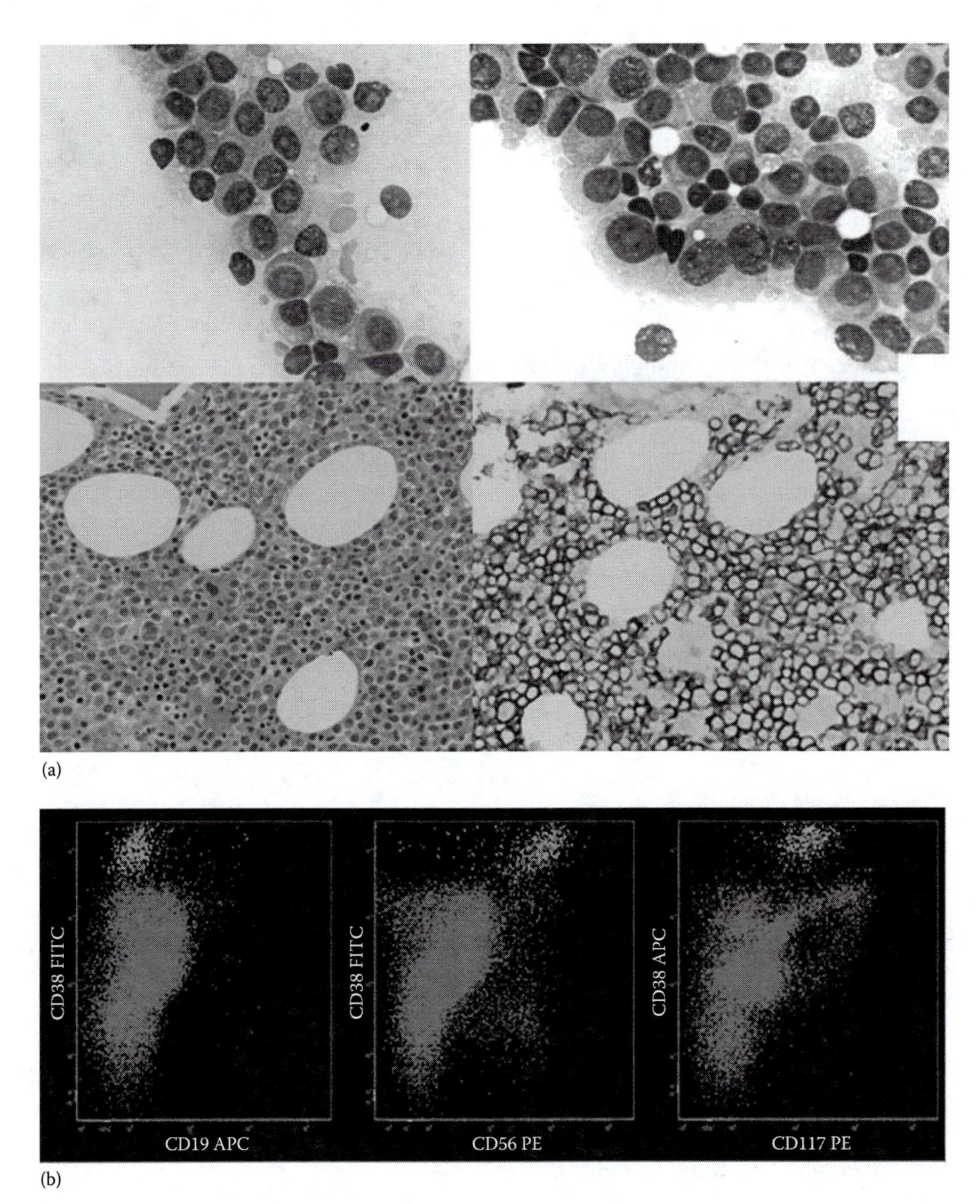

FIGURE 31.2 (See color insert.) The essentials for the diagnosis of MM: (a) The top panels show cell morphology of BM aspirate with sheets of atypical PCs displaying big nucleoli. The lower left panel is hypercellular BM with extensive involvement with myeloma as seen in BM biopsy. The right lower panel is IHC staining for CD138 of the same BMB. (b) This panel shows the results of flow cytometry analysis documenting the abnormal phenotype of $CD38^+$ myeloma cells, which include $CD56^+/CD19^-/CD117^+$ (photographs in a and b were generously provided by Dr. Samer Al-Quran, Department of Pathology, University of Florida).

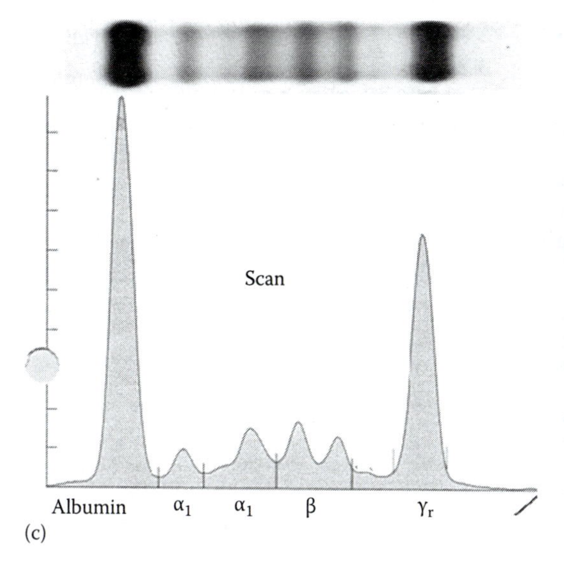

(c)

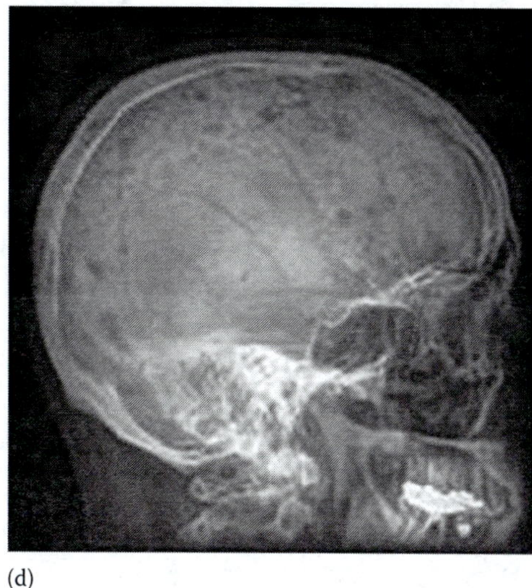

(d)

FIGURE 31.2 (continued) **(See color insert.)** The essentials for the diagnosis of MM: (c) This panel shows the results of SPEP. (This example was provided generously by Dr. Neil Harris, Department of Pathology and Laboratory Medicine, University of Florida.) (d) Skull plain x-ray as part of skeletal survey performed, and it shows multiple lytic lesions typical of MM.

important clinical test, providing valuable diagnostic and prognostic information. Several groups demonstrated that a high PCLI corresponds to a very short survival (Steensma et al., 2001; Larsen et al., 2011). Nevertheless, PCLI remains a technique available in only a few hematologic centers. It is simple and reproducible, with 100% specificity and about 55% sensitivity (Schambeck et al., 1995), but needs a lab staff well trained in myeloma research.

31.3.1.3 Chromosomal Abnormalities

Metaphase cytogenetics is routinely done at most centers and carries important prognostic information. Clinicians rely on this evaluation of the patient's cytogenetics, or karyotype, to guide management and counsel patients on disease outcomes. In most centers, chromosomal abnormalities are also assessed by fluorescent in situ hybridization (FISH), the results of which are usually reported in conjunction with those of the classic metaphase cytogenetics. Pending of both of these results, patients are divided into either standard-risk or high-risk categories, which may provide direction for counseling and guide treatment decisions (Table 31.1).

TABLE 31.1

Risk Stratification of Newly Diagnosed MM Patients according to Cytogenetics/FISH

Standard Risk [Involved Genes]	High Risk [Involved Genes]
Hyperdiploidy	Hypodiploidy
t(11;14) [CCND1]	Del 13 [RB1] (by cytogenetics)
t(6;14) [CCND3]	t(4;14) [FGFR3]
	t(14;16) [WWOX]
	Del 16q [CYLD]
	t(14;20) [MAFB]
	Del 17p [p53]
	1q gains/amplifications [PMSD4]

At the genetic level, MM is a heterogeneous disease that is broadly divided into two categories: hyperdiploid multiple myeloma (h-MM) and nonhyperdiploid MM (nh-MM) (Chng et al., 2005). This important distinction is based on the result of cytogenetics. Patients with h-MM have excess chromosomes with multiple chromosomal trisomies and a low prevalence of immunoglobulin heavy chain (IgH) translocations at the locus 14q32. As the predominant form of MM, 50%–60% of patients have this variant of the disease (Chng et al., 2005). Patients with h-MM may have anywhere from 48 to over 70 chromosomes on metaphase cytogenetics with the most frequently involved chromosomes being 3, 7, 9, 11, 15, and 19 (Chng et al., 2005). This form of the disease is generally associated with a more indolent course and more favorable prognosis. Within this group of patients, there exists a subgroup with a more aggressive variant of the disease (Carrasco et al., 2006; Chng et al., 2006) suggesting further that heterogeneity exists within this h-MM subtype.

Alternatively, patients with nh-MM may have high numbers of IgH translocations. This group is associated with a more aggressive subtype of MM and shortened survival (Fonseca et al., 2009). The three most common IgH translocations are t(11;14)(q13;q32), t(4;14)(p16;q32), and t(14;16)(q32;q23). There are identified molecular counterparts for these translocations (Table 31.1), and some of them have potential therapeutic implications such as the constitutive expression of FGFR3 with tyrosine kinase activity (see Section 31.5.5.3). While a patient's karyotype at the time of diagnosis carries important prognostic information, cytogenetic alterations during the disease course in patients with known h-MM have been associated with disease progression. These findings, particularly trisomy rearrangements, are tied to both cytogenetic and clinical progression in over 50% of h-MM cases and may represent a biomarker for h-MM progression (Alfaro et al., 2011).

The hemizygous deletion of 17p (del17p) has been correlated with similarly poor outcomes in MM patients (Boyd et al., 2011). This deletion results in the loss of p53, an important tumor suppressor and proapoptotic gene, and is associated with shortened OS (median OS 26.6 months vs. 48.5 months). Associations between del 17p and response to chemotherapy have also been discovered and will be explored later in this chapter.

Several newer chromosomal aberrations have been discovered in small cohorts of patients that also confer adverse risk. Among the abnormalities, the most frequent are those involving the long arm (q) of chromosome 1 (Chen et al., 2012). 1q gains/amplifications are present in 45% of MM—often at the 1q21 position. This finding, like the trisomy rearrangements, is indicative of a poor prognosis with accelerated disease progression. Also residing on chromosome 1q21 is the PSMD4 gene. Greater PSMD4 expression levels, along with higher 1q21 copy numbers (CNs), adversely affect clinical outcomes in patients with MM (Shaughnessy et al., 2011). Unfortunately, sensitivity and specificity for using PMSD4 in the prediction of MM prognosis have not been studied yet.

31.3.2 Noninvasive Biomarkers

31.3.2.1 Paraprotein in Blood and Urine

The initial diagnosis and staging of MM hinges on a variety biomarkers, many of which are well known and widely utilized. As a disease of PCs, the principal manifestations of MM are a result of the paraprotein and its sequelae in the circulation. The PCs secrete heavy chains and LCs separately, which are later constructed into an immunoglobulin. These clonal immunoglobulins can be appreciated on routine laboratory chemistries as a "protein gap" between the total protein and albumin. To evaluate for MM, a battery of long established testing is undertaken to confirm the diagnosis and to evaluate the extent of disease (Table 31.2). The most frequently affected immunoglobulin is immunoglobulin G (IgG). The others, in order of decreasing frequency, are IgA, IgM, IgD, and IgE. Patients with MM often also have either kappa (κ) or lambda (λ) LC involvement, which can occur in combination with or in the absence of the affected heavy chains. Rarely, patients secrete neither heavy chains nor LCs—these patients are said to have nonsecretory MM. The paraproteins (M-spikes) can be evaluated by serum and urine protein electrophoreses (SPEP and UPEP, respectively) and will frequently appear as a narrow spike in the beta

TABLE 31.2

Currently Used Tests and Biomarkers and Their Significance to the Diagnosis, Prognosis, and Staging of MM

Marker	Diagnosis	Prognosis	Disease Staging
Invasive	—	—	—
BM aspirate/biopsy	—	—	—
Morphology	% PCs	NA	Not applicable except for the differential diagnosis of MM from MGUS and smoldering myeloma
Flow cytometry	Abnormal phenotype	NA	
PCLI[a]	% proliferating PCs	Yes	
Cytogenetics	NA	Yes	
FISH	NA	Yes	
Plasmacytoma biopsy	Abnormal PCs	NA	
Noninvasive			
Serum: immunoglobulins	All serum and urine studies are required and done routinely at diagnosis. Help differentiate active myeloma from other PC dyscrasias.	NA	All serum and urine studies are used for the two staging systems mentioned in the text.
SPEP		NA	
IF		NA	
Serum-free LC		Yes	
β2-Microglobulin		Yes	
Albumin		NA	
LDH	Not routinely done. Required	Yes	NA
Urine: UPEP		NA	Required for staging
24 h urine protein		NA	
Whole blood: PCLI		Yes	
Skeletal survey		NA	

Abbreviations: BM, bone marrow; NA, not applicable; SPEP, serum protein electrophoresis; UPEP, urine protein electrophoresis; IF, immunofixation; LC, light chain; PCs, plasma cells; PCLI, plasma cell labeling index.

[a] PCLI is done in select medical center only.

or gamma zone (Figure 31.2c). These M-spikes are further quantified, and their types are recognized by immunofixation electrophoresis (IFE), which is usually used in conjunction with SPEP and UPEP at the initial diagnosis and again with relapses or to determine complete remission. Thus, the essentials for the diagnosis of MM are summarized in Figure 31.2 including BM morphology and flow cytometry, detection of paraprotein, and lytic lesions by skeletal survey (Figure 31.2d).

For reasons that are not well understood, PCs produce higher numbers of LC than heavy chains. In patients with MM, the monoclonal production of LCs, or an imbalance in LC versus heavy chain synthesis, results in an excess of LCs after immunoglobulin synthesis. These unbound LCs are referred to as free light chains (FLCs). In healthy patients, excess FLCs from immunoglobulin synthesis enter into peripheral circulation where they are filtered by the kidneys, reduced into amino acids, and recycled within the body. When the number of FLCs is significant, as in MM, the absorptive capabilities of the nephron are challenged and the LCs are excreted into the urine resulting in proteinuria and kidney damage. These LCs, after secretion in the urine, are referred to as the Bence-Jones protein (Chauveau and Choukroun, 1996). SPEP and IFE are not very sensitive in detecting the free LCs in the serum, but UPEP and IFE done on the urine are able to detect the LCs and identify kappa or lambda excess. The 24 h urine protein quantitation is needed to determine the quantity of abnormal protein secreted by the kidney in mg/24 h. Newer assays to directly measure the serum FLCs have been developed over the last decade (Bradwell et al., 2001; Drayson et al., 2001). The Freelite assay (The Binding Site Inc., Birmingham, United Kingdom) is the only assay system validated for routine serum measurements and is based on the use of specific latex-conjugated antibodies to each of the LCs and provides higher sensitivity (the lowest limit of detection) as shown in Table 31.3.

TABLE 31.3

Comparison of Sensitivity of the Serum FLC Assay to Existing Assays for Detection of M-Spike

Test	Kappa (mg/L)	Lambda (mg/L)	Diagnostic Requirement
SPE	500–2000	500–2000	Monoclonal band
IFE	150–500	150–500	Monoclonal band
Serum FLC	1.5	3.0	Abnormal κ/λ ratio

TABLE 31.4

Differentiating between MGUS, Smoldering Myeloma, and Active Myeloma

Disease Category	Serum Paraprotein (g/L)	BM% Clonal PCs (%)	End-Organ Damage (CRAB)[a]
MGUS	<30	<10	Absent
SMM	>30	>10	Absent
Active myeloma	>30	>10	Present

Abbreviations: BM, bone marrow; PCs, plasma cells; MGUS, monoclonal gammopathy of undetermined significance.

[a] CRAB stands for C, hypercalcemia; R, renal involvement; A, anemia; B, bone disease.

The International Myeloma Working Group (IMWG) has suggested the following diagnostic criteria for distinguishing patients with MGUS from patients with asymptomatic myeloma (Table 31.4) (Kyle et al., 2010):

MGUS

- Serum paraprotein is <30 g/L.
- Clonal PCs on BM biopsy is <10%.

Asymptomatic myeloma

- Serum paraprotein >30 g/L.
- Clonal PCs on BM biopsy is >10%.

These biomarkers and the previously mentioned classification system are widely used in the diagnosis and staging of MM patients. They are also used to monitor disease response or progression at intervals between treatment cycles. The most frequently used response classification is the one recommended by the IMWG (Durie et al., 2006).

31.3.2.2 Markers for Prognosis

A few noninvasive markers are currently available for predicting prognosis. First is the stage of the disease that is determined by the tests mentioned earlier. Although stage by either one of the staging systems was shown to predict different survival rates for each stage, however, it is a very limited tool due to the heterogeneity of myeloma.

B2-microglobulin (β2M) and albumin carry important prognostic information in MM patients and are integral components of the staging of these patients. The International Staging System (ISS) for myeloma, published in 2005, relies on these two laboratory values to stratify patients into one of three stages (Greipp et al., 2005). The ISS, however, is not without limitations. The β2M, a major component of this scoring system, is renally excreted. For this reason, patients with non-MM-induced renal dysfunction may have artificially elevated β2M levels that do not reflect their true MM risk (i.e., they are inappropriately upstaged) by the ISS. Another criticism of this scoring system is that it does not accurately characterize the volume of disease. For these reasons, the ISS is often used in conjunction with the Durie–Salmon staging system (Durie and Salmon, 1975), which incorporates the serum and urine paraprotein levels. Another consideration in the Durie–Salmon staging system is the presence of end-organ dysfunction such as anemia, bony findings, or hypercalcemia, which more accurately describes the volume of the disease process.

31.4 Recently Added Invasive and Noninvasive Biomarkers

31.4.1 Free Light Chain Measurements

As mentioned earlier, serum FLC assay is now available and being used routinely to assess patient at diagnosis, response, and prognosis (Dispenzieri et al., 2009). It is also the only tumor marker available for monitoring the treatment and disease progression in patients with nonsecretory or oligosecretory MM (Drayson et al., 2001). It provides measurements for kappa and lambda FLC and the K/L ratio. The diagnostic sensitivity and specificity of the K/L ratio are 98% and 95%, respectively (Katzmann et al., 2002). Furthermore, the ratio was able to predict malignant transformation from SMM to active MM within 2 years of diagnosis with sensitivity of 97% and specificity of 16% (Larsen et al., 2012). Table 31.5 shows the manufacturers and developers of other similar assays in urine as well and for research use only.

31.4.2 Microarray Gene Panels

On the molecular level, MM is characterized by significant heterogeneity in terms of chromosomal aberrations and abnormal gene expression (Zhan et al., 2006; Meissner et al., 2011). This molecular heterogeneity translates into a wide range of survival and can be used for the design of new targeted therapies. Gene expression profiling (GEP) is an ideal tool to assess this molecular heterogeneity in terms of gene expression–based classifications of distinct biologic entities (Bergsagel and Kuehl, 2005; Bergsagel et al., 2005; De Vos et al., 2006; Broyl et al., 2010a,b). Publications from different myeloma groups published prognostic classifications based on GEP or gene expression–based proliferation index (GPI) (Shaughnessy et al., 2007; Decaux et al., 2008; Hose et al., 2011). The GEP reported from the University of Arkansas for Medical Sciences (UAMS; Little Rock, AR) uses the 70 most prognostic and relevant genes to MM (GEP70) and is now marketed as MyPRS Plus test from Signal Genetics LLC (New York). This was compared to GEP15, using 15 instead of 70 genes, reported by the Intergroupe Francophone du Myelome (Decaux et al., 2008). The comparison was performed in MM patients receiving their initial therapy with lenalidomide and dexamethasone prior to ASCT (Kumar et al., 2011), and the results confirmed the prognostic values of both GEP scoring systems.

Another gene expression profile with prognostic significance was developed by a Dutch group (Kuiper et al., 2012) and is called EMC-92 gene signature (uses a set of 92 genes). There are overlapping probe sets between all the published signatures, but few differences were found in the ability of each one to define high-risk MM patients (Kuiper et al., 2012). According to Kuiper et al., approximately 13% of patients were classified as high risk by either EMC-92 or GEP70, and 8% by combining the two signatures.

However, the limitations of these approaches include the need to purify myeloma cells from BM samples and the fact that the data provided may not be actionable in terms of initial treatment choice since none of the available treatment options have been demonstrated to be more effective in the high-risk MM groups. Bortezomib has been shown to be more effective in the presence of certain chromosomal abnormalities, and if bortezomib regimens are used for all newly diagnosed patients, then such prognostic classification may have only an academic value. Furthermore, one of the main difficulties remaining for prospective use of GEP in clinical routine is an affordable (i.e., academic) reporting tool giving

TABLE 31.5

Comparison of Different FLC Immunoassays

Assay	Serum/Urine/Others	Manufacturer	Clinical/Research Use
Freelite	Serum	Binding Site, United Kingdom	Clinical and research
FLCs	Urine, CSF	New Scientific Company, Italy	Clinical and research
Sandwiched ELISA	Serum, plasma, urine	BioVendor, Czech Republic	Research only

quality-controlled, validated, and clinically digestible information that can be used by clinicians without extensive bioinformatics training. Gene expression–based report (GEP-R) was described as one way to overcome the problem (Meissner et al., 2011), and it includes molecular classification, risk stratification, and assessment of target gene expression. The GEP-R is a noncommercial software framework adaptable to other cancer entities that can be freely downloaded (http://code.google.com/p/gep-r). Within the GEP R, an implemented metascore integrates current expression based and conventional prognostic factors into one superior prognostic classification (HM-metascore). The resulting HM-metascore is defined as the sum over the weighted factor gene expression–based risk assessment (UAMS-, IFM-score), proliferation, ISS stage, t(4;14), and expression of prognostic target genes (AURKA, IGF1R) for which clinical grade inhibitors exist. The HM-score delineates three significantly different groups of 13.1%, 72.1%, and 14.7% of MM patients with a 6-year survival rate of 89.3%, 60.6%, and 18.6%, respectively.

Overall, these assays are still not recommended for routine use on all MM patients according to consensus and expert opinions from different relevant medical societies (Fonseca et al., 2009; Fonseca and Braggio, 2011).

31.5 Future Invasive and Noninvasive Biomarkers

Beyond the well-known routinely used biomarkers, recent research has led to the discovery of numerous small molecules and signaling pathways, which may hold promise in the future prognostication and treatment of MM patients. Some of these genes and molecules are discussed later for the rest of the chapter. Intense research over the last decade has shown that MM is an inflammatory disease characterized by elevations of proinflammatory cytokines in affected patients. These inflammatory changes result in a rich microenvironment, or niche, where inflammation is allowed to persist unchecked and myeloma tumor cells thrive. Within this milieu, neoplastic PCs are shielded from the effects of cytotoxic chemotherapy, are allowed to multiply, and may eventually develop drug resistance.

Establishing new noninvasive biomarkers that can be detected in the peripheral blood or serum will be preferable and more convenient for patients and their physicians. However, detecting molecular biomarkers in the myeloma cells themselves seems to be the more frequently studied area. The recent advances in proteomics may change that trend and allow the discovery of specific biomarkers in the serum. Proteomics profiling analysis on the serum of myeloma patients in comparison to control patients has been reported to identify four novel biomarkers that achieved high sensitivity and specificity with validation (He et al., 2012). This was accomplished using CLINPROT, which is an integrated set of tools provided by Bruker Daltonics Inc. (Billerica, MA) for preparation, measurement, and visualization of peptide and protein biomarkers in context to clinical proteomics. This system is consisted of magnetic bead-based sample preparation, matrix-assisted laser desorption/ionization (MALDI)-TOF mass spectrometry (MS) acquisition, and a bioinformatics package for inspection and comparison of data sets as well as for the discovery of complex biomarker pattern models, which greatly facilitate the clinical proteomic studies (Ketterlinus et al., 2005).

While many of these developments discussed in the succeeding text are limited to small patient samples or cell culture/animal work, they represent exciting advances in improving care for patients with MM. We will discuss these new potential biomarkers later and their relevance to diagnosis, prognosis, prediction of response to different treatments, and complications of therapy. Summaries are provided for in tables dealing with invasive and noninvasive markers separately with the disease and commercial relevant information about each potential marker.

31.5.1 Biomarkers for Diagnosis/Progression/Disease Activity

31.5.1.1 Microenvironment Factors

Significant interest has focused on the mesenchymal stromal cell (MSC), cells that are an important functional component of the BM niche. The MSCs secrete interleukin-6 (IL-6) and interleukin-10 (IL-10), in addition to a number of other growth factors including vascular endothelial growth factor (VEGF), stem cell factor, and tumor necrosis factor-alpha (TNF-α) (Podar and Anderson, 2007). These proinflammatory cytokines, particularly IL-6, are key constituents in MM growth. In vivo levels of IL-6 are tightly correlated with disease stage suggesting an important role for IL-6 in MM cell growth and survival (Tsirakis et al., 2011). At the cellular level, elevated levels of IL-6 facilitate inflammation, B-cell differentiation, monoclonal protein secretion, and inhibition of albumin synthesis in the liver. These changes drive the pathophysiology of MM and underscore the importance of IL-6 in the pathogenesis of MM.

Hepatocyte growth factor (HGF), a ligand that binds with the tyrosine kinase receptor (TCR) c-Met, also works in concert with a number of these proinflammatory cytokines to further promote tumorigenesis in MM patients. Confirming this association is the finding that elevated serum levels of soluble c-Met are associated with higher disease burden in MM patients (Wader et al., 2011).

Further supporting the significance of IL-6 in the pathogenesis of MM is the finding that primary bone marrow stromal cells (BMSCs) from MM patients display elevated levels of endogenous X-box binding protein 1 spliced (XBP1s) compared to those from healthy donors. During times of stress, XBP1 mRNA is unconventionally spliced to generate XBP1s mRNA. The transcription factor drives the expression of a wide variety of gene targets seen in physiologic processes such as lipogenesis and adipogenesis. Importantly, XBP1s overexpression in B-lineage cells results in PC differentiation and ultimately the upregulation of IL-6. Levels of XBP1s mRNA from MM patients were 4.6 times higher than those from healthy donors, while Xbp1 ratios of spliced versus unspliced mRNA (XBP1u) remained normal between the two groups of patients. This suggests that XBP1s signaling is activated in MM MSCs and that its overexpression is likely involved in PC pathogenesis. Increased ratios of XBP1s versus XBP1u predict poor survival in MM patients (Xu et al., 2012). Furthermore, there is evidence that blockade of XBP1 can have therapeutic benefit in MM (Mimura et al., 2012; Ri et al., 2012).

Interactions between TNF-α and the MSCs result in the secretion of vascular cell adhesion molecule 1 (VCAM-1), which leads to the secretion of several proinflammatory cytokines including IL-6 and receptor activator of nuclear factor kappa-B ligand (RANKL). Elevated levels of XBP1s, discussed previously, further upregulate VCAM-1, which results in greater cellular adhesion within the niche, cellular growth, and chemoresistance. This suggests an important role for IRE1/XBP1s in PC growth and survival. Additionally, XBP1 signaling has been implicated in bony disease through its disruption of osteoclast regulation (Xu et al., 2012). Its unique activities, elevation in patients with MM, and normal values in healthy controls make it an attractive biomarker for the diagnosis of MM. Further, its role in osteoclast function suggests that it may have a purpose as a marker for skeletal events as well as a target for future therapeutics.

Enhancing the production of these proinflammatory cytokines (particularly VEGF, MMP-9, HGF, and RANKL) and driving tumor progression is heparanase (HPSE) (Kelly et al., 2003; Mahtouk et al., 2007). HPSE, which is associated with aggressive MM tumor subtypes, is a protein encoded by the SDC-1 gene. High levels of HPSE result in a reduction of the levels of syndecan-1, an intranuclear protein with heparan sulfate chains. Reduced levels of syndecan-1, through the reduction of HPSE side chains, allow for an increase in the activity of histone acetyltransferase (HAT) and ultimately an increase in gene activation and protein transcription that appear to drive a more active MM subtype. There is a positive correlation between increased HPSE, HAT activity, and protein transcription that ultimately results in a more aggressive MM subtype (Purushothaman et al., 2011). The quantification of HPSE or HAT may provide information regarding prognosis in MM patients. Similar to cytokines, whose levels appear to fluctuate with the disease course, levels of HPSE or HAT may provide similarly useful information. This dramatic cytokine-mediated increase in protein synthesis, which is further bolstered by HPSE and HAT, is central to the pathogenesis of MM. Increases in gene activation, cellular signaling, and cytokine production ultimately result in increased protein transcription within the cell. These increased demands require enhanced protein folding and trafficking that is referred to as the unfolded protein response (UPR).

31.5.1.2 Surface Cell Markers

Overexpression of CD28, a T-cell costimulatory receptor, has been reported during disease progression and in patients with adverse risk MM (Robillard et al., 1998; Almeida et al., 1999; Bahlis et al., 2007). CD28+ myeloma cells were detected in 21 of 79 (26%) MM cases at diagnosis, 13 of 22 (59%) at medullary relapse ($P < 0.009$), and 14 of 15 (93%) at extramedullary relapse ($P = 0.05$), including 10 of 10 (100%) secondary PC leukemias ($P = 0.05$). The binding of CD28+ myeloma PCs to the ligand

CD80/CD86 on BM stromal cells results in the development of chemoresistance and protection against cell death (Nair et al., 2011). Blocking of the CD28 receptor may result in improved chemosensitivity with heightened susceptibility to death. Furthermore, reduced levels of IL-6, as a result of this blockade, could have additional antimyeloma effects. Recent study showed that engagement by CD28 to its ligand CD80/CD86 on stromal dendritic cell directly transduces a prosurvival signal to myeloma cell, protecting it against chemotherapy and growth factor withdrawal-induced death. Simultaneously, CD28-mediated ligation of CD80/CD86 induces the stromal dendritic cell to produce the prosurvival cytokine IL-6 (involving novel cross talk with the Notch pathway) and the immunosuppressive enzyme IDO. These findings identify CD28 and CD80/CD86 as important molecular components of the interaction between myeloma cells and the BM microenvironment and point to similar interaction for normal PCs.

Soluble CD40 ligand (sCD40L) is a member of the TNF family, which binds to CD40 receptor expressed on myeloma PCs. Such binding triggers immune response against the tumor and induces apoptosis. Yet high levels in the serum could predict poorer outcomes in hematologic malignancies including MM (Hock et al., 2006). The serum levels of sCD40L have been correlated with other cytokines discussed previously including VEGF, HGF, and IL-6. A correlation also exists between sCD40L, the Ki-67 proliferation index (Ki-67 PI), and BM PC infiltration (Tsirakis et al., 2012). Elevated sCD40L concentration also significantly correlates with advanced disease stage and is significantly higher in patients with partial remission or less. Pretreatment levels of sCD40L were higher in MM patients compared to the values seen in healthy controls. Values significantly fell in patients after receiving effective antimyeloma therapy lending further credence to this finding (Tsirakis et al., 2012).

31.5.1.3 Angiogenesis Biomarkers

Angiogenesis is part of the normal processes in the BM environment that could be affected significantly through interaction between myeloma PCs and their niche in the BM. A positive correlation has been established between microvessel density (MVD) and myeloma progression (Sezer et al., 2000) as evidence mounts that increased BM vascularization is associated with poorer risk disease. VEGF and IL-8 are key players in angiogenesis and promote the increased MVD and subsequent tumor progression. The biologically active splice variants VEGF165 and VEGF121 were expressed and secreted by myeloma cell lines and PCs isolated from the marrow of patients with MM. There is mutual stimulation between IL-6 and VGEF, which suggests paracrine interactions between myeloma and marrow stromal cells triggered by these two cytokines (Dankbar et al., 2000).

The ELR+ CXC chemokines are important mediators of tumorigenesis, related to their angiogenic properties. Serum concentrations of angiogenesis-related chemokines ELR+ motif, such as interleukin-8 (IL-8), epithelial neutrophil-activating protein-78 (ENA-78), and growth-related gene-alpha (GRO-α), as well the BM MVD, were studied in patients with MM at diagnosis and after treatment, in plateau phase. In addition, serum levels of other known angiogenic factors, HGF, VEGF, and TNF-α, were determined in 63 newly diagnosed MM patients, 30 in plateau phase and in 20 healthy controls. IL-8, ENA-78, and GRO-α were found to correlate with angiogenic growth factors and may play a role in the progression of MM. However, further studies are still needed to determine their prognostic and predictive significance (Pappa et al., 2011). Multiple other studies have been previously published on such correlation between angiogenic cytokine serum levels, and the clinical course of MM has been published; however, none of these findings have been incorporated into the clinical practice of treating these patients.

The matrix protein osteopontin is also a potent regulator of angiogenesis. Higher serum osteopontin levels were observed in patients with more aggressive forms of myeloma, whereas lower values correlated with patients who had less aggressive forms of disease. Furthermore, osteopontin levels decreased after treatment with antimyeloma therapy. Osteopontin levels correlate with VEGF and BM MVD—both of which are linked to advanced forms of MM, chemoresistance, and shortened survival (Sfiridaki et al., 2011).

31.5.1.4 Bone Disease Biomarkers

Bone lytic lesions or severe osteopenia are common complications of MM and represent a significant source of morbidity in these patients. At the fundamental level, it represents an imbalance between bone remodeling through suppression of osteoblasts and a loss of osteoclast regulation. While the mechanisms behind this tightly regulated process are not yet fully understood, recent advances have suggested that CCL3 (MIP-1α in the old terminology), an osteoclast growth factor, through interactions with CC chemokine receptors (CCRs), CCR1 and CCR5, stimulate bone resorption by regulating osteoclast differentiation and inhibiting osteoblast function (Vallet et al., 2011). CCL3, IL-1β, and other cytokines have been studied in the serum and may represent biomarkers of patients at increased risk of developing bony complications from their MM. The serum levels of these cytokines also correlate to other markers of disease activity (Tsirakis et al., 2011). Similarly associated with MM bony lesions is tartrate-resistant acid phosphatase (TRAcP). TRAcP is highly specific and closely related to the extent of myeloma bone lesions (Chao et al., 2010; Terpos et al., 2003). Osteopontin, discussed previously as a regulator of angiogenesis, is also a marker of osteoclastic activity. Osteopontin levels correlate with the N-terminal propeptide of procollagen type I (NTx), a bone turnover marker. Due to its association with osteoclastic activity, it may also serve a marker of skeletal events (Sfiridaki et al., 2011).

Sclerostin, which is expressed by osteocytes, reduces bone production through the inhibition of osteoblasts. Its primary effect is through the inhibition of Wnt signaling via Wnt inhibitors such as DKK1, SFRP-2, and SFRP-3 (Brunetti et al., 2011) as well is Int-1 inhibition. Like other markers such as osteopontin and TRAcP, circulating levels of sclerostin correlate with disease activity and skeletal events. Sclerostin levels from four groups of patients ranging from healthy controls to patients with relapsed disease were compared. Patients with active MM had higher sclerostin levels than healthy controls. Patients with fractures had higher levels yet. Like other markers discussed previously, sclerostin levels fell after treatment with bortezomib (Terpos et al., 2012). Sclerostin may have implications as a prognostic biomarker but may also represent a marker of patients at risk for developing skeletal events.

Tissue inhibitor of metalloproteinases 1 (TIMP-1) is a matrix metalloproteinase (MMP)-independent regulator of growth and apoptosis in various cell types. TIMP-1 and similar proteins help regulate bone turnover including resorption and ossification. Excess of TIMP-1 contributes to tumor development because it directly encourages cell growth and inhibits apoptosis, encourages angiogenesis, and thus fuels tumor growth. Tissue inhibitor of TIMP-1 was evaluated in the pretreatment serum of 55 newly diagnosed patients with symptomatic myeloma. TIMP-1 was elevated in 47% of patients and correlated with lytic bone disease and increased bone resorption. In fact, TIMP-1 levels in MM patients were more than double that in healthy controls (431.9 vs. 201 ng/mL). Importantly, TIMP-1 correlated with ISS stage ($P = 0.005$) and was an independent prognostic covariate for survival ($P = 0.004$) in these patients who were all treated with novel agents (bortezomib and/or immunomodulatory drug [IMiD]) during their disease course. This study provides evidence that pretreatment serum TIMP-1 is associated with advanced myeloma and suggests the further evaluation of this molecule to better determine its predictive and prognostic potential as a biomarker in MM (Terpos et al., 2010).

31.5.1.5 Other Genetic Markers

B-cell activating factor (BAFF), or B lymphocyte stimulator (BLys), is a B-cell growth factor, member of the TNF superfamily, and functions as a costimulator of immunoglobulin production. Serum BAFF levels correlate with TNF-α activity, LDH, β2M, proliferating cell nuclear antigen (PCNA), and BM MVD. Its role in oncogenesis, mediated through the effects of NF-KB, is diverse and involves cellular proliferation, differentiation, migration, and angiogenesis. Elevated BAFF levels have been linked to patients with advanced disease compared to those in the plateau phase as well as the development of drug resistance (Jiang et al., 2009; Fragioudaki et al., 2012). Elevations in BAFF are associated with shortened survival making its detection and quantification attractive as a prognostic marker and target for future therapy.

31.5.2 MGUS, Smoldering Myeloma and Progression to MM

31.5.2.1 Current Models for Risk Assessment

MGUS is asymptomatic premalignant stage in the development of MM with a 1% annual risk of transformation into a malignant tumor including active MM. Although certain clinical markers of MGUS progression have been identified, it is currently not possible to accurately determine individual risk of progression. A better understanding of the pathogenesis will allow us to define the biologic high-risk precursor disease and, ultimately, to develop early intervention strategies designed to delay and prevent full-blown MM. Unfortunately, at this time, we lack reliable markers to predict the risk of MM progression for individual patients with MGUS (Mailankody et al., 2010). There are two major models for the assessment of the risk of progression of MGUS: one by the Mayo Clinic (Rochester, MN) and the other by the Spanish study group. The Mayo Clinic model focuses on serum protein abnormalities. The following features are considered as adverse risk factors: non-IgG isotype, M-protein concentration >1.5 g/dL, and an abnormal serum FLC ratio (normal reference 0.26–1.65) (Rajkumar et al., 2005). For patients with asymptomatic or SMM, the risk factors for progression are serum M-protein concentration >3 g/dL, BM PCs >10%, and an abnormal FLC ratio. The cumulative risk of progression at 10 years with one, two, and three of the risk factors was 50%, 65%, and 84%, respectively (Landgren et al., 2011). The Spanish study group model uses multiparametric flow cytometry of BM aspirates to differentiate aberrant from normal PCs (Perez-Persona et al., 2007). The ratio of phenotypically abnormal PCs to total BM PCs at diagnosis allowed the risk stratification of patients with MGUS and SMM progression to overt MM (Perez-Persona et al., 2007).

31.5.2.2 Genetic Biomarkers

Recently, some investigators have attempted to identify GEP signatures and microRNA (miRNA) profiles that might predict progression of MGUS to MM (Zhang et al., 2007; Korde et al., 2011). There are limitations to the use of GEP in MGUS because it is done on purified PCs from BM aspirate and, according to the MGUS definition, there will be low number of abnormal PCs contaminated by normal PCs. MiRNA profiling may have the same problems. One study showed that, unlike MGUS, miR-32 and the cluster miR-17*92 (in particular miR-19a and b) were significantly upregulated only in MM samples, thus suggesting a possible predictive role in the progression of MGUS to MM (Pichiorri et al., 2008). Circulating miRNAs in the serum of various cancer patients have been analyzed for the feasibility to detect early cancer development (Brase et al., 2010). Two recent reports described such unique circulating miRNAs in MGUS and MM patients (Huang et al., 2012; Jones et al., 2012). However, clinical studies for validation of the predictive value of miRNAs have not been done yet. A group of investigators at the University of Sussex (Brighton, United Kingdom) have developed a miRNA-based biomarker blood test (the Sussex multiple myeloma biomarker assay) ready for marketing and are seeking commercial partners. The purpose of the tests is to help differentiate between MM and MGUS and disease monitoring without the need for BM biopsies (http://www.sinc.co.uk/home/index.html).

31.5.2.3 Epigenetic Biomarkers

DNA methylation is an epigenetic process of methylating specific CpG dinucleotides in the genome. These "CpG islands" are usually associated with the promoter region, and their methylation usually is inhibitory for gene expression. A number of studies have been conducted to assess the role of promoter methylation in patients with MGUS and MM. For example, one study found that there is significant difference in the p16 methylation status in MGUS and MM (Ng et al., 1997), while others have shown that there is no such difference (Gonzalez-Paz et al., 2007). Thus, in summary, and although p16 methylation has been associated with worse prognosis in other solid tumors, there is no evidence that p16 methylation in MM is associated with worse outcomes.

DNA methylation and acetylation are parallel processes and may need to study both for better understanding the pathogenesis of transformation and to be able to deliver effective treatment (see succeeding text).

31.5.3 Biomarkers for Prognosis/Survival

Clinically, the stratification of patients with high-risk disease versus those with standard-risk disease has important implications for both counseling and treatment. Patients at high risk of relapse may be offered more aggressive therapy upfront, while patients who appear to have a more indolent disease course may be offered maintenance therapy instead. Due to the considerable heterogeneity and shortcomings of our current scoring systems, there has been a push in recent years to evaluate for biomarkers, which may be associated with higher- versus standard-risk disease.

31.5.3.1 Protein and Proteomic Markers

The ratio of albumin to monoclonal protein provides additional important prognostic information. A ratio of <1 at the time of diagnosis correlates to adverse outcomes at 2 years and at 5 years in patients treated with proteasome inhibitors and anti-angiogenic therapy compared to patients with ratios >1 (Kádár et al., 2012).

Overexpression of dicer and drosha, two key enzymes in the miRNA-processing pathway, was evaluated by real-time quantitative PCR done on RNA isolated from selected CD138-positive PCs in patients with MGUS, asymptomatic myeloma, and MM. Dicer expression was significantly higher ($P < 0.1$) in patients with MGUS than patients with smoldering or symptomatic MM. Furthermore, the median progression-free survival was significantly longer ($P = 0.2$) in symptomatic myeloma patients with high dicer expression suggesting a role in progression and prognosis of monoclonal gammopathies. On the other hand, there were no differences between the groups in the expression of drosha (Sarasquete et al., 2011).

31.5.3.2 Genetic Biomarkers

The transcription factor, interferon regulatory factor-4 (IRF4) is required during an immune response for lymphocyte activation and the generation of immunoglobulin-secreting PCs (Klein et al., 2006; Sciammas et al., 2006; Shaffer et al., 2007). Overexpression of IRF4, which is common in MM, is associated with poor prognosis. Patients with higher IRF4 expression have significantly poorer overall survival than those with low IRF4 expression (Lopez-Girona et al., 2011). Lenalidomide is an IMiD that has both tumouricidal and immunomodulatory activities in MM. This study showed that lenalidomide downregulated IRF4 levels in MM cell lines and BM samples within 8 h of drug exposure. This was associated with a decrease in MYC levels, as well as an initial G1 cell cycle arrest, decreased cell proliferation, and cell death by day 5 of treatment. In eight MM cell lines, high IRF4 levels correlated with increased lenalidomide sensitivity. The clinical significance of this observation was investigated in 154 patients with MM. Among MM patients with high levels of IRF4 expression, treatment with lenalidomide led to a significantly longer overall survival than other therapies in a retrospective analysis. These data confirm the central role of IRF4 in MM pathogenesis, indicate that this is an important mechanism by which lenalidomide exerts its antitumor effects, and may provide a mechanistic biomarker to predict response to lenalidomide (Lopez-Girona et al., 2011). This effect of lenalidomide was confirmed by another publication. Double antigen labeling immunohistochemistry (IHC) studies to assess IRF4 expression in $CD138^+$ PCs were performed on bone marrow biopsy (BMB) sections. The study also reported translational relationship between IRF-4 and CCAAT/enhancer-binding protein (C/EBPβ) (Li et al., 2011) and effect on cell proliferation.

31.5.3.3 Epigenetic Biomarkers

Recent studies have shown that epigenetic changes such as DNA methylation play a role by silencing various cancer-related genes in MM (Moreaux et al., 2012). Most of these studies have been performed on limited number of genes using methylation specific PCR. Among the genes identified with promoter hypermethylation in MM, cyclin-dependent kinase inhibitor 2A (*CDKN2A*) and transforming growth factor beta receptor 2 (*TGFBR2)* have been shown to be associated with a poor prognosis in MM patients with discrepant results for *CDKN2A* (de Carvalho et al., 2009). Heller at al. have identified several cancer-related genes inactivated through methylation in three human myeloma cell lines (HMCLs) and validated the relevance of 10 of these genes in six additional HMCLs, premalignant PCs from 24 MGUS patients, and MM cells from 111 patients with MM (Heller et al., 2008).

A global view of methylation in myeloma was performed by Heller et al. (2008), using expression arrays to document genes upregulated by the demethylating agent 5-azacytidine. This investigation identified two genes, SPARC and BNIP3, whose methylation was associated with poor overall survival. A more recent study using the same strategy identified RASD1 as a candidate gene suppressed by methylation to be linked to dexamethasone resistance (Nojima et al., 2009). Furthermore recent studies have identified alterations in promoter hypermethylation that correlate with disease stage and progression. The hypermethylation of TGFBR2 has been shown to correlate with poor outcome in patients (de Carvalho et al., 2009), and hypermethylation of the MGMT promoter is associated with extramedullary disease (Yuregir et al., 2010). The hypermethylation of the maternally imprinted gene MEG3 was associated with disease progression and subtype, with a high percentage of advanced-stage disease and IgG/IgM subtype patients found to have differentially methylated MEG3 (Benetatos et al., 2008).

Myeloma is linked to the overexpression of a histone methyltransferase multiple myeloma SET (suppressor of variegation, enhancer of zeste, and trithorax) domain (MMSET) and inactivating mutations of a histone demethylase (UTX), suggesting that the regulation of histone methylation is a potential therapeutic target (Smith et al., 2010).

31.5.4 Biomarkers Predictive of Response to Treatment

31.5.4.1 In Nontransplant Therapies

As newer novel biologic agents have shown promise in the treatment of MM, there has been a shift away from conventional cytotoxic therapy. The trend has been combining the old cytotoxic drugs with novel drugs in order to achieve more responses and durable remissions. Some of the same markers that predict MM prognosis can predict response to certain drug or combination of drugs and direct us in the initial choice of therapy.

31.5.4.1.1 Response to Proteasome Inhibitors

Overexpression of cyclin kinase subunit 1B (CKS1B), as detected by IHC done on decalcified BM biopsy, is associated with shortened PFS and OS in relapsed/refractory MM patients being treated with the biologic agent bortezomib, a reversible inhibitor of the 26S proteasome (Chen et al., 2012b). Furthermore, CKS1B was found to predict the chromosome 1p21 amplification and adverse outcome for MM patients (Zhan et al., 2007; Chang et al., 2010). The percentage of PCs with amplification of CKS1B and the level of amplification were also shown to be significantly increased in relapsed marrows in comparison to marrows done at diagnosis (Chang et al., 2006).

In a clinical comparison of bortezomib and thalidomide, patients treated with bortezomib effectively had an increase of the serum alkaline phosphatase (ALP) level. Since serum ALP elevation was observed in many patients for whom bortezomib was effective, ALP may be considered a predictor of bortezomib efficacy (Satoh et al., 2011). In another study, the percentage of ALP increments in responders (complete and partial response) and nonresponders was analyzed at different thresholds and time points. For all bortezomib-treated patients enrolled in the trial ($N = 333$), at least a 25% increase in ALP from the baseline at 6 week was the most powerful predictor of treatment response ($P < 0.0001$) and time to progression (206 vs. 169 days) relative to patients with less than a 25% increase in ALP ($P = 0.01$). Such relationship is explained by bortezomib-induced osteoblastic activation in MM patients (Zangari et al., 2007).

To better demarcate the subset of patients that respond favorably to bortezomib, an IHC staining was performed on paraffin-fixed BMBs collected from patients enrolled in a clinical trial aimed at assessing the efficacy of bortezomib in patients with relapsed or refractory MM (Dawson et al., 2009). The IHC panel was chosen to include markers of cell cycle activity, apoptosis, and angiogenesis. IHC was done on an automated immunostainer (Lab Vision Autostainer 360-2D; Lab Vision) according to the manufacturer's protocols. Paraffin-embedded BMB sections were decalcified and sequentially cut (3 Am thick sections), mounted, dewaxed, and immunostained. Peroxidase staining was done using Lab Vision UltraVision LP Large Volume Detection System HRP Polymer (ready to use). Antibodies were used according to the manufacturers' instructions and included anti-CD138 (clone MI15; DAKO), anticyclin D1 (clone SP4; Lab Vision), anti-Bcl-2 (clone 124; DAKO), anti-Bcl-xL (clone 2H12; Zymed), anti-p53 (clone DO-7; Novocastra), anti-p16INK4A (clone 3G5D5; Zymed), anti-p21CIP/WAF1 (clone EA10; Zymed), anti-RelA (sc-109; Santa Cruz Biotechnology), anti-VEGF receptor-1 (clone VG1; Zymed), and anti-FGFR3 (sc-13121; Santa Cruz Biotechnology). The results showed that patients who expressed cyclin D1 were more likely to achieve a response. In contrast, patients who expressed p16INK4A, cytoplasmic p53, and the highest intensity of Bcl-2 staining had a poor response. Patients who achieved a response to bortezomib and those patients who expressed cyclin D1 at baseline showed a significant survival advantage. Patients who expressed FGFR3, a poor prognostic marker, responded equally well and had similar outcomes with bortezomib compared with FGFR3-negative patients (Dawson et al., 2009).

In another study, using liquid chromatography coupled to MS (LC/MS) with similar objective of identifying biomarkers in order to predict patient response to bortezomib sooner and more accurately compared to serum M-protein levels. The plasma LC/MS biomolecular/biochemical profiles, comprised of thousands of endogenous small molecules, peptides, and proteins, were determined for 10 MM patients at predose and 24 h after initial dosing with bortezomib. The comparative analysis of the metabolic profiles of nonresponders and partial responders provided an opportunity to investigate mechanisms related to disease progression and identify biomarkers related to drug response. The plasma levels of two potential efficacy response markers were significantly more abundant in the nonresponsive patients compared to the responders at 24 h postdose. The potential response biomarkers, apolipoprotein C-I and apolipoprotein C-I', were identified by mass spectral analyses and confirmed by authentic protein standards based on MALDI-TOF MS/MS sequencing of proteolytic peptides. There was no apparent relationship between the plasma levels of apoC-I and apoC-I' (at predose or 24 h postdose bortezomib) with the incidence of peripheral neuropathy under the conditions of this study. ApoC-I and apoC-I' were not drug-response predictive markers if these patients were not treated with bortezomib (i.e., predose). ApoC-I and apoC-I' are not appropriate, however, for disease diagnostics in MM because patients may have baseline plasma levels that are similar to healthy subjects (Hsieh et al., 2009) (Nextcea, Inc., Woburn, MA).

Genomic studies supported by the developing companies of bortezomib have been performed in collaboration with medical centers performing phase II and III clinical trials with bortezomib and have been reported and showed that patients with increase expression of genes in the NFκ-B and adhesion molecule pathways may be more sensitive to bortezomib therapy, but these biomarkers did not predict sensitivity to dexamethasone therapy (Mulligan et al., 2007).

31.5.4.1.2 Response to IMiDs

The impact of del(17p) was discussed previously as an adverse cytogenetic marker. Patients with del(17p) were treated with conventional therapy versus thalidomide-based induction therapy. Within the del(17p) group, thalidomide-based therapy was associated with better response rates but did not favorably impact on OS compared to conventional therapy (Boyd et al., 2011).

In patients with overexpression of IRF4, discussed earlier as a poor prognostic marker, lenalidomide reduced IRF4 levels in MM cell lines and BM samples from MM patients. This downregulation in IRF4 was associated with a decrease in c-MYC levels, G1 cell cycle arrest, slowed cellular proliferation, and cell death. Clinically, MM patients with high levels of IRF4 expression who were treated with lenalidomide had significantly longer OS suggesting that the antitumor effects of lenalidomide are exerted through its effects on IRF4, which in turn can become a mechanistic biomarker to identify patients who will respond favorably to lenalidomide (Lopez-Girona et al., 2011).

Proteomic analysis was performed on 39 newly diagnosed MM patients treated with a thalidomide-based regimen (22 responders, 17 nonresponders) using immunodepletion, 2-D DIGE analysis, and MS. Patients who did not respond to chemotherapy were found to have elevations in zinc-α-2-glycoprotein (ZAG), vitamin D-binding protein (VDB), serum amyloid-A protein (SAA), and β2M, while haptoglobin levels were lower. The results were validated by enzyme-linked immunosorbent assay (ELISA) using unfractionated serum from another group of 51 newly diagnosed MM patients. The patients found resistant to thalidomide went on to respond to second-line therapy suggesting that this panel of biomarkers is unique to predicting sensitivity to thalidomide (Patent EP 2467723 by University of Dublin City, 2012) (Rajpal et al., 2011).

E3 ligase protein cereblon (CRBN) is one of the primary teratogenic targets of thalidomide, which, after binding, leads to inactivation. Previous studies demonstrated that thalidomide, lenalidomide, and another IMiD drug pomalidomide bound endogenous CRBN and recombinant CRBN-DNA damage binding protein-1 (DDB1) complexes (Lopez-Girona et al., 2012). While CRBN depletion is initially cytotoxic to the PCs, surviving cells with stable CRBN reductions become resistant to both pomalidomide and lenalidomide but remain sensitive to other agents such as bortezomib, melphalan, and dexamethasone. Thus, thalidomide requires a minimal level of CRBN activity in order to exert its antimyeloma effect. Downstream from CRBN is IRF4, which has been discussed previously as a target of lenalidomide. Patients with lenalidomide resistance had lower CRBN levels after therapy suggesting resistance to thalidomide as well. CRBN is essential for thalidomide sensitivity and may be used as a biomarker for assessment of patients who will respond to therapy with thalidomide as well as pomalidomide and lenalidomide (Zhu et al., 2011).

31.5.4.1.3 Other Disease Response Predictors

A cohort of Danish MM patients whose functional polymorphisms in the promoter region of IL-1β were studied underwent treatment with high-dose therapy (HDT), interferon-α maintenance, or thalidomide versus bortezomib. The wild-type C-allele of IL-1β and absence of the IL-1β promoter resulting in high IL-1β promoter activity were associated with increased time-to-treatment failure (TTF) and OS after high-dose treatment. Patients carrying the wild-type C-allele of IL-1β who were treated with IFN-α showed a trend toward better TTF. Further study showed a fourfold increase in TTF for homozygous carriers of the wild-type alleles at both loci when compared to patients carrying variant alleles. There was no correlation between genotype and clinical outcome in the relapsed patients treated with thalidomide or bortezomib. This work indicates that populations of patients with the WT allele of IL-1β, and absence of the IL-1β promoter (resulting in high IL-1β activity), lead to increased TTF and better OS after treatment with HDT. The WT allele was also associated with a trend toward better TTF in patients treated with IFN-α suggesting that patients with this genotype should be treated with HDT or IFN-α (Vangsted et al., 2011).

Multidrug resistance (MDR) is a clinical challenge most patients and physicians will encounter at some point in their treatment course. MDR is thought to be a result of substrate transport of adenosine triphosphate binding cassette (ABC) transport proteins. Of the ABC genes encoding these transport proteins, ABCB4 may be a prominent mediator of PC MDR in MM. The single-nucleotide polymorphism (SNP), rs1045642, is within the highly studied gene ABCB1 and negatively affects OS. Microarray testing for this polymorphism may provide important information about patients unlikely to respond to therapy (Drain et al., 2011).

Searching the Internet through Google for myeloma-related patents revealed several potential predictors of therapeutic response in MM described through the Technology Venture Development of the University of Utah. Expression of the parathyroid hormone receptor (PTHR1) in BMBs is associated with a statistically significant impact on overall survival (P = 0.002) and event free survival (P = 0.001). PTHR1 is reported to be predictive of therapeutic response to proteasome inhibitors and other drugs. Another gene, protein kinase NeK2, is reported to be associated with poor prognosis and resistance to therapy in MM cases with overexpression of the gene (no related citation in PubMed). Furthermore, a new gene model for MM survival index14 (MMSI14) was recently reported from a group of investigators at the University of Utah, which can separate MM patients into low- and high-risk groups and predict response to therapy and long-term outcomes. MMSI14 was developed from GEP data sets from a public archive of Gene Expression Omnibus (GEO) and includes 14 common genes: CHRDL1, DENND1B, FAM20B, HIST1H1C, IFI16, MAD2L1, NEK2, NOL11, PMS2L5, PPP3CC, RFC4, SGK3, TRIM25, and TYROBP. Applying MMSI14 to independent data sets, we were able to classify 39% of patients as low risk, with a survival probability of more than 90% at 60 months (Chen et al., 2012a).

New treatments undergoing investigation target both the malignant PCs and the BM microenvironment—the protective niche that provides the conditions for the survival, migration, and proliferation of the PCs and, at the same time, confers drug resistance. These include hypomethylating agents and histone deacetylase inhibitors (HDACIs). Relatively little is known about the degree of CpG methylation in myeloma. With the advent of commercially available CpG arrays, this is a rapidly changing field. An important objective for optimizing these clinical trials will be the identification of biomarkers predictive for sensitivity of MMCs to DNMT inhibitors (DNMTis). In a recent study, the authors reported the building of a DNA methylation score (DM score) predicting for the efficacy of decitabine, an inhibitor of DNA methyltransferase (DNMT), targeting methylation-regulated gene expression. DM score was built by identifying 47 genes regulated by decitabine in HMCLs and whose expression in primary MM PCs of previously untreated patients is predictive for overall survival. A high DM score predicts for patients' poor survival and, of major interest, for high sensitivity of primary MM PCs or human myeloma cell lines to decitabine in vitro. Thus, DM score could be useful to design novel treatments with DNMTi in MM and has highlighted 47 genes whose gene products could be important for MM disease development (Moreaux et al., 2012).

Another study showed high frequency at which the gene DLC1 was found to be methylated (43/44 myeloma cell lines), suggesting that it may be useful as a clinical biomarker following epigenetic treatment; subsequent to exposure to demethylating agent and an HDACI, gene silencing was relieved and the gene reexpressed (Ullmannova-Benson et al., 2009).

31.5.4.2 In Transplant Therapy

Despite an armamentarium of cytotoxic chemotherapy and biologic agents, ASCT and allogeneic stem cell transplantation (allo-SCT) remain important in the treatment of MM. However, due to toxicity and increased of mortality, it would be helpful to have biomarkers that can help choose the appropriate patient candidates for either type of transplant and the likely benefit they are going to reap from one type of transplant or another. For example, if a biomarker exists that predicts short PFS and/or OS after ASCT, then allo-SCT may be the preferred type for first transplant, provided that an appropriate donor has been identified. Few such markers have been studied.

In ASCT, stem cells are mobilized and harvested from patients prior to receiving a high-dose chemotherapy conditioning regimens followed by stem cell infusion. The vast majority of patients will eventually relapse and require salvage therapy. Recent work has focused on predicting which patients are at highest risk of relapse. Some have shown that a patient's disease response after ASCT is an important predictor of both progression-free survival and overall survival (Samaras et al., 2011; Kumar et al., 2012). Others have worked to identify molecular markers that can provide important prognostic information in this group of patients.

The qualities/characteristics of the autograft used during ASCT have implications on OS. CD44 is a transmembrane glycoprotein that exists in at least 20 different isoforms due to splicing variants and posttranslational modifications. The most commonly found isoform on hematopoietic cells is CD44H. Soluble CD44 is a cleaved fragment, which is found in the serum of patients with metastasized epithelial and hematologic malignancies and in some other cancers, and has been demonstrated to be correlated with clinical outcome. Thus, the CD44 content of autologous grafts was measured using an ELISA kit (Bender Med Systems, Vienna, Austria). Briefly, intact cell suspension samples from stem cell products were added in duplicate to the wells of the microtiter plate coated with an antibody against CD44. CD44 present in the ASCT graft (from patients with hematologic malignancies including MM patients) was detected with a horseradish peroxidase–conjugated monoclonal antibody against CD44. Patients with autograft CD44 levels of <22,000 ng/mL had superior survival compared to those with higher levels. This information suggests that autograft CD44 levels can predict outcomes in MM patients undergoing ASCT (Krause et al., 2010). Along the same lines, MM patients with more than 100,000 peripheral blood CD34+ cells/mL on the day of stem cell collection had a better post-ASCT OS and PFS than patients with CD34+ cell counts below this threshold (Raschle et al., 2011).

The role of IL-6 is central to the pathogenesis and progression of MM leading some to question if there is upregulation of the IL-6 receptor (IL-6R). The amplification of IL-6R, evaluated for by FISH, was detected in over half of MM patients. The 5-year OS was similar between patients with IL-6R gene amplification and those without the amplification. Alternatively, in patients who received high-dose conventional chemotherapy followed by autoHCT, those with ≥3.1 CNs of the IL-6R showed adverse 5-year OS compared to those with <2.1 copies of the gene suggesting an independent marker of poor prognosis for MM patients undergoing autoHCT (Kim et al., 2011).

31.5.5 Biomarkers as Targets for New Therapies

While transplants, both autologous and allogeneic, remain important in the treatment of MM, the treatment paradigm is transitioning toward more specific and targeted therapies such as immunotherapy and demethylating agents. The use of newer technologies such as genetic and epigenetic profiling has resulted in the discovery of new targets for such treatments. With the push toward individualized medicine, the role of biomarkers as targets in immunotherapy is substantial. Targeting molecular markers in MM actually goes beyond those genes that are known to be dysregulated, and the list is much longer than is presented here (X and target-specific therapies). In general, combination regimens are the most effective considering the multiple pathways involved in the pathogenesis of MM.

31.5.5.1 Plasma Cell Surface Markers

Cancer–testis antigens (CTAs) are a diverse group of genes of which more than 40 families have been identified during the past 15 years. CTAs have been considered promising targets for immunotherapy of human malignancies based on their tumor-restricted expression and on their immunogenicity in cancer patients. Some of them are restricted to expression on the cell surface. Several of them have been used to develop adoptive immunotherapy to treat MM patients. The type I melanoma antigen gene (MAGE) proteins CT7 (MAGE-C1) and MAGE-A3 are commonly expressed in MM, and their expression correlates with increased PC proliferation and poor clinical outcome. MAGE-C1/CT7 seems to be related to disease progression, and functional studies suggest that this CTA might play a role in cell cycle and mainly in survival of malignant PCs, protecting myeloma cells against spontaneous as well as drug-induced apoptosis (de Carvalho et al., 2012). Other studies also showed significant association of the CTA expression in myeloma and prognosis (CTA as prognostic). Data also indicate that CTAs can elicit cellular (CT7) and humoral (MAGE-A1, SSX1) immune responses in MM patients and further support investigation of vaccine strategies targeting these proteins (Lendvai et al., 2010). Other popular target for immunotherapy is NY-ESO-1 (NYESO1) and ropporin. Ropporin is a testis-specific protein located in the flagella of sperm but is not normally expressed in healthy tissues. Ropporin expression was found on the surface of PCs in 44% of MM patient samples suggesting its role as a novel target. Further, the development of human leukocyte antigen class I-restricted cytotoxic lymphocytes was able to kill autologous MM cells lending further credence to ropporin as a potential target in immune therapy (Chiriva-Internati et al., 2011).

Cell surface CS1 is a novel MM antigen. CS1 mRNA and protein were highly expressed in $CD138^+$ purified primary tumor cells from the majority of MM patients (more than 97%) with low levels of circulating CS1 detectable in MM patient sera but not in healthy donors. CS1 was also found to be expressed at adhesion-promoting uropod membranes of polarized MM cells (Tai et al., 2008). Elotuzumab, a humanized anti-CS1 monoclonal antibody, used in conjunction with lenalidomide or bortezomib, has shown clinically significant responses in patients with relapsed/refractory MM (van Rhee et al., 2009; Richardson et al., 2011; Jakubowiak et al., 2012; Zonder et al., 2012).

The chemokine receptor CXCR4 and its ligand CXCL12 are involved in MM progression. The binding of CXCL12 to CXCR4 activates an intracellular signaling cascade, which regulates cell proliferation, chemotaxis, and apoptosis among a number of other functions. 4F-benzoyl-TN14003 (BKT140), a CXCR4 antagonist, stimulates MM apoptotic cell death through phosphatidylserine externalization, caspase-3 activation, sub-G1 arrest, and DNA double-stranded breaks. BKT140, in xenograft models, reduced MM tumor volumes (Beider et al., 2011; Schmidt-Hieber et al., 2011).

Daratumumab, an anti-CD38 human monoclonal antibody, has potent antibody-mediated cytotoxicity in CD38-expressing lymphoma and MM cell lines including patient MM cells. In addition to the antibody-mediated cytotoxicity, daratumumab also induces complement-mediated cytotoxicity in patient MM cells. This dual mechanism of action gives daratumumab a considerable advantage over other CD38 monoclonal antibodies. Significantly, its antimyeloma effects do not appear to be dampened by the BMSCs/BM microenvironment—a significant limitation of most of our current antimyeloma therapies (de Weers et al., 2011).

The IL-6 receptor represents one of the most important receptors present on PCs. The ligand, IL-6, is a known growth factor for MM cells, and its levels correlate with tumor mass and overall prognosis. An anti-IL-6R chimeric antibody was developed by Centocor Ortho Biotech (Horsham, PA), CNTO 328, which is given intravenously every 2 weeks. Again, CNTO 328 (siltuximab) was not active as a single agent, but responses were seen when given with bortezomib or dexamethasone (Chanan-Khan et al., 2010).

CD56 is a cell surface molecule typically found on abnormal PCs in about 75% of MM patients. A new humanized monoclonal antibody, HuN901-DM1 (developed by ImmunoGen Inc. and British Biotech) and immunoconjugated with maytansinoid, is given weekly for the treatment of myeloma. In phase I study, only one patient out of 12 MM patients had minor response (Ocio et al., 2008).

CD40 is expressed on cells with high proliferative activity and in all antigen-presenting cells. A humanized monoclonal antibody against CD40 receptor was developed by Seattle Genetics Inc. It is called SGN-40 or dacetuzumab, and it is in early phases of clinical testing (Ocio et al., 2008).

31.5.5.2 Epigenetic Biomarkers

Myeloma is linked to the overexpression of a histone methyltransferase (MMSET) and inactivating mutations of a histone demethylase (UTX), suggesting that the regulation of histone methylation is a potential therapeutic target (Smith et al., 2010). There is now evidence that histone acetylation and DNA methylation should not be considered as isolated epigenetic events but are coordinated processes that cooperate to determine gene expression patterns.

Despite the recent description of altered histone methylation in myeloma discussed earlier, the most widely studied histone modification in this regard remains the acetylation of specific histone lysine residues, regulated by HATs and HDACs. Early observations found increased histone acetylation resulted in more open, transcriptionally active regions of the chromatin (euchromatin) (Adler et al., 1974). The opposing activity of HDACs, a family of 18 members, is associated with gene silencing in neoplastic cells and the subsequent downregulation of tumor suppressor genes. While there are currently no data supporting abnormal HDAC expression or activity in myeloma, there are many reports of HDACIs having potent antimyeloma activity both in vitro and in vivo. At least six relevant HDACIs are available and have been tested for activity against MM in clinical trials (Smith et al., 2010). HDACIs, including the most advanced agents in clinical trials vorinostat (Merck & Co. Inc., Whitehouse Station, NJ) and panobinostat (Novartis AG, Basel, Switzerland), represent a novel class of drugs targeting enzymes involved in epigenetic regulation of gene expression, which have been evaluated also for the treatment of MM. Although the clinical role in this setting is evolving and their precise utility remains to be determined, to date, that single-agent anti-MM activity is modest. More importantly, HDACIs appear to be synergistic both in vitro and in vivo when combined with other anti-MM agents, mainly proteasome inhibitors including bortezomib (Zain, 2012).

Methylation of DNA cytosine residues is another epigenetic event associated with gene silencing, characterized by the transfer of a methyl group to the C-5 position of cytosine in a CpG dinucleotide and catalyzed by DNA methyl transferase enzymes (DNMTs). There are three mammalian DNMT enzymes: DNMT1, DNMT3a, and DNMT3b. As discussed earlier, there are many genes found to be hypermethylated in myeloma samples and cell lines, providing a good panel of potential biomarkers to measure the success of treatment (Smith et al., 2010). 5-Azacytidine (azacytidine)/5-Aza-2′-deoxycytidine (decitabine) are both nucleoside analogues with FDA approval for use in myelodysplastic syndrome. Clinical trials in myeloma combining these demethylating agents with chemotherapy or other agents are underway.

DNMT1 is associated with deacetylase activity and is found to co-immunoprecipitate with HDAC1 indicating a direct interaction between these epigenetic processes (Fuks et al., 2000). Although no formal studies have been performed in myeloma as yet, the future of epigenetic treatments may lie in a coordinated therapeutic approach targeting multiple epigenetic mechanisms.

31.5.5.3 Tyrosine Kinase Receptors

TCRs are very frequently expressed in cancer, including MM, and consequently several drugs have been designed to block their beneficial effects in promoting cancer proliferation and survival. The abnormality is either in the receptor itself becoming constitutively activated or its ligand being overexpressed by either the myeloma cells or the BMSCs. C-KIT is expressed on myeloma cells in about a third of MM patients, while platelet-derived growth factor receptor and SRC are found constitutively activated in MM cells (Coluccia et al., 2008; Mateo et al., 2008). Based on that, dasatinib and imatinib, approved drugs for the treatment of chronic myelogenous leukemia, were entered clinical trials for MM.

Imatinib was not active, while dasatinib as a single agent resulted in disease stabilization and potentiated other drugs when given in combination (Ocio et al., 2008).

The t(4;14) translocation is present in 15% of MM patients and results in the constitutive activation of FGFR3 in MM cells. More specific TK inhibitors (TKIs), such as dovitinib (Novartis) and AB1010 (AB Science, S.A., Paris, France), were tried in phase II studies but without significant clinical activity (Ocio et al., 2008). Another target is VEGFR with several TKIs available that have shown in vitro activity. Unfortunately, so far, the expectations have not been confirmed clinically. Pazopanib was ineffective in phase II. Bevacizumab, a humanized antibody against VEGF, has been tested in combination with lenalidomide and dexamethasone with 7/10 patients achieving partial remission (Ocio et al., 2008). Another target is the insulin growth factor-1 (IGF-1), the receptor of which has been identified on most MM cell lines and patient samples, and its activation stimulates proliferation and promotes drug resistance (Mitsiades et al., 2004). An anti-IGF-1R monoclonal antibody, AVE-1642 (Sanofi-Aventis/Immunogen, Vitry sur Seine, France), was used as single agent in 14 MM patients and only one minor response seen. The alternative is to use TKIs specific to the IGF-1R. NVP-AEW541 (Novartis) is such an inhibitor that was shown to potentiate the efficacy of other antimyeloma drugs, but it is no longer on the pipeline (Ocio et al., 2008).

31.5.5.4 Signaling Pathways

There are several known signaling pathways affected in myeloma cells. Studies have shown specific mutations in genes that regulate the NF-κB pathway in 80% of patients with MM. Bortezomib and carfilzomib target this pathway, but other inhibitors for NF-κB are being developed. Another target is the RAS pathway since mutations of N-RAS and K-RAS are frequently seen in relapsed MM (Fonseca et al., 2004). Tipifarnib (Zarnestra), a farnesyltransferase inhibitor, is the only drug widely tested for the aim of blocking the RAS pathway, but no significant activity was seen when used as a single agent in MM (Alsina et al., 2004). The drug was not given FDA approval for the treatment of AML in an application by Johnson & Johnson pharmaceutical company submitted in 2005.

31.5.6 Biomarkers Predictive of Treatment-Related Complications

31.5.6.1 Bisphosphonate-Induced Osteonecrosis of the Jaw

Intravenous bisphosphonates (BPs) such as zoledronic acid and pamidronate are considered standard treatment for MM patients with bone disease. Bisphosphonate-induced osteonecrosis of the jaw (BONJ) is a complication in patients taking not only the intravenous but to a lesser degree also the oral BPs (Marx, 2003; Epstein et al., 2012). The occurrence of exposed bone (Figure 31.3) in the jaw might be asymptomatic or painful and may be associated with swelling and fractured jaw (Ruggiero et al., 2009). According to the American Association of Oral and Maxillofacial Surgery (AAOMS), the staging of BONJ is as follows (Ruggiero et al., 2009):

Stage 1: Exposed/necrotic bone in patients who are asymptomatic and have no evidence of infection

Stage 2: Exposed/necrotic bone in patients with pain and clinical evidence of infection

Stage 3: Exposed/necrotic bone in patients with pain, infection, and one or more of the following: pathologic fracture, extraoral fistula, or osteolysis extending to the inferior border

The affected sites may include the mandible, the maxilla, or both and may occur following dental procedures such as tooth extraction, implant placement, root canal therapy, or oral trauma associated with dentures (Tennis et al., 2012). In about 30%–50% of the cases, BONJ lesions occur spontaneously (Marx et al., 2007). Risk factors include length and type of BP therapy, smoking, the presence of dental tori, and the presence of periodontitis (Marx et al., 2007). Although suggested by few authors, diabetes was not proven to pose a higher risk for the development (Khamaisi et al., 2007; Lazarovici et al., 2009). BONJ was first described by Marx (2003). Since then, hundreds of cases have been reported. Most incidences are related to intravenous BP use in cancer patients, but several cases have also been reported in association with oral BPs (Lazarovici et al., 2009) and biologic bone resorption blocking agents (Epstein et al., 2012).

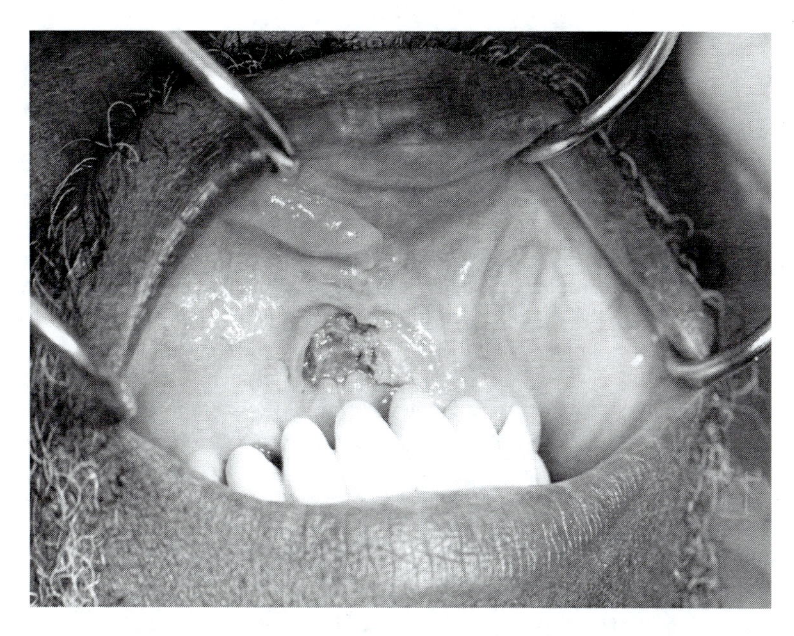

FIGURE 31.3 **(See color insert.)** This photograph is of an MM patient who developed bisphosphonate-induced osteonecrosis of the upper jaw while receiving monthly intravenous zoledronic acid as part of his MM treatment.

Not all patients receiving BPs develop BONJ, suggesting that environmental and/or genetic variation between individuals may confer susceptibility or resistance to developing BONJ (Katz et al., 2011). In a genome-wide association study of 22 BONJ patients and 65 matched controls, only the cytochrome P450 2C8 gene (*CYP2C8*) showed a significantly different distribution between cases and controls (Sarasquete et al., 2008). This finding has not been replicated in an independent study (English et al., 2010). BPs are not metabolized by P450 enzymes so such an association was presumed to be through other metabolic pathways that may be affected by *CYP2C8* (Sarasquete et al., 2008). In a cohort study of MM patients that we published (JSM and JK), a trend for higher odds for BONJ was found for SNPs in five genes: *COL1A1* (rs1800012), *RANK* (rs12458117), *MMP2* (rs243865), *OPG* (rs2073618), and *OPN* (rs11730582). Considering all five SNPs together, patients with genotype scores $\geq$5 had a BONJ event rate of 57%; those with scores <5 had a rate of 10%. The adjusted odds ratio was 11.2 (Katz et al., 2011). This work was supported by Micromedic (Tel Aviv, Israel), and patent application was submitted.

Other studies have been published on the same issue that reported other findings. A polymorphism in the VEGF gene and elevated levels of its protein are reported to be associated with BONJ (Arduino et al., 2011; Vincenzi et al., 2012). An isolated study reported of aromatase polymorphism (g.132810C>T) as a predictor of risk factor for BONJ (La Ferla et al., 2011). Polymorphism of gene encoding for the farnesyl pyrophosphate synthase (FDPS) with ONJ was recently reported in patients treated with zoledronic acid for MM and metastatic mammary and prostate cancer. The AA and CC genotypes were highly differently distributed among ONJ patients and controls, matched for sex and type of malignant disease (Marini et al., 2010). Other investigators have identified N-telopeptide of type I collagen (NTX) and serum C-terminal cross-linking telopeptide of type I collagen (CTX) as potential predictors of BONJ onset; however, these findings were not found to be consistent (Marx et al., 2007; Morris et al., 2012). It is obvious that more studies are needed to better identify predictive biomarkers for this complication. Our group is working on validating our findings in a larger group of patients.

31.5.6.2 Bortizomib-Induced Neuropathy

The introduction of bortezomib (Millennium Pharmaceuticals, Cambridge, MA) has greatly improved the management of MM (Richardson et al., 2005). The dose-limiting toxicity of bortezomib is peripheral neuropathy, which frequently requires a dose reduction or treatment discontinuation

(Richardson et al., 2005). Bortezomib-induced peripheral neuropathy (BiPN) differs from preexisting peripheral neuropathy associated with 10% of untreated MM patients. BiPN, described in detail by Delforge et al. (2010) is predominantly sensory, reversible in most cases, and characterized by distal paresthesias, numbness, and neuropathic pain.

A number of studies have looked at the pharmacogenetic characterization of BiPN (Broyl et al., 2010a; Delforge et al., 2010). In the study carried out by Broyl et al. (2010), the comparison between early onset (within one treatment cycle) BiPN and late onset (after two or three treatment cycles) BiPN revealed that genes for apoptosis contribute to early onset BiPN, whereas genes that have a role in inflammatory pathways and DNA repair contribute to the development of late onset BiPN, indicating that distinct genetic factors are involved in the development of early onset and late onset forms of this side effect. Recently, Favis et al. from the Johnson & Johnson Pharmaceutical Research and Development section (Raritan, NJ) reported on the association between SNPs and the time to BiPN within the VISTA trial with associated SNPs including genes associated with immune function (CTLA4, CTSS), reflexive coupling within Schwann cells (GJE1), drug binding (PSMB1), and neuron function (TCF4, DYNC1I1) (Favis et al., 2011).

Another recent pharmacogenetic association study by Corthals et al. (2011) using a discovery set (IFM 2005–01; n = 238) and a validation set (HOVON65/GMMG-HD4 and a Czech data set; n = 231) revealed SNP with pointwise significance: rs619824 in *CYP17A1*. Previous studies showed that bortezomib is primarily metabolized by cytochrome P450 isoforms *CYP3A4*, *CYP2C19*, *CYP1A2*, with a minor contribution of *CYP2D6* and *CYP2C9* (Uttamsingh et al., 2005). The results of this study showed an enrichment of the major bortezomib metabolizing genes within the top 56 SNPs ($P = 0.0013$).

31.6 Imaging Biomarkers

There are no new imaging techniques for MM. The standard method for the initial evaluation of bone lytic lesions has remained skeletal survey. Some modifications have been introduced on existing CT scan, MRI, and PET scans that can be applied to the diagnosis and disease monitoring in MM patients. These are reviewed somewhere else (Mena et al., 2011; Tan et al., 2011). The dynamic contrast-enhanced MRI (DCE MRI) can be used to asses response (Lin et al., 2010). In addition, there are few patents on the use of arterial spin labeling (ASL) with MRI apparatus, which can potentially provide better information about changes in the BM structure as well as provide earlier signs of response and anti-angiogenic effects (Lin et al., 2010). On the other hand, there has been development of new imaging techniques relying on biomarkers associated with amyloidosis (Wall et al., 2010; Chen and Dilsizian, 2012). These, however, are still investigative and in preclinical development.

31.7 Ethnic-Specific Markers

To date, no markers specific to patients' ethnicity have been developed. However, racial disparities exist in incidence and outcome of MM (Waxman et al., 2010), the reasons for which have not been elucidated. The same is true for the incidence of MGUS (Weiss et al., 2011). The results of a large-scale, population-based study to assess differences in incidence and survival patterns in MM among blacks and whites in the United States indeed showed younger age of onset among blacks and better survival between 1973 and 2005. The black to white incidence rate ratio was 3.1 for patients <50-year-old and 2.1 in patients >70-year-old ($P = 0.002$), thus confirming genetic basis for myelomagenesis. Studies attempted to explain these differences were reviewed before (Benjamin et al., 2003), and the results can be summarized as follows: Obesity is likely a risk factor for myeloma, in both blacks and whites, but obesity is more prevalent in the black population, which may help explain some of the increased incidence of myeloma in blacks; genetic factors such as HLA antigens and family history seem to be important in explaining the differential risk of myeloma; exposure to immunological challenges, especially urinary tract infections in black men, seems important in explaining some of the excess risk in blacks. On the other hand, factors such as socioeconomic status, dietary preferences, vitamin intake, and alcohol and tobacco use either lack a consensus finding or may not play a role in explaining the increased myeloma morbidity and mortality in blacks. Equal treatment yields equal outcome among black and white patients with equivalent disease. Indeed, a recent study by Hari et al. (2010) from the Center for International Bone Marrow Transplantation on 91 patients receiving ASCT in an equal access health system showed no difference in survival.

The search for ethnicity-specific polymorphisms and genetic markers for MM has been the focus of very few previous investigations (Pottern et al., 1992; Cao et al., 1995; Patel et al., 2002). However, and as summarized in recent review (Greenberg et al., 2012), these studies were too small, and further investigation is critically needed to determine the specific cytogenetic types of MGUS and MM and the genetic mechanisms involved in the racial disparity, so that we can better assess patient risk in blacks and develop better management strategies that will improve outcomes for all races and ethnicities.

31.8 Patent Information

A number of patents exist for novel methods to aid in the initial diagnosis and treatment of patients with MM. These methods represent a broad spectrum of laboratory techniques, gene targets, and biomarkers that collectively depict an advancing field for patients diagnosed with MM. Granted patents that were filed from 2003 to 2013 that are specific to MM have been included in Table 31.6. Patents with utility in MM, as well as a number of other malignancies, have been excluded from this discussion for the purpose of clarity. All information was obtained from Patent Lens (www.patentlens.net) and is organized by categories according to their use as diagnostic, prognostic, or therapeutic patents. Invasive and noninvasive biomarkers have been labeled where appropriate.

The majority of the patents listed have therapeutic implications as antimyeloma agents through a variety of unique pathways and targets. Two of the patents, those involving DKK1 and osteoprotegerin variant proteins (OVPs), are potential targets for the prevention of bony disease and its complications in MM. The remainder represents novel methods of diagnosing and predicting disease outcomes through gene expression assays and proteins such as DKK1, FRZB, and JAG2.

31.9 Concluding Remarks and Future Perspective

MM is preceded by a premalignant precursor MGUS. MM is a heterogeneous disease, and genetic abnormalities have been identified in both MGUS and active myeloma. From a clinical standpoint, the identification of biologic and molecular markers will be crucial to identify MGUS with high risk of progression and allow defining risk groups (high vs. others) among myeloma patients, with the possibility of translating the information into specific therapeutic interventions. The current genetic classification of MM is still mainly dependent on cytogenetics and FISH analysis done on BM aspirate. However, considering the fact that these myeloma cells have initially low proliferative activity, the metaphase cytogenetics reflects mostly normal hematopoiesis. The low proliferative activity of the tumor cells is an important limitation of conventional cytogenetics, since only dividing cells can be analyzed. Even within cells with an abnormal karyotype, some aberrations are cryptic to metaphase analysis; for example, the t(4;14)(p16;q32) translocation is a submicroscopic aberration and cannot be detected with conventional banding techniques (Sawyer, 2011). Other techniques such as FISH, multicolor FISH, spectral karyotyping, and array comparative genomic hybridization (aCGH) offer new information that can overcome the shortcomings of conventional cytogenetics and provide new evidence for the heterogeneity of MM with more genomic defects discovered. Furthermore, a large amount of secondary chromosomal aberrations is detected with disease progression, which highlights the challenges of treatment resistance and the need for continual adjustment to the prognosis and risk-adapted therapy.

Whole genome molecular profiling techniques include GEP that has enabled the simultaneous analysis of RNA expression patterns of thousands of different genes pertinent to biologic functions. A high-resolution aCGH and SNP-based arrays detected DNA CN abnormalities, which are important in the molecular classification of MM. Several groups have attempted to define new molecular classification

TABLE 31.6

List of MM-Related Patents over the Last 10 Years (Obtained from Patent Lens)

Patent Number	Title	Category	Patent Assignee	Year Filed
US 7308364	Diagnosis of MM on GEP (expression of 14–24 genes)	Diagnostics; invasive	Board of Trustees of the University of Arkansas, Little Rock, AR	2003
US 7449303	Use of JAG2 expression in diagnosis of PC disorders	Diagnostic; invasive	Health Research, Inc., Buffalo, New York	2004
US 7811750	Molecular determinants of myeloma bone disease and use thereof (DKK1 and FRZB)	Diagnostic; invasive. bony disease	Board of Trustees of the University of Arkansas, Little Rock, AR	2006
7983850	Diagnosis, prognosis, identification, and classification of MM based on GEP (15-gene model)	Diagnostic and prognostic; invasive	Board of Trustees of the University of Arkansas, Little Rock, AR	2008
EP 1204683 B1	Ovarian cancer cell and myeloma cell surface glycoproteins, antibodies thereto, and uses thereof (monoclonal antibody VAC69)	Diagnostic and therapeutic; invasive	Molecular Discoveries, L.L.C, New York, United States	2000
US 7741035	Use of GEP to predict survival in cancer patient (ASPM, OPN3, and CKS1B)	Prognosis; invasive	Board of Trustees of the University of Arkansas, Little Rock, AR	2005
US 7935679	GEP-based identification of CKS1B as a potential therapeutic target in MM	Prognostic and therapeutic; invasive	Board of Trustees of the University of Arkansas, Little Rock, AR	2005
US 7341721	β2-Microglobulin (β2m) and anti-β2m binding agents as anticancer therapeutics	Therapeutic; antimyeloma	Board of Trustees of the University of Arkansas, Little Rock, AR	2003
US 8232101	Identification of antigenic peptides from MM cells (activated cytotoxic T lymphocytes)	Therapeutic; antimyeloma	Janssen Pharmaceutica NV, Beerse, Belgium	2011
US 8168404	Methods to treat cancer with 10-propargyl-10-deazaaminopterin and methods for assessing cancer for increased sensitivity to 10-propargyl-10-deazaaminopterin	Therapeutic; antimyeloma	Sloan-Kettering Institute for Cancer Research, New York, United States	2009
US 7842293	Compositions and methods using anti-CS1 antibodies to treat MM	Therapeutic; antimyeloma	Facet Biotech Corporation, Redwood City, CA	2007
US 7838041	Method for treating MM (KI-121 like antibody)	Therapeutic; antimyeloma	Immune System Therapeutics Ltd, Ultimo, Australia	2008
US 7825088	Methods for the treatment of MM (CXCR4 inhibition)	Therapeutic; antimyeloma	The CBR Institute for Biomedical Research, Inc., Boston, MA	2006
US 7825132	Inhibition of FGFR3 and treatment of MM	Therapeutic; antimyeloma	Novartis Vaccines and Diagnostics, Inc., Emeryville CA	2004
US 7820167	IL1-β: a new target for myeloma therapy (IL1-β inhibition)	Therapeutic; antimyeloma	Mayo Foundation for Medical Education and Research, Rochester, MN	2005

TABLE 31.6 (continued)

List of MM-Related Patents over the Last 10 Years (Obtained from Patent Lens)

Patent Number	Title	Category	Patent Assignee	Year Filed
US 7691392	Method of treating MM using 17-AAG or 17-AG or a prodrug of either	Therapeutic; antimyeloma	Kosan Biosciences Incorporated, Princeton, NJ	2006
US 7371736	GEP-based identification of DKK1 as a potential therapeutic targets for controlling bone loss	Therapeutic; bony disease	Board of Trustees of the University of Arkansas, Little Rock, AR	2004
US 7612169	OVPs	Therapeutic; bony disease	EvoGenix, Ltd., Melbourne, Australia	2005

systems based on selected information extracted from these genomic studies. The advent of even newer technologies, such as high-throughput proteomics, miRNA profiling, whole genome methylation profiling, and whole genome sequencing, will provide additional new molecular diagnostic and prognostic markers that should aid in this task. In fact, the sequencing of MM whole genome has been accomplished, and the data are available for researchers (Chapman et al., 2011). Several new and unexpected oncogenic mechanisms were suggested by the pattern of somatic mutation across the data set, which now will be the basis of further investigation.

The ongoing question will be how to more precisely define the currently evolving molecular subgroups and validate these subgroups for integration into routine clinical use. It is possible that the approach to implementing such progress in favorable risk newly diagnosed MM patients versus the high-risk patients will need to be different (Morgan and Kaiser, 2012). Furthermore, the amount of primary and secondary genetic abnormalities that occur in MM, especially with progression/relapse, may make it impossible to use personalized medicine across the board, and further stratifications will be needed when it comes to relapsing patients.

There have been other effects to this evolving field of clinical biomarkers on other aspects of MM and the related disorders such as the discovery of potential new therapeutic targets, defining genetic predictors for response and therapy-related complications, and developing better predictive biomarkers for disease progression. All these discoveries will continue to affect our approach to treating MM in the next few years.

References

Adler AJ, Fasman GD, Wangh LJ, Allfrey VG. 1974. Altered conformational effects of naturally acetylated histone f2al (IV) in f2al-deoxyribonucleic acid complexes. Circular dichroism studies. *J Biol Chem* 249:2911–2914.

Alfaro R, Rosell J, Durán MA et al. 2011. Structural rearrangements of trisomies are a risk marker of clinical progression in hyperdiploid multiple myeloma. *Anticancer Res* 31:1599–1602.

Almeida J, Orfao A, Ocqueteau M et al. 1999. High-sensitive immunophenotyping and DNA ploidy studies for the investigation of minimal residual disease in multiple myeloma. *Br J Haematol* 107:121–131.

Alsina M, Fonseca R, Wilson EF et al. 2004. Farnesyltransferase inhibitor tipifarnib is well tolerated, induces stabilization of disease, and inhibits farnesylation and oncogenic/tumor survival pathways in patients with advanced multiple myeloma. *Blood* 103:3271–3277.

Arduino PG, Menegatti E, Scoletta M et al. 2011. Vascular endothelial growth factor genetic polymorphisms and haplotypes in female patients with bisphosphonate-related osteonecrosis of the jaws. *J Oral Pathol Med* 40:510–515.

Bahlis NJ, King AM, Kolonias D et al. 2007. CD28-mediated regulation of multiple myeloma cell proliferation and survival. *Blood* 109:5002–5010.

Beider K, Begin M, Abraham M et al. 2011. CXCR4 antagonist 4F-benzoyl-TN14003 inhibits leukemia and multiple myeloma tumor growth. *Exp Hematol* 39:282–292.

Benetatos L, Dasoula A, Hatzimichael E, Georgiou I, Syrrou M, Bourantas KL. 2008. Promoter hypermethylation of the MEG3 (DLK1/MEG3) imprinted gene in multiple myeloma. *Clin Lymphoma Myeloma* 8:171–175.

Benjamin M, Reddy S, Brawley OW. 2003. Myeloma and race: A review of the literature. *Cancer Metastasis Rev* 22:87–93.

Bergsagel PL, Kuehl WM. 2005. Molecular pathogenesis and a consequent classification of multiple myeloma. *J Clin Oncol* 23:6333–6338.

Bergsagel PL, Kuehl WM, Zhan F, Sawyer J, Barlogie B, Shaughnessy J. 2005. Cyclin D dysregulation: An early and unifying pathogenic event in multiple myeloma. *Blood* 106:296–303.

Boyd KD, Ross FM, Tapper WJ et al. 2011. NCRI Haematology Oncology Studies Group. The clinical impact and molecular biology of del (17p) in multiple myeloma treated with conventional or thalidomide-based therapy. *Genes Chromosomes Cancer* 50:765–774.

Bradwell AR, Carr-Smith HD, Mead GP et al. 2001. Highly sensitive, automated immunoassay for immunoglobulin free light chains in serum and urine. *Clin Chem* 47:673–680.

Brase JC, Wuttig D, Kuner R, Sültmann H. 2010. Serum microRNAs as non-invasive biomarkers for cancer. *Mol Cancer* 9:306.

Broyl A, Corthals SL, Jongen JL et al. 2010a. Mechanisms of peripheral neuropathy associated with bortezomib and vincristine in patients with newly diagnosed multiple myeloma: A prospective analysis of data from the HOVON-65/GMMG-HD4 trial. *Lancet Oncol* 11:1057–1065.

Broyl A, Hose D, Lokhorst H et al. 2010b. Gene expression profiling for molecular classification of multiple myeloma in newly diagnosed patients. *Blood* 116:2543–2553.

Brunetti G, Oranger A, Mori G et al. 2011. Sclerostin is overexpressed by plasma cells from multiple myeloma patients. *Ann NY Acad Sci* 1237:19–23.

Cao J, Hong C, Rosen L et al. 1995. Deletion of genetic material from a poly (ADP-ribose) polymerase-like gene on chromosome 13 occurs frequently in patients with monoclonal gammopathies. *Cancer Epidemiol Biomarkers Prev* 4:759–763.

Carrasco DR, Tonon G, Huang Y et al. 2006. High-resolution genomic profiles define distinct clinico-pathogenetic subgroups of multiple myeloma patients. *Cancer Cell* 9:313–325.

Chanan-Khan AA, Borrello I, Lee KP, Reece DE. 2010. Development of target-specific treatments in multiple myeloma. *Br J Haematol* 151:3–15.

Chang H, Jiang N, Jiang H et al. 2010. CKS1B nuclear expression is inversely correlated with p27Kip1 expression and is predictive of an adverse survival in patients with multiple myeloma. *Haematologica* 95:1542–1547.

Chang H, Qi X, Trieu Y et al. 2006. Multiple myeloma patients with CKS1B gene amplification have a shorter progression-free survival post-autologous stem cell transplantation. *Br J Haematol* 135:486–491.

Chang H, Trieu Y, Qi X et al. 2007. Bortezomib therapy response is independent of cytogenetic abnormalities in relapsed/refractory multiple myeloma. *Leuk Res* 31:779–782.

Chao TY, Wu YY, Janckila AJ. 2010. Tartrate-resistant acid phosphatase isoform 5b (TRACP 5b) as a serum maker for cancer with bone metastasis. *Clin Chim Acta* 411:1553–1564.

Chapman MA, Lawrence MS, Keats JJ et al. 2011. Initial genome sequencing and analysis of multiple myeloma. *Nature* 2011;471:467–472.

Chauveau D, Choukroun G. 1996. Bence Jones proteinuria and myeloma kidney. *Nephrol Dial Transplant* 11:413–415.

Chen MH, Qi C, Reece D, Chang H. 2012b. Cyclin kinase subunit 1B nuclear expression predicts an adverse outcome for patients with relapsed/refractory multiple myeloma treated with bortezomib. *Hum Pathol* 43:858–864.

Chen T, Berno T, Zangari M. 2012a. Low-risk identification in multiple myeloma using a new 14-gene model. *Eur J Haematol* 89:28–36.

Chen W, Dilsizian V. 2012. Molecular imaging of amyloidosis: Will the heart be the next target after the brain? *Curr Cardiol Rep* 14:226–233.

Chiriva-Internati M, Mirandola L, Yu Y et al. 2011. Cancer testis antigen, ropporin, is a potential target for multiple myeloma immunotherapy. *J Immunother* 34:490–499.

Chng WJ, Santana-Dávila R, VanWier SA et al. 2006. Prognostic factors for hyperdiploid-myeloma: Effects of chromosome 13 deletions and IgH translocations. *Leukemia* 20:807–813.

Chng WJ, VanWier SA, AhmannGJ et al. 2005. A validated FISH trisomy index demonstrates the hyperdiploid and nonhyperdiploid dichotomy in MGUS. *Blood* 106:2156–2161.

Coluccia AM, Cirulli T, Neri P et al. 2008. Validation of PDGFRbeta and c-Src tyrosine kinases as tumor/vessel targets in patients with multiple myeloma: Preclinical efficacy of the novel, orally available inhibitor dasatinib. *Blood* 112:1346–356.

Corthals SL, Kuiper R, Johnson DC et al. 2011. Genetic factors underlying the risk of bortezomib induced peripheral neuropathy in multiple myeloma patients. *Haematologica* 96:1728–1732.

Dankbar B, Padró T, Leo R et al. 2000. Vascular endothelial growth factor and interleukin-6 in paracrine tumor-stromal cell interactions in multiple myeloma. *Blood* 95:2630–2636.

Dawson MA, Opat SS, Taouk Y et al. 2009. Clinical and immunohistochemical features associated with a response to bortezomib in patients with multiple myeloma. *Clin Cancer Res* 15:714–722.

de Carvalho F, Colleoni GW, Almeida MS, Carvalho AL, Vettore AL. 2009. TGFbetaR2 aberrant methylation is a potential prognostic marker and therapeutic target in multiple myeloma. *Int J Cancer* 125:1985–1991.

de Carvalho F, Vettore AL, Colleoni GW. 2012. Cancer/Testis Antigen MAGE-C1/CT7: New target for multiple myeloma therapy. *Clin Dev Immunol* 2012:257695.

De Gruttola VG, Clax P, DeMets DL et al. 2001. Considerations in the evaluation of surrogate endpoints in clinical trials. Summary of a National Institutes of Health workshop. *Control Clin Trials* 22:485–502.

De Vos J, Hose D, Rème T et al. 2006. Microarray-based understanding of normal and malignant plasma cells. *Immunol Rev* 210:86–104.

Decaux O, Lode L, Magrangeas F et al. 2008. Prediction of survival in multiple myeloma based on gene expression profiles reveals cell cycle and chromosomal instability signatures in high-risk patients and hyperdiploid signatures in low-risk patients: A study of the Intergroupe Francophone du Myelome. *J Clin Oncol* 26:4798–4805.

Delforge M, Blade J, Dimopoulos MA et al. 2010. Treatment-related peripheral neuropathy in multiple myeloma: The challenge continues. *Lancet Oncol* 11:1086–1095.

de Weers M, Tai YT, van der Veer MS et al. 2011. Daratumumab, a novel therapeutic human CD38 monoclonal antibody, induces killing of multiple myeloma and other hematological tumors. *J Immunol* 186:1840–1848.

Dispenzieri A, Kyle R, Merlini G et al. 2009. International Myeloma Working Group guidelines for serum-free light chain analysis in multiple myeloma and related disorders. *Leukemia* 23:215–224.

Drain S, Flannely L, Drake MB et al. 2011. Multidrug resistance gene expression and ABCB1 SNPs in plasma cell myeloma. *Leuk Res* 35:1457–1463.

Drayson M, Tang LX, Drew R, Mead GP, Carr-Smith H, Bradwell AR. 2001. Serum free light-chain measurements for identifying and monitoring patients with nonsecretory multiple myeloma. *Blood* 97:2900–2902.

Durie BG, Harousseau JL, Miguel JS et al. 2006. International uniform response criteria for multiple myeloma. *Leukemia* 20:1467–1473.

Durie BG, Salmon SE. 1975. A clinical staging system for multiple myeloma. Correlation of measured myeloma cell mass with presenting clinical features, response to treatment, and survival. *Cancer* 36:842–854.

Egan JB, Shi CX, Tembe W et al. 2012. Whole-genome sequencing of multiple myeloma from diagnosis to plasma cell leukemia reveals genomic initiating events, evolution, and clonal tides. *Blood* 120:1060–1066.

English BC, Baum CE, Adelberg DE et al. 2010. SNP in CYP2C8 is not associated with the development of bisphosphonate-related osteonecrosis of the jaw in men with castrate-resistant prostate cancer. *Ther Clin Risk Manag* 6:579–583.

Engstrom PF, Bloom MG, Demetri GD et al. 2011. NCCN molecular testing white paper: Effectiveness, efficiency, and reimbursement. *J Natl Compr Canc Netw* 9(Suppl 6):S1–S16.

Epstein MS, Ephros HD, Epstein JB. 2012. Review of current literature and implications of RANKL inhibitors for oral health care providers. *Oral Surg Oral Med Oral Pathol Oral Radiol* (August 15) [Epub ahead of print].

Favis R, Sun Y, van de Velde H et al. 2011. Genetic variation associated with bortezomib-induced peripheral neuropathy. *Pharmacogenet Genom* 21:121–129.

Fonseca R, Barlogie B, Bataille R et al. 2004. Genetics and cytogenetics of multiple myeloma: A workshop report. *Cancer Res* 64:1546–1558.

Fonseca R, Bergsagel PL, Drach J et al. 2009. International Myeloma Working Group molecular classification of multiple myeloma: Spotlight review. *Leukemia* 23:2210–2221.

Fonseca R, Braggio E. 2011. The use of genetic markers and signatures in multiple myeloma risk stratification. *ASCO Educational Book*. pp. 357–361.

Fragioudaki M, Boula A, Tsirakis G et al. 2012. B cell-activating factor: Its clinical significance in multiple myeloma patients. *Ann Hematol* 91:1413–1418.

Frank R, Hargreaves R. 2003. Clinical biomarkers in drug discovery and development. *Nat Rev Drug Discov* 2:566–580.

Fuks F, Burgers WA, Brehm A, Hughes-Davies L, Kouzarides T. 2000. DNA methyltransferase Dnmt1 associates with histone deacetylase activity. *Nat Genet* 24:88–91.

Gonzalez-Paz N, Chng WJ, McClure RF et al. 2007. Tumor suppressor p16 methylation in multiple myeloma: Biological and clinical implications. *Blood* 109:1228–1232.

Greenberg AJ, Vachon CM, Rajkumar SV. 2012. Disparities in the prevalence, pathogenesis and progression of monoclonal gammopathy of undetermined significance and multiple myeloma between blacks and whites. *Leukemia* 26:609–614.

Greipp PR, Lust JA, O'Fallon WM, Katzmann JA, Witzig TE, Kyle RA. 1993. Plasma cell labeling index and beta 2-microglobulin predict survival independent of thymidine kinase and C-reactive protein in multiple myeloma. *Blood* 81:3382–3387.

Greipp PR, San Miguel J, Durie BG et al. 2005. International staging system for multiple myeloma. *J Clin Oncol* 23:3412–3420.

Hari PN, Majhail NS, Zhang MJ et al. 2010. Race and outcomes of autologous hematopoietic cell transplantation for multiple myeloma. *Biol Blood Marrow Transplant* 16:395–402.

He A, Bai J, Huang C et al. 2012. Detection of serum tumor markers in multiple myeloma using the CLINPROT system. *Int J Hematol* 95:668–674.

Heller G, Schmidt WM, Ziegler B et al. 2008. Genome-wide transcriptional response to 5-aza-2'¢-deoxycytidine and trichostatin a in multiple myeloma cells. *Cancer Res* 68:44–54.

Hervé AL, Florence M, Philippe M et al. 2011. Molecular heterogeneity of multiple myeloma: Pathogenesis, prognosis, and therapeutic implications. *J Clin Oncol* 29:1893–1897.

Hock BD, McKenzie JL, Patton NW et al. 2006. Circulating levels and clinical significance of soluble CD40 in patients with hematologic malignancies. *Cancer* 106:2148–2157.

Hose D, Reme T, Hielscher T et al. 2011. Proliferation is a central independent prognostic factor and target for personalized and risk-adapted treatment in multiple myeloma. *Haematologica* 96:87–95.

Hsieh FY, Tengstrand E, Pekol TM, Guerciolini R, Miwa G. 2009. Elucidation of potential bortezomib response markers in multiple myeloma patients. *J Pharm Biomed Anal* 49:115–122.

Huang JJ, Yu J, Li JY, Liu YT, Zhong RQ. 2012. Circulating microRNA expression is associated with genetic subtype and survival of multiple myeloma. *Med Oncol* 29:2402–2408.

Kádár K, Wolf K, Tábori J, Karádi I, Várkonyi J. 2012. The albumin and monoclonal protein ratio as prognostic marker for multiple myeloma in the era of novel agents. *Pathol Oncol Res* 18:557–561.

Katz J, Gong Y, Salmasinia D et al. 2011. Genetic polymorphisms and other risk factors associated with bisphosphonate induced osteonecrosis of the jaw. *Int J Oral Maxillofac Surg* 40:605–611.

Katzmann JA, Clark RJ, Abraham RS et al. 2002. Serum reference intervals and diagnostic ranges for free kappa and free lambda immunoglobulin light chains: Relative sensitivity for detection of monoclonal light chains. *Clin Chem* 48:1437–1444.

Keats JJ, Chesi M, Egan JB et al. 2012. Clonal competition with alternating dominance in multiple myeloma. *Blood* 120:1067–1076.

Kelly T, Miao HQ, Yang Y et al. 2003. High heparanase activity in multiple myeloma is associated with elevated microvessel density. *Cancer Res* 63:8749–8756.

Ketterlinus R, Hsieh SY, Teng SH, Lee H, Pusch W. 2005. Fishing for biomarkers: Analyzing mass spectrometry data with the new ClinProTools software. *Biotechniques* 37–40.

Khamaisi M, Regev E, Yarom N et al. 2007. Possible association between diabetes and bisphosphonate-related jaw osteonecrosis. *J Clin Endocrinol Metab* 92:1172–1175.

Kim SY, Min HJ, Park HK et al. 2011. Increased copy number of the interleukin-6 receptor gene is associated with adverse survival in multiple myeloma patients treated with autologous stem cell transplantation. *Biol Blood Marrow Transplant* 17:810–820.

Klein U, Casola S, Cattoretti G et al. 2006. Transcription factor IRF4 controls plasma cell differentiation and class-switch recombination. *Nat Immunol* 7:773–782.

Korde N, Kristinsson SY, Landgren O. 2011. Monoclonal gammopathy of undetermined significance (MGUS) and smoldering multiple myeloma (SMM): Novel biological insights and development of early treatment strategies. *Blood* 117:5573–5581.

Krause DS, Spitzer TR, Stowell CP. 2010. The concentration of CD44 is increased in hematopoietic stem cell grafts of patients with acute myeloid leukemia, plasma cell myeloma, and non-Hodgkin lymphoma. *Arch Pathol Lab Med* 134:1033–1038.

Kumar L, Cyriac SL, Tejomurtula TV et al. 2012. Autologous stem cell transplantation for multiple myeloma: Identification of prognostic factors. *Clin Lymphoma Myeloma Leuk* 13:32–41.

Kumar S, Rajkumar SV, Greipp PR, Witzig TE. 2004. Cell proliferation of myeloma plasma cells: Comparison of the blood and marrow compartments. *Am J Hematol* 77:7–11.

Kumar SK, Uno H, Jacobus SJ et al. 2011. Impact of gene expression profiling-based risk stratification in patients with myeloma receiving initial therapy with lenalidomide and dexamethasone. *Blood* 118:4359–4362.

Kuiper R, Broyl A, de Knegt Y et al. 2012. A gene expression signature for high-risk multiple myeloma. *Leukemia* 26:2406–2413.

Kyle RA, Durie BG, Rajkumar SV et al. 2010. Monoclonal gammopathy of undetermined significance (MGUS) and smoldering (asymptomatic) multiple myeloma: IMWG consensus perspectives risk factors for progression and guidelines for monitoring and management. *Leukemia* 24:1121–1127.

Jakubowiak AJ, Benson DM, Bensinger W et al. 2012. Phase I trial of anti-CS1 monoclonal antibody elotuzumab in combination with bortezomib in the treatment of relapsed/refractory multiple myeloma. *J Clin Oncol* 30:1960–1965.

Jiang P, Yueguo W, Huiming H, Hongxiang Y, Mei W, Ju S. 2009. B-Lymphocyte stimulator: A new biomarker for multiple myeloma. *Eur J Haematol* 82:267–276.

Jones CI, Zabolotskaya MV, King AJ et al. 2012. Identification of circulating microRNAs as diagnostic biomarkers for use in multiple myeloma. *Br J Cancer* 107:1987–1996.

La Ferla F, Paolicchi E, Crea F et al. 2011. An aromatase polymorphism (g.132810C>T) predicts risk of bisphosphonate-related osteonecrosis of the jaw. *Front Biosci (EliteEd)* 3:364–370.

Landgren O, Kyle RA, Rajkumar SV. 2011. From myeloma precursor disease to multiple myeloma: New diagnostic concepts and opportunities for early intervention. *Clin Cancer Res* 17:1243–1252.

Larsen JT, Chee CE, Lust JA, Greipp PR, Rajkumar SV. 2011. Reduction in plasma cell proliferation after initial therapy in newly diagnosed multiple myeloma measures treatment response and predicts improved survival. *Blood* 118:2702–2707.

Larsen JT, Kumar SK, Dispenzieri A et al. 2012. Serum free light chain ratio as a biomarker for high-risk smoldering multiple myeloma. *Leukemia* 27:941–946.

Lazarovici TS, Yahalom R, Taicher S, Elad S, Hardan I, Yarom N. 2009. Bisphosphonate-related osteonecrosis of the jaws: A single-center study of 101 patients. *J Oral Maxillofac Surg* 67:850–855.

Lendvai N, Gnjatic S, Ritter E et al. 2010. Cellular immune responses against CT7 (MAGE-C1) and humoral responses against other cancer-testis antigens in multiple myeloma patients. *Cancer Immun* 10:4.

Lesko LJ, Atkinson AJ Jr. 2001. Use of biomarkers and surrogate endpoints in drug development and regulatory decision making: Criteria, validation, strategies. *Annu Rev Pharmacol Toxicol* 41:347–366.

Li S, Pal R, Monaghan SA et al. 2011. IMiD immunomodulatory compounds block C/EBP{beta} translation through eIF4E down-regulation resulting in inhibition of MM. *Blood* 117:5157–5165.

Lin C, Luciani A, Belhadj K et al. 2010. Multiple myeloma treatment response assessment with whole body dynamic contrast-enhanced MR imaging. *Radiology* 254:521–531.

Lopez-Girona A, Heintel D, Zhang LH et al. 2011. Lenalidomide downregulates the cell survival factor, interferon regulatory factor-4, providing a potential mechanistic link for predicting response. *Br J Haematol* 154:325–336.

Lopez-Girona A, Mendy D, Ito T et al. 2012. Cereblon is a direct protein target for immunomodulatory and antiproliferative activities of lenalidomide and pomalidomide. *Leukemia* 26:2326–2335.

Mahtouk K, Hose D, Raynaud P et al. 2007. Heparanase influences expression and shedding of syndecan-1, and its expression by the bone marrow environment is a bad prognostic factor in multiple myeloma. *Blood* 109:4914–4923.

Mailankody S, Mena E, Yuan CM, Balakumaran A, Kuehl WM, Landgren O. 2010. Molecular and biologic markers of progression in monoclonal gammopathy of undetermined significance to multiple myeloma. *Leuk Lymphoma* 51:2159–2170.

Marini F, Tonelli P, Cavalli L et al. 2010. Pharmacogenetics of bisphosphonate-associated osteonecrosis of the jaw. *Ther Clin Risk Manag* 6:579–583.

Marx RE. 2003. Pamidronate (Aredia) and zoledronate (Zometa) induced avascular necrosis of the jaws: A growing epidemic. *J Oral Maxillofac Surg* 61:1115–1117.

Marx RE, Cillo JE Jr, Ulloa JJ. 2007. Oral bisphosphonate-induced osteonecrosis: Risk factors, prediction of risk using serum CTX testing, prevention, and treatment. *J Oral Maxillofac Surg* 65:2397–2394.

Mateo G, Montalbán MA, Vidriales MB et al. 2008. Prognostic value of immunophenotyping in multiple myeloma: A study by the PETHEMA/GEM cooperative study groups on patients uniformly treated with high-dose therapy. *J Clin Oncol* 26:2737–2744.

McCarthy PL, Owzar K, Hofmeister CC et al. 2012. Lenalidomide after stem-cell transplantation for multiple myeloma. *N Engl J Med* 366:1770–1781.

Meissner T, Seckinger A, Rème T et al. 2011. Gene expression profiling in multiple myeloma—Reporting of entities, risk, and targets in clinical routine. *Clin Cancer Res* 17:7240–7247.

Mena E, Choyke P, Tan E, Landgren O, Kurdziel K. 2011. Molecular imaging in myeloma precursor disease. *Semin Hematol* 48:22–31.

Mimura N, Fulciniti M, Gorgun G et al. 2012. Blockade of XBP1 splicing by inhibition of IRE1α is a promising therapeutic option in multiple myeloma. *Blood* 119:5772–5781.

Mitsiades CS, Mitsiades NS, McMullan CJ et al. 2004. Inhibition of the insulin-like growth factor receptor-1 tyrosine kinase activity as a therapeutic strategy for multiple myeloma, other hematologic malignancies, and solid tumors. *Cancer Cell* 5:221–230.

Moreaux J, Rème T, Leonard W et al. 2012. Development of gene expression-based score to predict sensitivity of multiple myeloma cells to DNA methylation inhibitors. *Mol Cancer Ther* 11:2685–2692.

Morgan GJ, Kaiser MF. 2012. How to use new biology to guide therapy in multiple myeloma. *Hematol Am Soc Hematol Educ Program* 2012:342–349.

Morris PG, Fazio M, Farooki A et al. 2012. Serum N-telopeptide and bone-specific alkaline phosphatase levels in patients with osteonecrosis of the jaw receiving bisphosphonates for bone metastases. *J Oral Maxillofac Surg* 70:2768–2775.

Mulligan G, Mitsiades C, Bryant B et al. 2007. Gene expression profiling and correlation with outcome in clinical trials of the proteasome inhibitor bortezomib. *Blood* 109:3177–3188.

Nair JR, Carlson LM, Koorella C et al. 2011. CD28 expressed on malignant plasma cells induces a prosurvival and immunosuppressive microenvironment. *J Immunol* 187:1243–1253.

Ng MH, Chung YF, Lo KW, Wickham NW, Lee JC, Huang DP. 1997. Frequent hypermethylation of p16 and p15 genes in multiple myeloma. *Blood* 89:2500–2506.

Nojima M, Maruyama R, Yasui H et al. 2009. Genomic screening for genes silenced by DNA methylation revealed an association between RASD1 inactivation and dexamethasone resistance in multiple myeloma. *Clin Cancer Res* 15:4356–4364.

Ocio EM, Mateos MV, Maiso P, Pandiella A, San-Miguel JF. 2008. New drugs in multiple myeloma: Mechanisms of action and phase I/II clinical findings. *Lancet Oncol* 9:1157–1165.

Pappa CA, Tsirakis G, Kanellou P et al. 2011. Monitoring serum levels ELR + CXC chemokines and the relationship between microvessel density and angiogenic growth factors in multiple myeloma. *Cytokine* 56:616–620.

Patel M, Wadee A, Galpin J et al. 2002. HLA class I and class II antigens associated with multiple myeloma in southern Africa. *Clin Lab Haematol* 24:215–219.

Perez-Persona E, Vidriales MB, Mateo G et al. 2007. New criteria to identify risk of progression in monoclonal gammopathy of uncertain significance and smoldering multiple myeloma based on multiparameter flow cytometry analysis of bone marrow plasma cells. *Blood* 110:2586–2592.

Pichiorri F, Suh SS, Ladetto M et al. 2008. MicroRNAs regulate critical genes associated with multiple myeloma pathogenesis. *Proc Natl Acad Sci USA* 105:12885–12890.

Podar K, Anderson KC. 2007. Inhibition of VEGF signaling pathways in multiple myeloma and other malignancies. *Cell Cycle* 6:538–542.

Pottern L, Gart J, Nam J et al. 1992. HLA and multiple myeloma among black and white men: Evidence of a genetic association. *Caner Epidemiol Biomarkers Prev* 1:177–182.

Purushothaman A, Hurst DR, Pisano C, Mizumoto S, Sugahara K, Sanderson RD. 2011. Heparanase-mediated loss of nuclear syndecan-1 enhances histone acetyltransferase (HAT) activity to promote expression of genes that drive an aggressive tumor phenotype. *J Biol Chem* 286:30377–30383.

Rajkumar SV, Kyle RA, Therneau TM et al. 2005. Serum free light chain ratio is an independent risk factor for progression in monoclonal gammopathy of undetermined significance. *Blood* 106:812–817.

Rajpal R, Dowling P, Meiller J et al. 2011. A novel panel of protein biomarkers for predicting response to thalidomide-based therapy in newly diagnosed multiple myeloma patients. *Proteomics* 11:1391–1402.

Raschle J, Ratschiller D, Mans S, Mueller BU, Pabst T. 2011. High levels of circulating CD34 + cells at autologous stem cell collection are associated with favourable prognosis in multiple myeloma. *Br J Cancer* 105:970–974.

Ri M, Tashiro E, Oikawa D et al. 2012. Identification of Toyocamycin, an agent cytotoxic for multiple myeloma cells, as a potent inhibitor of ER stress-induced XBP1 mRNA splicing. *Blood Cancer J* 2:e79.

Richardson PG, Lonial S, Jakubowiak AJ, Harousseau JL, Anderson KC. 2011. Monoclonal antibodies in the treatment of multiple myeloma. *Br J Haematol* (July 21) 154:745–754.

Richardson PG, Sonneveld P, Schuster MW et al. 2005. Bortezomib or high-dose dexamethasone for relapsed multiple myeloma. *N Engl J Med* 352:2487–2498.

Robillard N, Jego G, Pellat-Deceunynck C et al. 1998. CD28, a marker associated with tumoral expansion in multiple myeloma. *Clin Cancer Res* 4:1521–1526.

Rolan P, Atkinson AJ Jr, Lesko LJ, Scientific Organizing Committee, Conference Report Committee. 2003. Use of biomarkers from drug discovery through clinical practice: Report of the Ninth European Federation of Pharmaceutical Sciences Conference on Optimizing Drug Development. *Clin Pharmacol Ther* 73:284–291.

Ruggiero SL, Dodson TB, Assael LA, Landesberg R, Marx RE, Mehrotra B. 2009. American Association of Oral and Maxillofacial Surgeons position paper on bisphosphonate-related osteonecrosis of the jaws—2009 update. *J Oral Maxillofac Surg* 67(Suppl 5):2–12.

Samaras P, Blickenstorfer M, Haile SR et al. 2011. Validation of prognostic factors and survival of patients with multiple myeloma in a real-life autologous stem cell transplantation setting: A Swiss single centre experience. *Swiss Med Wkly* 141:w13203.

Sarasquete ME, García-Sanz R, Marín L et al. 2008. Bisphosphonate-related osteonecrosis of the jaw is associated with polymorphisms of the cytochrome P450 CYP2C8 in multiple myeloma: A genome-wide single nucleotide polymorphism analysis. *Blood* 112:2709–2712.

Sarasquete ME, Gutiérrez NC, Misiewicz-Krzeminska I et al. 2011. Upregulation of Dicer is more frequent in monoclonal gammopathies of undetermined significance than in multiple myeloma patients and is associated with longer survival in symptomatic myeloma patients. *Haematologica* 96:468–471.

Satoh M, Oguro R, Yamanaka C et al. 2011. Clinical assessment of bortezomib for multiple myeloma in comparison with thalidomide. *J Pharm Pharm Sci* 14:78–89.

Sawyer JR. 2011. The prognostic significance of cytogenetics and molecular profiling in multiple myeloma. *Cancer Genet* 204:3–12.

Schambeck CM, Wick M, Bartl R, Lamerz R, Fateh-Moghadam A. 1995. Plasma cell proliferation in monoclonal gammopathies: Measurement using BU-1 antibody in flow cytometry and microscopy: Comparison with serum thymidine kinase. *J Clin Pathol* 48:477–481.

Schmidt-Hieber M, Pérez-Andrés M, Paiva B et al. 2011. CD117 expression in gammopathies is associated with an altered maturation of the myeloid and lymphoid hematopoietic cell compartments and favorable disease features. *Haematologica* 96:328–332.

Sciammas R, Shaffer AL, Schatz JH, Zhao H, Staudt LM, Singh H. 2006. Graded expression of interferon regulatory factor-4 coordinates isotype switching with plasma cell differentiation. *Immunity* 25:225–236.

Sezer O, Niemöller K, Eucker J et al. 2000. Bone marrow microvessel density is a prognostic factor for survival in patients with multiple myeloma. *Ann Hematol* 79:574–577.

Sfiridaki A, Miyakis S, Pappa C et al. 2011. Circulating osteopontin: A dual marker of bone destruction and angiogenesis in patients with multiple myeloma. *J Hematol Oncol* 4:22.

Shaffer AL, Emre NC, Lamy L et al. 2007. IRF4 addiction in multiple myeloma. *Nature* 454:226–231.

Shaughnessy JD Jr, Qu P, Usmani S et al. 2011. Pharmacogenomics of bortezomib test-dosing identifies hyperexpression of proteasome genes, especially PSMD4, as novel high-risk feature in myeloma treated with Total Therapy 3. *Blood* 118:3512–3524.

Shaughnessy JD, Zhan F, Burington BE et al. 2007. A validated gene expression model of high-risk multiple myeloma is defined by deregulated expression of genes mapping to chromosome 1. *Blood* 109:2276–2284.

Smith EM, Boyd K, Davies FE. 2010. The potential role of epigenetic therapy in multiple myeloma. *Br J Haematol* 148:702–713.

Steensma DP, Gertz MA, Greipp PR et al. 2001. A high bone marrow plasma cell labeling index in stable plateau-phase multiple myeloma is a marker for early disease progression and death. *Blood* 97:2522–2523.

Tai YT, Dillon M, Song W et al. 2008. Anti-CS1 humanized monoclonal antibody HuLuc63 inhibits myeloma cell adhesion and induces antibody-dependent cellular cytotoxicity in the bone marrow milieu. *Blood* 112:1329–1337.

Tan E, Weiss BM, Mena E, Korde N, Choyke PL, Landgren O. 2011. Current and future imaging modalities for multiple myeloma and its precursor states. *Leuk Lymphoma* 52:1630–1640.

Tennis P, Rothman KJ, Bohn RL et al. 2012. Incidence of osteonecrosis of the jaw among users of bisphosphonates with selected cancers or osteoporosis. *Pharmacoepidemiol Drug Saf* 21:810–817.

Terpos E, Christoulas D, Katodritou E et al. 2012. Elevated circulating sclerostin correlates with advanced disease features and abnormal bone remodeling in symptomatic myeloma: Reduction post-bortezomib monotherapy. *Int J Cancer* 131:1466–1471.

Terpos E, de la Fuente J, Szydlo R et al. 2003. Tartrate-resistant acid phosphatase isoform 5b: A novel serum marker for monitoring bone disease in multiple myeloma. *Int J Cancer* 106:455–457.

Terpos E, Dimopoulos MA, Shrivastava V et al. 2010. High levels of serum TIMP-1 correlate with advanced disease and predict for poor survival in patients with multiple myeloma treated with novel agents. *Leuk Res* 34:399–402.

Tsirakis G, Pappa CA, Kaparou M et al. 2011. Assessment of proliferating cell nuclear antigen and its relationship with proinflammatory cytokines and parameters of disease activity in multiple myeloma patients. *Eur J Histochem* 55:e21.

Tsirakis G, Pappa CA, Psarakis FE et al. 2012. Serum concentrations and clinical significance of soluble CD40 ligand in patients with multiple myeloma. *Med Oncol* 29:2396–2401.

Ullmannova-Benson V, Guan M, Zhou X et al. 2009. DLC1 tumor suppressor gene inhibits migration and invasion of multiple myeloma cells through RhoA GTPase pathway. *Leukemia* 23:383–390.

Uttamsingh V, Lu C, Miwa G, Gan LS. 2005. Relative contributions of the five major human cytochromes P450, 1A2, 2C9, 2C19, 2D6, and 3A4, to the hepatic metabolism of the proteasome inhibitor bortezomib. *Drug Metab Dispos* 33:1723–1728.

Vallet S, Pozzi S, Patel K et al. 2011. A novel role for CCL3 (MIP-1α) in myeloma-induced bone disease via osteocalcin downregulation and inhibition of osteoblast function. *Leukemia* 25:1174–1181.

van Rhee F, Szmania SM, Dillon M et al. 2009. Combinatorial efficacy of anti-CS1 monoclonal antibody elotuzumab (HuLuc63) and bortezomib against multiple myeloma. *Mol Cancer Ther* 8:2616–2624.

van Rhee F, Szymonifka J, Anaissie E et al. 2010. Total Therapy 3 for multiple myeloma: Prognostic implications of cumulative dosing and premature discontinuation of VTD maintenance components, bortezomib, thalidomide, and dexamethasone, relevant to all phases of therapy. *Blood* 116:1220–1227.

Vangsted AJ, Klausen TW, Abildgaard N et al. 2011. Single nucleotide polymorphisms in the promoter region of the IL1B gene influence outcome in multiple myeloma patients treated with high-dose chemotherapy independently of relapse treatment with thalidomide and bortezomib. *Ann Hematol* 90:1173–1181.

Vincenzi B, Napolitano A, Zoccoli A et al. 2012. Serum VEGF levels as predictive marker of bisphosphonate-related osteonecrosis of the jaw. *Biomark Med* 6:201–209.

Wader KF, Fagerli UM, Holt RU, Børset M, Sundan A, Waage A. 2011. Soluble c-met in serum of patients with multiple myeloma: Correlation with clinical parameters. *Eur J Haematol* 87:394–399.

Wall JS, Kennel SJ, Stuckey AC et al. 2010. Radioimmunodetection of amyloid deposits in patients with AL amyloidosis. *Blood* 116:2241–2244.

Waxman AJ, Mink PJ, Devesa SS et al. 2010. Racial disparities in incidence and outcome in multiple myeloma: A population-based study. *Blood* 116:5501–5506.

Weiss BM, Minter A, Abadie J et al. 2011. Patterns of monoclonal immunoglobulins and serum free light chains are significantly different in black compared to white monoclonal gammopathy of undetermined significance (MGUS) patients. *Am J Hematol* 86:475–478.

Xu G, Liu K, Anderson J et al. 2012. Expression of XBP1s in bone marrow stromal cells is critical for myeloma cell growth and osteoclast formation. *Blood* 119:4205–4214.

Yuregir OO, Yurtcu E, Kizilkilic E, Kocer NE, Ozdogu H, Sahin FI. 2010. Detecting methylation patterns of p16, MGMT, DAPK and E-cadherin genes in multiple myeloma patients. *Int J Lab Hematol* 32:142–149.

Zain J. 2012. Role of histone deacetylase inhibitors in the treatment of lymphomas and multiple myeloma. *Hematol Oncol Clin North Am* 26:671–704.

Zangari M, Esseltine D, Cavallo F et al. 2007. Predictive value of alkaline phosphatase for response and time to progression in bortezomib-treated multiple myeloma patients. *Am J Hematol* 82:831–833.

Zhan F, Colla S, Wu X et al. 2007. CKS1B, overexpressed in aggressive disease, regulates multiple myeloma growth and survival through SKP2- and p27Kip1-dependent and -independent mechanisms. *Blood* 109:4995–5001.

Zhan F, Huang Y, Colla S et al. 2006. The molecular classification of multiple myeloma. *Blood* 108:2020–2028.

Zhang B, Pan X, Cobb GP, Anderson TA. 2007. Micro-RNAs as oncogenes and tumor suppressors. *Dev Biol* 302:1–12.

Zhu YX, Braggio E, Shi CX et al. 2011. Cereblon expression is required for the antimyeloma activity of lenalidomide and pomalidomide. *Blood* 118:4771–4779.

Zonder JA, Mohrbacher AF, Singhal S et al. 2012. A phase 1, multicenter, open-label, dose escalation study of elotuzumab in patients with advanced multiple myeloma. *Blood* 120:552–559.

Part VIII

Melanoma

32

Diagnostic and Prognostic Biomarkers in Cutaneous Melanoma

Eijun Itakura and Alistair J. Cochran

CONTENTS

ABSTRACT Biomarkers of cutaneous malignant melanoma now guide certain aspects of clinical practice and have a great potential for early detection of cancer. This chapter will review biomarkers that have a role in the clinical management of malignant melanoma. Pathological parameters such as tumor thickness, ulceration, and mitosis are important factors for staging of melanoma. Elevated serum LDH is correlated with poorer prognosis and is now introduced into the AJCC staging system.

S100B is also a useful prognostic biomarker. Molecular diagnostics of melanoma has become widely accepted to detect metastatic melanoma cells. mRNA for melanoma-associated genes such as MART-1 (*MELANA*) are utilized to detect metastatic melanoma cells in serum and sentinel nodes. The benefits and pitfalls of molecular diagnostics will be discussed. We will also discuss other prognostic biomarkers as well as immunological biomarkers indicating the tumor-induced immunosuppression.

Abbreviations

5-S-CD	5-*S*-cysteinyldopa
6H5M12C	6-hydroxy-5-methoxyindole-2-carboxylic acid
AJCC	American Joint Committee on Cancer
CRP	C-reactive protein
FDA	United States Food and Drug Administration
GalNAc-T	β-1,4 *N*-acetylgalactosaminyltransferase 1
gp100	glycoprotein 100
IC	immune complexes
ICAM-1	intercellular adhesion molecule 1
IL	interleukin
LDH	lactate dehydrogenase
MAGE	melanoma-associated antigen
MALDI-TOF	matrix-assisted laser desorption/ionization time-of-flight mass spectrometry
MART-1	melanoma antigen recognized by T-cells 1
MIA	melanoma-inhibitory activity
mRNA	messenger RNA
miRNA	microRNA
PAX3	paired box 3
qRT–PCR	quantitative reverse transcription–polymerase chain reaction
RT–PCR	reverse transcription–polymerase chain reaction
SAA	serum amyloid A
TA90	tumor-associated antigen 90
TRP	tyrosinase-related protein
VCAM-1	vascular cell adhesion molecule 1

32.1 Introduction

Cutaneous malignant melanoma has a high potential for metastases and accounts for more than 8000 deaths per year in the United States [1]. The incidence of melanoma has also increased over the past decades [2]. The principle treatment of primary melanoma remains surgical wide excision. Sentinel lymph node biopsy [3] has been recently developed and becomes widely used in the management of melanoma patients. The histological status of the sentinel lymph node is the main predictor of prognosis and survival in melanoma patients [4]. In the clinical management of cutaneous melanoma, it is critical to determine which patients are cured by surgery alone and which should be treated with adjuvant therapy. To assist in this decision, biomarkers are needed that would help to refine the risk of progression and assess the outcome.

Biomarkers in cutaneous melanoma now guide certain aspects of clinical practice and have a great potential for early detection of cancer [5–7]. These biomarkers offer the possibility of improved tumor staging through the molecular detection of circulating tumor cells and micrometastases to sentinel lymph nodes that are not visible on routine histological examination [8,9]. Here, we present an overview of the advances in biomarkers with diagnostic, prognostic, and therapeutic implications in cutaneous melanoma.

32.2 Clinical and Pathological Parameters in Melanoma

32.2.1 TNM Staging System and Biomarkers

A biomarker is defined as any characteristic that can be objectively measured and evaluated as a diagnostic indicator of pathogenic process to detect the presence of disease or to assess severity of disease. In this term, cancer staging and pathological parameters such as tumor thickness and ulceration can be in some way regarded as biomarkers. The principal factors determining surgical strategy in melanoma treatment or predicting prognosis include tumor thickness (Breslow thickness) and ulceration. In its most recent version, the American Joint Committee on Cancer (AJCC) staging system for cutaneous melanoma considers sentinel lymph node biopsy results along with primary tumor thickness, mitosis, and the presence or absence of ulceration of the primary tumor. In addition to these pathological parameters, elevated serum lactate dehydrogenase (LDH) is introduced into the AJCC staging system (Tables 32.1 and 32.2) [10,11].

TABLE 32.1

TNM Classification for Cutaneous Melanoma (AJCC)

Tis		**Melanoma In Situ**	
Primary Tumor (T)			
T1		≤1.0 mm in thickness	
	T1a		Without ulceration and mitosis <1/mm^2
	T1b		With ulceration or mitoses ≥1/mm^2
T2		1.01–2.0 mm	
	T2a		
	T2b		
T3		2.01–4.0 mm	
	T3a		Without ulceration
	T3b		With ulceration
T4		>4.0 mm	
	T4a		Without ulceration
	T4b		With ulceration
Regional lymph nodes (N)			
N0		No regional lymph node metastasis	
N1		1 node	
	N1a		Micrometastasis[a]
	N1b		Macrometastasis[b]
N2		2–3 nodes	
	N2a		Micrometastasis[a]
	N2b		Macrometastasis[b]
	N2c		In transit metastases/satellites without metastatic nodes
N3		4 or more metastatic nodes, or matted nodes, or in transit met(s)/satellite(s) with metastatic nodes	
Distant metastasis (M)			
M0		No distant metastasis	
M1		Distant metastasis	
	M1a		Metastases to skin, subcutaneous tissues, or distant lymph nodes
	M1b		Metastases to lung
	M1c		Metastases to all other visceral sites or distant metastases to any site combined with an elevated serum LDH

[a] Micrometastases are diagnosed after sentinel lymph node biopsy and completion lymphadenectomy (if performed).
[b] Macrometastases are defined as clinically detectable nodal metastases confirmed by therapeutic lymphadenectomy or when nodal metastasis exhibits gross extracapsular extension.

TABLE 32.2

Cutaneous Melanoma Staging (AJCC)

Stage	T	N	M
0	Tis	N0	M0
IA	T1a	N0	M0
IB	T1b	N0	M0
	T2a	N0	M0
IIA	T2b	N0	M0
	T3a	N0	M0
IIB	T3b	N0	M0
	T4a	N0	M0
IIC	T4b	N0	M0
IIIA	T1-4a	N1a	M0
	T1-4a	N2a	M0
IIIB	T1-4b	N1a	M0
	T1-4b	N2a	M0
	T1-4a	N1b	M0
	T1-4a	N2b	M0
	T1-4a	N2c	M0
IIIC	T1-4b	N1b	M0
	T1-4b	N2b	M0
	T1-4b	N2c	M0
	Any T	N3	M0
IV	Any T	Any N	M1

The T staging of melanoma is mostly based on tumor thickness (Breslow thickness). Breslow thickness is the micrometer-measured thickness of invasive primary melanoma. It is measured from the granular layer of the epidermis to the deepest portion of the tumor [12]. For each T classification, there is a subclassification based on the absence or presence of ulceration. The survival rates of patients with an ulcerated melanoma are proportionately lower than those of patients with a nonulcerated melanoma of equivalent T category. The 10-year survival was 92% in T1 melanomas (≤1.0 mm in thickness), while it was 80% in melanomas (1.01–2.0 mm in thickness), 63% in T3 melanomas (2.01–4.0 mm in thickness), and 50% in T4 melanomas (>4.0 mm in thickness) [13]. Mitotic index, a number of mitoses in a square millimeter, should be taken into consideration when subclassifying T1 melanomas. The recent analysis of the AJCC melanoma staging database demonstrated a significant inverse correlation between primary tumor mitotic rate and survival. The 10-year survival ranged from 93% for patients whose tumors had 0 mitosis/mm^2 to 48% for those with ≥20/mm^2 [14]. Ulceration is also correlated with a higher mitotic rate [14,15].

Tumor thickness is one of the most important factors in determining surgical strategy in the treatment of melanoma. Additional resection and sentinel lymph node biopsy should be taken into consideration if melanoma is greater than 1.0 mm in thickness. Advances in ultrasound technology allow more accurate noninvasive assessment of the characteristics of primary melanoma, such as tumor thickness and blood flow [16]. Recent studies showed that sonographic measurements of tumor thickness were well correlated with Breslow thickness [17–19]. A more commonly available 10 MHz scanner was capable of differentiating between melanomas ≤1 mm in thickness and those >1 mm in thickness with good accuracy [19].

The N staging describes degree of spread to regional lymph nodes. Metastasis to one regional lymph node is classified into N1. Metastasis to two to three regional lymph nodes are classified into N2. For N1 and N2 subclassification, micrometastases are metastatic lymph nodes that are diagnosed after sentinel node biopsy, and macrometastases are metastatic lymph nodes that are clinically detectable and confirmed by therapeutic lymphadenectomy or nodal metastases exhibiting gross extracapsular extension. In-transit metastasis or satellite with metastatic lymph node, or 4 or more metastatic lymph nodes are classified into N3 (Table 32.1) [11]. The 5-year survival rates were 78%, 59%, and 40% for stage IIIA

(T1–T4a N1a or T1–T4a N2a), IIIB (T1–T4b N1a, T1–T4b N2a, T1–T4a N1b, T1–T4a N2b, or T1–T4a N2c), and IIIC (T1–T4b N1b, T1–T4b N2b, T1–T4b Nc, T1–T4a N3, or any T N3) melanomas, respectively [13]. Morphometric parameters based on the tumor extent in the sentinel lymph node have been suggested to predict recurrent disease and prognosis [20–24]. The invasion depth and diameter of sentinel lymph node metastasis best predict metastases to nonsentinel lymph nodes [24].

There are attempts to identify lymph node metastasis in clinically node-negative melanoma using preoperative ultrasound [25–28]. However, routine preoperative ultrasound in clinically node-negative melanoma is still not practical at this time. It requires continuous effort to refine the technique and criteria involved in the detection of lymph node metastasis of melanoma by preoperative ultrasound.

The M staging describes distant metastasis. Metastases to skin, subcutaneous tissues, or distant lymph nodes are classified into M1a. Metastases to lung are classified into M1b, and metastases to all other visceral sites or distant metastases to any site combined with elevated serum LDH are classified into M1c (Table 32.1) [11]. LDH has consistently found to be the most predictive factor for a poor outcome in stage IV melanoma [13,29]. The 1-year survival rates were 62% for M1a, 53% for M1b, and 33% for M1c melanomas [13].

32.2.2 Other Pathological Parameters

Clark level describes the level of anatomical invasion of melanoma in the skin. Melanoma confined to the epidermis (melanoma in situ) is classified into level I. Invasion into the papillary dermis is classified into level II. Clark level III is defined as spreading through the papillary dermis but not into the reticular dermis. Invasion into the reticular dermis is classified into level IV. Invasion into the subcutaneous adipose tissue is classified into level V [30]. Clark level is a related staging system similar to Breslow thickness. Perhaps, Clark level is a characteristic that is not objectively measured and evaluated. The measurement and evaluation of Clark level may vary among pathologists because of the difficulty in accurately measuring stromal invasion. Determining whether melanoma invasion is Clark level III or IV is often difficult. In this term, Breslow thickness is more reliable, because tumor thickness can be most accurately measured. Breslow thickness is also correlated more closely with prognosis than Clark level [14]. The seventh edition of the AJCC Staging Manual replaces the Clark level of invasion.

Ki-67 is widely used as a proliferation marker in immunohistochemistry. Ki-67 protein is present during active phases of the cell cycle (G1, G2, and mitosis). Ki-67 labeling index is a fraction of Ki-67-positive tumor cells and is often used for evaluation of cell proliferation. Ki-67 immunoreactivity in primary melanoma is correlated to increasing tumor thickness [31–33] and metastatic activity [32]. In lymph node metastases, high Ki-67 expression is correlated with multiple lymph node involvement [33]. A systematic review of tissue biomarkers in melanoma reported that elevated Ki-67 is correlated with increased risk of both all-cause mortality and melanoma-specific mortality [34].

32.3 Blood and Serum Biomarkers for Melanoma

32.3.1 Detection of Circulating Tumor Cells

The ability to measure circulating tumor cells represents a potentially powerful tool for monitoring patients with melanoma. Many studies have demonstrated the diagnostic and prognostic value of circulating tumor cells in melanoma [35–47]. The currently Food and Drug Administration (FDA)-approved laboratory test for circulating tumor cells is CellSearch® circulating tumor cell test (Veridex) to detect metastatic breast cancer, colorectal cancer, or prostate cancer, but not melanoma. Most experimental studies to detect circulating cells have been conducted using reverse transcription–polymerase chain reaction (RT–PCR) or quantitative RT–PCR (qRT–PCR) for mRNA for various melanoma-associated genes. Important antigens include melanin synthesis enzymes (tyrosinase, tyrosinase-related protein-1 [TRP-1], TRP-2/dopachrome tautomerase [DCT]), the melanocyte lineage/differentiation antigens (MART-1/Melan-A, gp100/Pmel17), and cancer/testis antigens (MAGE family) (Table 32.3). Due to heterogeneous expression in advanced melanomas, single-biomarker assays are often limited. The careful selection of biomarkers and multiple biomarkers assays are necessary to increase the sensitivity of circulating tumor cell detection and reduce

TABLE 32.3

Biomarkers Used for the Detection of Melanoma Cells in Sentinel Lymph Nodes and Blood Using RT–PCR/qRT–PCR

Biomarker	Abbreviation	Gene	Characteristics
Tyrosinase		*TYR*	A rate-limiting enzyme in melanin synthesis
Tyrosinase-related protein-1	TRP-1	*TYRP1*	A melanosomal enzyme for melanin synthesis
Tyrosinase-related protein-2/dopachrome tautomerase	TRP-2/DCT	*DCT*	A melanosomal enzyme for melanin synthesis
Microphthalmia-associated transcription factor	MITF	*MITF*	A transcription factor regulating gene expression of tyrosinase, TRP-1, TRP-2, and MART-1
Melanoma antigen recognized by T-cells 1/Melan-A	MART-1	*MLANA*	A cell-surface antigen specific for the melanocyte lineage
Glycoprotein 100/melanocyte protein Pmel17	gp100/Pmel17	*PMEL*	A melanocyte lineage-specific cell-surface glycoprotein
Melanoma-associated antigen 3	MAGE-A3	*MAGEA3*	A cancer–testis antigen
High molecular weight–melanoma-associated antigen/melanoma-associated chondroitin sulfate proteoglycan/chondroitin sulfate proteoglycan 4	HMW–MAA/MCSP/CSPG4	*CSPG4*	An integral membrane chondroitin sulfate proteoglycan expressed by melanoma cells
Melanotransferrin/p97/CD228		*MFI2*	A cell-surface glycoprotein on melanoma cells. A member of the transferrin superfamily
MUC18/melanoma cell adhesion molecule/CD146	MCAM	*MCAM*	A cell adhesion molecule
β-1,4 *N*-acetylgalactosaminyltransferase 1	GalNAc-T	*B4GALNT1*	An enzyme in the synthesis of GM2 and GD2 glycosphingolipids
Paired box 3	PAX3	*PAX3*	A member of the paired box (PAX) family of transcription factors

false-negative results. The utility of the multiple biomarker assay in monitoring adjuvant therapy for stage III melanomas was demonstrated using MART-1, MAGE-A3, GalNAc-T, and PAX3 [45].

32.3.2 Diagnostic and Prognostic Biomarkers (Table 32.4)

32.3.2.1 LDH

Elevated serum LDH is one of the strongest prognostic factors in metastatic melanoma [5,6]. LDH is involved in the conversion of pyruvate and lactate. An elevated serum level is thought to be due to spillage of LDH from melanoma cells. LDH is in the whole body, and almost every type of cancer as well as many other diseases can elevate serum LDH levels. Thus, there is the potential for false-positive results secondary to factors that may not be related to melanoma metastases. To avoid such false-positive results, the use of an elevated serum LDH should be used only when there are two or more determinations obtained more than 24 h apart [10]. There is a nonspecific pattern of elevation among the various LDH isoenzymes. Elevated serum LDH correlates with poor prognosis in patients with advanced melanoma [10,29,48,49]. As mentioned earlier, elevated serum LDH is introduced into the AJCC staging system. Distant metastases to any site combined with elevated serum LDH are classified into M1c [10,11]. The 1- and 2-year survival rates for stage IV melanomas with a normal serum LDH were 65% and 40%, respectively, while those were 32% and 18%, respectively, for stage IV melanomas with an elevated serum LDH [13]. Serum LDH may also be useful to monitor post-surgery adjuvant therapy [50,51]. In a randomized study of dacarbazine with or without oblimersen, elevated LDH levels were correlated with poorer prognosis, and LDH was highly predictive of oblimersen effect [52].

TABLE 32.4

Serological Biomarkers for Cutaneous Melanoma

LDH
S100B
MIA
TA90
5-S-CD
CRP
Soluble IL-2R
IL-10
Soluble ICAM-1
Soluble VCAM-1

32.3.2.2 S100B

S100 protein is a family of low molecular weight calcium-binding protein. S100 protein mostly exists as dimmers within cells. S100 protein has been widely used as an immunohistochemical marker of pigmented skin lesions including melanoma. S100B is a protein of the S100 protein family. The gene of S100B (*S100B*) is localized at 21q22.3 [53,54], while other S100 genes are located on chromosome 1. S100B is most abundant in glial cells of the central and peripheral nervous system and is also well expressed in melanocytes and melanoma cells. S100B functions in proliferation of melanoma cells. S100B is regarded to be useful in many aspects of the clinical management of melanoma [55]. Serum levels of S100B are increased in many melanomas. This protein has been shown to be of use in staging melanoma, in establishing prognosis, in evaluating treatment success and in predicting relapse [55]. Several reports have indicated that increased serum S100B levels correlate with more aggressive disease and reduced survival [56–64], indicating a role for its use as a prognostic marker [6]. A recent meta-analysis of 22 studies involving a total of 3393 melanomas has concluded that serum S100B levels are a clinically valuable independent prognostic indicator, with particular regard to stage I–III melanoma [65].

Serum S100B levels can also be useful for monitoring treatment in melanoma. Unsuccessful treatment can be detected early if there is a marked rise in serum S100B level [55,66,67]. Lower serum S100B levels at baseline and during follow-up are correlated with longer survival. A changing S100B from low at baseline to high on follow-up are correlated with poorer prognosis [67]. Serum S100B may be more suitable for prediction and monitoring of response to chemotherapy and immunotherapy for metastatic melanoma, because the recent study revealed that S100B assessment was superior to LDH in the identification of early distant metastasis [51].

32.3.2.3 MIA

Melanoma Inhibitory Activity (MIA) is an 11 kDa, soluble protein, which is secreted by melanoma cells [68,69]. The name of the protein is very confusing. In fact, overexpression of MIA is correlated with increased invasiveness, extravasation, and metastasis [70]. Serum MIA levels are increased in many advanced melanomas [71–74]. Particularly, elevated serum MIA levels are correlated with metastases to visceral organs and poorer prognosis [74]. However, in a subsequent study that evaluated the combination of S100B, MIA, and LDH, MIA had lower sensitivity compared with S100B and lower specificity compared with both S100B and LDH [75]. It is also noted that MIA may not be specific to melanoma. MIA mRNA can be detected in other neoplastic and normal cells. Low levels of serum MIA mRNA is also detectable in patients with other than melanoma and healthy subjects [76].

32.3.2.4 TA90

Tumor-associated antigen 90 (TA90) is a 90 kDa glycoprotein tumor-associated complex. Serum TA90 immune complexes (TA90-IC) is detected in stage I–III melanomas, and positivity for TA90-IC is correlated with recurrence and poorer prognosis [77]. Positive TA90-IC is also correlated with poorer

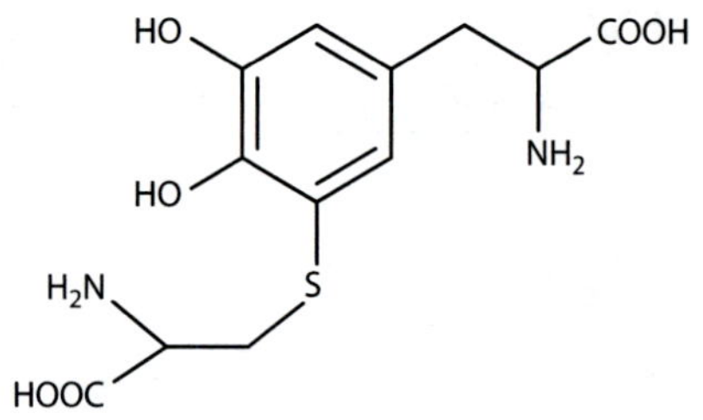

FIGURE 32.1 The chemical formula of 5-S-CD. Elevation of serum and urine levels of 5-S-CD, a metabolite in melanin synthesis, is correlated with advanced melanomas.

prognosis after surgery and adjuvant immunotherapy in stage IV melanomas [78]. In a subsequent study, TA90-IC was compared with MIA and S100B in stage III melanomas undergoing adjuvant vaccine immunotherapy. TA90-IC was the earliest elevated marker in 57% of recurrences. Multivariate regression analysis revealed that TA90-IC was an independent predictor of survival when elevation occurred between 2 weeks and 3 months [79].

32.3.2.5 5-S-CD

5-*S*-cysteinyldopa (5-S-CD) is a metabolite in melanin synthesis. 5-S-CD is formed by binding of cysteine and dopaquinone, which is a highly reactive molecule and is converted from tyrosine by catalysis of tyrosinase enzyme (Figure 32.1). Oxidation of cysteinyldopa leads to the production of pheomelanin (red/yellow melanin). Some 5-S-CD leaks into circulation and is eventually excreted in the urine [80]. Elevated levels of serum 5-S-CD are correlated with advanced melanomas [63,81–85]. The specificity of elevated serum 5-S-CD levels in detecting distant metastasis is very high [85]. 5-S-CD levels tend to remain low when metastases are amelanotic [82,85]. Elevation of serum 5-S-CD often precedes clinical detection of visceral metastases, and the serum level of 5-S-CD may be useful in following up patients with high-risk melanoma [85].

32.3.2.6 CRP

C-reactive protein (CRP) is a protein produced by hepatocytes in acute inflammation. It is released in response to infection, injury, or other inflammatory conditions. CRP is a nonspecific inflammatory parameter but may have a role in the detection of melanoma progression [86]. High serum CRP levels of are correlated with poorer prognosis in metastatic melanoma [87,88]. In a study that compared CRP and LDH, CRP showed better sensitivity and specificity than LDH in stage IV melanomas [87]. CRP may also be useful to monitor adjuvant therapy for metastatic melanoma [89–92]. It is noted that interferon-alpha (IFN-α) treatment may decrease serum CRP levels [93].

32.3.2.7 miRNAs

MicroRNAs (miRNAs) are small, noncoding RNAs that function in the posttranscriptional regulation of gene expression. miRNAs have emerged as novel diagnostic and prognostic markers in many hematologic and solid malignant tumors. There have been reports on the diagnostic and prognostic utility of miRNAs in melanoma [94–97]. miR-221 is abnormally expressed in melanoma cells, and it is associated with the induction of the malignant phenotype through downmodulation of p27Kipl/CDKN1B and the c-KIT [94]. Serum miR-221 levels were significantly higher in stage I–IV melanomas compared to melanoma in situ, and serum miR-221 levels were correlated to tumor thickness [95]. In a study in screening 355 miRNAs in serum from patients with melanoma, 5 miRNAs (miR-15b, miR-33a, miR-150, miR-199a-5p, miR-424) were identified to classify melanoma patients into high- and low-recurrence risk groups [96].

32.3.2.8 BRAF Mutation

BRAF has attracted great interest in recent years in melanoma. B-Raf protein plays a role in regulating the MAPK/ERK signaling pathway in cell division and differentiation. *BRAF* mutation is identified in various cancers. The frequency of *BRAF* mutation is higher in melanomas and nevi, too. Most frequent *BRAF* mutation is a single nucleotide substitution at position 1799 in exon 15, leading to the V600E amino-acid substitution [98]. A selective B-Raf inhibitor, vemurafenib, has received approval from FDA for treatment and diagnosis of melanoma with *BRAF* V600E mutation. Detection of mutant *BRAF* in serum can potentially be used as a marker of prognosis and/or a surrogate for assessment of clinical response. It has been shown that the *BRAF* V600E mutation is more frequently found in metastatic melanoma than in primary melanoma [99], suggesting *BRAF* mutation may be acquired during melanoma progression to distant metastasis, and it may not always occur at initiation of melanoma [9]. *BRAF* mutation can be detected in circulating tumor cells in blood in stage IV melanomas [100].

32.3.2.9 Angiogenic Proteins

Angiogenesis promoters such as vascular endothelial growth factor (VEGF) may be associated with melanoma progression. Increased levels of serum VEGF is correlated with advanced melanomas [101]. An analysis of multiple angiogenic promoters showed that elevated serum levels of VEGF, angiogenin, basic fibroblast growth factor (bFGF), and interleukin-8 (IL-8) were correlated with advanced disease stage and disease burden. VEGF, bFGF, and IL-8 were independent predictors of overall survival [102].

32.3.2.10 Biomarkers for Early Melanoma

There are few biomarkers useful for diagnosis of melanoma in the early stage. Glypican-3 is a cell-surface heparan sulfate proteoglycan and its functions include regulating cell growth and controlling cell division. Serum glypican-3 is detected in 40% of melanomas, especially stage 0–II melanomas [103,104]. Secreted protein, acidic, cysteine-rich (SPARC) (also known as osteonectin) is detected in serum of patients with stage 0–II melanomas [104]. Glypican-3 and SPARC may be potential biomarkers for melanoma in the early stage.

32.3.3 Immunological Biomarkers

32.3.3.1 Soluble IL-2R

IL-2 exerts its biological effects via signaling through its receptor, IL-2R. IL-2 and IL-2R are required for T-cell proliferation and other fundamental functions in the immune response. Serum-soluble IL-2 receptor is elevated in patients with metastatic melanoma and elevated serum IL-2 receptor levels are correlated with poorer prognosis [83,105–108]. The source of soluble IL-2R in serum of patients with melanoma and the function of soluble IL-2R in melanoma remain to be defined. IL-2R can be derived from the tumor as well as from the host cells such as T-cells and B-cells. In the later stages, with established cancer, the activation of the IL-2/IL-2R pathway on tumor cells and lymphocytes may reflect a failure of immune protection and may stimulate the growth of melanoma cells through autocrine/paracrine mechanisms, while in the early stage, IL-2/IL-2R activation can induce an anticancer immune response [108].

32.3.3.2 IL-10

IL-10 is a Th2 cytokine that impedes immune functions, including T-cell proliferation and cytotoxicity. IL-10 is secreted by melanoma cells, including metastatic melanoma cells [109–112] and tumor infiltrating lymphocytes and macrophages [112]. Elevated levels of serum IL-10 are correlated with advanced melanomas [106,113,114]. In an analysis of peripheral blood mononuclear cells from patients with melanoma undergoing adjuvant vaccine immunotherapy, CD14+ monocytes were the dominant cellular source of IL-10, and increasing IL-10 levels were correlated with poorer prognosis [115].

32.3.3.3 Immunological Responses to IFN-α 2b Treatment

Immunological responses to IFN-α 2b treatment have been reported. In patients with melanoma treated with the combination of chemotherapy and IL-2 and IFN-α 2b, increased levels of serum IL-6 and IL-10 were correlated with patient response [116]. In a multiplex analysis of cytokine and chemokine responses in melanoma undergoing IFN-α 2b treatment, proinflammatory cytokines IL-1β, IL-1α, IL-6, and TNF-α and chemokines CCL3 and CCL4 were correlated with longer relapse-free survival [117].

32.3.3.4 Cell Adhesion Molecules

Cell adhesion molecules may act as mediators in the metastatic process and can be released into circulation. Serum-soluble intercellular adhesion molecule-1 (ICAM-1) and soluble vascular cell adhesion molecule 1 (VCAM-1) are associated with advanced melanomas [82,106,107,118]. High levels of serum soluble ICAM-1 are more correlated with liver and bone metastases than with lung and soft tissue metastases [107].

32.3.3.5 Macrophage Markers

Macrophage markers in serum may also be a prognostic marker. In a study with stage I–II melanomas, serum levels of soluble CD163 (sCD163) and the presence of CD68 macrophage infiltration at the tumor invasive front were independent predictors of survival [119].

32.3.4 Proteomics in Melanoma: Matrix-Assisted Laser Desorption/Ionization Time-of-Flight Mass Spectrometry

Proteomics is a powerful screening method for protein expression patterns. Matrix-assisted laser desorption/ionization time-of-flight mass spectrometry (MALDI-TOF) is a recently developed technique in mass spectrometry, allowing the analysis of biomolecules such as DNA and proteins. MALDI-TOF analysis has yielded novel and promising data to assist in the detection and identification of diagnostic and prognostic biomarkers from tissue, serum, and plasma samples. Protein profiling by MALDI-TOF combined with artificial neural network analysis and modeling artificial neural may be more useful to identify high-risk melanomas. Eighty percent of serum samples from stage III melanomas were correctly assigned as progressors or nonprogressors, and progressors were correctly identified by MALDI-TOF combined with artificial neural network analysis in 82% of progressors in stage III melanomas, while serum S100B was detected in only 21% of progressors in stage III melanomas [120]. Serum amyloid A (SAA) is also identified by proteomic profiling as a prognostic marker. SAA combined with CRP may be used as prognostic serological biomarkers in stage I–III melanomas [88]. A recent study with MALDI-TOF combined with artificial neural network analysis and modeling has identified peptides derived from α1-acid glycoprotein precursors 1/2 and complement C3 component precursor 1 as biomarkers for metastatic melanoma. Serum α1-acid glycoprotein precursors levels are elevated in stage IV melanomas [121]. In a melanoma lung metastasis mouse model, MALDI-TOF analysis identified several candidate peptides derived from complement C3, fibrinogen β chain, zyxin, bradykinin, α2-macroglobulin, apolipoprotein A-I, hemoglobin subunit β, transferrin, and albumin [88]. MALDI-TOF is also utilized for detection of the mutant V600E allele of *BRAF* [6].

32.4 Urinary Biomarkers for Melanoma

Urinary biomarkers for melanoma diagnosis received much greater interest, but for now, urinary biomarkers are not of much account, because the analysis of urine may lack the sensitivity required for a diagnostic biomarker. In advanced melanomas, melanin synthesis is upregulated, and metabolites in melanin synthesis including 5-S-CD are increased in the serum and a large amount of such metabolites are eventually excreted in the urine. Initial studies focused on urine 5-S-CD. Urine 5-S-CD levels in patients with metastatic melanoma (stage IV melanomas) are much higher than those of nonmetastatic melanoma [81,122–125]. However, serum 5-S-CD is superior to urinary 5-S-CD to detect progression of metastatic melanoma [81]. An increase in 5-S-CD in urine may also be correlated with tumor progression and poorer prognosis in stage I–III melanomas [59]. Another melanin metabolite, 6H5MI2C, can be detected in the urine of patients with melanoma [59,126,127], but the sensitivity of urine 5-S-CD is higher than urine 6H5MI2C [126,127]. In a study that evaluated the combination of serum S100B and urine 5-S-CD and 6H5MI2C, the overall survival rate in stage I–III melanomas was associated most strongly with serum S100B and, to a lesser extent, with urine 5-S-CD. High levels of urine 6H5MI2C was found in a very few patients [59].

32.5 Biomarkers to Detect Metastasis in Sentinel Lymph Nodes

Sentinel lymph node evaluation permits accurate staging and determines the need for complete lymphadenectomy. Approximately 20% of patients with melanoma ≥1 mm in thickness have metastatic tumor in the sentinel lymph nodes [4,128]. Accurate determination of tumor status in the sentinel lymph nodes requires evaluation of multiple sections and immunohistochemistry for multiple melanocyte lineage-associated antigens [129]. Yet, micrometastases may be missed if the wrong part of a node is examined or if tumor cells do not express melanoma-associated markers detectable by immunohistochemistry. Molecular analyses including the RT–PCR have been reported to detect mRNA for melanoma-associated genes that may indicate micrometastases in sentinel lymph nodes [128,130–133] (Table 32.3). The use of multiple melanoma markers including MART-1 and MAGE family with qRT–PCR can significantly improve the specificity of molecular testing [134,135]. A meta-analysis of qRT–PCR upstaging of sentinel lymph nodes in stage I and II melanomas showed that qRT–PCR status was correlated with TNM stage, disease recurrence, and poor prognosis [136]. These findings have been considered to indicate the presence of occult melanoma cells that are difficult to detect microscopically or missed by limited sampling. However, it is possible that such molecular techniques may be more sensitive but less specific and may augment signals for melanoma-associated markers from cells other than melanoma cells, providing results that are thus "false positive" [137]. When attempting to detect micrometastases in sentinel lymph nodes by molecular analyses, attention should be paid to the possibility of downregulation of tumor-associated antigens.

References

1. Jemal A, Siegel R, Xu J, Ward E. Cancer statistics. *CA Cancer J Clin* 2010;60:277–300.
2. Markovic SN, Erickson LA, Rao RD et al. Malignant melanoma in the 21st century, part 1: Epidemiology, risk factors, screening, prevention, and diagnosis. *Mayo Clin Proc* 2007;82:364–380.
3. Morton DL, Wen DR, Wong JH et al. Technical details of intraoperative lymphatic mapping for early stage melanoma. *Arch Surg* 1992;127:392–399.
4. Morton DL, Thompson JF, Cochran AJ et al. Sentinel-node biopsy or nodal observation in melanoma. *N Engl J Med* 2006;355:1307–1317.
5. Gogas H, Eggermont AM, Hauschild A et al. Biomarkers in melanoma. *Ann Oncol* 2009;20(Suppl 6):vi8–vi13.
6. Palmer SR, Erickson LA, Ichetovkin I, Knauer DJ, Markovic SN. Circulating serologic and molecular biomarkers in malignant melanoma. *Mayo Clin Proc* 2011;86:981–990.
7. Mori T, Kang JH. *Biomarkers for Melanoma Diagnosis and the Technologies Used to Identify Them.* In: Tanaka Y, (ed). *Breakthroughs in Melanoma Research.* Rijeka, Croatia: InTech;2011. pp. 389–412.
8. Larson AR, Konat E, Alani RM. Melanoma biomarkers: Current status and vision for the future. *Nat Clin Pract Oncol* 2009;6:105–117.

9. Tanaka R, Koyanagi K, Narita N, Kuo C, Hoon DSB. Prognostic molecular biomarkers for cutaneous malignant melanoma. *J Surg Oncol* 2011;104:438–446.
10. Balch CM, Buzaid AC, Soong SJ et al. Final version of the American Joint Committee on Cancer staging system for cutaneous melanoma. *J Clin Oncol* 2001;19:3635–3648.
11. Edge SB, Byrd DR, Compton CC (eds). *AJCC Cancer Staging Manual*. 7th edn., New York: Springer;2010.
12. Breslow A. Thickness, cross-sectional areas and depth of invasion in the prognosis of cutaneous melanoma. *Ann Surg* 1970;172:902–908.
13. Balch CM, Gershenwald JE, Soong SJ et al. Final version of 2009 AJCC melanoma staging and classification. *J Clin Oncol* 2009;27:6199–6206.
14. Thompson JF, Soong SJ, Balch CM et al. Prognostic significance of mitotic rate in localized primary cutaneous melanoma: An analysis of patients in the multi-institutional American Joint Committee on Cancer melanoma staging database. *J Clin Oncol* 2011;29:2199–2205.
15. Paek SC, Griffith KA, Johnson TM et al. The impact of factors beyond Breslow depth on predicting sentinel lymph node positivity in melanoma. *Cancer* 2007;109:100–108.
16. Wortsman X. Sonography of the primary cutaneous melanoma: A review. *Radiol Res Pract* 2012;2012:814396.
17. Lassau N, Lamuraglia M, Koscielny S et al. Prognostic value of angiogenesis evaluated with high-frequency and colour Doppler sonography for preoperative assessment of primary cutaneous melanomas: Correlation with recurrence after a 5 year follow-up period. *Cancer Imaging* 2006;6:24–29.
18. Guitera P, Li LX, Crotty K et al. Melanoma histological Breslow thickness predicted by 75-MHz ultrasonography. *Br J Dermatol* 2008;159:364–369.
19. Vilana R, Puig S, Sanchez M et al. Preoperative assessment of cutaneous melanoma thickness using 10-MHz sonography. *Am J Roentgenol* 2009;193:639–643.
20. Starz H, Balda BR, Kramer KU, Buchels H, Wang H. A micromorphometry-based concept for routine classification of sentinel lymph node metastases and its clinical relevance for patients with melanoma. *Cancer* 2001;91:2110–2121.
21. Cochran AJ, Wen DR, Huang RR et al. Prediction of metastatic melanoma in nonsentinel nodes and clinical outcome based on the primary melanoma and the sentinel node. *Mod Pathol* 2004;17:747–755.
22. Dewar DJ, Newell B, Green MA et al. The microanatomic location of metastatic melanoma in sentinel lymph nodes predicts nonsentinel lymph node involvement. *J Clin Oncol* 2004;22:3345–3349.
23. Scolyer RA, Li LX, McCarthy SW et al. Micromorphometric features of positive sentinel lymph nodes predict involvement of nonsentinel nodes in patients with melanoma. *Am J Clin Pathol* 2004;122:532–539.
24. van der Ploeg IM, Kroon BB, Antonini N, Valdes Olmos RA, Nieweg OE. Comparison of three micromorphometric pathology classifications of melanoma metastases in the sentinel node. *Ann Surg* 2009;250:301–304.
25. Voit C, Kron M, Schafer G et al. Ultrasound-guided fine needle aspiration cytology prior to sentinel lymph node biopsy in melanoma patients. *Ann Surg Oncol* 2006;13:1682–1689.
26. Sibon C, Chagnon S, Tchakerian A et al. The contribution of high-resolution ultrasonography in preoperatively detecting sentinel-node metastases in melanoma patients. *Melanoma Res* 2007;17:233–237.
27. Ulrich J, van Akkooi AJ, Eggermont AM, Voit C. New developments in melanoma: Utility of ultrasound imaging (initial staging, follow-up and pre-SLNB). *Expert Rev Anticancer Ther* 2011;11:1693–1701.
28. Chai CY, Zager JS, Szabunio MM et al. Preoperative ultrasound is not useful for identifying nodal metastasis in melanoma patients undergoing sentinel node biopsy: Preoperative ultrasound in clinically node-negative melanoma. *Ann Surg Oncol* 2012;19:1100–1106.
29. Deichmann M, Benner A, Bock M et al. S100-Beta, melanoma-inhibiting activity, and lactate dehydrogenase discriminate progressive from nonprogressive American Joint Committee on Cancer stage IV melanoma. *J Clin Oncol* 1999;17:1891–1896.
30. Clark WH, Jr., From L, Bernardino EA, Mihm MC. The histogenesis and biologic behavior of primary human malignant melanomas of the skin. *Cancer Res* 1969;29:705–727.
31. Talve LA, Collan YU, Ekfors TO. Nuclear morphometry, immunohistochemical staining with Ki-67 antibody and mitotic index in the assessment of proliferative activity and prognosis of primary malignant melanomas of the skin. *J Cutan Pathol* 1996;23:335–343.
32. Moretti S, Spallanzani A, Chiarugi A, Fabiani M, Pinzi C. Correlation of Ki-67 expression in cutaneous primary melanoma with prognosis in a prospective study: Different correlation according to thickness. *J Am Acad Dermatol* 2001;44:188–192.

33. Pearl RA, Pacifico MD, Richman PI et al. Ki-67 expression in melanoma. A potential method of risk assessment for the patient with a positive sentinel node. *J Exp Clin Cancer Res* 2007;26:109–115.
34. Gould Rothberg BE, Bracken MB, Rimm DL. Tissue biomarkers for prognosis in cutaneous melanoma: A systematic review and meta-analysis. *J Natl Cancer Inst* 2009;101:452–474.
35. Stevens GL, Scheer WD, Levine EA. Detection of tyrosinase mRNA from the blood of melanoma patients. *Cancer Epidemiol Biomarkers Prev* 1996;5:293–296.
36. Hoon DSB, Wang Y, Dale PS et al. Detection of occult melanoma cells in blood with a multiple-marker polymerase chain reaction assay. *J Clin Oncol* 1995;13:2109–2116.
37. Kunter U, Buer J, Probst M et al. Peripheral blood tyrosinase messenger RNA detection and survival in malignant melanoma. *J Natl Cancer Inst* 1996;88:590–594.
38. Palmieri G, Strazzullo M, Ascierto PA et al. Polymerase chain reaction-based detection of circulating melanoma cells as an effective marker of tumor progression. Melanoma Cooperative Group. *J Clin Oncol* 1999;17:304–311.
39. de Vries TJ, Fourkour A, Punt CJ et al. Reproducibility of detection of tyrosinase and MART-1 transcripts in the peripheral blood of melanoma patients: A quality control study using real-time quantitative RT-PCR. *Br J Cancer* 1999;80:883–891.
40. Tsukamoto K, Ueda M, Hirata S et al. gp100 mRNA is more sensitive than tyrosinase mRNA for RT-PCR amplification to detect circulating melanoma cells in peripheral blood of melanoma patients. *J Dermatol Sci* 2000;23:126–131.
41. Mellado B, Del Carmen Vela M, Colomer D et al. Tyrosinase mRNA in blood of patients with melanoma treated with adjuvant interferon. *J Clin Oncol* 2002;20:4032–4039.
42. Gogas H, Kefala G, Bafaloukos D et al. Prognostic significance of the sequential detection of circulating melanoma cells by RT-PCR in high-risk melanoma patients receiving adjuvant interferon. *Br J Cancer* 2002;87:181–186.
43. Palmieri G, Ascierto PA, Perrone F et al. Prognostic value of circulating melanoma cells detected by reverse transcriptase-polymerase chain reaction. *J Clin Oncol* 2003;21:767–773.
44. Mocellin S, Del Fiore P, Guarnieri L et al. Molecular detection of circulating tumor cells is an independent prognostic factor in patients with high-risk cutaneous melanoma. *Int J Cancer* 2004;111:741–745.
45. Koyanagi K, O'Day SJ, Gonzalez R et al. Serial monitoring of circulating melanoma cells during neoadjuvant biochemotherapy for stage III melanoma: Outcome prediction in a multicenter trial. *J Clin Oncol* 2005;23:8057–8064.
46. Nowecki ZI, Rutkowski P, Kulik J, Siedlecki JA, Ruka W. Molecular and biochemical testing in stage III melanoma: Multimarker reverse transcriptase-polymerase chain reaction assay of lymph fluid after lymph node dissection and preoperative serum lactate dehydrogenase level. *Br J Dermatol* 2008;159:597–605.
47. Koyanagi K, O'Day SJ, Boasberg P et al. Serial monitoring of circulating tumor cells predicts outcome of induction biochemotherapy plus maintenance biotherapy for metastatic melanoma. *Clin Cancer Res* 2010;16:2402–2408.
48. Finck SJ, Giuliano AE, Morton DL. LDH and melanoma. *Cancer* 1983;51:840–843.
49. Sirott MN, Bajorin DF, Wong GY et al. Prognostic factors in patients with metastatic malignant melanoma. A multivariate analysis. *Cancer* 1993;72:3091–3098.
50. Bedikian AY, Millward M, Pehamberger H et al. Bcl-2 antisense (oblimersen sodium) plus dacarbazine in patients with advanced melanoma: The Oblimersen Melanoma Study Group. *J Clin Oncol* 2006;24:4738–4745.
51. Egberts F, Hitschler WN, Weichenthal M, Hauschild A. Prospective monitoring of adjuvant treatment in high-risk melanoma patients: Lactate dehydrogenase and protein S-100B as indicators of relapse. *Melanoma Res* 2009;19:31–35.
52. Agarwala SS, Keilholz U, Gilles E et al. LDH correlation with survival in advanced melanoma from two large, randomised trials (Oblimersen GM301 and EORTC 18951). *Eur J Cancer* 2009;45:1807–1814.
53. Allore R, O'Hanlon D, Price R et al. Gene encoding the beta subunit of S100 protein is on chromosome 21: Implications for Down syndrome. *Science* 1988;239:1311–1313.
54. Duncan AM, Higgins J, Dunn RJ, Allore R, Marks A. Refined sublocalization of the human gene encoding the beta subunit of the S100 protein (S100B) and confirmation of a subtle t(9;21) translocation using in situ hybridization. *Cytogenet Cell Genet* 1989;50:234–235.

55. Harpio R, Einarsson R. S100 proteins as cancer biomarkers with focus on S100B in malignant melanoma. *Clin Biochem* 2004;37:512–518.
56. Guo HB, Stoffel-Wagner B, Bierwirth T, Mezger J, Klingmuller D. Clinical significance of serum S100 in metastatic malignant melanoma. *Eur J Cancer* 1995;31A:1898–1902.
57. von Schoultz E, Hansson LO, Djureen E et al. Prognostic value of serum analyses of S-100 beta protein in malignant melanoma. *Melanoma Res* 1996;6:133–137.
58. Abraha HD, Fuller LC, Du Vivier AW, Higgins EM, Sherwood RA. Serum S-100 protein: A potentially useful prognostic marker in cutaneous melanoma. *Br J Dermatol* 1997;137:381–385.
59. Karnell R, von Schoultz E, Hansson LO et al. S100B protein, 5-S-cysteinyldopa and 6-hydroxy-5-methoxyindole-2-carboxylic acid as biochemical markers for survival prognosis in patients with malignant melanoma. *Melanoma Res* 1997;7:393–399.
60. Bonfrer JM, Korse CM, Nieweg OE, Rankin EM. The luminescence immunoassay S-100: A sensitive test to measure circulating S-100B: Its prognostic value in malignant melanoma. *Br J Cancer* 1998;77:2210–2214.
61. Hauschild A, Engel G, Brenner W et al. S100B protein detection in serum is a significant prognostic factor in metastatic melanoma. *Oncology* 1999;56:338–344.
62. Mohammed MQ, Abraha HD, Sherwood RA, MacRae K, Retsas S. Serum S100 beta protein as a marker of disease activity in patients with malignant melanoma. *Med Oncol* 2001;18:109–120.
63. Bánfalvi T, Gilde K, Gergye M et al. Use of serum 5-S-CD and S-100B protein levels to monitor the clinical course of malignant melanoma. *Eur J Cancer* 2003;39:164–169.
64. Kruijff S, Bastiaannet E, Kobold AC et al. S-100B concentrations predict disease-free survival in stage III melanoma patients. *Ann Surg Oncol* 2009;16:3455–3462.
65. Mocellin S, Zavagno G, Nitti D. The prognostic value of serum S100B in patients with cutaneous melanoma: A meta-analysis. *Int J Cancer* 2008;123:2370–2376.
66. Hamberg AP, Korse CM, Bonfrer JM, de Gast GC. Serum S100B is suitable for prediction and monitoring of response to chemoimmunotherapy in metastatic malignant melanoma. *Melanoma Res* 2003;13:45–49.
67. Tarhini AA, Stuckert J, Lee S, Sander C, Kirkwood JM. Prognostic significance of serum S100B protein in high-risk surgically resected melanoma patients participating in Intergroup Trial ECOG 1694. *J Clin Oncol* 2009;27:38–44.
68. Bogdahn U, Apfel R, Hahn M et al. Autocrine tumor cell growth-inhibiting activities from human malignant melanoma. *Cancer Res* 1989;49:5358–5363.
69. Blesch A, Bosserhoff AK, Apfel R et al. Cloning of a novel malignant melanoma-derived growth-regulatory protein, MIA. *Cancer Res* 1994;54:5695–5701.
70. Guba M, Bosserhoff AK, Steinbauer M et al. Overexpression of melanoma inhibitory activity (MIA) enhances extravasation and metastasis of A-mel 3 melanoma cells in vivo. *Br J Cancer* 2000;83:1216–1222.
71. Bosserhoff AK, Kaufmann M, Kaluza B et al. Melanoma-inhibiting activity, a novel serum marker for progression of malignant melanoma. *Cancer Res* 1997;57:3149–3153.
72. Bosserhoff AK, Lederer M, Kaufmann M et al. MIA, a novel serum marker for progression of malignant melanoma. *Anticancer Res* 1999;19:2691–2693.
73. Stahlecker J, Gauger A, Bosserhoff A et al. MIA as a reliable tumor marker in the serum of patients with malignant melanoma. *Anticancer Res* 2000;20:5041–5044.
74. Meral R, Duranyildiz D, Tas F et al. Prognostic significance of melanoma inhibiting activity levels in malignant melanoma. *Melanoma Res* 2001;11:627–632.
75. Krahn G, Kaskel P, Sander S et al. S100 beta is a more reliable tumor marker in peripheral blood for patients with newly occurred melanoma metastases compared with MIA, albumin and lactate-dehydrogenase. *Anticancer Res* 2001;21:1311–1316.
76. de Vries TJ, Fourkour A, Punt CJ et al. Melanoma-inhibiting activity (MIA) mRNA is not exclusively transcribed in melanoma cells: Low levels of MIA mRNA are present in various cell types and in peripheral blood. *Br J Cancer* 1999;81:1066–1070.
77. Kelley MC, Gupta RK, Hsueh EC et al. Tumor-associated antigen TA90 immune complex assay predicts recurrence and survival after surgical treatment of stage I-III melanoma. *J Clin Oncol* 2001;19:1176–1182.
78. Hsueh EC, Gupta RK, Qi K et al. TA90 immune complex predicts survival following surgery and adjuvant vaccine immunotherapy for stage IV melanoma. *Cancer J Sci Am* 1997;3:364–370.

79. Faries MB, Gupta RK, Ye X et al. A comparison of 3 tumor markers (MIA, TA90IC, S100B) in stage III melanoma patients. *Cancer Invest* 2007;25:285–293.
80. Ito S, Wakamatsu K, Ozeki H. Chemical analysis of melanins and its application to the study of the regulation of melanogenesis. *Pigment Cell Res* 2000;13(Suppl 8):103–109.
81. Horikoshi T, Ito S, Wakamatsu K, Onodera H, Eguchi H. Evaluation of melanin-related metabolites as markers of melanoma progression. *Cancer* 1994;73:629–636.
82. Hirai S, Kageshita T, Kimura T et al. Serum levels of sICAM-1 and 5-S-cysteinyldopa as markers of melanoma progression. *Melanoma Res* 1997;7:58–62.
83. Hasegawa M, Takata M, Hatta N et al. Simultaneous measurement of serum 5-S-cysteinyldopa, circulating intercellular adhesion molecule-1 and soluble interleukin-2 receptor levels in Japanese patients with malignant melanoma. *Melanoma Res* 1997;7:243–251.
84. Wimmer I, Meyer JC, Seifert B et al. Prognostic value of serum 5-S-cysteinyldopa for monitoring human metastatic melanoma during immunochemotherapy. *Cancer Res* 1997;57:5073–5076.
85. Wakamatsu K, Kageshita T, Furue M et al. Evaluation of 5-S-cysteinyldopa as a marker of melanoma progression: 10 years experience. *Melanoma Res* 2002;12:245–253.
86. Bouwhuis MG, ten Hagen TL, Eggermont AM. Immunologic functions as prognostic indicators in melanoma. *Mol Oncol* 2011;5:183–189.
87. Deichmann M, Kahle B, Moser K, Wacker J, Wust K. Diagnosing melanoma patients entering American Joint Committee on Cancer stage IV, C-reactive protein in serum is superior to lactate dehydrogenase. *Br J Cancer* 2004;91:699–702.
88. Findeisen P, Zapatka M, Peccerella T et al. Serum amyloid A as a prognostic marker in melanoma identified by proteomic profiling. *J Clin Oncol* 2009;27:2199–2208.
89. Tartour E, Blay JY, Dorval T et al. Predictors of clinical response to interleukin-2—Based immunotherapy in melanoma patients: A French Multiinstitutional Study. *J Clin Oncol* 1996;14:1697–1703.
90. Guida M, Ravaioli A, Sileni VC et al. Fibrinogen: A novel predictor of responsiveness in metastatic melanoma patients treated with bio-chemotherapy: IMI (Italian melanoma inter-group) trial. *J Transl Med* 2003;1:13.
91. Sarnaik AA, Yu B, Yu D et al. Extended dose ipilimumab with a peptide vaccine: Immune correlates associated with clinical benefit in patients with resected high-risk stage IIIc/IV melanoma. *Clin Cancer Res* 2011;17:896–906.
92. Tarhini AA, Cherian J, Moschos SJ et al. Safety and efficacy of combination immunotherapy with interferon alfa-2b and tremelimumab in patients with stage IV melanoma. *J Clin Oncol* 2012;30:322–328.
93. Stam TC, Swaak AJ, Kruit WH, Eggermont AM. Regulation of ferritin: A specific role for interferon-alpha (IFN-alpha)? The acute phase response in patients treated with IFN-alpha-2b. *Eur J Clin Invest* 2002;32(Suppl 1):79–83.
94. Garofalo M, Di Leva G, Romano G et al. miR-221&222 regulate TRAIL resistance and enhance tumorigenicity through PTEN and TIMP3 downregulation. *Cancer Cell* 2009;16:498–509.
95. Kanemaru H, Fukushima S, Yamashita J et al. The circulating microRNA-221 level in patients with malignant melanoma as a new tumor marker. *J Dermatol Sci* 2011;61:187–193.
96. Friedman EB, Shang S, de Miera EV et al. Serum microRNAs as biomarkers for recurrence in melanoma. *J Transl Med* 2012;10:155.
97. Segura MF, Greenwald HS, Hanniford D, Osman I, Hernando E. MicroRNA and cutaneous melanoma: From discovery to prognosis and therapy. *Carcinogenesis* 2012;33:1823–1832.
98. Davies H, Bignell GR, Cox C et al. Mutations of the BRAF gene in human cancer. *Nature* 2002;417:949–954.
99. Shinozaki M, O'Day SJ, Kitago M et al. Utility of circulating B-RAF DNA mutation in serum for monitoring melanoma patients receiving biochemotherapy. *Clin Cancer Res* 2007;13:2068–2074.
100. Kitago M, Koyanagi K, Nakamura T et al. mRNA expression and BRAF mutation in circulating melanoma cells isolated from peripheral blood with high molecular weight melanoma-associated antigen-specific monoclonal antibody beads. *Clin Chem* 2009;55:757–764.
101. Osella-Abate S, Quaglino P, Savoia P et al. VEGF-165 serum levels and tyrosinase expression in melanoma patients: Correlation with the clinical course. *Melanoma Res* 2002;12:325–334.
102. Ugurel S, Rappl G, Tilgen W, Reinhold U. Increased serum concentration of angiogenic factors in malignant melanoma patients correlates with tumor progression and survival. *J Clin Oncol* 2001;19:577–583.
103. Nakatsura T, Kageshita T, Ito S et al. Identification of glypican-3 as a novel tumor marker for melanoma. *Clin Cancer Res* 2004;10:6612–6621.

104. Ikuta Y, Nakatsura T, Kageshita T et al. Highly sensitive detection of melanoma at an early stage based on the increased serum secreted protein acidic and rich in cysteine and glypican-3 levels. *Clin Cancer Res* 2005;11:8079–8088.
105. Boyano MD, Garcia-Vazquez MD, Gardeazabal J et al. Serum-soluble IL-2 receptor and IL-6 levels in patients with melanoma. *Oncology* 1997;54:400–406.
106. Boyano MD, Garcia-Vazquez MD, Lopez-Michelena T et al. Soluble interleukin-2 receptor, intercellular adhesion molecule-1 and interleukin-10 serum levels in patients with melanoma. *Br J Cancer* 2000;83:847–852.
107. Vuoristo MS, Laine S, Huhtala H et al. Serum adhesion molecules and interleukin-2 receptor as markers of tumour load and prognosis in advanced cutaneous melanoma. *Eur J Cancer* 2001;37:1629–1634.
108. Ottaiano A, Leonardi E, Simeone E et al. Soluble interleukin-2 receptor in stage I-III melanoma. *Cytokine* 2006;33:150–155.
109. Chen Q, Daniel V, Maher DW, Hersey P. Production of IL-10 by melanoma cells: Examination of its role in immunosuppression mediated by melanoma. *Int J Cancer* 1994;56:755–760.
110. Krüger-Krasagakes S, Krasagakis K, Garbe C et al. Expression of interleukin 10 in human melanoma. *Br J Cancer* 1994;70:1182–1185.
111. Gerlini G, Tun-Kyi A, Dudli C et al. Metastatic melanoma secreted IL-10 down-regulates CD1 molecules on dendritic cells in metastatic tumor lesions. *Am J Pathol* 2004;165:1853–1863.
112. Itakura E, Huang RR, Wen DR et al. IL-10 expression by primary tumor cells correlates with melanoma progression from radial to vertical growth phase and development of metastatic competence. *Mod Pathol* 2011;24:801–809.
113. Dummer W, Becker JC, Schwaaf A et al. Elevated serum levels of interleukin-10 in patients with metastatic malignant melanoma. *Melanoma Res* 1995;5:67–68.
114. Dummer W, Bastian BC, Ernst N et al. Interleukin-10 production in malignant melanoma: Preferential detection of IL-10-secreting tumor cells in metastatic lesions. *Int J Cancer* 1996;66:607–610.
115. Torisu-Itakura H, Lee JH, Huynh Y et al. Monocyte-derived IL-10 expression predicts prognosis of stage IV melanoma patients. *J Immunother* 2007;30:831–838.
116. Grimm EA, Smid CM, Lee JJ et al. Unexpected cytokines in serum of malignant melanoma patients during sequential biochemotherapy. *Clin Cancer Res* 2000;6:3895–3903.
117. Yurkovetsky ZR, Kirkwood JM, Edington HD et al. Multiplex analysis of serum cytokines in melanoma patients treated with interferon-alpha2b. *Clin Cancer Res* 2007;13:2422–2428.
118. Franzke A, Probst-Kepper M, Buer J et al. Elevated pretreatment serum levels of soluble vascular cell adhesion molecule 1 and lactate dehydrogenase as predictors of survival in cutaneous metastatic malignant melanoma. *Br J Cancer* 1998;78:40–45.
119. Jensen TO, Schmidt H, Moller HJ et al. Macrophage markers in serum and tumor have prognostic impact in American Joint Committee on Cancer stage I/II melanoma. *J Clin Oncol* 2009;27:3330–3337.
120. Mian S, Ugurel S, Parkinson E et al. Serum proteomic fingerprinting discriminates between clinical stages and predicts disease progression in melanoma patients. *J Clin Oncol* 2005;23:5088–5093.
121. Matharoo-Ball B, Ratcliffe L, Lancashire L et al. Diagnostic biomarkers differentiating metastatic melanoma patients from healthy controls identified by an integrated MALDI-TOF mass spectrometry/bioinformatic approach. *Proteomics Clin Appl* 2007;1:605–620.
122. Agrup G, Agrup P, Andersson T et al. Urinary excretion of 5-S-cysteinyldopa in patients with primary melanoma or melanoma metastasis. *Acta Derm Venereol* 1975;55:337–341.
123. Agrup G, Agrup P, Andersson T et al. Five years experience of 5-S-cysteinyldopa in melanoma diagnosis. *Acta Derm Venereol* 1979;59:381–388.
124. Yamada K, Walsh N, Hara H et al. Measurement of eumelanin precursor metabolites in the urine as a new marker for melanoma metastases. *Arch Dermatol* 1992;128:491–494.
125. Sasaki Y, Shimizu H, Naka W, Takeshita E, Nishikawa T. Evaluation of the clinical usefulness of measuring urinary excretion of 5-S-cysteinyldopa in melanoma: 10 Years experience of 50 patients. *Acta Derm Venereol* 1997;77:379–381.
126. Karnell R, Kagedal B, Lindholm C et al. The value of cysteinyldopa in the follow-up of disseminated malignant melanoma. *Melanoma Res* 2000;10:363–369.
127. Wakamatsu K, Takasaki A, Kagedal B, Kageshita T, Ito S. Determination of eumelanin in human urine. *Pigment Cell Res* 2006;19:163–169.

128. Morton DL, Hoon DSB, Cochran AJ et al. Lymphatic mapping and sentinel lymphadenectomy for early-stage melanoma: Therapeutic utility and implications of nodal microanatomy and molecular staging for improving the accuracy of detection of nodal micrometastases. *Ann Surg* 2003;238:538–549.
129. Cochran AJ, Roberts A, Wen DR et al. Update on lymphatic mapping and sentinel node biopsy in the management of patients with melanocytic tumours. *Pathology* 2004;36:478–484.
130. Bostick PJ, Morton DL, Turner RR et al. Prognostic significance of occult metastases detected by sentinel lymphadenectomy and reverse transcriptase-polymerase chain reaction in early-stage melanoma patients. *J Clin Oncol* 1999;17:3238–3244.
131. Blaheta HJ, Ellwanger U, Schittek B et al. Examination of regional lymph nodes by sentinel node biopsy and molecular analysis provides new staging facilities in primary cutaneous melanoma. *J Invest Dermatol* 2000;114:637–642.
132. Goydos JS, Patel KN, Shih WJ et al. Patterns of recurrence in patients with melanoma and histologically negative but RT-PCR-positive sentinel lymph nodes. *J Am Coll Surg* 2003;196:196–204.
133. Hilari JM, Mangas C, Xi L et al. Molecular staging of pathologically negative sentinel lymph nodes from melanoma patients using multimarker, quantitative real-time RT-PCR. *Ann Surg Oncol* 2009;16:177–185.
134. Takeuchi H, Morton DL, Kuo C et al. Prognostic significance of molecular upstaging of paraffin-embedded sentinel lymph nodes in melanoma patients. *J Clin Oncol* 2004;22:2671–2680.
135. Rutkowski P, Nowecki ZI, van Akkooi AC et al. Multimarker reverse transcriptase-polymerase chain reaction assay in lymphatic drainage and sentinel node tumor burden. *Ann Surg Oncol* 2010;17:3314–3323.
136. Mocellin S, Hoon DSB, Pilati P, Rossi CR, Nitti D. Sentinel lymph node molecular ultrastaging in patients with melanoma: A systematic review and meta-analysis of prognosis. *J Clin Oncol* 2007;25:1588–1595.
137. Itakura E, Huang RR, Wen DR, Cochran AJ. "Stealth" melanoma cells in histology-negative sentinel lymph nodes. *Am J Surg Pathol* 2011;35:1657–1665.

Index

F

I

K

L

N

O

Q

R

T

U